# Textbook of Endodontics





*System requirement:*
- Windows XP or above
- Power DVD player (Software)
- Windows media player 10.0 version or above (Software)

*Accompanying DVD ROM is playable only in Computer and not in DVD player.*

Kindly wait for few seconds for CD to autorun. If it does not autorun then please do the following:
- Click on my computer
- Click the **CD/DVD** drive and after opening the drive, kindly double click the file **Jaypee**

# CONTENTS OF DVD

DVD 1

1. Access, cleaning, shaping and obturation of root canal in extracted mandibular molar using step back techniques
2. Access, cleaning, shaping and filling of a canal in an acrylic block using crown down technique

DVD 2

1. Access, cleaning, and shaping of root canal using hand ProTaper instruments
2. Access preparation, cleaning and shaping of root canal using rotary ProTaper instruments

# Textbook of Endodontics

**SECOND EDITION**


**Nisha Garg**
MDS (Conservative Dentistry and Endodontics)

Ex Resident, PGIMER, Chandigarh
Ex Resident, Government Dental College, Patiala
Presently at, Manav Rachna Dental College
Faridabad, Haryana, India

**Amit Garg**
MDS (Oral and Maxillofacial Surgery)

Ex Resident, Government Dental College
PGIMS, Rohtak
Presently at, Manav Rachna Dental College
Faridabad, Haryana, India

*Foreword*

**Sanjay Tewari**



**JAYPEE BROTHERS MEDICAL PUBLISHERS (P) LTD**

New Delhi • St Louis (USA) • Panama City (Panama) • London (UK) • Ahmedabad
Bengaluru • Chennai • Hyderabad • Kochi • Kolkata • Lucknow • Mumbai • Nagpur

*Published by*

Jitendar P Vij
**Jaypee Brothers Medical Publishers (P) Ltd**

***Corporate Office***
4838/24 Ansari Road, Daryaganj, **New Delhi** - 110002, India
Phone: +91-11-43574357, Fax: +91-11-43574314

***Registered Office***
B-3 EMCA House, 23/23B Ansari Road, Daryaganj, **New Delhi** - 110 002, India
Phones: +91-11-23272143, +91-11-23272703, +91-11-23282021
+91-11-[illegible], Fax: +91-11-23276490, +91-11-23245683
[illegible] Website: www.jaypeebrothers.com

# CONTRIBUTORS

**Poonam Bogra**
Professor
Department of Conservative Dentistry and Endodontics
DAV Dental College
Yamuna Nagar, Haryana

**Ravi Kapoor**
Professor and Head of Department
Department of Conservative Dentistry and Endodontics
MM College of Dental Sciences
Mullana, Ambala, Haryana

**Arundeep Singh**
Professor and Head of the Department
Department of Conservative Dentistry and Endodontics
MR Dental College
Faridabad, Haryana

**Manav Nayyar**
Associate Professor
Department of Conservative Dentistry and Endodontics
Seema Dental College
Rishikesh, Uttranchal

**Dheeraj Sehgal**
Professor
Department of Conservative Dentistry and Endodontics
Laxmi Bai Dental College
Patiala, Punjab

**Navjot Singh Khurana**
Lecturer
Department of Conservative Dentistry and Endodontics
Govt. Dental College
Patiala, Punjab

**Sandhya Kapoor Punia**
Asst. Professor
Department of Conservative Dentistry and Endodontics
Darshan Dental College
Udaipur, Rajasthan

**Manoj Hans**
Asst. Professor
Department of Conservative Dentistry and Endodontics
KD Dental College
Mathura, Uttar Pradesh

**Pankaj Dhawan**
Professor and Head of the Department
Department of Prosthodontics
MR Dental College
Faridabad, Haryana

**Dax**
Reader
Department of Conservative Dentistry and Endodontics
IDST, Modinagar
Uttar Pradesh

# FOREWORD

It gives me great pleasure in writing this foreword for the second edition of the book *Textbook of Endodontics* which is quite popular among the undergraduate and postgraduate students across the globe. It is reflection of a book's success when its second edition is made available in short span of time. The first edition of this book has proved to be a best seller largely due to emergence as comprehensive textbook on the subject of endodontics when there was actual need for the same.

The hallmark of this book is an extensive picture-wise coverage of the vast subject of endodontics in accordance with syllabus of Dental Council of India. When going through the pages of this book, I found that authors have made sincere attempt to present a concise panorama of various aspects of endodontics. I am sure that owing to its umpteen illustrations, clinical photographs, simple language and in-depth explanation of every aspect of subject including the recent advances, this book is definitely appropriate for a thorough knowledge in the field of endodontics.

This edition deserves a hearty congratulations for all the efforts and hard work, the authors have undertaken. I am sure that this book will guide the students in gaining an insight into the vast field of endodontics. It is with great pride that I wish Dr Nisha Garg and Dr Amit Garg all that's best for the success of this venture.

**Sanjay Tewari**
Principal and Head of the Department
Department of Conservative Dentistry and Endodontics
Government Dental College, PGIMS
Rohtak, Haryana, India

# PREFACE TO THE SECOND EDITION

It gives us great pleasure and sense of satisfaction to present you the second edition of our book, *Textbook of Endodontics*. This has been possible due to overwhelming response given by students and teachers to the first edition of the book and its reprints. So, a very big thanks to all of them. This has encouraged us to revise, reorganize and update the book and present it to you in the form of second edition.

The new edition has been updated by adding nine new chapters, keeping in mind the present scenario and the curriculum of all universities. The new chapters are on rationale of endodontics, tissue engineering, geriatric endodontics, magnification, etc.

Many of the old chapters have been revised and upgraded in view of latest developments and researches happening in the field of endodontics. A lot of new illustrations, radiographs, tables and flow charts have been added so as to have a clear understanding and grasp of the subject. In this edition, self-assessment questions have been added at the end of each chapter to increase the utility for students appearing in university examination. Also, the bibliography has been added at the end of chapter for referring the main articles in that area.

We gratefully acknowledge the support given by Dr OP Bhalla (President) and Dr Amit Bhalla (Vice-President, MRIU) during the completion of this task.

We also acknowledge the support given by Dr AK Kapoor (Director–Principal, MRDC) and Dr SK Mangal (Medical Superintendent, MRDC) during this project.

We would like to thank all our contributors and supporters who helped us in improving the first edition of the book in more refined form along with extensive details of the subject.

We would like to express our thanks to staff of Department of Conservative Dentistry and Endodontics, MRDC, Faridabad, Dr Manish Gupta, Dr Sarika and Dr Babita, for their “ready to help” attitude, constant guidance and positive criticism which helped in improvement of this book.

We would like to thank, particularly Mr Manoj Dwivedi (Marketing Manager) and Company “Dentsply”, for providing illustrations and videos for benefit of students and teachers across the globe.

We are also thankful to Mr Shammi Gambhir and his company, Unicorn Denmart for providing us photographs of loupes and endomicroscopes.

We are thankful to Dr Vivek Hegde and Dr Gurkirat Singh for providing us video of crown down technique.

We would like to thank Dr Vishal Juneja for providing us radiographs for better presentation of the text.

We are thankful to Shri Jitendar P Vij (Chairman and Managing Director), Mr Tarun Duneja (Director-Publishing) and staff of Jaypee Brothers Medical Publishers (P) Ltd, New Delhi for all encouragement as well as for bringing out this book in an excellent form.

Last but not the least, we are thankful to the students of this country, who appreciated our previous textbooks, *Textbook of Operative Dentistry* and *Review of Endodontics and Operative Dentistry*. Please send us reviews and suggestions to incorporate in further edition of this book to make it more student friendly.

**Nisha Garg**
drnishagarg1@gmail.com

**Amit Garg**
dramitgarg1@gmail.com

# PREFACE TO THE FIRST EDITION

The amount of literature available in dentistry today is vast. Endodontics being no exception. However, during both our graduation as well as postgraduation we always felt the need for a book which would help us to revise and update our knowledge. When we were doing undergraduation, there were no Indian authored books on Endodontics. We were thus motivated to frame a specialized, precise, concise, easy to read and remember yet, up-to-date Textbook of Endodontics.

The line diagrams are in an expressive interpretation of endodontic procedures, which are worked upon and simplified to render them more comprehensive and comparable with real photographs. These illustrations (around 1200) are easy to remember and reproduce during examinations.

Emphasis is laid upon the language which is simple, understandable and exclusively designed for undergraduates, postgraduates, general practitioners and teachers in the field.

It took us more than three years to accomplish the arduous task of writing this book. This thrust for knowledge led us to link everywhere, where we could medline journals, books and more.

Nevertheless, a never-ending approach and internal craving of mind and soul finally resulted in publication of this book. God perhaps gave us some ability and showered His light on us, guiding us for this task.

Till the last week before the publication of this book, we were frantically looking for loopholes, missing information and any important updates we might have missed out. To the best of our knowledge, we did everything we could. But for knowledge, one life is not enough. The sky is the limit.

We await the response of this first edition, which would improve us in the next editions to come.

**Nisha Garg**
**Amit Garg**

# CONTENTS

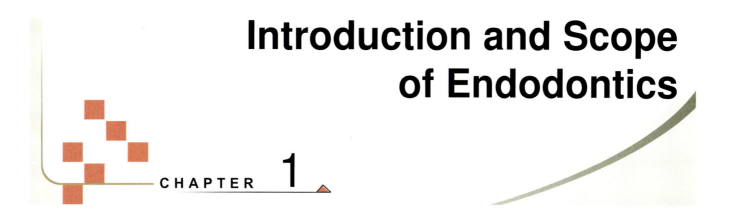

# Introduction and Scope of Endodontics

CHAPTER 1



## INTRODUCTION

Endo is a Greek word for "Inside" and Odont is Greek word for "Tooth". Endodontic treatment treats inside of the tooth.

Endodontics is the branch of clinical dentistry associated with the prevention, diagnosis and treatment of the pathosis of the dental pulp and their sequelae.

That is, the *main aim of the endodontic therapy involves to*:

i. Maintain vitality of the pulp.
ii. Preserve and restore the tooth with damaged and necrotic pulp.
iii. Preserve and restore the teeth which have failed to the previous endodontic therapy, to allow the tooth to remain functional in the dental arch.

Thus we can say that the primary goal of endodontic therapy is to create an environment within the root canal system which allows the healing and continued maintenance of the health of the periradicular tissue.

Since nothing is as good as the natural teeth, one should take care of them. The endodontic therapy is a necessary treatment to cure a damaged or diseased tooth.

Endodontics has been defined as art as well as science of clinical dentistry because in spite of all the factual scientific foundation on which the endodontics is based, to provide an ideal endodontic treatment is an art in itself.

Before understanding what is root canal therapy, how and when it is performed and other facts regarding endodontic therapy, we should be familiar with the *history of endodontics*.

## HISTORY OF ENDODONTICS (TABLE 1.1)

Endodontics has been practiced as early as second or third century BC. The history of endodontics begins in 17th century and since then many advances, developments and research work has been proceeded continuously.

Though advances in endodontics have been made continuously, but especially after Pierre Fauchard (1678-1761) [Founder of modern dentistry] in his textbook "Le Chirugien Dentiste" described the pulp very precisely.

Later in 1725, Lazare Rivere introduced the use of clove oil as sedative and in 1746, Pierre Fauchard demonstrated the removal of pulp tissue. Dr Grossman, the pioneer of endodontics divided the evolution of endodontics in four eras from 1776 to 1976, each consisting of 50 years.

| | | |
|---|---|---|
| Pre science | : | 1776 to 1826 |
| Age of discovery | : | 1826 to 1876 |
| Dark age | : | 1876 to 1926 |
| The renaissance | : | 1926 to 1976 |
| Innovation Era | : | 1977 till date |

***Pre science (1776 to 1826)***: In this era, endodontic therapy mainly consisted of crude modalities like abscesses were being treated with poultices or leeches and pulps were being cauterized using hot cauteria.

***Age of discovery (1826 to 1876)***: In this era there occurred the development of anesthesia, gutta-percha and barbed broaches. Also the medications were created for treating pulpal infections and the cements and pastes were discovered to fill them.

***The dark age (1876 to 1926)***: In spite of introduction of X-rays and general anesthesia, extractions was the choice of treatment than endodontics in most of the cases of damaged teeth because theory of the focal infection was main concern at that time.

***The renaissance (1926 to 1976)***: In this era, endodontics was established as science and therapy, forming its golden era. It showed the improvement in anesthesia and radiographs for better treatment results. The theory of focal infection was also fading out, resulting in more of endodontics being practiced and in 1943, because of growing interest in endodontics, the AAE, that is, the American Association of Endodontists was formed.

**Table 1.1: History of endodontics**

| | | | |
|---|---|---|---|
| 1725 | L. Riverie | - | Introduced clove oil for sedative property |
| 1746 | Pierre Fauchard | - | Described of removal of pulp tissue |
| 1820 | L. Koecker | - | Cauterized exposed pulp with heated instrument and protected it with lead foil |
| 1836 | S. Spooner | - | Suggested arsenic trioxide for pulp devitalization |
| 1838 | Edwards Maynard | - | Introduced first root canal instrument |
| 1847 | E. Truman | - | Introduced gutta-percha. |
| 1864 | S.C. Barnum | - | Prepared a thin rubber leaf to isolate the tooth during filling |
| 1867 | Bowman | - | Used gutta-percha cones for filling of root canals |
| 1867 | Magitot | - | Use of electric current for testing pulp vitality |
| 1879 | G.A. Mills | - | Etiologic factor of pulp sequelae was lack of vitality in the tooth |
| 1885 | Lepkoski | - | Substituted formations for arsenic to dry the nonvital pulp. |
| 1890 | | - | Introduced gold plated copper points for filling |
| 1891 | Otto Walkhoff | - | Introduced camphorated chlorophenol as a medication |
| 1895 | Roentgen | - | Introduced formocresol |
| 1901-1905 | | - | Introduction of k-instrument |
| 1914 | Callahan | - | Introduction of lateral compaction technique |
| 1918 | Cluster | - | Use of electrical current for determination of working length |
| 1920 | Hermann | - | Introduced calcium hydroxide |
| 1936 | Walker | - | Sodium hypochlorite |
| 1942 | Suzuki | - | Presented scientific study on apex locator |
| 1944 | Johnson | - | Introduced profile instrument system |
| 1957 | Nygaard Ostby | - | Introduced EDTA |
| 1958 | Ingle and Levine | - | Gave standardizations and guidelines for endodontic instruments |
| 1961 | Sparser | - | Walking bleach technique |
| 1962 | Sunanda | - | Calculated electrical resistance between periodontium and oral mucous membrane |
| 1967 | Ingle | - | Introduced standardized technique |
| 1971 | Weichman Johnson | - | Use of lasers |
| 1979 | Mullaney et al | - | Use of step-back technique |
| 1979 | | - | McSpadden technique |
| 1980 | Marshall and Pappin | - | Introduction of Crown down pressureless technique |
| 1985-86 | Roane, Sabala and Powell | - | Introduction of Balanced force technique |
| 1988 | Munro | - | Introduced first commercial bleaching product |
| 1989 | Haywood and Heymann | - | Nightguard vital bleaching |
| 1990 | | - | Introduction of microscope in endodontics |
| 1993 | Torabinejad | - | Introduced MTA |
| 2004 | Pentron clinical laboratory | - | Introduced Resilon |

***Innovation era***: It is the period from 1977 onwards in which tremendous advancements at very fast rate are being introduced in the endodontics. The better vision, better techniques of biomechanical preparations, and obturation are being developed resulting in the simpler, easier and faster endodontics with more of the successful results.

Also the concept of single visit endodontics is now globally accepted in contrast to multiple visits.

## MODERN ENDODONTICS

As we have seen, over the years, there has been a great improvement in the field of endodontics. Many researches have been conducted and papers are being presented regarding the advances, modifications and change in attitude regarding endodontic therapy. In the past two decades, extensive studies have been done on microbial flora of pulp and the periapical tissue. The biological changes, role of innate and acquired immunological factors are being investigated in dental pulp after it gets infected, healing of the periapical tissue after undergoing root canal therapy is also being investigated.

Various ways to reduce the levels of microbial infection *viz.* chemical, mechanical and their combination have led to development of newer antimicrobial agents and techniques of biomechanical preparation for optimal cleaning and shaping of the root canals.

To increase the efficiency of root canal instrumentation, introduction of engine driven rotary instruments is made. Introduction of Nickel Titanium multitapered instruments with different types of cutting tips have allowed the better, easier and efficient cleaning and shaping of the root canals.

The advent of endomicroscope in the field of endodontics has opened the great opportunities for an endodontist. It is used in every phase of the treatment, i.e. from access opening till the obturation of root canals. It makes the images both magnified and illuminated, thus helps in making the treatment more predictable and eliminating the guess work.

Introduction of newer obturation systems like system B Touch and heat have made it possible to fill the canal three dimensionally. Material like MTA (Mineral Trioxide Aggregate), a root canal repair material has made the procedures like apexification, perforation repair to be done under moist field. Since endodontics is based on the principles of inflammation, pulp and periapical disease processes and the treatment available, future of endodontics lies to redefine the rationale of endodontic therapy using newer modalities and to meet the set of standards of excellence in the future.

## SCOPE OF ENDODONTICS

Scope of endodontics includes following:

a. Vital pulp therapy (pulp capping, pulpotomy)
b Diagnosis and differential diagnosis of oral pain.
c. Root canal treatment of teeth with or without periradicular pathology of pulpal origin.
d. Surgical management of pathology resulting form pulpal pathosis.
e. Management of avulsed teeth (replantation)
f. Endodontic implants
g. Root end resections, hemisections and root resections
h. Retreatment of teeth previously treated endodontically
i. Bleaching of discolored teeth.
j. Coronal restorations of teeth using post and cores.

## PATIENT EDUCATION

Most of the patient who are given endodontic treatment, are often curious and interested in their treatment. For such patients following information should be transferred to the patient in anticipation of frequently asked questions.

### Who Performs an Endodontic Therapy?

Generally, all dentists receive basic education in endodontic treatment but an endodontist is preferred for endodontic therapy. General dentists often refer patients needing endodontic treatment to endodontists.

### Who is an Endodontist?

An endodontist is a dentist who undergoes a special training in diagnosing and treating the problems associated with inside of the tooth. To become specialists, they complete dental school and an additional two or more years of advanced training in endodontics. They perform routine as well as difficult and very complex endodontic procedures, including retreatment of previous root canals that have not healed completely, as well as endodontic surgery.

### What is Endodontics?

Endodontics is the diagnosis and treatment of inflamed and damaged pulps. Teeth are composed of protective hard covering (enamel, dentin and cementum) encasing a soft living tissue called pulp (Fig. 1.1). Pulp contains blood vessels, nerves, fibers and connective tissue. The pulp extends from the crown of the tooth to the tip of the roots where it connects to the tissues surrounding the root. The pulp is important during a tooth's growth and development. However, once a tooth is fully mature it can survive without the pulp, because the tooth continues to be nourished by the tissues surrounding it.

### How does Pulp Become Damaged?

Number of ways which can damage the pulp include tooth decay (Figs 1.2 and 1.3), gum diseases, injury to the tooth by accident.

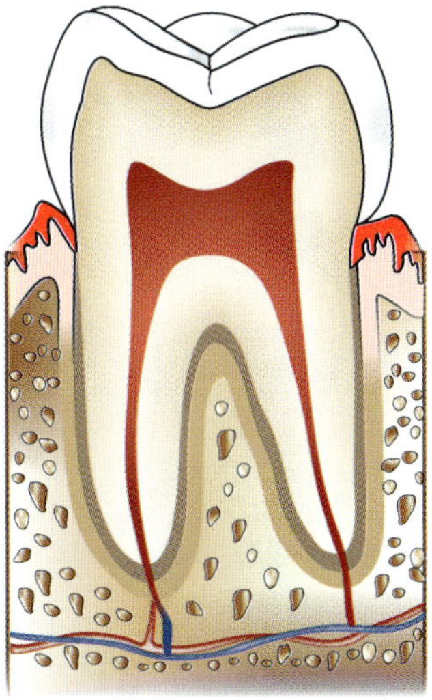

Fig. 1.1: Normal anatomy of a tooth showing enamel, dentin, cementum and pulp

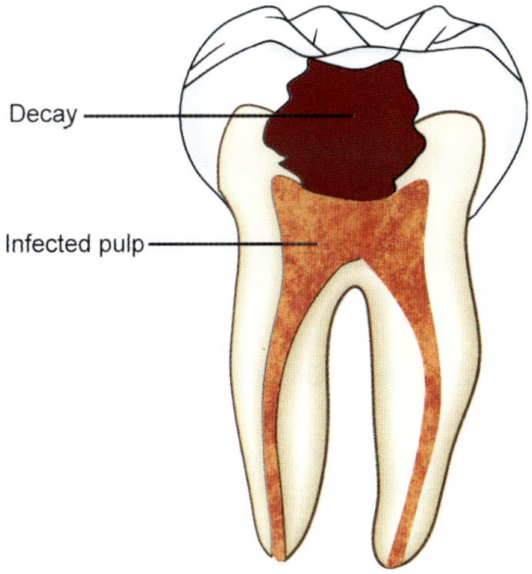


Fig. 1.2: Tooth decay causing damage to pulp

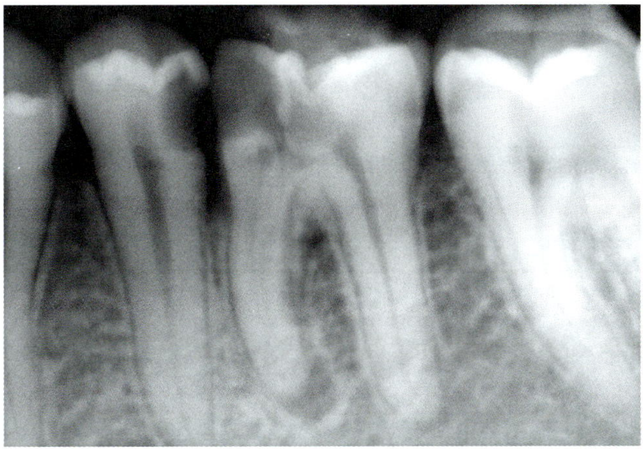

Fig. 1.3: Radiograph showing carious exposure of pulp

### Why do I Feel Pain?

When pulp becomes infected, it causes increased blood flow and cellular activity, and pressure cannot be relieved from inside the tooth. This causes pain. Pulp can even die without causing significant pain.

### How can You Tell if Pulp is Infected?

When pulp gets inflamed, it may cause toothache on taking hot or cold, spontaneous pain, pain on biting or on lying down. on occasion a damaged pulp is noticed by drainage, swelling, and abscess at the root end (Fig. 1.4). Sometimes, however, there are no symptoms.

### Why do I Need Root Canal Therapy?

Because tooth will not heal by itself, the infection may spread around the tissues causing destruction of bone and supporting tissue (Fig. 1.5). This may cause tooth to fall out. Root canal treatment is done to save the damaged pulp by thorough cleaning and shaping of the root canal system and then filling it with gutta-percha (rubber like) material to prevent recontamination of the tooth. Tooth is permanently restored with crown with or without post.

### What are Alternatives to Root Canal Therapy?

If tooth is seriously damaged and its support is compromised, then extraction is only alternative.

### What is Root Canal Procedure?

Once the endodontic therapy is recommended, your endodontist will numb the area by injecting local anesthetic. After this a rubber sheet is placed around the tooth to isolate it. Then the opening is made in the crown of the tooth and very small sized instruments are used to clean the pulp from pulp chamber and root canals (Fig. 1.6). After thorough cleaning and shaping of root canals (Fig. 1.7), they are filled with rubber like material called gutta-percha, which will prevent the bacteria from entering this space again (Figs 1.8 and 1.9).

After completion of endodontic therapy, the endodontist places the crown or other restoration so as to restore the tooth to full function (Figs 1.10 and 1.11).

### What are Risks and Complications?

It has been seen that more than 95 percent cases of endodontic therapy are successful. However sometimes because of unnoticed canal malformations, instrument errors a root canal therapy may fail.

### Does the Tooth need any Special Care after Endodontic Therapy?

Since unrestored tooth is more prone to fracture so you should not chew hard until it has been completely restored, otherwise you should continue your regular oral hygiene routine including brushing, flossing and regular check-up.

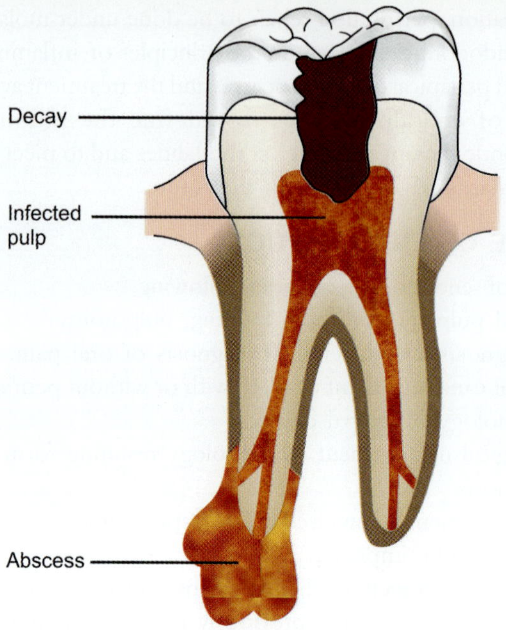


**Fig. 1.4:** Tooth with infected pulp and abscess formation

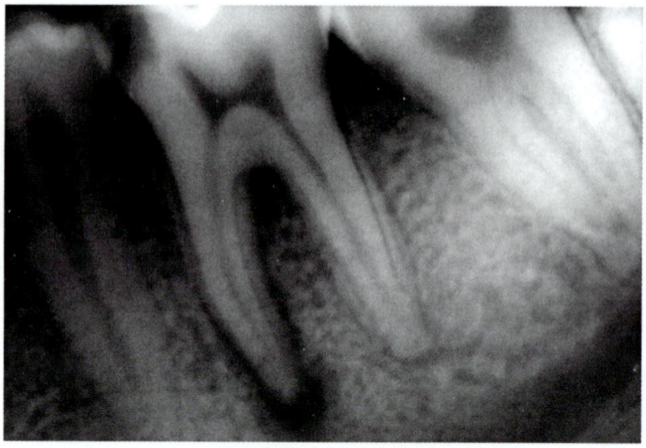

**Fig. 1.5:** Radiograph showing periapical lesion due to carious exposure

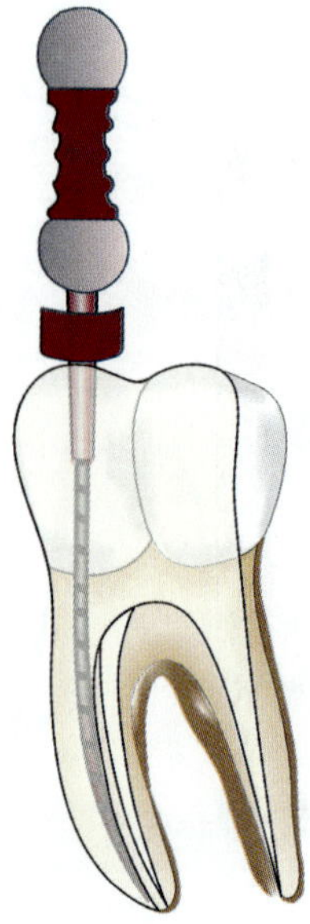

**Fig. 1.6:** Cleaning and shaping of root canal system

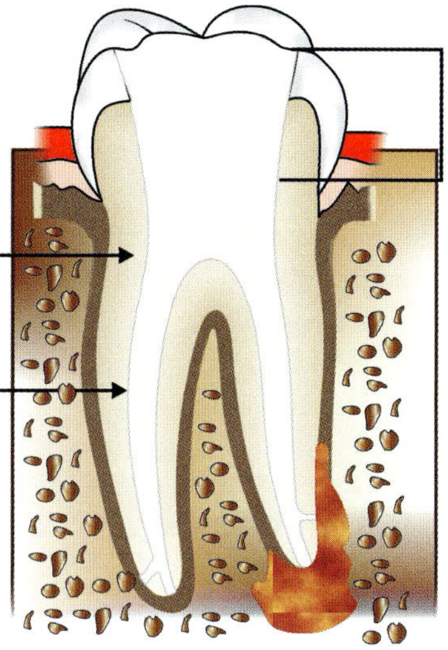


**Fig. 1.7:** Cleaned and shaped tooth

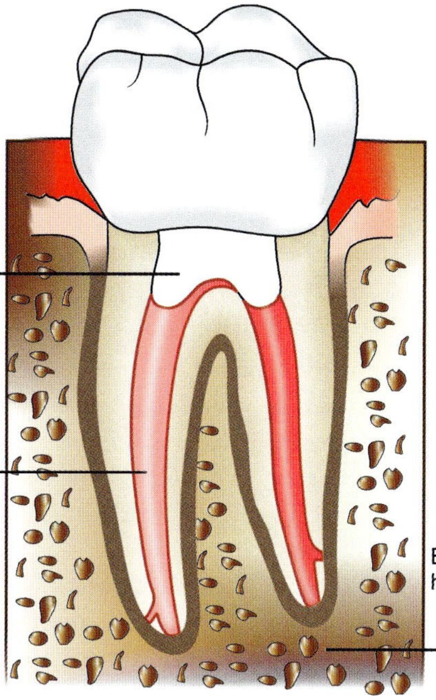


**Fig. 1.10:** Complete restoration of tooth with crown placed over the restored tooth

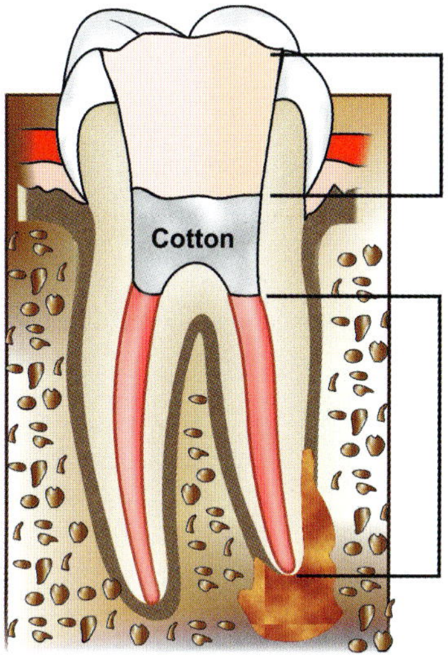


**Fig. 1.8:** Obturation of root canal system

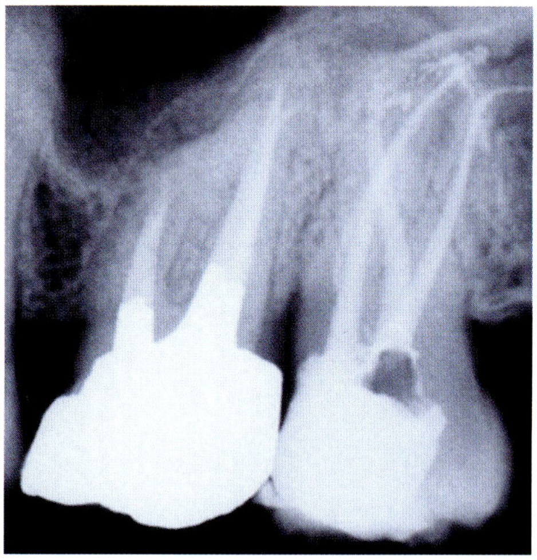

**Fig. 1.11:** Complete endodontic treatment with root canal obturation and crown placement

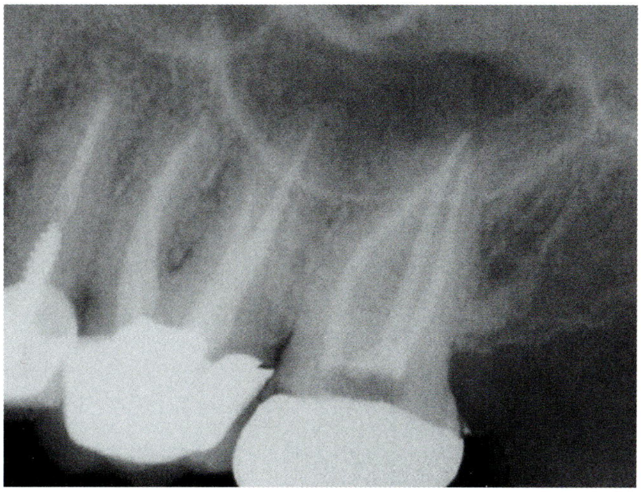

**Fig. 1.9:** Radiograph showing obturated canals

## How many Visits will it Take to Complete this Treatment?

Nowadays most of the treatment can be completed in 1-2 visits. But treatment time can vary according to condition of the tooth.

## Will I Feel Pain during or after Treatment?

Nowadays with better techniques, and better understanding of anesthesia most of the patients feel comfortable during the treatment. But for first few days after therapy, you might feel sensation especially if pain and infection was present prior to the procedure. This pain can be relieved by medication. If continuous severe pain or pressure remains, consult your endodontist.

## Will I have a Dead Tooth after Root Canal Therapy?

No, since tooth is supplied by blood vessels present in periodontal ligament. It continues to receive the nutrition and remains healthy.

## Will the Tooth Need Any Special Care or Additional Treatment after Endodontic Treatment?

You should not chew or bite on the treated tooth until you have had it restored by your dentist. The unrestored tooth is susceptible to fracture, so you should visit your dentist for a full restoration as soon as possible. Otherwise, you need only practice good oral hygiene, including brushing, flossing, and regular check-ups and cleanings.

Most endodontically treated teeth last as long as other natural teeth. In a few cases, a tooth that has undergone endodontic treatment does not heal or the pain continues. Occasionally, the tooth may become painful or diseased months or even years after successful treatment. Often when this occurs, redoing the endodontic procedure can save.

## Can All Teeth be Treated Endodontically?

Most of the teeth can be treated endodontically. But sometimes when root canals are not accessible, root is severely fractured, tooth cannot be restored or tooth doesn't have sufficient bone support, it becomes difficult to treat the tooth endodontically. However, advances in endodontics are making it possible to save the teeth that even a few years ago would have been lost.

Newer researches, techniques and materials have helped us to perform the endodontic therapy in better way with more efficiency. Since introduction of rotary instruments and other technologies reduce the treatment time, the concept of single visit is gaining popularity nowadays. It has been shown that success of endodontic therapy depends on the quality of root canal treatment and not the number of visits. In the modern world single visit endodontics is becoming quite popular.

## QUESTION

**Q. What is scope of endodontics?**

## BIBLIOGRAPHY

1. Balkwill FH. On the treatment of pulpless teeth. Br Dent J 1883;4:588-92.
2. Gatchel RJ. The prevalence of dental fear and avoidance expanded adult and recent adolescent surveys. J Am Dent Assoc 1989;118:591.
3. Harding WE. A few practical observations on the treatment of the pulp. J Brit Dent Assoc 1883;4:318-21.
4. Landers RR, Calhoun RL. One-appointment endodontic therapy: A nationwide survey of endodontists. J Am Dent Assoc 1970;80:1341.
5. Soltanoff W. Comparative study of the single visit and multiple visit endodontic procedure. J Endod 1978;4:278.
6. Skillen WG. Morphology of root canals. J Am Dent Assoc 1932;19:719-35.
7. Wolch I. The one-appointment endodontic technique. J Can Dent Assoc 1975;41:613.

# Pulp and Periradicular Tissue

CHAPTER 2



## INTRODUCTION

The dental pulp is soft tissue of mesenchymal origin located in the center of the tooth. It consists of specialized cells, odontoblasts arranged peripherally in direct contact with dentin matrix. This close relationship between odontoblasts and dentin is known as "pulp-dentin complex" (Fig. 2.1). The pulp is connective tissue system composed of cells, ground substances, fibers, interstitial fluid, odontoblasts, fibroblasts and other cellular components. Pulp is actually a microcirculatory system consists of arterioles and venules as the largest vascular component. Due to lack of true collateral circulation pulp is dependent upon few arterioles entering through the foramen. Due to presence of the specialized cells, i.e. odontoblasts as well as other cells which can differentiate into hard tissue secreting cells; the pulp retains its ability to form dentin throughout the life. This enables the vital pulp to partially compensate for loss of enamel or dentin occurring with age. The injury to pulp may cause discomfort and the disease.

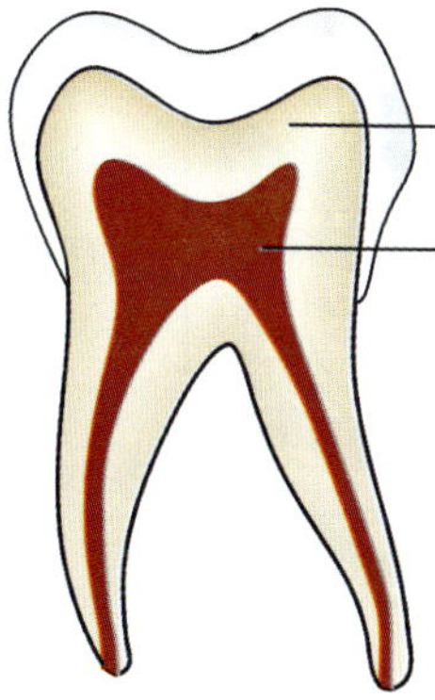


Fig. 2.1: Pulp dentin complex

Consequently, the health of pulp is important to successful completion of the restorative procedures. Because the symptoms as well as radiographic and clinical signs of pulp diseases are not always differentiated from sign and symptoms of other dental diseases, knowledge of biology of pulp is essential for development of rational treatment plan. In this chapter, we would discuss the comprehensive description of pulp embryology, anatomy, histology, physiology and pulp changes with age.

**Features of pulp which distinguish it from tissue found elsewhere in the body:**

a. Pulp is surrounded by rigid walls and so is unable to expand in response to injury as a part of the inflammatory process. Therefore, pulpal tissue is susceptible to a change in pressure affecting the pain threshold.
b. There is minimal collateral blood supply to pulp tissue which reduces its capacity for repair following injury.
c. The pulp is composed almost entirely of simple connective tissue, yet at its periphery there is a layer of highly specialized cells, the odontoblasts. Secondary dentin is gradually deposited as a physiological process which reduces the blood supply and therefore, the resistance to infection or trauma.
d. The innervation of pulp tissue is both simple and complex. Simple in that there are only free nerve endings and consequently the pulp lacks proprioception. Complex because of innervation of the odontoblast processes which produces a high level of sensitivity to thermal and chemical change.

## DEVELOPMENT OF DENTAL PULP

The pulp originates from ectomesenchymal cells of dental papilla. Dental pulp is identified when these cells mature and dentin is formed.

Before knowing the development of pulp we should understand the development of the tooth. Basically the development of tooth is divided into bud, cap and bell stage.

The **bud stage** (Fig. 2.2) is initial stage where epithelial cells of dental lamina proliferate and produce a bud like projection into adjacent ectomesenchyme.

The **cap stage** (Fig. 2.3) is formed when cells of dental lamina proliferate to form a concavity which produces cap like appearance. It shows outer and inner enamel epithelia and stellate reticulum. The rim of the enamel organ, i.e. where inner and outer enamel epithelia are joined is called cervical loop. As the cells of loop proliferate, enamel organ assumes **bell shape** (Fig. 2.4).

The differentiation of epithelial and mesenchymal cells into ameloblasts and odontoblasts occur during bell stage. The pulp is initially called as dental papilla; it is designated as pulp only when dentin forms around it. The differentiation of odontoblasts from undifferentiated ectomesenchymal cells is accomplished by interaction of cell and signaling molecules mediated through basal lamina and extracellular matrix. The dental papilla has high cell density and the rich vascular supply as a result of proliferation of cells within it.

The cells of dental papilla appear as undifferentiated mesenchymal cells, gradually these cells differentiate into fibroblasts. The formation of dentin by odontoblasts heralds the conversion of dental papilla into pulp. The boundary between inner enamel epithelium and odontoblast form the future dentinoenamel junction. The junction of inner and outer enamel epithelium at the basal margin of enamel organ represent the future cementoenamel junction. As the crown formation with enamel and dentin deposition continues, growth and organization of pulp vasculature occurs. According to Saunders (1966) and Cutright (1970), the blood supply of the developing tooth bud originates from an oval or circular reticulated plexus in the alveolar bone. Series of blood vessels arise from the plexus, which then grows into dental papilla.

At the same time as tooth develops unmyelinated sensory nerves and autonomic nerves grow into pulpal tissue. Myelinated fibers develop and mature at a slower rate, plexus of Raschkow does not develop until after tooth has erupted.

## HISTOLOGY OF DENTAL PULP

When pulp is examined histologically, it can be distinguished into four distinct zones from periphery to center of the pulp (Fig 2.5). The zones are as following:

a. Odontoblastic layer at the pulp periphery
b. Cell free zone of Weil
c. Cell rich zone
d. Pulp core

A. ***Odontoblastic layer:*** Odontoblasts consists of cell bodies and cytoplasmic processes. The odontoblastic cell bodies form the odontoblastic zone whereas the odontoblastic processes are located within predentin matrix. Capillaries, nerve fibers (unmyelinated) and dendritic cells may be found around the odontoblasts in this zone.

B. ***Cell free zone of Weil:*** Central to odontoblasts is subodontoblastic layer, termed cell free zone of Weil. It

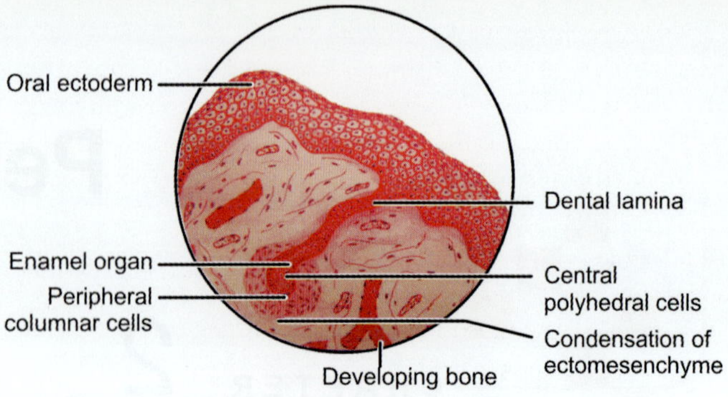


**Fig. 2.2:** Development of tooth showing bud stage

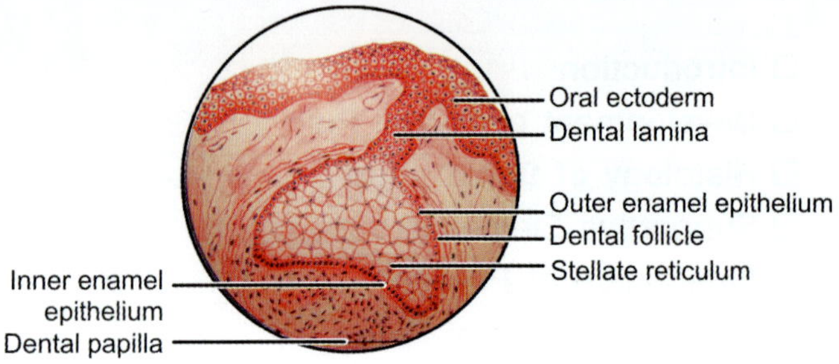


**Fig. 2.3:** Development of tooth showing cap stage

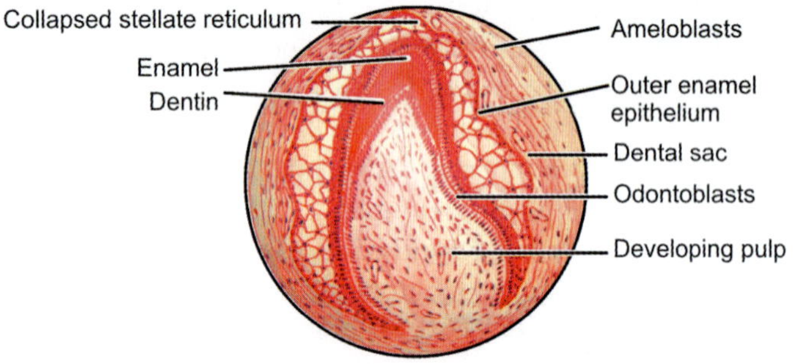


**Fig. 2.4:** Development of tooth showing "Bell stage"

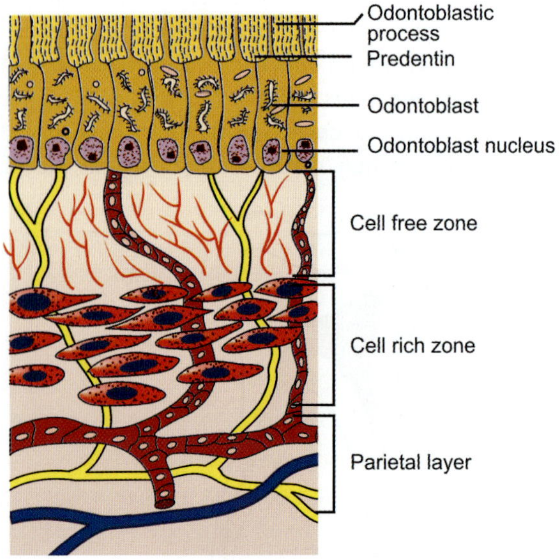


**Fig. 2.5:** Zones of pulp

contains plexuses of capillaries and small nerve fibers ramification.

C. ***Cell rich zone:*** This zone lies next to subodontoblastic layer. It contains fibroblasts, undifferentiated cells which maintain number of odontoblasts by proliferation and differentiation.

D. ***Pulp core:*** It is circumscribed by cell rich zone. It contains large vessels and nerves from which branches extend to peripheral layers. Principal cells are fibroblasts with collagen as ground substance.

**Contents of the pulp**

| | | | |
|---|---|---|---|
| I. Cells | 1. Odontoblasts | | |
| | 2. Fibroblasts | | |
| | 3. Undifferentiated mesenchymal cells | | |
| | 4. Defense cells | - | Macrophages |
| | | | Plasma cells |
| | | | Mast cells |
| II. Matrix | 1. Collagen fibers | - | Type I |
| | | | Type II |
| | 2. Ground Substance | - | Glycosaminoglycans |
| | | - | Glycoproteins |
| | | - | Water |
| III. Blood Vessels | - Arterioles, Venules, Capillaries | | |
| IV. Lymphatics | - Draining to submandibular, submental and deep cervical nodes | | |
| V. Nerves | - Subodontoblastic plexus of Raschkow | | |
| | - Sensory afferent from Vth nerve and Superior cervical ganglion | | |

## Structural or Cellular Elements

1. ***Odontoblasts (Fig. 2.6):*** They are first type of cells encountered as pulp is approached from dentin. The number of odontoblasts has been found in the range of 59,000 to 76,000 per square millimeter in coronal dentin, with a lesser number in root dentin. In the crown of the fully developed tooth, the cell bodies of odontoblasts are columnar and measure approximately 500 µm in height, whereas in the midportion of the pulp, they are more cuboidal and in apical part, more flattened.

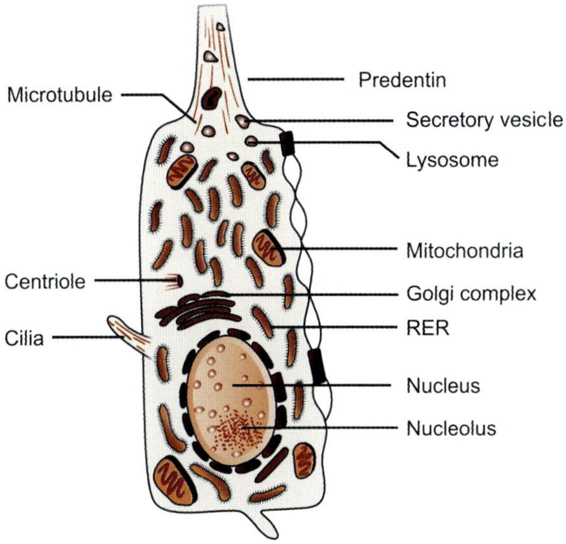


**Fig. 2.6:** Diagram showing odontoblasts

The morphology of odontoblasts reflects their functional activity and ranges from an active synthetic phase to a quiescent phase. Ultrastructure of the odontoblast shows large nucleus which may contain up to four nucleoli. Nucleus is situated at basal end. Golgi bodies are located centrally. Mitochondria, rough endoplasmic reticulum (RER), ribosome are also distributed throughout the cell body.

Odontoblasts synthesize mainly type I collagen, proteoglycans. They also secrete sialoproteins, alkaline phosphatase, phosphophoryn (phosphoprotein involved in extracellular mineralization).

Irritated odontoblast secretes collagen, amorphous material, and large crystals into tubule lumen which result in dentin permeability to irritating substance.

**Similar characteristic features of odontoblasts, osteoblasts and cementoblasts**

1. They all produce matrix composed of collagen fibers and proteoglycans capable of undergoing mineralization.
2. All exhibit highly ordered RER, golgi complex, mitochondria, secretory granules, rich in RNA with prominent nucleoli.

**Difference between odontoblasts, osteoblasts and cementoblasts**

1. Odontoblasts are columnar in shape while osteoblasts and cementoblast are polygonal in shape.
2. Odontoblasts leave behind cellular processes to form dentinal tubules while osteoblasts and cementoblast are trapped in matrix as osteocytes and cementocytes.

2. ***Fibroblasts:*** The cells found in greatest numbers in the pulp are fibroblasts. "Baume" refers them to mesenchymal cells/ pulpoblasts or pulpocytes in their progressive levels of maturation. These are particularly numerous in the coronal portion of the pulp, where they form the cell-rich zone. These are spindle shaped cells which secrete extracellular components like collagen and ground substance (Fig. 2.7). They also eliminate excess collagen by action of lysosomal enzymes. Fibroblasts of pulp are much like ***"Peter Pan"*** because they "never grow up" and remain in relatively undifferentiated state.

3. ***Reserve cells/undifferentiated mesenchymal cells:*** Undifferentiated mesenchymal cells are descendants of undifferentiated cells of dental papilla which can dedifferentiate and then redifferentiate into many cell types.

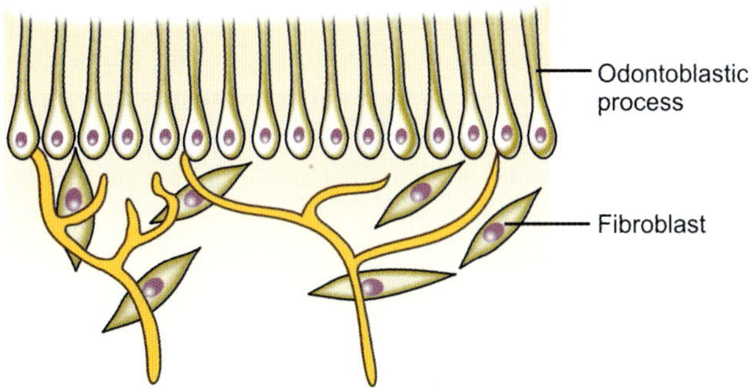


**Fig. 2.7:** Histology of pulp showing fibroblasts

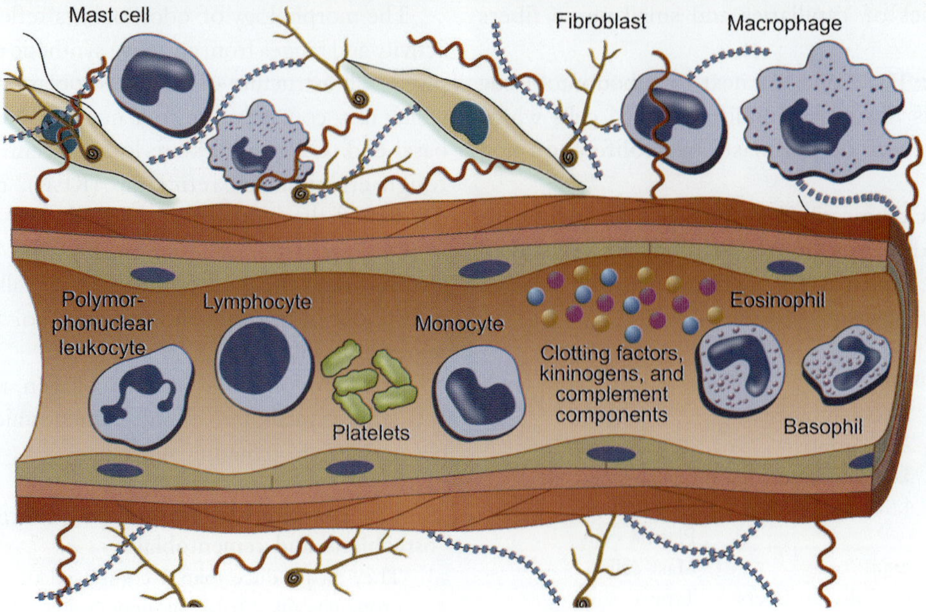


**Fig. 2.8:** Cells taking part in defence of pulp

Depending on the stimulus, these cells may give rise to odontoblasts and fibroblasts. These cells are found throughout the cell-rich area and the pulp core and often are related to blood vessels. When these cells are examined under light microscope, they appear as large polyhedral cells possessing a large, lightly stained, centrally placed nucleus and displays abundant cytoplasm and peripheral cytoplasm extensions. In older pulps, the number of undifferentiated mesenchymal cells diminishes, along with number of other cells in the pulp core. This reduction, along with other aging factors, reduces the regenerative potential of the pulp.

4. ***Defence cells:*** (Fig. 2.8)
   I. ***Histiocytes and macrophages:*** They originate from undifferentiated mesenchymal cells or monocytes. They appear as large oval or spindle shaped cells which are involved in the elimination of dead cells, debris, bacteria and foreign bodies, etc.
   II. ***Polymorphonuclear leukocytes:*** Most common form of leukocyte is neutrophil, though it is not present in healthy pulp. They are major cell type in micro abscesses formation and are effective at destroying and phagocytising bacteria and dead cells.
   III. ***Lymphocytes:*** In normal pulps, mainly T- lymphocytes are found but B-lymphocytes are scarce. They appear at the site of injury after invasion by neutrophils. They are associated with injury and resultant immune response. Thus their presence indicates presence of persistent irritation.
   IV. ***Mast cells:*** On stimulation, degranulation of mast cells release histamine which causes vasodilatation, increased vessel permeability and thus allowing fluids and leukocytes to escape.

## Extracellular Components

The extracellular components include fibers and the ground substance of pulp:

***Fibers:*** The fibers are principally type I and type III collagen. Collagen is synthesized and secreted by odontoblasts and fibroblasts. The overall collagen content of the pulp increases with age, while the ratio between types I and III remains stable. Fibers produced by these cells differ in the degree of cross-linkage and variation in hydroxyline content. Fibers secreted by fibroblasts don't calcify. Collagen with age becomes coarser and can lead to formation of pulp stones.

In peripheral pulp, collagen fibers have unique arrangement forming Von korff's fibers. These are corkscrew like originating between odontoblasts and pass into dentin matrix.

> Fibers are more numerous in radicular pulp than coronal and greatest concentration of collagen generally occurs in the most apical portion of the pulp. This fact is of practical significance when a pulpectomy is performed during the course of endodontic treatment. Engaging the pulp with a barbed broach in the region of the apex affords a better opportunity to remove the tissue intact than does engaging the broach more coronally, where the pulp is more gelatinous and liable to tear.

## Ground Substance

The ground substance of the pulp is part of the system of ground substance in the body. It is a structureless mass with gel like consistency forming bulk of pulp. ***Chief components of ground substance*** are:

a. Glycosaminoglycans
b. Glycoproteins
c. Water

Functions of ground substance:

1. Forms the bulk of the pulp.
2. Supports the cells.
3. Acts as medium for transport of nutrients from the vasculature to the cells and of metabolites from the cells to the vasculature.

Depolymerization by enzymes produced by microorganisms found in pulpal inflammation may change ground substance of the pulp. Alexander et al in 1980 found that these enzymes can degrade the ground substance of the pulp by disrupting the glycosaminoglycan – collagen linkage. Alterations in the composition of ground substance caused by age or disease interfere with metabolism, reduced cellular function and irregularities in mineral deposition. Thus, the ground substance plays an important role in health and diseases of the pulp and dentin.

## SUPPORTIVE ELEMENTS

### Pulpal Blood Supply

Teeth are supplied by branches of maxillary artery (Flow Chart 2.1). Mature pulp has an extensive and unique vascular pattern that reflects its unique environment. Blood vessels which are branches of dental arteries consisting of arterioles enter the dental pulp by way of apical and accessory foramina. One or sometimes two vessels of arterioler size (about 150 μm) enter the apical foramen with sensory and sympathetic nerve bundles. The arterioles course up through radicular pulp and give off branches which spread laterally towards the odontoblasts layer and form capillary plexus. As they pass into coronal pulp, they diverge towards dentin, diminish in size and give rise to capillary network in sub-odontoblastic region (Fig. 2.9). This network provides odontoblasts with rich source of metabolites.

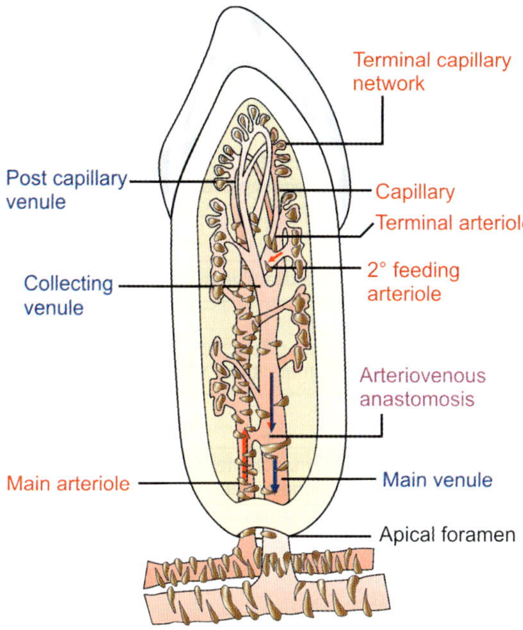


**Fig. 2.9:** Diagram showing circulation of pulp

Blood passes from capillary plexus into venules which constitute the efferent (exit) side of the pulpal circulation and are slightly larger than corresponding arterioles. Venules enlarge as they merge and advance toward the apical foramen (Flow Chart 2.2). Efferent vessels are thin walled and show only scanty smooth muscle.

### *Lymphatic Vessels (Flow Chart 2.3)*

Lymphatic vessels arise as small, blind, thin-walled vessels in the coronal region of the pulp and pass apically through middle

**Flow Chart 2.1:** Arterial supply of teeth

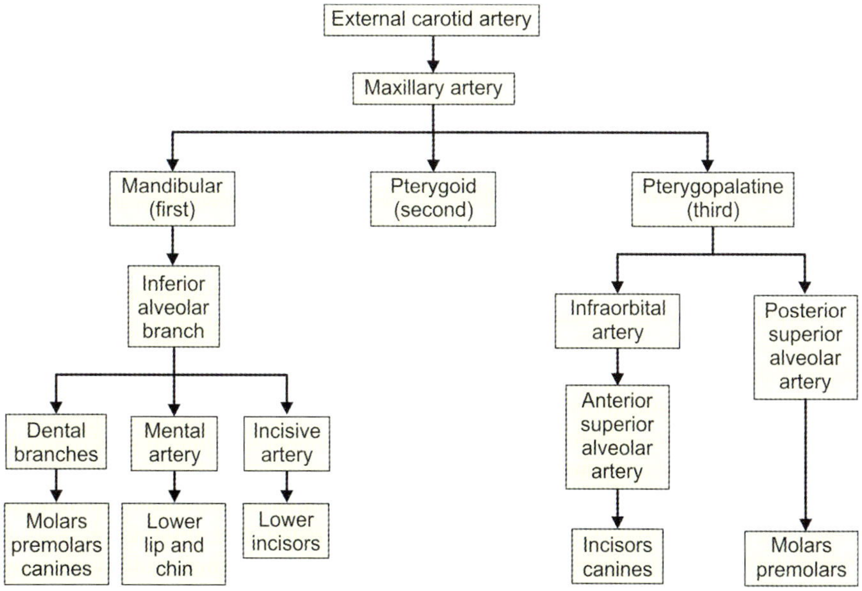

absent. The unmyelinated nerves are usually found in autonomic nervous system. The nerve fibers are classified according to their diameter, velocity of conduction and function. The fibers having largest diameter are classified as A fibers while those having smallest diameter are classified as C-fibers (Fig. 2.13). The A delta fibers are faster conducting and are responsible for localized, sharp dentinal pain. The C fibers are slower conducting fibers and are considered responsible for dull and throbbing pain. The pain receptors transmit their message to the central nervous system at different rates depending upon size, diameter and coating of the nerves.

Thermal, chemical or mechanical stimuli stimulate C fibers resulting in dull, poorly localized and throbbing pain.

Electrical pulp tester stimulates A delta fibers first because of their lower threshold. As the intensity of stimulus is increased along with A-delta fibers, some of the C-fibers also get stimulated resulting in strong unpleasant sensation.

## Basic Structure of a Neuron

The basic unit of nervous system is the neuron (Fig. 2.14). The cell membrane of the neuron is composed of bimolecular layer of lipid between two layers of protein. The physiology of nerve conduction is related to changes in cell membrane. The resting potential of the neuron depends on the selective permeability of plasma membrane and sodium pump of the cell. Stimulation of a neuron causes it to depolarize in the region of stimulus and subsequently adjacent areas of cell membrane are also depolarized. This depolarization during passage of excitation along the neuron constitutes the action potential or a nerve impulse. The cell information, in form of action potential is transduced into chemical message. When the nerve is at rest, the $Na^+$ are more concentrated in extracellular fluid than cytoplasm of the nerve itself and the $K^+$ ions are more concentrated in cytoplasm rather in extracellular fluid. Because of this, unequal concentration of ion, nerve fiber membrane is polarized. During excitation, there is rapid increase of $Na^+$ in the cell and $K^+$ ion flow out to lesser extent. As the impulse moves away, the membrane is recharged by outward movement. Subsequently, $Na^+$ ion are expelled into extracellular fluid while $K^+$ pump return $K^+$ into the intracellular fluid (Fig. 2.15). When the impulse arrives at synaptic terminals, neurotransmitters are released form the synaptic vesicles. These neurotransmitters generate an electrical impulse in the receptors of the dendrite of other neurons.

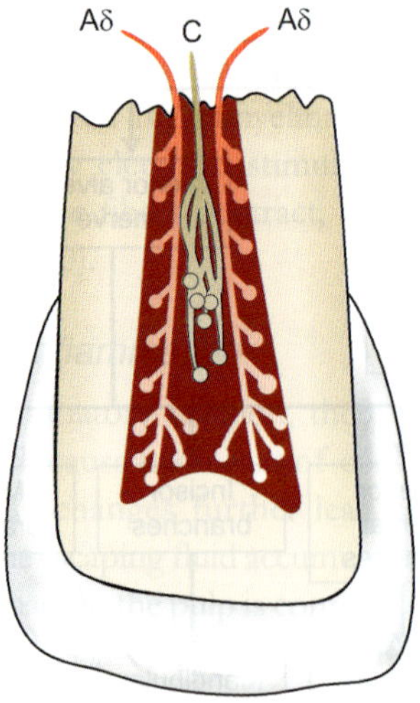

Fig. 2.13: Diagram showing nerve fibers of pulp

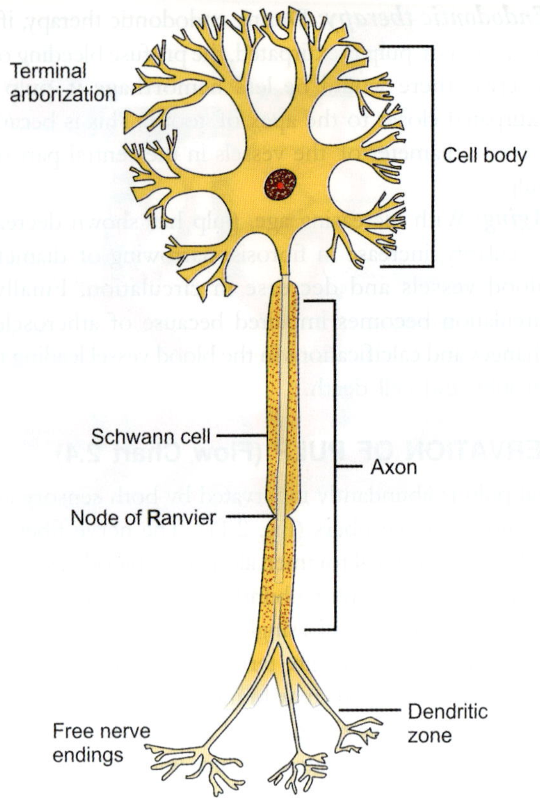

Fig. 2.14: Diagram showing structure of a neuron

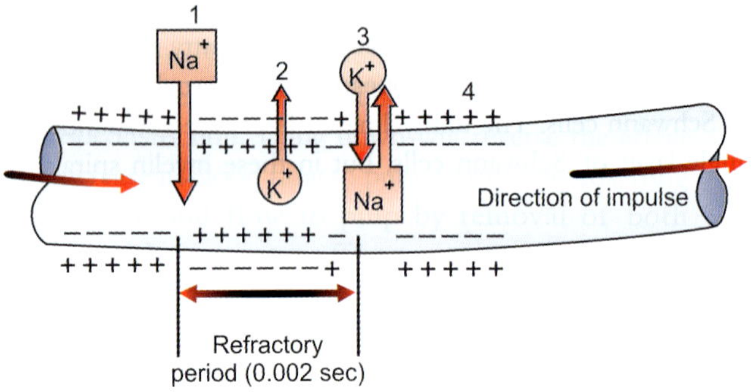

Fig. 2.15: Physiology of nerve conduction

**Difference between A-delta and C-fibers**

| *A-delta fibers* | *C-fibers* |
|---|---|
| 1. High conduction velocity (6-30 m/sec) | 1. Slow conduction velocity (0.5-2 m/sec) |
| 2. Myelinated | 2. Unmyelinated |
| 3. Pain is well localized | 3. Not well localized |
| 4. Have low threshold | 4. Have high threshold |
| 5. Sharp, quick and momentary pain | 5. Dull throbbing |

**A-delta nerve fibers**

- Most of myelinated nerve fibers are A-delta fibers.
- At the odontoblastic layer, they lose their myelin sheath and anastomose forming network of nerves called "Plexuses of Raschkow". The send free nerve endings into dentinal tubules.
- These are large fibers with fast conduction velocities.
- Pain transmitted through there fibers is perceived as sharp, quick and momentary pain.
- Pain disappears quickly on removal of stimulus

**A-beta nerve fibers**

- These fibers have fastest conduction velocities
- Extreme cold and hydrodynamic changes stimulate these fibers.
- A-delta fibers act as mechanoreceptors.

**C-nerve fibers**

- C-nerve fibers are small unmediated nerves.
- They have slow conduction velocities and high threshold.
- They are stimulated by intense cold or hot stimuli or mechanical stimulation.
- Even in presence of radiographic lesion, C-fibers can show response because these are more resistant to hypoxic conditions or compromised blood flow, when compared to A-delta fibers.
- These are responsible for pain occurring during instrumentation of teeth.

## ANATOMY OF DENTAL PULP

Pulp lies in the center of tooth and shapes itself to miniature form of tooth. This space is called pulp cavity which is divided into pulp chamber and root canal (Fig. 2.16).

In the anterior teeth, the pulp chamber gradually merges into the root canal and this division becomes indistinct (Fig. 2.17). But in case of multirooted teeth, there is a single pulp chamber and usually two to four root canals (Figs 2.18 and 2.19). As the external morphology of the tooth varies from person to person, so does the internal morphology of crown and the root. The change in pulp cavity anatomy results from age, disease, trauma or any other irritation.

## PULP CHAMBER

It reflects the external form of enamel at the time of eruption, but anatomy is less sharply defined. The roof of pulp chamber consists of dentin covering the pulp chamber occlusally. Canal orifices are openings in the floor of pulp chamber leading into the root canals (Fig. 2.20).

A specific stimulus such as caries leads to the formation of irritation dentin. With time, pulp chamber shows reduction in size as secondary or tertiary dentin is formed (Fig. 2.21).

## ROOT CANAL

Root *canal* is that portion of pulp cavity which extends from canal orifice to the apical foramen. The shape of root canal varies with size, shape, number of the roots in different teeth. A straight root canal throughout the entire length of root is uncommon. Commonly curvature is found along its length which can be gradual or sharp in nature (Fig. 2.22). In most cases, numbers of root canals correspond to number of roots but a root may have more than one canal.

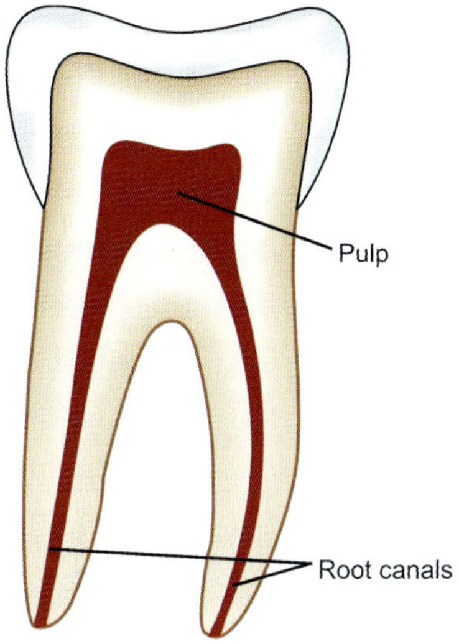


Fig. 2.16: Diagram showing pulp cavity

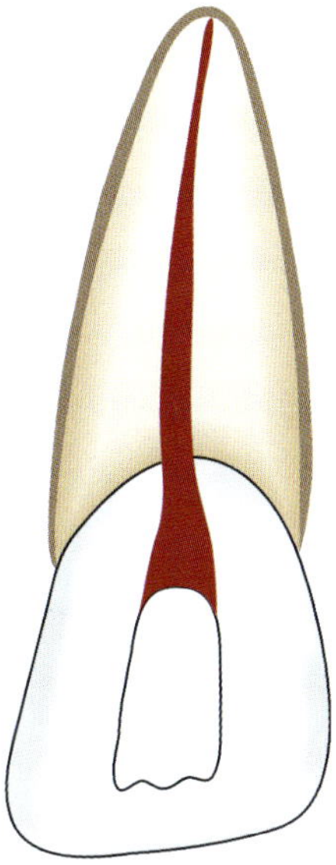

Fig. 2.17: Diagram showing pulp anatomy of anterior tooth

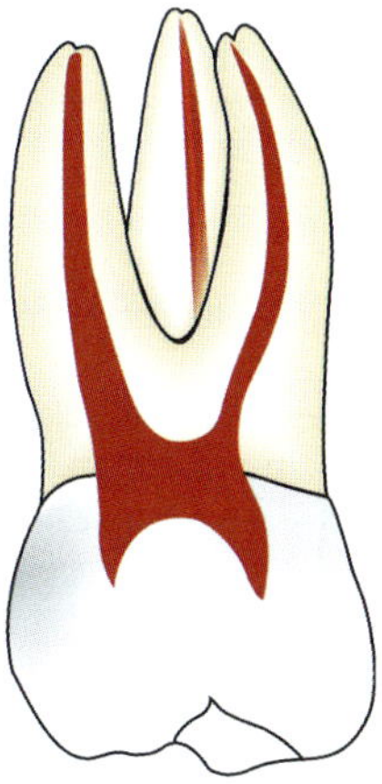

Fig. 2.18: Diagram showing pulp cavity of posterior tooth

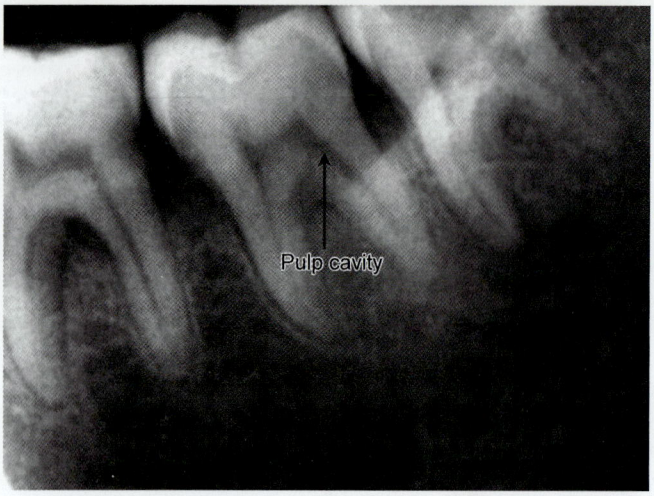


**Fig. 2.19:** Radiographic appearance of pulp cavity

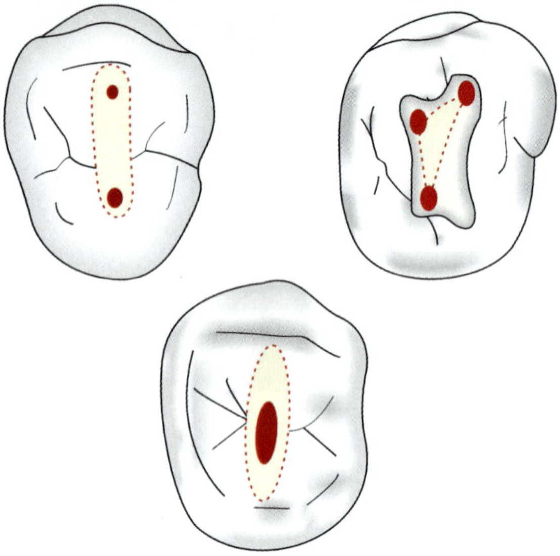

**Fig. 2.20:** Diagram showing opening of canal orifices in the pulp chamber

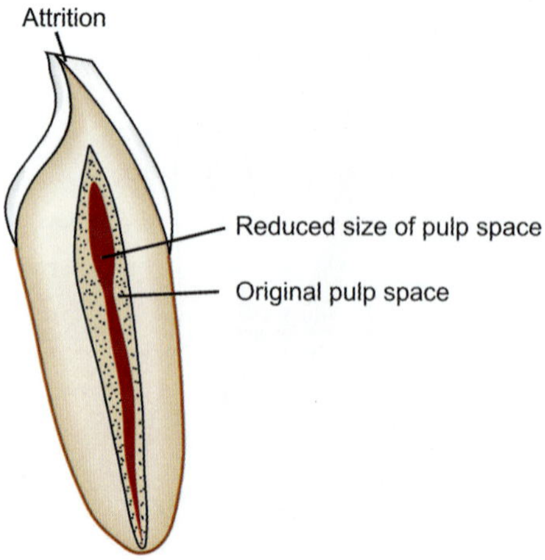


**Fig. 2.21:** Reduction in size of pulp cavity because of formation of secondary and tertiary dentin

According to Orban, the shape of the canal to large extent is largely determined by the shape of the root. Root canals can be round, tapering elliptical, broad, thin, etc.

"MEYER" stated that roots which are round and cone shaped usually contain one canal but roots which are elliptical with flat or concave surface frequently have more than one canal (Fig. 2.23).

Change in shape and location of foramen is seen during post-eruptive phase due to functional forces (tongue pressure, mesial drift) acting on the tooth which leads to cementum resorption and deposition on the walls of foramen. This whole process resulted in new foramen away from the apex. The total volume of all permanent pulp organs is 0.38 cc with mean of 0.02 cc.

***The apical foramen*** is an aperture at or near the apex of a root through which nerves and blood vessels of the pulp enter or leave the pulp cavity (Fig. 2.24). Normally, it is present near the apex but sometimes, opening may be present on the accessory and lateral canals of root surface forming the accessory foramina.

In young newly erupted teeth, it is wide open but as the root develops, apical foramen becomes narrower. The inner surface of the apex becomes lined with the cementum which may extend for a short distance into the root canal. Thus we can say that dentinocemental junction does not necessarily occur at the apical end of root, but may occur within the main root canal (Fig. 2.25).

Multiple foramina are frequent phenomenon in multirooted teeth. Majority of single rooted teeth have single canal which terminate in a single foramina. Continuous deposition of new layers of cementum causes change in foramen anatomy. Average size of maxillary teeth is 0.4 mm and of mandibular teeth is 0.3 mm.

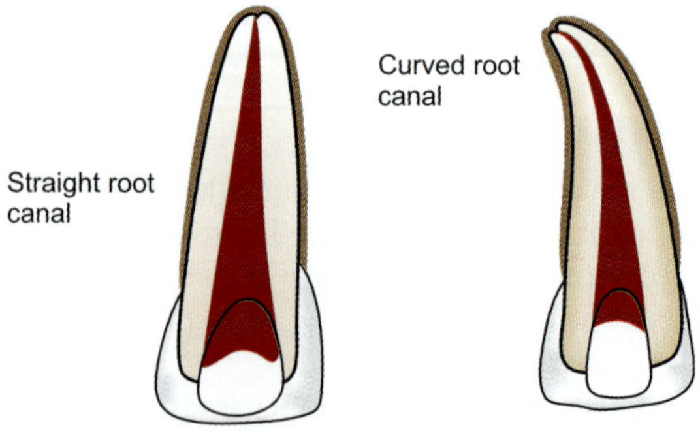


**Fig. 2.22:** Straight and curved root canal

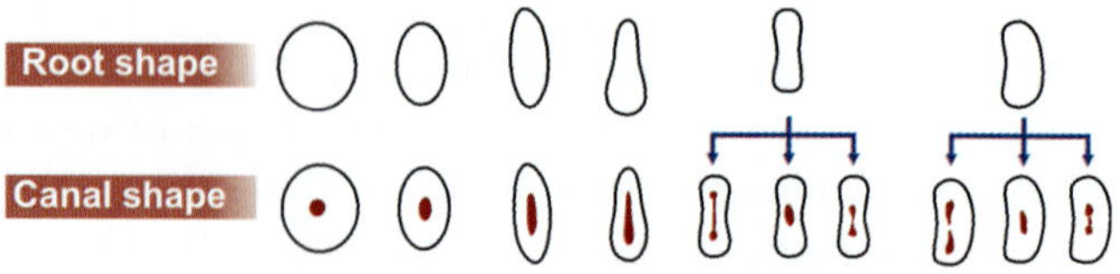


**Fig. 2.23:** Diagram showing relationship between shape of root and number of root canals

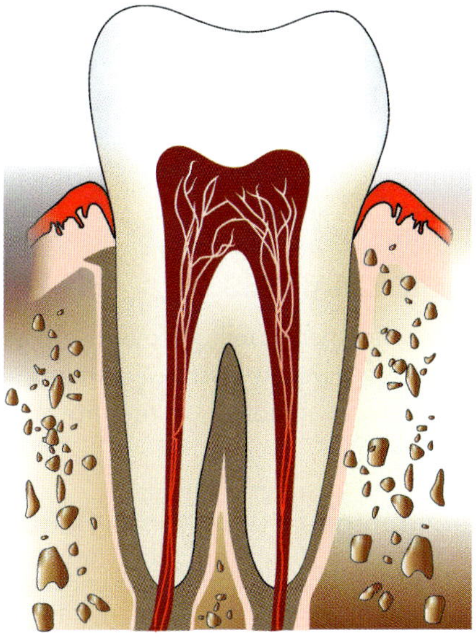

Fig. 2.24: Apical foramen through which nerves and blood vessels enter or leave the pulp cavity

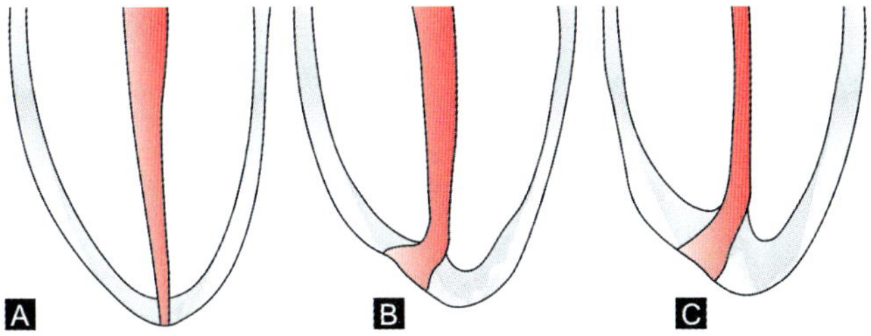


Fig. 2.25: Diagram showing variation in position of cementodentinal junction

*Accessory canals:* They are lateral branches of the main canal that form a communication between the pulp and periodontium. Accessory canals contain connective tissue and vessels and can be seen anywhere from furcation to apex but tend to more common in apical third and in posterior teeth (Fig. 2.26).

In other words, more apical and farther posterior the tooth, the more likely the accessory canals will be present.

Exact mechanism of their formation is not known but they occur in areas where there is premature loss of root sheath cells because these cells induce formation of odontoblasts. They also develop where developing root encounters a blood vessel. If vessel is located in this area, where dentin is forming; hard tissue may develop around it making a lateral canal from radicular pulp.

## FUNCTION OF PULP

The pulp lives for Dentin and the Dentin lives by the grace of the pulp.

**Pulp performs four basic functions i.e.:**
1. Formation of dentin
2. Nutrition of dentin
3. Innervation of tooth
4. Defense of tooth

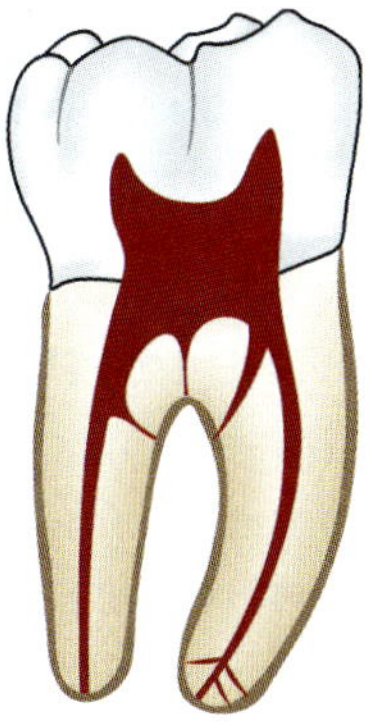

Fig. 2.26: Diagram showing accessory and lateral canals

### 1. Formation of Dentin

It is primary function of pulp both in sequence and importance. Odontoblasts are differentiated from the dental papilla adjacent to the basement membrane of enamel organ which later deposits dentin. Pulp primarily helps in:

- Synthesis and secretion of organic matrix.
- Initial transport of inorganic components to newly formed matrix.
- Creates an environment favorable for matrix mineralization.

### 2. Nutrition of Dentin

Nutrients exchange across capillaries into the pulp interstitial fluid. This fluid travels into the dentin through the network of tubules formed by the odontoblasts to contain their processes.

### 3. Innervation of Tooth

Through the nervous system, pulp transmits sensations mediated through enamel or dentin to the higher nerve centers. Pulp transmits pain, also senses temperature and touch.

Teeth are supplied by the maxillary and mandibular divisions of the trigeminal (V) nerve. The dental nerve divides into multiple branches as it traverses the bone. At the apical alveolar plate, the A delta and C axons enter the periodontal ligament. Then the nerves enter the apical foramina and unite to form common pulpal nerve. This nerve proceeds coronally with afferent blood vessels and later divides into cuspal nerves at the coronal portion of the tooth. On approaching the cell free zone of pulp, a mixture of myelinated and non-myelinated axons branch repeatedly forming overlapping network of nerves plexus of Raschkow. The nerve twigs either end among the stroma of the pulp or terminate among the odontoblasts.

### 4. Defense of Tooth

Odontoblasts form dentin in response to injury particularly when original dentin thickness has been compromised as seen in caries, attrition, trauma or restorative procedure. Odontoblasts also have the ability to form dentin at sites when dentin continuity has been lost.

The formation of reparative dentin and sclerotic dentin are defense mechanisms of the tooth.

Pulp also has the ability to elicit an inflammatory and immunologic response in an attempt to neutralize or eliminate invasion of dentin by caries causing micro-organisms and their byproducts.

## AGE CHANGES IN THE PULP

Pulp like other connective tissues, undergoes changes with time. These changes can be natural or may be result of injury such as caries, trauma or restorative dental procedure. Regardless of the cause, the pulp shows changes in appearance (morphogenic) and in function (physiologic).

## MORPHOLOGIC CHANGES

1. Continued deposition of intratubular dentin- reduction in tubule diameter.
2. Reduction in pulp volume due to increase in secondary dentin deposition (Fig. 2.27) – root canal appears very thin or seem to totally obliterated (Fig. 2.28).
3. Presence of dystrophic calcification and pulp stones (Fig. 2.29).
4. Decrease in the number of pulp cells-between 20 and 70 years. Cells density decreases by 50 percent.
5. Degeneration and loss of myelinated and unmyelinated axons–decrease in sensitivity.
6. Reduction in number of blood vessels- displaying arteriosclerotic changes.
7. Once believed that collagen content with age reduces, but recent studies prove that collagen stabilizes after completion of tooth formation. With age, collagen forms bundle making its presence more apparent.

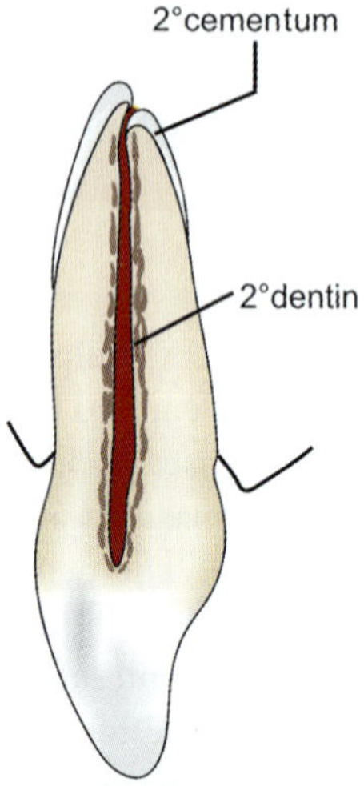


**Fig. 2.27:** Reduction in size of pulp volume

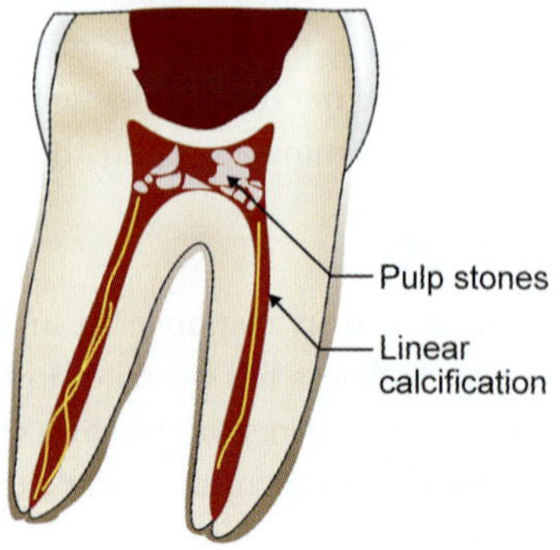


**Fig. 2.28:** Diagram showing pulp stones and reduced size of pulp cavity

## PHYSIOLOGIC CHANGES

1. Decrease in dentin permeability provides protected environment for pulp - reduced effect of irritants.
2. Possibility of reduced ability of pulp to react to irritants and repair itself.

### Pulpal Calcifications/Pulp Stones/Denticles

Pulp stones are nodular calcified masses appearing in either coronal and radicular pulp or both of these. The larger calcifications are called denticles. It is seen that pulp stones are present in at least 50 percent of teeth. Pulp stones may form either due to some injury or a natural phenomenon (Fig. 2.30).

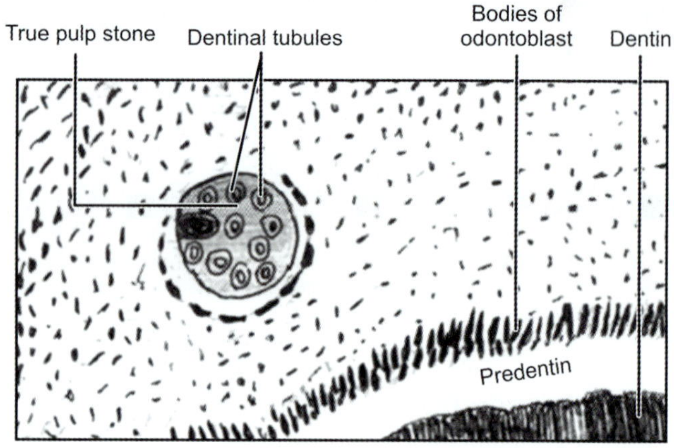


**Fig. 2.29:** Diagram showing true denticle

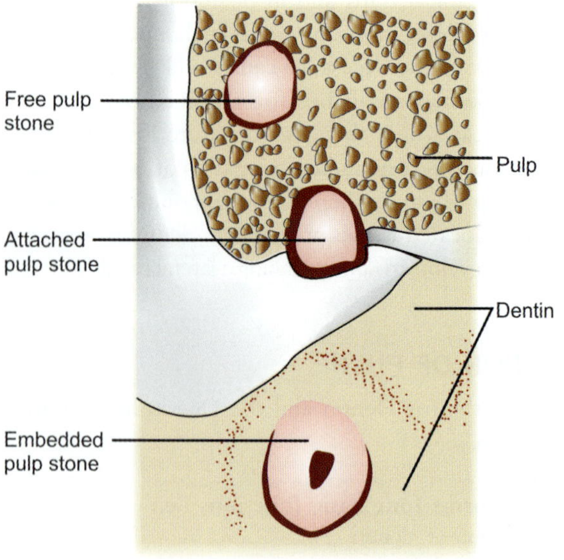


**Fig. 2.30:** Free, attached and embedded pulp stones

Sometimes denticles become extremely large, almost obliterating the pulp chamber or the root canal.

Pulp stones may be classified (1) according to structure (2) according to size (3) according to location.

**Classification of pulp stone**

1. According to structure
   a. True
   b. False
2. According to size
   a. Fine
   b. Diffuse
3. According to location
   a. Free
   b. Attached
   c. Embedded

## According to Structure

They can be classified into true and false denticles. The difference between two is only morphologic and not chemical.

### a. True Denticle

A true denticle is made up of dentin and is lined by odontoblasts. These are rare and are usually located close to apical foramen. Development of true denticle is caused by inclusions of remnants of epithelial root sheath within the pulp (Fig. 2.28) These epithelial remnants induce the cells of pulp to differentiate into odontoblast which form dentin masses called true pulp stones.

### b. False Denticles

Appear as concentric layers of calcified tissue. These appear within bundles of collagen fibers. They may arise around vessels. Calcification of thrombi in blood vessels called, phleboliths, may also serve as nidi for false denticles. All denticles begin as small nodules but increase in size by incremental growth on their surface.

## According to Size

According to size, there are fine and diffuse mineralizations. Diffuse calcifications are also known as fibrillar or linear calcifications because of their longitudinal orientation. They are found more frequently in the root canals, but can also be present in the coronal portion of the pulp. They are aligned closely to the blood vessels, nerves or collagen bundles.

### *According to Location they can be Classified as:*

- Free
- Attached
- Embedded

***Free denticles*** are entirely surrounded by pulp tissue.

***Attached denticles*** are partially fused dentin (Fig. 2.30).

***Embedded denticles*** are entirely surrounded by dentin calcifications, are seen more in older pulps. This may be due to increase in extent of cross linking between collagen molecules.

## Clinical Significance of Pulp Stones

Presence of pulp stones may alter the internal anatomy of the pulp cavity. Thus, making the access opening of the tooth difficult. They may deflect or engage the tip of endodontic instrument. Since the pulp stone can originate in response to chronic irritation, the pulp chamber which appears to have diffuse and obscure outline may represent large number of irregular pulp stones which may indicate chronic irritation of the pulp.

## Calcific Metamorphosis

Calcific metamorphosis is defined as a pulpal response to trauma that is characterized by deposition of hard tissue within the root canal space. It has also been referred to as pulp canal obliteration.

Calcific metamorphosis occurs commonly in young adults because of trauma. It is evident usually in the anterior region of the mouth and can partially or totally obliterate the canal space radiographically.

The ***clinical picture*** of calcific metamorphosis has been described by Patterson and Mitchell as a tooth that is darker in hue than the adjacent teeth and exhibits a dark yellow color because of a decrease in translucency from a greater thickness of dentin under the enamel.

The ***radiographic appearance*** of calcific metamorphosis is partial or total obliteration of the pulp canal space with a normal periodontal membrane space and intact lamina dura. Complete radiographic obliteration of the root canal space, however, does not necessarily mean the absence of the pulp or canal space; in the majority of these cases there is a pulp canal space with pulpal tissue.

The pulps of 20 maxillary permanent incisors were evaluated microscopically by Lundberg and Cvek. The teeth were treated endodontically because of progressive hard tissue formation in the canal space. The tissue changes were characterized by a varied increase in collagen content and a marked decrease in the number of cells. Osteoid tissue with included cells was found adjacent to mineralized areas in the pulp, with only one pulp showing moderate lymphocytic inflammatory infiltrate because of further trauma. They concluded that tissue changes in the pulps of teeth with calcific metamorphosis do not indicate the necessity for root canal treatment.

***The mechanism of hard tissue formation during calcific metamorphosis*** is characterized by an osteoid tissue that is produced by the odontoblasts at the periphery of the pulp space or can be produced by undifferentiated pulpal cells that undergo differentiation as a result of the traumatic injury. This results in a simultaneous deposition of a dentin-like tissue along the periphery of the pulp space and within the pulp space proper. These tissues can eventually fuse with one another, producing the radiographic appearance of a root canal space that has become rapidly and completely calcified.

The ***management of canals*** with calcific metamorphosis is similar to the management of pulpal spaces with any form of calcification.

## PERIRADICULAR TISSUE

Periradicular tissue consists of cementum, periodontal ligament and alveolar bone.

### Cementum

Cementum can be defined as hard, avascular connective tissue that covers the roots of the teeth (Fig. 2.31). It is light yellow in color and can be differentiated from enamel by its lack of luster and darker hue. It is very permeable to dyes and chemical agents, from the pulp canal and the external root surface.

### Types

There are two main types of root cementum
1. Acellular (Primary)
2. Cellular (Secondary)

### Acellular Cementum

1. Covers the cervical third of the root
2. Formed before the tooth reaches the occlusal plane.
3. As the name indicated, it does not contain cells.
4. Thickness is in the range 30-230 μm.
5. Abundance of sharpey's fibers.
6. Main function is anchorage.

### Cellular Cementum

1. Formed after the tooth reaches the occlusal plane.
2. It contains cells.
3. Less calcified than acellular cementum.
4. Sharpey's fibers are present in lesser number as compared to acellular cementum.
5. Mainly found in apical third and interradicular region
6. Main function is adaptation.

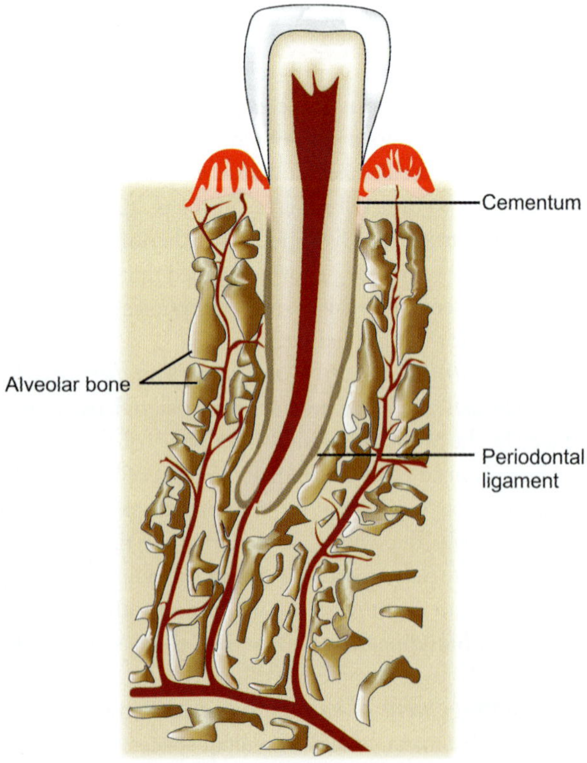


**Fig. 2.31:** Diagram showing periradicular tissue

### Periodontal Ligament

Periodontal ligament is a unique structure as it forms a link between the alveolar bone and the cementum. It is continuous with the connective tissue of the gingiva and communicates with the marrow spaces through vascular channels in the bone. Periodontal ligament houses the fibers, cells and other structural elements like blood vessels and nerves.

The periodontal ligament comprises of the following components
- I. Periodontal fibers
- II. Cells
- III. Blood vessels
- IV. Nerves

### Periodontal Fibers

The most important component of periodontal ligament is principal fibers. These fibers are composed mainly of collagen type I while reticular fibers are collagen type III. The principal fibers are present in six arrangements (Fig. 2.32).

#### *Horizontal Group*

These fibers are arranged horizontally emerging form the alveolar bone and attached to the root cementum.

#### *Alveolar Crest Group*

These fibers arise from the alveolar crest in fan like manner and attach to the root cementum. These fibers prevent the extrusion of the tooth.

#### *Oblique Fibers*

These fibers make the largest group in the periodontal ligament. They extend from cementum to bone obliquely. They bear the occlusal forces and transmit them to alveolar bone.

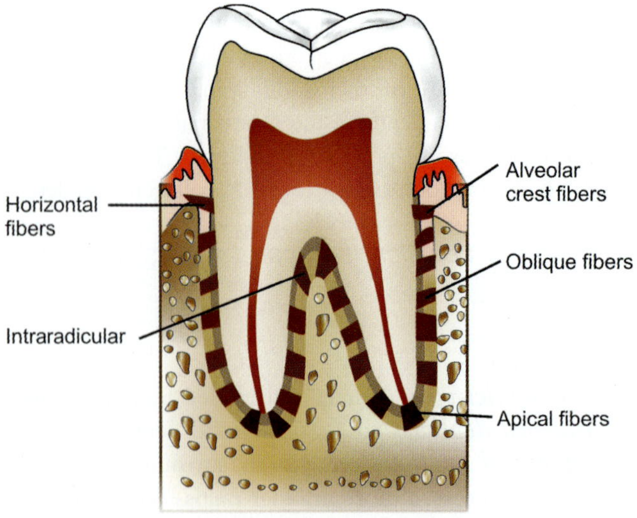


**Fig. 2.32:** Principal fibers of periodontal ligament

### *Transeptal Fibers*

These fibers run from the cementum of one tooth to the cementum of another tooth crossing over the alveolar crest.

### *Apical Fibers*

These fibers are present around the root apex.

### *Interradicular Fibers*

Present in furcation areas of multirooted teeth.

Apart from the principal fibers, oxytalan and elastic fibers are also present.

## Cells

The cells present in periodontal ligament are

a. Fibroblast
b. Macrophages
c. Mast cells
d. Neutrophils
e. Lymphocytes
f. Plasma cells
g. Epithelial cells rests of Mallassez.

## Nerve Fibers

The nerve fibers present in periodontal ligament, is either of myelinated or non-myelinated type.

## Blood Vessels

The periodontal ligament receives blood supply form the gingival, alveolar and apical vessels.

## Functions

### *Supportive*

Tooth is supported and suspended in alveolar socket with the help of periodontal ligament.

### *Nutritive*

Periodontal ligament has very rich blood supply. So, it supplies nutrients to adjoining structures such as cementum, bone and gingiva by way of blood vessels. It also provides lymphatic drainage.

### *Protective*

These fibers perform the function of protection absorbing the occlusal forces and transmitting to the underlying alveolar bone.

### *Formative*

The cells of PDL help in formation of surrounding structures such as alveolar bone and cementum.

## Resorptive

The resorptive function is also accomplished with the cells like osteoclasts, cementoclasts and fibroblasts provided by periodontal ligament.

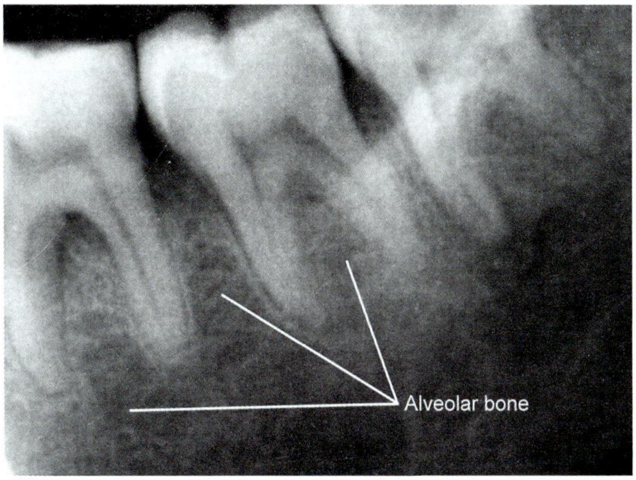


**Fig. 2.33:** Radiographic appearance of alveolar bone

## Alveolar Bone (Fig. 2.33)

Bone is specialized connective tissue which comprises of inorganic phases that is very well designed for its role as load bearing structure of the body.

## Cells

Cells present in bone are:

a. Osteocytes
b. Osteoblasts
c. Osteoclasts

## Intercellular Matrix

Bone consists of two third inorganic matter and one third organic matter. Inorganic matter is composed mainly of minerals calcium and phosphate along with hydroxyl apatite, carbonate, citrate etc. while organic matrix is composed mainly of collagen type I (90%).

Bone consists of two plates of compact bone separated by spongy bone in between. In some area there is no spongy bone. The spaces between trabeculae of spongy bone are filled with marrow which consists of hemopoietic tissue in early life and fatty tissue later in life. Bone is a dynamic tissue continuously forming and resorbing in response to functional needs. Both local as well as hormonal factors play an important role in metabolism of bone. In healthy conditions the crest of alveolar bone lies approximately 2-3 mm apical to the cemento-enamel junction but it comes to lie more apically in periodontal diseases. In periapical diseases, it gets resorbed easily.

## QUESTION

**Q. Write short notes on:**

a. Zones of dental pulp
b. Odontoblasts
c. Accessory and lateral canals
d. Innervation of pulp
e. Functions of pulp
f. Age changes in the pulp
g. Pulp stones/denticles/pulpal calcifications

## BIBLIOGRAPHY


1. Bernick S. Differences in nerve distribution between erupted and non-erupted human teeth. J Dent Res 1964;43:406.
2. Byers MR. The development of sensory innervations in dentine. J Comp Neurol 1980;191:413.
3. Heverass KJ. Pulpal, microvascular, and tissue pressure. J Dent Res 1985;64:585.
4. Johnsen DC. Innervations of teeth: qualitative, quantitative and developmental assessment. J Dent Res 1985;64:555.
5. Kim S. Regulation of pulpal blood flow. J Dent Res 1983;64:590.
6. Linde A. The extracellular matrix of the dental pulp and dentin. J Dent Res 1985;64:523.
7. Mjör IA. Dentin-predentin complex and its permeability: pathology and treatment overview. J Dent Res 1985;64:621.
8. Närhi MVO. The characteristics of intradental sensory units and their responses to stimulation. J Dent Res 1985;64:564.
9. Olgart LM. The role of local factors in dentin and pulp in intradental pain mechanisms. J Dent Res 1985;64:572.
10. Pashley DH. Dentin-predentin complex and its permeability: Physiologic overview. J Dent Res 1985;64:613.
11. Ruch JV. Odontoblast differentiation and the formation of odontoblas layer. J Dent Res 1985;64:489.
12. Thomas HF. The dentin-predentin complex and its permeability; anatomical overview. J Dent Res 1985;64:607.
13. Veis A. The role of dental pulp—thoughts on the session on pulp repair processes. J Dent Res 1985;64:552.
14. Yamamura T. Differentiation of pulpal cells and inductive influences of various matrices with reference to pulpal wound healing. J Dent Res 1985;64:530.

# Pathologies of Pulp and Periapex

CHAPTER 3



## INTRODUCTION

Dental pulp consists of vascular connective tissue contained within the rigid dentin walls. It is the principle source of pain within the mouth and also a major site of attention in endodontics and restorative treatment.

**Some important features of pulp are as follows (Fig. 3.1)**

- Pulp is located deep within the tooth, so defies visualization
- It gives radiographic appearance as radiolucent line
- Pulp is a connective tissue with several factors making it unique and altering its ability to respond to irritation
- Normal pulp is a coherent soft tissue, dependent on its normal hard dentin shell for protection. Therefore once exposed, it is extremely sensitive to contact and to temperature but this pain does not last for more than 1-2 seconds after the stimulus removed.
- Pulp is totally surrounded by a hard dental tissue, dentin which limits the area for expansion and restricts the pulp's ability to tolerate edema.
- The pulp has almost a total lack of collateral circulation, which severely limits its ability to cope with bacteria, necrotic tissue and inflammation
- The pulp consists of unique cells the odontoblasts, as well as cells that can differentiate into hard-tissue secreting cells. These cells form dentin and/or irritation dentin in an attempt to protect pulp from injury (Fig. 3.2).
- Pulpal responses are unpredictable, "Some pulps die if you look at them cross eyes, while others would not die even if you hit them with an axe".
- Correlation of clinical signs and symptoms with corresponding specific histological picture is often difficult.
- Thus the knowledge to pulp is essential not only for providing dental treatment, but also to know the rationale behind the treatment provided.

After all, "This little tissue has created a big issue".

## ETIOLOGY OF PULPAL DISEASES

I. Etiology of pulpal diseases can be broadly classified into:
   1. Physical
      - Mechanical
      - Thermal
      - Electrical
   2. Chemical

3. Bacterial
4. Radiation

II. *WEIN* classifies the causes of pulpal inflammation, necrosis or dystrophy in a logical sequence beginning with the most frequent irritant, microorganisms.

1. *Bacterial*

***Bacterial irritants:*** In 1891, WD Miller said that bacteria are a possible cause of pulpal inflammation (Fig. 3.3). Most common cause for pulpal injury-bacteria or their products may enter pulp through a break in dentin either from:

- Caries (Fig. 3.4)
- Accidental exposure
- Fracture
- Percolation around a restoration
- Extension of infection from gingival sulcus
- Periodontal pocket and abscess (Fig. 3.5)
- Anachoresis (Process by which microorganisms get carried by the bloodstream from another source localize on inflamed tissue).

Bacteria most often recovered from infected vital pulps are:

- Streptococci
- Staphylococci
- Diphtheroids, etc.

2. *Traumatic*

- Acute trauma like fracture, luxation or avulsion of tooth (Fig. 3.6).
- Chronic trauma including para-functional habits like bruxism.

3. *Iatrogenic* (Pulp inflammation for which the dentists own procedures are responsible is designated as Dentistogenic pulpitis). *Various iatrogenic causes of pulpal damage can be*:
   a. *Thermal changes* generated by cutting procedures, during restorative procedures, bleaching of enamel, electrosurgical procedures, laser beam, etc. can cause severe damage to the pulp if not controlled.
   b. Orthodontic movement
   c. Periodontal curettage
   d. Periapical curettage

*A use of chemicals* like temporary and permanent fillings, liners and bases and use of cavity desiccants such as alcohol.

4. *Idiopathic*
   a. Aging
   b. Resorption internal or external (Fig. 3.7).

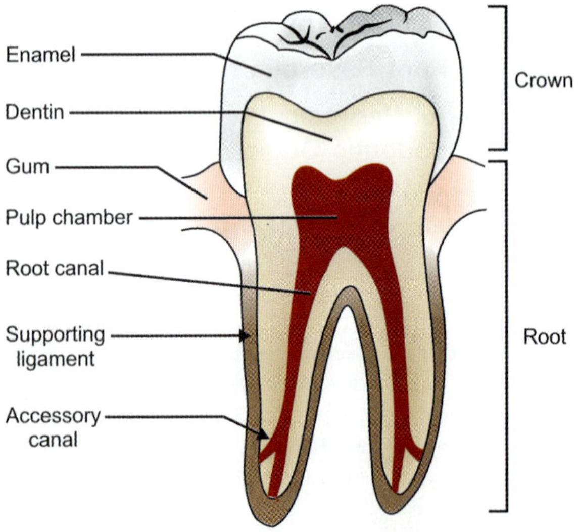


**Fig. 3.1:** Relation of pulp with its surrounding structures

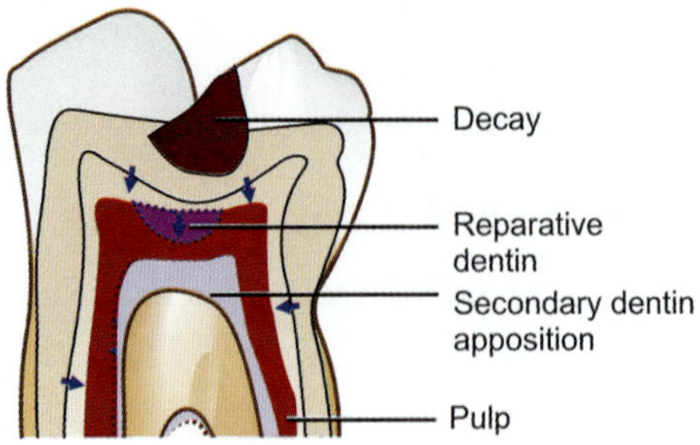


**Fig. 3.2:** Formation of irritation dentin

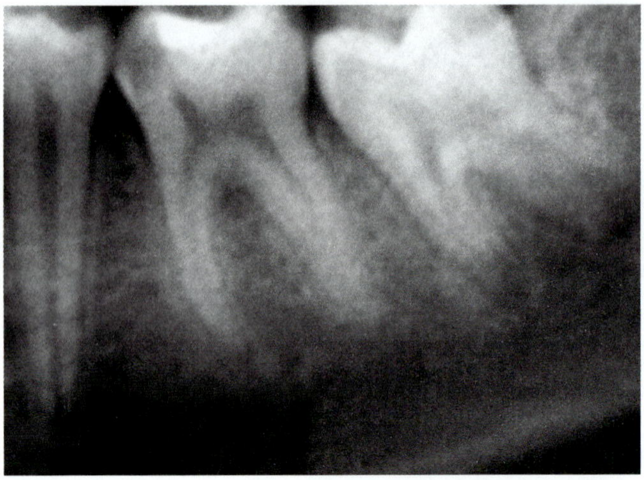

**Fig. 3.3:** Radiograph showing carious exposure of pulp in first molar

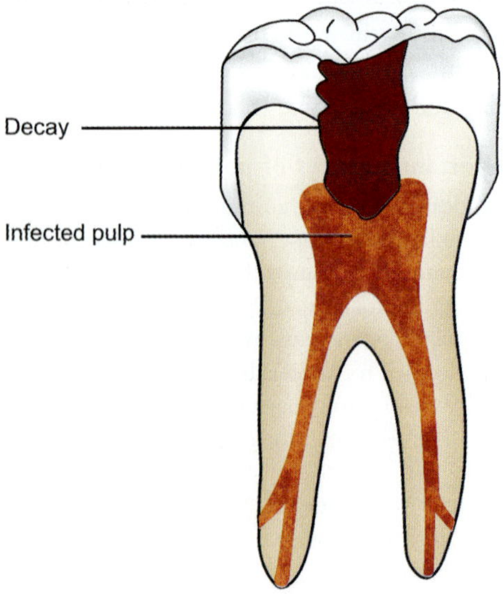


**Fig. 3.4:** Tooth decay causing pulpal inflammation

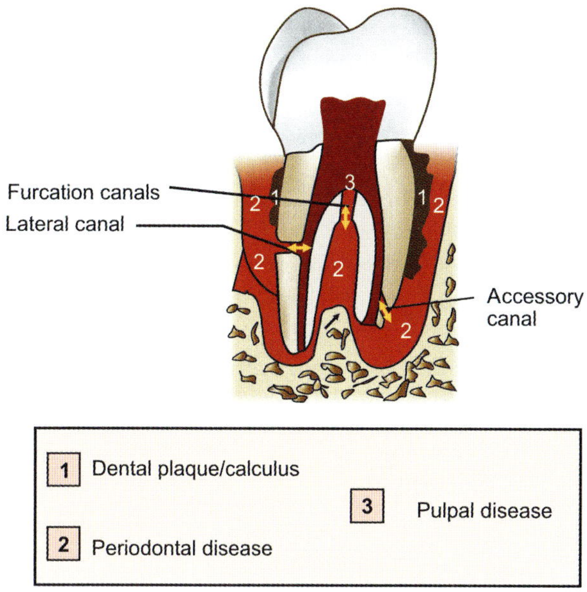


Fig. 3.5: Periodontal disease causing pulpal inflammation

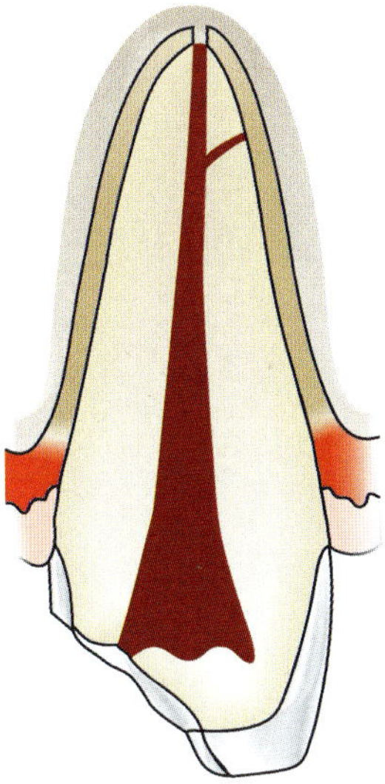

Fig. 3.6: Fracture of tooth can also cause pulpal inflammation

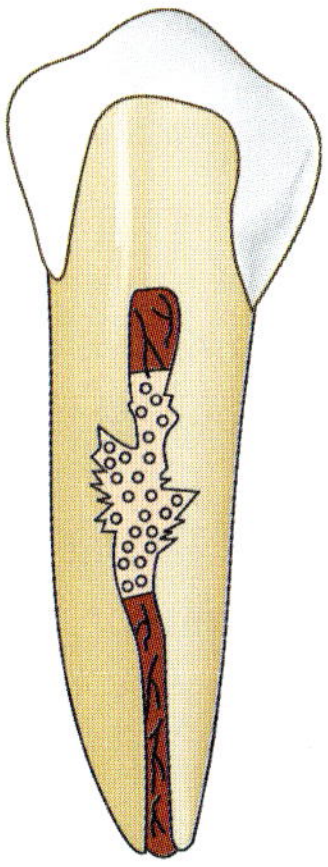

Fig. 3.7: Resorption of tooth involving pulp

## RADIATION INJURY TO PULP

Radiation therapy affect pulps of fully formed teeth in patients exposed to radiation therapy. The pulp cells exposed to ionizing radiation may become necrotic, there may occur vascular damage and the interference in mitosis of cells. Irradiations also affect the salivary glands causing decreased salivary flow, thereby increased disposition to dental caries and pulp involvement. Radiation damage to teeth depends on dose, source, type of radiation, exposure factor and stage of tooth development at the time of irradiation.

## PROGRESSION OF PULPAL PATHOLOGIES

Pulp reacts to above mentioned irritants as do other connective tissues. Degree of inflammation is proportional to intensity and severity of tissue damage. For example, slight irritation like incipient caries or shallow tooth preparation cause little or no pulpal inflammation, whereas extensive operative procedures may lead to severe pulpal inflammation.

Depending on condition of pulp, severity and duration of irritant, host response, pulp may respond from mild inflammation to pulp necrosis (Fig. 3.8).

These changes may not be accompanied by pain and thus may proceed unnoticed.

**Pulpal reaction to microbial irritation (Fig. 3.9)**

Carious enamel and dentin contains numerous bacteria
↓
Bacteria penetrate in deeper layers of carious dentin
↓
Pulp is affected before actual invasion of bacteria via their toxic byproducts
↓
Byproducts cause local chronic cell infiltration
↓
When actual pulp exposure occurs pulp tissue gets locally infiltrated by PMNs to form an area of liquefaction necrosis at the site of exposure
↓
Eventually necrosis spreads all across the pulp and periapical tissue resulting in severe inflammatory lesion.

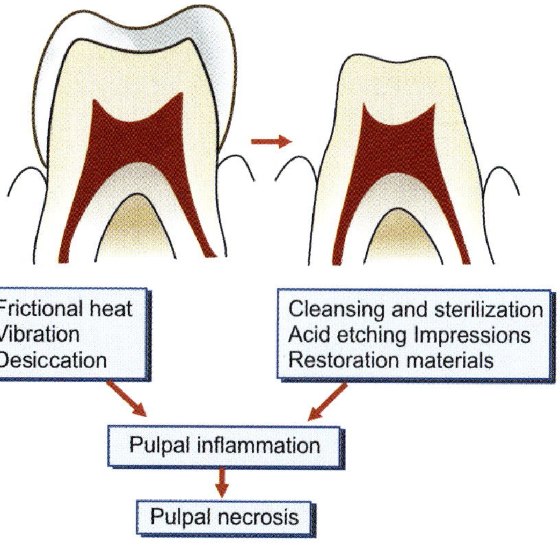


Fig. 3.8: Response of pulp to various irritants

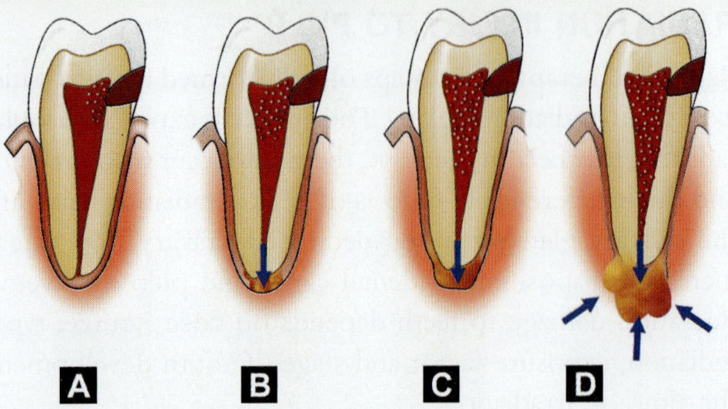


**Fig. 3.9:** Gradual response of pulp to microbial invasion

**Degree and nature of inflammatory response caused by microbial irritants depends upon**

1. Host resistance
2. Virulence of microorganisms
3. Duration of the agent
4. Lymph drainage
5. Amount of circulation in the affected area
6. Opportunity of release of inflammatory fluids

## DIAGNOSTIC AIDS FOR PULPAL PATHOLOGY

- Subjective symptoms—most common being pain
- Objective symptoms
  1. Visual and tactile inspection — 3**C**s –
     - i. **C**olor
     - ii. **C**ontour
     - iii. **C**onsistency
  2. Thermal tests
     - i. *Heat tests* — isolation of tooth — use of:
       - Warm air
       - Hot water
       - Hot burnisher
       - Hot gutta-percha stick
     - ii. *Cold tests*:
       - Ethyl chloride spray
       - Ice pencils
       - $CO_2$ snow — temperature 18°C
  3. Electrical pulp testing
  4. Radiographs
  5. Anesthetic tests
  6. Test cavity

Recent advances in diagnostic aids for pulpal pathology include:

1. Laser Doppler flowmetry
2. Liquid crystal testing
3. Hughes probeye camera
4. Infrared thermography
5. Thermocouples
6. Pulpoximetry
7. Dual wavelength spectrophotometry
8. Plethysmography
9. Xenon-133 radioisotopes

## CLASSIFICATION OF PULPAL PATHOLOGIES

- ***Baume's classification:*** Based on clinical symptoms
  1. Asymptomatic, vital pulp which has been injured or involved by deep caries for which pulp capping may be done.
  2. Pulps with history of pain which are amenable to pharmacotherapy.
  3. Pulps indicated for extirpation and immediate root filling.
  4. Necrosed pulps involving infection of radicular dentin accessible to antiseptic root canal therapy.
- ***Seltzer and Bender's classification:*** Based on clinical tests and histological diagnosis.
  1. *Treatable*
     - a. Intact uninflamed pulp
     - b. Transition stage
     - c. Atrophic pulp
     - d. Acute pulpitis
     - e. Chronic partial pulpitis without necrosis
  2. *Untreatable*
     - a. Chronic partial pulpitis with necrosis
     - b. Chronic total pulpitis
     - c. Total pulp necrosis

### *Engel's classification*

1. *Inflammatory changes*
   - a. Hyperreactive pulpalgia
     - Hypersensitivity
     - Hyperemia.
   - b. Acute pulpalgia
     - Incipient
     - Moderate
     - Advanced
   - c. Chronic pulpalgia
   - d. Hyperplastic pulpitis
   - e. Pulp necrosis
2. Retrogressive changes
   - a. Atrophic pulposis.
   - b. Calcific pulposis

- Grossman's clinical classification
  1. Pulpitis
     - a. Reversible
       - Symptomatic (Acute)
       - Asymptomatic (Chronic)
     - b. Irreversible pulpitis
     - i. Acute
       - a. Abnormally responsive to cold
       - b. Abnormally responsive to heat
     - ii. Chronic
       - a. Asymptomatic with pulp exposure
       - b. Hyperplastic pulpitis
       - c. Internal resorption
  2. Pulp degeneration
     - a. Calcific (Radiographic diagnosis)
     - b. Other (Histopathological diagnosis)
  3. Necrosis

## NORMAL PULP AND PULPITIS

***A normal pulp*** gives moderate response to pulp test and this response subsides when the stimulus is removed. The tooth is free of spontaneous pain. Radiograph shows an intact lamina dura, absence of any pulpal abnormality, calcifications, and resorption (Fig. 3.10).

***Pulpitis*** is inflammation of the dental pulp resulting from untreated caries, trauma, or multiple restorations. Its principal symptom is pain. Diagnosis is based on clinical finding and in confirmed in X-ray. Treatment involves removing decay, restoring the damaged tooth, and, sometimes, performing root canal therapy or extracting the tooth.

Pulpitis can occur when caries progresses deeply into the dentin, when a tooth requires multiple invasive procedures, or when trauma disrupts the lymphatic and blood supply to the pulp. It starts as a reversible condition in which the tooth can be saved by a simple filling. If untreated, it progresses as swelling inside the rigid encasement of the dentin compromising the circulation, making the pulp necrotic, which predisposes to infection.

Infectious sequelae of pulpitis include apical periodontitis, periapical abscess cellulitis, and osteomyelitis of the jaw (Fig. 3.11). Spread from maxillary teeth may cause purulent sinusitis, meningitis, brain abscess, orbital cellulitis, and cavernous sinus thrombosis. Spread from mandibular teeth may cause Ludwig's angina, parapharyngeal abscess, mediastinitis, pericarditis and empyema (Fig. 3.12).

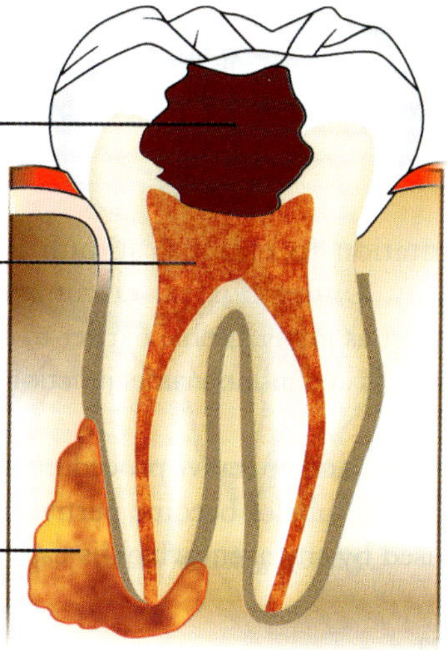


Fig. 3.11: Infectious sequelae of pulpitis

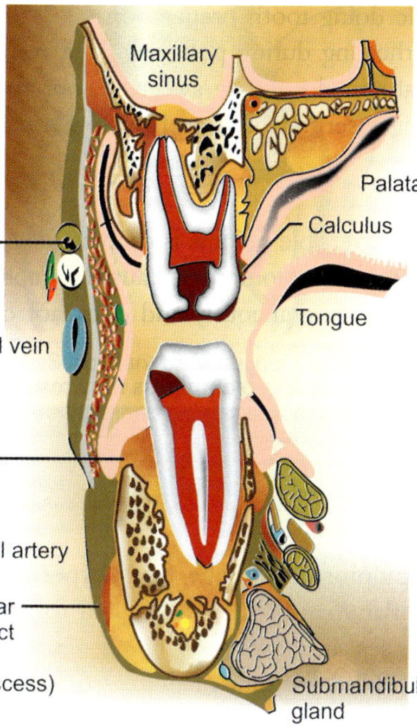


Fig. 3.12: Spread of pulpal inflammation to surrounding tissues

## BARODONTALGIA/AERODONTALGIA

It is pain experienced in a recently restored tooth during low atmospheric pressure. Pain is experienced either during ascent or descent. Chronic pulpitis which appears asymptomatic in normal conditions, may also manifests as pain at high altitude because of low pressure.

Rauch classified barodontalgia according to chief complaint:

**Class I:** In acute pulpits, sharp pain occurs for a moment on ascent

**Class II:** In chronic pulpitis, dull throbbing pain occurs on ascent.

**Class III:** In necrotic pulp, dull throbbing pain occurs on descent but it is asymptomatic on ascent.

**Class IV:** In periapical cyst or abscess, pain occurs with both ascent and descent.

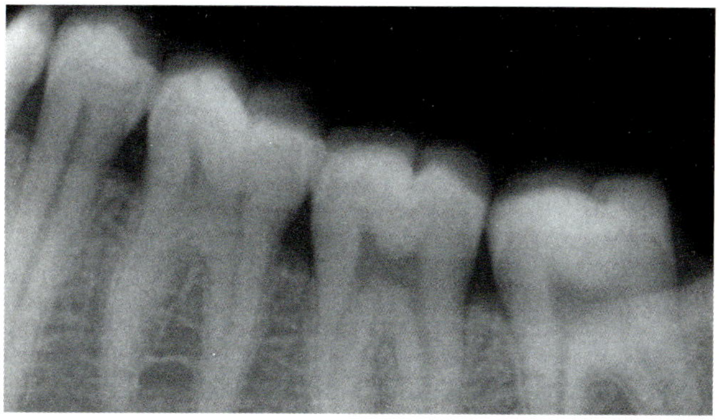

Fig. 3.10: Radiographic picture of normal teeth

## REVERSIBLE PULPITIS/HYPEREMIA/ HYPERACTIVE PULPALGIA

This is the first stage where the pulp is symptomatic. There is a sharp hypersensitive response to cold, but the pain subsides when stimulus is removed. The patient may describe symptoms of momentary pain and is unable to locate the source of pain. This stage can last for month or years.

### Definition

"Reversible pulpitis is the general category which histologically may represent a range of responses varying from dentin hypersensitivity without concomitant inflammatory response to an early phase of inflammation."

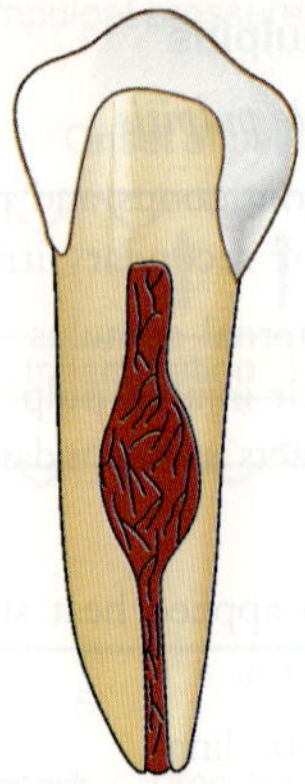

Fig. 3.23: Diagram showing internal resorption of the tooth

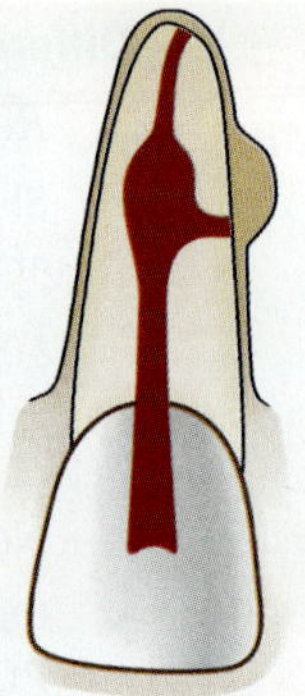

Fig. 3.24: Internal resorption of tooth causing perforation of root

**Mechanism of resorption**

Pulp inflammation due to infection
↓
Alteration or loss of predentine and odontoblastic layer
↓
Undifferentiated mesenchymal cells come in contact with mineralized dentin
↓
Differentiate into dentinoclasts
↓
Resorption results

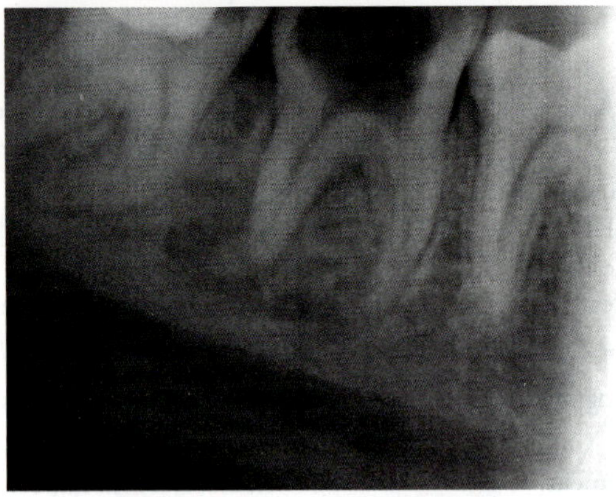

Fig. 3.25: Tooth decay resulting in pulpal necrosis

## Symptoms

- Usually asymptomatic, recognized clinically through routine radiograph
- Pain occurs in cases of perforation of crown (Fig. 3.24)
- "Pink Tooth" is the pathognomic feature of internal root resorption.

## Diagnosis

- ***Clinically:*** "Pink Tooth" appearance
- ***Radiographic changes:***
  - Radiolucent enlargement of pulp canal
  - Original root canal outline distorted
  - Bone changes are seen only when root perforation into periodontal ligament takes place.
- ***Pulp tests*:** Positive, though coronal portion of pulp is necrotic, apical pulp could be vital.

## Treatment

- Pulp extirpation stops internal root resorption.
- Surgically treatment is indicated if conventional treatment fails.

# PULP NECROSIS

Pulp necrosis or death is a condition following untreated pulpitis. The pulpal tissue becomes dead and if the condition is not treated, noxious materials will leak from pulp space forming the lesion of endodontic origin (Fig. 3.25).

Necrosis may be partial or total, depending on extent of pulp tissue involvement.

The pulp necrosis is of ***two types***:

- ***Coagulation necrosis:*** In coagulation necrosis protoplasm of all cells becomes fixed and opaque. Cell mass is recognizable histologically, intracellular details lost.
- ***Liquefaction necrosis:*** In liquefaction necrosis the entire cell outline is lost. The liquefied area is surrounded by dense zone of PMNL (dead or drying), chronic inflammatory cells.

## Etiology

Necrosis is caused by noxious insult and injuries to pulp by bacteria, trauma, and chemical irritation.

## Symptoms

- Discoloration of tooth—First indication of pulp death (Fig. 3.26)
- History from patient
- Tooth might be asymptomatic.

## Diagnosis

1. ***Pain:*** It is absent in complete necrosis.
2. ***History of patient*** reveals past trauma or past history of severe pain which may last for some time followed by complete and sudden cessation of pain.
3. ***Radiographic changes:*** Radiograph shows a large cavity or restoration (Fig. 3.27) or normal appearance unless there is concomitant apical periodontitis or condensing osteitis.
4. ***Vitality test:*** Tooth is nonresponding to vitality tests. But multirooted teeth may show mixed response because only one canal may have necrotic tissue.

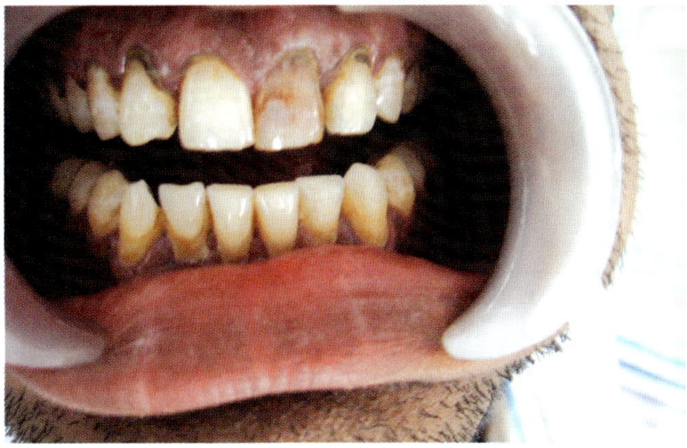

Fig. 3.26: Pulpal necrosis of 21 resulting in discoloration

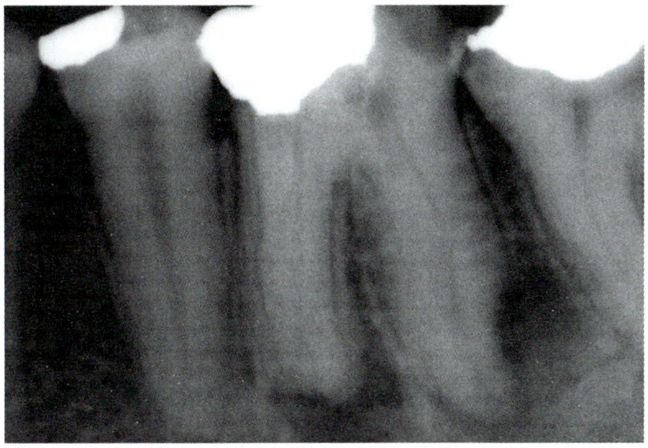

Fig. 3.27: Radiograph showing a large restoration in molar resulting in pulpal irritation

Sometimes teeth with liquefaction necrosis may show positive response to electric test when electric current is conducted through moisture present in a root canal.

5. ***Visual examination:*** Tooth shows color change like dull or opaque appearance due to lack of normal translucency (Fig. 3.28).
6. ***Histopathology:*** Necrotic pulp tissue, cellular debris and microorganisms are seen in pulp cavity. If there is concomitant periodontal involvement, there may be presence of slight evidence of inflammation.

### Treatment

Complete removal of pulp followed by restoration or extraction of nonrestorable tooth.

## PULP DEGENERATION

Pulp degeneration is generally present in older people. It may be the result of persistent mild irritation in the teeth of younger people. Usually pulp degeneration is induced by attrition, abrasion, erosion, bacteria, operative procedures, caries, pulp capping and reversible pulpitis.

It may occur in following forms:

1. ***Atrophic degeneration and fibrosis***
   - It is wasting away or decrease in size which occurs slowly as tooth grows old (Fig. 3.29). There is gradual shift in ratio and quality of tissue elements. In this condition number of collagen fibers/unit area increases leading to fibrosis. Number of pulp cells and size of cells decreases so the cells appear as "shrunken solid particles in a sea of dense fibers"
   - Fibroblastic processes are lost, cells have round and pyknotic nuclei
   - Dentinoblasts decrease in length, appear cuboidol or flattened.

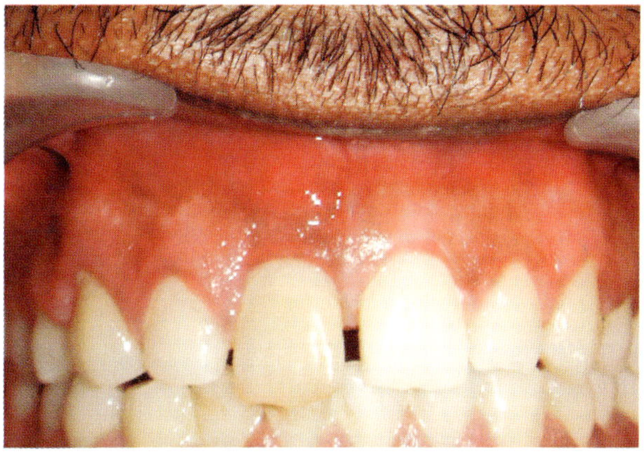

Fig. 3.28: Lack of normal translucency in nonvital

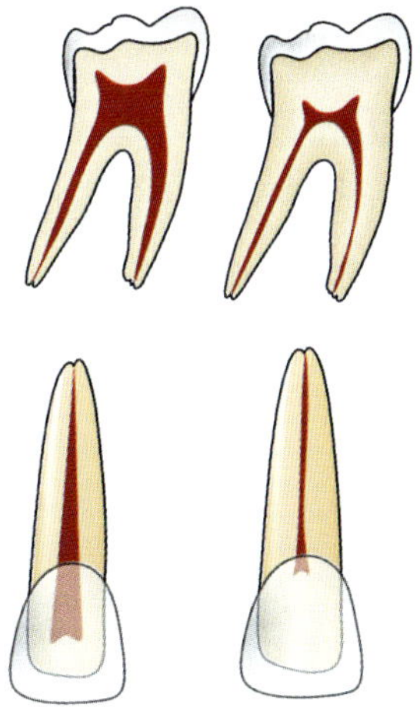

Fig. 3.29: Atrophic changes of pulp with age

2. ***Calcifications***

   In calcific degeneration, part of the pulp tissue is replaced by calcific material (Fig. 3.30). Mainly three types of calcifications are seen in pulp:
   - Dystrophic calcification
   - Diffuse calcification
   - Denticles/pulp stones.

### Dystrophic Calcifications

They occur by deposition of calcium salts in dead or degenerated tissue. The local alkalinity of destroyed tissues attracts the salts. They occur in minute areas of young pulp affected by minor circulatory disturbances, in blood clot or around a single degenerated cell. It can also begin in the connective tissue walls of blood vessels and nerves and follow their course.

### Diffuse Calcifications

They are generally observed in root canals. The deposits become long, thin and fibrillar on fusing.

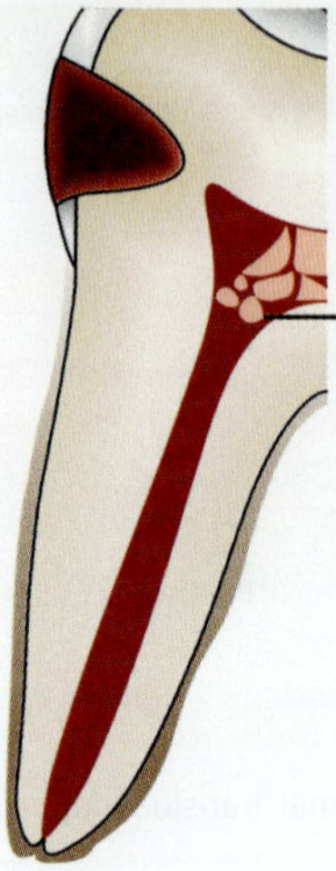


Fig. 3.30: Calcifications present in pulp

### Denticles/Pulp Stone

These are usually seen in pulp chamber.

### Classification

*According to location* (Fig. 3.31)
- Free
- Embedded
- Attached

*According to structure*
- True
- False

***True denticles:*** It is composed of dentin formed from detached odontoblasts or fragments of Hertwig's enamel root sheath which stimulate and undifferentiated cells to assume dentinoblastic activity.

***False denticles:*** Here degenerated tissue structures act as nidus for deposition of concentric layers of calcified tissues.

## PERIRADICULAR PATHOLOGIES

Periradicular tissue contains apical root cementum, periodontal ligament and alveolar bone (Fig. 3.32).

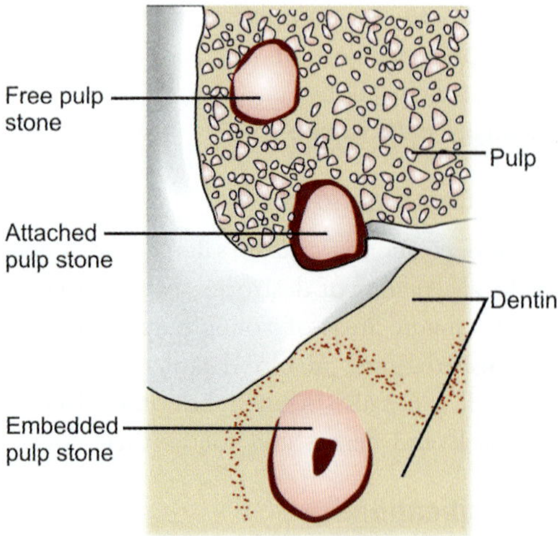


Fig. 3.31: Types of pulp stones

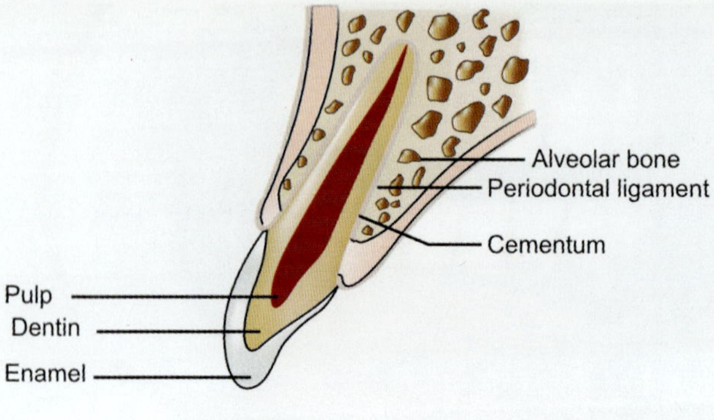


Fig. 3.32: Diagram showing periodontium

Apical periodontium consists of cellular and extracellular components. Fibroblasts, cementoblasts, osteoblasts, undifferentiated mesenchymal cells, epithelial cells rests of Malassez, blood vessels, lymphatics, sensory and motor nerve fibers form its components.

Alveolar bone proper lines the alveolus. It consists of:
- *Bundle bone*: Peripheral bone
- *Lamellated*: Center of alveolar process

Lamina Dura is radiographic image of alveolar bone proper.

*Cementum*: Two types of collagen fibers are present in cementum.

a. *Matrix fibers*—parallel to root surface; inter woven, mainly consists of cementoblasts.
b. *Sharpey's fibers*—fibroblast are the main component of Sharpey's fibers.

## ETIOLOGY OF PERIRADICULAR DISEASES

### Bacterial

- Untreated pulpal infection leads to total pulp necrosis. If left untreated, irritants leak into periapical region forming periapex pathologies (Fig. 3.33). Severity of periapical inflammation is related to microorganisms in root canals and the length of exposure to infecting microorganisms. Anachoresis also accounts for microbial infection in teeth. Microorganisms may invade pulp from periodontal pocket and accessory canals leading to development of lesion of endodontic origin

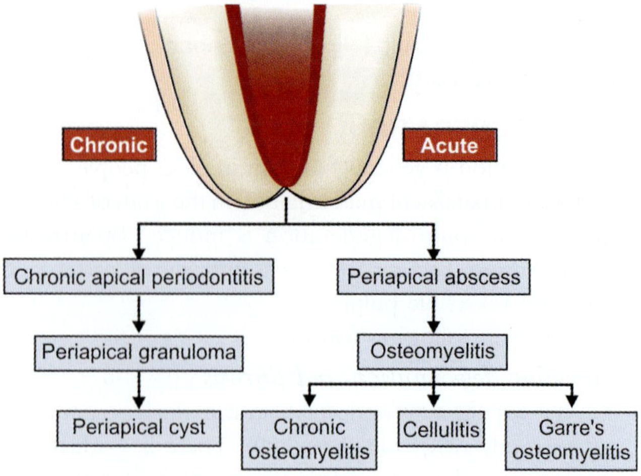


Fig. 3.33: Sequelae of pulpal inflammation

**Different features of pulpitis**

| *No.* | | *Reversible pulpitis* | *Acute pulpitis* | *Chronic pulpitis* | *Hyperplastic pulpitis* | *Pulp necrosis* |
|---|---|---|---|---|---|---|
| 1. | Pain and stimulus | Mid pain lasting for a moment | Constant to severe pain caused by hot or cold stimuli | Mild and intermittent | Pain not present but it bleeds due to presence of rich network of blood vessels in granulomatous tissue into carious cavity | Not present |
| 2. | Stimulus | Heat, cold or sugar | • Hot or cold<br>• Spontaneous | • Spontaneous<br>• Dead/injured pulp tissue acts as secondary stimulus | | |
| 3. | Pulp test | | | | | |
| | i. Thermal | Readily responds to cold | Acute pain to hot stimuli | No response | No response | No response |
| | ii. Electric | Normal response | Normal to elevated response | More current is required<br>with electric tester | More current is required<br>response is seen | In cases of liquefaction necrosis, positive |
| 4. | Radiograph | Deep caries, Defective restoration | Deep caries Defective restoration | i. Chronic apical periodontitis<br>ii. Local condensing osteitis | Same<br>Same | • Large restoration<br>• Sometimes apical periodontitis or condensing osteitis |
| 5. | Treatment | Removal of decay, restoration with pulp protection, occlusal adjustment | • Pulpotomy<br>• Root canal therapy | • RCT<br>• Extraction of nonrestorable tooth | • Removal of polypoid tissue with curette/ spoon excavator followed by RCT | • RCT/extraction |

- Root canal is unique, stringent ecological niche for bacterial growth because of lack of oxygen. For bacteria present here the primary nutrient sources is host tissues and tissue fluids.
- Microorganisms in chronically infected root canals are mainly anaerobic and gram-negative type. Most common micro-organisms are:
  - *Streptococcus*
  - *Peptostreptococcus*
  - *Provotella*

    Black pigmented microorganisms
  - *Porphyromonas*
  - *Enterococcus*
  - *Campylobacter*
  - *Fusobacterium*
  - *Eubacterium*
  - *Propionibacterium*

## Trauma

- Physical trauma to tooth, or operative procedures which results in dental follicle desiccation or significant heat transfer causes sufficient damage to pulp and its blood supply. It results in inflammation with immediate response involving the production of endogenous inflammatory mediators which cause increase in vascular permeability, stasis and leukocyte infiltration
- In cases of severe trauma to tooth resulting in immediate interruption of blood supply, pulp becomes necrotic but is not infected
- Persistent periapical tissue compression from traumatic occlusion leads to apical inflammatory response.

## Factors Related to Root Canal Procedures

Several complications can arise from improper endodontic technique which can cause periapical diseases:

1. It is impossible to extirpate pulp without initiating an inflammatory response because a wound is created.
2. Using strong or excessive amounts of intracanal medicaments between appointments may induce periapical inflammation.
3. Improper manipulation of instruments within root canal or over instrumentation can force dentinal debris, irrigating solution and toxic components of necrotic tissue in the periapex.
4. Overextended endodontic filling material may induce periapical inflammation by directly inducing foreign body reaction which is characterized by presence of leukocyte infiltration, macrophages and other chronic inflammatory cells (Fig. 3.34).

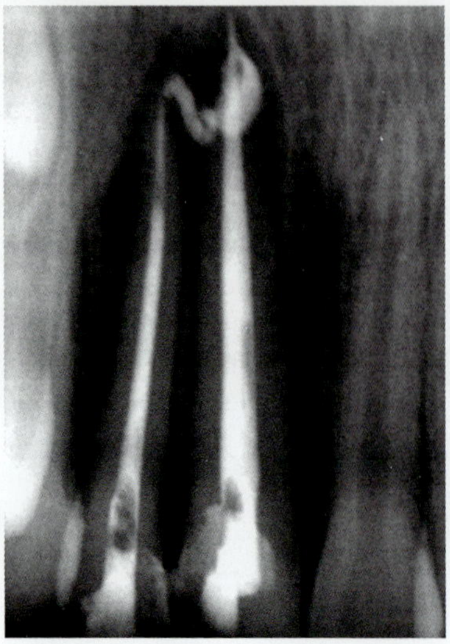

**Fig. 3.34:** Inflammation of periradicular tissue resulting from overextension of obturation material

## DIAGNOSIS OF PERIRADICULAR PATHOLOGIES

1. ***Chief complaint*:** Patient usually complains of pain on biting, pain with swelling, pus discharge, etc.
2. ***Dental history*:** Recurring episodes of pain, swelling with discharge, swelling which reduces on its own.

## OBJECTIVE EXAMINATION

1. ***Extraoral examination:*** General appearance, skin tone, facial asymmetry, swelling, extraoral sinus, sinus-tract, tender or enlarged cervical lymph nodes.
2. ***Intraoral examination:*** It includes examination of soft tissues and teeth to look for dicoloration, abrasion, caries, restoration, etc.

## CLINICAL PERIAPICAL TESTS

1. ***Percussion:*** Indicates inflammation of periodontium (Fig. 3.35).
2. ***Palpation:*** Determines how far the inflammatory process has extended periapically.
3. ***Pulp vitality:***
   i. Thermal tests which can be heat or cold
   ii. Electrical pulp testing
4. ***Periodontal examination:*** It is important because periapical and periodontal lesion may mimic each other and require differentiation.
   a. ***Probing:*** Determines the level of connective tissue attachment. Probe can penetrate into an inflammatory periapical lesions that extends cervically (Fig. 3.36).
   b. ***Mobility:*** Determines the status of periodontal ligament.
5. ***Radiographic examination*** (Fig. 3.37): Periradicular lesions of pulpal origin have four characteristics:
   - Loss of lamina dura apically.
   - Radiolucency at apex regardless of cone angle.
   - Radiolucency resembles a hanging drop.
   - Cause of pulp necrosis is usually evident.

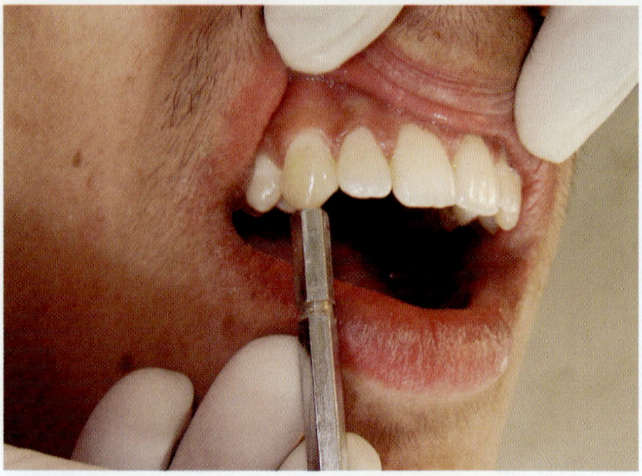

**Fig. 3.35:** Pain on percussion indicates inflamed periodontium

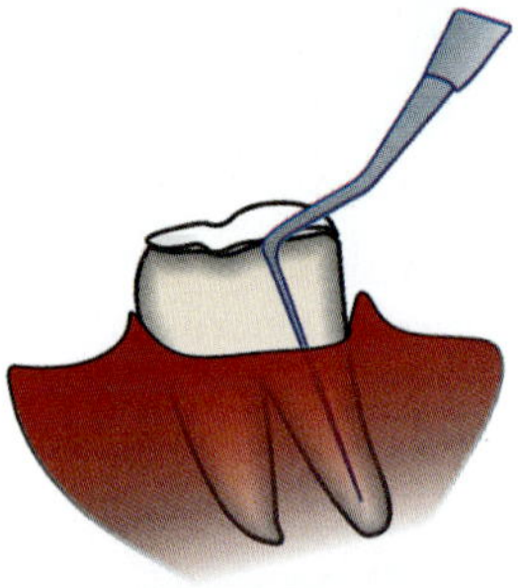

**Fig. 3.36:** Probing of tooth determines the level of connective tissue attachment

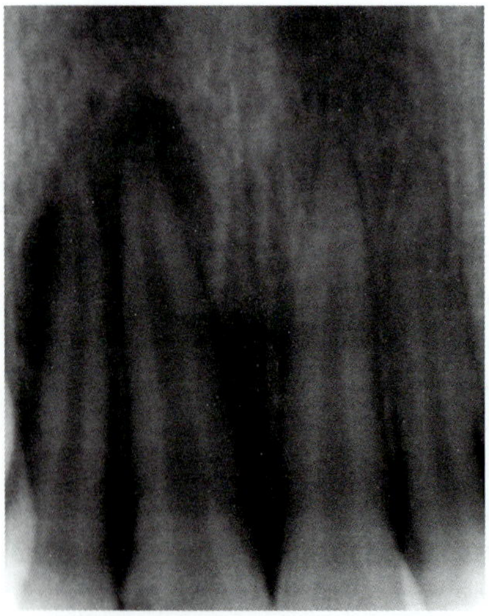

**Fig. 3.37:** Radiograph showing periapical lesion associated with 21

*Recent advances in radiography*:
- Digital substraction radiography
- Xeroradiography
- Digital radiometric analysis
- Computed tomography
- Radiovisiography
- Magnetic resonance imaging.

## CLASSIFICATION OF PERIRADICULAR PATHOLOGIES

I. *Grossman's classification*

1. Acute periradicular disease
   a. Acute alveolar abscess
   b. Acute apical periodontitis
      i. Vital
      ii. Nonvital
2. Chronic periradicular disease with areas of rarefaction:
   a. Chronic alveolar abscess
   b. Granuloma
   c. Cyst
3. Condensing osteitis
4. External root resorption
5. Disease of the periradicular tissues of nonendodontic origin.

II. *WHO classification*

K 04.4 - Acute apical periodontitis
K 04.5 - Chronic apical periodontitis (apical granuloma)
K 04.6 - Periapical abscess with sinus
K 04.60 - Periapical abscess with sinus to maxillary antrum
K 04.61 - Periapical abscess with sinus to nasal cavity
K 04.62 - Periapical abscess with sinus to oral cavity
K 04.63 - Periapical abscess with sinus to skin
K 04.7 - Periapical abscess without sinus
K 04.8 - Radicular cyst (periapical cyst)
K 04.80 - Apical and lateral cyst
K 04.81 - Residual cyst
K 04.82 - Inflammatory paradental cyst.

III. *Ingle's classification of pulpoperiapical pathosis:*

A. *Painful pulpoperiapical pathosis*:
1. Acute apical periodontitis
2. Advanced apical periodontitis
   a. Acute apical abscess
   b. Phoenix abscess
   c. Suppurative apical periodontitis (chronic apical abscess)

B. *Nonpainful pulpoperiapical pathosis*
1. Condensing osteitis
2. Chronic apical periodontitis both incipient and advanced stages.
3. Chronic apical periodontitis
   a. Periapical granuloma
   b. Apical cyst
   c. Suppurative apical periodontitis.

## ACUTE APICAL PERIODONTITIS (AAP)

Acute apical periodontitis is defined as painful inflammation of the periodontium as a result of trauma, irritation or infection, through the root canal, regardless of whether the pulp is vital or nonvital. It is an inflammation around the apex of a tooth. The distinctive features of AAP are microscopic rather than roentgenographic, symptomatic rather than visible.

### Etiology

a. In vital tooth, it is associated with occlusal trauma, high points in restoration or wedging or forcing object between teeth.
b. In nonvital tooth, AAP is associated with sequelae to pulpal diseases.
c. Iatrogenic causes can be over instrumentation of root canal pushing debris and microorganisms beyond apex, overextended obturation and root perforations.

### Signs and Symptoms

- Tooth is tender on percussion
- Dull, throbbing and constant pain
- Pain occurs over a short period of time
- Negative or delayed vitality test
- No swelling
- Pain on biting
- Cold may relieve pain or no reaction
- Heat may exacerbate pain or no reaction
- No radiographic sign; sometimes widening of periodontal ligament space.

### Histopathology

Inflammatory reaction occur in apical periodontal ligament
↓
Dilatation of blood vessels
↓
Initiation of inflammatory response due to presence of polymorphonuclear leukocytes and round cells
↓
Accumulation of serous exudate
↓
Distention of periodontal ligament and extrusion of tooth, slight tenderness
↓
If continued irritation occurs
↓
Loss of alveolar bone.

### *Treatment*

*Management of acute apical periodontitis:*
- Endodontic therapy should be initiated on the affected tooth at the earliest (Fig. 3.38)
- To control postoperative pain following initial endodontic therapy, analgesics are prescribed
- Use of antibiotics, either alone or in conjunction with root canal therapy is not recommended
- If tooth is in hyperocclusion, relieve the occlusion
- For some patients and in certain situations, extraction is an alternative to endodontic therapy.

## ACUTE APICAL ABSCESS (FIG. 3.39)

It is a localized collection of pus in the alveolar bone at the root apex of the tooth, following the death of pulp with extension of the infection through the apical foramen into periradicular tissue (Fig. 3.40).

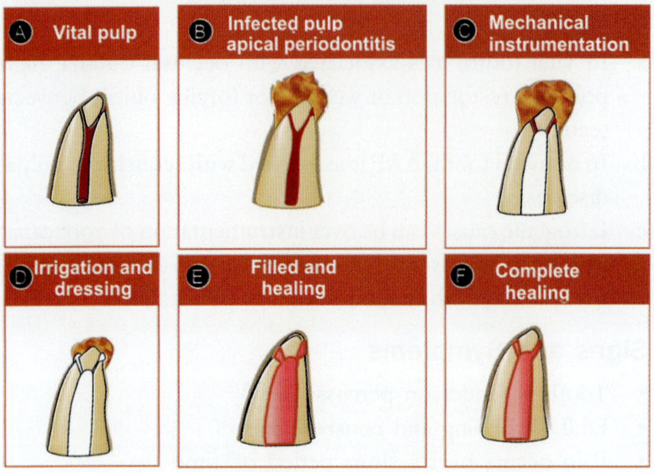


**Fig. 3.38:** Management of acute apical periodontitis

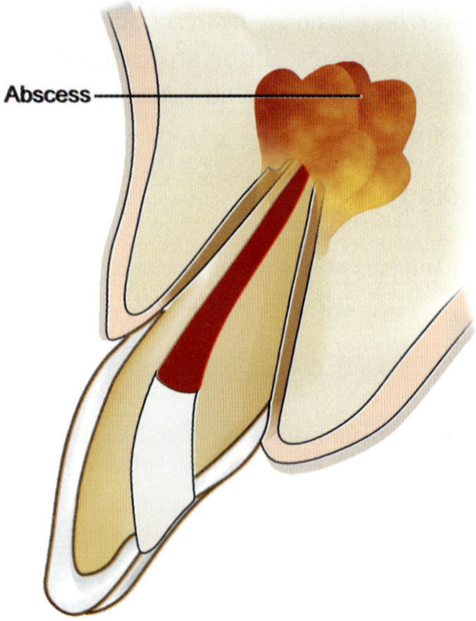


**Fig. 3.39:** Diagram showing periapical abscess

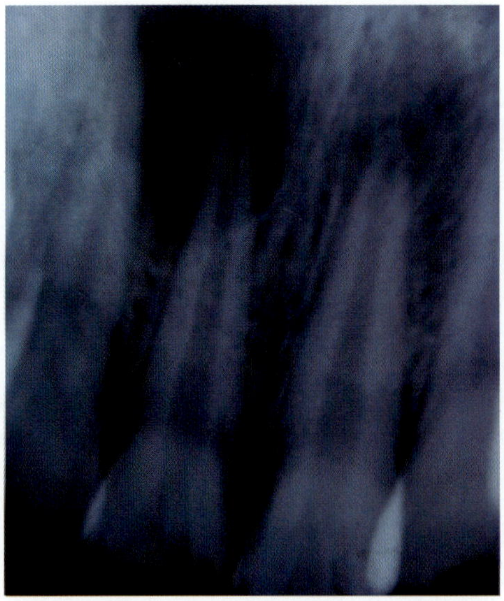

**Fig. 3.40:** Radiograph showing periapical abscess in relation to 21

## Etiology

- Most common cause is invasion of bacteria from necrotic pulp tissue.
- trauma, chemical or any mechanical injury resulting in pulp necrosis.
- Irritation of periapical tissue by chemical or mechanical treatment during root canal treatment.

Tissue at surface of swelling appears taut and inflamed and pus starts to form underneath it. Surface tissue may become inflated from the pressure of underlying pus and finally rupture from this pressure. Initially, the pus comes out in the form of a small opening but latter it may increase in size or number depending upon the amount of pressure of pus and softness of the tissue overlying it. This process is beginning of chronic abscess.

**Pathophysiology of apical abscess formation**

Increase in pulpal pressure
↓
Collapse in venous circulation
↓
Hypoxia and anoxia of local tissue
↓
Localized destruction of pulp tissue
↓
Formation of pulpal abscess because of breakdown of PMNs, bacterias and lysis of pulp remnants

**Features of acute apical abscess**

- Tooth is nonvital
- Pain
  - Rapid onset
  - Readily localized as tooth becomes increasingly tender to percussion
  - Slight tenderness to intense throbbing pain
  - Marked pain to biting
- Swelling
  - Palpable, fluctuant
  - Localized sense of fullness
- Mobility
  May or may not be present
- Tooth may be in hyperocclusion
- Radiographic changes
  No change to large periapical radiolucency

## Symptoms

In early stage, there is tenderness of tooth which is relieved by continued slight pressure on extruded tooth to push it back into alveolus. Later on throbbing pain develops with diffuse swelling of overlying tissue. Tooth becomes more painful, elongated and mobile as infection increases in latter stages. Patient may have systemic symptoms like fever, increased WBC count. Spread of lesion towards a surface may take place causing erosion of cortical bone or it may become diffuse and spread widely leading to formation of cellulitis (Fig. 3.41). Location of swelling is determined by relation of apex of involved tooth to adjacent muscle attachment (Fig. 3.42).

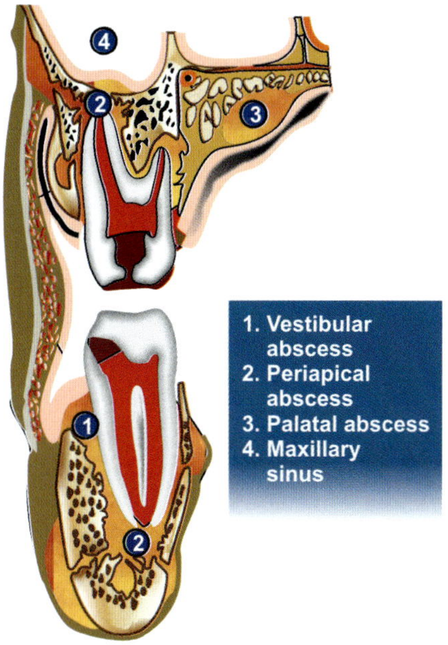


**Fig. 3.41:** Spread of apical abscess to surrounding tissues, if it is not treated

## Diagnosis

- Clinical examination
- Initially locating the offending tooth is difficult due to the diffuse pain. Location of the offending tooth becomes easier when tooth gets slightly extruded from the socket.
- Pulp vitality tests give negative response
- Tenderness on percussion and palpation.
- Tooth may be slightly mobile and extruded from its socket.
- Radiography helpful in determining the affected tooth as it shows a cavity or evidence of bone destruction at root apex.

**Differential diagnosis of acute alveolar abscess and periodontal abscess**

| *Features* | *Acute alveolar abscess* | *Periodontal abscess* |
|---|---|---|
| 1. Pain Type | Pulsating, pounding, continuous | Dull |
| 2. Pain Localization | Easily localized due to percussive tenderness | Upon probing |
| 3. Pain at night/ Postural | Pain continuous | No |
| 4. Mobility | Yes | Sometimes |
| 5. Pulp tests | | |
| I. EPT | No response | Normal |
| II. Cold | No response | Normal |
| III. Heat | No response | Normal |
| 6. Swelling | Yes – often to large size | Occasionally |
| 7. Radiograph | Caries, defective restorations | Possible foreign body or vertical bone loss |
| 8. Treatment | • Establish drainage (Incision and drainage)<br>• Antibiotics<br>• NSAIDs | • Removal of foreign body<br>• Scaling<br>• Curettage if necessary |

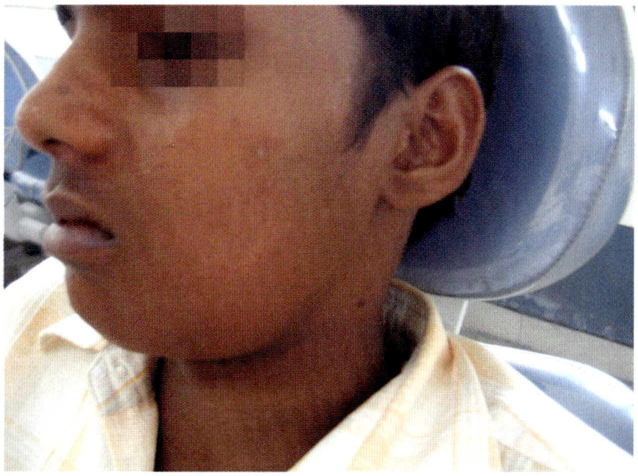

**Fig. 3.42:** Patient showing swelling of mandibular area because of apical abscess

## Histopathology

Polymorphonuclear leukocytes infiltrate and initiate inflammatory response
↓
Accumulation of inflammatory exudates in response to active infection
↓
Distention of periodontal ligament
↓
Elongation of tooth
↓
If the process continues, separation of periodontal ligament
↓
Tooth becomes mobile
↓
Bone resorption at apex
↓
Localized lesion of liquefaction necrosis containing polymorphonuclear leukocytes, debris, cell remnants and purulent exudates

## Management of an Acute Apical Abscess

- Drainage of the abscess should be initiated as early as possible. This may include:
  a. Non-surgical endodontic treatment (Root canal therapy) (Fig. 3.43)
  b. Incision and drainage
  c. Extraction
- Considerations regarding the treatment should be dependent on certain factors:
  a. Prognosis of the tooth
  b. Patient preference
  c. Strategic value of the tooth
  d. Economic status of the patient
- In case of localized infections, systemic antibiotics provide no additional benefit over drainage of the abscess
- In the case of systemic complications such as fever, lymphadenopathy, cellulitis or patient who is immunocompromised, antibiotics should be given in addition to drainage of the tooth
- Relieve the tooth out of occlusion in hyperocclusion cases

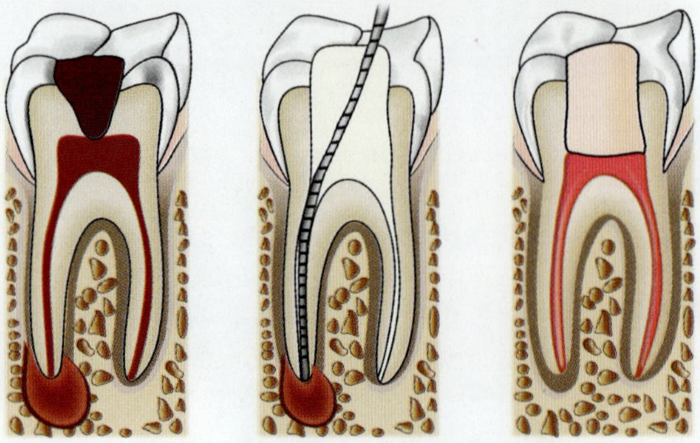

Fig. 3.43: Management of periapical abscess

- To control postoperative pain following endodontic therapy, nonsteroidal anti-inflammatory drugs should be given.

## PHOENIX ABSCESS/RECRUDESCENT ABSCESS

Phoenix abscess is defined as an acute inflammatory reaction superimposed on an existing chronic lesion, such as a cyst or granuloma; acute exacerbation of a chronic lesion.

### Etiology

Chronic periradicular lesions such as granulomas are in a state of equilibrium during which they can be completely asymptomatic. But sometimes, influx of necrotic products from diseased pulp or bacteria and their toxins can cause the dormant lesion to react. This leads to initiation of acute inflammatory response. Lowered body defenses also trigger an acute inflammatory response.

### Symptoms

- Clinically often indistinguishable from acute apical abscess
- At the onset—tenderness of tooth and elevation of the tooth from socket
- Tenderness on palpating the apical soft tissue.

### Diagnosis

- Associated with initiation of root canal treatment most commonly
- History from patient
- Pulp tests show negative response
- Radiographs show large area of radiolucency in the apex created by inflammatory connective tissue which has replaced the alveolar bone at the root apex
- Histopathology of phoenix abscess shows areas of liquefaction necrosis with disintegrated polymorphonuclear leukocytes and cellular debris surrounded by macrophages, lymphocytes, plasma cells in periradicular tissues
- Phoenix abscess should be differentiated from acute alveolar abscess by patient's history, symptoms and clinical tests results.

### Treatment

- Establishment of drainage
- Once symptoms subside—complete root canal treatment.

## PERIAPICAL GRANULOMA

Periapical granuloma is one of the most common sequelae of pulpitis. It is usually described as a mass of chronically inflamed granulation tissue found at the apex of nonvital tooth (Fig. 3.44).

### Etiology of Periapical Granuloma

Periapical granuloma is a cell mediated response to pulpal bacterial products. Bacterial and toxins cause mild irritation of periapical tissues. This leads to cellular proliferation and thus granuloma formation.

### Clinical Features

- Most of the cases are asymptomatic but sometimes pain and sensitivity is seen when acute exacerbation occurs
- Tooth is not sensitive to percussion
- No mobility
- Soft tissue overlying the area may/may not be tender
- No response to thermal or electric pulp test
- Mostly, lesions are discovered on routine radiographic examination.

### Radiographic Features

- Mostly discovered on routine radiographic examination
- The earliest change in the periodontal ligament is found to be thickening of ligament at the root apex
- Lesion may be well circumscribed or poorly defined
- Size may vary from small lesion to large radiolucency exceeding more than 2 cm in diameter.
- Some amount of root resorption has been reported.

### Histopathologic Features (Fig. 3.45)

- It consists of inflamed granulation tissue that is surrounded by a fibrous connective tissue wall

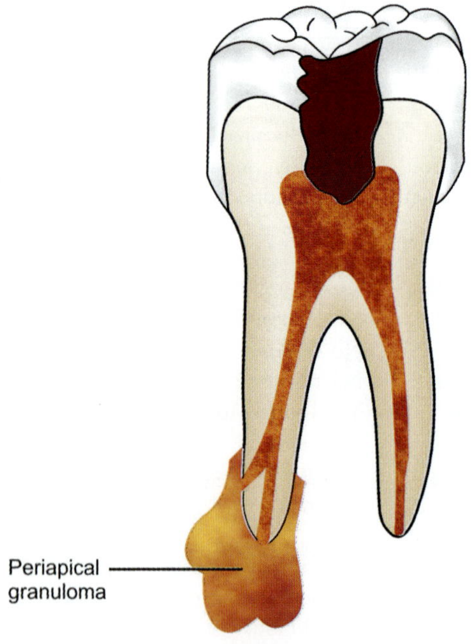


Fig. 3.44: Periapical granuloma present at the apex of nonvital tooth

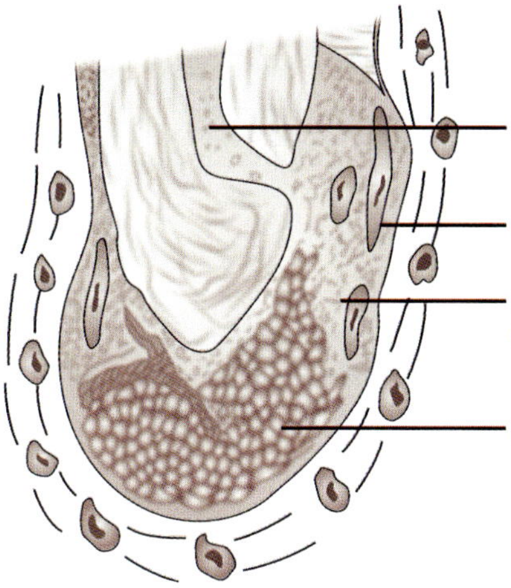


Fig. 3.45: Histopathology of periapical granuloma

- The granulation consists of dense lymphocytic infiltrate which further contains neutrophils, plasma cells, histiocytes and eosinophils
- Sometimes, Russel bodies may also be present.

### Treatment and Prognosis

Main objective in treatment is to reduce and eliminate offending organisms and irritants from the periapical area.
- In restorable tooth, root canal therapy is preferred
- In non-restorable tooth, extraction followed by curettage of all apical soft tissue.

## RADICULAR CYST

The radicular cyst is an inflammatory cyst which results because of extension of infection from pulp into the surrounding periapical tissues.

### Etiology

- Caries
- Irritating effects of restorative materials
- Trauma
- Pulpal death due to development defects.

### Clinical Features

- The cyst is frequently asymptomatic and sometimes it is discovered when periapical radiographs are taken of teeth with nonvital pulps
- Incidence - Males are affected more than females.
- Age - Peak incidence in third or fourth decades.
- Site - Highest in anterior maxilla
  - In mandibular posterior teeth, separate small cysts arise from each apex of multi-rooted teeth.
- Slowly enlarging swelling sometimes attains a large size.
- As the cyst enlarges in size, the covering bone becomes thin in size and exhibits springiness due to fluctuation.
- In maxilla, palatal expansion is mainly seen in case of maxillary lateral incisor.
- The involved tooth/teeth usually found to be nonvital, discolored, fractured or failed root canal.

### Pathogenesis

Periapical granulomas are initiated and maintained by the degradation products of necrotic pulp tissue. Stimulation of the resident epithelial rests of Malassez occurs in response to the products of inflammation. Cyst formation occurs as a result of epithelial proliferation, which helps to separate the inflammatory stimulus from the surrounding bone. When proliferation occurs within the body of the granuloma, it plugs the apical foramen which limits the egress of bacteria (Fig. 3.46). Sometimes, epithelial plugs protrude out from the apical foramen resulting in a pouch connected to the root and continuous with the root canal. This is termed as ***pocket or bay cyst*** (Fig. 3.47).

- Breakdown of cellular debris within the cyst lumen raises the protein concentration, producing an increase in osmotic pressure. The result is fluid transport across the epithelial lining into the lumen from the connective tissue side. Fluid ingress assists in outward growth of the cyst. With osteoclastic bone resorption, the cyst expands. Other bone-resorbing factors, such as prostaglandins, interleukins, and proteinases, from inflammatory cells and cells in the peripheral portion of the lesion permit additional cyst enlargement.

### Radiographic Features (Fig. 3.48)

Radiographically radicular cyst appears as round, pear or ovoid shaped radiolucency, outlined by a narrow radiopaque margin (Fig. 3.49).

### Treatment

Different options for management of residual cyst are:
- Endodontic treatment
- Apicoectomy
- Extraction (severe bone loss)
- Enucleation with primary closure
- Marsupilization (in case of large cysts).

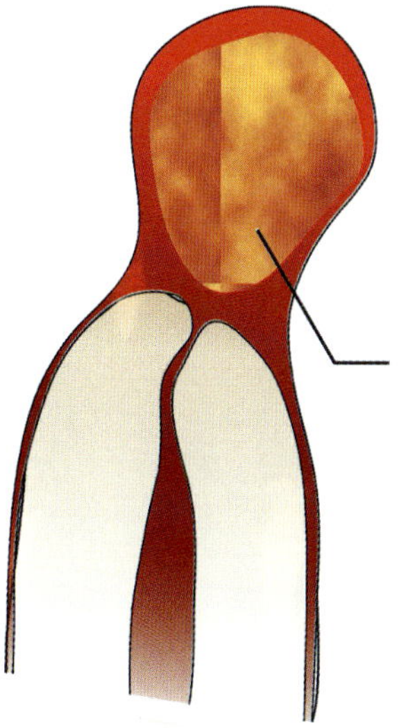


Fig. 3.46: Cyst formation in periapical area

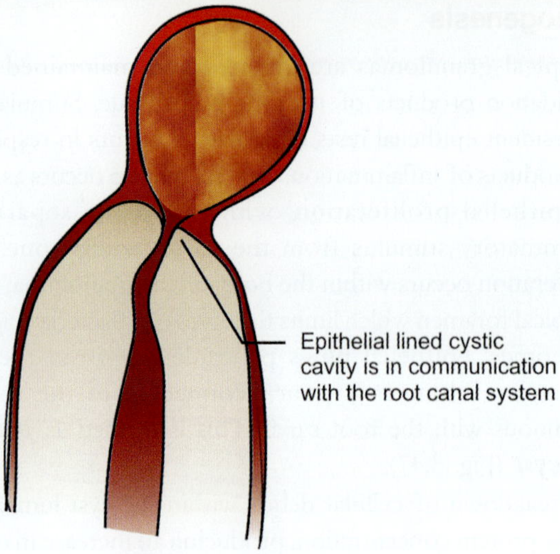


**Fig. 3.47:** Pocket or bay cyst

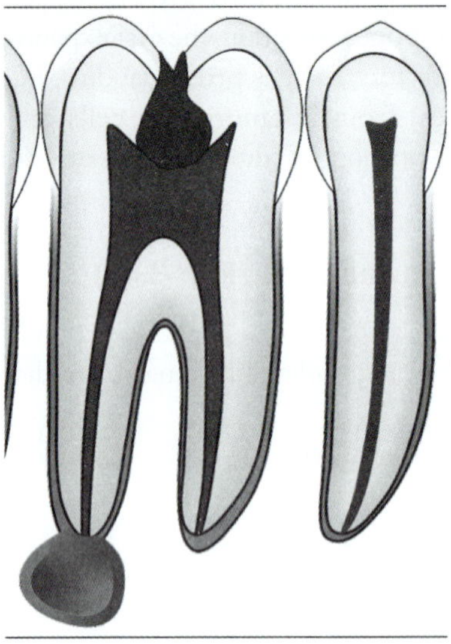

**Fig. 3.48:** Radiographic picture of a periapical cyst

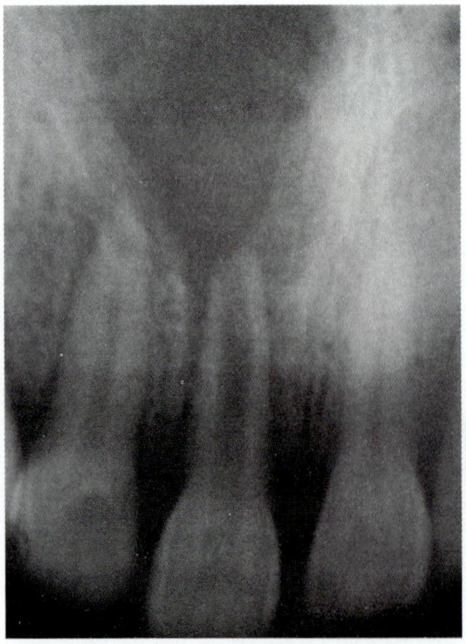

**Fig. 3.49:** Radiograph showing periapical cyst in relation to 11

## CHRONIC ALVEOLAR ABSCESS

Chronic alveolar abscess is also known as suppurative apical periodontitis which is associated with gradual egress of irritants from root canal system into periradicular area leading to formation of an exudate.

### Etiology

It is similar to acute alveolar abscess. It also results from pulpal necrosis and is associated with chronic apical periodontitis that has formed an abscess. The abscess has burrowed through bone and soft tissue to form a sinus react stoma on the oral mucosa (Fig. 3.50).

### Symptoms

- Generally asymptomatic
- Detected either by the presence of a sinus tract or on routine radiograph
- In case of open carious cavity—drainage through root canal sinus tract prevents swelling or exacerbation of lesion—can be traced to apex of involved tooth.

### Diagnosis

Chronic apical abscess may be associated with asymptomatic or slightly symptomatic tooth. Patient may give history of sudden sharp pain which subsided and has not reoccurred. Clinical examination may show a large carious exposure, a restoration of composite, acrylic, amalgam or metal, or discoloration of crown of tooth.

It is associated symptoms only if sinus drainage tract become blocked. Vitality tests show negative response because of presence of necrotic pulps.

*Radiographic examination* shows diffuse area of rarefaction (Fig 3.51). The rarefied area is so diffuse as to fade indistinctly into normal bone.

### Differential Diagnosis

Chronic alveolar abscess must be differentially diagnosed from a granuloma or cyst, in which accurate diagnosis is made by

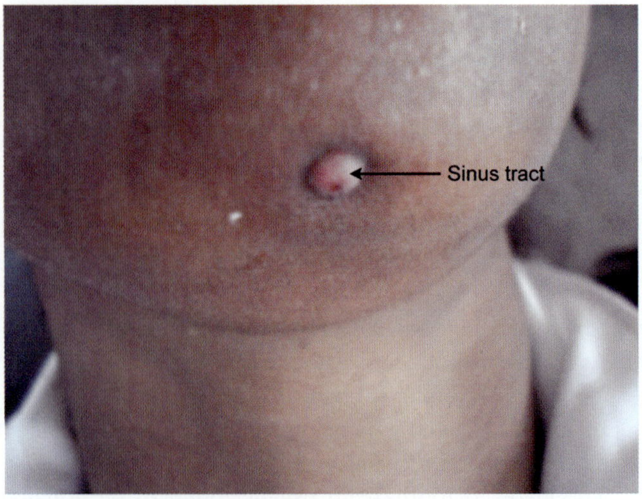


**Fig. 3.50:** Sinus tract

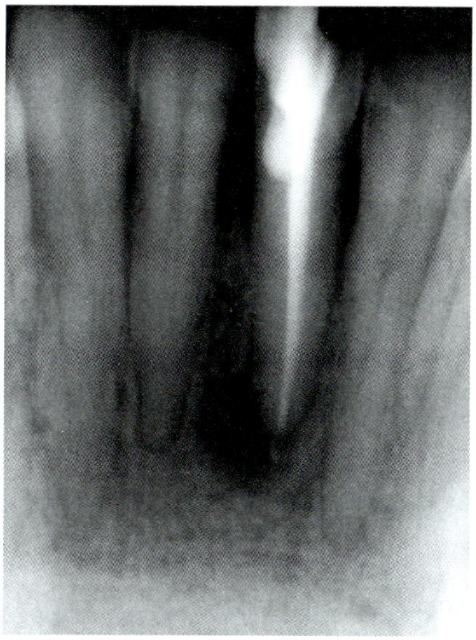

Fig. 3.51: Radiograph showing chronic alveolar abscess

studying the tissue microscopically. It should also be differentiated with cementoma which is associated with vital tooth.

### Treatment

Removal of irritants from root canal and establishing drainage is main objective of the treatment. Sinus tract resolve following root canal treatment removing the irritants.

## EXTERNAL ROOT RESORPTION

*Resorption* is a condition associated with either physiologic or a pathologic process that results in loss of substance from a tissue such as dentin, cementum or alveolar none (Fig. 3.52).

In external root resorption, root resorption affects the cementum or dentin of the root of tooth. It can be:

- Apical root resorption
- Lateral root resorption
- Cervical root resorption.

### Etiology

Periradicular inflammation due to

- Infected necrotic pulp
- Over instrumentation during root canal treatment
- Trauma
- Granuloma/cyst applying excessive pressure on tooth root
- Replantation of teeth
- Adjacent impacted tooth.

### Symptoms

- Asymptomatic during development
- When root is completely resorbed, tooth becomes mobile
- When external root resorption extends to crown, it gives "Pink tooth" appearance
- When replacement resorption/ankylosis occur, tooth becomes immobile with characteristic high percussion sound (Fig. 3.53).

### Radiographic Features

Radiograph shows:

- Radiolucency at root and adjacent bone
- Irregular shortening or thinning of root lip
- Loss of Lamina dura.

### Treatment

- Remove stimulus of underlying inflammation.
- Nonsurgical endodontic treatment should be attempted before surgical treatment is initiated.

## DISEASES OF PERIRADICULAR TISSUE OF NONENDODONTIC ORIGIN

Periradicular lesions may arise from the remnants of odontogenic epithelium.

### Benign Lesions

1. Early stages of periradicular cemental dysplasia
2. Early stages of monostatic fibrous dysplasia

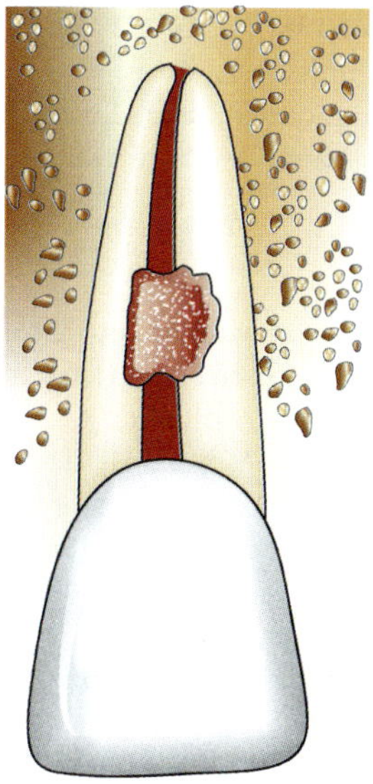

Fig. 3.52: External root resorption

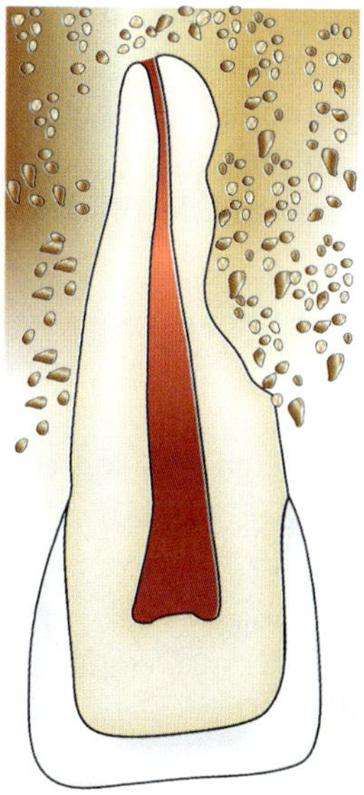

Fig. 3.53: Replacement resorption

3. Ossifying fibroma
4. Primordial cyst
5. Lateral periodontal cyst
6. Dentigerous cyst
7. Traumatic bone cyst
8. Central giant cell granuloma
9. Central hemangioma
10. Hyperparathyroidism
11. Myxoma
12. Ameloblastoma.

### Radiographic Features of Lesions of Nonodontogenic Origin

- Radiolucent areas
- Intact lamina dura.

### Diagnosis

Teeth associated with nonodontogenic lesions are usually vital. Final diagnosis is based on surgical biopsy and histopathological examination.

## Malignant Lesions

*They simulate endodontic periradicular lesions and are often meta static in nature*

1. Squamous cell carcinoma.
2. Osteogenic sarcoma
3. Chondrosarcoma
4. Multiple myeloma.

### Diagnosis

- ***Involved tooth is vital.*** Occasionally disruption of pulp and sensory nerve may cause no response
- ***Radiographic features***: Lesions are associated with rapid and extensive loss of hard tissue, bone and tooth
- ***Biopsy***: Histological evaluation of diagnosis.

## QUESTIONS

**Q. Enumerate etiology of pulpal diseases. Write in detail about reversible pulpitis.**

**Q. Classify pulpal pathologies. What are clinical features of irreversible pulpitis.**

**Q. Explain the etiology and classification of periradicular pathologies.**

**Q. Write short notes on:**

a. Phoenix abscess
b. Radicular cyst
c. Differentiate acute abscess and chronic abscess
d. Chronic hyperplastic pulpitis/pulp polyp.

## BIBLIOGRAPHY


1. Abou-Rass M, Bogen G. Microorganisms in closed periapical lesions. Int Endod J 1997;31:39-47.
2. Ando N, Hoshino E. Predominant obligate anaerobes invading the deep layers of root canal dentine. Int Endod J 1990;23:20-27.
3. Andreasen JO, Rud J. A histobacteriologic study of dental and periapical structure after endodontic surgery. Int J Oral Surg 1972;1:272-81.
4. Barbakow F, Cleaton-Jones P, Friedman D. Endodontic-treatment of teeth with periapical radiolucent areas in a general practice. Oral Surg Oral Med Oral Pathol 1981;51:552-9.
5. Baume LJ. Diagnosis of diseases of the pulp. Oral Surg Oral Med Oral Pathol 1970;29:102-16.
6. Baumgartener JC, Khemaleelkul SU, Xia T. Identification of spirochetes (treponemas) in endodontic infections. J Endod 2003;29:794-7.
7. Baumgartner JC, Falkler WA. Bacteria in the apical 5 mm of infected root canals. J Endod 1991;17:380-83.
8. Baumgartner JC, Watkins BJ, Bae K-S, Xia T. Association of black-pigmentated bacteria with endodotic infections. J Endod 1999;25:413-5.
9. Bender IB. Reversible and irreversible painful pulpitides: diagnosis and treatment. Aust Endod J 2000;26:10-14.
10. Bergenholtz G. Microorganisms from necrotic pulp of traumatized teeth. Odont Rev 1974;25:347-58.
11. Bhasker SN. Periapical lesion: Types, incidence and clinical features. Oral Surg Oral Med Oral Pathol 1966;21:657-71.
12. Brännström M, Gola G, Nordenvall KJ. Invasion of microorganisms and some structural changes in incipient enamel caries. Caries Res 1980;14:276.
13. Browne RM, O Riordan BC. Colony of actinomyces-like organism in a periapical granuloma. Br Dent J 1966;120:603-6.
14. Byström A, Happonen RP, Sjögren U, Sundqvist G. Healing of periapical lesions of pulpless teeth after endodontic treatment with controlled asepsis. Endod Dent Taumotol 1987;3:58-63.
15. Cotti E, Torabinejad M. Detection of leukotrience C4 in human periradicular lesions. Int Endod J 1994;27:82-6.
16. Dubrow H. Silver points and gutta-percha and the role of root canal fillings. J Am Dent Assoc 1976;93:976-80.
17. Dummer PMH, Hicks R, Huws D. Clinical signs and symptoms in pulp disease. Int Endod J 1980;13:27-35.
18. Engström B, Frostell G. Bacteriological studies of the non-vital pulp in cases with intact pulp cavities. Acta Odont Scand 1961;19:23-39.
19. Garfunkel A, Sela J, Almansky M. Dental Pulp pathosis: Clinicopathologic correlation based on 109 cases. Oral Surg Oral Med Oral Pathol 1987;35:110-17.
20. Hancock H, Sigurdsson A, Trope M, Moiseiwitsch J. Bacteria isolated after unsuccessful endodontic treatment in a North American population. Oral Surg Oral Med Oral Pathol 2001; 91:579-86.
21. Hasler JE, Mitchell DF. Painless pulpitis. J Am Dent Assoc 1970;81:671-7.
22. Head MA. Foreign body reaction to inhalation of lentil soup: giant cell pneumonia. Dtsch Zschr Tiermed 1879;5(2 Suppl): 125-10.
23. Holland Rm De Souza V, Nery MJ, de Mello W, Brnabé PEE, Filho JAO. Tissue reactions following apical plugging of the root canal with infected dentine chips. Oral Surg Oral Med Oral Pathol 49:366-9.
24. Horiba N, Maekawa Y, Matsumoto T, Nakamura H. A study of the detection of endotoxin in the dental wall of infected root canals. J Endod 1990;16:331-4.
25. Iwu C, MacFarlane TW, MacKenzie D, Stenhouse D. The microbiology of periapical granulomas. Oral Surg Oral Med Oral Pathol 1990;69:502-5.

26. Koppang HS, Kopping R. Solheim T, Aarmes H, Stølen SØ. Cellulose fibers from endodontic paper points as an etiologic factor in postendodontic periapical granulomas and cysts. J Endod 1989;15:369-72.
27. Lalonde ER. A new rationale for the management of periapical granulomas and cysts: An evaluation of histopathological and radiographic findings. J Am Dent Assoc 1970;80:1056-9.
28. Langeland MA, Block RM, Grossman LI. A histopathologic and histobacteriologic study of 35 periapical endodontic surgical specimens. J Endod 1977;3:8-23.
29. Laux M, Abbott P, Pajarola G, Nair PNR. Apical inflammatory root resoption: A correlative radiographic and histological assessment. Int Endod J 2000;33:483-93.
30. Lin LM, Pascon EA, Skribner J, Gängler P, langeland K. Clinical, radiographic, and histologic study of endodontic treatment failures. Oral Surg Oral Med Oral Pathol 1991;71: 603-11.
31. Martin IC, Harrison JD. Periapical actinomycosis. Br Dent J 1984;156:169-70.
32. Marton IJ, Kiss C. Characterization of inflammatory cell infiltrate in dental periapical lesions. Int Endod J 1993;26:131-6.
33. Michaelson PL, Holland GR. Is pulpitis painful? Int Endod J 2002;35:829-32.
34. Morse DR, Seltzer S, Sinai I, Biron G. Endodontic Classification. J Am Dent Assoc 1977;94:685-9.
35. Nagaoka S, Miyazaki Y, Liu HJ, Iwamoto Y, Kitano M, kawagoe M. Bacterial invasion into dentinal tubules in human vital and nonvital teeth. J Endod 1995;21:70-73.
36. Nair PNR, Pajarola G, Schroeder HE. Types and incidence of Human periapical lesions obtained with extracted teeth. Oral Surg Oral Med Oral Pathol 1996;81:93-102.
37. Nair PNR, Sundqvist G, Sjögren U. Experimental evidence support the abscess theory of development of radicular cysts. Oral Surg Oral Med Oral Pathol Oral Radiol Endod 2008;106: 294-303.
38. Nair PNR. Cholesterol as an aetiological agent in endodontic failures: A review. Aust Endod J 1999;25:19-3-26.
39. Nair PNR. New perspectives on radicular cysts: do they heal? Int Endod J 1998;31:155-60.
40. Nobuhara WK, Del Rio CE. Incedence of periradicular pathoses in endodontic treatment failures. J Endod 1993; 19:315-8.
41. Patterson SS, Shafer WG, Healey HJ. Periapical lesions associated with endodontically treated teeth. J Am Dent Assoc 1964;68:191-4.
42. Peters LB, Wesselink PR, Moorer WR. The fate and the role of bacteria left in root dentinal tubules. Int Endod J 1995;28:95-9.
43. Pitt Ford TR. The effects of the periapical tissues of bacterial contamination of filled root canal. Int Endod J 1982;15:16-22.
44. Reeves R, Stanley HR. The relationship of bacterial penetration and pulpal pathosis in carious teeth. Oral Surg 1966;22:59.
45. Robinson HBG, Boling LR. The anachoretic effect in pulpitis. Bacteriologic studies. J Am Dent Assoc 1941;28:268-82.
46. Sabeti M, Slots J. Herpesviral-bacterial coinfection in periapical pathosis. J Endod 2004;30:69-72.
47. Sakellariou PL. Periapical actinomycosis: Report of a case and review of the literature. Endod Dent Traumatol 1996;12:151-4.
48. Seltzer S, Bender IB, Turkenkopf S. Factors affecting successful repair after root canal treatment. J Am Dent Assoc 1963; 67:651-62.
49. Seltzer S, Bender IB, Zionitz M. The dynamics of pulp inflammation: Correlation between diagnostic data and actal histologic findings in the pulp. Oral Surg Oral Med Oral pathol 1963;16:846-71.
50. Seltzer S. Classification of pulpal pathosis. Oral Surg Oral Med Oral Pathol 1972;34:269-80.
51. Sigurdsson A, Maixner W. Effects of experimental and clinical noxious counter irritants on pain perception. Pain 1994;57:265-75.
52. Simon JHS. Incidence of periapical cysts in relation to the root canal. J Endod 1980;6:845-8.
53. Stockdale CR, Chandler NP. The nature of the periapical lesion—A review of 1108 cases. J Dent 1988;16:123-9.
54. Storms JL. Factors that influence the success of endodontic treatment. J Can Dent Assoc 1969;35:83-97.
55. Sunde PT, Olsen J, Debelian GJ, Tronstad L. Microbiota of periapical lesions refractory to endodontic therapy. J Endod 2002;28:304-10.
56. Sundqvist G, Reuterving CO. Isolation of actinomyces israelii from periapical lesion. J Endod 1980;6:602-6.
57. Sundqvist G. Ecology of the root canal flora. J Endod 1992;18: 427-30.
58. Swerdlow H, Stanley HR. 'Reaction of the human dental pulp to cavity preparation. I. Effect of water spray at 20,000 rpm'. J Am Dent Assoc 1958;56:317.
59. Szajkis S, Tagger M. Periapical healing in spite of incomplete root canal debridement and filling. J Endod 1983;9:203-9.
60. Torabinejad M, Cotti E, Jung T. Concentration of leucotriene B4 in symptomatic and asymptomatic periapical lesions. J Endod 1992;18:205-8.
61. Torabinejad M. The role of immunological reactions in apical cyst formation and the fate of the epithelial cells after root canal therapy: a theory. Int J Oral Surg 1983;12:14-22.
62. Trott JR, Chebib F, Galindo Y. Factors related to cholesterol formation in cysts and granulomas. J Cand Dent Assoc 1973; 38:76-48.
63. Wayman BE, Murata M, Almeida RJ, fowler CB. A bacteriological and histological evaluation of 58 periapical lesions. J Endod 1992;18:152-5.
64. Yamazaki K, Nakajima T, Gemmell E, Polak B, Seymour GJ, Hara K. IL-4 and IL-6-producing cells in human periodontal disease tissue. J Oral Pathol Med 1994;23:347-53.
65. Yanagisawa W. Pathologic study of periapical lesions. I. periapical granulomas: Clinical, histologic and immunohistopathologic studies. J Oral Pathol 1980;9:288-300.
66. Young G, Turner S, Davis JK, Sundqvist G, Figdor D. Bacterial DNA persists for extended periods after cell death. J Endod 2007;33:1417-20.

# Endodontic Microbiology

CHAPTER 4



## INTRODUCTION

Most of the pathologies of pulp and the periapical tissues are directly or indirectly related to the microorganisms. Therefore to effectively diagnose and treat endodontic infection, one should have the knowledge of bacteria associated with endodontic pathology. Since many years, the interrelationship of microorganisms and the root canal system have been proved. Leeuwenhoek observed infected root canal of a tooth and found "cavorting beasties". After this, it took 200 years for WD Miller to make the correlation between microorganisms and pulpal or periradicular pathologies.

Then in 1965, Kakehashi et al found that bacteria are the main etiological factors in the development of pulpal and periradicular diseases. Kakehashi et al proved that without bacterial involvement only minor inflammation occurred in exposed pulp.

So we have seen that a strong relationship occurs between microorganisms and pulpal or periradicular diseases. All the surfaces of human body are colonized by microorganisms. Colonization is the establishment of bacteria in a living host. It occurs if biochemical and physical conditions are available for growth. Permanent colonization in symbiotic relationship with host tissue results in establishment of normal flora.

Infection results if microorganisms damage the host and produce clinical signs and symptoms. The degree of pathogenicity produced by microorganisms is called as virulence.

**History of microbiology in association to endodontics**

17th century: AV Leeuwenhoek. First described oral microflora.
1890: WD Miller. Father of oral microbiology authorized book "Microorganisms of human mouth"
1904: F. Billings described theory of focal infection as a circumscribed area of tissue with pathognomic microorganisms.
1909: EC Rosenow described theory of focal infection as localized or generalized infection caused by bacteria traveling via bloodstream from distant focus of infection.
1939: Fish observed four distinct zones of periapical reaction in response to infection.
1965: Kakehashi, et al proved that bacteria are responsible for pulpal and periapical disease.
1976: Sundqvist used different culturing techniques for identification of both aerobic and anaerobic organisms and concluded that root canal infections are multibacterial.

## PORTALS OF ENTRY FOR MICROORGANISMS

Microorganisms may gain entry into pulp through several routes. Most common portal of entrance for microorganisms to dental pulp is dental caries.

They can also gain entry into pulp cavity via mechanical or traumatic injury, through gingival sulcus and via bloodstream.

**Entry of microorganisms into pulp through**

1. Open cavity
2. Open dentinal tubules
3. Periodontal ligament or gingival sulcus
4. Anachoresis
5. Faulty restorations

### Entry Through Open Cavity

This is the most common way of entry of microorganisms into the dental pulp. When enamel and dentin are intact, they act as barrier to microorganisms (Fig. 4.1). But when these protective layers get destroyed by caries, bacteria gain entry into the pulp (Fig. 4.2).

This protective barrier of enamel and dentine also gets destroyed by traumatic injuries, fractures, cracks or restorative procedures, thus allowing the access of microorganisms to the pulp (Fig. 4.3).

### Through Open Dentinal Tubules

It has been seen that microorganisms can pass into the dentinal tubules and subsequently to the pulp. Bacterial penetration into dentinal tubules has been shown to be greater in teeth with necrotic pulp (Fig. 4.4). Bacteria are preceded in the course of the tubules by their breakdown products which may act as pulp irritants.

### Through the Periodontal Ligament or the Gingival Sulcus

Microorganisms also gain entry into pulp via accessory and lateral canals which connect pulp and the periodontium. If periodontal disease or therapy destroys the protective covering, canal may get exposed to the microorganisms present in the gingival sulcus (Fig. 4.5). The removal of cementum during periodontal therapy also exposes dentinal fluids to oral flora.

### Anachoresis

A transient bacteremia is usually associated with many activities in a healthy individual. Anachoresis refers to the attraction of blood-borne bacteria in the areas of inflammation. In other words anachoresis is a process by which microorganisms are transported in the blood to an area of inflammation where they establish an infection. But whether anachoresis contributes to pulpal or periradicular infection has not been determined.

### Through Faulty Restorations

It has been seen that faulty restoration with marginal leakage can result in contamination of the pulp by bacteria. Bacterial contamination of pulp or periapical area can occur through broken temporary seal, inadequate final restoration and unused post space (Figs 4.6 to 4.10).

## CLASSIFICATION OF MICROORGANISMS (FIG. 4.11)

Microbial flora can be classified on the basis of:

1. Gram stain technique
   i. Gram-positive organisms, e.g. *Streptococcus, Enterococcus, Treponema, Candida, Actinomyces, Lactobacillus,* etc.
   ii. Gram-negative organisms, e.g. *Fusobacterium, Campylobacter, Bacteroides, Veillonella, Neisseria,* etc.

I. *Obligate aerobes:* The organisms which require oxygen for their growth. Example: *Tubercle bacilli.*

II. *Facultative anaerobes:* These organisms can grow in the presence or absence of oxygen, e.g. *Staphylococcus.*

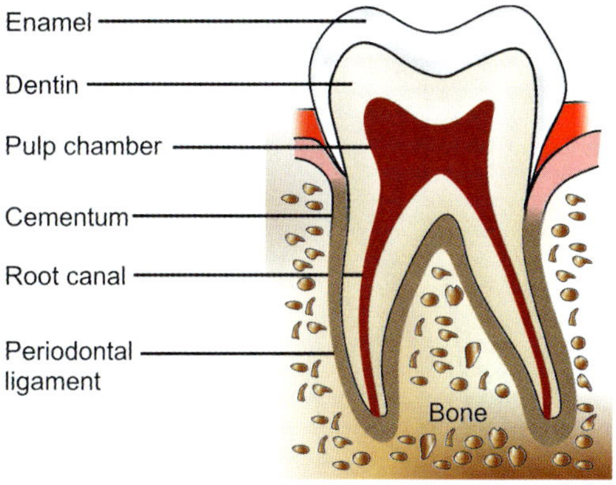


**Fig. 4.1:** Normal tooth anatomy with protective layers of the pulp

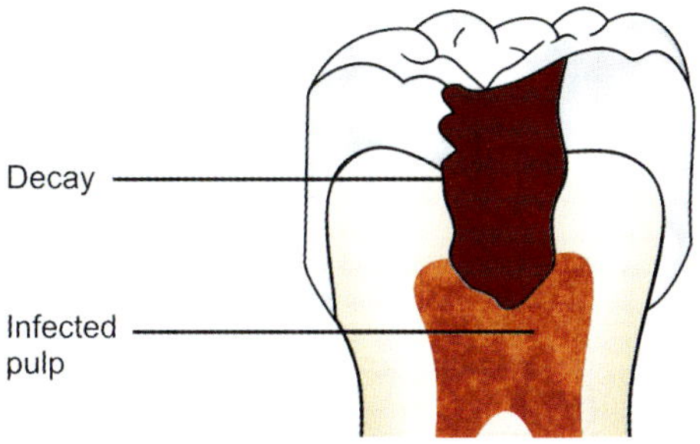


**Fig. 4.2:** Pulp infection from tooth decay

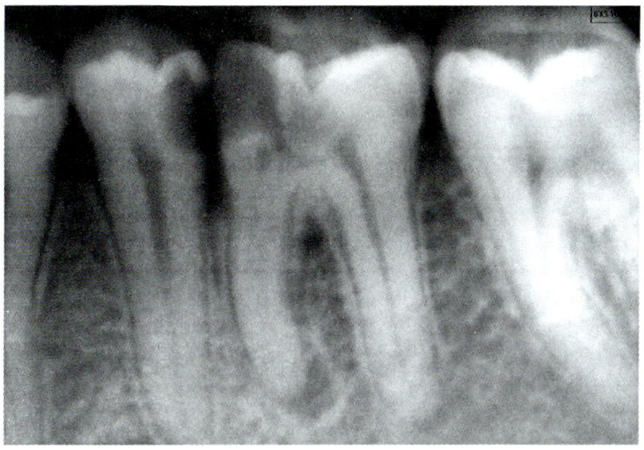

**Fig. 4.3:** Radiograph showing deep carious lesion infecting the pulp

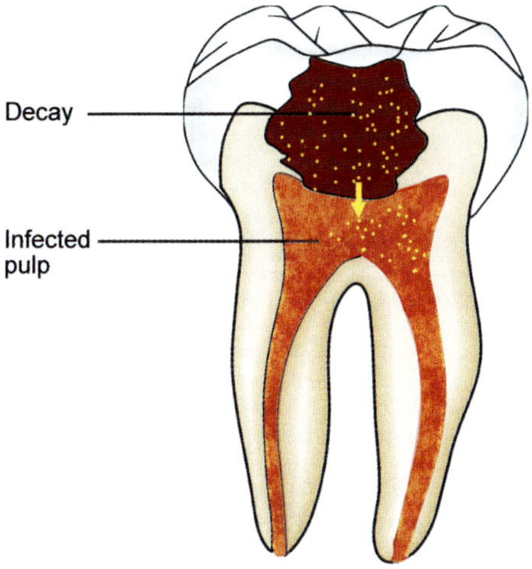


**Fig. 4.4:** Entry of bacteria through decay into pulp

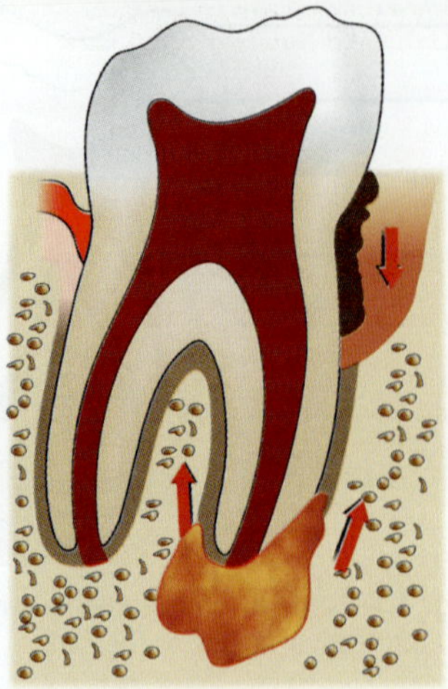

Fig. 4.5: Periodontal lesions causing inflammation of pulp

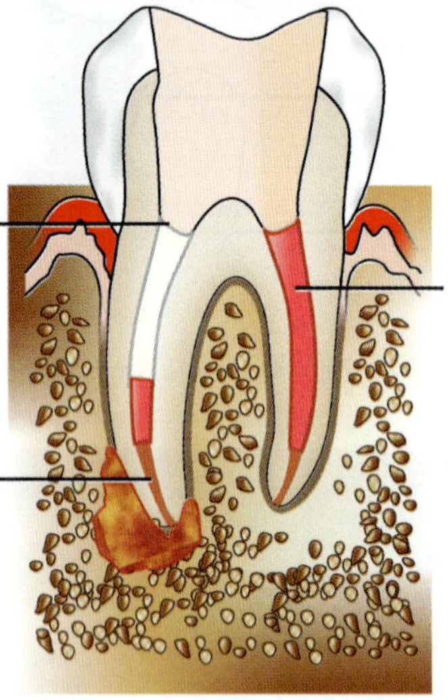


Fig. 4.6: Untreated canal and empty post space causing root canal failure

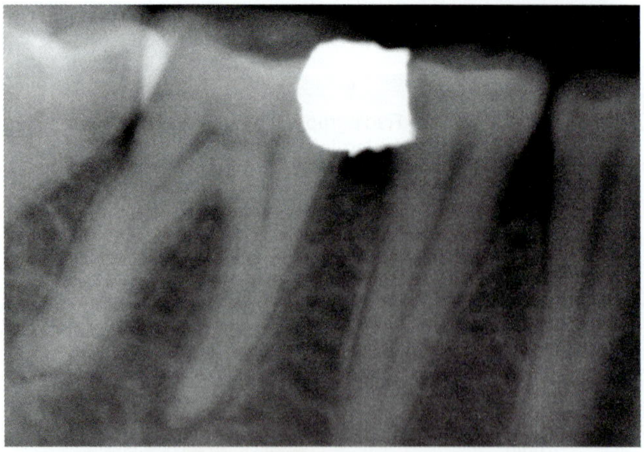

Fig. 4.7: Radiograph showing faulty restoration

III. *Microaerophilic:* They grow in an oxygen environment but derive their energy only from fermentative pathways that occur in absence of oxygen, e.g *Streptococcus,* etc.
IV. *Obligate anaerobes:* These bacteria can grow only in absence of oxygen. E.g. *Bacteroides, Fusobacterium.*

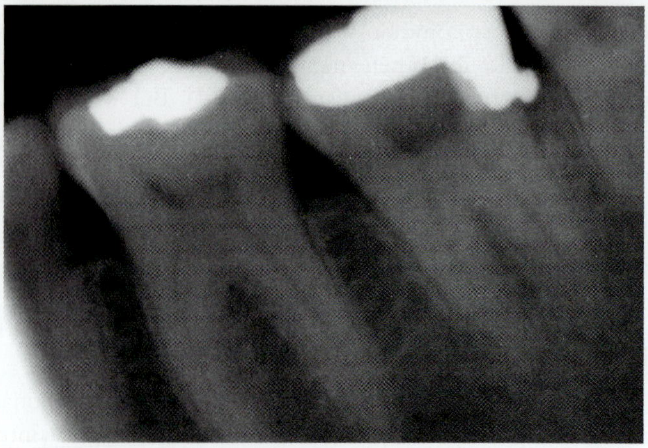

Fig. 4.8: Deep restoration may irritate the pulp

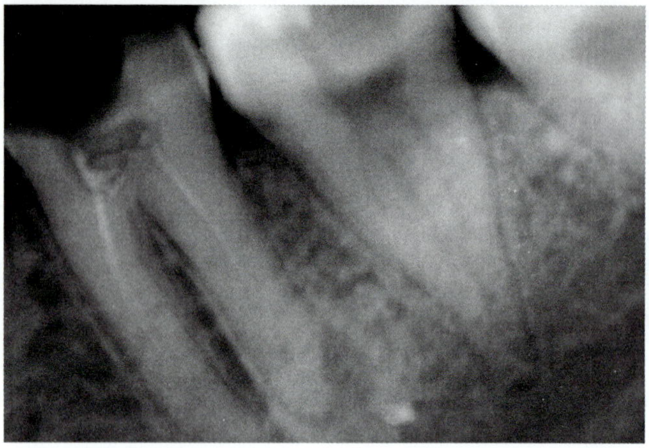

Fig. 4.9: Periradicular infection as a result of poorly obturated canal

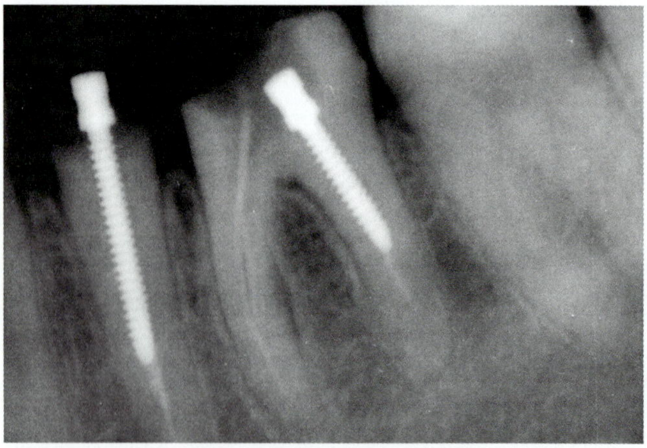

Fig. 4.10: Poorly obturated canals resulting in root canal failure

## MICROBIAL VIRULENCE AND PATHOGENICITY

Under normal conditions pulp and periapical tissues are sterile in nature, when microorganisms invade and multiply in these tissues, endodontic infections result.

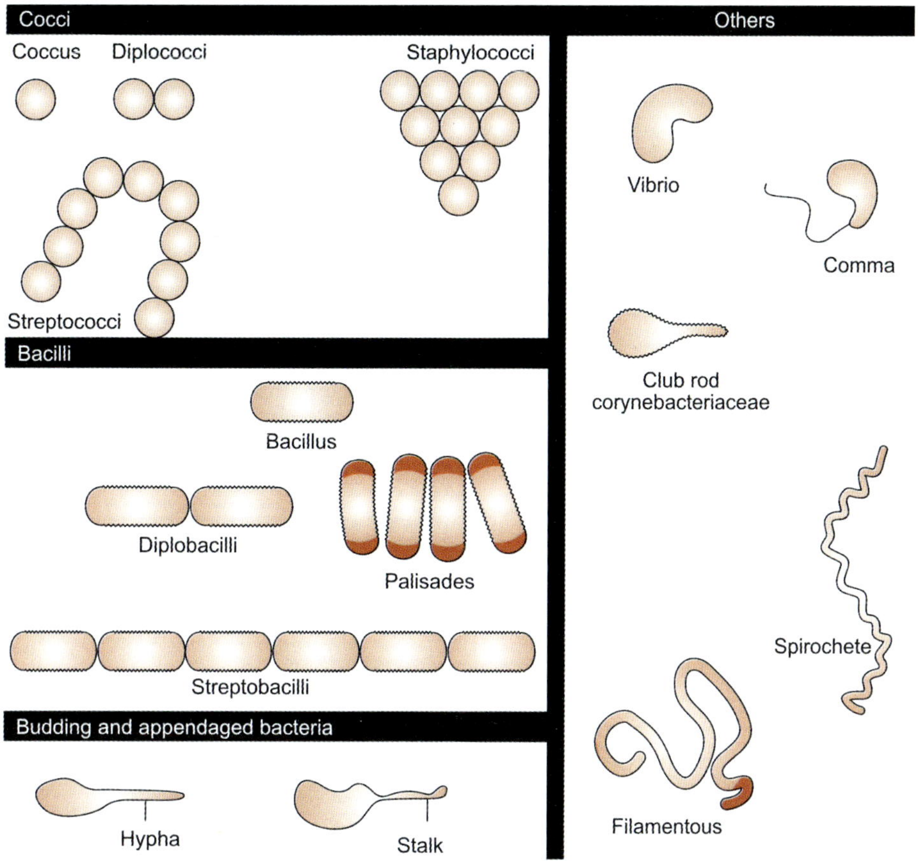


**Fig. 4.11:** Different types of microorganisms

*Pathogenicity* is ability of microorganisms to produce a disease.

*Virulence* is degree of pathogenicity.

Bacterial virulence factors include fimbriae, capsules, lipopolysaccharides, enzymes (collagenase, hyaluronidase, proteases), extracellular vesicles, short chain fatty acids, polyamines and low molecular weight products such as ammonia and hydrogen sulfide. Virulence factors may vary from strain to strain. Virulence is directly related to pathogenicity.

In 1965, Hobson gave an equation showing the relation of number of microorganisms, their virulence, resistance of host and severity of the disease.

$$\frac{\text{Number of microorganisms} \times \text{Virulence of microorganisms}}{\text{Resistance of host}} = \text{Severity of the disease}$$

We can see that along with number of microorganisms, their virulence is also directly related to the severity of the disease.

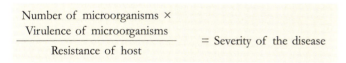

**Various virulent factors**
1. Lipopolysaccharides (LPS)
2. Extracellular vesicles
3. Enzymes
4. Fatty acids
5. Polyamines
6. Capsule
7. Pilli

## Lipopolysaccharides (LPS)

Lipopolysaccharides are present on the surface of gram- negative bacteria. LPS have nonspecific antigens which are not neutralized by antibodies. They exert numerous biologic functions when released from cells in the form of endotoxins. Endotoxins have capability to diffuse into the dentin. Various studies have shown the relationship between the endotoxins and the periradicular inflammation.

## Extracellular Vesicles

Extracellular vesicles are produced by gram-negative bacteria in the form of endotoxins, outer membrane fragments or blebs. They have trilaminar structure similar to outer membrane of the parent bacteria. These vesicles contain various enzymes and toxic products which are responsible for hemagglutination, hemolysis and bacterial adhesion. Since they have antigenic properties similar to the parent bacteria, they may protect bacteria by neutralizing specific antibodies.

## Enzymes

Enzymes produced by bacteria have numerous activities like they help in spread of the infection, neutralization of immunoglobulin and the complement components. PMN leukocytes release hydrolytic enzymes which degenerate and lyse to form purulent exudates and have adverse effects on the surrounding tissues.

### Fatty Acids

Various short chain fatty acids like propionic acid, butyric acid are produced by anaerobic bacteria. These cause neutrophil chemotaxis, degranulation, phagocytosis, and stimulate interleukin-1 production which further causes bone resorption and periradicular diseases.

### Polyamines

These are biologically active chemicals found in the infected canals. Some of polyamines such as cadaverine, putrescine, spermidine help in regulation of the cell growth, regeneration of tissues and modulation of inflammation.

Other virulent factors like capsules present in gram- negative black pigmented bacteria, enable them to avoid phagocytosis. Pilli may play an important role in attachment of bacteria to surfaces and interaction with other bacteria.

## FACTORS INFLUENCING THE GROWTH AND COLONIZATION OF MICROORGANISMS

### Influence of Oxygen

A factor highly selective for the microbial flora of root canal is low availability of oxygen in infected root canals. In the initial stages, there is predominance of facultative organisms but later they are replaced by anaerobic bacteria.

### Nutritional Factors

Bacterias obtain their nutrition from tissue fluid and the breakdown products of necrotic pulp tissue. These nutrients are rich in polypeptides and amino acids, which are essential for growth of the bacteria. Other source of nutrition for bacterias is inflammatory exudates containing serum and blood factors discharged from related inflammatory processes in the remaining pulp or the periapical tissues.

### Bacteriocins

Some bacterias produce bacteriocins, which are antibiotic like proteins produced by one species of bacteria to inhibit another species of bacteria.

### Coaggregation

It is the existence of "symbiotic relationship" between some bacterias which may result in an increase in virulence by the organisms in that ecosystem.

### Bacterial Interrelationships

Interrelationships between certain bacteria can be commensal or antagonistic which affect their survival.

## MICROBIAL ECOSYSTEM OF THE ROOT CANAL

Since many years, various papers have been published regarding the microbial flora of the root canals, normal and infected both. But over past 5-10 years, difference in flora has reported because of improved technology in sampling, culture techniques, culture media as well as more advanced technology regarding isolation and identification of the microorganism.

Most commonly gram-positive organisms are found in the root canals, but gram-negative and obligate anaerobes have also been found in the root canals. Usually the microorganisms which can survive in environment of low oxygen tension and can survive the rigors of limited pabulums are found in root canals. Variety of microorganisms enters the root canal system through various portals of entry but only those which fit for survival in such environment do survive. Most commonly seen bacteria in root canals is streptococci, others can be *Staphylococcus*, gram-negative and anaerobic bacteria.

In necrotic pulp, a mix of bacterial species is found. In necrotic pulp, there is lack of circulation with compromised host defense mechanism; this makes pulp as a reservoir for invading microbes.

**New nomenclature of bacteroids species**

1. *Porphyromonas* - Dark-pigmented (asaccharolytic Bacteroides species)
   - *Porphyromonas asaccharolyticus*
   - *Porphyromonas gingivalis**
   - *Porphyromonas endodontalis**
2. *Prevotella*-Dark-pigmented (saccharolytic Bacteroides species)
   - *Prevotella melaninogenica*
   - *Prevotella denticola*
   - *Prevotella intermedia*
   - *Prevotella nigrescens**
   - *Prevotella corporis*
   - *Prevotella tannerae*
3. *Prevotella* - Nonpigmented (saccharolytic *Bacteroides* species)
   - *Prevotella buccae**
   - *Prevotella bivia*
   - *Prevotella oralis*
   - *Prevotella olurum*

*Most commonly isolated species of black-pigmented bacteria

In necrotic pulps, tissue fluids and disintegrated cells from necrotic tissue, low oxygen tension and bacterial interactions are the main factors which determine which bacteria will predominate. The growth of one bacterial species may be dependent on the other bacterial species which supplies the essential nutrients. In the similar way, antagonistic relationship may occur in bacteria, i.e. byproducts of some bacterial species may kill or retard the growth of others species. In other words, some byproducts can act either as nutrient or as toxin depending on bacterial species (Fig. 4.12).

Naidorf summarized the few generalizations in relation to organisms isolated from the root canals:

1. Mixed infections are more common than single organisms.
2. Pulp contains flora almost similar to that of oral cavity.
3. Approximately 25 percent of isolated organisms are anaerobes.
4. Organisms isolated from flare-up as well as asymptomatic cases are almost similar.
5. Various researchers have identified wide variety of microorganisms in the root canals which is partially related to personal interest and culture techniques used by them.

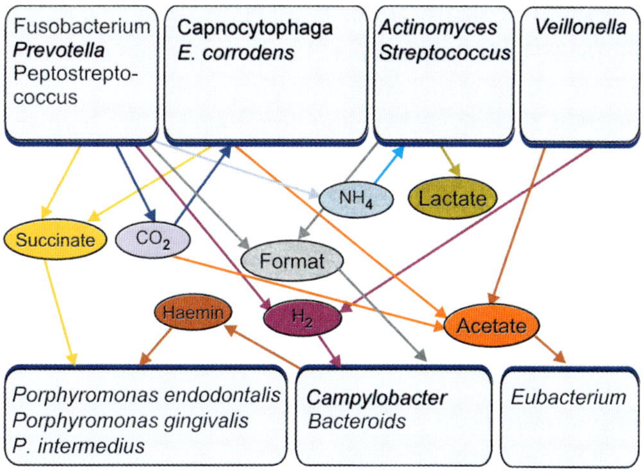


**Fig. 4.12:** Interrelationship of various root canal microorganisms

## PRIMARY ENDODONTIC INFECTIONS

In 1890, Miller first investigated the association of presence of bacteria with pulpal diseases. Later in 1965, Kakehashi et al proved the bacteria as main causative factor for endodontic diseases. It has been shown by various studies that endodontic infections are polymicrobial, though facultative bacteria predominate in early root canal infections, in latter stages they are replaced by strict anaerobic organisms.

A root canal containing a necrotic pulp becomes a selective habitat that allows some species of bacteria to grow in preference to others. The nutrients provided by the breakdown products of a necrotic pulp, tissue fluid and serum from surrounding tissues along with low oxygen tension, and bacterial byproducts support the growth of selected microorganisms. The coronal portion of a root canal may harbor organisms different from those in the apical portion.

Some species of black-pigmented bacteria, peptostreptococci, *Fusobacterium* and *Actinomyces* species have been found related to clinical signs and symptoms. But because of polymicrobial nature of the endodontic infections, no absolute correlation has been found between bacterial species and severity of endodontic infections.

Coaggregation of different species of bacteria or self aggregation of the same species may present the organisms protection from the host's defenses and supply nutrients from the surrounding bacteria. The combination of *Fusobacterium nucleatum* with dark-pigmented bacteria Prevotella intermedia and *Porphyromonas gingivalis* has been shown to be more virulent than when the bacteria are in pure culture. This supports the concept that there is a synergistic relationship between bacteria in an endodontic infection.

Traditional methods of identifying microorganisms were based on gram staining, colonial morphology and biochemical tests, etc. Nowadays newer technologies like DNA method, molecular techniques like PCR (Polymerase chain reaction) SDS-PAGE have helped to identify various microorganisms. For example using DNA studies, black pigmented bacteria previously in génesis *Bacteroids* now have been placed in the genesis *Porphyromonas* and *Prevotella*. PCR technique has been used to show that geographical differences exist among the endodontic infections.

The virulence potential of dark-pigmented bacteria has been studied in animals. Strains of cultivable bacteria have been shown to possess the ability to resist phagocytosis, degrade immunoglobulins, and increase pathogenesis when in combination with other specific strains of *bacteroids*.

**Microbiology of infected root canal**

| Obligate anaerobes | Facultative anaerobes |
|---|---|
| Gram negative bacilli | Gram negative bacilli |
| *Porphyromonas** | Capnocytophaga |
| *Prevotella*** | *Eikenella* |
| *Fusobacterium* | |
| *Campylobacter* | |
| *Bacteroides* | |
| Gram-negative cocci | Gram-negative cocci |
| *Veillonella* | *Neisseria* |
| Gram-positive bacilli | Gram-positive bacilli |
| *Actinomyces* | *Actinomyces* |
| *Lactobacillus* | *Lactobacillus* |
| *Proprionibacterium* | |
| Gram-positive cocci | Gram-positive cocci |
| *Streptococcus* | *Streptococcus* |
| *Peptostreptococcus* | *Enterococcus* |
| Spirochetes | Fungi |
| *Treponema* | *Candida* |

*Dark pigmented bacteria
**Dark pigmented bacteria and nonpigmenting bacteria

The pathogenicity of *Bacteroides* is mainly related to the presence of lipopolysaccharides and peptidoglycans. These:

i. Induce hormones like cytokinins which play an important role in inflammations
ii. Stimulate B-lymphocytes.
iii. Activate complement cascade
iv. Release various enzymes like collagenase
v. Enhance production of various pain mediators like bradykinin, histamine and prostaglandins.
vi. LPS once released (as endotoxin) causes biological effects including inflammation and bone resorption.

Certain gram-positive bacteria have also been found associated with endodontic infections. *Actinomyces* may colonize periapical tissues. Aggregates of organisms may be recognized in periradicular biopsy sections as sulfur granules. A recent study using the PCR detected species of *Actinomyces* (israelii, naeslundii, viscosus) in 80 percent of the infected root canals and 46 percent of periradicular abscesses.

*A. israelii* is a bacterial species of endodontic infections which is resistant to conventional endodontic treatment. But at present combination of sodium hypochlorite and calcium hydroxide has proved to be an effective method in killing them. Surgery is another option to eliminate *A. israelii* from the periapical region.

Other gram-positive bacteria often cultured from endodontic infections include Peptostreptococci, *Streptococcus, Enterococcus,* and *Eubacterium.* Using PCR, Peptostreptococci was detected in 28 percent of the infected root canals tested. Recently DNA hybridization and PCR have been used for screening spirochetes.

Fungi have been cultivated and detected using molecular methods in infected root canal. When using PCR, *Candida albicans* was detected in 21 percent of infected root canals.

Viruses may also be associated with endodontic disease. Bacteriocins are viruses that infect bacteria and carry DNA into the genome of the bacteria. Usually the HIV, cytomegalovirus and Epstein Barr virus are seen to be associated with periapical pathologies.

Molecular methods such as DNA hybridization and PCR detect and identify many more microorganism than the so-called "gold standard" of culturing. Molecular methods are much more sensitive and offer precise identification at the DNA level. A disadvantage of molecular methods is not knowing whether the DNA was from an alive or dead organism. Currently antibiotic susceptibility tests cannot be accomplished without viable organisms. In the future, probes may be used to identify antimicrobial resistant genes in the DNA samples without need of growing the organisms for susceptibility tests.

## MICROBIOLOGY OF PERIRADICULAR ENDODONTIC INFECTIONS

Once a necrotic pulp is infected, the root canal system becomes storehouse of microorganisms (Fig. 4.13). At the apical foramen and at the root ends of infected canal, plaque like biofilms have been found.

Extraradicular bacteria are usually associated with acute symptoms, the presence of a sinus tract, an infected cyst, or in cases not responding to endodontic treatment. Both acute and chronic periradicular abscesses are polymicrobial infections with large numbers of bacteria.

Periapical inflammatory lesions contain macrophages, lymphocytes (T-cells and B-cells), plasma cells and neutrophils. Their function is to prevent microorganisms from invading periradicular tissues. Both the pulp and periradicular inflammatory tissues have been shown to produce cellular and humoral responses to the microorganisms. Microbial invasion of periradicular tissues results in production of an abscess or cellulitis which presents the signs and symptoms because of both specific and nonspecific inflammation.

Several studies have shown that polymicrobial infections are found both in acute and chronic stages of periradicular infections. In many asymptomatic patients with chronic infection, sinus tracts have also been found. It has been seen that sinus tracts are associated with chronic periradicular abscess that always encompass a polymicrobial infection. They are relatively asymptomatic because the sinus tract provides a pathway of drainage.

Invasion of periradicular tissues is related to the virulence of the microorganisms and the host's resistance. Periapical inflammatory lesions are dynamic inflammatory events and may contain an abscess with bacteria, a cyst and surrounding inflammatory tissue simultaneously.

It is seen that most common cause of persistent periradicular infections is incomplete debridement of the root canal system (Fig. 4.8). Therefore three-dimensional sealing of the root canal system is necessary for resolution of periapical pathologies.

## MICROBIOLOGY OF ROOT CANAL FAILURES

The lack of periradicular healing following root canal treatment seems to be related to the persistence of microbes in the root canal system (Fig. 4.14). This would appear to be related to an inability to effectively shape, clean, and seal the complete root canal system (Fig. 4.15). Interestingly, the microflora cultured from previously filled root canals with persistent apical lesions differs significantly for the microbes in untreated necrotic canals. Various researches have shown that microbiology of untreated canals is different from previously obturated canals.

Bacteria isolated from canals previously obturated but still associated with radiographic lesions tend to have more facultative bacteria rather than strict anaerobes. Instead of having approximately equal amounts of gram-negative and gram-positive bacteria, the bacteria isolated from previously obturated canals tend to have only one to two cultivable strains of mainly gram-positive bacteria. In several studies, previously filled canals had a relative increase in the presence of *Enterococcus faecalis.*

Recently a study using PCR found the presence of *E. faecalis, Propionibacterium alactolyticus, P. propionicum* in previously filled root canal failure cases.

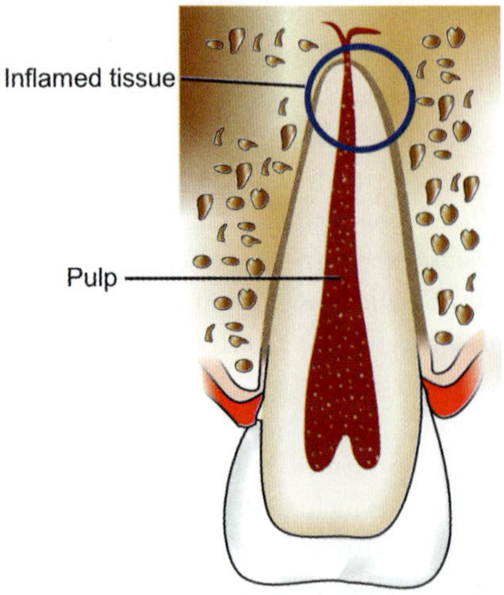


**Fig. 4.13:** Microorganisms in infected root canal

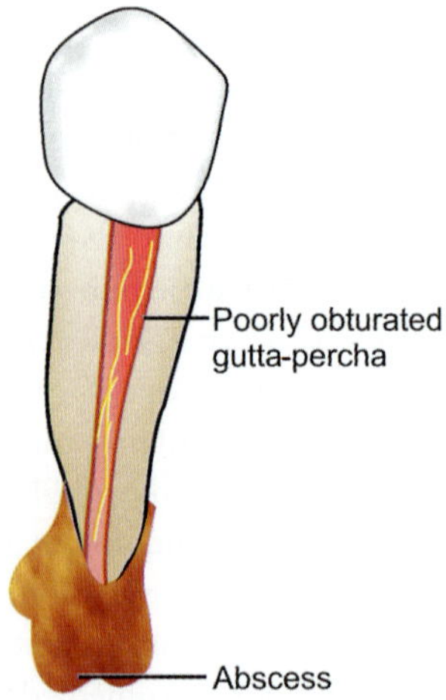


**Fig. 4.14:** Abscess formation due to poorly obturated canal

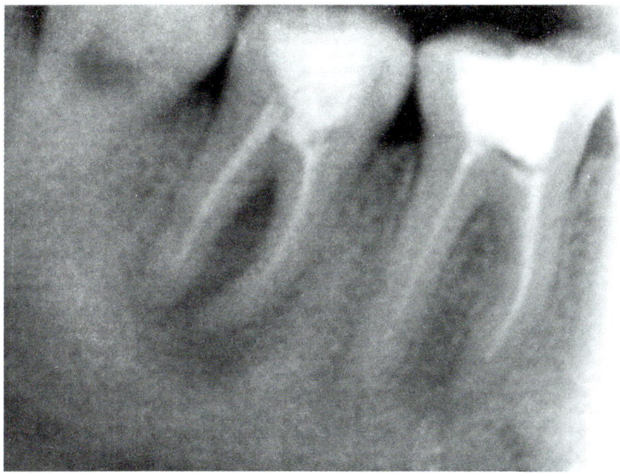

Fig. 4.15: Periapical lesion due to root canal failure of 47

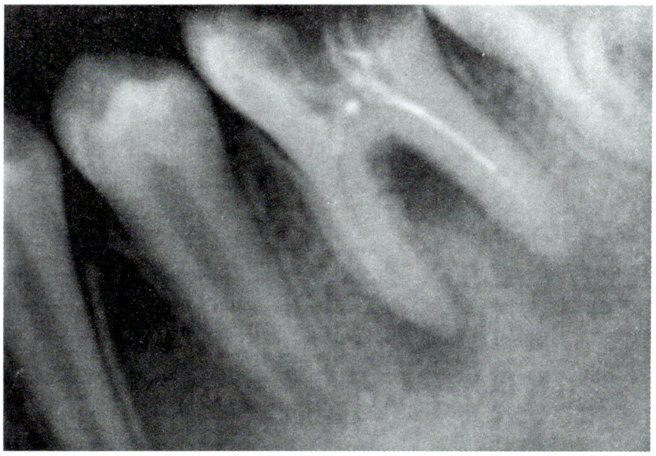

Fig. 4.16: Non-healing of periapical lesion because of untreated canal

Filifactor alocis and *Dialister pneumosintes* have not been isolated from previously filled root canals with periradicular lesions. They are anaerobic bacteria recently shown to be prevalent in untreated root canals. The presence of bacteria in all of the failed root canals supports the assertion that the vast majority of endodontic treatment failures are caused by intraradicular infections.

## ENDODONTIC ABSCESSES AND CELLULITIS (FIG. 4.16)

The extent of endodontic infections beyond the root canal system is related to virulence of the bacteria, host response, and associated anatomy. Infections may localize or continue to spread. An abscess is a cavity of purulent exudates consisting primarily of bacteria, bacterial byproducts, inflammatory cells, lysed cells and their contents. The content of inflammatory cells includes enzymes, which are damaging to the surrounding tissues. Endodontic abscesses are polymicrobial infections with organisms similar to those found in infected root canals. A diffuse cellulitis may have foci of abscesses. The spread of infection and ensuing edema associated with inflammation often produces an indurated swelling. Over the time, neutrophils accumulate and produce a fluctuant abscesses. This concept supports the rationale for early incision for drainage to provide a pathway for the drainage of bacteria, bacterial byproducts, and inflammatory mediators.

## ENTEROCOCCUS FAECALIS

*E. faecalis* is considered to be most common reason for failed root canals and in canals with persistent infection.

It is a gram-positive cocci and is facultative anaerobe. Due to presence of following features, it can stay in root canals even in adverse conditions:

a. It can persist in poor nutrient environment of root canal treated teeth.
b. It can survive in presence of medicaments like calcium hydroxide.
c. It can stay alive in presence of irrigants like sodium hypochlorite.
d. It can convert into viable but non-cultivable state.
e. It can form biofilm in medicated canals.
f. It can penetrate and utilize fluid present in dentinal tubules.
g. It can survive in prolonged periods of starvation and utilize tissue fluid that flow from periodontal ligament.
h. It can survive in low pH and high temperature.
i. It can acquire gene encoding resistance combined with natural resistance to antibiotics.
j. It can establish monoinfections in medicated root canals.

## IDENTIFICATION OF THE BACTERIA

Following tests can be done to detect microorganisms and to test which antibiotic they are sensitive to.

1. *Gram's stain*: It was developed by Christian Gram in 1884. It helps in differentiating bacterias in Gram-positive and Gram-negative organisms.
2. *Culture*: Culture taking method though done less these days, but it still holds its importance because of wide range of bacteria found in the endodontic infections. The empirical administration of antibiotics may not produce satisfactory results, in such cases, culturing may provide a valuable information for better antibiotic selection. Thus we can say that with supportive information from culturing, an intelligent alteration in antibiotic therapy can be made.

### Principle of Culturing

Culturing of root canals is done for two main reasons:

1. In cases of persistent infection, to grow and isolate the microbial flora for antibiotic sensitivity and resistance profiles.
2. To assess the bacteriologic status of root canal system before obturation and determine the effectiveness of debridement procedure.

#### Types of tissue cultures

**Cell culture:** It is an *in vitro* growth of cells although the cells proliferate they do not organize into tissue.

**Anaerobic culture:** It is the culture which is carried out in the absence of air.

**Pure culture:** It is a culture of a single cell species, without presence of any contaminants.

**Primary culture:** Refers to cultures prepared from tissues taken directly from animals.

**Secondary culture:** It refers to a subculture derived from a primary culture.

**Plate culture:** It refers to the culture which is grown on a medium, usually agar or gelatin, on a Petri dish.

**Streak culture:** It refers to the culture one in which the medium is inoculated by drawing an infected wire across it.

**Suspension culture:** It refers to a culture in which cells multiply while suspended in a suitable medium.

**Slant culture:** This culture is made on the surface of solidified medium in a tube which has been tilted to provide a greater surface area for growth.

**Stab culture:** In theis culture, the medium is inoculated by thrusting a needle deep into its substance.

**Tissue culture:** It refers to the culture in which maintenance or growth of tissue, organ primordia, or the whole or part of an organ *in vitro* is done so as to preserve its architecture and function.

## Types of Culture Medium

1. Liquid (broth)
2. Solid (agar)
3. Semisolid

## Liquid Culture Medium

The original liquid media developed by Louis Pasteur contained wine or meat broth. In liquid media, nutrients are dissolved in water and bacterial growth is indicated by a change in the broth's appearance from clear to turbid. Minimum of $10^6$ bacteria per milliliter of broth are required for turbidity to be detected with unaided eye. More of the bacterial growth is indicated by greater turbid appearance.

## Solid Media

It was developed by Robert Koch in 1881. It contained pieces of potato, gelatin, and meat extract. Since gelatin used to liquefy at 24°C, so he substituted it with agar.

## Bacteriological Media

It consists of water, agar, growth enriching constituents like yeast extract, and blood.

*Anaerobic culture method:* An anaerobic bacteria culture is a method used to grow anaerobes from a clinical specimen. Anaerobic bacterial culture is performed to identify bacteria that grow only in the absence of oxygen. The methods of obtaining specimens for anaerobic culture and the culturing procedure are performed to ensure that the organisms are protected from oxygen.

## Culture Technique

For culturing, samples can be obtained from either from an infected root canal or from a periradicular abscess.

## Sample from Draining Root Canal

1. Isolate the tooth with a rubber dam. Disinfect the surface of the tooth and surrounding area with betadine, chlorhexidine or NaOCl.
2. Gain access to the root canals using sterile burs and instruments.
3. If there is drainage, collect the sample using a sterile needle and syringe or with use of sterile absorbent paper points. Place the aspirate in anaerobic transport media.

## Sample from Dry Canal

To sample a dry canal, use a sterile syringe to place transport media into canal. Take the sample using a syringe or paper points and place the aspirate in anaerobic media.

## Sample from the Abscess

Palpate the fluctuant abscess and determine the most dependent part of swelling. Disinfect the surface of mucosa with alcohol or iodophor. Penetrate a sterile 16-20 gauge needle in the surface and aspirate the exudates. Inject this aspirate into anaerobic transport media.

## Culture Reversal

Sometimes negative culture becomes positive after 24-48 hours. So it is advised to allow more than 48 hours between taking culture and obturation.

### *Advantages of Culturing Techniques*

- Culture helps to determine bacteriological status of root canal.
- It helps to isolate microbial flora for resistant profiles and for antibiotic sensitivity.
- Helps in identification of broad range of microorganisms.

### *Disadvantages of Culturing Method*

1. Unable to grow several microorganisms which can give false negative results.
2. Strictly depend on mode of sample transport which must allow growth of anaerobic bacteria.
3. Low sensitivity and specificity.
4. Time consuming.
5. Expensive and laborious.

## Molecular Diagnostic Methods

To overcome these disadvantages, various molecular diagnostic methods have developed. Molecular diagnostic methods identify the microorganisms using gene as a target which are unique for each species. These include DNA-DNA hybridization method, polymerase chain reaction method.

## DNA-DNA Hybridization Method

This method uses DNA probes which target genomic DNA or individual genes. This method helps in simultaneous determination of the presence of a multitude of bacterial species in single or multiple clinical samples and is especially useful for large scale epidemiologic research. In this method, segments of labeled, single strand DNA locate and bind to their complementary nucleic acid sequences. After washing, the presence of bound label indicates the presence of the target DNA sequence.

### *Advantages of DNA-DNA Hybridization Method*

- Can be used for large scale epidemiological research.
- Allows simultaneous detection of multiple species.
- Microbial contaminants are not cultivated and their DNA is not amplified.

### *Disadvantages of DNA-DNA Hybridization Method*

- Cross reaction can occur on non-target microorganisms.
- Identifies only cultivable microorganisms.
- Does not detect unexpected.
- Detects only target microorganisms.

## Polymerase Chain Reaction Method (PCR Method)

PCR method involves *in vitro* replication of DNA, therefore it is also called as "genetic xeroxing" method. Multiple copies of specific region of DNA are made by repeated cycles or heating and cooling.

PCR has remarkable sensitivity and specificity because each distinct microbial species has unique DNA sequences.

PCR can be used to detect virtually all bacterial species in a sample. It is also used to investigate microbial diversity in a given environment. Clonal analysis of microorganisms can also be done by PCR method.

### *Disadvantages of PCR*

- Identify microorganisms qualitatively not quantitatively.
- Detect only target microorganisms.
- Difficult in microorganisms with thick wall like fungi.
- Possibility of false positive and negative results.

### *Advantages of Molecular Methods*

Molecular methods have following advantages over the culturing methods:

- They are helpful in detection of both cultivable and uncultivable microbial species.
- They are more sensitive tests.
- Molecular methods have greater specificity.
- They are less time consuming.
- Do not need special control for anaerobic bacteria.
- Are useful when a large number of samples are needed to be analyzed for epidemiologic studies.
- They do not require cultivation.
- They can be identified even when they are viable.
- They can be used during antimicrobial treatment.
- Large number of samples can be stored at low temperature and surveyed at once.

## HOW TO COMBAT MICROBES IN THE ENDODONTIC THERAPY

The microbial ecosystem of an infected root canal system and inflammatory response caused by it will persist until source of irritation is completely removed. The main factor which is needed for successful treatment of pulp and periradicular inflammation is complete removal of the source of infection such as microorganisms and their byproducts, etc.

Following measures should be taken to completely rid of these irritants:

1. *Thorough cleaning and shaping of the root canal system:* Root canal system is thoroughly cleaned and shaped to remove the bacteria and substrates which can support microorganisms. Thorough cleaning and shaping followed by three dimensional obturation of the root canals have shown to produce complete healing of periradicular tissue (Figs 4.17A to C). Complete debridement of canal should be done with adjunctive use of irrigants like sodium hypochlorite which efficiently removes bacteria as well as their substrate from irregularities of canal system where instruments cannot reach such as fins, indentations, cul-de-sacs, etc.
   NaOCl is considered an excellent antimicrobial agent with tissue dissolving properties. It can be used alone or in combination with other irrigants like chlorhexidine, EDTA, hydrogen peroxide, etc.
2. Oxygenating a canal simply by opening it is detrimental to anaerobes. Use of oxygenating agents as glyoxide can be of great help but care should be taken to avoid inoculation of these oxygenating agents into periapical tissues.
3. A tooth with serous or purulent or hemorrhagic exudate should be allowed to drain with rubber dam in place for a time under supervision. An abscess which is a potent irritant, has an elevated osmotic pressure. This attracts more tissue fluid and thus more edema and pain. Drainage by canal or by soft tissues decrease discomfort caused by inflammatory mediators.
4. Antibiotics should also be considered as adjunctive in severe infections. The choice of antibiotic agent should be done on the knowledge of microorganisms associated with the endodontic infections. The drug of choice for endodontic infections is the Penicillin VK because of its spectrum of microbial activity against most of the bacteria associated with endodontic infections and also because of its low toxicity.

   Other antibiotics which can be given to combat endodontic infections include amoxicillin because of its wider spectrum than penicillin, clarithromycin, azithromycin and metronidazole for their action against most of the anaerobes found in root canals. If patient is allergic to penicillin, clindamycin is recommended. It is effective against anaerobic bacteria, both obligate as well as facultative.

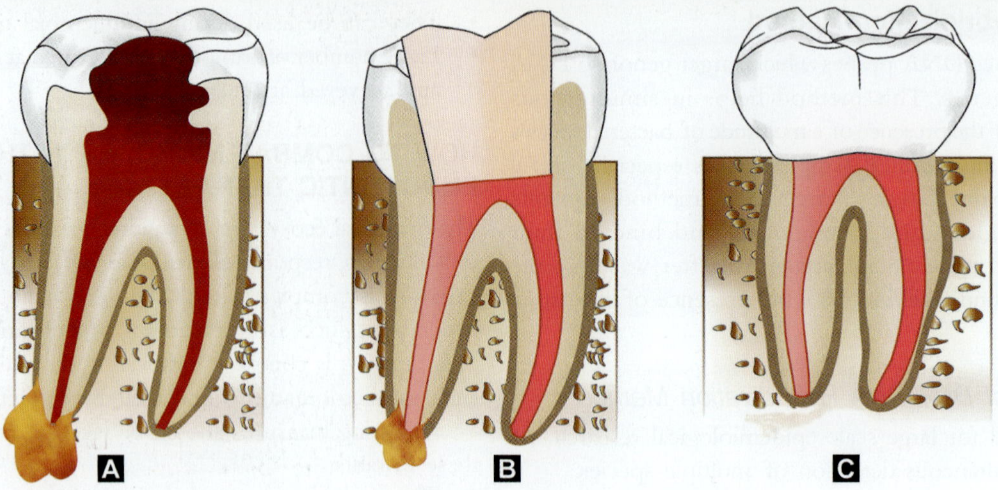


**Figs 4.17A to C:** (A) Infection of pulp which has progressed to alveolar abscess; (B) Complete cleaning and shaping of root canal system; (C) Successful root canal therapy and healed periapical bone

5. Intracanal medicaments play an important role in combating the microorganisms.
6. Use of calcium hydroxide in canals with necrotic pulps after instrumentation have shown to provide the beneficial results. Intracranial use of calcium hydroxide have shown to increase the efficiency of sodium hypochlorite and also the effectiveness of antimicrobial agent. Calcium hydroxide powder is mixed with water or glycerin to form a thick paste which is placed in pulp chamber with amalgam carrier or a syringe. This paste is covered with a sterile cotton pellet and access is sealed with temporary restoration.

Thus, we can say that for successful endodontic outcome, one must have awareness of the close relationship between endodontic infections and microorganisms.

## QUESTIONS

**Q. What are different methods used for identification of bacteria. Write in detail about culture method?**

**Q. Write short notes on:**

a. Anachoresis
b. Microbial virulence and pathogenicity
c. Explain microbiology of infected root canals.

## BIBLIOGRAPHY

1. Akpata E Blecjman H. Bacterial invasion of pulpal dentin wall in vitro. J Dent Res 1982;61:435-8.
2. Baumgartner JC, Falkler WA Jr. Bacteria in the apical 5 mm of infected root canals. JOE 1991;17:380.
3. Baumgartner JC, Heggers J, Harrison. The incidence of bacteremias related to endodontic procedures. I. Nonsurgical endodontics. JOE 1976;2:135.
4. Bender IB, Seltzer S, Yermish M. The incidence of bacteremia in endodontic manipulation. Oral Surg 1960;13:353.
5. Bibel D. The discovery of the oral flora: a 300-year retrospective. J Am Dent Assoc 1983;107:569.
6. Bibel DJ. The discovery of oral flora-300-year retrospective. J Am Dent Assoc 1983;10:569-70.
7. Byström A, Happonen RP, Sjögren U, Sundqvist G. Healing of periapical lesions of pulpless teeth after endodontic treatment with controlled asepsis. Endod Dent Traumator 1987;3:58.
8. Bystrom A, Sandqvist G. The antibacterial action of sodium hypochlorite and EDTA in 60 cases of endodontic therapy. Int Endod J 1985;1:35.
9. Bystrom A, Sundqvist G. Bacteriologic evaluation of the efficacy of mechanical root canal instrumentation in endodontic therapy. Scand J Dent Res 1981;89:321.
10. Czarnecki RT, Schilder H. A histological evaluation of the human pulp in teeth with varying degrees of periodontal desease. Joe 1979;5:242.
11. David A Spratt. Significance of bacterial identification by molecular biology methods; Endodontic Topics 2004;9:5-14.
12. Debelian GJ, Olsen I, Tonstad L. Bacteremia in conjunction with endodontic therapy. Endod dent trumatol 1995;11:142.
13. Denis P Lych. Oral candiasis-History, classification, and clinical presentation; Oral Surg Oral Med Oral Patho 1994;78:189-93.
14. Drucker D, Lilly J, Tucker D, Gibbs C. The endodontic microflora revisited Microbios 1992;71:225.
15. Easlick K. An evaluation of the effect of dental foci of infection on health. J Am Dent Assoc 1951;42:694.
16. Ehrmann. Focal infection—The endodontic point of view; Surg Oral Med Oral Path 1997;44(4).
17. Fish EW. Bone infection. J Am Dent Assoc 1939;26:691.
18. Gilberto J Debelian. Systemic diseases caused by oral microorganisms; Endod Dent Traumatol 1994;10:57-65.
19. Glick M, Trope M, Pliskin M. Detection of HIV in the dental pulp of a patient with AIDS. J Am Dent Assoc 1989;119:649.
20. Gomes BPFA, Drucker DB, Lilley JD. Association of specific bacteria with some endodontic signs and symptoms. Int Endod J 1994;27:291.
21. Goran sundquist. Taxonomy, ecology, and pathogenicity of the root canal flora; Oral Surg Med Oral pathol 1994;78;522-30.
22. Grossman LI. Focal infection: Are oral foci of infection related to systemic disease? Dent Clin North Am 1960;4:749.
23. Guven Kayaglu. Virulence factors of Enterococcus faecalis. Relationship to endodontic disease. Crit Rev Oral Bio Med 2004;15(5):308-20.

24. Haapasalo M, Udnaes T, Endal U. Persistent, recurrent, and acquired infection of the root canal system post-treatment. Endod Topics 2003;6:29-56.
25. Haapasalo M. Bacteroides spp. In dental root canal infections. Endod Dent Traumatol 1989;5:1.
26. Haapassalo HK, et al. Inactivation of local root canal medicaments by dentine: An in vitro study. Int Endo J 2000;33:126-31.
27. Happonen RP. Periapical actinomycosis a follow-up Study of 16 surgically treated cases. Endod Dent Traumatol 1986;2:205.
28. Hashioka K, Yamasaki M, Nakane A, et al. The relationship between clinical symptoms and anaerobic bacteria from infected root canals. JOE 1992;18:558.
29. Horiba N, Markawa Y, Abe Y, et al. Correlations between endotoxin and clinical symptoms or radiolucent areas in infected root canals. Oral Surg 1991;71:492.
30. Howard K Kuramitsu. Virulence factors of mutans streptococci: Role of molecular genetics; Crit Rev Oral Bio Med 1993;4(2);159-76.
31. Isabelle Portenier, Tuomos MT. Waltimo: Enterococcus faecalis-the root canal survivor and 'star' in post-treatment disease. Endodontic Topics 2003;6:135-59.
32. Jose F Siqueira (Jr), Isabela N Rocas. Clinical implications and microbiology of bacterial persistence after treatment procedures'. J Endod 2008;34:1291-301.
33. Jose F Siqueira Jr. Exploiting the molecular methods to explore endodontic infections: Part I-current molecular technologies for microbial diagnosis. J Endodon 2005;31(6): 411-21.
34. Jose F Siqueira Jr. Fungi in endodontic infection. Oral Surg Oral Med Oral Patho 2004;97:632-41.
35. Jose F Siqueira Jr. PCR methodology as a valuable tool for identification of endodontic pathogen. J Dent 2004;31:333-9.
36. Jose F Siqueira Jr. Taxododontic changes of bacteria associated with endodontic infections. J. endodon 2003;29(10):619-23.
37. Kakehashi S, Stanley HR, Fitzgerald RJ. The effects of surgical exposures of dental pulps in germ free and conventional laboratory rats. Oral Surg 1965;20:340.
38. Kaufman B, Spångberg L, Barry J, Fouad AF. Enterococcus spp. In endodontically treated teeth with and without periradicular lesions. J Endod 2005;31:851-56.
39. Langeland K, Rodrigues H, Dowden W. Periodontal disease, bacteria, and pulpal histopathology. Oral Surg 1974;37:257.
40. Love RM. Enterococcus faecalis-a mechanism for its role in endodontic Failure. Int Endod J 2001;34:399-405.
41. Marshall K. Dental workspace contamination and the role of rubber dam. CPD Dentistry 2001;2:48-50.
42. Mazur B, Massler M. Influence of periodontal disease on the dental pulp. Oral Surg 1964;17:592.
43. Moksha Nayak, Mithra Hegde. Molecular diagnostic methods in endodontics. Endodontology 2006;18(2):35-42.
44. Molander A, Reit C, Dehlén G. Microbiological evaluation of clindamycin as a root canal dressing in teeth with apical periodontitis. Int Endod J 1990;23:113-18.
45. Molander A, Reit C, et al. T. Microbiological status of root-filled teeth with apical periodontitis. Int Endod J 1998;31:1-7.
46. Muerman. Dental infections and general health; Quintessence into 1997;28(12):807-10.
47. Murray, Saunders. Root canal treatment and general health. Int Endodo J 2000;33:1-18.
48. Nair PNR, Sjögren U, et al. Intraradicular bacteria and fungi in root-filled, asymptomatic human teeth with therapy-resistant periapical lesions: A long-term light and electron microscopic follow-up. J Endod 1990;16:580-68.
49. Nair PNR. Light and electron microscopic studies of root canal flora and periapical lesions. J Endod 1987;13:29-39.
50. Orstavik D, Haapasalo M. Disinfection by endodontic irrigants and dressings of experimentally infected dentinal tubules. Endod Dent Traumatol 1990;6:142-49.
51. Robert J, Berkowitz. Acquisition and transmission of mutans streptococci. Journal of California Dental Association 2003;31(2):135.
52. Rocas Jose F, Siquiera Jr. Association of Enterococcus faecalis with different forms of periradicular diseases; J Endodon 2005;30(5):315-20.
53. Safavi KE, Spånberg LSW, Langeland K. Root canal dentinal tubule disinfection. J Endod 1990;16:207-10.
54. Siqueira (Jr) JF. Microbial causes of endodontic flare-ups. Int Endod J 2003;36:453-63.
55. Sjögren U, Figdor D, persson S, Sundqvist G. Influence of infection at the time of root filling on the outcome of endodontic treatment of teeth with apical periodontitis. Int Endod J 1997;30(5):297-306.
56. Suchitra U. Enterococcus faecalis: An endodontic pathogen; Endodontology 2006;18(2):11-13.
57. Thomas J. Pallasch: Focal infection:New age or ancient history;endodontic topics 2003;4:32-45.
58. Torabinejad M, Kigar RD. A histologic evaluation of dental pulp tissue of a patient with periodontal disease. Oral Surg 1985;59:198.
59. Torabinejad. M, Ung B, Kettering J. In vitro bacterial penetration of coronally unsealed endodontically treated teeth. J Endod 1990;16:566-69.
60. Tronstad L, Sunde PT. The evolving new understanding of endodontic infections. Endod Topics 2003;6:57-77.
61. Trope M, Rosenberg E, Tronstad L. Darkfield microscopic spirochete count in the differentiation of endodontic and periodontal abscesses. JOE 1992;18:82.
62. Waltimo T, Siren E, Orstavik D, Haapasalo MP. Fungi in therapy resistant apical periodontitis. Int Endod J 1997;30: 96-101.
63. Wong R, Hirsch RS, Clarke NG. Endodontic effects of root planning in humans. Endod Dent Traumatol 1989; 5:193.
64. Wu Mk, Dummer PMH, Wesselink PR. Consequences of and strategies to deal with residual post-treatment root canal infection. Int Endod J 2006;39:343-56.
65. Yoshiba M, Fukushima H, Yamamoto K, et al. Correlation between clinical symptoms and microorganisms isolated from root canals of teeth with periapical pathosis. JOE 1987;13:24.

# Rationale of Endodontic Treatment

CHAPTER 5



Endodontic pathology is mainly caused by injury to the tooth which can be physical, chemical or bacterial. Such injury can results in reversible or irreversible changes in the pulp and periradicular tissues. These resultant changes depend on the intensity, duration, pathogenicity of the stimulus and the host defense mechanism. The changes that occur are mediated by a series of inflammatory and immunological reactions (in the vascular, lymphatics and connective tissue). All these reactions take place to eliminate the irritant and repair any damage.

However, certain conditions are beyond the reparative ability of the body and need to be treated endodontically to aid the survival of tooth.

Rationale of endodontic therapy is complete debridement of root canal system followed by three-dimensional obturation.

## THEORIES OF SPREAD OF INFECTION

### Focal Infection

*Definition:* It is localized or general infection caused by the dissemination of microorganisms or toxic products from a focus of infection.

### Focus of Infection

*Definition:* This refers to a circumscribed area of tissue, which is infected with exogenous pathogenic microorganisms and is usually located near a mucous or cutaneous surface.

### Theory Related to Focal Infection

About a century ago, William Hunter first suggested that oral microorganisms and their products involved in number of systemic diseases, are not always of infectious origin.

In year 1940, Reimann and Havens criticized the theory of focal infection with their recent findings.

### Mechanism of Focal Infection

There are generally two most accepted mechanisms considered responsible for initiation of focal infection:

1. Metastasis of microorganisms from infected focus by either hematogenous or lymphogenous spread.
2. Carrying of toxins or toxic byproducts through bloodstream and lymphatic channel to site where they may initiate a hypersensitive reaction in tissues.

   *For example:* In scarlet fever, erythrogenic toxin liberated by infected streptococci is responsible for cutaneous features of this disease.

### Oral Foci of Infection

Possible sources of infection in oral cavity which later on may set up distant metastases are:

1. Infected periapical lesions such as:
   i. Periapical granuloma
   ii. Periapical abscess
   iii. Periapical cyst
2. Teeth with infected root canals.
3. Periodontal diseases with special reference to tooth extraction.

## CULPRIT OF ENDODONTIC PATHOLOGY

Many studies have shown that root canal infections are multibacterial in nature. In 1965, Kakehashi found that when dental pulps of conventional and germ free rats were exposed to their own oral microbial flora, the conventional rats showed pulpal and periapical lesions whereas the germ free rats did not show any development of lesion. So he described importance of microorganisms for the development of pulpal and periapical pathologies.

## PORTALS FOR ENTRY OF MICROORGANISMS (FIGS 5.1 AND 5.2)

Though microorganisms may gain entry into pulp through several routes, most common route for entering of micro-organisms to dental pulp is dental caries. They can also gain entry into pulp cavity via mechanical or traumatic injury, through gingival sulcus and via bloodstream.

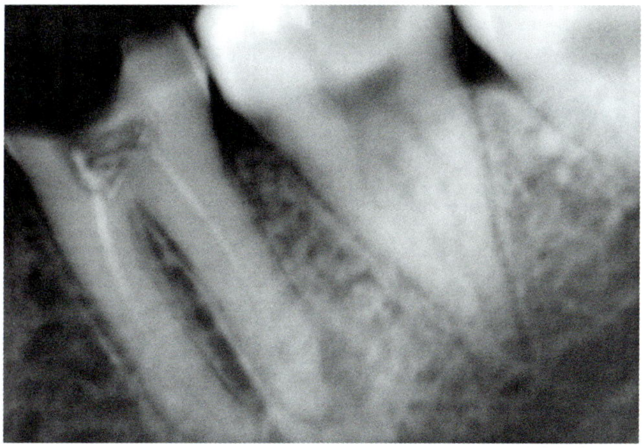

Fig. 5.1: Radiograph showing poorly obturated canals

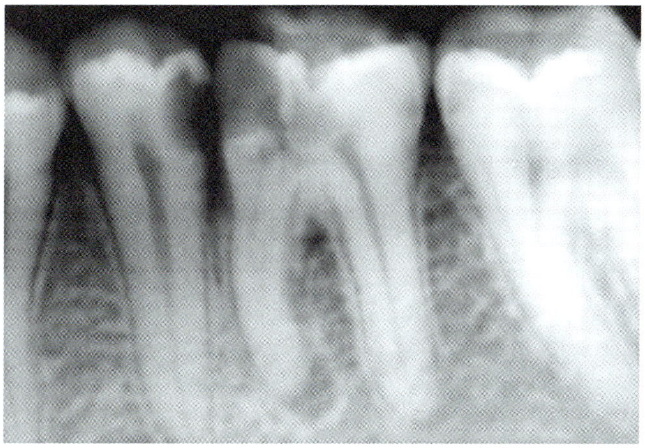

Fig. 5.2: Deep carious lesion resulting in pulp necrosis and periapical lesion

### Entry of Microorganisms into Pulp Through

*Dental caries*—Caries is the most common way of entry of microorganisms into the dental pulp.

Through open dentinal tubules-Microorganisms can pass into the dentinal tubules and subsequently to the pulp resulting in its necrosis.

Through the periodontal ligament or the gingival sulcus, microorganisms can enter into the pulp via accessory and lateral canals which connect pulp and the periodontium.

*Anachoresis*—Anachoresis refers to the attraction of blood borne bacteria in the areas of inflammation. In other words, anachoresis is a process by which microorganisms are transported in the blood to an area of inflammation where they establish an infection.

Through defective restorations, faulty restoration with marginal leakage can result in contamination of the pulp by bacteria.

## INFLAMMATION

Inflammation is defined as the local response of living mammalian tissue to injury due to any agent.

It is a body defense reaction in order to limit the spread or eliminate it or to remove consequent necrosed cells and tissues. Following agents cause inflammation:

a. Physical agents like cold, heat, mechanical trauma or radiation.
b. Chemical agents like organic and inorganic poisons.
c. Infective agents like bacteria, viruses and their toxins.
d. Immunological agents like antigen-antibody cell mediated reactions.

Therefore, we can say that inflammation is distinct from infection. Inflammation is the protective response by the body, while infection is invasion into the body by harmful microbes and their resultant ill effects by toxins.

### Signs of Inflammation

The roman writer celsus in 1st century AD gave four cardinal signs of inflammation:

1. Rubor i.e. redness
2. Tumor i.e. swelling
3. Color i.e. heat
4. Dolor i.e. pain

Virchow later added the fifth sign function lasea, i.e. loss of function.

### Inflammation is of Two Types

- Acute inflammation dominated by PMNLs (Polymorpho-nuclear lymphocytes) and few macrophages
- Chronic inflammation dominated by lymphocytes, macrophages and plasma cells.

The balance between the host defense and microbial factor determines the formation of lesion. In an infected canal, the microbes are usually confined within the canal. As the blood supply is compromised, the host defense mechanisms do not totally eliminate the bacteria. These bacteria release certain enzymes that stimulate the inflammatory process in the periapical tissue.

## TISSUE CHANGES FOLLOWING INFLAMMATION

As a result of inflammation, tissues exhibit two types of changes viz degenerative changes and proliferative changes.

1. **Degenerative changes** in the pulp can be:
   - Fibrous
   - Resorptive
   - Calcific.

   Continuous degeneration of the tissue results in necrosis. Suppuration is another form of degeneration which is due to injury to polymorphonuclear cells. This injury causes release of proteolytic enzymes with resulting liquefaction of dead tissues thus leading to formation of pus or suppuration.

**Three requisites which are necessary for suppuration**
- Tissue necrosis
- Polymorphonuclear leukocytes
- Digestion of the necrotic material by proteolytic enzymes released by injured polymorphonuclear cells.

*Clinical significance:* An abscess can result even in absence of microorganisms because of chemical or physical irritation. It results in formation of sterile abscess.

2. **Proliferative changes (Fig. 5.3)** are produced by irritants which are mild enough to act as stimulants. These irritants may act as both irritant and stimulant, such as calcium hydroxide and its effect on adjacent tissues.

   In the approximation of the inflamed area, the irritant may be strong enough to produce degeneration or destruction, whereas at the periphery, the irritant may be mild enough to stimulate proliferation. The principal cells of proliferation or repair are the fibroblasts, which lay down cellular fibrous tissues. In some cases collagen fibers may be substituted by a dense acellular tissue. In either case it results in formation of fibrous tissue.

   In an infected canal, the microbes are usually confined within the canal. As the blood supply is compromised, the host defense mechanisms do not totally eliminate the bacteria. These bacteria release certain enzymes that stimulate the inflammatory process in the periapical tissue.

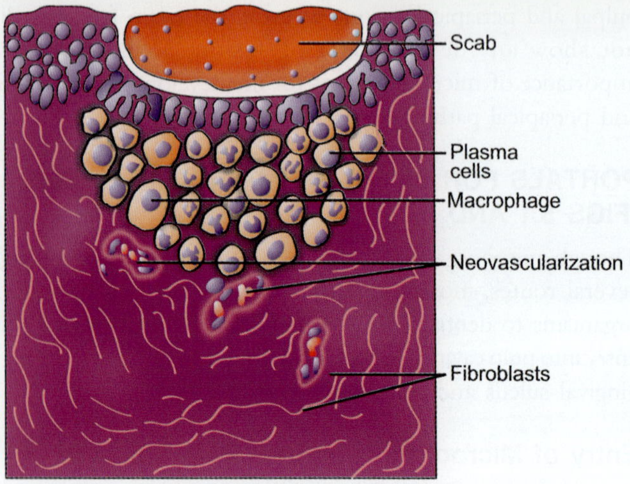


**Fig. 5.3:** Inflammatory cells present at the healing site

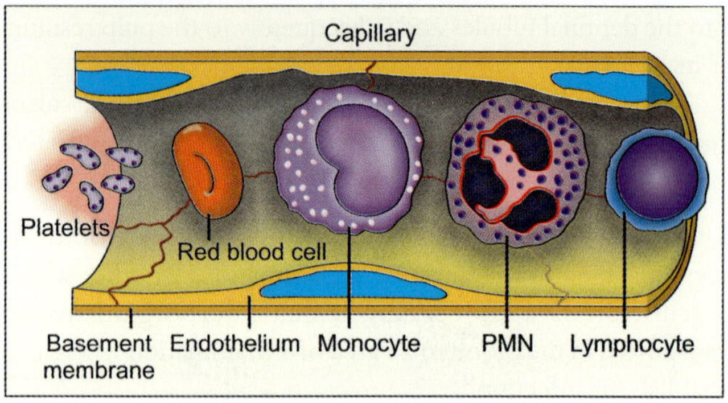


**Fig. 5.4:** Inflammatory cells

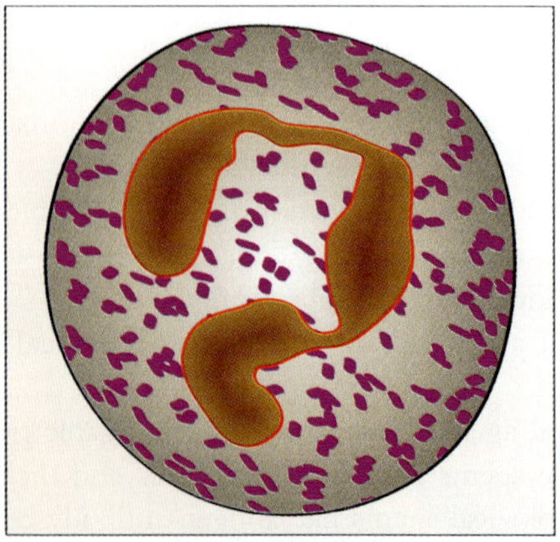

**Fig. 5.5:** Neutrophil

## INFLAMMATORY CELLS (FIG. 5.4)

1. **Neutrophils (PMNLs) (Fig. 5.5):** Along with basophils and eosinophils, polymorphonuclear neutrophils are called granulocytes because of presence of granules in the cytoplasm. Neutrophils are attracted to the site of injury within 24 hours and phagocytose the bacteria and cellular debris releasing lactic acid. Because of its low pH, this lactic acid results in death of the PMNLs and release of proteolytic enzymes (pepsin and cathepsin) prostaglandins and leukotrienes. All these changes result in breaks down of the tissue resulting in the formation of an abscess (dead PMNLs + debris).
2. **Eosinophils (Fig. 5.6):** They have many functional and structural similarities with neutrophils like their formation in bone marrow, phagocytosis, presence of granules in the cytoplasm, bactericidal and toxic action against many parasites. However, granules of eosinophils lack lysozyme and they are richer in myeloperoxidase than neutrophils. Number of eosinophils increase in following conditions:

- Allergic conditions
- Skin diseases
- Parasitic infestations

**Macrophages (Fig. 5.7):** When the PMNLs fail to remove the bacteria, the circulating monocytes reach the site of inflammation and change into macrophages. These macrophages are slow moving and remain at the site of inflammation for a longer time (approximately 2 months). This result in development of chronic inflammation.

Macrophages perform following functions:
- They help in phagocytosis and pinocytosis
- Perform immunological function
- Secrete lysosomal enzymes
- Secrete complement protein and prostaglandins

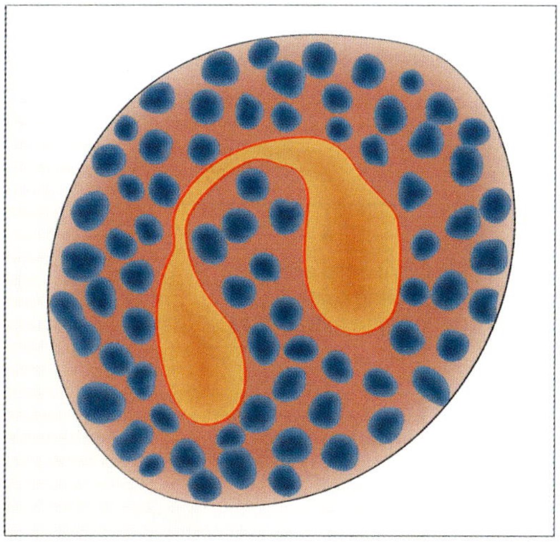

Fig. 5.6: Eosinophil

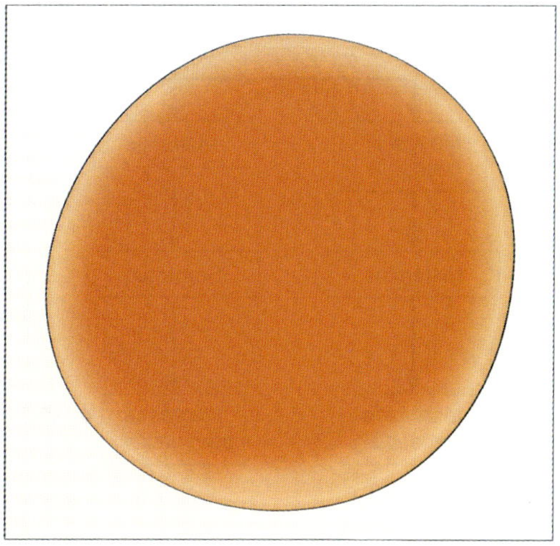

Fig. 5.8: Lymphocyte

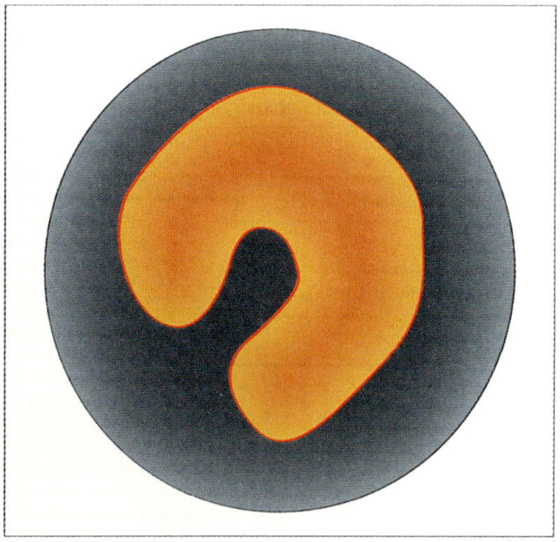

Fig. 5.7: Macrophage

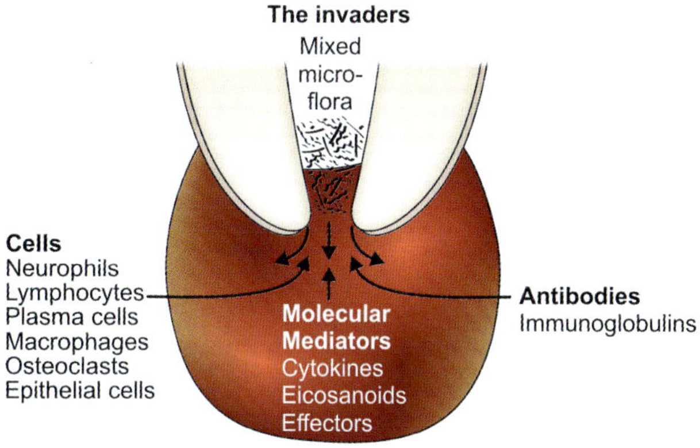


Fig. 5.9: Inflammatory response to periapical lesion

- Provide antigen to the immunocomplement cells
- They act as scavenger of dead cells, tissues and foreign bodies
- They fuse with other macrophages to produce multinucleated giant cells like osteoclasts, dentinoclasts and foreign body giant cells.

3. **Lymphocytes (Fig. 5.8):** They are the most numerous cells (20-45%) after neutrophils. There are two types of lymphocytes seen in apical periodontitis:
   a. *T-lymphocytes*
      – T-helper cells (Th): They are present in the acute phase of lesion expansion.
      – T-suppressor cells (Ts): They predominate in later stages preventing rapid expansion of the lesion.
   b. *B-lymphocytes* – On getting signals from antigens and T-helper cells, they transform into plasma cells and secrete antibodies. Their number increases in following conditions:
      – hypersensitivity state
      – prolonged infection with immunological response.
4. **Osteoclasts:** In the physiologic state, the preosteoclasts remain dormant as monocytes in the periradicular bone. In case of apical periodontitis, they proliferate and fuse on stimulation by cytokines and other mediators to form osteoclasts. These osteoclasts are responsible for demineralization of the bone and enzymatic dissolution of organic matrix at the osteoclast-bone interface. This results in bone resorption.
5. **Epithelial cells:** Cytokines and other mediators stimulate the dormant cell rests of malassez. These cells undergo division and proliferation which results in inflammatory hyperplasia.

## INFLAMMATORY RESPONSE TO PERIAPICAL LESION (FIG. 5.9)

### Nonspecific Mediators of Periradicular Lesions

Nonspecific mediators can be classified into following types:

1. Cell derived mediators:
   – Neuropeptides
   – Eicosanoids/arachidonic acid derivatives
   – Cytokines
   – Lysosomal enzymes

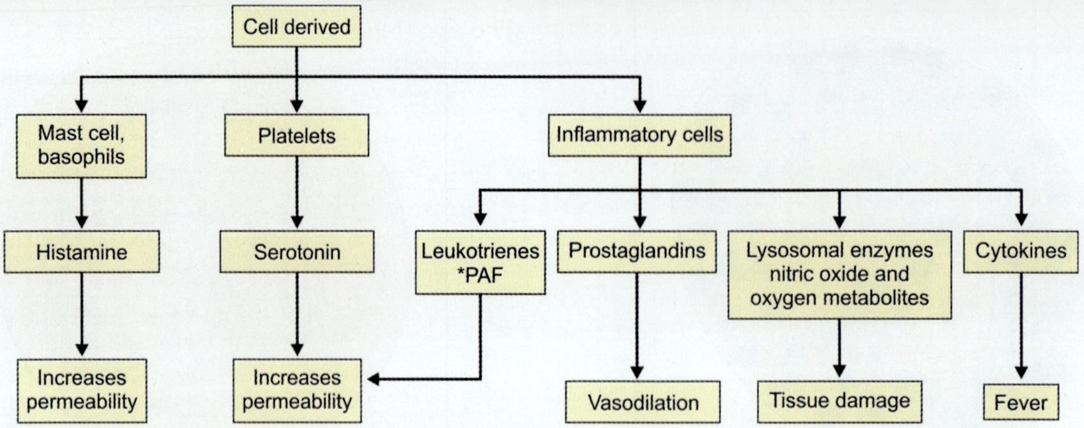


**Fig. 5.10:** Cell derived mediators

- Platelet activating factor
- Vasoactive amines
- Prostaglandins

2. Plasma derived mediators
   - The fibrinolytic system
   - The complement system
   - The kinin system
3. Extracellular matrix derived mediators
   - Effector molecules

## Cell Derived Mediators (Fig. 5.10)

1. **Neuropeptides:** These are generated following tissue injury by the somatosensory and autonomic nerve fibers. Neuropeptides include:
   - Substance P (SP): Causes vasodilation, increased vascular permeability and increased blood flow.
   - Calcitonin-gene related peptide (CGRP): results in vasodilation.
2. **Eicosanoids:** The injury to cells results in release membrane phospholipid, arachidonic acid which is metabolized by either cyclooxygenase pathway or lipoxygenase pathway to form prostaglandins (PGs) or leukotrienes (LTs) respectively, which are involved in inflammatory process.
   a. Prostaglandins are of various types:
   - $PGE_2$,
   - $PGD_2$,
   - $PGF_{2a}$,
   - $PGI_2$

   In cases of acute apical periodontitis and areas of bone resorption, $PGE_2$ and $PGI_2$ are commonly observed.

   Action of PGs can be inhibited by administration of indomethacin which inhibits the enzyme cyclooxygenase thus inhibiting formation of prostaglandins.

   b. *Leukotrienes:* These are produced by activation of lipoxygenase pathway of arachidonic acid metabolism. Studies have shown the presence of $LTB_4$, $LTC_4$, $LTD_4$ and $LTE_4$ in periradicular lesions which cause different effects on the tissues as shown in (Fig. 5.11).

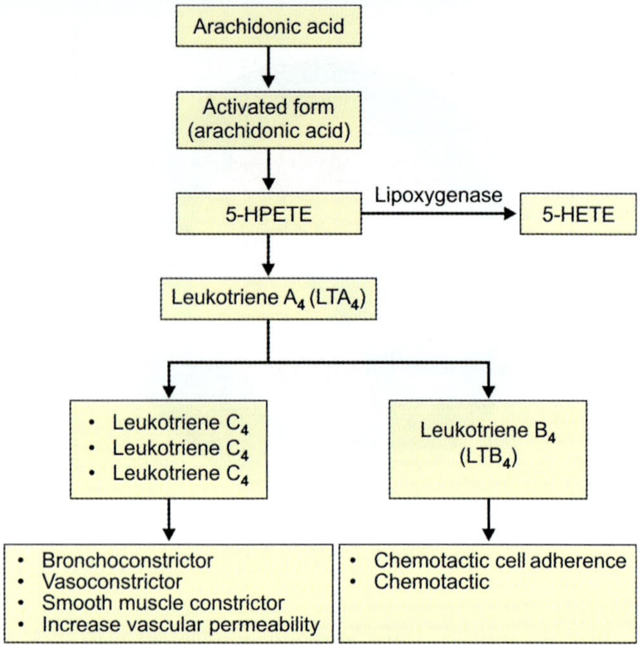


**Fig. 5.11:** Leukotrienes

3. **Cytokines –** These are low molecular weight polypeptides secreted by activated structural and hematopoietic cells. Different cytokines such as interleukins and tumor necrosis factor (TNF) cause development and perpetuation of periradicular lesions.

   They are of two types:

| | |
|---|---|
| a. Proinflammatory cytokines (Interleukins) | – IL1 α and β,<br>– IL6 α and β,<br>– IL8 α and β. |
| b. Chemotactic cytokines (Tumor necrosis factor) | – TNFα (macrophage derived)<br>– TNFβ (T-lymphocyte derived)<br>– TNFγ. |

*a. Proinflammatory cytokines*

IL1 – The local effects of IL1 are –

- Enhanced leukocyte adhesion to endothelial walls.
- Stimulate PMNLs and lymphocytes.
- Activates production of prostaglandins and proteolytic enzymes.
- Enhances bone resorption.
- Inhibits bone formation.

IL1 β is predominant in cases of periapical pathology.
IL6 – It is secreted by lymphoid and non-lymphoid cells and causes inflammation under the influence of IL1, TNF α and interferon γ (IFN). It is seen in periapical lesions.
IL8 – It is produced by macrophages and fibroblasts under the influence of IL1 β and TNF α and is associated with acute apical periodontitis.

***b. Chemotactic cytokines***

TNF – They are seen in chronic lesions associated with cytotoxic and debilitating effect. TNF α is seen in chronic apical lesions and root canal exudates.

1. Colony stimulating factor (CSF) – They are produced by osteoblasts and regulate the proliferation of PMNLs and preosteoclasts.
2. Growth factors (GF) – They are the proteins produced by normal and neoplastic that regulate the growth and differentiation of non- hematopoietic cells. They can transform a normal cells to neoplastic cells and are known as transforming growth factors (TGF).
   They are of two types -
   a. TGF α (produced by malignant cells) – not seen in periapical lesions.
   b. TGF β (produced by normal cells and platelets).
   They counter the adverse effects of inflammatory host response by:
   – Activating macrophages.
   – Proliferation of fibroblasts.
   – Synthesis of connective tissue fibers and matrices.

### *Lysosomal Enzymes*

Lysosomal enzymes such as alkaline phosphatase, lysozyme, peroxidases, collagenase cause increase in vascular permeability, leukocytic chemotaxis, bradykinin formation and activation of complement system.

### *Platelet Activating Factor*

It is released from IgE—sensitized basophils or mast cells. Its action include increase in vascular permeability, chemotaxis, adhesion of leukocytes to endothelium and broncho-constriction.

### *Vasoactive Amines*

Vasoactive amines such as histamine, serotonin are present in mast cells, basophils and platelets. Their release cause increase in tissue permeability, vasodilation used vascular permeability (Fig. 5.9).

### *Prostaglandins*

These are produced by activation of cyclooxygenase pathway of arachidonic acid metabolism. Studies have shown high levels of $PGE_2$ in periradicular lesions. Torbinejad et al found that periradicular bone resorption can be inhibited by administration of indomethacin, an antagonist of PGs. This indicates that prostaglandins are also involved in the pathogenesis of periradicular lesions.

### *Plasma Derived Mediators (Fig. 5.12)*

1. ***The fibrinolytic system:*** The fibrinolytic system is activated by Hageman factor which causes activation of plasminogen. This results in release of fibrinopeptides and fibrin degradation products which cause increase in vascular permeability and leukocytic chemotaxis.
2. ***The complement system:*** Trauma to periapex can result in activation of kinin system which in turn activates complement system. Several studies have shown elevated levels of kinins and $C_3$ complement component in periradicular lesions. Products released from activated complement system cause swelling, pain and tissue destruction.
3. ***The kinin system:*** These are produced by proteolytic cleavage of kininogen. Release of kinins cause smooth muscle contraction, vasodilation and increase in vascular permeability (Fig. 5.13).

## Effector Molecules

The inflammatory process causes not only the destruction of the cells but also the extracellular matrix in the periapical pathosis. The extracellular matrix is degraded by enzymatic effector molecules by various pathways like

- Osteoclast regulated pathway,
- Phagocyte regulated pathway,
- Plasminogen regulated pathway and

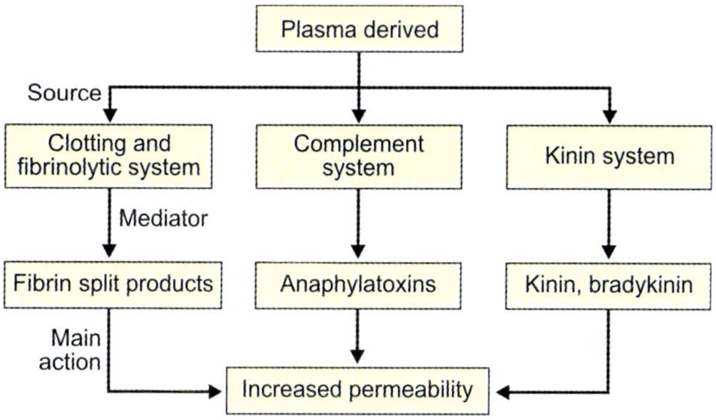


**Fig. 5.12:** Plasma derived mediators

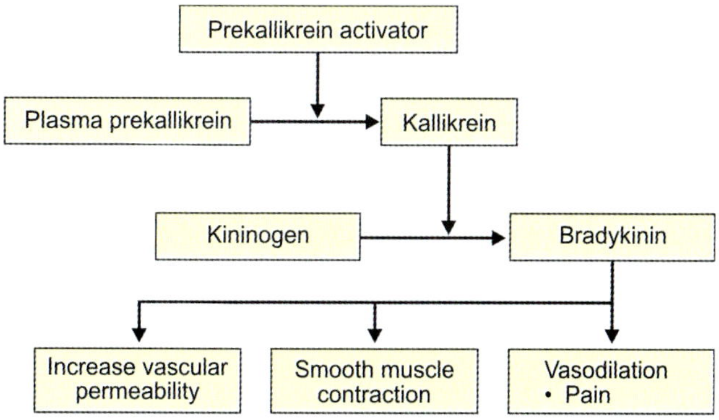


**Fig. 5.13:** Kinin system

- Metalloenzyme regulated pathway (Matrix Metallo Proteases-MMPs)

  The collagen (proteins) based matrices are degraded by MMPs.

## ANTIBODIES (SPECIFIC MEDIATORS OF IMMUNE REACTIONS)

These are produced by plasma cells and are of two types:

- Polyclonal antibodies – are nonspecific like IgE mediated reactions which interact with antigen resulting in release of certain chemical mediators like histamine or serotonin.
- Monoclonal antibodies – like IgG and IgM, interact with the bacteria and its by-products to form antigen-antibody complexes that bind to the platelets resulting in release vasoactive amines thus increasing the vascular permeability and chemotaxis of PMNs.

  The monoclonal antibodies exhibit antimicrobial effect.
- In acute abscess, the complex enters the systemic circulation. The concentration of these complexes return to normal levels after endodontic treatment.
- In chronic lesions, the Ag-Ab complexes are confined within the lesion and do not enter into the systemic circulation.

> **The response of periapical/host tissue is controlled by:**
> - Cells
> - Molecular mediators (Nonspecific mediators of inflammation), and
> - Antibodies (Specific mediators of inflammation)

## ROLE OF IMMUNITY IN ENDODONTICS

The immune system of human being is a complex system consisting of cells, tissues, organs as well as molecular mediators that act together to maintain the health and well-being of the individual. The cells and microbial irritants interact with each other via a number of molecular mediators and cell surface receptors to result in various defense reactions.

Immunity is of two types:

- Innate immunity
- Acquired/adaptive immunity

**Innate immunity:** It consists of cells and molecular elements which act as barriers to prevent dissemination of bacteria and bacterial products into the underlying connective tissue. The innate immunity is responsible for the initial nonspecific reactions.

Cells providing innate immunity are neutrophils, monocytes, eosinophils, basophils, NK cells, dendritic cells, and odontoblasts.

**Acquired/Adaptive immunity:** It involves release of specific receptor molecules by lymphocytes which recognize and bind to foreign antigens.

Adaptive immunity is provided by:

- T-Lymphocytes that release T-cell antigen receptors
- B-Lymphocytes that release B-cell antigen receptors or immunoglobulins.

### Histopathology of Periapical Tissue Response to Various Irritants

Root canal of teeth contains numerous irritants because of some pathologic changes in pulp. Penetration of these irritants from infected root canals into periapical area can lead to formation and perpetuation of periradicular lesions. In contrast to pulp, periradicular tissue have unlimited source of undifferentiated cells which can participate in inflammation and repair in inflammation and repair. Also these tissues have rich collateral blood supply and lymph drainage.

Depending upon severity of irritation, duration and host, response to periradicular pathosis may range from slight inflammation to extensive tissue destruction. Reactions involved are highly complex and are usually mediated by nonspecific and specific mediators of inflammation.

## ENDODONTIC IMPLICATIONS (PATHOGENESIS OF APICAL PERIODONTITIS AS EXPLAINED BY FISH) (FIG. 5.14)

FISH described the reaction of the periradicular tissues to bacterial products, noxious products of tissue necrosis, and antigenic agents from the root canal. He established an experimental foci of infection in the guinea pigs by drilling openings in the jaw bone and packing it with wool fibers saturated with a broth culture of microorganisms. FISH in 1939 theorised that the zones of infection are not an infection by themselves but the reaction of the body to infection. Thus he concluded that the removal of this nidus of infection will result in resolution of infection.

Four well defined zones of reaction were found during the experiment:

a. Zone of infection or necrosis *(PMNLs)*
b. Zone of contamination ***(Round cell infiltrate – lymphocytes)***

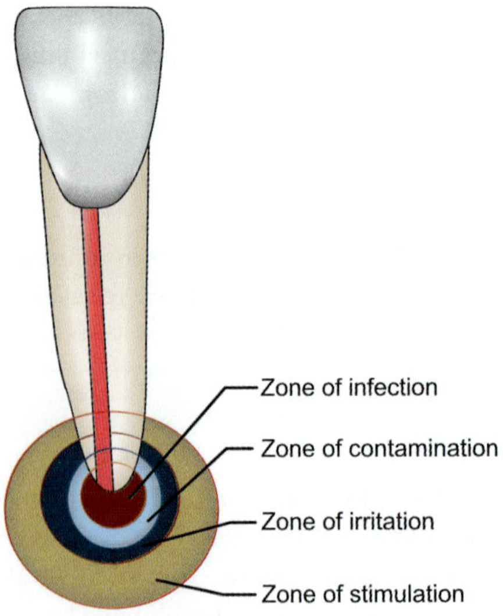


**Fig. 5.14:** FISH zones

c. Zone of irritation ***(Histiocytes and osteoclasts)***
d. Zone of stimulation ***(Fibroblasts, capillary buds and Osteoblasts).***

### Zone of Infection

In FISH study, infection was confined to the center of the lesion. This zone is characterized by polymorphonuclear leukocytes and microorganisms along with the necrotic cells and detructive components released from phagocytes.

### Zone of Contamination

Around the central zone, FISH observed the area of cellular destruction. This zone was not invaded by bacteria, but the destruction was from toxins discharged from the microorganisms in the central zone. This zone is characterized by round cell infiltration, osteocyte necrosis and empty lacunae. Lymphocytes were prevalent everywhere.

### Zone of Irritation

FISH observed evidence of irritation further away from the central lesion as the toxins became more diluted. This is characterized by macrophages, histocytes and osteoclasts. The degradation of collagen framework by phagocytic cells and macrophages was observed while osteoclasts attack the bone tissue. ***The histologic picture is much like preparatory to repair.***

### Zone of Stimulation

FISH noted that, at the periphery, the toxin was mild enough to act as stimulant. This zone is characterized by fibroblasts and osteoblasts. In response to this stimulatory irritant, fibroblasts result in secretion of collagen fibers, which acted both as wall of defense around the zone of irritation and as a scaffolding on which the osteoblasts synthesize new bone.

So the knowledge gained in FISH study can be applied for better understanding of reaction of periradicular tissues to a nonvital tooth.

The root canal is the main source of infection. The microorganisms present in root canal are rarely motile. Though they do not move from the root canal to the periapical tissues; but they can proliferate sufficiently to grow out of the root canal. The metabolic byproducts of these microorganisms or the toxic products of tissue necrosis may also get diffused to the periradicular tissues. As the microorganisms enter in the periradicular area, they are destroyed by the polymorphonuclear leukocytes. But if microorganisms are highly virulent, they overpower the defensive mechanism and result in development of periradicular lesion.

The toxic byproducts of the microorganisms and the necrotic pulp in the root canal are irritating and destructive to the periradicular tissues. These irritants along with proteolytic enzymes (released by the dead polymorphonuclear leukocytes) result in the formation of pus. This results in development of chronic abscess.

At the periphery of the destroyed area of osseous tissue, toxic bacterial products get diluted sufficiently to act as stimulant. This results in formation of a granuloma.

After this fibroblasts come in the play and build fibrous tissue and osteoblasts restrict the area by formation of sclerotic bone. Along with these if epithelial rests of Malassez are also stimulated, it results in formation of a cyst.

## KRONFELD'S MOUNTAIN PASS THEORY (FIG. 5.15)

Kronfeld explained that the granuloma does not provide a favorable environment for the survival of the bacteria. He employed the FISH concept so as to explain the tissue reaction in and around the granulomatous area.

*Zone A:* He compared the bacteria in the infected root canal with the invaders entrenched behind high and inaccessible "mountains", the foramina serving as mountain passes.

*Zone B:* The exudative and granulomatous (proliferative) tissue of the granuloma represents a mobilized army defending the plains (periapex) from the invaders (bacteria). When a few invaders enter the plain through the mountain pass, they are destroyed by the defenders (leukocytes). A mass attack of invaders results in a major battle, analogous to acute inflammation.

*Zone C:* Only complete elimination of the invaders from their mountainous entrenchment will eliminate the need for a defense forces in the "plains". Once this is accomplished, the defending army of leukocytes withdraws, the local destruction created by the battle is repaired (granulation tissue) and the environment returns to its normal pattern.

This explains the rationale for the non-surgical endodontic treatment for teeth with periapical infection. The complete elimination of pathogenic irritants from the canal followed by the three-dimensional fluid impervious obturation will result in complete healing of periapical area.

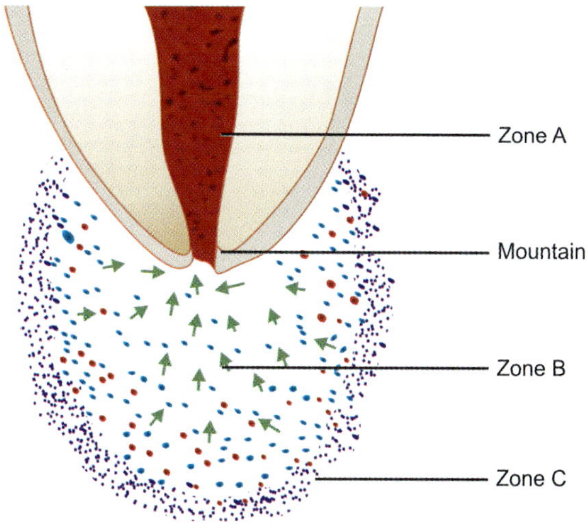


Fig. 5.15: Kronfeld's mountain pass theory

## RATIONALE OF ENDODONTIC THERAPY

The rationale of root canal treatment relies on the fact that the nonvital pulp, being avascular, has no defense mechanisms. The damaged tissue within the root canal undergoes autolysis and the resulting breakdown products will diffuse into the surrounding tissues and cause periapical irritation associated with the portals of exit even in the absence of bacterial contamination. It is essential therefore, that endodontic therapy must seal the root canal system three-dimensionally so as to prevent tissue fluids from percolating in the root canal and toxic byproducts from both necrotic tissue and microorganisms regressing into the periradicular tissues.

Endodontic therapy includes:

- Non-surgical endodontic treatment
- Surgical endodontic treatment

Non-surgical endodontic treatment includes three phases:

- *Access preparation:* The rationale for this is to create a straight line path for the canal orifice and the apex.
- *Shaping and cleaning:* The rationale for this is the complete elimination of vital or necrotic pulp tissue, microorganisms and their byproducts.
- *Obturation:* Main objective of obturation is to have a three dimensional well fitted root canal with fluid tight seal so as to prevent percolation and microleakage of periapical exudate into the root canal space and also to prevent infection by completely obliterating the apical foramen and other portals of communication.

### Surgical Endodontic Treatment

The rationale of surgical endodontics is to remove the diseased tissue present in the canal and around the apex, and retrofil the root canal space with biologically inert material so as to achieve a fluid tight seal.

## QUESTION

**Q. What is rationale of endodontics? Explain in detail about fish zones.**

## BIBLIOGRAPHY


1. Abou-Rass, Bogen G. Microorganisms in closed periapical lesions. Int Endod J 1998;31:39.
2. Alavi AM, Gulabivala K, Speight PM. Quantitative analysis of lymphocytes and their subsets in periapical lesions. Int Endod J 1998;31:233.
3. Baumgartner JC, Falkler (Ir) WA. Detection of immunoglobulin from explant cultures of periapical lesions. J Endod 1991;17:105.
4. Brännström M, Astrom A. The hydrodynamics of the dentin; its possible relationship to dentinal pain. Int Dent J 1972;22:219.
5. Dippel HW, et al. Morphology and permeability of the dentinal smear layer. J Prosthet Dent 1984;52:657.
6. FISH EW. Bone infection. J Am Dent Assoc 1939;26:691.
7. Goldman LB, Goldman M, Kronnman JH, Lin PS. The efficacy of several irrigating solutions for endodontics:a scanning electron micriscopic stody. Oral Surg 1981;52:197.
8. Jontell M, Bergenholtz G, Scheynius K, Ambrose W. Dendritic cells and macrophages expressing class I antigens in normal rat incisor pulp. J Dent Res 1988;67:1263.
9. Kuo M, Lamster I, Hasselgren G. Host mediators in endodontic exudates. J Endod 1998;24:598.
10. Lukic A, Arsenijevic N, Vujanic G, Ramic Z. Quantitative analysis of immunocompetent cells in periapical granuloma: Correlation with the histological characteristics of the lesions. J Endod 1990;16:119.
11. Michelich VJ, Schuster GS, Pashley DH. Bacterial penetration of human dentin, in vitro. J Dent Res 1980;59:1398.
12. Ogilvie RW, et al. Physiologic evidence for the presence of vasoconstrictor fibers in the dental pulp. J Dent Res 1966;45:980.
13. Pashley DH, Michelich V, Kehl T. Dentin permeability: Effect of smear layer removal. J Prosthet Dent 1981;46:531.
14. Robinson HB, Boling LR. The anachoretic effect in pulpitis. J Am Dent Assoc 1949;28:268.
15. Stern MH, Driezen S, Mackler BF, Selbst AG, Levy BM. Quantitative analysis of cellular composition of human periapical granuloma. J Endod 1981;7:117.
16. Torabinejad M, Kigar RD. Histological evaluation of a patient with periodontal disease. Oral Surg 1985;59:198.
17. Trope M, Rosenberg E, Tronsdat L. Dark field microscope spirochete count in the differentiation of endodontic and periodontal abscesses. J Endod 1992;18:82.
18. Wayman BE, Murata SM, almeida RJ, Fowler CB. A bacteriological and histological evaluation of 58 periapical lesions. J Endod 1992;18:152.

# Diagnostic Procedures

CHAPTER 6



## INTRODUCTION

*Diagnosis is defined as utilization of scientific knowledge for identifying a diseased process and to differentiate from other disease process.* In other words, literal meaning of diagnosis is determination and judgment of variations from the normal.

It is the procedure of accepting a patient, recognizing that he/she has a problem, determining the cause of problem and developing a treatment plan which would solve the problem. There are various diagnostic tools, out of all these, art of listening is most important. It also establishes patient-doctor rapport, understanding and trust.

Although diagnostic testing of some common complaints may produce classic results but sometimes tests may produce wrong results, which need to be carefully interpreted by clinician.

The diagnostic process actually consists of *four steps:*

*First step:* Assemble all the available facts gathered from chief complaints, medical and dental history, diagnostic tests and investigations.

*Second step:* Analyze and interpret the assembled clues to reach the tentative or provisional diagnosis.

*Third step:* Make differential diagnosis of all possible diseases which are consistent with signs, symptoms and test results gathered.

*Fourth step:* Select the closet possible choice.

The importance of making an accurate diagnosis cannot be overlooked. Many a time even after applying all the knowledge, experience and diagnostic tests, a satisfactory explanation for patient's symptoms is not determined. In many cases, nonodontogenic etiology is also seen as a source of chief complaint. To avoid irrelevant information and to prevent errors of omission in clinical tests, the clinician should establish a routine for examination, consisting of chief complaint, past medical and dental history and any other relevant information in the form of case history.

## CASE HISTORY

The purpose of case history is to discover whether patient has any general or local condition that might alter the normal course of treatment. As with all courses of treatment, a comprehensive medical and previous dental history should be recorded. In addition, a description of the patient's symptoms in his or her own words should be noted.

### Chief Complaint

It consists of information which promoted patient to visit a clinician. Phenomenon symptoms or signs of deviation from normal are indicative of illness. The form of notation should be in patient's own words.

### History of Present Illness

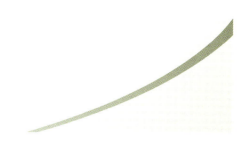

Once the patient completes information about his/her chief complaint, a report is made which provides more descriptive analysis about this initial information. It should include signs and symptoms, duration, intensity of pain, relieving and exaggerating factors, etc. Examples of type of the questions which may be asked by the clinician in recording the patient's complaints are as below:

1. How long have you had the pain?
2. Do you know which tooth it is?
3. What initiates pain?
4. How would you describe the pain?
   a. Quality—Dull, Sharp, Throbbing, Constant
   b. Location—Localized, Diffuse, Referred, Radiating
   c. Duration—Intermittent lasting for seconds, minutes or hours, Constant
   d. Onset—Stimulation Required, Intermittent, Spontaneous
   e. Initiated—Cold, Heat, Palpation, Percussion
   f. Relieved—Cold, Heat, Any medications, Sleep

In other words, history of present illness should indicate severity and urgency of the problem.

If a chief complaint is toothache but symptoms are too vague to establish a diagnosis, then analgesics should be prescribed to help the patient in tolerating the pain until the toothache localizes. A history of pain which persists without exacerbation may indicate problem of nonodontogenic origins.

The most common toothache may arise from either pulp or periodontal ligament. Pulpal pain can be sharp piercing if A delta fibers are stimulated. Dull, boring or throbbing pain occurs if there is stimulation of C-fibers. Pulp vitality tests are usually done to reach the most probable diagnosis. If pain is from periodontal ligament, the tooth will be sensitive to percussion, chewing and palpation. Intensity of pain gives an indication that pain is of pulpal origin. Patient is asked to mark the imaginary ruler with grading ranging from 0-10.

0—No pain 10—Most painful

Mild to moderate pain can be of pulpal or periodontal origin but acute pain is commonly a reliable sign that pain is of pulpal origin. Localization of pain also tells origin of pain since pulp does not contain proprioceptive fibers; it is difficult for patient to localize the pain unless it reaches the periodontal ligament.

## Medical History

There are no medical conditions which specifically contraindicate endodontic treatment, but there are several which require special care. **Scully** and **Cawson** have given a checklist of medical conditions which are needed to be taken a special care.

**Checklist for medical history (Scully and Cawson)**

- Anemia
- Bleeding disorders
- Cardiorespiratory disorders
- Drug treatment and allergies
- Endocrine disease
- Fits and faints
- Gastrointestinal disorders
- Hospital admissions and attendance
- Infections
- Jaundice
- Kidney disease
- Likelihood of pregnancy or pregnant itself

| | *Type of pain* | *Reason for pain* | *Provisional diagnosis* |
|---|---|---|---|
| Location | a. Localized pain | Due to presence of proprioceptive A-beta fibers present in periodontal ligament | Periodontal pain |
| | b. Diffuse pain | Due to lack of proprioceptive fibers in pulp. | Pulpal pain |
| Duration | a. Momentary pain on stimulation | | Reversible pulpitis |
| | b. Spontaneous pain for long duration | | Irreversible pulpitis |
| Nature | a. Sharp, shooting momentary pain on provoking | Due to stimulation of A-delta fibers because of movement of dentinal fluid present in odontoblastic processes | • Dentinal pain<br>• Reversible pulpitis |
| | b. Sharp shooting pain on mastication | | • Irreversible pulpitis<br>• Fracture of tooth |
| | c. Spontaneous dull, throbbing pain for long duration | Stimulation of C-fibers | Irreversible pulpitis |
| Stimulus | a. Sweet and sour | Due to stimulation of A-delta fibers present in odontoblastic processes | Reversible pulpitis |
| | b. Heat | Vasodilatation caused by heat stimulates C-fibers of pulp | Irreversible pulpitis |
| | c. Cold | Stimulation of A-delta fibers due to fluid movement in odontoblastic processes | Dentin hypersensitivity |
| | d. Heat and cold | | Early stages of irreversible pulpitis |
| | e. Stimulated by heat and relieved by cold | | Late stages of irreversible pulpitis |
| | f. On lying down or sleep | | Acute irreversible pulpitis |

If there is any doubt about the state of health of patient, consult medical practitioner before initiating endodontic treatment. Care should also be taken whether patient is on medication such as corticosteroids or anticoagulant therapy.

According to standards of American heart association, patient should be given antibiotic prophylaxis if there is high rise of developing bacterial endocarditis for example in cardiac conditions like prosthetic heart valves, rheumatic heart disease, previous bacterial endocarditis and complex cyanotic heart diseases.

## Extraoral Examination

Extraoral examination begins as soon as patient enters in the clinic and patient should be observed for unusual gait, habits, etc. which may suggest underlying systemic disease, drug or alcohol abuse, if any.

Patient should be looked for any facial asymmetry or distention of tissues (Fig. 6.1). Dentist must examine any localized swelling, presence of bruises, abrasions, scars or any other signs of trauma if present. Patient should be looked for size of pupils which may signify systemic disease, premedication or fear.

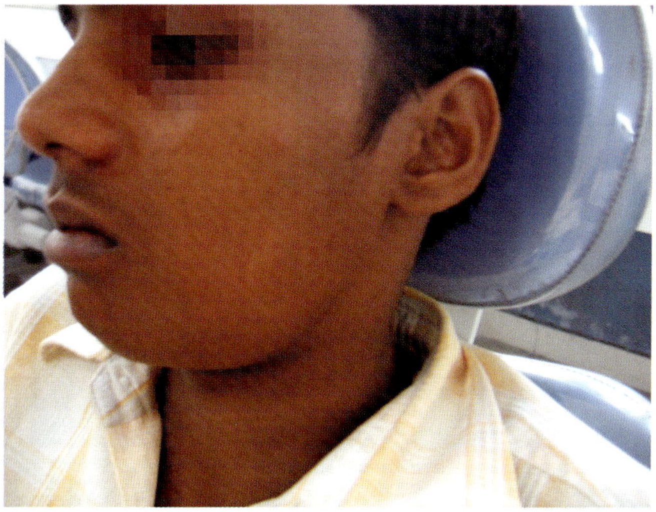

Fig. 6.1: Patient should be examined for facial asymmetry and swelling

After extraoral examination of head and neck region, one should go for extraoral palpation. If any localized swelling is present, then look for:

- Local rise in temperature
- Tenderness
- Extent of lesion
- Induration
- Fixation to underlying tissues, etc.

***Palpation of salivary glands*** should be done extraorally. Submandibular gland should be differentiated from lymph nodes in the submandibular region by bimanual palpation (Fig. 6.2).

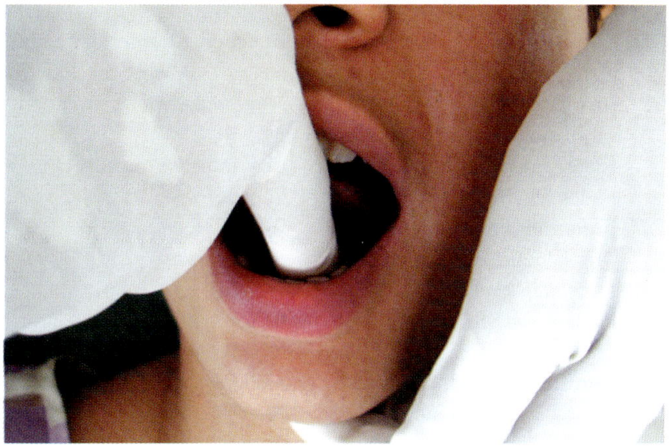

Fig. 6.2: Bimanual palpation of submandibular gland

***Palpation of TMJ*** can be done by standing in front of the patient and placing the index fingers in the preauricular region. The patient is asked to open the mouth and perform lateral excursion to notice (Fig. 6.3):

- Any restricted movement
- Deviation in movement
- Jerky movement
- Clicking
- Locking or crepitus

***Palpation of lymph nodes*** should be done to note any lymph node enlargement, tenderness, mobility and consistency (Fig. 6.4). The lymph nodes frequently palpated are preauricular, submandibular, submental and cervical.

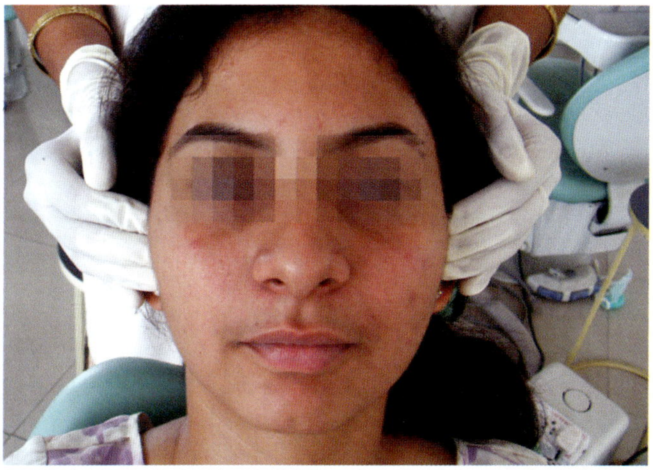

Fig. 6.3: Examination of TMJ

## Intraoral Examination

Before conducting intraoral examination check the degree of mouth opening. For a normal patient it should be at least two fingers (Fig. 6.5). During intraoral examination, look at the following structures systematically:

1. The buccal, labial and alveolar mucosa
2. The hard and soft palate
3. The floor of the mouth and tongue
4. The retromolar region
5. The posterior pharyngeal wall and facial pillars
6. The salivary gland and orifices

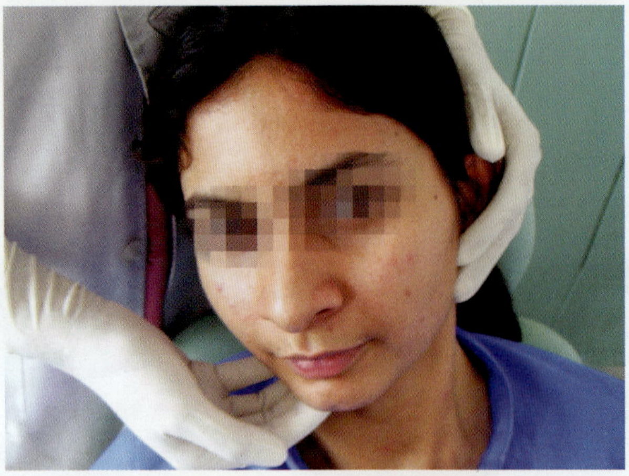

**Fig. 6.4:** Examination of lymph nodes

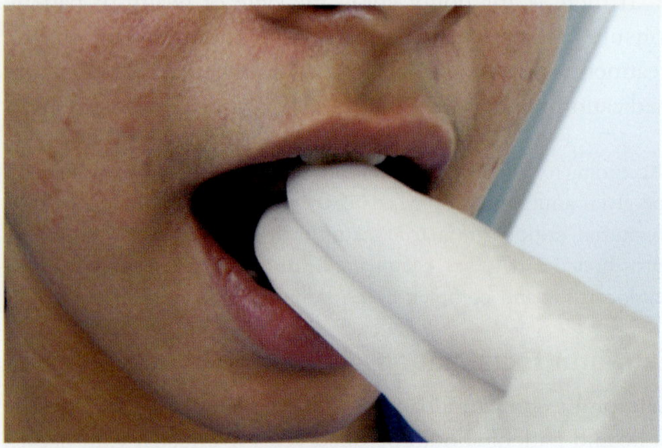

**Fig. 6.5:** Degree of mouth opening in a normal patient should be at least two fingers

**Provisional diagnosis after examination of lymph nodes**

| *Examination* | *Provisional diagnosis* |
|---|---|
| 1. Enlargement of submental lymph nodes | Infection of anterior teeth |
| 2. Involvement of submandibular lymph nodes | Mandibular molar infection |
| 3. Enlargement of lymph nodes at angle of mandible | May indicate tonsillar infection |
| 4. Firm and tender palpable lymph nodes associated with fever and swelling | Acute infection |
| 5. Palpable lymph node not associated with pain | Chronic infection |
| 6. Hard-fixed lymph node with stone-like consistency | Malignancy |
| 7. Matted, nontender lymph nodes | Tuberculosis |

After examining this, ***general dental state*** should be recorded, which includes:

a. Oral hygiene status
b. Amount and quality of restorative work
c. Prevalence of caries
d. Missing tooth
e. Presence of soft or hard swelling
f. Periodontal status
g. Presence of any sinus tracts
h. Discolored teeth
i. Tooth wear and facets

If patient's chief complaint includes symptoms which occur following specific events like chewing and drinking cold liquids, then specific intraoral examination should include tests which reproduce these symptoms. This will be helpful in establishing the diagnosis. For accurate diagnosis, evaluation of history, examination and clinical tests should be done properly. Clinical examination of tissue is done by palpation, percussion and other endodontic clinical tests.

***Palpation*** is done using digital pressure to check any tenderness in soft tissue overlying suspected tooth (Fig. 6.6). Sensitivity may indicate inflammation in periodontal tissues surrounding the affected tooth. Further palpation can tell any other information about fluctuation or fixation or induration of soft tissue, if any (Fig. 6.7).

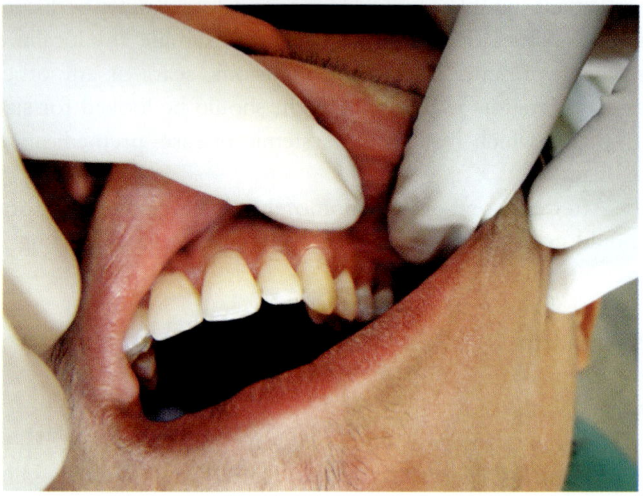

**Fig. 6.6:** Palpation of soft tissue using digital pressure

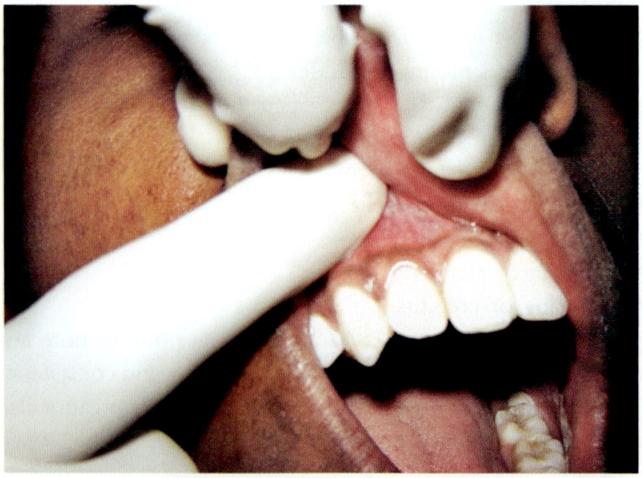

**Fig. 6.7:** Palpation of soft tissues

***Percussion of tooth*** indicates inflammation in periodontal ligament which could be due to trauma, sinusitis and/or PDL disease.

Percussion can be carried out by gentle tapping with gloved finger (Fig. 6.8) or blunt handle of mouth mirror (Fig. 6.9). Each tooth should be percussed on all the surfaces of tooth until the patient is able to localize the tooth with pain. Degree of response to percussion is directly proportional to degree of inflammation.

**Percussion:** Dull sound on percussion indicates abscess formation while sharp indicates inflammation.

Pain on percussion is indicative of possibility of following conditions:

a. Periodontal abscess
b. Pulp necrosis (Partial or total)
c. High points in restorations
d. During orthodontic treatment

***Periodontal evaluation*** can be assessed from palpation, percussion, mobility of tooth and probing (Figs 6.10 and 6.11). The mobility of a tooth is tested by placing a finger (Fig. 6.12) or blunt end of the instrument (Fig. 6.13) on either side of the crown and pushing it and assessing any movement with other finger.

Mobility can be graded as:

1. Slight (Normal)
2. Moderate mobility within a range of 1 mm.
3. Extensive movement (More than 1 mm) in mesiodistal or lateral direction combined with vertical displacement in alveolus.

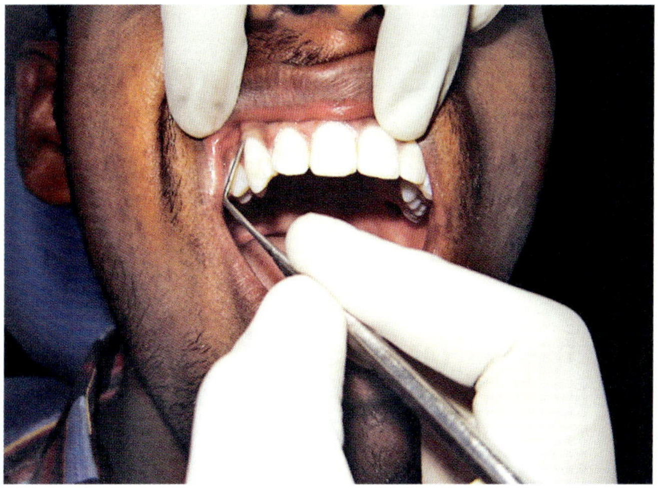

**Fig. 6.10:** Probing of a tooth determines the level of connective tissue attachment

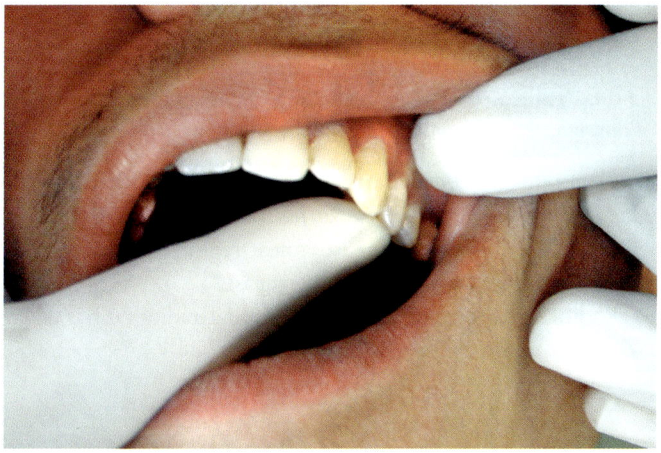

**Fig. 6.8:** Percussion of tooth using gloved finger

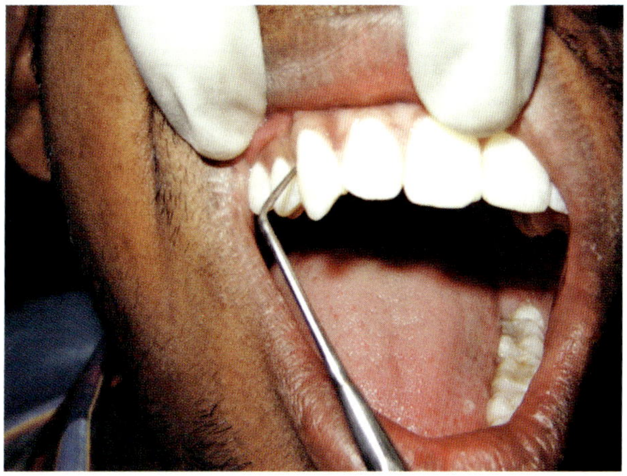

**Fig. 6.11:** Probing interdentally can identify any rough or overextended proximal restoration

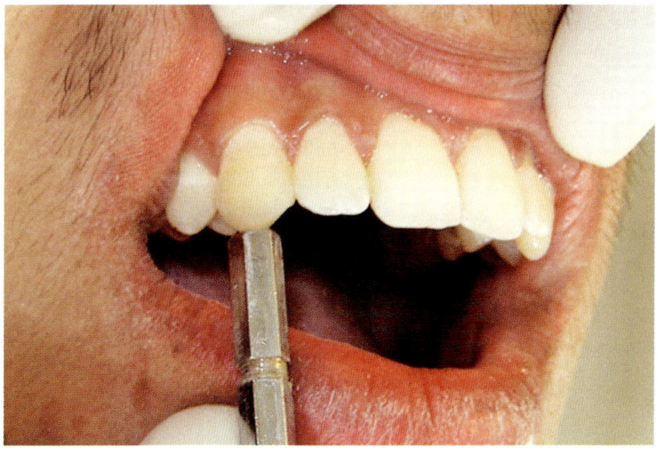

**Fig. 6.9:** Percussion of tooth using blunt handle of mouth mirror

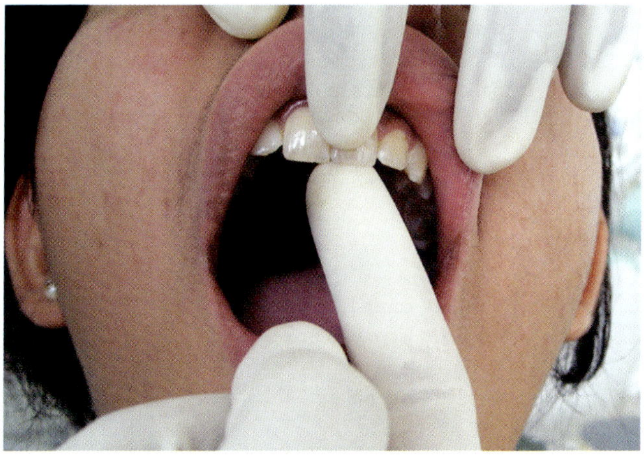

**Fig. 6.12:** Checking mobility of a tooth by palpating with fingers

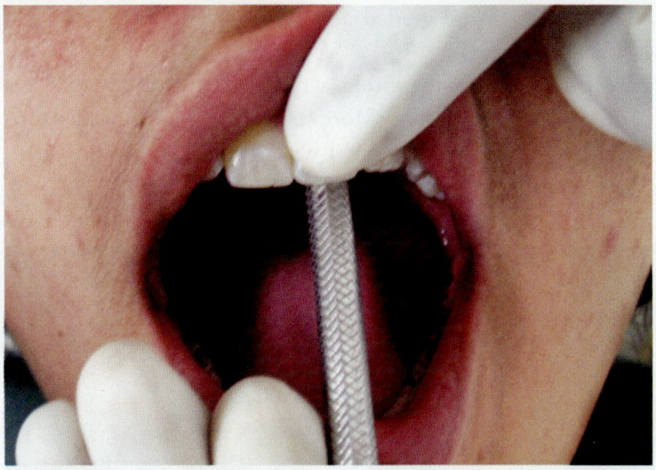

**Fig. 6.13:** Checking mobility of a tooth using blunt end of instrument

## DIFFERENTIAL DIAGNOSIS

Sometimes clinical signs and symptoms mimic each other they, so have to be enumerated in different clinical conditions this is known as differential diagnosis. It can include two or more conditions. After differential diagnosis to reach at definitive diagnosis, the clinician should get investigations done which include lab investigations, radiographs, pulp vitality tests.

**Diagnostic perplexities**

There are certain conditions in which it is difficult to reach proper diagnosis even after detailed history and examination. These conditions can be:

- Idiopathic tooth resorption
- Treatment failures
- Cracked tooth syndrome
- Persistent discomfort
- Unusual radiographic appearances
- Paresthesia

## RADIOGRAPH

The radiograph is one of most important tools in making a diagnosis. Without radiograph, case selection, diagnosis and treatment would be impossible as it helps examination of oral structure that would otherwise be unseen by naked eye.

In all endodontic cases, a good intraoral radiograph is mandatory as it gives excellent details and helps in diagnosis and treatment planning. They help to diagnose tooth-related problems like caries, fractures, root canal treatment or any previous restorations, abnormal appearance of pulp cavity or periradicular tissues, periodontal diseases and the general bony pattern. Sometimes the normal anatomic landmarks like maxillary antrum, foraminas, tori, inferior alveolar canal, etc. may be confused with endodontic pathologies which may result in wrong diagnosis and thus improper treatment.

**Interpretation of radiograph according to appearance**

| *Appearance* | *Tentative finding* |
|---|---|
| Black/Grey area | It can be:<br>a. Decay<br>b. Pulp<br>c. Gum in the space between teeth<br>d. Abscess<br>e. Cyst |
| White area | a. Enamel<br>b. Restoration<br>(Metal, gutta-percha, etc.) |
| Creamy white area | Dentin appears as creamy white area |
| White line around teeth | Lamina dura around teeth |

Generally the ***periapical lesions of endodontic origin have following characteristic features (Fig. 6.14):***

- Loss of lamina dura in the apical region
- Apparent etiology of pulpal necrosis
- Radiolucency remains at the apex even if radiograph is taken by changing the angle.

**Sites of localization of acute dental infections**

| *S.No.* | *Teeth* | *Usual exit from bone* | *Site of localization* |
|---|---|---|---|
| 1. | Mandibular incisors | Labial | • Submental space<br>• Oral vestibule |
| 2. | Mandibular canine | Labial | • Oral vestibule |
| 3. | Mandibular premolars | Buccal | • Oral vestibule |
| 4. | Mandibular first molar | • Buccal<br>• Lingual | • Oral vestibule<br>• Buccal space<br>• Sublingual space |
| 5. | Mandibular second molar | • Buccal<br>• Lingual | • Oral vestibule<br>• Buccal space<br>• Sublingual space<br>• Submandibular space |
| 6. | Maxillary central incisor | Labial | • Oral vestibule |
| 7. | Maxillary lateral incisor | • Labial<br>• Palatal | • Oral vestibule<br>• Palatal |
| 8. | Maxillary premolars | • Buccal<br>• Palatal | • Oral vestibule<br>• Palatal |
| 9. | Maxillary molars | • Buccal<br>• Palatal | • Oral vestibule<br>• Buccal space<br>• Palatal |

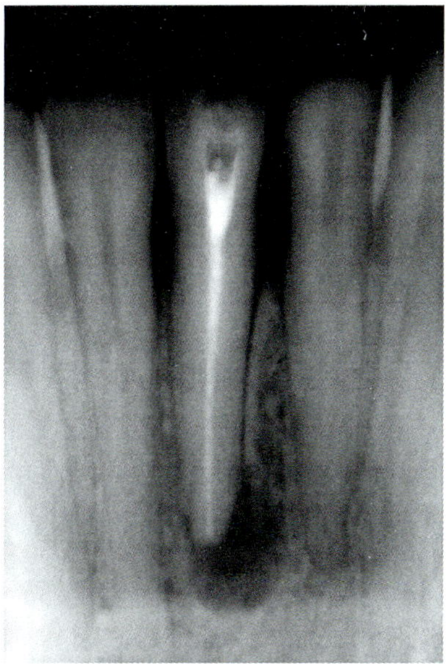

Fig. 6.14: Radiograph showing periapical lesion

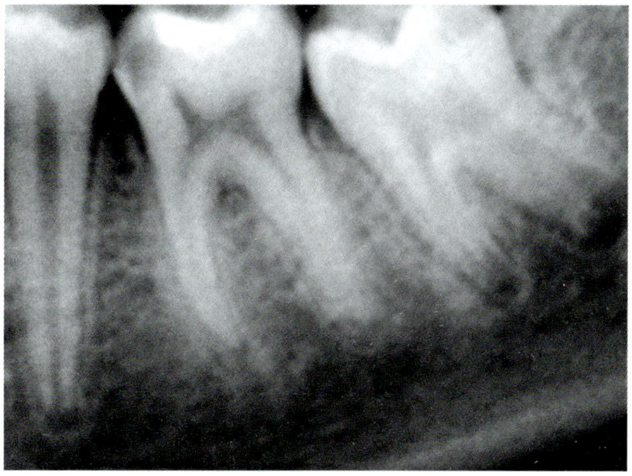

Fig. 6.16: Radiograph showing canal configuration of premolar and molars

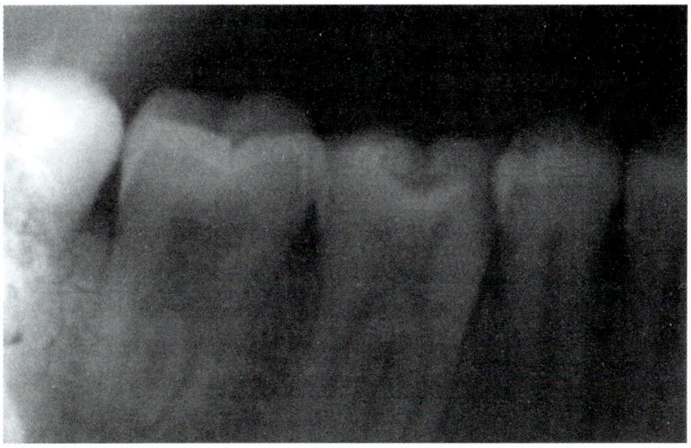

Fig. 6.15: Radiograph showing extent of caries in premolar and molar

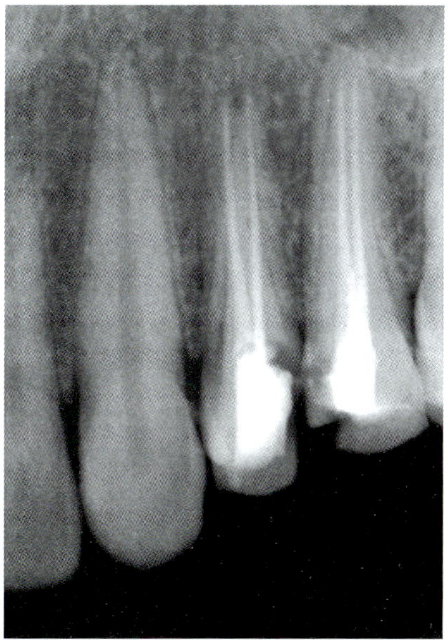

Fig. 6.17: Radiograph showing endodontic treatment of premolars

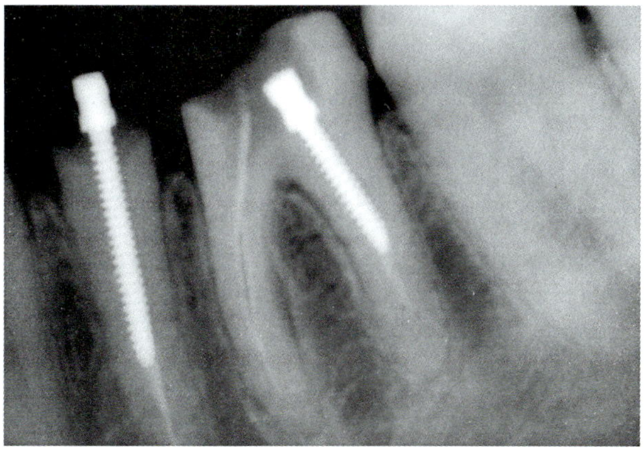

Fig. 6.18: Radiograph showing pins and posts

***Radiographs help us in following ways:***

a. Establishing diagnosis
b. Determining the prognosis of tooth
c. Disclosing the presence and extent of caries (Fig. 6.15)
d. Check the thickness of periodontal ligament
e. To see continuity of lamina dura
f. To look for any periodontal lesion associated with tooth
g. To see the number, shape, length and pattern of the root canals (Fig. 6.16)
h. To check any obstructions present in the pulp space.
i. To check any previous root canal treatment if done (Fig. 6.17)
j. To look for presence of any intraradicular pins or posts (Fig. 6.18)
k. To see the quality of previous root canal filling (Fig. 6.19)
l. To see any resorption present in the tooth
m. To check the presence of calcification in pulp space
n. To see rootend proximal structures
o. Help in determining the working length, length of master gutta-percha cone and quality of obturation
p. During the course of treatment they help in knowing the level of instrumental errors like perforation, ledging and instrumental separation.

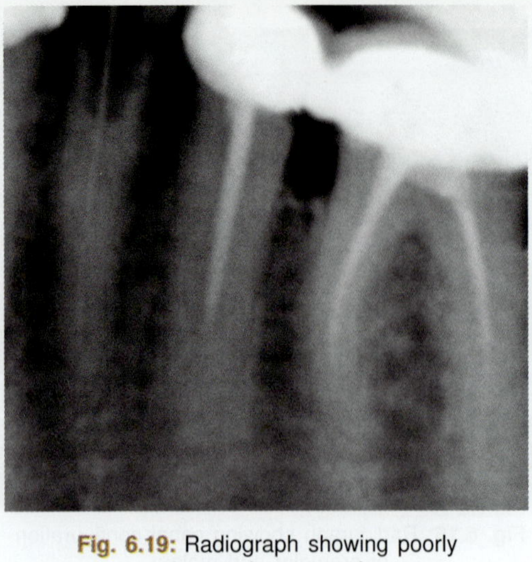

Fig. 6.19: Radiograph showing poorly obturated root canals

Lesions which commonly involve the periodontal ligament space include the periapical lesions which can be evident at apical part or at the lateral surface of the root, perforation lesions and fractured root lesions.

***Following lesions should be differentiated from the lesions of endodontic origin while interpreting radiographs:***

- Periodontal abscess
- Idiopathic osteosclerosis
- Cementomas
- Giant cell lesions
- Cysts
- Tumors

Though the radiographs play an important role in dentistry, they have a few ***shortcomings:***

a. They are only two-dimensional picture of a three-dimensional object.
b. Pathological changes in pulp are not visible in radiographs
c. The initial stages of periradicular diseases produce no changes in the radiographs.
d. They do not help in exact interpretation for example radiographic picture of an abscess, inflammation and granuloma is almost same.
e. Misinterpretation of radiographs can lead to inaccurate diagnosis.
f. Radiographs can misinterpret the anatomical structures like incisive and mental foramen with periapical lesions
g. To know the exact status of multirooted teeth, multiple radiographs are needed at different angles which further increase the radiation exposure.

It must be emphasized that though radiographs play a critical role in diagnosis of an endodontic case, a poor quality radiograph not only fails to yield diagnostic information but also causes unnecessary radiation to the patient.

## PULP VITALITY TESTS

Pulp testing is often referred to as vitality testing. Pulp vitality tests play an important role in diagnosis because these tests determine not only the vitality of tooth but also the pathological status of pulp. Pulp testers should only be used to assess the vital or nonvital pulp as they do not quantify the disease, nor do they measure the health and thus, should not be used to assess the degree of pulpal disease.

### Uses of Pulp Vitality Testing

1. It is done before carrying out restorative or orthodontic treatment so as to know status of the tooth/teeth even if teeth are asymptomatic and with normal radiographic appearance.
2. To confirm whether radiolucent area present at apical part of tooth is because of:
   - Pulpal origin
   - Other pathological reasons
   - Or it is a normal anatomic structure
3. To diagnose oral pain whether it is of pulpal or periodontal origin or because of other reason.
4. To assess vitality of traumatized teeth (however, vitality testing of traumatized teeth is controversial).
5. To check the status of tooth especially which has past history of pulp capping or deep restoration.

Various types of pulp tests performed are:

1. Thermal test
   a. Cold test
   b. Heat test
2. Electrical pulp testing
3. Test cavity
4. Anesthesia testing
5. Bite test

### 1. Thermal Test

In thermal test, the response of pulp to heat and cold is noted. The basic principle for pulp to respond to thermal stimuli is that patient reports sensation but it disappears immediately. Any other type of response, i.e. painful sensation even after removal of stimulus or no response are considered abnormal.

#### *a. Cold Test*

It is the most commonly used test for assessing the vitality of pulp. It can be done in a number of ways. The basic step of the pulp testing, i.e. individually isolating the tooth with rubber dam is mandatory. Use of rubber dam is especially recommended when performing the test using the ice-sticks because melting ice will run on to adjacent teeth and gingivae resulting in false-positive result.

1. The most commonly used method for performing pulp testing is ***spray with cold air*** directed against the isolated tooth.
2. The other frequently used method is ***use of ethyl chloride*** in form of:
   - Cotton pellet saturated with ethyl chloride (Fig. 6.20).
   - Spray of ethyl chloride. After isolation of tooth with rubber dam, ethyl chloride spray is employed. The ethyl chloride evaporates so rapidly that it absorbs heat and thus, cools the tooth.
3. The ***frozen carbon dioxide (dry ice)*** is reliable method of cold pulp testing. The frozen $CO_2$ is available in the form of solid sticks which is applied to the facial surface of the

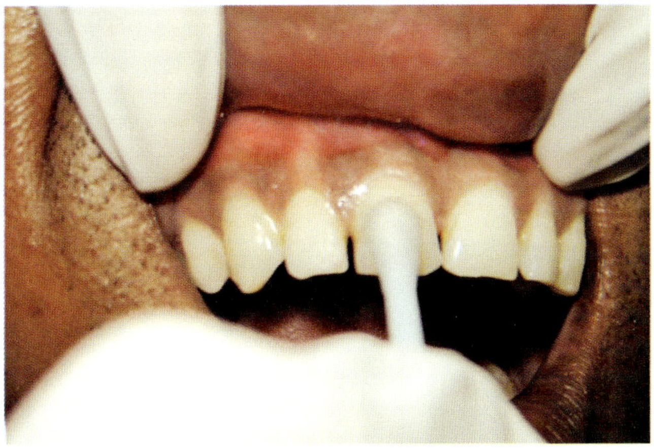

**Fig. 6.20:** Application of cotton pellet saturated with ethyl chloride

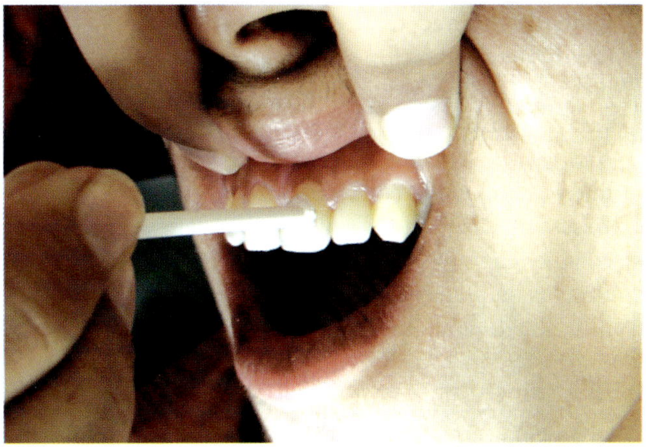

**Fig. 6.21:** Application of heated gutta-percha stick on tooth for heat test

tooth. While testing with carbon dioxide, precaution should be taken to properly isolate the oral soft tissue and teeth with gauge or cotton roll so that $CO_2$ does not come into contact with these structures, because of extremely low temperature of carbon dioxide, soft tissue burns may occur. The use of dry ice for pulp testing has been described by 'Ehrmann'. The advantage of using dry ice is that it can penetrate the full coverage restoration and can elicit a pulpal reaction to the cold because of its very low temperature (–69 to –119°F/–56 to –98°C).

4. One of the easy methods for cold test is to ***wrap an ice piece in the wet gauge*** and apply to the tooth. The ice sticks can also be prepared by filling the discarded anesthetic carpules with water and placing them in refrigerator.
5. ***Dichlorodifluoromethane (Freon)*** and the recently available material 1, 1, 1, 2-tetrafluoroethane are also used as cold testing material.

### *b. Heat Test*

Heat test is most advantageous in the condition where patient's chief complaint is intense dental pain upon contact with any hot object or liquid. It can be performed using different techniques. Isolation of the area to be tested is the basic step for all the techniques.

1. The easiest method is to direct the ***warm air*** to the exposed surface of tooth and note the patient response.
2. If a higher temperature is needed to illicit a response, other options like heated stopping stick, hot burnisher, hot water, etc. can be used.

Among these, ***heated gutta-percha stick*** (Fig. 6.21) is most commonly used method for heat testing. In this method, tooth is coated with a lubricant such as petroleum jelly to prevent the gutta-percha from adhering to tooth surface. The heated gutta-percha is applied at the junction of cervical and middle third of facial surface of tooth and patient's response is noted. While using gutta-percha stick, precautions should be taken not to overheat it because in this state, it is at higher temperature than required for pulp testing and may result in pulpal injury.

3. The ***hot burnisher, hot compound*** or any other heated instrument may also be used for heat test (Fig. 6.22).

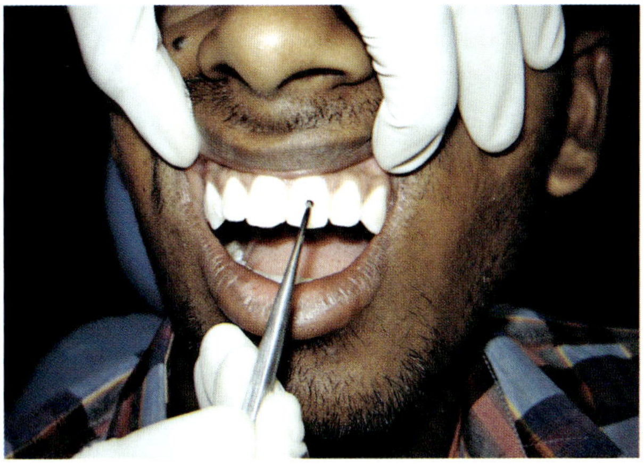

**Fig. 6.22:** Application of hot burnisher to check vitality of tooth

4. The other methods of heat testing is the use of ***frictional heat produced by rotating polishing rubber disc*** against the tooth surface.
5. One more method of heat test is to ***deliver warm water*** from a syringe on to the isolated tooth to determine the pulpal response. This method is especially useful for teeth with porcelain or full-coverage restoration. It also stimulates the existing conditions experienced by patient on taking hot foods or liquids.
6. ***Use of laser beam*** is also employed for thermal testing of teeth, In this, Nd: YAG laser is used to stimulate pulp. In case of normal pulp the pain produced by laser disappears on removal of stimulus while in case of acute pulpitis pain persists even after removal of stimulus.

*[The preferred temperature for heat test is 150°F (65.5°C)]*

The patient may respond to heat or cold test in following possible ways:

Mild, transitory response to stimulation shows normal pulp. Absence of response in combination with other tests indicates pulp necrosis. An exaggerated and lingering response indicates irreversible pulpitis.

But there are certain ***conditions which can give false negative response***, i.e. the tooth shows no response but the pulp could be possibly vital. These conditions can be:

1. Recently erupted teeth with immature apex—due to incompletely developed plexus of Rashkow. Hence, incapable of transmitting pain.
2. Recent trauma—injury to nerve supply at the apical foramen or because of inflammatory exudates around the apex may interfere the nerve conduction.
3. Excessive calcifications may also interfere with the nerve conduction.
4. Patients on premedication with analgesics or tranquillizers may not respond normally.

## 2. Electric Pulp Testing

Electric pulp tester is used for evaluation of condition of the pulp by electrical excitations of neural elements within the pulp. The pulp tester is an instrument which uses the gradations of electrical current to excite a response from the pulpal tissue. Pulp testers are available with cord which plug into electric outlets for power source (Fig. 6.23). They can also be available as battery operated instrument (Fig. 6.24). A positive response indicates the vitality of pulp. No response indicates nonvital pulp or pulpal necrosis.

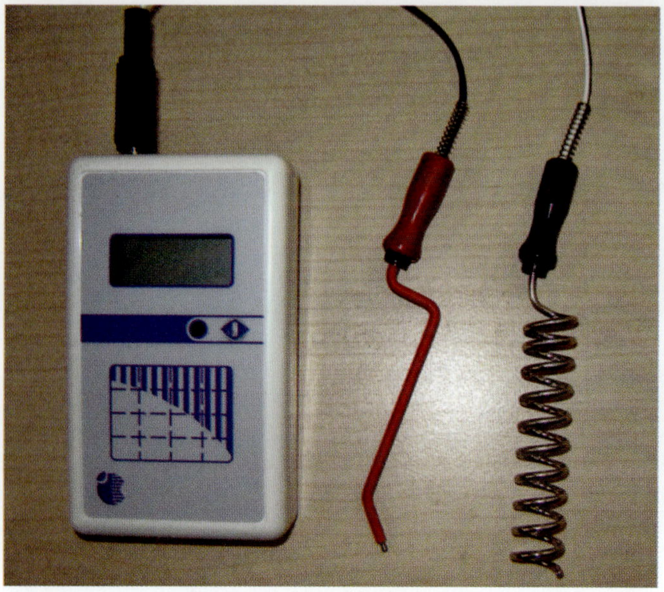

**Fig. 6.23:** Electric pulp tester

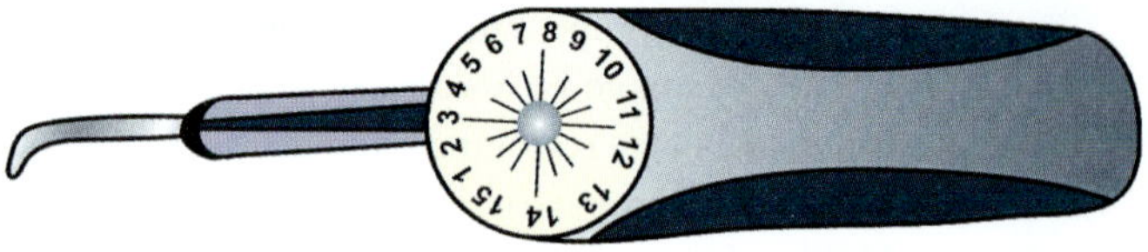

**Fig. 6.24:** Battery operated pulp tester

### *Procedure*

1. Before starting the procedure, patient must be explained about the method. This will be helpful in reducing the anxiety of patient.
2. Isolation of the teeth to be tested is one of the essential steps to avoid any type of false positive response. This can be done by using 2″ × 2″ gauge piece.
3. Apply an electrolyte on the tooth electrode and place it on the facial surface of tooth (Fig. 6.25). Precaution should be taken to avoid it contacting adjacent gingival tissue or restorations; this will cause false positive response.
4. One should note that there should be a complete circuit from electrode through the tooth, to the body of the patient and then back to the electrode. If gloves are not used, the circuit gets completed when clinician's finger contact with electrode and patient's cheeks. But with gloved hands, it can be done by placing patient's finger on metal electrode handle or by clipping a ground attachment on to the patient's lip.
5. Once the circuit is complete, slowly increase the current and ask the patient to point out when the sensation occurs.
6. Each tooth should be tested 2-3 times and the average reading is noted. If the vitality of a tooth is in question, the pulp tester should be used on the adjacent teeth and the contralateral tooth, as control.

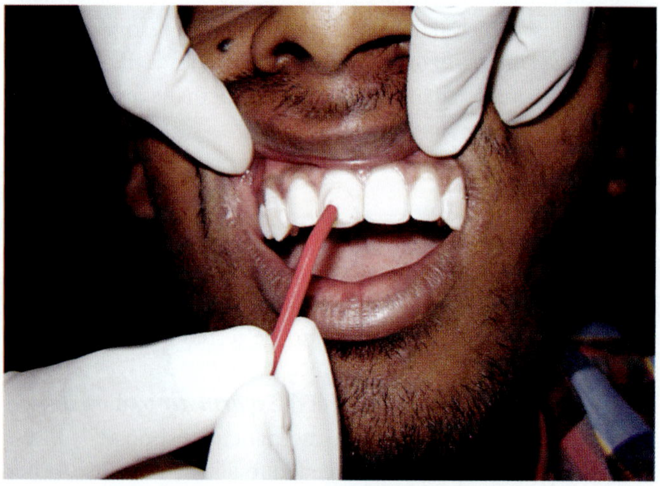

**Fig. 6.25:** Checking vitality of tooth using electric pulp tester

### *Disadvantages of Electric Pulp Testing*

Electric pulp testing should not be considered solely for determination of pulp vitality; it should be used in combination with other tests. Various conditions can give rise to wrong results and thus misdiagnosis. These conditions can be as follows:

1. In teeth with acute alveolar abscess, false positive response is seen because gaseous or liquefied products within the pulp canal can transmit electric current.
2. Electrode may contact gingival tissue thus giving the false positive response.
3. In multirooted teeth, pulp may be vital in one or more root canals and necrosed in others, thus eliciting a false positive response.
4. In certain conditions, it can give false negative response, for example:
   a. Recently traumatized tooth
   b. Recently erupted teeth with immature apex
   c. Patients with high pain threshold

d. Calcified canals
e. Poor battery or electrical deficiency in plug in pulp testers.
f. Teeth with extensive restorations or pulp protecting bases under restorations
g. Patients premedicated with analgesics or tranquilizers, etc.
h. Partial necrosis of pulp sometimes is indicated as totally necrosis by electric pulp tester.

### 3. Test Cavity

This method should be used only when all other test methods are inconclusive in results. Here a test cavity is made with high speed number 1 or 2 round burs with appropriate air and water coolant. The patient is not anesthetized while performing this test. Patient is asked to respond if any painful sensation occurs during drilling. The sensitivity or the pain felt by the patient indicates pulp vitality. Here the procedure is terminated by restoring the prepared cavity. If no pain is felt, cavity preparation may be continued until the pulp chamber is reached and later on endodontic therapy may be carried out.

### 4. Anesthesia Testing

When patient is not able to specify the site of pain and when other pulp testing techniques are inconclusive, the selective anesthesia may be used. The main objective of this test is to anesthetize a single tooth at a time until the pain is eliminated. It should be accomplished by using intraligamentary injection. Injection is administered to the most posterior tooth in the suspected quadrant. If the pain persists, even after tooth has been fully anesthetized, repeat the procedure to the next tooth mesial to it. It is continued until the pain disappears. If source of pain cannot be determined, repeat the same technique on the opposite arch.

### 5. Bite Test

This test helps if patient complains of pain on mastication. Tooth is sensitive to biting if pulpal necrosis has extended to the periodontal ligament space or if a crack is present in a tooth. In this test patient is asked to bite on a hard object such as cotton swab, tooth pick or orange wood stick with suspected tooth and the contralateral tooth (Fig. 6.26). Tooth slooth is another commercially available device for bite test. It has a small concave area on its top which is placed in contact with the cusp to be tested (Fig. 6.27). Patient is asked to bite on it. Pain on biting may indicate a fractured tooth.

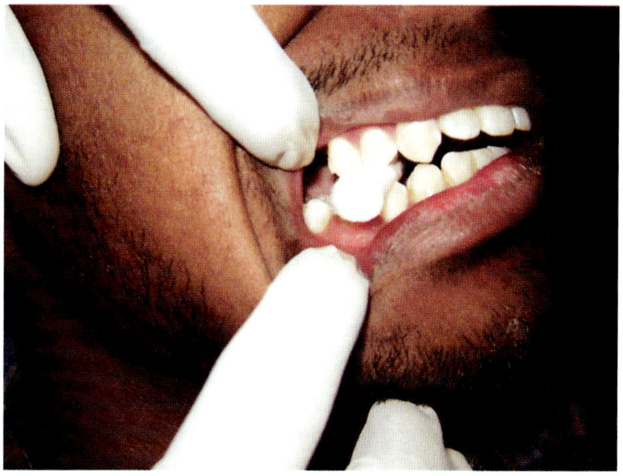

**Fig. 6.26:** Patient is asked to bite on cotton swab or hard object for bite test

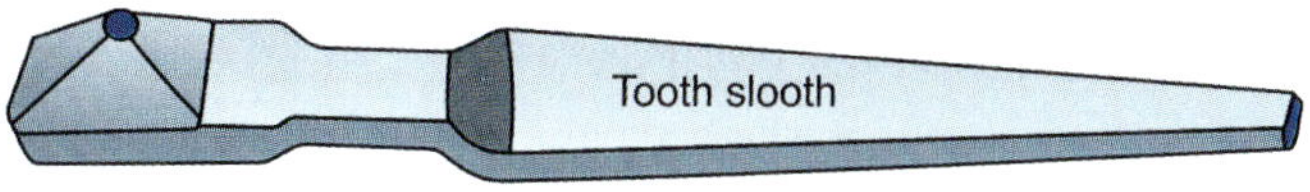


**Fig. 6.27:** Tooth slooth

## RECENT ADVANCES IN PULP VITALITY TESTING

The assessment of pulp vitality is a crucial diagnostic procedure in the practice of dentistry. Current routine methods rely on stimulation of A-delta nerve fibers and give no direct indication of blood flow within the pulp. These include thermal stimulation, electrical or direct dentine stimulation. These testing methods have the potential to produce an unpleasant and occasionally painful sensation and inaccurate results. In addition, each is a subjective test that depends on the patient's perceived response to a stimulus as well as the dentist's interpretation of that response.

Recent studies have shown that blood circulation and not innervation is the most accurate determinant in assessing pulp vitality as it provides an objective differentiation between necrotic and vital pulp tissue.

**Recently available pulp vitality tests are:**
- Laser Doppler flowmetry (LDF)
- Pulp oximetry
- Dual wavelength spectrophotometry
- Measurement of temperature of tooth surface
- Transillumination with fiber-optic light
- Plethysmography
- Detection of interleukin—1 beta
- Xenon—133
- Hughes probeye camera
- Gas desaturation
- Radiolabeled microspheres
- Electromagnetic flowmetry

### Laser Doppler Flowmetry (LDF)

Laser Doppler flowmeter was developed by Tenland in 1982 and later by Holloway in 1983. The technique depends on Doppler principle in which a low power light from a monochromatic laser beam of known wavelength along a fiberoptic cable is directed to the tooth surface, where the light passes along the direction of enamel prisms and dentinal tubules to the pulp.

The light that contacts a moving object is Doppler shifted, and a portion of that light will be back scattered out of tooth into a photodetector. Some light is reflected off moving red blood cells in pulpal capillaries and as a consequence frequency broadened. The reflected light is passed back to the flowmeter where the frequency broadened light, together with laser light scattered from static tissue, is photo-detected for strength of signal and pulsatility (Fig. 6.28).

Since, red blood cells represent the majority of moving objects within the tooth, measurements of Doppler shifted back scattered light may be interpreted as an index of pulpal blood flow.

The resulting photocurrent is processed to provide a blood flow measurement. The blood flow measured by laser Doppler technique is termed as 'flux', which is proportional to the product of average speed of blood cells and their concentration.

Pulp is a highly vascular tissue, and cardiac cycle blood flow in the supplying artery is transmitted as pulsations. These pulsations are apparent on laser Doppler monitor of vital teeth and are absent in nonvital teeth. The blood flux level in vital teeth is much higher than nonvital teeth. Currently available flowmeters display the signal on a screen, from which the clinician can interpret whether pulp is vital or nonvital.

**Advantages of laser Doppler flowmetry**

1. An objective test
2. Accurate to check vitality

**Disadvantages of laser Doppler flowmetry**

1. Cannot be used in patients who cannot refrain from moving or if tooth to be tested cannot be stabilized
2. Medications used in cardiovascular diseases can affect the blood flow to pulp
3. Requires higher technical skills to achieve
4. Use of nicotine also affects the blood flow to pulp
5. Expensive

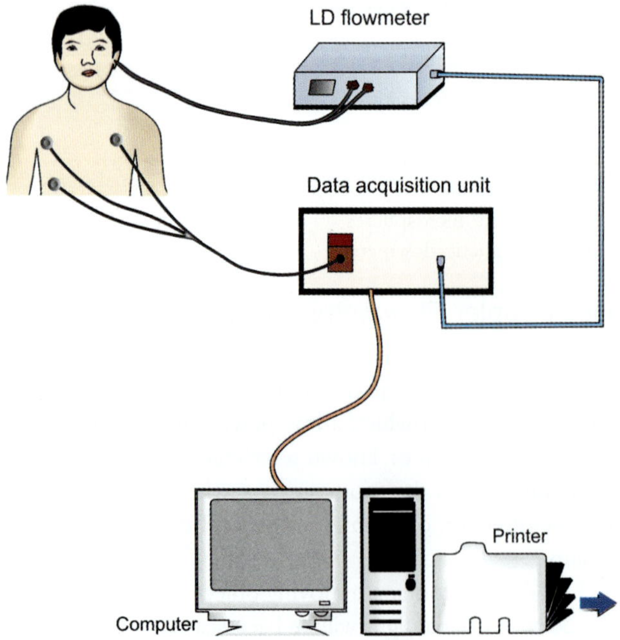


**Fig. 6.28:** Working of LDF

## Pulp Oximetry

Pulp oximetry is a non-invasive device for determining pulp vitality. The principle of this technology is based on modification of Beer's law and the absorbency characteristics of hemoglobin in red and infrared range.

The pulp oximeter is a non-invasive oxygen saturation monitor in which liquid crystal display oxygen saturation, pulse rate and plethysmographic wave form readings. The probe consists of red and infrared light-emitting diodes opposite a photoelectric detector. Clinically the detection of a pulse should be enough to establish pulp vitality or necrosis.

Pulp oximetry is especially helpful in cases of traumatic injury to the teeth during which nerve supply of the pulp may be injured, but the blood supply stays intact.

A distinctive advantage of this technique is its objectivity and lack of dependence on sensory response which eliminates the need for application of an unpleasant stimulus to the patient.

**Advantages of pulp oximetry**

1. Effective and objective method to evaluate pulp vitality
2. Useful in cases of traumatic injuries where the blood supply remains intact but nerve supply is damaged
3. Pulpal circulation can be detected independent of gingival circulation
4. Easy to reproduce pulp pulse readings
5. Smaller and cheaper pulp oximeters are now available

**Disadvantages of pulp oximetry**

1. Background absorption associated with venous blood

## Dual Wavelength Spectrophotometry

Dual wavelength spectrophotometry (DWLS) is a method independent of a pulsatile circulation. The presence of arterioles rather than arteries in the pulp and its rigid encapsulation by surrounding dentine and enamel make it difficult to detect a pulse in the pulp space. This method measures oxygenation changes in the capillary bed rather than the supply vessels and hence does not depend on a pulsatile blood flow.

DWLS detects the presence or absence of oxygenated blood at 760 nm and 850 nm. The blood volume or concentration channel (760 nm plus 850 nm) is arranged to respond linearly to the increase in light absorption. The oxygenation channel (760 nm minus 850 nm) senses the oxygenated blood because of the greater absorption at 850 nm as compared to 760 nm.

**Advantages of DWLS**

1. In case of avulsed and replanted teeth with open apices where the blood supply is regained within first 20 days but the nerve supply lags behind. Repeated readings for 40 days in such teeth reveal the healing process.
2. It uses visible light which is filtered and guided to the tooth by fiber optics, unlike laser light where eye protection is necessary for patient and the operator.
3. Non-invasive test
4. An objective test
5. Instrument is small, portable and inexpensive

### Measurement of Surface Temperature of Tooth

This method is based on the assumption that if pulp becomes nonvital, the tooth no longer has internal blood supply, thus should exhibit a lower surface temperature than that of its vital counterparts.

Fanibund in 1985 showed that it is possible to differentiate by means of crown surface temperature, distinct difference between vital and nonvital teeth. He used a thermistor unit consisting of two matched thermistors connected back to back, one measuring the surface temperature of the crown (measuring thermistor) while the other acting as a reference thermistor. The tooth to be tested was dried with gauze and the thermistor unit was positioned so that the measuring thermistor contacted the center of the buccal surface of the crown. The reference thermistor was suspended in air, close to it, but not touching either the measuring thermistor or the enamel surface.

Equilibrium was then achieved between the temperatures of the thermistors, the crown surface and the immediate environment by holding the measuring unit in the described position until a steady state was established for at least 20 seconds. Stimulation of the crown surface was carried out by means of a rubber-polishing cup fitted to a dental contra-angle hand piece. The recordings were continued for a period of time following the stimulation period. It was found that a difference was obtained between the critical period for vital and nonvital teeth and the difference corresponded with a specific temperature change.

### Transillumination with Fiberoptic Light

It is a system of illumination whereby light is passed through a finely drawn glass or plastic fibers by a process known as ***total internal reflection.***

By this method, a pulpless tooth that is not noticeably discolored may show a gross difference in translucency when a shadow produced on a mirror is compared to that of adjacent vital teeth.

### Detection of Interleukin-I Beta in Human Periapical Lesion

The inflammatory periapical lesions are common sequelae of infected pulp tissue. Numerous cell types including PMN leucocytes, T and B lymphocytes, macrophages and plasma cells are found in these tissues.

These inflammatory cells produce interleukin-I (IL-1), which acts as a mediator of various immunologic and inflammatory responses.

This lymphocyte activating factor IL-1 is responsible for osteoclast activation which results in bone resorption which is frequently a feature of inflammatory response.

### Plethysmography

It is a method for assessing the changes in volume and has been applied to the investigation of arterial disease because the volume of the limb or organ exhibits transient changes over the cardiac cycle. Plethysmography in limb or digit can be performed using air-filled cuffs or mercury in rubber strain gauges. As the pressure pulse passes through the limb segment, a wave form is recorded which relates closely to that obtained by intra-arterial cannulation. The same principle can be used to assess tooth vitality. Presence or absence of a wave form can indicate the status of the tooth.

## DIAGNOSTIC FINDINGS

Once the patient has been evaluated and the clinical examinations along with tests are completed, a diagnosis is made. The findings of examination are arranged in a rational manner so as to diagnose the pulpal or periapical diseases. Once the correct diagnosis is made, the treatment plan should be made. Basically the pulpal diseases can be reversible pulpitis, irreversible pulpitis or the necrotic pulp. The periapical diseases can be acute apical periodontitis, chronic apical periodontitis, acute or chronic apical abscess or condensing osteitis. These have been summarized in the table below.

## ROLE OF RADIOGRAPHS IN ENDODONTICS

Radiographs play an important role in diagnosis of the dental diseases. The interpretation of radiographs should be done in a systematic manner. The clinician should be familiar with normal radiographic landmarks.

***Normal radiographic landmarks are (Fig. 6.29):***

*Enamel:* It is the most radiopaque structure.

*Dentin:* Slightly darker than enamel

*Cementum:* Similar to dentin in appearance

*Periodontal ligament:* Appears as a narrow radiolucent line around the root surface.

*Lamina dura:* It is a radiopaque line representing the tooth socket.

*Pulp cavity:* Pulp chamber and canals are seen as radiolucent lines within the tooth.

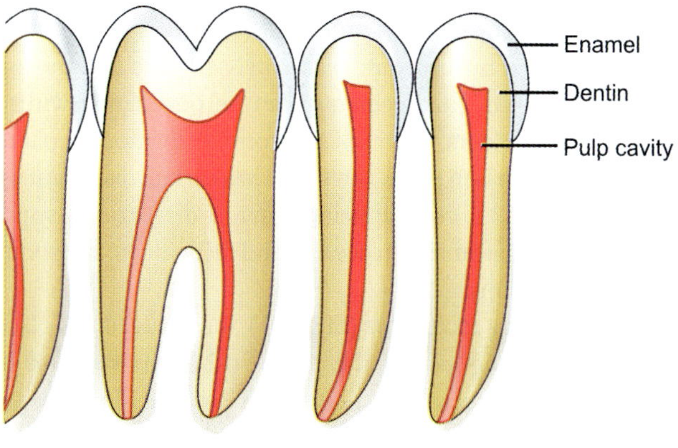


**Fig. 6.29:** Normal radiographic features of teeth

Though the radiographs play an important role in dentistry yet they have a few shortcomings. For example pathological changes in pulp are not visible in radiographs, also the initial stages of periradicular diseases produce no changes in the radiographs. They are only two-dimensional picture of a three-dimensional object. It must be emphasized that a poor quality radiograph not only fails to yield diagnostic information but also causes unnecessary radiation to the patient.

To reduce the amount of radiation exposure and to improve the quality of radiograph, continuous efforts have been made since the discovery of X-ray in 1895.

In order to decrease the radiation exposure, certain newer methods have been introduced which include:

a. Use the paralleling technique instead of bisecting angle technique.
b. Faster radiographic films.
c. Digital radiographic techniques.
d. Use of electronic apex locator to assist in endodontic treatment.

**History of dental radiology**

| | | |
|---|---|---|
| 1895 | WC Roentgen | Discovery of X-rays |
| 1896 | O Walkhoff | First dental radiograph |
| 1901 | WH Rollins | Presented first paper on dangers of X-rays |
| 1904 | WA Price | Introduction of bisecting technique |
| 1913 | Eastman Kodak company | Introduction of pre-wrapped dental films |
| 1920 | Eastman Kodak company | Introduction of machine made film packets |
| 1925 | HR Raper | Introduction of bitewing technique |
| 1947 | FG Fitzgerald | Introduction of paralleling cone technique |

## Principles of Radiography

For diagnostic purposes in endodontics, the number of radiographs required depends on situations. A properly placed film permits the visualization of approximately three teeth and at least 3-4 mm beyond the apex. In most of the cases, a single exposure is needed to get the information on root and pulp anatomy. Basically there are two types of techniques for exposing teeth viz; ***bisecting angle technique*** and ***paralleling technique.***

In ***bissecting angle technique*** (Fig. 6.30) the X-ray beam is directed perpendicular to an imaginary plane which bisects the angle formed by recording plane of X-ray film and the long axis of the tooth. This technique can be performed without the use of film holders, it is quick and comfortable for the patient when rubber dam is in place. But it also has certain disadvantages like incidences of cone cutting, image distortion, super-imposition of anatomical structures and difficulty to reproduce the periapical films.

In ***paralleling technique*** (Fig. 6.31), the X-ray film is placed parallel to the long axis of the tooth to be exposed and the X-ray beam is directed perpendicular to the film. Various advantages of paralleling technique are:

- Better accuracy of image
- Reduced dose of radiation
- Reproducibility
- Better images of bone margins, interproximal regions and maxillary molar region

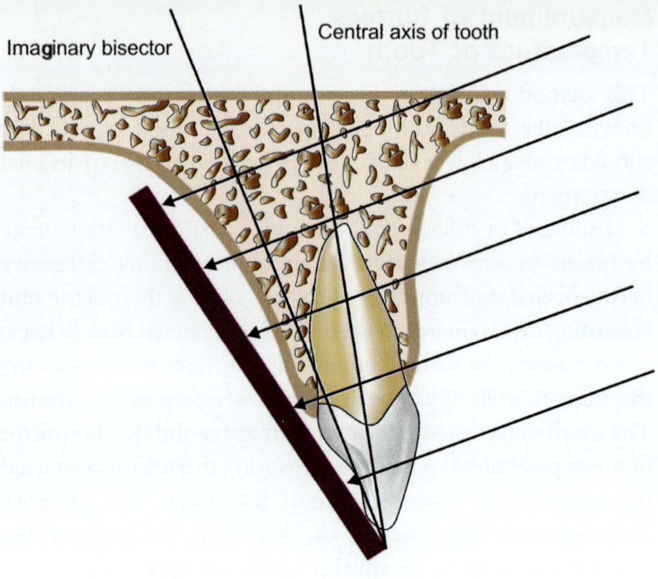


**Fig. 6.30:** Bissecting angle technique

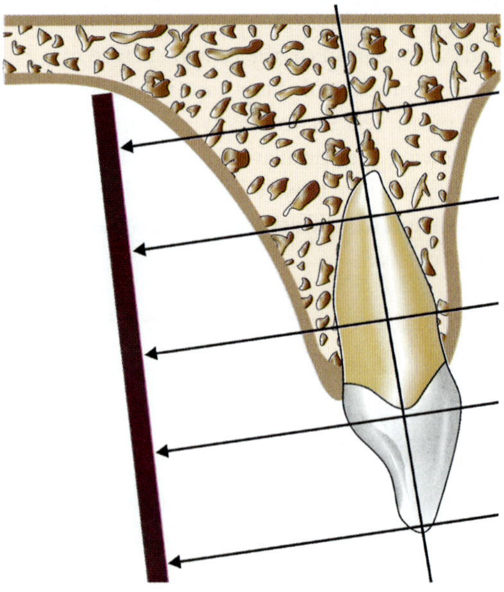

**Fig. 6.31:** Paralleling technique

Disadvantages associated with this technique are difficult to use in patients with shallow vault, gag reflex and when rubber dam is in place.

Cone angulation is one of the most important aspects of radiography because it affects the quality of image. We have seen that paralleling technique has been shown to be superior to bisecting angle technique, especially in reproduction of apical anatomy of the tooth. As the angle increases away from parallel, the quality of image decreases. This happens because as the angle is increased, the tissue that the X-rays must pass through includes greater percentage of bone mass thus anatomy becomes less predictable. To limit this problem, **Walton** gave a ***modified paralleling technique*** in which central beam is oriented perpendicular to radiographic film but not to teeth. Modified paralleling technique is also beneficial for some special situations in which paralleling technique is not feasible, for example shallow palatal vault, maxillary tori, extremely long roots, uncooperative and gagging patient.

There are some special situations during endodontic therapy which require special considerations to obtain best quality of radiographs. These radiographs are neither parallel nor bisecting angle, but in such radiograph some modifications are made by varying the horizontal cone angle, cone placement and modified film placement. Commonly, modified paralleling technique is used in such radiographs.

## Cone Image Shift Technique

An understanding of cone shift technique is essential to endodontic treatment. The proper application of this technique helps in distinguishing the objects which have been superimposed, differentiating the different types of resorption, and to locate additional number of roots or canals (Fig. 6.32). ***The main concept of technique*** is that as the vertical or horizontal angulations of X-ray tube head changes, the object buccal or closest to the tube head moves to opposite side of radiograph when compared to lingual object (Fig. 6.33). In other words, we can say that the cone image shift technique separates and identifies the facial and lingual structures.

As the cone position moves from parallel either towards horizontal or vertical, the object on the film shifts away from the direction of cone, i.e. in the direction of central beam.

In other words, when two objects and the film are in fixed position and the tube head is moved, images of both objects moving in opposite direction, the resultant radiograph shows lingual object that moved in the same direction as the cone and the buccal object moved in opposite direction. This is also known as "SLOB" rule (same lingual opposite buccal).

**Synonyms of cone image shift technique**
1. BOR (Buccal object rule)
2. SLOB (Same lingual opposite buccal)
3. BOMM (Buccal object moves most)
4. Clark's Rule
5. Walton's Projection

To simplify understanding of this rule, Walton gave an easy method. Place two fingers directly in front of open eyes so that one finger is superimposed on the other. By moving the head, from one way and the other, the position of finger, relative to each other shifts. The same effect is produced with two superimposed roots when central beam is shifted.

## Advantages of "SLOB" Rule

1. It helps in separation of overlapping canals for example in case maxillary premolars and mesial canals of mandibular molars.
2. The working length radiographs are better traced from orifice to the apex by this technique.
3. It helps to locate the root resorptive processes in relation to tooth.

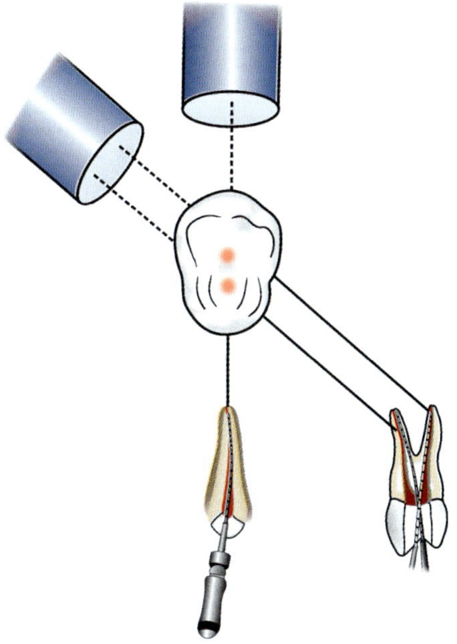

Fig. 6.32: Cone-shift technique

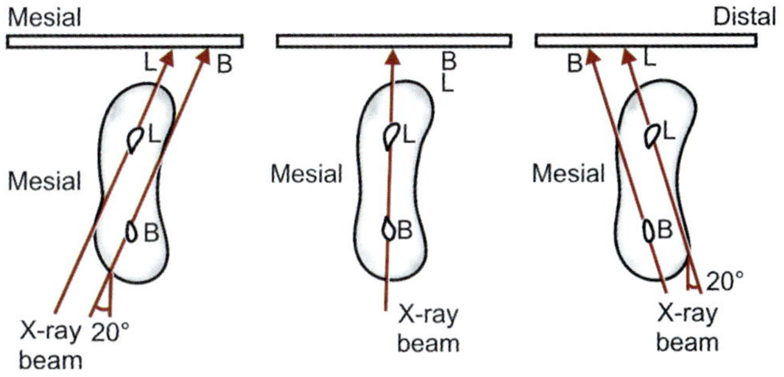


Fig. 6.33: As X-ray tube head changes, the object buccal or closest to the tube head moves to opposite side of radiograph when compared to lingual object

4. This technique is helpful in locating a canal in relation to radiopaque margin such as bur in the access opening.
5. It is useful in identification of anatomic landmarks and pathosis.
6. This rule is also used to increase the visualization of apical anatomy by moving anatomic landmarks such as zygomatic process or the impacted tooth.
7. It also helps to identify the angle at which particular radiograph was made, even if information was not recorded.
8. This technique is advantageous during access preparation. It helps to identify the missed canals or calcified canals and sometimes the canal curvature.

## Disadvantages of "SLOB" Rule

1. It results in blurring of the object which is directly proportional to cone angle. The clearest radiograph is achieved by parallel technique so when the central beam changes direction relative to object and the film, object become blurred.

2. It causes superimposition of the structures. Objects which have natural separation on parallel technique, with cone shift; they may move relative to each other and become superimposed. For example, in case of maxillary molars, all three separate roots are visible on parallel radiographs but an angled radiograph may move palatal root over the distobuccal or mesiobuccal root and thus decreasing the ability to distinguish apices clearly.

### Bitewing Radiographs

Bitewing radiographs include the crowns of maxillary and mandibular teeth and alveolar crest in the same film.

#### *Two Types*

i. Horizontal bitewing film: In this, beam is aligned between the teeth parallel to occlusal plane.
ii. Vertical bitewing film: In this, film is oriented vertically so as to record more of root area. It is done in cases of extensive bone loss.

#### *Advantages*

- Helps in detecting interproximal caries
- Evaluate periodontal conditions
- Evaluate secondary caries under restorations
- Help in assessing alveolar bone crest and changes in bone height by comparing it with adjacent teeth.

## FILM EXPOSURE AND QUALITY

Several choices are available regarding the film and processing. Studies have shown that there is no significant difference in the diagnostic quality of 'E' (EKTA speed) films when compared with 'D' films (Ultra speed). These, E plus films should be used to reduce the radiation exposure to the patient. The optimal setting for maximal contrast between their radiopaque and radiolucent structure is 70 kV. To maximize the clarity of the film, exposure time and milliamperage should be set individually on each machine. The rapid processing chemicals are also used in endodontic to expedite the development of the film for treatment radiograph.

**Safety concerns of X-rays**

- Though X-rays are harmful yet dental X-rays are safe because of their low level of radiation exposure. Moreover, to avoid excessive exposure, one should use lead apron to cover body and high speed film.
- To take X-ray of pregnant patient, lead shield should be used to cover body including the womb area. Moreover X-rays should be taken if necessary.

## FILM HOLDERS

Film holders are basically required for paralleling technique because their use decreases the distortion of X-rays caused by misorientation of film, tooth or X-ray beam (Fig. 6.34). The use of film holder has shown to provide more predictable results, this alignment device has following advantages:

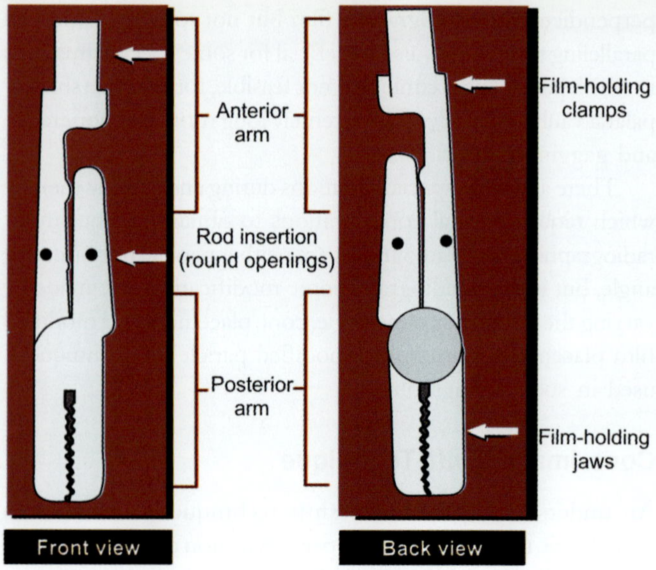


**Fig. 6.34:** Film holder

1. True image of tooth, its length and anatomical features can be obtained.
2. Subsequent films taken with same holder can be more accurately compared especially while assessing the degree of healing of periapical lesion.
3. Film holders reduce the cone cut, and improve the quality of radiograph.
4. They eliminate the patient's finger from the field of exposure and thus reduce the risk of displacing the film.

Commonly used device for holding X-ray film is hemostat, though various commercial devices are available as film holder like Endo Ray II, Snap-H-Ray, Uni Bite and the Stable disposable film holder.

## ADVANTAGES OF RADIOGRAPHS IN ENDODONTICS

In all the endodontic cases, a good intraoral periapical radiograph of the root and its related structures is mandatory. Radiography is the most reliable of all the diagnostic tests and provides the most valuable information.

In endodontics, the radiographs perform essential functions in three main areas that are diagnosis, treatment and recall.

### 1. Diagnosis

a. Radiographs help to know the presence of caries which may involve or on the verge of involving the pulp. Depth of caries, restoration, evidence of pulp capping or pulpotomy, etc. could be evaluated on seeing the radiograph (Fig. 6.35).
b. The radiographs help to know the root and pulpal anatomy, i.e. normal and abnormal root formation, curvature of the canal, number of roots and the canals, any calcifications if present in the canal and variation in the root canal system, i.e. presence of fused or extra roots and canals (Fig. 6.36), any bifurcation or trifurcation in the canal system if present.

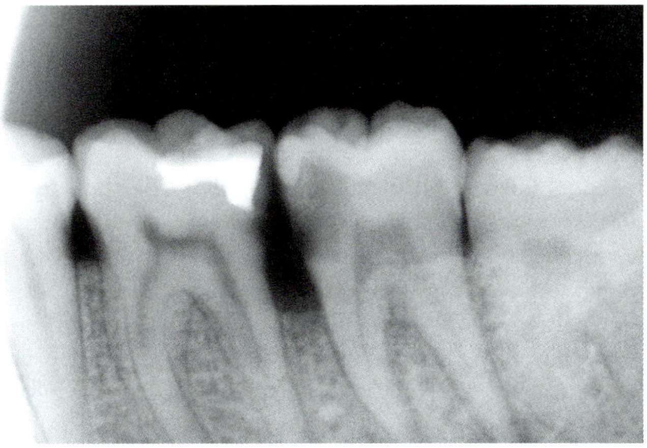

Fig. 6.35: Extent of caries/restoration can be seen on radiograph

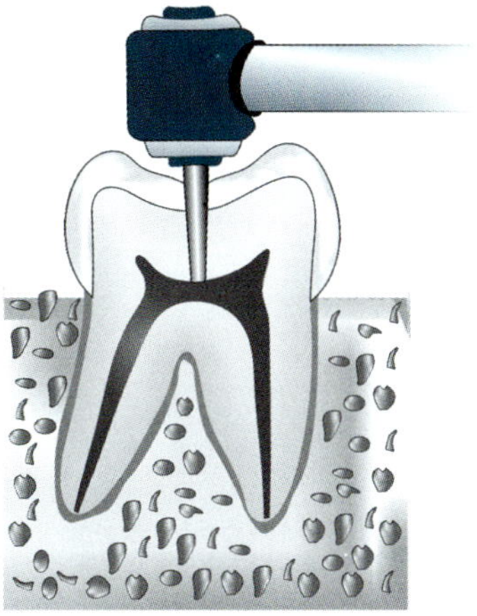

Fig. 6.37: Preoperative radiograph can provide information on orientation and depth of the angulation of handpiece

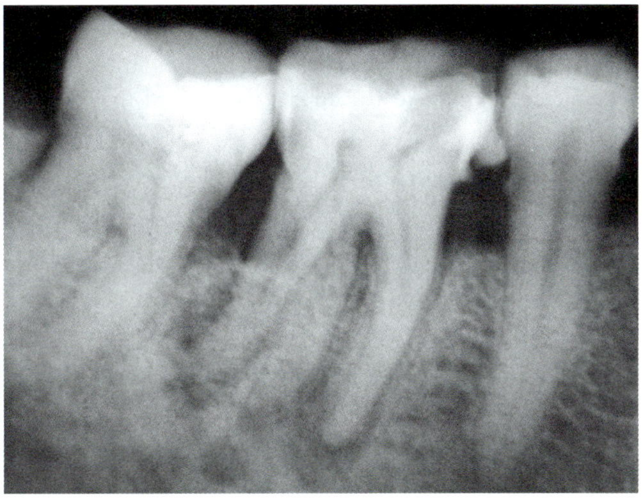

Fig. 6.36: Radiograph showing extra root in first molar

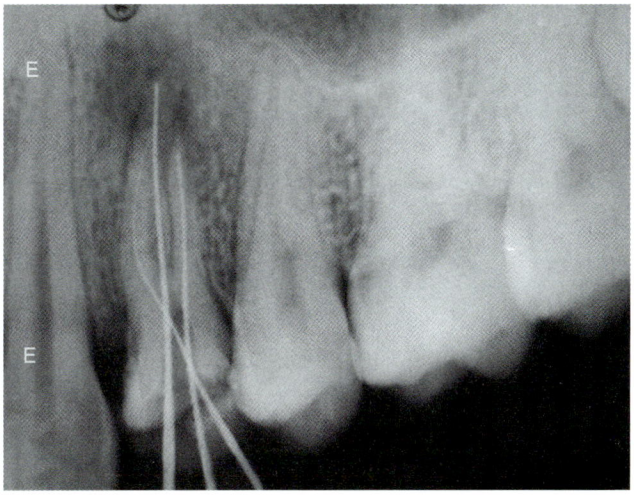

Fig. 6.38: Working length determination

c. Radiographs help to know the pulp conditions present inside the tooth like pulp stones, calcification, internal resorption, etc.
d. A good quality preoperative radiograph provides information on orientation and depth of bur relative to the pulp cavity (Fig. 6.37).
e. Other conditions like resorption from the root surface, i.e. external resorption, thickening of periodontal ligament and extent of periapical and alveolar bone destruction can be interpreted by viewing the radiographs.
f. They also help to identify the numerous radiolucent and radiopaque structures which often lie in the close proximity to the tooth. These must be distinguished and differentiated from the pathological lesions.

## 2. Treatment

The radiographs exposed during the treatment phase are known as ***working radiographs.*** Working radiographs are made while rubber dam is in place, i.e. these radiographs are exposed during treatment phase.

### a. Working Length Determination

In this, radiograph establishes the distance from the reference point to apex till which canal is to be prepared and obturated (Fig. 6.38). By using special cone angulations, some superimposed structures can be moved to give clear image of the apical region.

### b. Master Cone Radiographs

It is taken in the same way as with working length radiograph. Master cone radiograph is used to evaluate the length and fit of master gutta-percha cone (Fig. 6.39).

### c. Obturation

Radiographs help to know the length, density, configuration and the quality of obturation (Figs 6.40A and B).

## 3. Recall

1. Radiographs are essential to evaluate the post-treatment periapical status.

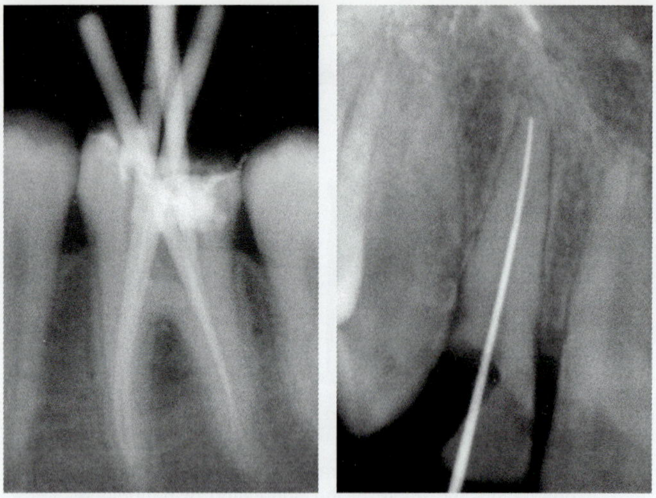

**Fig. 6.39:** Radiograph to check extent and fit of master cone before obturation

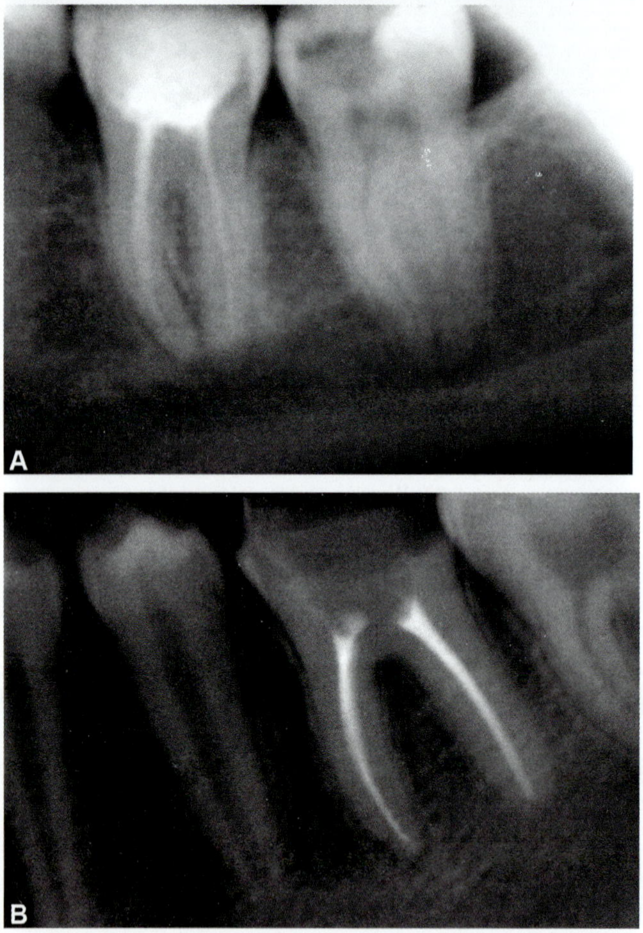

**Figs 6.40A and B:** Radiograph to see quality of obturation: (A) Poor quality obturation, (B) Good quality obturation

2. The presence and nature of lesion that have occurred after the treatment are best detected on radiographs. These lesions may be periapical, periodontal or non-endodontic.
3. Recall radiographs help to know the success of treatment by evaluating the healing process.

Thus, we can say that radiographs provide valuable information concerning the case selection, diagnosis, treatment planning and prognosis but one must not be totally dependent on the radiograph. In fact, radiographs can be misleading, thus must be viewed with caution and should be correlated with other clinical findings for example radiographs cannot differentiate granuloma, cyst or chronic abscess. For accurate diagnosis, histopathological examination is must. Similarly, presence of periapical radiolucencies on tooth does not indicate a diseased tooth. It could be due to normal anatomic structures like incisive or mental foramen or maxillary sinus or due to other odontogenic lesions such as ameloblastoma, early stages of cementoma or ossifying fibroma, etc. In ossifying fibroma, the pulp vitality confirms the diagnosis. It is associated with the vital tooth. Perplexity of radiograph is that it does not always the correct interpretation yet it has to be used as an important diagnostic tool. For reaching an accurate diagnosis, one should not rely only on radiographs but it has to be used in conjunction with other tests.

## DIGITAL RADIOGRAPHY

Most digital imaging in dentistry uses standard radiology techniques with film to record the image, and then subjects the finished image to digital processing to produce the final result.

The backlog film image is converted to a digital signal by a scanning device, such as videocamera. First the image is divided into a grid of uniformly sized pixels, each of which is assigned a grey scale value based on its optical diversity. This value is stored in computer. Once the image is in computer, a number of operations can be performed on computer program used.

One of the most useful operations is a comparison of images called digital substraction. The computers can compare two images, this property can be used to see the progression of disease over time and evaluation of treatment outcomes of endodontic therapy.

Another use is the detection of lesion on radiographs. This is where an endodontist can use this application for diagnosis. The computers can detect lesion with pattern recognition and boundary determination. Sometimes density changes on radiographs are so subtle that human eye has trouble identifying them, but machines are able to discriminate at density level beyond what human eye can see.

### Disadvantages

- The radiation dose to the patient is the same as that used for conventional radiographs.
- Requires equipment to print photographs or even for scanning of radiographs.

### Advantages

1. The amount of information available from these radiographs is greater than from radiographs that have not been digitized.
2. The storage of radiographs and quality of image is better.
3. Photographs of radiographs can be produced.

## DIGITAL DENTAL RADIOLOGY

Images in digital form can be readily manipulated, stored and retrieved on computer. Furthermore, technology makes the transmission of images practicable. The general principles of digital imaging are:

1. The chemically produced radiograph is represented by data that is acquired in a parallel and continuous fashion known as analog.
2. Computers use binary (0 or 1) language, where information is usually handled in 8 character words called bytes.
3. Each character can be either 0 or 1. This results in 28 possible combinations (words) that is 256 words. Thus digital dental images are limited to 256 shades of grey.
4. Digital images are made up of pixels (picture elements), each allocated a shade of grey.
5. The spatial resolution of a digital system is heavily dependent upon the number of pixels available per millimeter of image.

## Digital Dental Radiology is Possible with Two Methods

1. One uses charged couple devices.
2. Other uses photostimulable phosphorimaging plates.

Both methods can be used in dental surgery with conventional personal computers.

Digital imaging system requires an electronic sensor or detector, an analog to digital converter, a computer, and a monitor or printer for image of the components of imaging system. It instructs the X-ray generator when to begin and end the exposure, controls the digitizer, constructs the image by mathematical algorithm, determines the method of image display, and provides for storage and transmission of acquired data.

The most common sensor is the CCD, the other being phosphor image.

When a conventional X-ray unit is used to project the X-ray beam on to the sensor, an electronic charge is created, an analog output signal is generated and the digital converter converts the analog output signal from CCD to a numeric representation that is recognizable by the computer.

The radiographic image then appears on the monitor and can be manipulated electronically to alter contrast, resolution, orientation and even size.

## THE CCD SYSTEM

The CCD is a solid state detector containing array of X-ray or light sensitive phosphores on a pure silicon chip. These phosphors convert incoming X-rays to a wavelength that matches the peak response of silicon.

## RVG

RVG is composed of three major parts.

1. The "radio" part consists of a conventional X-ray unit, a precise timer for short exposure times and a tiny sensor to record the image. Sensor has a small (17 × 24 mm) receptor screen which transmits information via fiberoptic bundle to a miniature CCD. The sensor is protected from X-ray degradation by a fiberoptic shield and can be cold sterilized for infection control. Disposable latex sheath is also used to cover the sensor when it is in use (Fig. 6.41). Because the sensor does not need to be removed from mouth after each exposure, the time to take multiple images is greatly reduced.
2. The "visio" portion of the system receives and stores incoming signals during exposure and converts them point by point into one of 256 discrete gray levels. It consists of a video monitor and display processing unit (Fig. 6.42). As the image is transmitted to the processing unit, it is ***digitized*** and memorized by the computer. The unit magnifies the image four times for immediate display on video monitor and has additional capability of producing colored images (Figs 6.43 and 6.44). It can also display multiple images simultaneously, including a full mouth series on one screen. A zoom feature is also available to enlarge a portion of image upto face-screen size.
3. The "graphy" part of RVG unit consists of digital storage

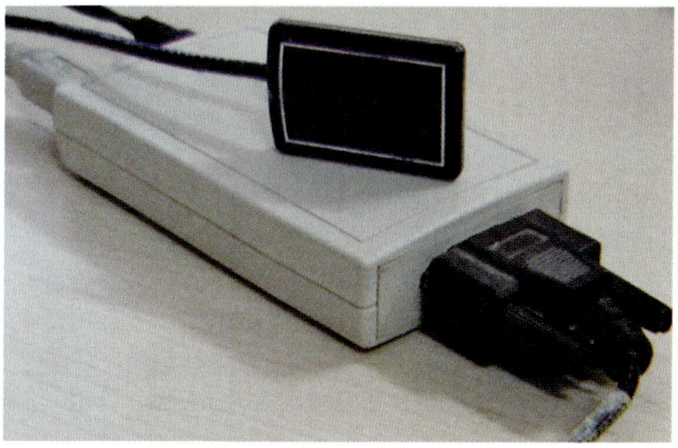

**Fig. 6.41:** Sensor used for RVG system

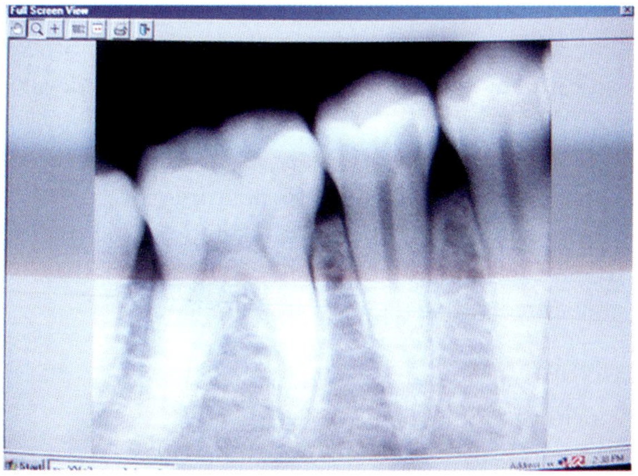

**Fig. 6.42:** Video monitor displaying image

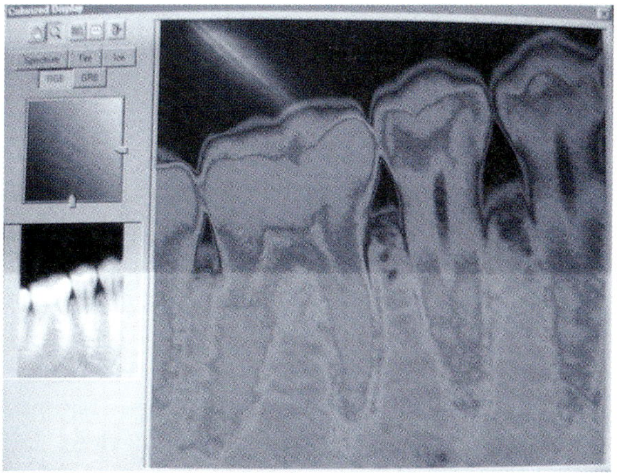

**Fig. 6.43:** Colored image produced in RVG

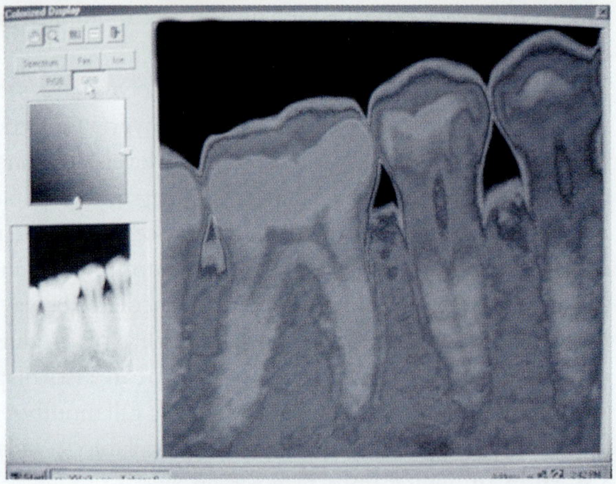

Fig. 6.44: Colored image produced in RVG

apparatus that can be connected to various print out or mass storage devices for immediate or later viewing.

### Advantages

1. Low radiation dose.
2. Increased diagnostic capability through digital enhancement and enlargement of specific areas for closer examination.
3. Elimination of image distortion from bent radiographic film.
4. Possible to alter contrast and resolution.
5. Instant display of images.
6. Filmless X-rays means, no dark room, no messy processing and no any problems/faults associated with developing of film.
7. Full mouth radiographs can be made within seconds.
8. Storages and archiving of patient information.
9. Transfer of images between institutions (teleradiology).
10. Infection control and toxic waste disposal problems associated with radiology are eliminated.

### Disadvantages

1. Expensive
2. Large disc space required to store images.
3. Bulky sensor with cable attachment, which can make placement in mouth difficult.
4. Soft tissue imaging is not very nice.

## PHOSPHOR IMAGING SYSTEM

Imaging which uses photostimulable phosphor is also called an indirect digital imaging technique. The image is captured on a phosphor plate as analogue information and is converted into a digital format when the plate is processed.

Two sizes of phosphor plates (size similar to conventional intraoral film) packets are provided. They have to be placed in plastic light-tight bags, before being placed in the mouth. They are then positioned in the same manner as film packets, using holders, incorporating beam-aiming devices, and are exposed using conventional dental X-ray equipment. The dose is highly reduced. The image is displayed and manipulated. A hard copy can be obtained if necessary.

### Advantages

- Low radiation dose (90% reduction)
- Almost instant image (20-30 seconds)
- Wide exposure latitude (almost impossible to burn out information)
- Same size receptor as films
- X-ray source can be remote from PC
- Image manipulation facilities.

### Disadvantages

- Cost
- Storage of images (same as with CCD systems)
- Inconvenience of plastic bags.

## QUESTION

**Q. Write short notes on:**

a. Pulp vitality tests
b. Thermal test for pulp vitality
c. Recent advances in pulp vitality testing
d. Role of radiograph in endodontics
e. Digital radiography
f. RVG/radiovisiography
g. Electric pulp testing

## BIBLIOGRAPHY


1. Barker BCW, Ehrmann EH. Human pulp reactions to a ducocorticosteroid antibiotic compound. Aust Dent J 1969;14:104-19.
2. Bender IB, Seltzer S. The effect of periodontal disease on the pulp. Oral Surg Oral Med Oral Pathol 1972;33:458-74.
3. Bender IB, Landau MA, et al. The optimum placement-site of the electrode in electric pulp testing of the 12 anterior teeth. J Am Dent Assoc 1989;118:305-10.
4. Bernick S, Nedelman C. Effect of ageing on the human pulp. J Endod 1975;1:88-94.
5. Bernick S. Differences in nerve distribution between erupted and non-erupted human teeth. J Dent Res 1969;43:406-11.
6. Bhasker SN, Rappaport HM. Dental vitality tests and pulp status J Am Dent Assoc 1973;86:409-11.
7. Brannstrom M. The hydrodynamic theory of dentinal pain: Sensation in preparations, caries and dentinal crack syndrome. J Endod 1986;12:453-57.
8. Cave SG, Freer TJ, Podlich HM. Pulp-test responses in orthodontic patients. Aust Orthodont J 2002;18:27-34.
9. Chilton NW, Fertig JW. Pulpal responses of bilateral intact teeth. Oral Surg Oral Med Oral Pathol 1972;33:797-800.
10. Cooley RL, Barkmeier WW. An alternative to electric pulp testing. Quint Int 1977;8:23-25.
11. Cooley RL, Robison EF. Variables associated with electric pulp testing. Oral Surg, Oral Med Oral Pathol 1980;50:66-73.
12. Degering CI. Physiological evaluation of dental pulp testing methods. J Dent Res 1962;41:695-700.
13. Dummer PMH, Tanner M. The response of caries-free, unfilled teeth to electrical Excitation: A comparison of two new pulp testers. Int Endod J 1986;19:172-77.

14. Dummer PMH, et al. A laboratory study of four electric pulp testes. Int Endod J 1986;19:161-71.
15. Dummer PMH, Hicks R, Huws D. Clinical signs and symptoms in pulp disease. Int Endod J 1980;13:27-35.
16. Cotti E, Campisi G, Garau V, Puddu G. A new technique for the study of periapical bone lesion; ultrasound real time imaging international Endodontic Journal 2002;148-52.
17. Ehrmann EH. Pulp testers and pulp testing with particular reference to the use of dry ice. Aust Dent J 1977;22:272-79.
18. Eli I. Dental Anxiety: A cause for possible misdiagnosis of tooth vitality. Int Endod J 1993;26:251-53.
19. Fanibunda KB. The feasibility of temperature measurement as a diagnostic procedure in human teeth. J Dent 1986;14:126-29.
20. Fuss Z, Trowbridge H, et al. Assessment of reliability of electrical and thermal pulp testing agents. J Endod 1986; 12:301-05
21. Garfunkel A, Sela A, Ulmansky M. Dental pulp pathosis. Oral Surg Oral Med Oral Pathol 1973;35:110-17.
22. Gazelius B, Olgart I, Edwali B, Edwali L. Nonincasive recording of blood flow in human dental pulp. Endod Dent traumatol 1986;2:219-21.
23. Harkins SW, Chapman CR. Detection and decision factors in pain perception in young and elderly men. Pain 1976;2:253-64.
24. Harris WE. Endodontic pain referred across the midline: Report of a case. J Am Dent Assoc 1973;87:1240-243.
25. Harris WE. Pseudoendodontic sinus tract; Report of a case. J Am Dent Assoc 1971;83:165-67.
26. Howell RM, Duell RC, Mulllaney TP. The determination of pulp vitality by thermographic means using cholesteric liquid crystals. A preliminary study. Oral Surg Oral Med Oral Pathol 1970;29:763-68.
27. Hyman JJ, Cohen ME, Lakes G. The predictive value of endodontic diagnostic tests. Oral Surg 1984;58:343-46.
28. JS Rhodes, TR Pitt Ford, JA Lynch, PJ Liepens, RV. Curtis microcomputerized tomography: A new tool in experimental endodontology. Int Endod J 1999;32:165-70.
29. Kahan RS, Gulabivala K, Snook M, Setchell DJ. Evaluation of a pulse oximeter and customized probe for pulp vitality testing. J Endod 1996;22.
30. Kaletsky T, Furedi A. Reliability of various types of pulp testers as diagnostic aid. J Am Dent Assoc 1935;22:1559-573.
31. Kells BE, Kennedy JG, Biagioni PA, Lamey PJ. Computerized infrared thermographic imaging and pulpal blood flow: Part 2. Rewarming of healthy human teeth following a controlled cold stimulus. Int Endod J 2000;33:448-62.
32. Kramer IR. The relationship between pain and changes in the dental pulp following the insertion of fillings. Br. Dent J 1954;96:9-13.
33. Krell KV. The effects of $CO_2$ ice on PFM restorations [Abstract]. JOE 1985;11:26.
34. Markowitz K, Kim S. Hypersensitive teeth. Experimental studies of dentinal desensitizing agents. Dent Clin North Am 1990;34:491-501.
35. Marshall FJ. Planning endodontic treatment. Dent Clin North Am 1979;23:495-518.
36. Mesaros SV, Trope M. Revascularization of traumatized teeth assessed by laser Doppler flowmetry: case report. Endod Dent Traumatol 1997;13:24-30.
37. Michaelson RE, Seidberg BH, Guttuso J. An in vivo evaluation of interface media used with the electric pulp tester. J Am Dent Assoc 1975;91:118-21.
38. Mickel AK, Lindquist KAD, Chogle S, Jones JJ, Curd F. Electric pulp tester conductance through various interface media. J Endod 2006;32:1178-80.
39. Mumford JM. Evaluation of gutta-percha and ethyl chloride in pulp-testing. Br Dent J 1964;116:338-43.
40. Myers JW. Demonstration of a possible source of error with an electric pulp tester. J Endod 1998;24:199-200.
41. Narhi MVO. The neurophysiology of the teeth. Dent Clin North Am 1990;34:439-48.
42. Naylor MN. Studies on sensation to cold stimulation in human teeth. Br Dent J 1964;117:482-86.
43. Odor TM, Pitt Ford TR, McDonald F. Effect of wavelength and bandwidth on the clinical reliability of laser Doppler recordings. Ended Dent Traumatol 1996;12:9-15.
44. P. Carrottem Endodontics: part 2 diagnosis and treatment planning. Br Den J 2004;197:231-38.
45. Pantera EA, Anderson RW, Pantera CT. Reliability of electric pulp testing after pulpal testing with dichlorodifluoromethane. J Endod 1993;19:312-14.
46. Peter DD. Evaluation of the effects of carbon dioxide used as a pulp test. Part III. In vivo effect on human enamel. JOE 1986;12:13.
47. Peters DD, Baumgartner JC, Lorton L. Adult pulpal diagnosis 1. Evaluation of the positive and negative responses to cold and electrical pulp tests. J Endod 1994;20:506-11.
48. Rickoff B, Trowbridge H, et al. Effects of thermal vitality tests on human dental pulp. J Endod 1988;14:482-85.
49. Rowe AHR, Pitt Ford TR. The assessment of pulpal vitality. Int Endod J 1990;23:77-83.
50. Rubach WC, Mitchell DE. Periodontal disease, age, and pulp status. Oral Surg Oral Med Oral Pathol 1965;19:482-93.
51. Schnettler JM, Wallace JA. Pulse oximeter as a diagnostic tool of pulp vitality. J Endod 1991;17:488-90.
52. Stark MM, Kempler D, Pelzner RB, Rosenfeld J, Leung RL, Mintatos S. Rationalization of electric pulp testing methods. Oral Surg Oral Med Oral Pathol 1977;43:598-606.
53. Steven A Held, Yi H Kao, Donald W Wells. Endoscope an endodontic application J. Endod 1996;22:327-29.
54. Teitler D, Tzadik D, Efliecer E, Chosack A. A clinical evaluation of vitality tests in anterior teeth following fractures of enamel and dentine. Oral Surg Oral Med Oral Pathol 1972;34:649-52.
55. Tronstad L. Root resorption—Etiology, terminology and clinical manifestations. Endod Dent Traumatol 1988;4:241-52.
56. Van Hassel HJ, Harrington GW. Localisation of pulpal sensation. Oral Surg Oral Med Oral Pathol 1969;28:753-60.
57. Wilder-Smith, PEEB. A new method for the non-invasive measurement of pulpal blood. Int Endod J 1988;21:307-12.
58. Y Kimura, P Wilder-Smithand K. Matsumoto: Lasers in endodontics: A review; international endodontic Journal, 2000;173-85.
59. Yanipiset K, Vongsavan N, Sigurdsson A, Trope M. The efficacy of laser Doppler flowmetry for the diagnosis of revascularization of reimplanted immature dog teeth. Dent Traumatol 2001;17:63-70.
60. Zadik D, Chosack A, Eidelman E. The prognosis of traumatized permanent anterior teeth with fracture of the enamel and dentine. Oral Surg Oral Med Oral Pathol 1979;47:173-75.

# CHAPTER 7

# Differential Diagnosis of Orofacial Pain



## INTRODUCTION

Orofacial pain is the field of dentistry related to diagnosis and management of chronic, complex facial pain and orofacial disorders. The dentist assumes a great responsibility for the proper management of pains in and around the mouth, face and neck. To do this, he or she must have accurate knowledge of pain problems arising from other than oral and maxillofacial area. This specialty in dentistry has been developed over a number of years for diagnosis of orofacial pain which did not seem to have a clearly defined medical problem.

Orofacial pain, like pain elsewhere in the body, is usually the result of tissue damage and the activation of nociceptors, which transmit a noxious stimulus to the brain. Orofacial disorders are complex and difficult to diagnose due to rich innervations in head, face and oral structures. Ninety percent of orofacial pain arises from teeth and adjoining structures. As a dentist, one must be trained to diagnose and treat acute dental pain problems.

After ruling out dental problems, myofacial and neuropathic pain conditions are the most common causes of dental pain. For accurate diagnosis and treatment planning, one must have thorough understanding of basic concepts of pain and its transmission.

## PAIN

***Dorland's Medical Dictionary defines pain as*** "A more or less localized sensation of discomfort, distress or agony resulting from the stimulation of nerve endings." It indicates that pain is a protective mechanism against injury. ***International Association for the Study of Pain (IASP) has defined pain as*** "an unpleasant sensory and emotional experience associated with actual or potential tissue damage, or described in terms of such damage".

It is usually found that the more severe the pain and the more distressed the patient more emotional are his responses leading to greater impact on his ability of function.

## DIAGNOSIS

The most important component of managing pain is in understanding the problem and establishing the proper diagnosis. For establishing the correct diagnosis, the dentist must record all relevant information regarding signs, symptoms, history of present complaint, past medical and dental history. The history is an important part of diagnosis, it should assess the present location of the pain, its causative and aggravating factors and a detailed description of the pain since its origin. The clinician should record all the factors related to the pain such as emotional, physical and influence of any prior trauma, infection or systemic illness. For establishing differential diagnosis, an accurate history taking is the most important aspect.

## HISTORY OF PAIN

History of pain includes the following:

### Chief Complaint

- Location
- Onset

- Chronology
- Quality
- Intensity
- Aggravating factors
- Precipitating factors
- Past medical and dental history
- Psychologic analysis
- Review of systems

### *Location*

The patient's ability to locate the pain usually helps in diagnosis but sometimes wrong localization of pain problems for clinician. The patient's description of the location of his or her complaint identifies only site of pain. So, it is the dentist's responsibility to determine whether it is the true source of pain or the referred pain.

### *Onset*

It is important to record the conditions associated with initial onset of pain. Sometimes, it may facilitate in recognizing the etiology of pain.

### *Chronology*

Chronology of pain should be recorded in a following pattern:

- Initiation
- Clinical course and temporal pattern
  A. Mode B. Periodicity
  C. Frequency D. Duration

### *Quality*

It should be classified according to how pain makes the patient feel.

- Dull, grawing or aching
- Throbbing, pounding or pulsating
- Sharp, recurrent or stabbing pain
- Squeezing or crushing pain.

### *Intensity*

Intensity of pain is usually established by distinguishing between mild, moderate and severe pain. A visual analog scale is used to assess the intensity of pain. The patient is given a line on which no pain is written on one end and at other end there is most severe pain which patient has experienced. A scale of 0-10 is used to assess the pain, 0-being no pain while 10-being the maximum pain possible.

- Pain index : 0-10 (Fig. 7.1)
- Pain classification : Mild
  Moderate
  Severe

## Aggravating Factors

Aggravating factors always help the clinician in diagnosis. These can be local or conditional. Local factors can be in form of irritants like heat, cold, sweets and pain on biting, etc. Conditional factors include change of posture, activities and hormonal changes, etc.

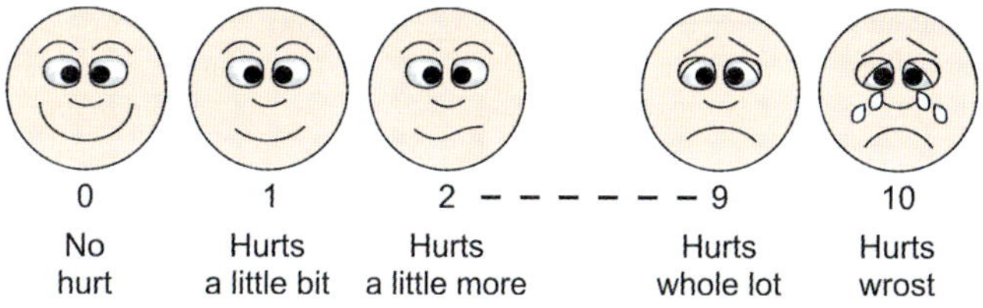


**Fig. 7.1:** Rating scale to check intensity of pain ranging from (0-10)

| *Local factors* | *Conditional factors* |
|---|---|
| • Sweets | • Change of posture |
| • Chewing | • Time of day |
| • Palpation | • Activities |
| • Heat | • Hormonal |
| • Cold | |
| • Percussion | |

## TRANSMISSION OF PAIN

Pain sensation from the intraoral and extraoral structures of the head and face are carried to central nervous system by trigeminal system. The term "***trigeminal system***" refers to complex arrangement of nerve fibers, synaptic connections and interneurons which process incoming information from three divisions of the trigeminal nerve. Sensory information from the face and oral cavity (except proprioception) is carried out by primary afferent neurons. These neurons further transmit information to higher centers by forming synapses on neurons located within the trigeminal brainstem complex, which span the midbrain and cervical spinal cord. This complex receives afferent input primarily from trigeminal nerve, it also receives afferent axons from the facial, glossopharyngeal, vagus and upper cervical nerves ($C_2$, $C_3$). The connection between the upper cervical nerves and trigeminal spinal tract nucleus may perhaps be a mechanism involved in facial pain and headaches. The trigeminal brainstem sensory nuclear complex can be separated into trigeminal main sensory nucleus and trigeminal spinal tract nucleus. The spinal tract nucleus is composed of three separate nuclei proceeding from superior to inferior (caudal) direction (Fig. 7.2).

- Subnucleus oralis
- Subnucleus interpolaris
- Subnucleus caudalis

***Subnucleus caudalis,*** the most inferior one is located in the medulla, at times extending to level of $C_2$ and $C_3$ and is the principal brain relay site of nociceptive information arising from the orofacial region (Fig. 7.3). Because the subnucleus caudalis is continuous and structurally similar to spinal cord dorsal horn and it also extends into the medulla. So, it is often referred to as the medullary dorsal horn. Both incoming nociceptive signals to subnucleus caudalis and projected nociceptive signals on their way to the thalamus can be modified by descending nerve fibers from higher levels of the central nervous system or by drugs.

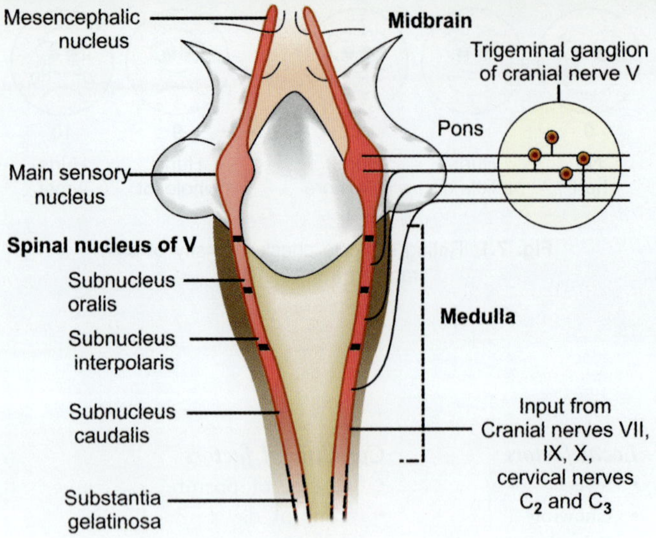


**Fig. 7.2:** Trigeminal brainstem sensory nuclear complex

### *Convergence of neurons with in the trigeminal spinal tract*

Primary nociceptors from both visceral and cutaneous neurons often converge onto the same second-order pain transmission neurons in the spiral cord. In many cases, the brain is unable to interpret the exact location of the original oral stimulus for example early stages of pulpal pain. In an inflammatory or pain process, a signal is sent only when a certain critical level of insult is reached, for example in cases of deep caries.

The brain may appreciate that there is toothache somewhere but cannot localize it and due to convergence factors, the brain may experience more difficulty in localizing the pain.

## Second Order Neurons

These neurons can be classified into three types of transmission cells (Fig. 7.4).

1. Wide dynamic range (WDR) neurons
2. Nociceptive-specific (NS) neurons
3. Low threshold mechanoreceptive (LTM) neurons

### *1. Wide Dynamic Range (WDR) Neurons*

These neurons are excited by both noxious stimuli and non-noxious tactile stimuli over a wide range of intensities.

### *2. Nociceptive-specific (NS) Neurons*

These neurons are excited by intense noxious mechanical and thermal stimuli by thin nociceptive fibers.

The WDR and NS neurons predominate in laminar I, II, V, and comprise the trigeminal nociceptive pathways. They all receive input from cutaneous structures and at least half of them receive input from deep structures of the mouth and face also (Fig. 7.5).

### *3. Low Threshold Mechanoreceptive (LTM)*

These neurons are normally non-nociceptive and respond to light tactile stimuli. They mainly lie in laminar III and IV. These neurons appear to be excited by strong electrical stimulation of tooth pulp and may involve in pathological conditions of pulp.

## Third Order Neurons

The next major synaptic transmission in pain transmission is in the thalamus where axons travelling in trigeminothalamic tract synapse with third order neurons. All sensory information from

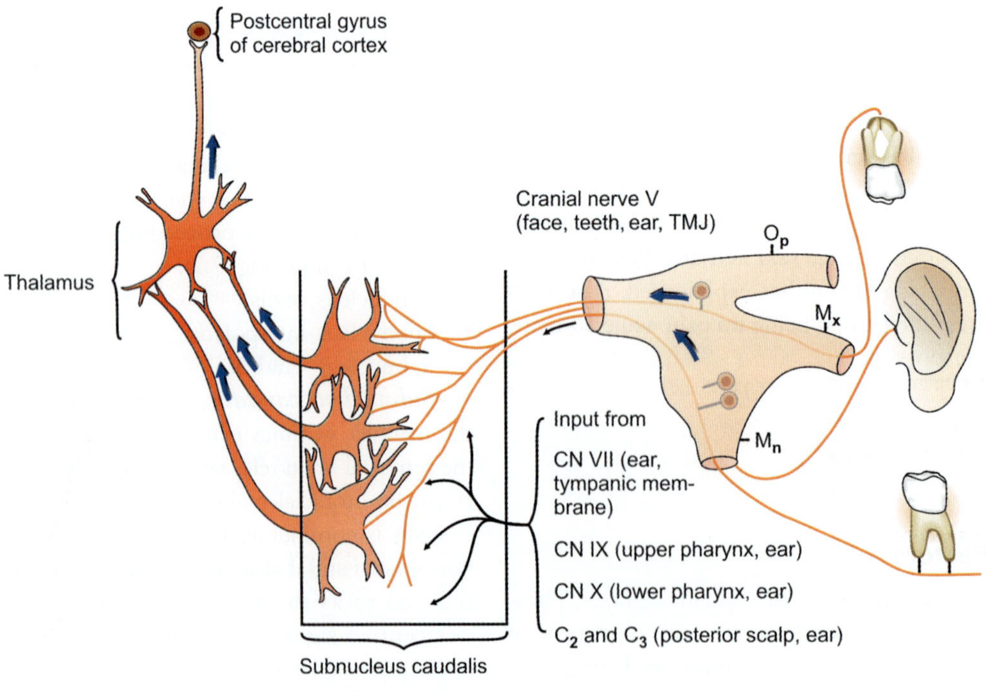


**Fig. 7.3:** Diagram showing subnucleus caudalis

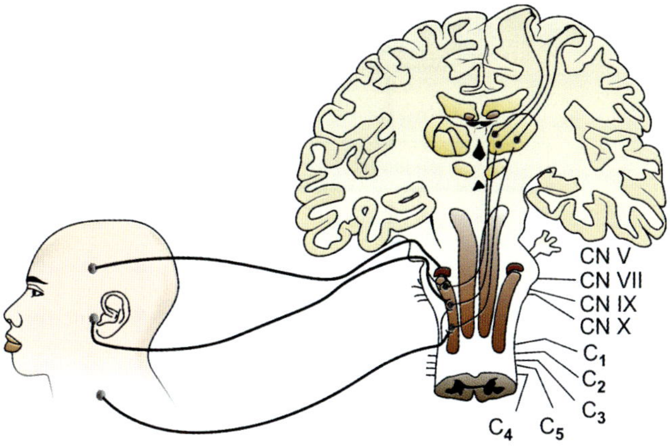


**Fig. 7.4:** Second order neurons showing pain transmission

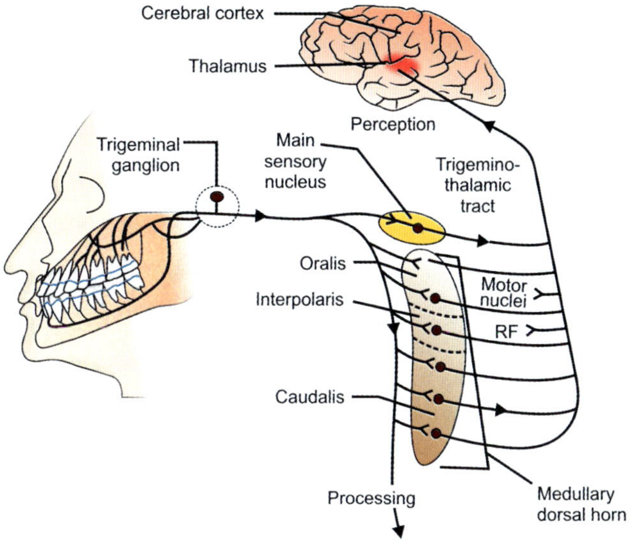


**Fig. 7.5:** Pathway of transmission of nociceptive signals from the orofacial region

spinal cord and brainstem passes through the thalamus making it one of the primary relay stations between the brainstem and different parts of the somatosensory cerebral cortex (Fig. 7.6). For all nerve pathways from the thalamus to the cerebral cortex, there are reciprocal connections from the cortex to the thalamus. Sensory information reaching the thalamus may also be relayed to several distinct nuclei in the thalamus.

At the thalamic level, the action potential will be subjected to extensive processing through interactions among its various nuclei and by interconnections with limbic, hypothalamic and cortical regions of the brain. It should be noted that until the nociceptive signal reaches the level of the thalamus, most of the reactions in the CNS are reflex in nature. Only when thalamus is involved, elements of consciousness and alertness introduced.

## PAIN MODULATION AND PERCEPTION

***Modulation is defined*** as the ability to alter the intensity of nociceptive signals and reduce the pain experience. In human nervous system, the key pathways start in periqueductal gray area of midbrain. The signals from this area descend to dorsal horn of spinal cord where neuron interactions further reduce the transmission of primary pain signal from the peripheral nociceptive receptors to the second order neuron.

Finally, the perception of pain takes place in the posterior parietal cortex of the brain. The differences in the size of sensory map on the brain reflect the differences in functional importance.

Orofacial pain can be basically divided into odontogenic (dental pain) and nonodontogenic pain (nondental). Dental pain may have origin in the pulpal tissue or the periradicular tissue. *Nondental pain can be in form of myofacial toothache, vascular headache, cluster headache, sinusitis, trigeminal neuralgia.*

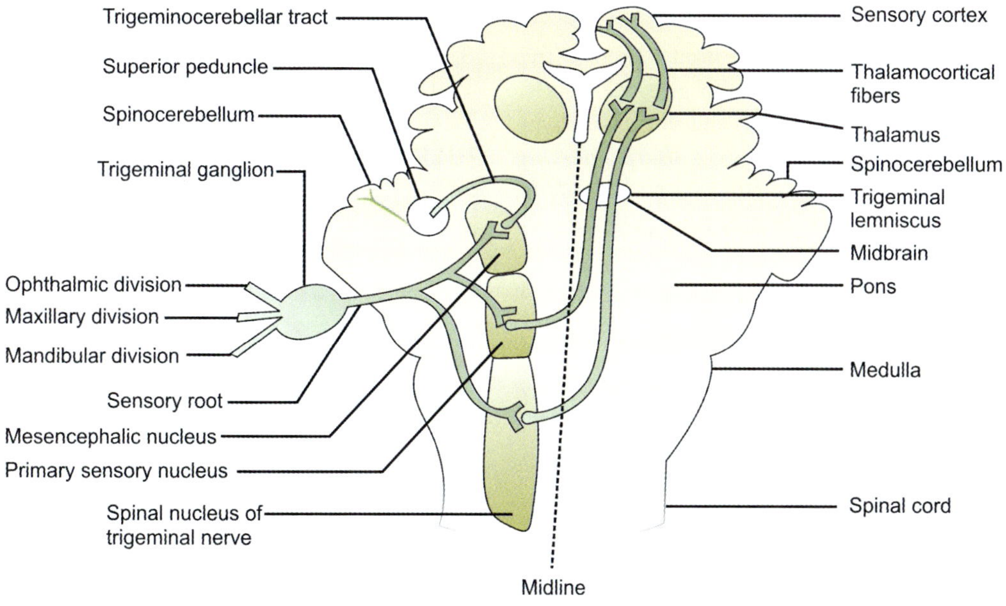


**Fig. 7.6:** Trigeminal pathway

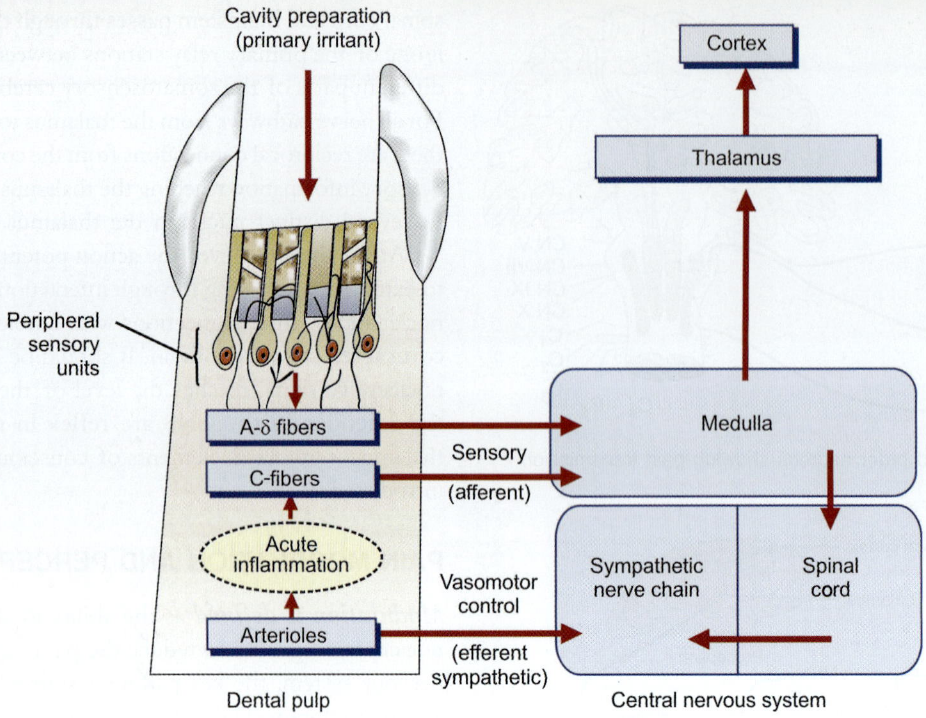


**Fig. 7.7:** Neurophysiology of pulpal pain

## SOURCES OF ODONTOGENIC PAIN

### a. Dental Pain of Pulpal Origin

Dental pulp is richly innervated by A and C nerve fibers. The nerves of the pulp include primary afferent fibers that are involved in pain transmission and sympathetic efferent fibers which modulate the microcirculation of the pulp. The sympathetic efferent fibers reduce the flow of the blood through pulp by stimulating smooth muscle cells encircling the arterioles. Also, four types of nerve endings are present in pulp:

a. Marginal fibers
b. Simple predentinal fibers
c. Complex predentinal fibers
d. Dentinal fibers

Both pain and touch sensations have been related to free nerve endings but stimulation of the pulp give rise only to pain. Fast pain is associated with A-fibers and slow pain is with C-fibers. ***Stimulation of A-fibers produce a sharp, piercing or stabbing sensation while C-fibers produce dull, burning, and aching sensation that is usually harder to endure*** (Fig. 7.7).

The pulpal pain is of threshold type, that is, no response occurs until threshold level is increased. Pulp may respond to chemical, mechanical, electrical or thermal stimulation but not to ordinary masticatory functions. Pulpal pain cannot be localized by the patient. A basic feature of pain of pulpal origin is that it does not remain the same for long periods. Generally it resolves, becomes chronic or involves the periodontal structure.

### b. Dental Pain of Periodontal Origin

Periodontal pain is deep somatic pain of the musculoskeletal type because of presence of proprioceptor fibers. Patient can localize the pain of periodontal origin. Therefore, periodontal pain presents no diagnostic problems because the offending tooth can be readily identified. This localization can be identified by applying pressure to the tooth axially and laterally.

When the periodontal pain involves many teeth, one may consider occlusal overstressing which could be due to occlusal interferences or parafunctional habits such as bruxism.

**Sources of odontogenic pain**

***Pulpal pain***

| | |
|---|---|
| 1. Dentinal sensitivity | 2. Reversible pulpitis |
| 3. Irreversible pulpitis | 4. Necrotic pulp |

***Periodontal pain***

| | |
|---|---|
| 1. Acute apical periodontitis | 2. Acute apical abscess |
| 3. Chronic apical periodontitis | 4. Pericoronitis |
| 5. Periodontal abscess | |

## PULPAL PAIN

### 1. DENTINAL SENSITIVITY

In the absence of inflammation, dentinal sensitivity is the mildest form of pulp discomfort. The pain is often characterized as a short, sharp, shock and it is brought on by some stimulating factor such as hot or cold, sweet, sour, acid or touch. It is not pathologic, but is rather, fluid flow in the dentinal tubules which stretches or compresses the nerve endings that pass alongside the tubular extensions of the pulp odontoblasts.

Dentinal sensitivity may also develop when dentin is exposed from gingival recession or following periodontal surgery. Nerves in these exposed tubules not only respond to hot, cold, sweet and sour but also to scratching with a finger nail or during tooth brushing.

### Diagnosis

1. Apply the irritant which starts the painful reaction-hot or cold, sweet or sour or scratching with an instrument.
2. All diagnostic tests such as electric pulp test, percussion and radiographs give normal response.

### Treatment

After diagnosis, dentinal hypersensitivity can be treated by home use of desensitizing dentifrices containing strontium chloride, fluorides and potassium nitrate. Since rapid movement of fluid in the dentinal tubules is responsible for pain by activating intradental sensory nerves, the treatment of hypersensitive teeth should be aimed at reducing the anatomical diameter of the tubules so as to limit the fluid movement. Various agents can be use to occlude the dentinal tubules like varnishes, calcium compounds, fluoride compounds like sodium fluoride, stannous fluoride, iontophoresis, restorative resins and dentin bonding agents.

## 2. REVERSIBLE PULPITIS

In reversible pulpitis, pain occurs when a stimulus (usually cold or sweets) is applied to the tooth. When the stimulus is removed, the pain ceases with in 1 to 2 second, i.e. it should return to normal with removal of cause. The common causes of reversible pulpitis are caries, faulty restorations, trauma or any recent restorative procedures. Pulpal recovery is usually seen if reparative cells in the pulp are adequate.

### Diagnosis

Diagnosis is made by careful history and clinical examination. If there is discrepancy between the patient's chief complaint, symptoms and clinical examination, obtain more information from the patient. It is important to note that both pulpal and periapical diagnosis should be made before treatment is initiated. If tooth is sensitive to percussion, then look for bruxism and hyperocclusion.

### Treatment

1. Removal of the cause if present (caries, fractured restoration, exposed dentinal tubules).
2. If recent operative procedure or trauma has taken place, then postpone the additional treatment and observe the tooth.
3. If pulp exposure is detected, go for root canal treatment.

## 3. IRREVERSIBLE PULPITIS

Irreversible pulpitis develops, if inflammatory process progresses to involve pulp. Patient may have history of spontaneous pain or exaggerated response to hot or cold that lingers even after the stimulus is removed. The involved tooth usually presents an extensive restoration and/or caries.

### Diagnosis

Diagnosis is usually made after taking thorough history and clinical examination of the patient.

1. Patient usually gives a history of spontaneous pain.
2. Tooth is hypersensitive to hot or cold that is prolonged in duration.
3. Pulp may be vital or partially vital.
4. In certain cases of irreversible pulpitis, the patient may arrive at the dental clinic with a glass of ice/cold water. In these cases, cold actually alleviates the patient's pain and thus, can be used as a diagnostic test. Cooling of the dentin and the resultant contraction of the fluid in the tubules relieves the pressure on pulpal nerve fibers caused by edema and inflammation of the pulp.

### Treatment

Complete removal of pulpal tissue should be done, i.e. endodontic therapy.

## 4. NECROTIC PULP

It results from continued degeneration of an acutely inflamed pulp. Literal meaning of necrosis is death, that is pulpal tissue becomes dead because of untreated pulpal inflammation. In pulpal necrosis, there is progressive breakdown of cellular organization with no reparative function. It is frequently associated with apical radiolucent lesion. In case of multirooted teeth, one root may contain partially vital pulp, whereas other roots may be nonvital.

### Diagnosis

1. Tooth is usually asymptomatic; may give moderate to severe pain on biting pressure (It is not symptom of necrotic pulp but it indicates inflammation).
2. Pulp tests show negative response but in case of multirooted teeth, it can give false positive results.

### Treatment

Complete removal of pulpal tissue that is root canal treatment.

## PERIODONTAL PAIN

## 1. ACUTE APICAL PERIODONTITIS

It is the inflammation of periodontal ligament which is caused by tissue damage, extension of pulpal pathology or occlusal trauma. Tooth may be elevated out of the socket because of the built up fluid pressure in the periodontal ligament. Pain remains until the bone is resorbed, fluid is drained or irritants are removed.

### Diagnosis

1. Check for decay, fracture lines, swelling, hyperocclusion or sinus tracts.
2. Patient has moderate to severe pain on percussion.
3. Mobility may or may not be present.
4. Pulp tests are essential and their results must be correlated with other diagnostic information in order to determine if inflammation is of pulpal origin or from occlusal trauma.
5. Radiographs may show no change or widening of periodontal ligament space in some cases.

### Treatment

1. Complete removal of pulp.
2. Occlusal adjustment.

## 2. ACUTE PERIAPICAL ABSCESS

Acute periapical abscess is an acute inflammation of periapical tissue characterized by localized accumulation of pus at the apex of a tooth. It is a painful condition that results from an advanced necrotic pulp. Patients usually relate previous painful episode from irreversible pulpitis or necrotic pulp. Swelling, tooth mobility and fever are seen in advanced cases.

### Diagnosis

1. Spontaneous dull, throbbing or persistent pain is present.
2. Tooth is extremely sensitive to percussion.
3. Mobility may be present.
4. On palpation, tooth may be sensitive.
5. Vestibular or facial swelling in seen in these patients.
6. Pulp tests show negative results.

### Treatment

1. Drainage
2. Complete extirpation of pulp.
3. Appropriate analgesics and antibiotics if necessary.

## 3. CHRONIC APICAL PERIODONTITIS

It is caused by necrotic pulp which results from prolonged inflammation that erodes the cortical plate making a periapical lesion visible on the radiograph. The lesion contains granulation tissue consisting of fibroblasts and collagen.

### Diagnosis

1. It is usually asymptomatic but in acute phase may cause a dull, throbbing pain.
2. Pulp tests show nonvital pulp.
3. There is no pain on percussion.
4. Radiographically, it is usually associated with periradicular radiolucent changes.

## 4. PERIODONTAL ABSCESS

Acute periodontal abscess develops from and virulent infection of an existing periodontal pocket. It can also occur because of apical extension of infection from gingival pocket.

### Diagnosis

- Tooth is tender to lateral percussion
- When sinus tract is traced using gutta-percha, it points towards the lateral aspect of the tooth.

### Treatment

- Root planning and curettage.

## 5. Pericoronitis

It is inflammation of the periodontal tissues surrounding the erupting third molar.

### Diagnosis

- Deep pain which radiates to ear and neck.
- May be associated with trismus.

### Treatment

Operculectomy and surgical removal of tooth if required.

## SOURCES OF NONODONTOGENIC PAIN

As dental pain is considered one of the commonest cause of orofacial pain, so dentist can be easily drawn to diagnosis of pain of odontogenic origin. Tooth aches of nondental origin are usually suspected when patient convincingly reports that pain is usually felt in this particular tooth. But dentist should be aware of this fact that some tooth aches felt in the tooth/teeth do not originate from these structures. There are many structures in the head and neck region which can stimulate pain. Such types of pain are classified under heterotrophic pain. Heterotrophic pain can be defined as any pain felt in an area other than its true source.

There are three general types of pain:

i. Central pain
ii. Projected pain
iii. Referred pain.

**Referred pain** is a heterotrophic pain that is felt in an area innervated by a different nerve, from the one that mediates the primary pain. Referred pain is wholly dependent upon the original source of pain. It cannot be provoked by stimulation where the pain is felt while it can be accentuated only by stimulation the area where primary source of pain is present. Referred pain can be of odontogenic or nonodontogenic origin.

### Odontogenic Referred Pain

In this pain originates from pulpally involved tooth and is referred to adjacent teeth/tooth or proximating deep and superficial structures. For example, pain from pulpal involvement of mandibular second or third molar is referred to ear. This pain is diagnosed by selective anesthesia technique.

### Nonodontogenic Referred Pain

In this pain originates from deep tissues, muscles, joints, ligaments, etc. and is perceived at a site away from its origin. Pain arising from musculoskeletal organs is deep, dull, aching and diffuse type. Pain form cutaneous origin is of sharp, burning and localized. (For example, pain of maxillary sinusitis and may result pain in maxillary premolars.)

## Myofascial Toothache

Any deep somatic tissue in the head and neck region has tendency to induce referral pain in the teeth. In these structures, pains of muscular origin appear to be the most common. Muscles which are commonly affected are masseter, temporalis but in some cases medial, and lateral pterygoid and digastric muscles are also affected.

***Characteristic Findings of Muscular Toothache are:***

1. Non-pulsatile, diffuse, dull and constant pain.
2. Pain increases with function of masticatory muscles. For example, pain is increased when chewing is done because of effect on masseter muscle.
3. Palpation of the involved muscles at specific points (trigger points) may induce pain.
   *Trigger points are hyperexcitable muscle tissues which may feel like taut bands or knots.
4. Usually arise with or without pulpal or periradicular pathology.
5. Tooth pain is not relieved by anesthetizing the tooth; rather local anesthesia given at affected muscle may reduce the toothache.

***Diagnosis*** of these muscular pains as nonodontogenic tooth is purely based on lack of symptoms after diagnostic tests such as pulp testing, percussion and local anesthesia block.

Several therapeutic options used in the ***management*** of these muscular pain are:

i. Restriction of functional activities within painless limit
ii. Occlusal rearrangement
iii. Deep massage
iv. Spray and stretch technique
v. Ultrasound therapy
vi. Local anesthesia at the site of trigger points
vii. Analgesics
viii. Anxiolytics.

### Neurovascular Toothache

The most common neurovascular pain in the mouth and face is migraine. This category of pain includes three subdivisions of primary headache. These are:

i. Migraine
ii. Tension type headache
iii. Cluster headache.

These neurovascular entities can produce relatively localized pains that match with sign and symptoms with the toothache. These accompanying toothaches are usually mistaken for true odontogenic pains and can be treated as separate entities. Unfortunately there are several clinical characteristics that could misguide clinician in diagnosis and treatment.

The ***following characteristics*** are usually found common in ***neurovascular toothache*** are:

1. The pain is ***deep, throbbing, spontaneous*** in onset, variable in nature and pulsatile. These are characteristics which simulate pulpal pain.
2. The ***pain*** is predominantly ***unilateral***.
3. Accompanying ***toothache*** shows periods of ***remission*** that imitates the pain-free episodes or temporal behavior found in neurovascular pain.
4. ***Headache*** is considered as the main symptom. It is most often accompanied by toothache.
5. ***Recurrence*** is characteristic finding in neurovascular pain. Sometimes, the pain may undergo remission after dental treatment has been performed in these teeth. It usually appears for certain period of time and may even spread to adjacent teeth, opposing teeth or the entire face.
6. ***Autonomic effects*** such as nasal congestion, lacrimation, rhinorrhea and edema of the eyelids and face is seen. Sometimes edema of the eyelids and face might lead to confusion in diagnosis as these features bear a resemblance to abscess.

#### Migraine

Migraine has been divided into two main types:

1. Migraine with aura.
2. Migraine without aura.

### Features of Migraine

- Commonly found between the age group ***20-40 years***.
- ***Visual auras*** are most common. These usually occur 10-30 minutes prior to the onset of headache pain. (Migraine with aura.)
- Pain is usually unilateral, pulsatile or throbbing in nature
- More common in ***females***
- Patient usually experiences nausea, vomiting, photophobia
- Various drugs used in the ***management*** of migraine are sumatriptan, β-blockers, tricyclic antidepressants and calcium channel blockers.

## CLUSTER HEADACHE

- Commonly found in the age group 20-50 years
- Cluster headaches derive their name from the temporal behavior and usually occur in series, i.e. one to eight attacks per day
- More common in males than females
- Pain is unilateral, excruciating and continuous in nature and usually found in orbital, supraorbital or temporal region
- Autonomic symptoms such as nasal stuffiness, lacrimation, rhinorrhea or edema of eyelids and face are usually found
- Standard treatment is inhalation of 100 percent oxygen.

The behavior of neurovascular variants should be well appreciated to avoid any unnecessary treatment and frustration felt by patient and clinician. Although the term neurovascular toothache is nondescriptive, but it has given the dentist an important clinical entity that has been misdiagnosed and mistreated in the past. Some sign and symptoms of neurovascular headache that mimic the toothache are:

- Periodic and recurrent nature
- Precise recognition of painful tooth
- Absence of local dental etiology.

## CARDIAC TOOTHACHE

Severe referred pain felt in mandible and maxilla from area outside the head and neck region is most commonly from the heart. ***Cardiac pain is clinically characterized by heaviness, tightness or throbbing pain in the substernal region which commonly radiates to left shoulder, arm, neck and mandible.*** Cardiac pain is most commonly experienced on the left side rather than right. In advanced stages, the patient may complain of severe pain and rubs the jaw and chest. In present time, dentist should be aware of incidence of jaw pain that is occurring in number of patients secondary to cardiac pain.

Sometimes, patient presents dental complaints as the chief complaint rather than having pain in substernal region, it creates confusion in diagnosis for dental pain. A lack of dental cause for dental pain should always be an alerting sign. Anesthetizing the lower jaw or providing dental treatment does not decrease the tooth pain, it indicates that primary source of pain is not the tooth. ***Usually the cardiac toothache is decreased by taking rest or a dose of sublingual nitroglycerin.*** A complete medical history should be taken when cardiac toothache is suspected and should be immediately referred to cardiac unit in hospital.

In brief, the following characteristics of cardiac toothache are:

1. Pain is of sudden in onset, gradually increasing in intensity, diffuse with cyclic pattern that vary in intensity from mild to severe.
2. Tooth pain is increased with physical activities.
3. Chest pain is usually associated.
4. Pain is not relieved by anesthesia of lower jaw or by giving analgesics.

## NEUROPATHIC PAIN

Neuropathic pain is usually caused by abnormalities in the neural structures themselves. Neuropathic pain is sometimes misdiagnosed as psychogenic pain because local factors cannot be visualized.

Neuropathic pain can be classified into different categories:

i. Neuralgia
ii. Neuritis
iii. Neuropathy

### Neuralgia

***Paroxysmal, unilateral, severe, stabbing or lancinating pain,*** usually are the characteristics of all ***paroxysmal neuralgias.*** The pain is usually of short duration and lasts for few seconds.

### Trigeminal Neuralgia

- It is also known as **"Tic Doulourex"** which has literal meaning of ***painful jerking***
- Usually characterized by paroxysmal, unilateral, sharp, lancinating pain typically confined to one or more branches of 5th cranial nerve
- Even slight stimulation of "Trigger points" may elicit sharp, shooting pain
- Sometimes trigger points are present intraorally. These are stimulated upon chewing which may led to diagnosis of odontogenic pain. Intraoral trigger points always create confusion in diagnosis if not properly evaluated
- Local anesthesia given at the trigger point reduces the attacks
- It rarely crosses midline
- Frequently occur in persons over the age of 50 years
- Attacks generally do not occur at night
- Absence of dental etiology along with symptoms of paroxysmal, sharp, shooting pain always alert the dentist to include neuralgia in the differential diagnosis
- ***Treatment*** includes surgical and medicinal. Usually medicinal approach is preferred. It includes administration of carbamazepine, baclofen, phenytoin sodium and gabapentin, etc.

### Neuritis

***Neuritis literally means inflammation of nerve.*** It is usually observed as heterotopic pain in the peripheral distribution of the affected nerve. It may be caused by traumatic, bacterial and viral infection. In neuritis, the inflammatory process elevates the threshold for pricking pain but lowers it for burning pain. The characteristics of pain in neuritis are:

1. Pain has a characteristic burning quality along with easily localization of the site.
2. It may be associated with other sensory effects such as hyperesthesia, hypoesthesia, paresthesia, dysesthesia and anesthesia.
3. Pain is non-pulsatile in nature.
4. Pain may vary in intensity.

***Peripheral neuritis*** is an inflammatory process occurring along the course of never trunk secondary to traumatic, bacterial, thermal or toxic causes. Neuritis of superior dental plexus has been reported when inflammation of sinus is present. The dental nerves frequently lie just below the lining mucosa or are separated by very thin osseous structure. These nerves are easily involved due to direct extension. Symptoms usually seen along with antral disease are pain, paresthesia and anesthesia of a tooth, gingiva or area supplied by infraorbital nerve. ***Mechanical nerve trauma*** is more common in oral surgery cases. It usually arises from inflammation of the inferior dental nerve either due to trauma or infection.

***Acute neuritis cases are always misdiagnosed and remain untreated***. Most of the times, dental procedures are done to decrease the symptoms of neuritis as these are difficult to diagnose. These unnecessary dental procedures further act as aggravating factors for neuritis, making it chronic.

## TREATMENT OF NEURITIS

- Treatment of acute neuritis is based on its etiology
- If bacterial source is present, antibiotics are indicated
- If viral infection is suspected, antiviral therapy should be started
- If there is no infections, steroids should be considered.

### Neuropathy

***This is the term used for localized and sustained pain secondary to an injury or change in neural structure***. Atypical odontalgia has been included in neuropathy. Atypical odontalgia means toothache of unknown cause. It is also known as ***"Phantom tooth pain"*** or ***"dental migraine"***. Most patients who report with atypical odontalgia usually have multiple dental procedures completed before reaching a final diagnosis.

**Different type of conditions along with nature of pain, aggravating factors and duration**

| *Condition* | *Nature of pain* | *Aggravating factors* | *Duration* |
|---|---|---|---|
| Odontalgia | Stabbing, throbbing intermittent | Hot, Cold, lying down, tooth percussion | Hours to days |
| Trigeminal neuralgia | Lancinating excruciating episodic | Light touch on skin or mucosa | Second to minutes |
| Cluster Headache | Severe ache, episodic retro-orbital component | Sleep, alcohol | Hours |
| Cardiogenic | Temporary pain in left side of mandible, episodic | Exertion | Minutes |
| Sinusitis | Severe ache, throbbing, nonepisodic involving multiple maxillary posterior teeth | Tooth percussion, lowering of head | Hours, days |

## Clinical Characteristics of Neuropathy (Atypical Odontalgia)

1. More common in women.
2. Frequently found in 4th or 5th decades of life.
3. Tooth pain remains constant or unchanged for weeks or months.
4. Constant source of pain in tooth with no local etiology.
5. Pain usually felt in these patients is – dull, aching and persistent.
6. Most commonly affected teeth are maxillary premolar and molar region.
7. Response to local anesthesia is equal in both pulpal toothache and atypical odontalgia.

## SINUS OR NASAL MUCOSAL TOOTHACHE

Sinus and Nasal Mucosal pain is also another source which can mimic toothache. It is usually expressed as pain throughout the maxilla and maxillary teeth.

Clinical characteristics of sinus or nasal mucosal toothache are:

1. Fullness or pressure below the eyes.
2. Increased pain when palpation is done over the sinus.
3. Increased pain sensation when head is placed lower than the heart.
4. Local anesthesia of referred tooth/teeth does not eliminated pain while topical anesthesia of nasal mucosa will eliminate the pain if etiology lies in nasal mucosa.
5. Different diagnostic aids used to diagnose sinus disease include paranasal sinus view, computed tomography imaging and nasal ultrasound.

## PSYCHOGENIC TOOTHACHE

***This is a category of mental disorders in which a patient may complain of physical condition without the presence of any physical signs.***

In these cases, always think of psychogenic toothache. No damage to local tissue is typical in heterotrophic pain entities.

It must be noted that psychogenic pain is rare. So, all other possible diagnoses must be ruled out before making the diagnosis of psychogenic pain.

The following features are usually found in these diseases are:

1. Pain is observed in multiple teeth.
2. Precipitated by severe psychological stress.
3. Frequent changes in character, location and intensity of pain.
4. Response to therapy varies which can include lack of response or unusual response.
5. Usually referred to ***psychiatrist*** for further management.

## QUESTION

**Q. Write short notes on:**

a. Dentin hypersensitivity
b. Enumerate sources of odontogenic pain
c. Acute periapical abscess
d. Enumerate sources of nonodontogenic pain
e. Trigeminal neuralgia
f. Referred pain.

## BIBLIOGRAPHY


1. Barber J. Rapid induction analgesia: A clinical report. Am J Clin Hypn 1977;19:138.
2. Fearnhead RW. Histological evidence for the innervation of human dentine. I Anat 1957;91(2):267-77.
3. Fordyce WE. An operant conditioning method for managing chronic pain. Postgrad Med 1973;53:123.
4. Hargreaves KM, et al. Adrenergic regulation of capsaicin-sensitive neurons in dental pulp J Endod 2003;29(6):397-9.
5. Henry MA, Hargreaves KM. Peripheral mechanism of odontogenic pain. Dent Clin North Am 2007;51(1):19-44.
6. Julius D, Basbaum AI. Molecular mechanisms of nociception. Nature 2001;413(6852):203-10.
7. Merrill RL. Central mechanisms of orofacial pain Dent Clin. North Am 2007;51(1):45-59.
8. Merrill RL. Orofacial pain mechanisms and their clinical application. Dent Clin North Am 1997;41:167-88
9. Nurmikko TJ. Mechanisms of central pain. Clin J Pain 2000;16:21.
10. Olgart L. Neural Control of pulpal blood flow. Crit Rev Oral Biol Med 1996;7(2):159-71.

# Case Selection and Treatment Planning

CHAPTER 8



## INTRODUCTION

In the past, injured or diseased teeth frequently were indicated for extraction. But now the trend has been changed. The teeth now can be saved through endodontic treatment, because in modern scenario, the clinician as well as the general population is becoming more aware of the importance of natural teeth. Now it has become common practice to make additional efforts to retain the teeth which are pulpally or periradicularly involved. The endodontic therapy has become the recent trend among general population. Infact during conversation the people proudly claim that they have got the root canal done. Especially for last 30-40 years, role of endodontics have broadened in scope. Many factors such as increased awareness among people, development of latest instruments and techniques which further added comfort to both patient as well as clinician, are responsible for this. Infact high predictability of endodontic success plays an important role for its growth. Various studies have shown that if properly done, the success rate of 95 percent can be achieved in endodontic therapy. To further success of endodontic therapy, continuous education programs and professional study along with clinical experience are required.

## WHEN TO DO ENDODONTIC THERAPY?

This is sometimes difficult to decide simply when there is doubt about the case selection for endodontic therapy. Sometimes patients come to clinic having no symptoms with large restorations on teeth which require crowns. But the clinician suggests that endodontic treatment is needed for that particular tooth. So one can say that sometimes decision to do endodontic therapy becomes complicated because of involvement of multiple factors are involved in deciding the need, treatment planning and prognosis of tooth.

Following factors are important in deciding the need and success of the overall endodontic therapy:

### i. Actual Reason for Endodontic Therapy

If there is pulp involvement due to caries, trauma, etc. (Figs 8.1 to 8.3) the tooth must be treated endodontically and restored with proper restoration.

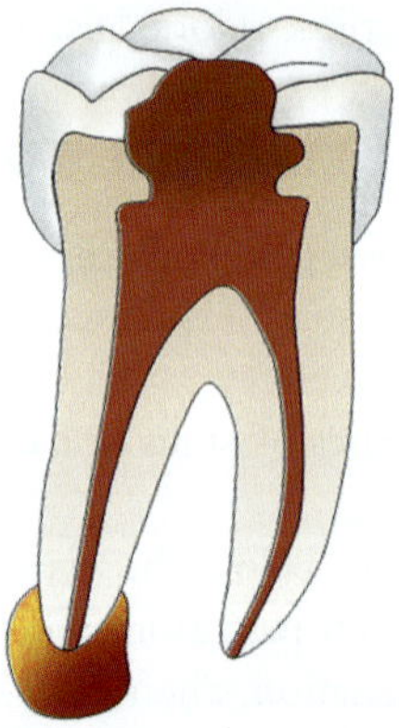

Fig. 8.1: Carious exposure of pulp resulting in pulp necrosis and periapical lesion

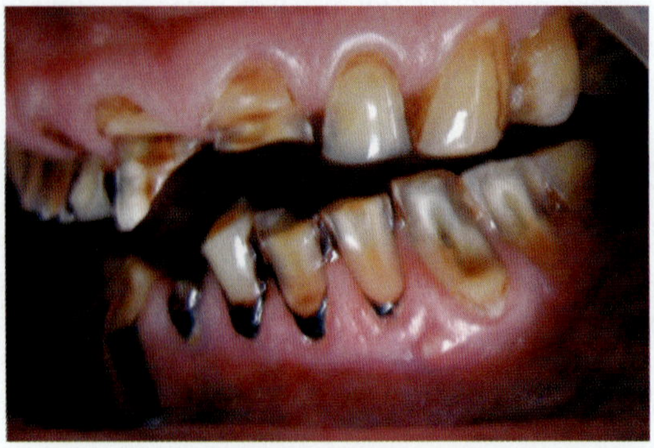

Fig. 8.2: Patient with multiple noncarious pulp exposures

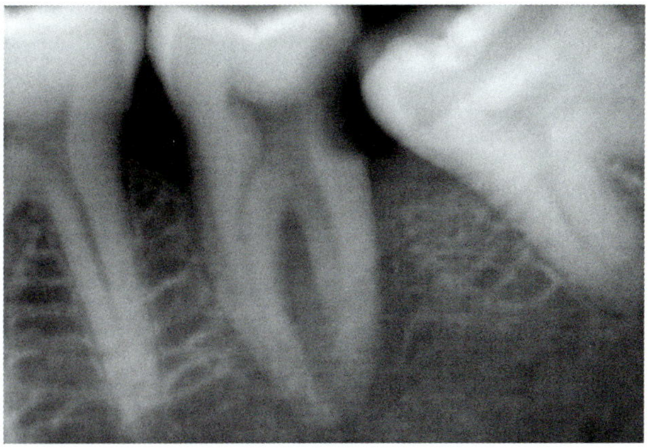

Fig. 8.3: Radiograph showing deep caries in 37 indicating root canal treatment

## ii. Elective Endodontics

Sometimes elective endodontic is done with crack or heavily restored tooth, to prevent premature loss of cusp during their restoration (usually crown preparation) and eliminate fear of pulp exposure (Figs 8.4A to C). Elective endodontics allows to do more predictable and successful restorative dentistry.

## iii. Inadequate Restorations

Patients with cracked or carious teeth having crowns, when want patch up of the crown margins or use pre-existing crown even after another restorative procedures show high degree of restorative failure. In such cases endodontic treatment followed by optimal restoration of the tooth provide high success rate.

## iv. Devitalization of Tooth

In patients with attrited teeth, rampant caries or recurrent decay and smooth surface defects, it is wise to do desensitization of the teeth so that patients do not feel discomfort to cold or sweets (Fig. 8.5).

## v. Endodontic Emergency

Sometimes patient comes with acute dental pain, in such cases endodontic therapy is often indicated before a complete examination and treatment plan has performed. It is important to place endodontic case in perspective with the needs of patient's entire mouth.

# CONTRAINDICATIONS OF ENDODONTIC THERAPY

There are only few true contraindications of the endodontic therapy. Otherwise any tooth can be treated by root canal treatment. Mainly there are following four factors which influence the decision of endodontic treatment:

a. Accessibility of apical foramen.
b. Restorability of the involved tooth.
c. Strategic importance of the involved tooth.
d. General resistance of the patient.

Therefore, before deciding the endodontic treatment, multiple factors should be considered. In general, following cases are considered poor candidates for endodontic treatment:

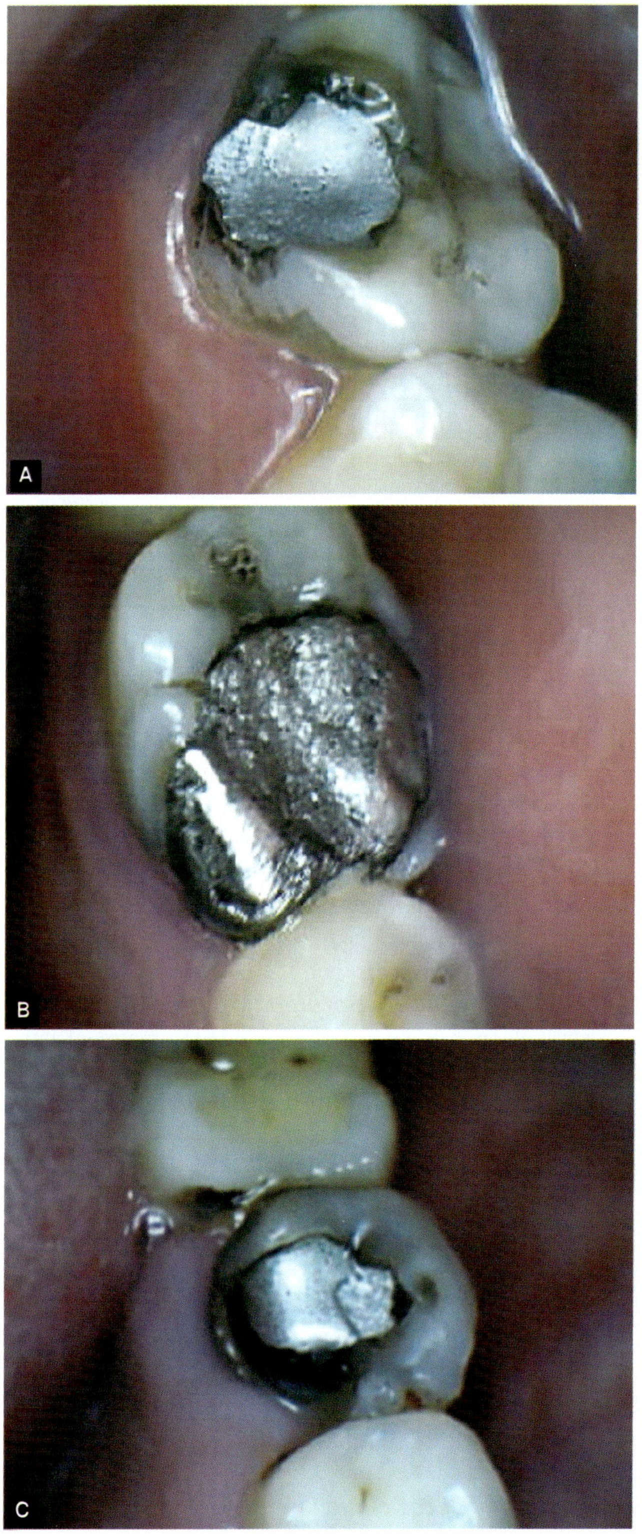


Figs 8.4A to C: Heavily restored teeth sometime indicate elective endodontic therapy

1. ***Non-restorable teeth:*** Such as teeth with extensive root caries, furcation caries, poor crown/root ratio and with fractured root are contraindicated for endodontic treatment. Because in such cases even the best canal filling is futile if it is impossible to place the restoration.
2. ***Teeth in which instrumentation is not possible:*** Such as teeth with sharp curves, dilacerations, calcifications,

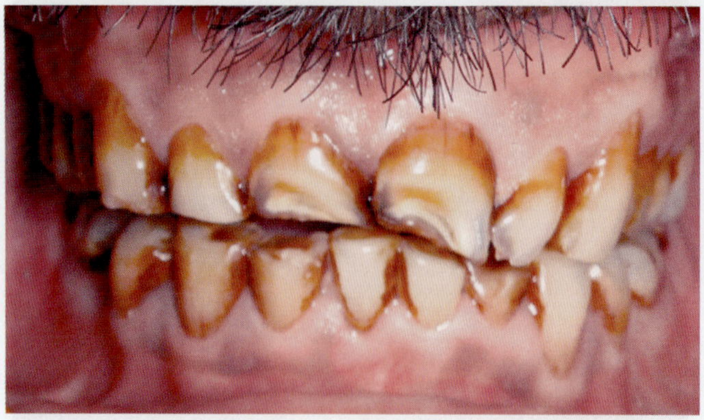

**Fig. 8.5:** When severe attrition of teeth results in sensitivity and discomfort, endodontic treatment is done for desensitization

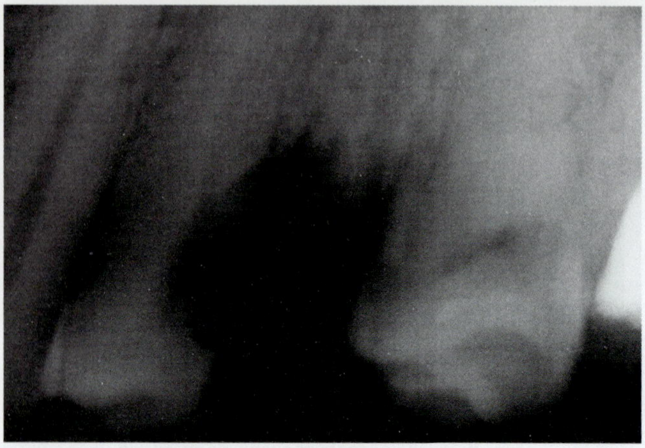

**Fig. 8.6:** Untreatable root resorption

dentinal sclerosis are treatment difficulties. Though use of recent instruments and techniques may help sometimes like NiTi files, anticurvature filing may help sometimes.

Several teeth with previous treatment show canal blockage by broken instruments, fillings, posts, ledges, and untreatable perforations and canal transportations. So, careful evaluation is needed before starting treatment in such teeth.

3. ***Poor accessibility:*** Occasionally trismus or scarring from surgical procedures or trauma, systemic problems, etc. may limit the accessibility due to limited mouth opening. These result in poor prognosis of the endodontic therapy.
4. ***Untreatable tooth resorption:*** Resorptions which are extremely large in size make the endodontic treatment almost impossible for such teeth (Fig. 8.6).
5. ***Vertical tooth fracture:*** Teeth with vertical root fractures pose the hopeless prognosis.
6. ***Non-strategic teeth:*** There are two major factors which relegate a strategic tooth to the hopeless status; restorability and periodontal support. The tooth that cannot be restored or that has inadequate, unmanageable periodontal support is hopeless. Evaluation of the oral cavity can decide whether tooth is strategic or not, for example, if a person has multiple missing teeth, root canal of third molar may be needed. But in case of well maintained oral hygiene with full dentition, an exposed third molar can be considered for extraction.
7. ***Evaluation of the clinician:*** Clinician should be honest while dealing with the case. Self evaluation should be done for his experience, capability to do the case, equipment he has or not for the completion of the case.
8. ***Systemic conditions:*** Most of the medical conditions do not contraindicate the endodontic treatment but patient should be thoroughly evaluated in order to manage the case optimally.

For predictable and successful endodontic therapy certain steps are needed and skipping a step may lead to the endodontic failure or less than desirable result.

These steps are as follows:

a. Take proper history and medical history of the patient
b. Make accurate diagnosis and treatment planning
c. Obtain adequate anesthesia
d. Isolate the tooth using rubber dam
e. Utilize adequate visualization and lighting
f. Obtain straight line access to the canals
g. Complete biomechanical preparation of the tooth
h. Efficient and safe use of nickel titanium files
i. Copiously irrigate at all stages
j. Obturate the canal three dimensionally
k. Give the coronal restoration to tooth.

## TREATMENT PLANNING

The treatment planning signifies the planning of the management of the patient's dental problems in systematic and ordered way that assumes a complete knowledge of patient needs, nature of problem and prognosis of the treatment to be done very rarely, both dentist and the patient have complete picture of considerations mentioned above.

Thus the stage of assessment of a complete picture overlaps with the stages of decision-making, treatment planning and treatment phase.

**The treatment planning consists of following phases**

- Establishing the nature of the problem
- Decision-making
- Planning required to deliver the selected treatment

A treatment plan for gaining the patient compliance and to have success in the pain management should progress as follows:

1. Treatment of acute problem which includes first step of endodontic treatment comprising of access opening, extirpation of pulp and allowing drainage through pulp space.

2. Oral hygiene instructions, diet instructions.
3. Temporary restoration of carious teeth, scaling and polishing.
4. Definitive restorations of carious teeth.
5. Complete root canal treatments of required teeth.
6. Do endodontic surgery if needed.
7. Evaluate the prognosis of treated teeth.
8. Provide postendodontic restorations.

## Factors Influencing the Treatment Planning

There are several factors which influence the treatment planning. The clinician must be aware of problems encountered during treatment, short and long-term goals of the treatment and patient's expectations about the treatment.

## Factors Affecting Treatment Planning

1. Chief complaint regarding pain and swelling requires urgent treatment and planning for definitive solution.
2. Previous history of dental treatment (solve the residual problems of previous dental treatment).
3. Medical history (identify factors which can compromise dental treatment).
4. Intraoral examination (to know the general oral condition first before focusing on site of complaint so as not to miss the cause).
5. Extraoral examination (to differentially diagnose the chief complaint).
6. Oral hygiene.
7. Periodontal status (to see the periodontal foundation for long-term prognosis of involved tooth).
8. Teeth and restorative status (to identify replacement of missing teeth, status of the remaining dentition).
9. Occlusion (to check functional relationship between opposing teeth, parafunctional habits, etc.).
10. Special tests (to explore the unseen tissues).
11. Diagnosis (repeat the series of conclusions).
12. Treatment options (evaluate various options to decide the best choice for long-term benefit of the patient).

## MEDICAL CONDITIONS INFLUENCING ENDODONTIC TREATMENT PLANNING

| *Medical condition* | *Modifications in treatment planning* |
|---|---|
| 1. **Patients with Valvular Disease and Murmers** | |
| Patients are susceptible to bacterial endocarditis secondary to dental treatment treatment | Prophylactic antibiotics are advocated before initiation of the endodontic |
| 2. **Patients with Hypertension** | |
| i. In these patients, stress and anxiety may further increase chances of myocardial infarction or cerebrovascular accidents | • Give premedication<br>• Plan short appointments |
| ii. Sometimes antihypertensive drugs may cause postural hypotension | • Use local anesthetic with minimum amount of vasoconstrictors |
| 3. **Myocardial Infarction** | |
| i. Stress and anxiety can precipitate myocardial infarction or angina | • Elective endodontic treatment is postponed if recent myocardial infarction is present, i.e. < 6 months |
| ii. Some degree of congestive heart failure may be present | • Reduce the level of stress and anxiety while treating patient |
| iii. Chances of excessive bleeding when patient is on aspirin | • Keep the appointments short and comfortable |
| iv. If pacemaker is present, apex locators can cause electrical interferences | • Use local anesthetics without epinephrine<br>• Antibiotic prophylaxis is given before initiation of the treatment |
| 4. **Prosthetic Valve or Implants** | |
| i. Patients are at high risk for bacterial endocarditis | • Prophylactic antibiotic coverage before initiation of the treatment |
| ii. Tendency for increased bleeding because of prolonged use of antibiotic therapy | • Consult physician for any suggestion regarding patient treatment |
| 5. **Leukemia** | |
| Patient has increased tendency for:<br>i. Opportunistic infections<br>ii. Prolonged bleeding<br>iii. Poor and delayed wound healing | • Consult the physician.<br>• Avoid treatment during acute stages<br>• Avoid long duration appointment<br>• Strict oral hygiene instructions<br>• Evaluate the bleeding time and platelet status<br>• Use of antibiotic prophylaxis |
| 6. **Cancer** | |
| Usually because of radiotherapy and chemotherapy,<br>i. These patients suffer from xerostomia, mucositis, trismus and excessive bleeding<br>ii. Prone to infections because of bone marrow suppression | • Consult the physician prior to treatment.<br>• Perform only emergency treatment if possible<br>• Symptomatic treatment of mucositis, trismus and xerostomia<br>• Optimal antibiotic coverage prior to treatment.<br>• Strict oral hygiene regimen |
| 7. **Bleeding Disorders** | |
| In cases of hemophilia, thrombocytopenia, prolonged bleeding due to liver disease, | • Take careful history of the patient<br>• Consult the physician |

*Contd...*

*Contd...*

| | |
|---|---|
| broadspectrum antibiotics, patients on anticoagulant therapy patient experiences<br>i. Spontaneous bleeding<br>ii. Prolonged bleeding<br>iii. Petechiae, ecchymosis and hematoma | for suggestions regarding the patient<br>• Avoid aspirin containing compounds and NSAIDs<br>• In thrombocytopenia cases, replacement of platelets is done before procedure<br>• Prophylactic antibiotic coverage to be given<br>• Incase of liver disease, avoid drugs metabolized by liver |
| 8. **Renal Disease** | |
| i. In this patient usually has hypertension and anemia<br>ii. Intolerance to nephrotoxic drugs<br>iii. Increased susceptibility to opportunistic infections<br>iv. Increased tendency for bleeding | • Prior consultation with physician<br>• Check the blood pressure before initiation of treatment.<br>• Antibiotic prophylaxis screen the bleeding time<br>• Avoid drugs metabolized and excreted by kidney |
| 9. **Diabetes Mellitus** | |
| i. Patient has increased tendency for infections and poor wound healing<br>ii. Patient may be suffering from diseases related to cardiovascular system, kidneys and nervous system like myocardial infarction, hypertension, congestive heart failure, renal failure and peripheral neuropathy. | • Take careful history of the patient<br>• Consult with physician prior to treatment<br>• Note the blood glucose levels.<br>• Patient should have normal meals before appointment<br>• If patient is on insulin therapy, he/she should have his regular dose of insulin before appointment<br>• Schedule the appointment early in the mornings<br>• Antibiotics may be needed<br>• Have instant source of sugar available in clinic<br>• Patient should be evaluated for the presence of hypertension, myocardial infarction or renal failure |
| 10. **Pregnancy** | |
| i. In such patients the harm to patient can occur via radiation exposures, medication and increased level of stress and anxiety | • Do the elective procedure in second trimester<br>• Use the principles of *ALARA while exposing patients to the radiation |
| ii. In the third trimester, chances of development of supine hypotension are increased | • Avoid any drugs which can cause harm to the fetus<br>• Consult the physician to verify the physical status of the patient and any precautions if required for the patient<br>• Reduce the number of oral microorganism (by chlorhexidine mouthwash)<br>• In third semesters, don't place patient in supine position for prolonged periods |
| 11. **Anaphylaxis** | |
| Patient gives history of severe allergic reaction on administration of:<br>i. Local anesthetics<br>ii. Certain drugs<br>iii. Latex gloves and rubber dam sheets | • Take careful history of the patient<br>• Avoid use of agents to which patient is allergic<br>• Always keep the emergency kit available<br>• In case the reaction develops:<br>– Identify the reaction<br>– Call the physician<br>– Place patient in supine position<br>– Check vital signs<br>– If vital signs are reduced, inject epinepherine tongue<br>– Provide CPR if needed<br>– Admit the patient |

*ALARA – As low as Reasonably Achievable

**Sequence of treatment delivery consists of three stages**

- Initial treatment
- Definitive treatment
- Patient recall check up

## Sequence of Treatment Delivery

a. ***Initial treatment:*** The initial treatment mainly aims at providing the relief from symptoms for example incision and drainage of an infection with severe pain and swelling, endodontic treatment of a case of acute irreversible pulpitis, etc.

Halting the progress of primary disease, i.e. caries or periodontal problem comes thereafter. Finally the patient is made to understand the disease and its treatment which further increases his/her compliance to the treatment. This approach is beneficial for the long-term prevention of the dental caries and periodontal disease.

b. ***Definite treatment:*** Definitive treatment involves root canal treatment, surgical treatment, endodontic retreatment or the extraction of teeth with hopeless prognosis. In this phase tooth is given endodontic treatment with final restoration to maintain its form, function and esthetics.

c. ***Patient recall check up:*** Regular patient recall is integral part of the planning process. It involves taking patient history, examination, diagnosing again for assessment of the endodontic treatment.

Before the clinician starts the endodontic therapy, a number of issues arise related to the treatment planning. These include maintaining asepsis of the operatory and infection control measures, premedication and administration of local anesthesia followed by review of radiographs and complete isolation of the operating site.

## Summary

Efficient and successful endodontics begins with proper case selection. The clinician must know his/her limitations and select cases accordingly. Since success of endodontic treatment depends upon many factors which can be modified to get better before initiating the treatment. Therefore accurate and thorough preparation of both patient as well as tooth to be treated should be carried out to achieve the successful treatment results.

## QUESTION

**Q. Write short notes on:**

a. Indications and contraindications of endodontic therapy
b. Role of medical history in endodontics

## BIBLIOGRAPHY


1. Brody HA, Nesbitt WR. Psychosomatic oral problem. J Oral Med 1967;22:43.
2. Brooks SL, Miles DA. Advances in diagnostic imaging in dentistry. Dent Clin N Amer 1993;37:91.
3. Chambers IG. The role and methods of pulp testing in oral diagnosis: a review. Int Endod J 1982;15:1.
4. Corah NL, Gale E, Illig S. Assessment of a dental anxiety scale. J Am Dent Assoc 1978;97:816.
5. Elfenbaum A. Causalgia in dentistry: An Abandoned pain sundrome. Oral Surg 1954;7:594.
6. Gier RE. Management of neurogenic and psychogenic problems. Dent Clin North Am, March 1968;177.
7. Harrigan WF. Psychiatric considerations in maxillofacial pain. J Am Dent Assoc 1955;51:408.
8. Kleinknecht R, et al. Factor analysis of the dental fear survey with cross-validation. J Am Dent Assoc 1984;108:59.
9. Murray CA, Saunders WP. Root canal treatment and general health: A review of literature. Int Endod J 2000;33:1.
10. Newton JT, Buck DJ. Anxiety and pain measures in dentistry: A guide to their quality and application. J Am Dent Assoc 2000;131:1449.
11. Weckstein MS. Basic psychology and dental practice. Dent Clin North Am 1970;14:379.
12. Weckstein MS. Practical applications of basic psychiatry to dentistry. Dent Clin North Am 1970;14:397.

CHAPTER 9

# Asepsis in Endodontics



## INTRODUCTION

Endodontics has long emphasized the importance of aseptic techniques using sterilized instruments, disinfecting solutions and procedural barriers like rubber dam. Dental professionals are exposed to wide variety of microorganisms in the blood and saliva of patients, making infection control procedures of utmost importance. The common goal of infection control is to eliminate or reduce number of microbes shared between the people. The procedures of infection control are designed to kill or remove microbes or to protect against contaminations.

## RATIONALE FOR INFECTION CONTROL

The deposition of organisms in the tissues and their growth resulting in a host reaction is called infection. The number of organisms required to cause an infection is termed as "the infective dose". Factors affecting infective dose are:

- Virulence of the organism
- Susceptibility of the host.
- Age, drug therapy, or pre-existing disease, etc.

*Microorganisms* can spread from one person to another via direct contact, indirect contact, droplet infection and airborne infection (Flow Chart 9.1). *Direct contact* occurs by touching soft tissues or teeth of patients. It causes immediate spread of infection by the source.

*Indirect contact* results from injuries with contaminated sharp instruments, needle stick injuries or contact with contaminated equipment and surfaces.

*Droplet infection* occurs by large particle droplets *spatter* which is transmitted by close contact. *Spatter* generated during dental procedures may deliver microorganisms to the dentist. Airborne infection involves small particles of $< 5\ \mu m$ size. These microorganisms remain airborne for hours and can cause infection when inhaled.

## CROSS-INFECTION

Cross-infection is transmission of infectious agents among patients and staff within a clinical environment. This source of infection can be:

- Patients suffering from infectious diseases
- Patients who are in the prodromal stage of infections
- Healthy carriers of pathogens.

### For an Infection to be Transmitted, the following Conditions are Required

- A pathogenic organism
- A source which allows pathogenic organism to survive and multiply
- Mode of transmission
- Route of entry
- A susceptible host.

### Different Routes of Spread of Infection

1. Patient to dental health care worker (DHCW)
2. DHCW to patient
3. Patient to patient
4. Dental office to community
5. Community to patient.

#### *Patient to Dental Health Care Worker*

*It can occur in following ways:*

- Direct contact through break in skin or direct contact with mucous membrane of DHCW
- Indirect contact via sharp cutting instruments and needle stick injuries
- Droplet injection by *spatter* produced during dental procedures and through mucosal surfaces of dental team.

Flow Chart 9.1: Chain of infection

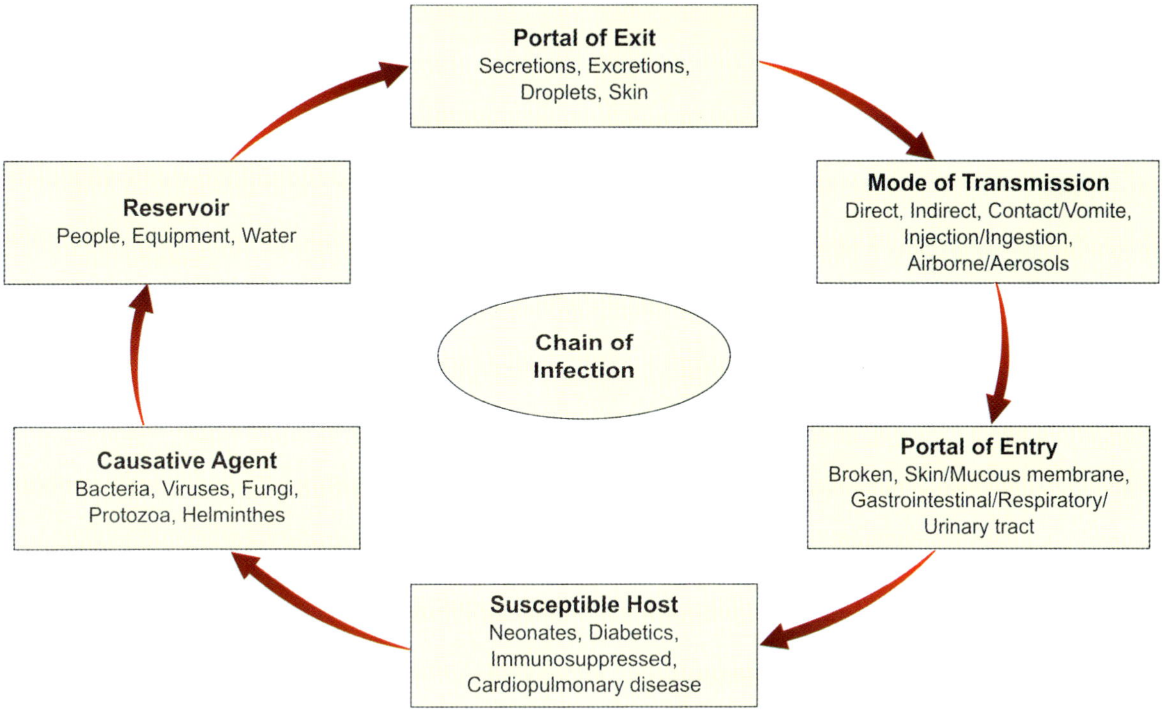


### *Dental Health Care Worker to the Patient*

*It occurs by:*

- Direct contact, i.e. through mucosal surfaces of the patient
- Indirect contact, i.e. via use of contaminated instruments and lack of use of disposable instruments
- Droplet infection via inhalation by the patient.

### *Patient to Patient*

It occurs by use of contaminated and nondisposable instruments.

### *Dental Office to the Community*

*It occurs:*

- When contaminated impression or other equipments contaminate dental laboratory technicians
- Via spoiled clothing and regulated waste.

### *Community to the Patient*

Community to the patient involves the entrance of microorganisms into water supply of dental unit. These microorganisms colonize inside the water lines and thereby form biofilm which is responsible for causing infection.

## OBJECTIVE OF INFECTION CONTROL

The main objective of infection control is elimination or reduction in spread of infection from all types of microorganisms. It is the duty of a clinician for implementing effective infection control to protect other patients and all members of the dental team.

Basically two factors are important in infection control:

- Prevention of spread of microorganisms from their hosts
- Killing or removal of microorganisms from objects and surfaces.

## UNIVERSAL PRECAUTIONS

Some strategies have to be followed in order to reduce the risk of infection and transmission caused by blood borne pathogens such as HBV and HIV. It is always recommended to follow some basic infection control procedures for all patients, termed as "universal precautions".

*These are as follows:*

- Immunization: All members of the dental team (who are exposed to blood or blood contaminated articles) should be vaccinated against hepatitis B
- Use of personal protective barrier techniques, that is use of protective gown, face mask, protective eyewear, gloves, etc. These reduce the risk of exposure to infectious material and injury from sharp instruments
- Maintaining hand hygiene.

### Personal Protection Equipment

### *Barrier Technique*

The use of barrier technique is very important, which includes gown, face mask, protective eyewear and gloves (Fig. 9.1).

***Protective gown:*** Protective gown should be worn to prevent contamination of normal clothing and to protect the skin of the clinician from exposure to blood and body substances.

- The clinician should change protective clothing when it becomes soiled and if contaminated by blood
- Gown can be reusable or disposable for use. It should have a high neck and long sleeves to protect the arms from splash and *spatter*
- Protective clothing must be removed before leaving the workplace
- Protective clothing should be washed in the laundry with health care facility. If it is not present, the gown should be washed separately from other clothing.

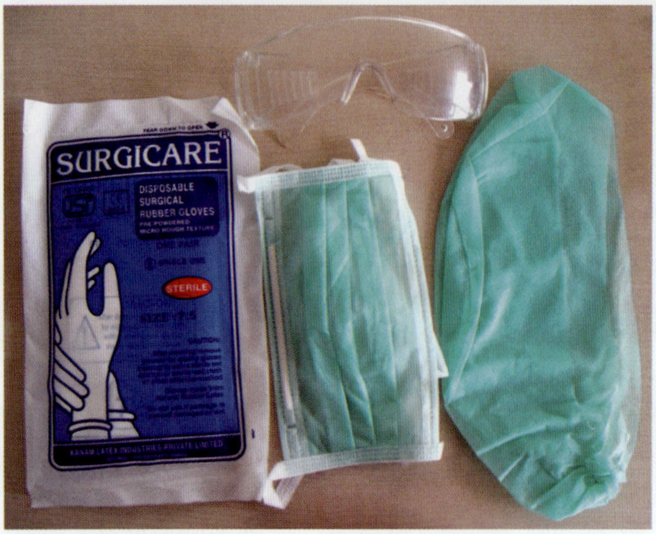


**Fig. 9.1:** Personal protective equipment showing face mask, gloves, eye wear, head cap

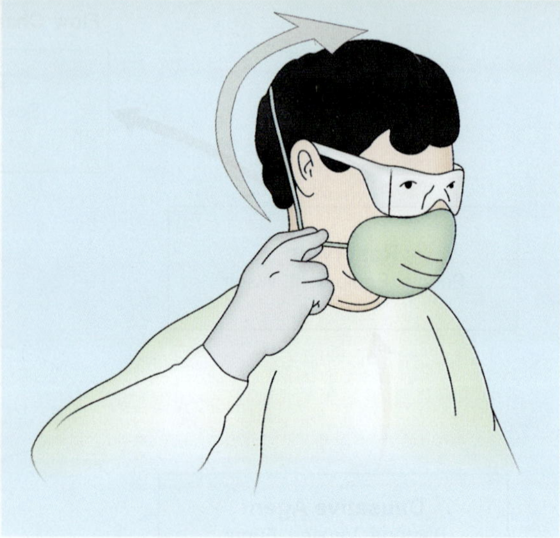

**Fig. 9.2:** Removal of facemask should be done by grasping it only by its strings, not by mask itself

***Facemasks:*** A surgical mask that covers both the nose and mouth should be worn by the clinician during procedures. Though facemasks do not provide complete microbiological protection but they prevent the *splatter* from contaminating the face. In other words, face masks provide protection against microorganisms generated during various procedures and droplet spatter that contain bloodborne pathogens.

Points to remember regarding facemasks:

- Masks should be changed regularly and between patients
- The outer surface of mask can get contaminated with infectious droplets from spray or from touching the mask with contaminated fingers, so should not be reused
- If the mask becomes wet, it should be changed between patients or even during patient treatment
- The maximum time for wearing masks should not be more than one hour, since it becomes dampened from respiration, causing its degradation
- In order to greater protection against *splatter*, a chin length plastic face shields must be worn, in addition to face masks
- To remove mask, grasp it only by its strings, not by the mask itself (Fig. 9.2).

***Head caps:*** Hair should be properly tied. Long hair should be either covered or restrained away from face. To prevent hair contamination head caps must be used.

***Protective eyewear:*** Clinician, helping staff and patient must protect their eyes against foreign bodies, splatter and aerosols which arise during operative procedures using protective glasses. Eyewear protects the eyes from injury and from microbes such as hepatitis B virus, which can be transmitted through conjunctiva.

Eyewear with solid side-shields or chin-length face shields must be used for optimal protection. Contaminated glasses should be washed in soapy water and disinfected with a product that does not cause irritation to the eyes. Do not touch the eyewear with ungloved hands, because it can be contaminated with spatter of blood and saliva during patient care.

***Gloves:*** Gloves should be worn to prevent contamination of hands when touching mucous membranes, blood, saliva and to reduce the chances of transmission of infected microorganisms from clinician to patient. All persons with direct patient contact must wear nonsterile gloves routinely. They must be worn for all dental procedures including extra and intraoral examination and not only for those procedures where there is a possibility of bleeding. It has been shown that working with bare hands results in the retention of microorganisms, saliva and blood under the fingernails for several days.

Ideally gloves should be:

- Good quality, sterile for all types of surgical procedures and non-sterile for all clinical procedures and changed after every patient
- Well fitted and non-powdered since the powder from gloves can contaminate veneers and radiographs and can interfere with wound healing
- Made up of "low extractable latex protein" to reduce the possibility of allergy.

Some important points regarding use of gloves:

- Gloves are manufactured as disposable items meant to be used for only one patient
- A new pair of gloves should be used for each patient and may need to be changed during a procedure
- Gloves should be changed between patients and when torn or punctured
- Overgloves or paper towels must be used for opening drawers, cabinets, etc.
- Handwashing should be performed immediately before putting on gloves. Similarly handwashing after glove removal is essential
- Gloves must be worn when handling or cleaning materials or surfaces contaminated with body fluids
- Some persons can show allergic reactions to gloves due to latex (polyisoprene) or antioxidants such as mercaptobenzothiazole. Ensure that latex free equipment and non latex

gloves (polyurethane or vinyl gloves) are used on patients who have a latex-allergy
- Person with skin problems (if related to use of glove) should be assessed properly
- Latex gloves should be used for patient examinations and procedures and should be disposed off thereafter
- Heavy utility gloves should be worn when handling and cleaning contaminated instruments and for surface cleaning and disinfection.

## Hand Hygiene

As in any clinical practice setting, hand hygiene plays a central role in the reduction of cross-contamination and in infection control. Hand hygiene significantly reduces potential pathogens on the hands and is considered the single most critical measure for reducing the risk of transmitting organisms to patients and dentists. The microbial flora of the skin consist of transient and resident microorganisms.

**Transient flora**, which colonize the superficial layers of the skin, are easier to remove by routine handwashing. They are acquired by direct contact with patients or contaminated environmental surfaces. These organisms are most frequently associated with health care associated infections.

**Resident flora** attached to deeper layers of the skin are more resistant to removal and less likely to be associated with such infections.

The preferred method for hand hygiene depends on the type of procedure, the degree of contamination and the desired persistence of antimicrobial action on the skin. For routine dental examinations and nonsurgical procedures, handwashing and hand antisepsis is achieved by using either a plain or antimicrobial soap with water. If the hands are not visibly soiled, an alcohol-based hand rub is adequate.

The purpose of surgical hand antisepsis is to eliminate transient flora and reduce resident flora for the duration of a procedure to prevent introduction of organisms in the operative wound, if gloves become punctured or torn. Skin bacteria can rapidly multiply under surgical gloves if hands are washed with soap that is not antimicrobial. Thus, an antimicrobial soap or alcohol hand rub with persistent activity should be used before surgical procedures.

For most routine dental procedures washing hands with plain, nonantimicrobial soap is sufficient. For more invasive procedures, such as cutting of gum or tissue, hand antisepsis with either an antiseptic solution or alcohol-based handrub is recommended. If available, waterless alcohol handrub/gel could be used in place of handwashing if hands are not visibly soiled.

### *Types of Hand Scrubs*

***Alcohol-based hand rub:*** An alcohol containing preparation help in reducing the number of viable microorganisms on the hands.

***Antimicrobial soap:*** A detergent containing an antiseptic agent.

***Antiseptic:*** It is a germicide used on living tissue for the purpose of inhibiting or destroying microorganisms.

### *Indications for Hand Hygiene*

*Handwashing should be done:*

- At the beginning of patient
- Between patient contacts
- Before putting on gloves
- After touching inanimate objects
- Before touching eyes, nose, face or mouth
- After completion of case
- Before eating, drinking
- Between each patient
- After glove removal
- After barehanded contact with contaminated equipment or surfaces and before leaving treatment areas
- At the end of the day.

### *Handwash Technique*

- Removal of rings, jewellery and watches
- Cover cuts and abrasions with waterproof adhesive dressings
- Clean fingernails with a plastic or wooden stick
- Scrub hands, nails and forearm using a good quality liquid soap preferably containing a disinfectant
- Rinse hands thoroughly with running water
- Dry hands with towel.

## CLASSIFICATION OF INSTRUMENTS

The center for disease control and prevention (CDC) classified the instrument into critical, semicritical and noncritical depending on the potential risk of infection during the use of these instruments. These categories are also referred to as Spaulding classification ***(by Spaulding in 1968).***

**Classification of instrument sterilization**

| *Category* | *Definition* | *Examples* |
|---|---|---|
| Critical | Where instruments enter or penetrate into sterile tissue, cavity or blood stream | • Surgical blades and instruments<br>• Surgical dental bur |
| Semicritical | Which contact intact mucosa or nonintact skin | • Amalgam condenser<br>• Dental handpieces<br>• Mouth mirror<br>• Saliva ejectors |
| Noncritical | Which contact intact skin | • Pulse oximeter<br>• Stethoscope<br>• Light switches<br>• Dental chair |

For complete sterilization, rule of universal sterilization should be followed. It means that all reusable instruments and handpieces are sterilized (not disinfected) between use on patient.

*CDC Recommends:*

- Critical and semicritical instruments are to be heat sterilized
- Semicritical items sensitive to heat should be treated with high level disinfectant after cleaning
- Noncritical items can be treated intermediate to low level disinfectant after cleaning.

### Definitions

***Cleaning:*** It is the process which physically removes contamination but does not necessarily destroy microorganisms. It is a prerequisite before decontamination by disinfection or sterilization of instruments since organic material prevents contact with microbes, inactivates disinfectants.

***Disinfection:*** It is the process of using an agent that destroys germs or other harmful microbes or inactivates them, usually referred to chemicals that kill the growing forms (vegetative forms) but not the resistant spores of bacteria.

***Antisepsis:*** It is the destruction of pathogenic microorganisms existing in their vegetative state on living tissue.

***Sterilization:*** Sterilization involves any process, physical or chemical, that will destroy all forms of life, including bacterial, fungi, spores and viruses.

***Aseptic technique:*** It is the method which prevents contamination of wounds and other sites, by ensuring that only sterile objects and fluids come into contact with them; and that the risks of air-borne contamination are minimized.

***Antiseptic:*** It is a chemical applied to living tissues, such as skin or mucous membrane to reduce the number of microorganisms present, by inhibition of their activity or by destruction.

***Disinfectant:*** It is a chemical substance, which causes disinfection. It is used on nonvital objects to kill surface vegetative pathogenic organisms, but not necessarily spore forms or viruses.

## INSTRUMENT PROCESSING PROCEDURES

Instrument processing is the collection of procedures which prepare the contaminated instruments for reuse. For complete sterilization process, prevention of the disease transmission and instruments should be processed correctly and carefully (Flow Chart 9.2).

### Steps of Instrument Processing

1. Presoaking (Holding)
2. Cleaning
3. Corrosion control
4. Packaging
5. Sterilization
6. Monitoring of sterilization
7. Handling the processed instrument.

**Flow Chart 9.2:** Instrument processing procedure

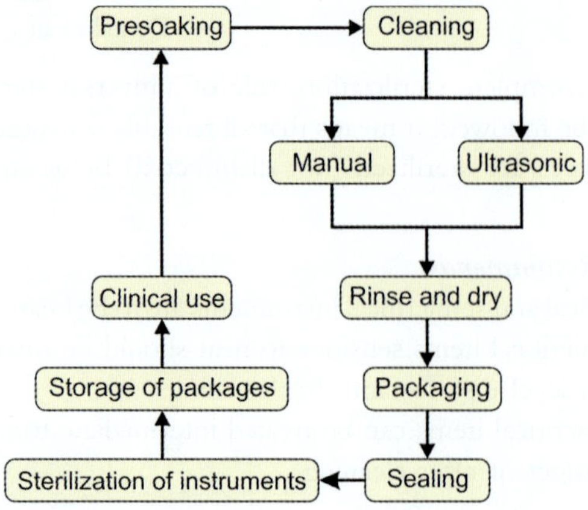


#### Presoaking (Holding)

It facilitates the cleaning process by preventing the debris from drying.

#### Procedure

- Wear puncture resistant heavy utility gloves and personnel protective equipments
- Place loose instruments in a perforated cleaning basket and then place the basket into the holding solution. Holding solution can be:
  a. Neutral pH detergents
  b. Water
  c. Enzyme solution.
- Perforated cleaning basket reduces the direct handling of instruments. So, chances of contamination are decreased
- Holding solution should be discarded atleast once a day or earlier if seems to be soiled
- Avoid instrument soaking for long time as it increases the chances of corrosion of instruments.

#### Cleaning

It aids in the subsequent cleaning process by removing gross debris. It is considered to be one of the important steps before any sterilization or disinfection procedure. The advantage of this procedure is that it reduces the bioburden, i.e. microorganisms, blood, saliva and other materials.

*Methods used for cleaning:*

1. Manual scrubbing
2. Ultrasonic cleaning
3. Mechanical – instrument washer

1. ***Manual scrubbing:*** It is one of the most effective method for removing debris, if performed properly. Now-a-days, this method is not recommended because of the risk-factors involved.

#### Procedure

a. Brush delicately all surfaces of instruments while submerged in cleaning solution.
b. Use long-handled stiff nylon brush to keep the scrubbing hand away from sharp instrument surfaces.
c. Always wear heavy utility gloves and personnel protective equipments.
d. Use neutral pH detergents while cleaning.
e. Instruments' surfaces should be visibly clean and free from stains and tissues.

*Disadvantages:* This procedure is not recommended as there are maximum chances of direct contact with instrument surfaces and also of cuts and punctures.

2. ***Ultrasonic cleaning (Fig. 9.3):*** It is excellent cleaning method as it reduces direct handling of instruments. So, it is considered safer and more effective than manual scrubbing.

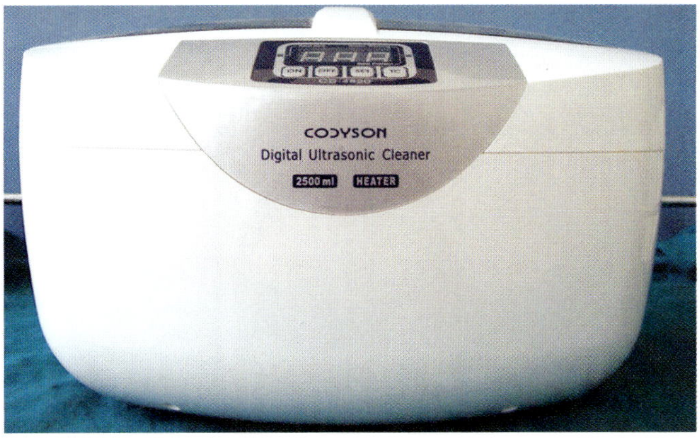


**Fig. 9.3:** Ultrasonic cleaner

### Procedure

a. *Mechanism of action:* Ultrasonic energy generated in the ultrasonic cleaner produces billions of tiny bubbles which, in further, collapse and create high turbulence at the surface of instrument. This turbulence dislodges the debris.
b. Maintain the proper solution level.
c. Use recommended cleaning solution.
d. Time may vary due to
   i. Nature of instrument
   ii. Amount of debris
   iii. Efficiency of ultrasonic unit.
   
   Usually the time ranges vary from 4-16 minutes.
e. After cleaning, remove the basket/cassette rack and wash under tap water. Use gloves while washing under tap water as the cleaning solution is also contaminated.
f. Discard the solution atleast daily.

3. ***Mechanical-instrument washer:*** These are designed to clean instruments in hospital setup. Instrument washer has also the advantage that it reduces the direct handling of the instrument.

### Control of Corrosion by Lubrication

It prevents damage of instruments because of drying. Some instruments or portions of instruments and burs (made up of carbon steel) will rust during steam sterilization, for example, grasping surfaces of forceps, cutting surfaces of orthodontic pliers, burs, scalers, hoes and hatchets.

For rust-prone instruments, use dry hot air oven/chemical vapor sterilization instead of autoclave. Use spray rust inhibitor (sodium nitrite) on the instruments.

### Packaging

It maintains the sterility of instruments after the sterilization. Unpacked instruments are exposed to environment when sterilization chamber is opened and can be contaminated by dust, aerosols or by improper handling or contact with contaminated surfaces.

Packaging is the procedure in which cleaned instruments are organized in functional sets, thereafter with wrapping, these are placed in sterilization pouches or bags. One may also add chemical and biological indicators of sterilization in the pouches or bags.

Varieties of packaging materials are available in the market such as self-sealing, paper-plastic and peel-pouches. Peel-pouches are the most common and convenient to use (Fig. 9.4).

*Packs should be stored with the following considerations:*

- Instruments are kept wrapped until ready for use
- To reduce the risk of contamination, sterile packs must be handled as little as possible
- Sterilized packs should be allowed to cool before storage; otherwise condensation will occur inside the packs
- Sterile packs must be stored and issued in correct date order. The packs, preferably, are stored in UV chamber (Fig. 9.5) or drums which can be locked.

### Methods of Sterilization

Sterilization is process by which an object, surface or medium is freed of all microorganisms either in the vegetative or spore state (Table 9.1).

**Table 9.1: Sterilization method and type of packaging material**

| *Sterilization method* | *Packaging material* |
|---|---|
| Autoclave<br>Wrapped cassettes | • Paper or plastic peel-pouches<br>• Plastic tubing (made up of nylon)<br>• Thin clothes (Thick clothes are not advised as they absorb too much heat)<br>• Sterilization paper (paper wrap) |
| Chemical vapor | • Paper or plastic pouches<br>• Sterilization paper |
| Dry heat | • Sterilization paper (paper wrap)<br>• Nylon plastic tubing (indicated for dry heat)<br>• Wrapped cassettes |

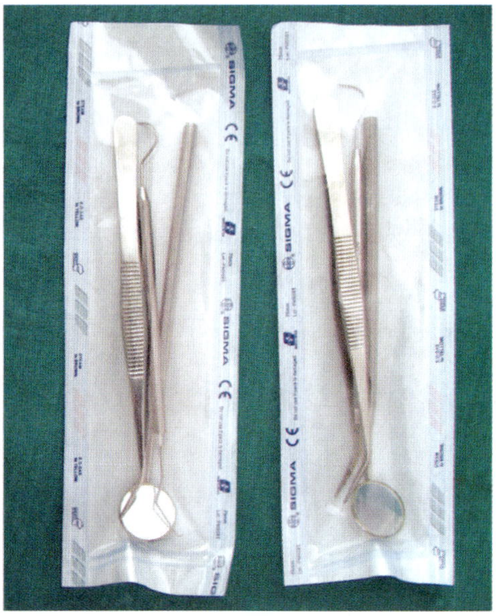

**Fig. 9.4:** Peel-pouches for packing instruments

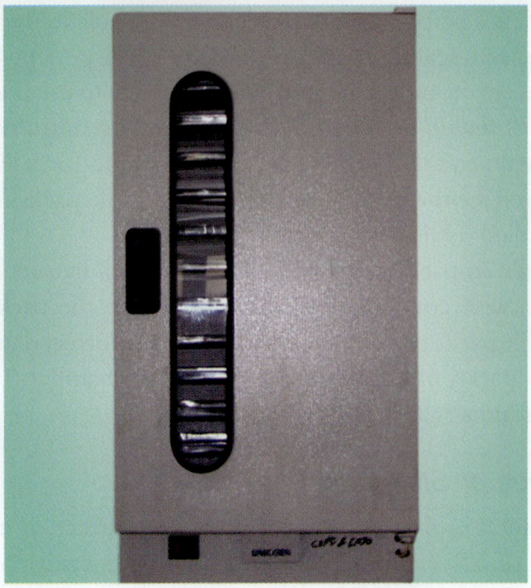

Fig. 9.5: UV chamber for storage of sterile instruments

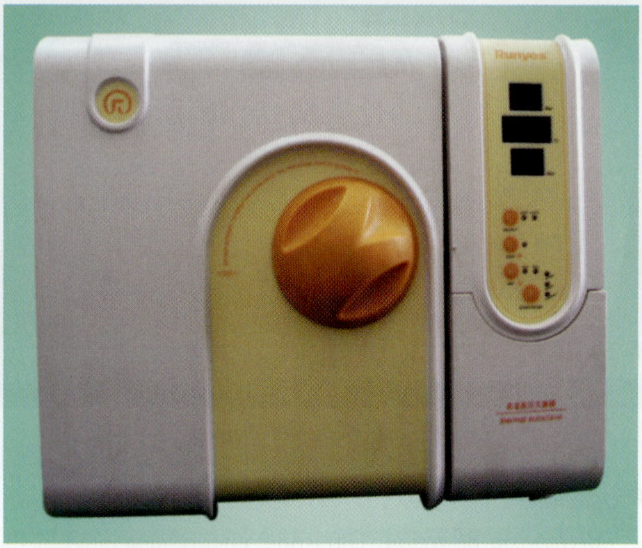

Fig. 9.6: Autoclave for moist heat sterilization

### Classification of Sterilizing Agents

*Physical agents:*

1. Sunlight
2. Drying
3. Cold
4. Dry heat
   a. Flaming
   b. Incineration
   c. Hot air oven
5. Moist heat
   a. Boiling
   b. Steam under pressure
   c. Pasteurization
6. Filtration
   a. Candles
   b. Membranes
   c. Asbestos pads
7. Radiation

*Chemical agents:*

1. Alcohols
   a. Ethanol
   b. Isopropyl alcohol
2. Aldehydes
   a. Formaldehyde
   b. Gluteraldehyde
3. Halogens
   a. Iodine
   b. Chlorine
4. Dyes
   a. Acridine
   b. Aniline
5. Phenols
   a. Cresol
   b. Carbolic acid
6. Metallic salts gases
   a. Ethylene oxide
   b. Formaldehyde
   c. Betapropiolactone
7. Surface active agents

The accepted methods of sterilization in our dental practice are:

1. Moist/steam heat sterilization.
2. Dry heat sterilization.
3. Chemical vapor pressure sterilization.
4. Ethylene oxide sterilization.

### Moist/Steam Heat Sterilization

***Autoclave:*** Autoclave provides the most efficient and reliable method of sterilization for all dental instruments. It involves heating water to generate steam in a closed chamber resulting in moist heat that rapidly kills microorganisms (Fig. 9.6).

Use of saturated steam under pressure is the most efficient, quickest, safest, effective method of sterilization because:

1. It has high penetrating power.
2. It gives up a large amount of heat (latent heat) to the surface with which it comes into contact and on which it condenses as water.

***Types of autoclaves:*** Two types of autoclaves are available:

1. Downward (gravitation) displacement sterilizer: This is non-vacuum type autoclave.
2. Steam sterilizers (autoclave) with pre and post vacuum processes.

***Steam sterilizers (Autoclave) with pre and post vacuum processes:*** In this, the sterilization process is composed of three main phases:

1. *Pre-treatment phase/heat-up cycle:* All air is virtually expelled by a number of pulses of vacuum and the introduction of steam, so that the saturated steam can affect the instruments during second phase.
2. *Sterilizing phase/sterilization cycle:* The temperature increases adequately upto the degree at which sterilization

is to take place. Actual sterilizing period (also called "Holding Time") starts when the temperature in all parts of the autoclave chamber and its contents has reached the sterilizing temperature. This should remain constant within specified temperature throughout the whole sterilization phase.
3. *Post-treatment phase/depressurization cycle:* In this phase either the steam or the revaporized condensed water is removed by vacuum to ensure that the goods are dried rapidly.

*Three main factors required for effective autoclaving:*
1. *Pressure:* It is expressed in terms of psi or kPa.
2. *Temperature:* For effective sterilization the temperature should be reached and maintained at 121°C. As the temperature and pressure increases, superheated steam is formed. This steam is lighter than air, thus rises to the upper portion of the autoclave. As more steam is formed, it eliminates air from autoclave. The reason of complete elimination of air is to help superheated steam to penetrate the entire load in the autoclave and remain in contact for the appropriate length of time.
3. *Time:* A minimum of 20 to 30 minutes of time is required after achieving full temperature and pressure.
   *Significance:* Higher the temperature and pressure, shorter is the time required for sterilization.
   - At 15 psi pressure, the temperature of 121°C, the time required is 15 minutes
   - At 126°C, time is 10 minutes
   - At 134°C, time is 3 minutes.

***Wrapping instruments for autoclaving:*** Packing instruments before sterilizing prevents them from becoming contaminated after sterilization till it is opened and used. For wrapping, closed containers such as closed metal trays, glass vials and aluminium foils should not be used, since they stop the steam from reaching the inner part of the packs.

For packaging of autoclaving instruments, one should use porous covering so as to permit steam to penetrate through and reach the instruments. The materials used for packaging can be fabric or sealed paper or cloth pouches (Fig. 9.7) and paper-wrapped cassettes. Finally the wrap is heat-sealed or sealed with tape.

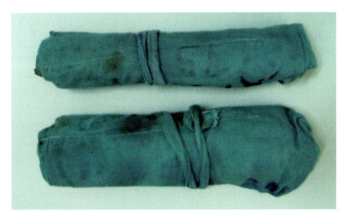

**Fig. 9.7:** Cloth pouches for instrument wrapping

If instruments are to be stored and not used shortly after sterilization, the autoclave cycle should end with a drying phase to avoid tarnish or corrosion of the instruments.

### Advantages of Autoclaving
1. Time efficient.
2. Good penetration.
3. The results are consistently good and reliable.
4. The instruments can be wrapped prior to sterilization.

### Disadvantages of Autoclaves
1. Blunting and corrosion of sharp instruments.
2. Damage to rubber goods.

### Dry Heat Sterilization
It is alternative method for sterilization of instruments. This type of sterilization involves heating air which on further transfers energy from air to the instruments. In this type of sterilization, higher temperature is required than steam or chemical vapor sterilization.

***Conventional hot air oven:*** The hot air oven utilizes radiating dry heat for sterilization as this type of energy does not penetrate materials easily. So, long periods of exposure to high temperature are usually required.

***Packaging of instruments for dry heat:*** Dry heat ovens usually achieve temperature above 320°F (160°C). The packs of instrument must be placed atleast 1 cm apart to air to circulate in the chamber. In conventional type of hot air oven, air circulates by gravity flow, thus it is also known as Gravity convection. The type of packaging or wrapping material used should be able to withstand high temperature otherwise it may get char.

### Packaging Material Requirements for Dry Heat
- Should not be destroyed by temperature used
- Should not insulate items from heat.

### Acceptable Materials
- Paper and plastic bags
- Wrapped cassettes
- Paper wrap
- Aluminum foil
- Nylon plastic tubing.

### Unacceptable Materials
Plastic and paper bags which are unable to withstand dry heat temperatures.

**Recommended temperature and duration of hot oven**

| | | *Hot air oven* | |
|---|---|---|---|
| *Temp °C* | *Time* | *Temp °C* | *Time* |
| 141°C | 3 hours | 170°C | 1 hour |
| 149°C | 2.5 hours | 180°C | 30 minutes |
| 160°C | 2 hours | | |

***Mechanism of action:*** The dry heat kills microorganisms by protein denaturation, coagulation and oxidation It is very important that organic matter such as oil or grease film must be removed from the instruments as this may insulate against dry heat.

Instruments which can be sterilized in dry hot oven are glassware such as pipettes, flasks, scissors, glass syringes, carbon steel instruments and burs. Dry heat does not corrode sharp instrument surfaces. Also it does not erode glassware surfaces. Before placing in the oven, the glassware must be dried. The oven must be allowed to cool slowly for about 2 hours as glassware may crack due to sudden or uneven cooling.

***Rapid heat transfer (forced air type):*** In this type of sterilizer, a fan or blower circulates the heated air throughout the chamber at a high velocity which, in turn, permits a more rapid transfer of heat energy from the air to instruments, thereby reducing the time.

### Temperature/Cycle Recommended

370-375°F - 12 minutes for wrapped instruments

370-375°F - 16 minutes for unwrapped instruments

### Advantages of Dry Heat Sterilization

1. No corrosion is seen in carbon-steel instruments and burs.
2. Maintains the sharpness of cutting instruments.
3. Effective and safe for sterilization of metal instrument and mirrors.
4. Low cost of equipment.
5. Instruments are dry after cycle.
6. Industrial forced draft types usually provide a larger capacity at reasonable price.
7. Rapid cycles are possible at higher temperatures.

### Disadvantages

1. Poor penetrating capacity of dry heat.
2. Long cycle is required because of poor heat conduction and poor penetrating capacity.
3. High temperature may damage heat sensitive items such as rubber or plastic goods.
4. Instruments must be thoroughly dried before placing them in sterilization.
5. Inaccurate calibration and lack of attention to proper settings often lead to errors in sterilization.
6. Heavy loads of instruments, crowding of packs and heavy wrapping easily defeat sterilization.
7. Generally not suitable for handpieces.
8. Cannot sterilize liquids.
9. May discolor and char fabric.

### Chemical Vapor Sterilization

Sterilization by chemical vapor under pressure is known as chemical vapor sterilization. In this, special chemical solution is heated in a closed chamber, producing hot chemical vapors that kill microorganisms.

*The various modes of action are:*

1. Coagulation of protein.
2. Cell membrane disruption.
3. Removal of free sulphydryl groups.
4. Substrate competition.

***Contents of chemical solution:*** The solution contains various ingredients which are as follows:

1. Active ingredient – 0.23% Formaldehyde
2. Other ingredient – 72.38% Ethanol + Acetone + Water and other alcohols

Temperature, pressure and time required for completion of one cycle is – 270°F (132°C) at 20 lb for 30 minutes. Chemical vapor sterilizer is also known as chemiclave. Usually four cycles are required for this sterilizer which is as follows:

1. Vaporization cycle.
2. Sterilization cycle.
3. Depressurization cycle.
4. Purge cycle (which collects chemicals from vapors in the chamber at the end of cycle).

### Advantage

Eliminates corrosion of carbon steel instruments, burs and pliers.

### Disadvantages

1. The instruments or items which are sensitive to elevated temperature are damaged.
2. Sterilization of liner, textiles, fabric or paper towels is not recommended.
3. Dry instruments should be loaded in the chamber.

### Precautions to be Taken

- Use gloves and protective eyewear while handling the chemical solution
- Use paper/plastic peel-pouches or bags recommended for use in chemiclave
- Use system in ventilated room
- Space should be given between the instruments that are to be sterilized in the chamber for better conduction and penetration
- Water should not be left on the instruments.

### Ethylene Oxide Sterilization (ETOX)

This sterilization method is best used for sterilizing complex instruments and delicate materials.

Ethylene oxide is highly penetrative, noncorrosive gas above 10.8°C with a cidal action against bacteria, spores and viruses. It destroys microorganisms by alkylation and causes denaturation of nucleic acids of microorganisms.

Since it is highly toxic, irritant, mutagenic and carcinogenic, thus should not be used on routine bases. It is suited for electric equipment, flexible-fiber endoscopes and photographic equipment.

The duration that the gas should be in contact with the material to be sterilized is dependent on temperature, humidity, pressure and the amount of material.

### Advantages

1. It leaves no residue.
2. It is a deodorizer.
3. Good penetration power.
4. Can be used at a low temperature.
5. Suited for heat sensitive articles, e.g. plastic, rubber, etc.

### Disadvantages

1. High cost of the equipment.
2. Toxicity of the gas.
3. Explosive and inflammable.

## Irradiation

Radiations used for sterilization are of two types:

1. Ionizing radiation, e.g. X-rays, gamma rays and high-speed electrons.
2. Non-ionizing radiation, e.g. ultraviolet light and infrared light.

### Ionizing Radiation

Ionizing radiations are effective for heat labile items. They are commonly used by the industry to sterilize disposable materials such as needles, syringes, culture plates, suture material, cannulas and pharmaceuticals sensitive to heat. High energy gamma rays from cobalt-60 are used to sterilize such articles.

### Non-ionizing Radiation

Two types of non-ionizing radiations are used for sterilization, i.e. ultraviolet and infrared.

1. ***Ultraviolet rays:*** UV rays are absorbed by proteins and nucleic acids and kill microorganisms by the chemical reactions. Their main application is purification of air in operating rooms to reduce the bacteria in air, water and on the contaminated surfaces. Care must be taken to protect the eyes while using U-V radiation for sterilization.
2. ***Infrared:*** It is used for sterilizing a large number of syringes sealed in metal container, in a short period of time. It is used to purify air in the operating room. Infrared is effective, however, it has no penetrating ability.

## Glass Bead Sterilizer

It is rapid method of sterilization which is used for sterilization of instruments (Fig. 9.8). It usually uses table salt which consists approximately of 1 percent sodium silico-aluminate, sodium carbonate or magnesium carbonate. So it can be poured more readily and does not fuse under heat. Salt can be replaced by glass beads provided the beads are smaller than 1 mm in diameter because larger beads are not efficient in transferring the heat to endodontic instruments due to presence of large air spaces between the beads.

The instruments can be sterilized in 5 to 15 seconds at a temperature of 437-465°F (260°C) even when inoculated with spores.

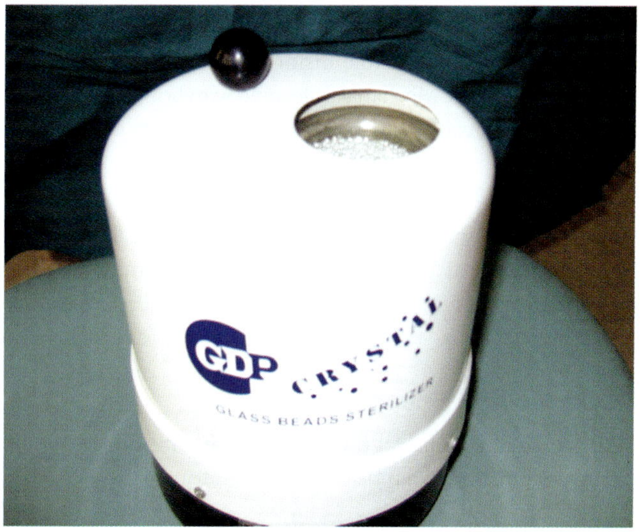


**Fig. 9.8:** Glass bead sterilizer

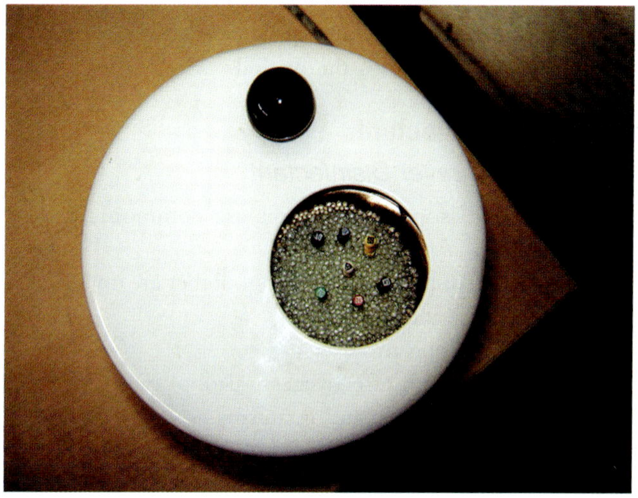

**Fig. 9.9:** Files placed in glass bead sterilizer

The specific disadvantage of these sterilizers is that the handle portion is not sterilized and therefore these articles are not entirely "sterile". These are not recommended unless absolutely required (Fig. 9.9).

### Advantages

- Commonly used salt is table salt which is easily available and cheap
- Salt does not clog the root canal. If it is carried into the canal, it can be readily removed by irrigation.

## DISINFECTION

It is the term used for destruction of all pathogenic organisms, such as, vegetative forms of bacteria, mycobacteria, fungi and viruses, but not bacterial endospores.

## Methods of Disinfection

### Disinfection by Cleaning

Cleaning with a detergent and clean hot water removes almost all pathogens including bacterial spores.

### Disinfection by Heat

Heat is a simple and reliable disinfectant for almost anything except living tissues. Mechanical cleaning with hot water provides an excellent quality of disinfection for a wide variety of purposes.

### Low Temperature Steam

Most vegetative microorganisms and viruses are killed when exposed to steam at a temperature of 73°C for 20 minutes below atmospheric pressure. This makes it a useful procedure to leave spoiled instruments safe to handle prior to sterilization.

### Disinfection by Chemical Agents

They are used to disinfect the skin of a patient prior to surgery and to disinfect the hands of the operator.

*Disadvantages of using chemicals*

- No chemical solution sterilizes the instruments immersed in it
- There is a risk of producing tissue damage if residual solution is carried into the wound.

## Levels of Disinfectant

### Alcohols Low Level Disinfectant

- Ethanol and isopropyl alcohols are commonly used as antiseptics
- Possess some antibacterial activity, but they are not effective against spores and viruses
- Act by denaturing proteins
- To have maximum effectiveness, alcohol must have a 10 minutes contact with the organisms
- Instruments made of carbon steel should not be soaked in alcoholic solutions, as they are corrosive to carbon steel
- Rubber instruments absorb alcohol thus their prolonged soaking can cause a reaction when material comes in contact with living tissue.

### Phenolic Compounds—Intermediate Level, Broad-spectrum Disinfectant

Phenol itself is toxic to skin and bone marrow. The phenolic compounds were developed to reduce their side effects but are still toxic to living tissues. These compounds, in high concentration, are protoplasmic poison and act by precipitating the proteins and destroy the cell wall.

Lawrence and Block (1968) reported that their spectrum of activity includes lipophilic viruses, fungi and bacteria but not spores. The newer synthetic combinations seem to be active against hydrophilic viruses; hence these are approved by ADA for use as surface or immersion disinfectant.

These compounds are used for disinfection of inanimate objects such as walls, floors and furniture. They may cause damage to some plastics and they do not corrode certain metals such as brass, aluminium and carbon steel. It has unique action that is it keeps working for longer period after initial application, known as "Residual Activity".

### Aldehyde Compounds—High Level Disinfectant

*Formaldehyde*

- Broad-spectrum antimicrobial agent
- Flammable and irritant to the eye, skin and respiratory tract
- Has limited sporicidal activity
- Used for large heat sensitive equipment such as ventilators and suction pumps excluding rubber and some plastics.

Not preferred due to its pungent odor and because 18 to 30 hours of contact is necessary for cidal action.

*Glutaraldehyde*

- Toxic, irritant and allergenic
- A high level disinfectant
- Active against most vegetative bacteria, fungi and bacterial spores
- Frequently used for heat sensitive material
- A solution of 2 percent glutaraldehyde (Cidex), requires immersion of 20 minutes for disinfection; and 6 to 10 hours of immersion for sterilization
- Safely used on metal instruments, rubber, plastics and porcelain
- Activated by addition of sodium bicarbonate, but in its activated form, it remains potent only for 14 days.

## Antiseptics (Fig. 9.10)

Antiseptic is a chemical disinfectant that can be diluted sufficiently to be safe for application to living tissues like intact skin, mucous membranes and wounds.

*Alcohols*

- Two types of alcohols are used ethyl alcohol and isopropyl alcohol
- Used for skin antisepsis
- Their benefit is derived primarily in their cleansing action
- The alcohols must have a prolonged contact with the organisms to have an antibacterial effect

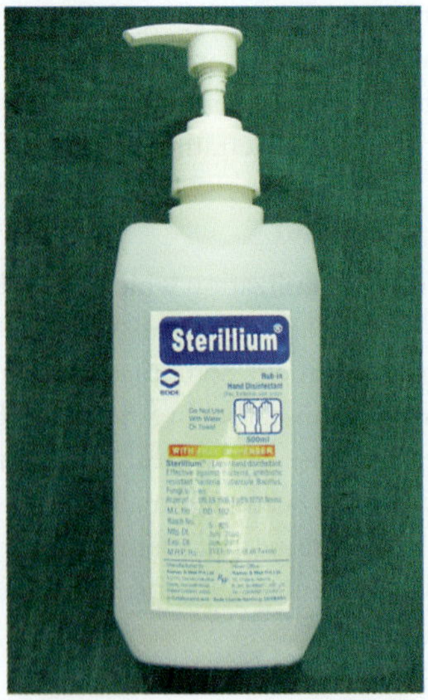


**Fig. 9.10:** Hand disinfectant

- Ethyl alcohol is used in the concentration of 70 percent as a skin antiseptic
- Isopropyl alcohol is used in the concentration of 60 to 70 percent for disinfection of skin.

### *Aqueous Quarternary Ammonium Compounds*

Benzalkonium chloride (Zephiran) is the most commonly used antiseptic. It is well tolerated by living tissues.

### *Iodophor Compounds*

- Used for surgical scrub, soaps and surface antisepsis
- Usually effective within 5-10 minutes
- Discolor surfaces and clothes
- Iodine is complexed with organic surface active agents such as polyvinyl-pyrrolidine (Betadine, Isodine). Their activity is dependent on the release of iodine from the complex.
- Concentrated solutions have less free iodine. Iodine is released as the solution is diluted
- These compounds are effective against most bacteria, spores, viruses and fungi.

### *Chloride Compounds*

- Commonly used are sodium hypochlorite and chlorine dioxide
- Sodium hypochlorite has rapid action
- A solution of 1 part of 5% sodium hypochlorite with 9 parts of water is used
- Chlorous acid and chlorine dioxide provides disinfection in 3 minutes.

### *Diguanides*

- Chlorhexidine is active against many bacteria
- Gets inactivated in the presence of soap, pus, plastics, etc.
- Mainly used for cleaning skin and mucous membrane
- As a 0.2 percent aqueous solution or 1 percent gel it can be used for suppression of plaque and postoperative infection.

## INFECTION CONTROL CHECKLIST

### Infection Control During the Pretreatment Period

- Utilize disposable items whenever possible.
- Ensure before treatment that all equipments has been sterilized properly.
- Remove avoidable items from the operatory area to facilitate a thorough cleaning following each patient.
- Identify those items that will become contaminated during treatment, for example, light handles, X-ray unit heads, tray tables, etc. Disinfect them when the procedure is complete.
- Review patient records before initiating treatment.
- Place radiographs on the X-ray view box before starting the patient.
- Preplan the materials needed during treatment to avoid opening of the cabinets and drawers once the work is started.
- Use separate sterilized bur blocks for each procedure to eliminate the contamination of other, unneeded burs.
- Always keep rubber dam kit ready in the tray.
- Follow manufacturer's directions for care of dental unit water lines (DUWL).

| | *Method of sterilization* | *Sterilizing conditions* | *Advantages* | *Disadvantages* |
|---|---|---|---|---|
| 1. Dry heat | i. Hot air oven | i. 160°C temp for 60-120 minutes | i. No corrosion<br>ii. Instruments are dry after cycle<br>iii. Low cost of equipment | i. Poor penetration of dry heat<br>ii. Long cycle of sterilization<br>iii. Damage to rubber and plastic<br>iv. Higher temperature may damage the instruments |
| | ii. Rapid heat transfer | ii. 190°C for 6-12 minutes | | |
| 2. Moist heat | i. Autoclave | i. 121°C at 15 psi for 15 minutes | i. Better penetration of moist heat<br>ii. Rapid and effective method of sterilization | i. Dulling and corrosion of sharp instruments<br>ii. Damage to plastic and rubber<br>iii. Instruments need to be air dried at the end of cycle |
| | ii. Flash autoclave | ii. 134°C for 3-10 minutes | iii. Does not destroy cotton or cloth products<br>iv. Use for most of instruments | |
| 3. Chemical | Chemical vapor pressure sterilization | 127-131°C at 20 Psi for 20 minutes | i. Short sterilization cycle<br>ii. Lack of corrosion of instrument<br>iii. Effective method | i. Requires adequate ventilation<br>ii. Instruments should be dried before sterilization<br>iii. May emit offensive vapor smell<br>iv. Chemical vapors can damage sensitive instruments |
| 4. Chemical | Ethylene oxide sterilization | | i. Good penetration<br>ii. Non toxic<br>iii. Heat sensitive articles can be sterilized | i. Expensive<br>ii. Explosive and inflammable<br>iii. Toxicity of gas |

| Disinfection of dental material | | |
|---|---|---|
| Material | Disinfectant | Technique |
| Cast | Iodophor | Soaking for 10 min |
| Wax records | Iodoform, NaOCl | Immersion |
| Alginate impression | Iodophors, NaOCl<br>Phenolic compound | Soaking for less than 10 min |

| Sterilization of the dental equipment | | |
|---|---|---|
| *S.No.* | *Instrument* | *Method* |
| 1. | Mouth Mirror Probes, Explorer | Autoclave |
| 2. | Endodontic Instruments—Files, reamers, broaches | Autoclave |
| 3. | Steel, burs | Disposable |
| 4. | Carbide and Diamond burs | Autoclave |
| 5. | Local anesthetic cartridges | Presterilized/disposable |
| 6. | Needles | Disposable |
| 7. | Rubber dam equipment | |
| | a. Carbon steel clamps and metal frames | Dry heat, ethylene oxide, autoclave |
| | b. Punch | Dry heat, ethylene oxide |
| 8. | Gutta-percha points | Dip in 5.2% sodium hypochlorite for 1 min and then rinse with ethyl alcohol |

- Clinician should be prepared before initiating the procedure, this includes the use of personal protective equipment (gown, eyewear, masks and gloves) and hand hygiene.
- Update patient's medical history.

## Chairside Infection Control

- Treat all patients as potentially infectious
- Take special precautions while handling syringes and needles
- Use a rubber dam whenever possible
- Use high volume aspiration
- Ensure good ventilation of the operatory area
- Be careful while receiving, handling, or passing sharp instruments
- Do not touch unprotected switches, handles and other equipments once gloves have been contaminated
- Avoid touching drawers or cabinets, once gloves have been contaminated. When it becomes necessary to do so, ask your assistant to do this or use another barrier, such as over glove to grasp the handle or remove the contaminated gloves and wash hands before touching the drawer and then reglove for patient treatment.

## Infection Control During the Post-treatment Period

- Remove the contaminated gloves used during treatment, wash hands and put on a pair of utility gloves before beginning the clean up
- Continue to wear protective eyewear, mask and gown during clean up
- Dispose of blood and suctioned fluids which have been collected in the collection bottles during treatment
- After disposing of blood and suctioned fluids, use a 0.5% chlorine solution to disinfect the dental unit collection bottle. Keep the solution in the bottle for atleast 10 minutes
- Clean the operatory area and disinfect all the items not protected by barriers
- Remove the tray with all instruments to sterilization area separate from the operatory area
- Never pick up instruments in bulk because this increases the risk of cuts or punctures. Clean the instruments manually or in an ultrasonic cleaner
- Sterilize the hand pieces whenever possible. In general hand piece should be autoclaved but the hand piece which cannot be heat sterilized, should be disinfected by the use of chemicals. Clean the handpiece with a detergent and water to remove any debris. Sterilize it
- Waste that is contaminated with blood or saliva should be placed in sturdy leak proof bags
- Handle sharps items carefully
- Remove personal protective equipment after clean-up. Utility gloves should be washed with soap before removal
- At the end, thoroughly wash hands.

## QUESTIONS

**Q. What is rationale of infection control? Mention different routes of infection transmission?**

**Q. Write short notes on:**

a. Glass bead sterilizer
b. Autoclave
c. Asepsis in endodontics

## BIBLIOGRAPHY


1. Association reports: Current status of sterilization instruments devices, and methods for the dental office; LADA 1981;102:683-89.
2. Charles H Stuart. Enterococcus faecalis: Its role in root canal treatment failure and current concepts in retreament;J endodon 2006;32(2):93-98.
3. Chris H Miller. Cleaning, sterilization and disinfection; JADA; 1993;24:48-56.
4. Chris H Miller. Sterilization and disinfection; JADA 1992;123:46-54.

# Isolation

CHAPTER 10



## INTRODUCTION

The complexities of oral environment present obstacles to the endodontic procedures starting from diagnosis till the final treatment is done. In order to minimize the trauma to these surrounding structures and to provide comfort to the patient the clinician needs to control that field. While performing any operative procedure, many structures require proper control so as to prevent them from interfering the operating field. These structures together constitute the oral environment.

Following components of oral environment need to be controlled during operative procedures.

1. Saliva
2. Moving organs
   - Tongue
   - Mandible
3. Lips and cheeks
4. Gingival tissue
5. Buccal and lingual vestibule

## ADVANTAGES OF MOISTURE CONTROL

### *Patient Related Factors*

- Provides comfort to patient.
- Protects patients from swallowing or aspirating foreign bodies.
- Protects patient's soft tissues–tongue, cheeks by retracting them from operating field.

### *Operator Related Factors*

The following are the operator related advantages of isolation of operating field.

- A dry and clean operating field
- Infection control by minimizing aerosol production.
- Increased accessibility to operative site
- Improved properties of dental materials, hence better results are obtained
- Protection of the patient and operator
- Improved visibility of the working field and diagnosis.
- Less fogging of the dental mirror.
- Prevents contamination of tooth preparation.
- Hemorrhage from gingiva does not enter operative site.

## ISOLATION WITH RUBBER DAM

Isolation of the tooth requires proper placement of the rubber dam/dental dam. It helps to isolate the pulp space from saliva and protects oral tissues from irrigating solutions, chemicals and other instruments. Rubber dam was introduced by ***Barnum, a New York dentist in 1863*** (Fig. 10.1).

***Rubber dam*** can be defined as a flat thin sheet of latex/non-latex that is held by a clamp and frame which is perforated to allow the tooth/teeth to protrude through the perforations while all other teeth are covered and protected by sheet (Fig. 10.1). The rubber dam eliminates saliva from the operating site, retracts the soft tissue and defines the operating field by isolation of one or more teeth from the oral environment.

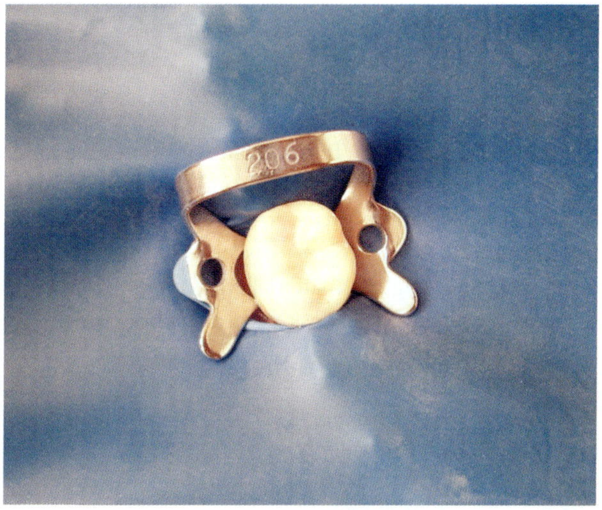


**Fig. 10.1:** A tooth isolated using rubber dam

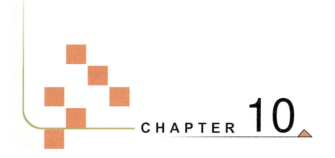

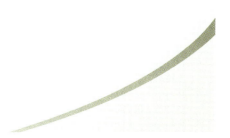

**Advantages of using a rubber dam**

1. It is raincoat for the teeth.
2. It helps in improving accessibility and visibility of the working area.
3. It gives a clean and dry field while working.
4. It protects the lips, cheeks and tongue by keeping them out of the way.
5. It helps to avoid unnecessary contamination through infection control.
6. It protects the patient from inhalation or ingestion of instruments and medicaments.
7. It helps in keeping teeth saliva free while performing a root canal so that tooth does not get decontaminated by bacteria present in saliva.
8. It improves the efficiency of the treatment.
9. It limits bacterial laden splash and splatter of saliva and blood.
10. It potentially improves the properties of dental materials.
11. It provides protection of patient and dentist.

**Disadvantages**

- Takes time to apply
- Communication with patient can be difficult
- Incorrect use may damage porcelain crowns/crown margins/ traumatize gingival tissues
- Insecure clamps can be swallowed or aspirated

**Contraindications of use of rubber dam**

- Asthmatic patients
- Allergy to latex
- Mouth breathers
- Extremely malpositioned tooth
- Third molar (in some cases)

**Rubber dam equipment**

1. Rubber dam sheet
2. Rubber dam clamps
3. Rubber dam forceps
4. Rubber dam frame
5. Rubber dam punch

**Rubber dam accessories**

1. Lubricant/petroleum jelly
2. Dental floss
3. Rubber dam napkin

### *Rubber Dam Sheet (Fig. 10.2)*

The rubber dam is available in size 6 × 6 squares and colors are usually green or black. It is available in three thicknesses, i.e. light, medium and heavy. The middle grade is usually preferred as thin is more prone to tearing and thickest more difficult to apply. Latex free dam is necessary as number of patients are increasing with latex allergy. ***Flexi Dam*** is latex free dam of standard thickness with no rubber smell.

**Thickness of rubber dam sheet**

| | | |
|---|---|---|
| Thin | - | 0.15 mm |
| Medium | - | 0.2 mm |
| Heavy | - | 0.25 mm |
| Extra heavy | - | 0.30 mm |
| Special heavy | - | 0.35 mm |

### *Rubber Dam Clamps*

Rubber dam clamps, to hold the rubber dam on to the tooth are available in different shapes and sizes (Fig. 10.3). Clamps mainly serve two functions:

1. They anchor the rubber dam to the tooth.
2. Help in retracting the gingivae.

Rubber dam clamps can be divided into two main groups on the basis of jaw design.

1. Bland
2. Retentive

*Bland clamps:* Bland clamps are usually identified by the jaws, which are flat and point directly towards each other. In these clamps, flat jaws usually grasp the tooth at or above the gingival margin. They can be used in fully erupted tooth where cervical constriction prevents clamp from slipping off the tooth.

*Retentive clamps:* As the name indicates, these clamps provide retention by providing four-point contact with the tooth. In these, jaws are usually narrow, curved and slightly inverted which displace the gingivae and contact the tooth below the maximum diameter of crown (Fig. 10.4).

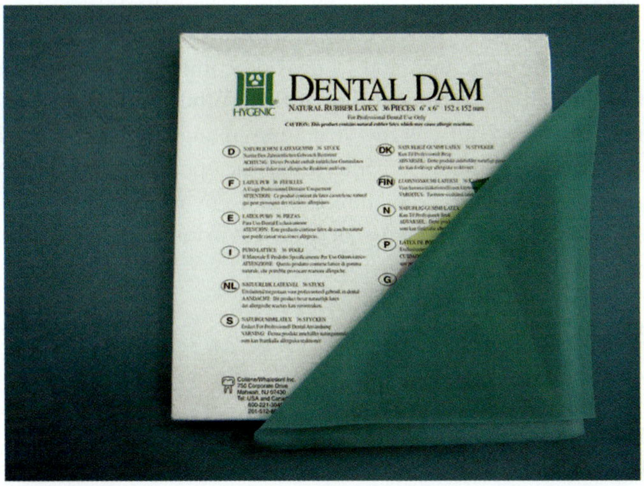


**Fig. 10.2:** Rubber dam sheet

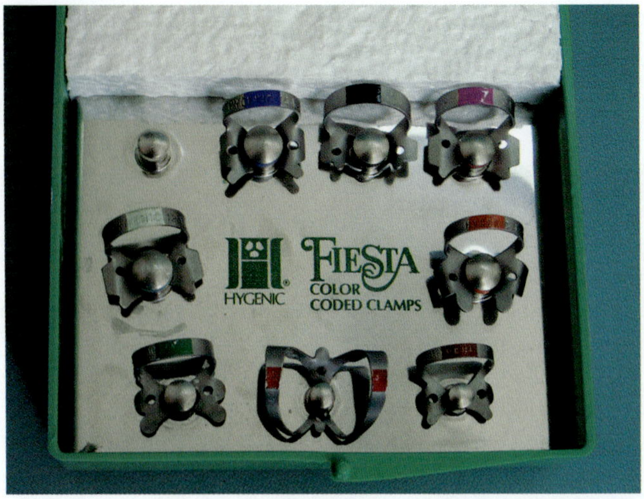


**Fig. 10.3:** Rubber dam clamps

Both flanges are further subdivided into:

- Winged
- Wingless

Rubber dam clamp can also be divided on the basis of material used.

1. Metallic
2. Non-metallic

*Metallic:* Traditionally, clamps have been made from tempered carbon steel and more recently from stainless steel.

*Non-metallic:* Non-metallic are made from polycarbonate plastic. An advantage of these clamps over metallic is radiolucency.

A good length of dental floss should always be passed through the holes in the clamp as a security in case it is dropped in the mouth or the bow fractures.

**Rubber dam clamps**

# 22 Similar to #207, but wingless
# 27 Similar to #206, but wingless, festooned
# 29 For upper and lower bicuspids, with broad beaks
# 206 For upper and lower bicuspids, with festooned beaks
# 207 For upper and lower bicuspids, with flat beaks
# 208 For bicuspids (large), with similar pattern to #207
# 209 For lower bicuspids, with flat beaks
# 0 For small bicuspids and primary central incisors
# 00 For very small bicuspids and primary central incisors
# 1 For roots, with deep festooned beaks
# 2 For lower bicuspids, with flat beaks
# 2A Similar to #2, but with large beaks
# W2A Similar to #2A, but wingless
# P-1,#P-2 For children's first molars

### Rubber Dam Forceps

Rubber dam forceps are used to carry the clamp to the tooth. They are designed to spread the two working ends of the forceps apart when the handles are squeezed together (Fig. 10.5). The working ends have small projections that fit into two corresponding holes on the rubber dam clamps. The area between the working end and the handle has a sliding lock device which locks the handles in positions while the clinician moves the clamp around the tooth. It should be taken care that forceps do not have deep grooves at their tips or they become very difficult to remove once the clamp is in place.

### Rubber Dam Frame

Rubber dam frames support the edges of rubber dam (Fig. 10.6). They have been improved dramatically since the old style with the huge "butterflies". Modern frames have sharp pins which easily grip the dam. These are mainly designed with the pins that slope backwards.

Rubber dam frames serve following purposes:

1. Supporting the edges of rubber dam
2. Retracting the soft tissues
3. Improving accessibility to the isolated teeth.

Rubber dam frames are available in either metal or plastic. Plastic frames have advantage of being radiolucent.

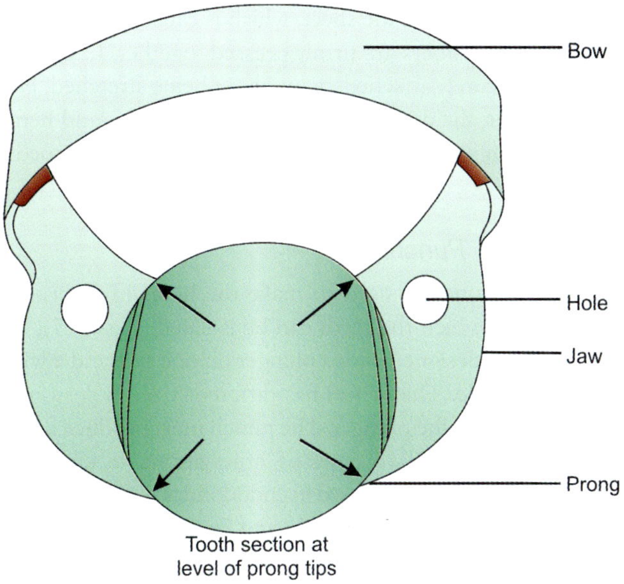


**Fig. 10.4:** A clamp should contact tooth from all sides

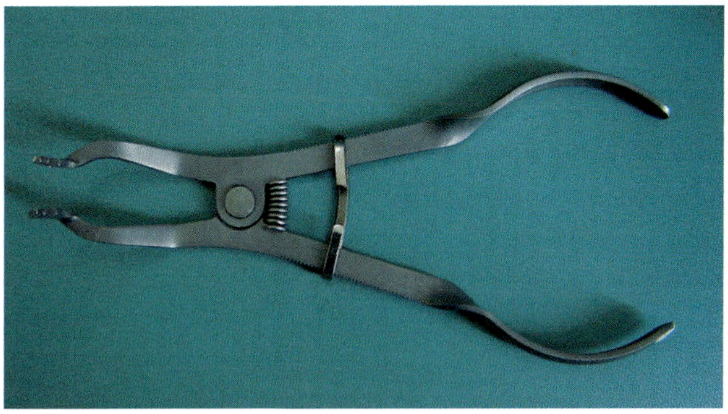

**Fig. 10.5:** Rubber dam forceps

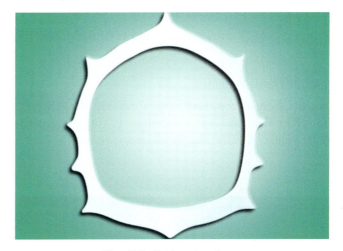

**Fig. 10.6:** Rubber dam frame

As we see when taut, rubber dam sheet exerts too much pull on the rubber dam clamps, causing them to come loose, especially clamps attached to molars. To overcome this problem, a new easy-to-use rubber dam frame ***(Safe-T-Frame)*** has been developed that offers a secure fit without stretching the rubber dam sheet. Instead, its "snap-shut" design takes advantage of the clamping effect on the sheet, which is caused when its two mated frame members are firmly pressed together. In this way, the sheet is securely attached, but without being stretched. Held in this manner, the dam sheet is under less tension, and hence, exerts less tugging on clamps—especially on those attached to molars.

### *Rubber Dam Punch*

Rubber dam punch is used to make the holes in the rubber sheet through which the teeth can be isolated (Fig. 10.7). The working end is designed with a plunger on one side and a wheel on the other side. This wheel has different sized holes on the flat surface facing the plunger. The punch must produce a clean cut hole every time. Two types of holes are made, single and multi-hole. Single holes are used in endodontics mainly. If rubber dam punch is not cutting cleanly and leaving behind a tag of rubber, the dam will often split as it is stretched out.

### *Rubber Dam Template (Fig. 10.8)*

It is an inked rubber stamp which helps in marking the dots on the sheet according to position of the tooth. Holes should be punched according to arch and missing teeth.

### *Rubber Dam Accessories*

A ***lubricant or petroleum jelly*** is usually applied on the undersurface of the dam. It is usually helpful when the rubber sheet is being applied to the teeth.

### *Dental Floss*

It is used as flossing agent for rubber dam in tight contact areas. It is usually required for testing interdental contacts.

### *Wedjets*

Sometimes wedjets are required to support the rubber dam (Fig. 10.9).

### *Rubber Dam Napkin*

This is a sheet of absorbent materials usually placed between the rubber sheet and soft tissues (Fig. 10.10). It is generally not recommended for isolation of single tooth.

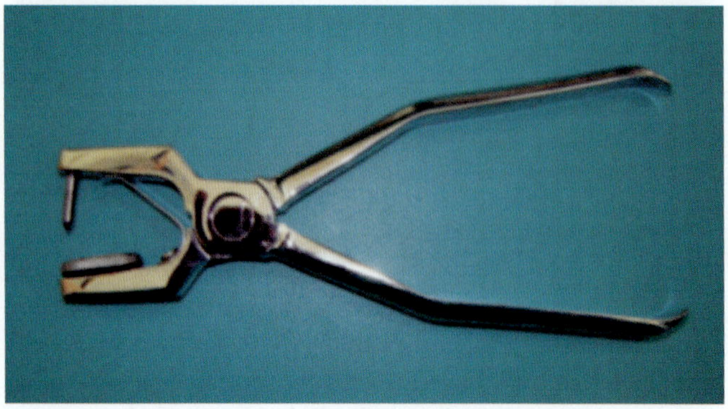

**Fig. 10.7:** Rubber dam punch

## Recent Modifications in the Designs of Rubber Dam

### *Insti-dam*

It is recently introduced rubber dam for quick, convenient rubber dam isolation.

### *Salient Features of Insti-dam*

- It is natural latex dam with prepunched hole and built-in white frame.
- Its compact design is just the right size to fit outside the patient's lips.
- It is made up of stretchable and tear-resistant, medium gauge latex material.
- Radiographs may be taken without removing the dam.

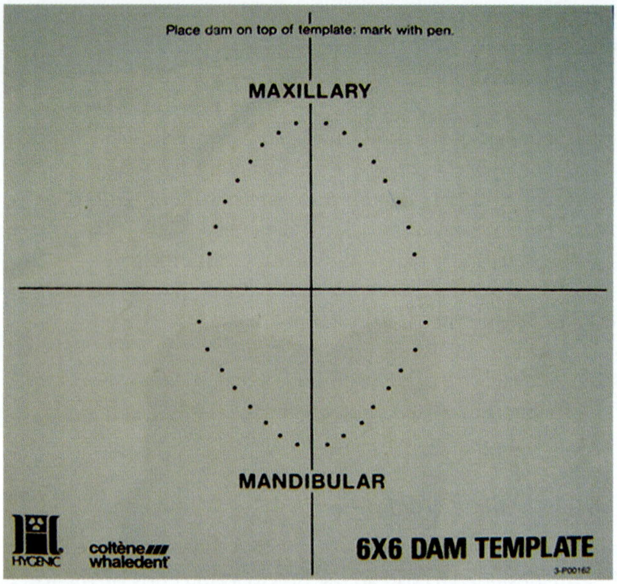


**Fig. 10.8:** Rubber dam template

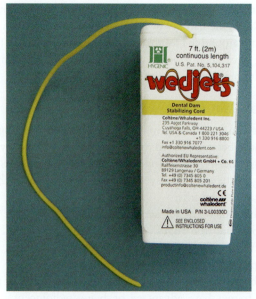


**Fig. 10.9:** Wedjets

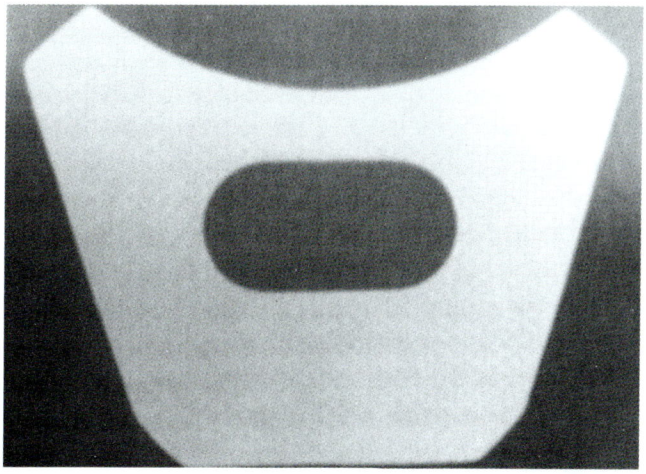

Fig. 10.10: Rubber dam napkin

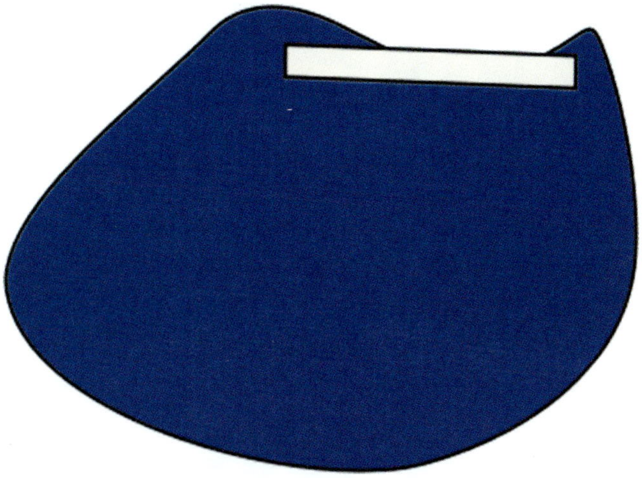

Fig. 10.11: Handi dam

- Built-in flexible nylon frame eliminates bulky frames and sterilization.
- Off-center, prepunched hole customizes fit to any quadrant—add more holes if desired.

### Handi Dam

Another recently introduced dam is **Handi dam**. This is preframed rubber dam, eliminates the need for traditional frame (Fig. 10.11).

Handi dam is easy to place and saves time of both patient as well as doctor. It allows easy access to oral cavity during the procedure.

### Dry Dam

Another newer type of rubber dam is also available which does not require a frame **"dry dam"**.

## Placement of Rubber Dam

Before placement of rubber dam, following procedures should be done:

1. Thorough prophylaxis of the oral cavity.
2. Check contacts with dental floss.
3. Check for any rough contact areas.
4. Anesthetize the gingiva if required.
5. Rinse and dry the operated field.

### Methods of Rubber Dam Placement

**Method I: Clamp placed before rubber dam (Figs 10.12A to C):**

- Select an appropriate clamp according to the tooth size.
- Tie a floss to clamp bow and place clamp onto the tooth.
- Larger holes are required in this technique as rubber dam has to be stretched over the clamp. Usually two or three overlapping holes are made.
- Stretching of the rubber dam over the clamps can be done in the following sequence:
  – Stretch the rubber dam sheet over the clamp
  – Then stretch the sheet over the buccal jaw and allow to settle into place beneath that jaw
  – Finally, the sheet is carried to palatal/lingual side and released.

This method is mainly used in posterior teeth in both adults and children except third molar.

**Method II: Placement of rubber dam and clamp together (Figs 10.13A to C):**

1. Select an appropriate clamp according to tooth anatomy.
2. Tie a floss around the clamp and check the stability.
3. Punch the hole in rubber dam sheet.
4. Clamp is held with clamp forceps and its wings are inserted into punched hole.
5. Both clamp and rubber dam are carried to the oral cavity and clamp is tensed to stretch the hole.
6. Both clamp and rubber dam is advanced over the crown. First, jaw of clamp is tilted to the lingual side to lie on the gingival margin of lingual side.
7. After this, jaw of the clamp is positioned on buccal side.
8. After seating the clamp, again check stability of clamp.
9. Remove the forceps from the clamp.
10. Now, release the rubber sheet from wings to lie around the cervical margin of the tooth.

**Method III: Split dam technique:** This method is *"Split dam technique"* in which rubber dam is placed to isolate the tooth without the use of rubber dam clamp. In this technique, two overlapping holes are punched in the dam. The dam is stretched over the tooth to be treated and over the adjacent tooth on each side. Edge of rubber dam is carefully teased through the contacts of distal side of adjacent teeth.

This technique is indicated:

- To isolate anterior teeth.
- When there is insufficient crown structure.
- When isolation of teeth with porcelain crown is required. In such cases placement of rubber dam clamp over the crown margins can damage the cervical porcelain.

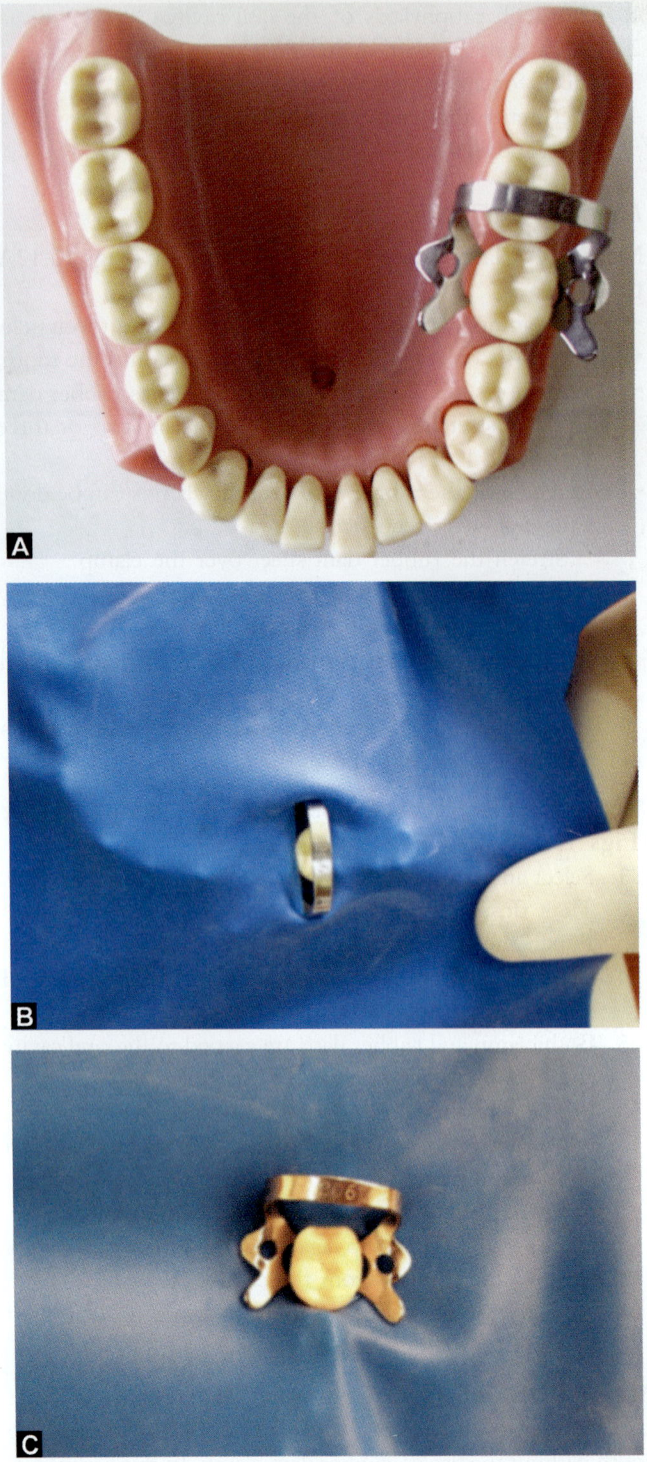


**Figs 10.12A to C:** Placement of rubber dam; (A) Placing clamp on selected tooth; (B) Stretching rubber dam sheet over clamp; (C) After complete stretching tooth is isolated

## MANAGEMENT OF DIFFICULT CASES

### *Malpositioned Teeth*

To manage these cases, following *modifications* are done.

a. Adjust the spacing of the holes.
b. In tilted teeth, estimate the position of root center at gingival margin rather than the tip of the crown.

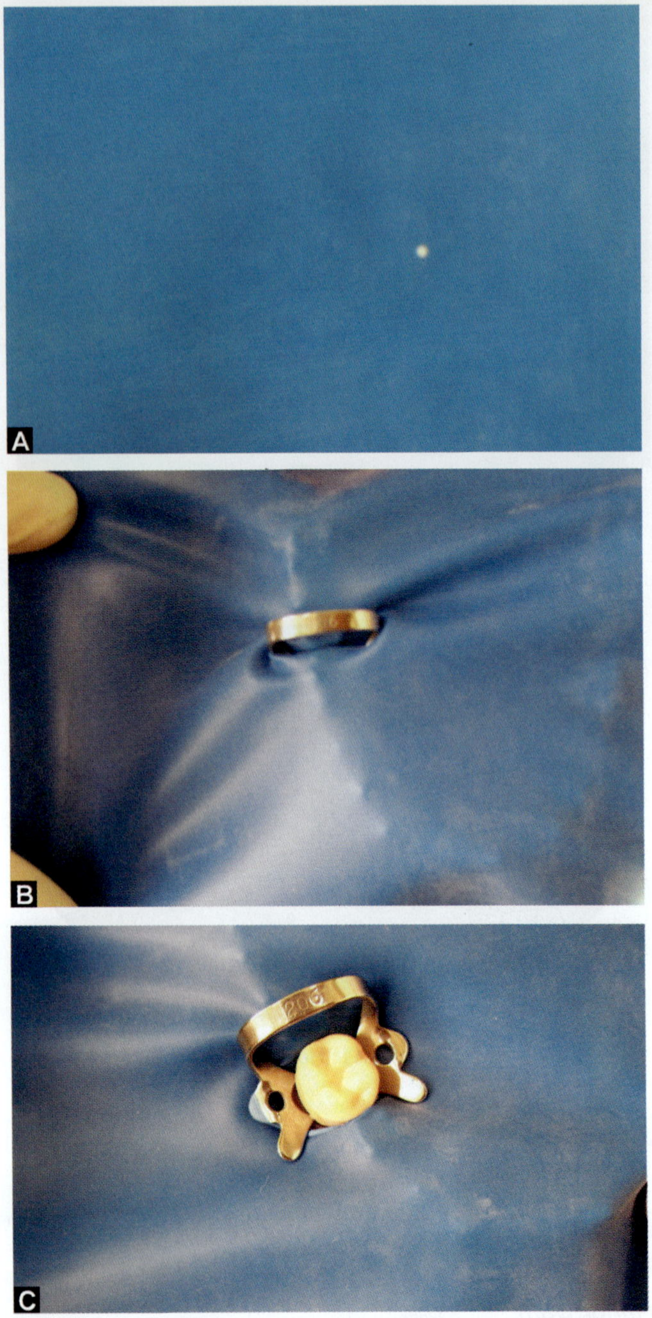


**Figs 10.13A to C:** (A) Punch hole in the rubber dam sheet according to selected tooth; (B) Clamp and its wings are inserted in the punched hole; (C) Carry both clamp and rubber dam over the crown and seat it

c. Another approach is to make a customized cardboard template.
d. Tight broad contact areas can be managed by:
   i. Wedging the contact open temporarily for passing the rubber sheet
   ii. Use of lubricant

### *Extensive Loss of Coronal Tissue*

When sound tooth margin is at or below the gingival margin because of decay or fracture, the rubber dam application becomes difficult. In such cases, to isolate the tooth:

**Commonly encountered problems during application of rubber dam**

| *Problem* | *Consequences* | *Correction* |
|---|---|---|
| 1. Improper distance between holes | | |
| a. Excessive distance between holes | i. Wrinkling of dam<br>ii. Interference in accessibility | Proper placement of holes by accurate use of rubber dam punch and template |
| b. Too short distance between holes | i. Overstretching of dam<br>ii. Tearing of dam<br>iii. Poor fit | |
| 2. Off-center arch form | i. Obstructs breathing<br>ii. Makes patient uncomfortable | Folding of extradam material under the nose and proper punching of holes |
| 3. Torn rubber dam | i. Leakage<br>ii. Improper isolation | Replacement of dam<br>Use of cavit, periodontal packs or liquid rubber dam |

1. Use retentive clamps
2. Punch a bigger hole in the rubber dam sheet so that it can be stretched to involve more teeth, including the tooth to be treated.
3. In some cases, the modification of gingival margin can be tried so as to provide supragingival preparation margin. This can be accomplished by gingivectomy or the flap surgery.

### *Crowns with Poor Retentive Shapes*

Sometimes anatomy of teeth limits the placement of rubber dam (lack of undercuts and retentive areas). In such cases, following can be done:
1. Placing clamp on another tooth.
2. By using clamp which engages interdental spaces below the contact point.
3. By building retentive shape on the crown with composite resin bonded to acid etched tooth surface.

### *Teeth with Porcelain Crowns*

In such cases, placing a rubber dam may cause damage to porcelain crown. To avoid this:
1. Clamp should be placed on another tooth.
2. Clamp should engage below the crown margin.
3. Do not place clamp on the porcelain edges.
4. Place a layer of rubber dam sheet between the clamp and the porcelain crown which acts as a cushion and thus minimizes and localized pressure on the porcelain.

### *Leakage*

Sometimes leakage is seen through the rubber dam because of the accidental tears or holes. Such leaking gaps can be sealed by using cavit, periodontal packs, liquid rubber dam or ora-seal. Nowadays, the rubber dam adhesive can be used which can adhere well to both tooth as well as rubber dam. For sealing the larger gaps, the rubber dam adhesives in combination with orabase can be tried. If leakage persists inspite of these efforts, the rubber dam sheet should be replaced with new one.

Depending upon clinical condition, isolation of single or multiple teeth can be done with the help of rubber dam. Table 10.1 entails problems commonly encountered during application of rubber dam.

## Removal of Rubber Dam

Before the rubber dam is removed, use the water syringe and high volume evacuator to flush out all debris that collected during the procedure. Cut away tied thread from the neck of the teeth. Stretch the rubber dam facially and pull the septal rubber away from the gingival tissue and the tooth. Protect the underlying soft tissue by placing a fingertip beneath the septum. Free the dam from the interproximal space, but leave the rubber dam over the anterior and posterior anchor teeth. Use the clamp forceps to remove the clamp. Once the retainer is removed, release the dam from the anchor tooth and remove the dam and frame simultaneously. Wipe the patient's mouth, lips, and chin with a tissue or gauze to prevent saliva from getting on the patient's face.

Check for any missing fragment after procedure. If a fragment of the rubber dam is found missing, inspect interproximal area because pieces of the rubber dam left under the free gingival can result in gingival irritation.

## QUESTIONS

**Q. Write in detail about rubber dam isolation**

**Q. Write short notes on:**

a. Rubber dam application in teeth with porcelain crowns.
b. Insti-dam

## BIBLIOGRAPHY


1. Cohen S, et al. Endodontic complications and the law. J Endod 1987;13:191-7.
2. Govila CP. Accident Swallowing of an endodontic instrument. A report of two cases. Oral Surg. Oral Med. Oral Pathol Oval Radiol Endod 1979;48:269-71.
3. Kosti E, et al. Endodontic treatment in cases of allergic reaction to rubber dam. J Endod 2002;28:787-9.
4. Lambrianides T, et al. Accident swallowing of endodontic instruments. Endod Dent Tramatol 1996;12:301-4.
5. Miller CH. Infection control. Dent clin. North Am 1996; 40:437-56.
6. Weisman MI. Remedy for dental dam leakage problems. J Endod 1991;17:88-9.

# Pharmacology in Endodontic

CHAPTER 11



## INTRODUCTION

In field of endodontics, dentist commonly faces the problems regarding pain, anxiety and infection. Accordingly clinician has to be well prepared to use drugs, which help to solve these problems. Pain and anxiety though are entirely different problems, yet they are closely related. In endodontics, pain control often proves to be more of a difficult problem than management of anxiety, but because of this difficulty in achieving effective pain control, patients often anticipate the experience with great deal of anxiety.

Pain management is an integral part of endodontics. Pain from a pulpitis or apical periodontitis that produces the need for endodontic therapy may be unbearable without analgesic. Also a similar degree of pain may follow appointments in which canals are enlarged or filled, particularly when the apical constriction is violated or following a surgical procedure. Analgesics may be necessary before an emergency appointment. Practice of endodontics requires a thorough understanding of pain mechanism and management. In addition to pharmacological effectiveness of drugs many people have a positive psychological reaction to the prescription.

Because of common belief that root canal treatment is very complex in nature and there may be severe pain as nerve removal will take place from root canal, patient may suffer from mild to severe apprehension. Also, dental incident or the stories told by other persons about their dental experience causes further dental fear in patient's mind. When this reaches a degree that produced alteration of physiologic and psychological functions, preoperative sedation is required usually in the form of sedatives or tranquilizers. In the present day pharmacological drugs are available that work directly against anxiety without much of side effects, making dental treatment easier for the patient and the practitioner, enabling more patients to receive optimal dental care.

## ANXIETY CONTROL

Certain patients enter the office in such a state of nervousness or agitation that they even find taking of radiographs almost unbearable. Some of them who outwardly appear normal may also be suffering from severe inner apprehension. A kind, supportive and understanding attitude together with suggestion for control of such feelings will be greatly appreciated and usually yield acceptable response.

When an apprehensive patient is rested in the dental chair, clinician should try to recognize the cause of anxiety. Doctor should spend some time at each visit speaking with the patient, anxiety may be expressed at that time.

A variety of techniques for management of anxiety are available. Together these techniques are termed as spectrum of pain and anxiety control. They represent a wide range from non drug technique to general anesthesia.

On the whole there are two major types of sedation, first, requiring administration of the drugs (pharmacosedation) and second, requiring no administration of drugs (Iatrosedation).

### Pharmacosedation

Sedatives and tranquilizers are drugs that are CNS depressants and decrease cortical excitability. Both have similar actions reducing abnormal and excessive response to environmental situations that produce agitation, tension and anxiety.

*Sedative* is a drug that subdues excitement and calms the subject without inducing sleep but drowsiness may be produced. Sedation refers to decreased responsiveness to any level of stimulation and is associated with some decrease in motor activity and sedation. At higher doses sleep may occur.

*Tranquilizers* do not produce sleep and serves effectively to block intolerant and overly aggressive reactions. With tranquilizer use, no attendant is required to the clinic as driving is not contraindicated with tranquilizers. It also eliminates more objectionable types of patient defense reactions and produce acceptable relaxation. Ambulatory patient for whom sedatives are prescribed must be warned against driving at the completion of appointment. Tranquilizer themselves do not produce sleep but may relax the patient to such a degree that extreme drowsiness will develop. This is particularly true where stress or lack of sleep is caused by some emotional factors. Therefore, sedatives and tranquilizers both should be prescribed in lower dosages for patient without prior experience of ingestion until some indication as to the degree of relaxation produced by a given dose is determined.

Short acting barbiturates and their substitutes are excellent for use with endodontic therapy. Initial dose should be given the night before the appointment to ensure restful night, with another taken 30 min before the patient is seated for the treatment. Patients requiring sedatives should be seen in the morning.

## Barbiturates

Barbiturates depress all areas of CNS but reticular activating system is most sensitive, its depression is primarily responsible for inability to maintain wakefulness. Barbiturates don't have selective antianxiety action. They can impair learning, short-term memory and judgment.

**Short acting barbiturates are used in endodontics which are:**

a. Butobarbitone
b. Secobarbitone
c. Pentobarbitone

Barbiturates are well absorbed from gastrointestinal tract. The rate and entry of the drug in CNS depends on lipid solubility.

| *Drugs* | *Dosage* |
|---|---|
| A. Pentobarbital (Nembutal) | a. For relaxed patient: 30 mg night before appointment and 30-60 mg 30 min. before appointment<br>b. For heavier sedation: 30 mg night before appointment and 90 mg 30 min before appointment. |
| B. Secobarbital (Seconal) | 50 mg night before appointment and 50 mg before appointment |
| C. Ethinamate (Valmid) | 1-2 tab night before appointment and 1 tab. 20-30 min before appointment. |

## Contraindications of use of Barbiturates

1. Acute Intermittent porphyria: By inducing microsomal enzyme (8 aminolevulinic acid synthetase) and increases porphyrin synthesis.
2. Liver and kidney disease.
3. Severe pulmonary insufficiency.
4. Obstructive sleep apnea.

## Benzodiazepines

Antianxiety benzodiazepines are:

- Diazepam
- Chlordiazepoxides
- Oxazepam
- Lorazepam
- Alprazolam

Benzodiazepines have a high therapeutic index. Benzodiazepines act preferentially on midbrain ascending reticular formation and on limbic system. Muscle relaxation is produced by a primary medullary site of action.

Benzodiazepines have different oral bioavailability and intramuscular bioavailability. It depends on lipid solubility and plasma protein binding capacity.

## Diazepam

The active metabolites of diazepam are desmethyl diazepam and oxazepam.

With prolonged use, its accumulation occurs which results in anxiolytic effects. Its withdrawal phenomena are mild.

### *Doses*

Oral Route – 5, 10 mg tab. night before appointment and 1 tab. before appointment.
i.m. Route – 10 mg/2 ml syringe before appointment.

## Triazolam

Half-life of about 3 hours, so popular for dental procedures.

- Very potent, peak effect occurs in 1 hour
- Does not accumulate on repeated use
- Higher doses can alter sleep architecture, produce anta grade amnesia and anxiety the following day.

## Midazolam

- Extremely rapid absorption.
- Peak in 20 min.
- Also used as an IV anesthetic.

## Chlordiazepoxide

5 mg capsule therapy to start day before appointment, 1 capsule 3 times daily and 1 capsule morning of appointment.

## Iatrosedation

It is a non-drug technique of causing sedation. A relaxed and pleasant doctor patient relationship has favorable influence on action of the sedative drugs. A patient, who is comfortable with doctor, responds well to the drugs than to patient who are anxious about the doctor and treatment to be done. An effective effort should be done by all the members of dental clinic to help allay the anxiety of patients.

## PAIN CONTROL

Odontogenic pain is usually caused by either noxious physical stimuli or the release of inflammatory mediators that stimulate receptors located on terminal endings of nociceptive afferent nerve fibers.

There are two type of nociceptors:

a. C-fibers
b. A-delta fibers

In human dental pulp C-fibers are found 8-10 times more than A-delta fibers. These are unmyelinated fibers. C-fibers are thought to have a predominant role for encoding inflammatory pain arising from dental pulp and periradicular tissues. After activation, C-and A-delta fibers transmit nociceptive signals primarily via trigeminal nerves to the trigeminal nucleus caudalis located in Medulla. Hyperalgesia is caused by both peripheral and central mechanisms.

Pain control in endodontics though is not very difficult but sometimes it becomes almost impossible to control pain. In endodontics procedures the control of pain becomes difficult mostly at the first appointment. Once the pulp has been extirpated, the pain comes under control. But before initiating the procedure, to avoid discomfort or pain and for soft tissue anesthesia for rubber dam application, local anesthesia injection is needed.

Analgesic can be taken either while local anesthesia is still effective or if no anesthesia was used, as soon as possible after treatment. When a local anesthesia is used and analgesic is prescribed the dentist must calculate the anticipated duration of remaining anesthesia effectiveness. The analgesic should be ingested 30-60 minutes prior to the wearing off of anesthetic so the drug will have sufficient opportunity to take effect. Highly nervous or fidgety patients may metabolize rapidly, and thus the anesthesia lasts for less than the anticipated duration.

Pain control can be achieved through:

1. Opioid drugs
2. Non-opioid drugs
3. Local anesthesia

## 1. OPIOID DRUGS

Generally narcotic (opioid) analgesics are used to relieve acute, severe pain and slight to moderate pain. Clinician's therapeutic judgment determines which analgesic should be prescribed. He must decide the strength of the drug, whether it is to be used alone or in compound form, the frequency of use and side effects associated with it. The drugs used most often are the mild, non-opioid analgesics.

The opioid receptors are located at several important sites in brain, and their activation inhibits the transmission of nociceptive signals from trigeminal nucleus to higher brain regions. Opioids also activate peripheral opioid receptors.

### Classification

a. Natural opium alkaloids:
   - Morphine
   - Codeine
b. Semisynthetic opiates:
   - Diacetyl morphine (Heroin)
   - Pholcodeine
c. Synthetic opioids:
   - Pethidine (Meperidine)
   - Fentanyl
   - Methadone
   - Dextropropoxyphene
   - Tramadol
   - Etoheptazine

Others – Alfentanil, Sufentanil, Lenorphanel, Dextromoranride.

Generally Codeine, Morphine, Tramadol, Propoxyphene, Hydrocodeine and Oxycodeine are used in endodontic pain management.

### *Codeine*

- It is methyl morphine
- Occurs naturally in opium, partly converted into morphine in body
- Good activity by oral route
- It is less potent than morphine and also less efficacious. Codeine is 1/6 to 1/10 as analgesic to morphine
- Comparative to aspirin it is more potent. 60 mg Codeine = 600 mg Aspirin.

**Side effects** – Constipation.

### *Morphine*

- It has site specific depressant and stimulant actions in CNS
- Degree of analgesia increases with dose
- Dull poorly localized visceral pain is relieved better than sharply defined somatic pain
- Calming effects on mood, inability to concentrate
- Depress respiratory centers, death in poisoning is due to respiratory failure
- Oral bioavailability averages ¼ of parenterally administered drug
- About 30% bound to plasma protein and high first pass metabolism present
- Plasma $t\frac{1}{2}$ = 2-3 hours
- Morphine is non cumulative.

**Doses–** 10-15 mg IM or SC.

### Side Effects

- Sedation
- Constipation
- Respiratory depression
- Blurring of vision
- Urinary retention
- Nausea and vomiting
- Blood pressure fall in hypovolemic patients
- Urticaria, itching and swelling of lips

**Antidote – Naloxone** 0.4-0.8 mg IV repeated every 2-3 min till respiration picks up; used in acute morphine poisoning.

### *Dextropropoxyphene*

- Half as potent as codeine
- Has a low oral : parenteral activity ratio
- t½ is 4-12 hours
- Abuse liability is lower than codeine
- Mild oral analgesic
- Combination with aspirin and paracetamol is supra-additive

**Doses**—60-120 mg three times a day.

### *Tramadol*

- Centrally acting analgesic; relieves pain by opioid as well as additional mechanism
- Injected IV 100 mg tramadol is equianalgesic to 10 mg morphine
- Oral bioavailability is good (oral : parentral ratio is 1:2)
- t½ is 3-5 hours, effects last 4-6 hours
- Indicated for medium intensity short lasting pain due to diagnostic procedures, injury, surgery, etc. as well as for chronic pain including cancer pain
- Abuse potential is low.

**Side effects—** Dizziness, nausea, sleepiness, dry mouth, sweating

- It inhibits reuptake of serotonin and norepinephrine, a monoamine, hence, concomitant administration with monoamine oxidase inhibitor drugs is not recommended.
- Narcotics can cause addiction, with characteristics unique from other types of addiction. Both physical and psychological addiction occurs. Narcotics are central nervous system, depressants and work synergistically with all other CNS depressants. Alcohol is contraindicated with narcotics. Narcotics patient must not drive or operate machinery. Narcotics are combined with acetaminophen or aspirin or an NSAID to make them more effective without excessive narcotic side effects.

## 2. NON-OPIOID DRUGS

- Weaker analgesic
- They act primarily on peripheral pain mechanism also in CNS to raise pain threshold.

Non-opioid analgesics interfere with membrane phospholipid metabolism. Mild analgesics interfere with cyclooxygenase pathway and reduce synthesis of prostaglandin and result is the reduction or elimination of pain. More frequently used non-narcotic analgesics are aspirin, acetaminophen, diflunisal, naproxen and ibuprofen, etc.

**Classification**

a. *Analgesic and anti-inflammatory*
   1. Salicylates → Aspirin
   2. Pyrazolone derivatives → Phenylbutazone, Oxyphenbutazone
   3. Indole derivatives → Indomethacin
   4. Propionic acid derivatives → Ibuprofen, Naproxen
   5. Anthranilic acid derivatives → Mephenamic acid
   6. Aryl-acetic acid derivatives → Diclofenac
   7. Oxicam derivatives → Piroxicam, Meloxicam
   8. Pyrrolopyrrole derivative → Ketorolac
   9. Sulfonanilide derivative → Nimesulide
   10. Alkanones → Nabumetone.

b. *Analgesic but poor anti-inflammatory*:
   1. Para-aminophenol derivatives → Paracetamol (Acetaminophen)
   2. Pyrazolone derivative → Metamizol
   3. Benzoxazocine derivative → Nefopam.

**Selective COX-2 inhibitors**

- Rofecoxib
- Celecoxib
- Etocoxib, etc.

NSAIDs are very effective for managing pain of inflammatory origin and by virtue of binding to plasma proteins actually exhibits increased delivery to inflamed tissue.

### Aspirin

- Rapidly converted in the body to salicylic acid which is responsible for most of actions
- Aspirin inhibits COX irreversibly. Return of COX activity depends on synthesis of fresh enzymes
- Analgesic action is mainly due to obtunding of peripheral pain receptors and prevention of prostaglandin mediated sensitization of nerve endings
- It has antipyretic action by promoting heat loss
- Absorbed from stomach and small intestines
- Plasma t½ = 15-20 min

  t½ of anti-inflammatory dose – 8-12 hours.
- Analgesic dose – 600 mg three times a day
- Anti-inflammatory dose – 3-6 g/day or 100 mg/kg/day.

### Side Effects

- Gastric upset
- Irreversibly inhibits $TXA_2$ synthesis by platelets thus it interferes with platelet aggregation and prolong bleeding time
- Hypersensitivity and Idiosyncrasy.

### Contraindications

- Peptic ulcer patient
- Bleeding disorders
- Chronic liver disease
- Pregnancy.

### Precaution

Aspirin should be stopped 1 week before elective surgery.

Aspirin can be buffered with chemicals such as magnesium, calcium or aluminum compounds to decrease stomach complaint.

### Ibuprofen

- Better tolerated alternative to aspirin
- Side effects are milder than aspirin
- Gastric discomfort, nausea and vomiting are less than aspirin.

### Contraindications

- Pregnancy
- Peptic ulcer
  Dose—400-800 mg TDS.

### Piroxicam

- It is a long acting potent NSAID
- Rapidly and completely absorbed, 99 percent plasma protein bound
- Plasma t½ is 2 days
- Suitable for use as short term analgesic as well as long term anti-inflammatory drug
- Single daily administration is sufficient.
  Dose—20 mg BD

### Diclofenac Sodium

- Well absorbed orally
- Plasma t½ is 2 hours
- Epigastric pain, nausea, headache, dizziness, rashes are side effects
- Gastric ulceration and bleeding are less common
- Used in postoperative inflammatory condition.
  Dose—50 mg eight hourly

### Nimesulides

- Selective COX-2 inhibitor
- Weak inhibitory action on prostaglandin synthesis
- Used primarily for short lasting painful inflammatory conditions like sports injury, sinusitis, dental surgery, postoperative pain
- Almost completely absorbed orally
  Dose—100 mg BD.

#### *Para-amino Phenol Derivative (Paracetamol or Acetaminophen)*

- Central analgesic action, it raises pain threshold
- Weak peripheral anti-inflammatory component
- Poor ability to inhibit COX in the presence of peroxides which are generated at site of inflammation
- Well absorbed orally
- Plasma t½ is 2-3 hours
- Paracetamol is one of the most commonly used "over the counter" analgesia where anti-inflammatory action is not required
- One of the best drugs to be used as antipyretic
- Much safer analgesic
  Dose—500-1000 mg TDS
- Should be used cautiously in patients with liver disease or chronic alcohol use.

### Choice of NSAIDs

a. Mild to moderate pain with little inflammation – Paracetamol or low dose ibuprofen.
b. Acute musculoskeletal/injury associated inflammation – Diclofenac or piroxicam, ibuprofen.
c. Short lasting painful condition with minimal inflammation – Ketorolac, nefopam.
d. Exacerbation of acute pain – High dose aspirin, indomethacin, piroxicam.
e. Severe pain – Aspirin, or combination with narcotic drugs.

## 3. LOCAL ANESTHESIA

#### *Definition*

It is defined as a loss of sensation in a circumscribed area of the body caused by depression of excitation in nerve endings or an inhibition of the conduction process in peripheral nerves.

#### *Classification of Local Anesthetic Agents*

All local anesthetics except cocaine are synthetic. They are broadly divided into two groups, i.e. ester and amide (non ester) group.

### A. Based on Chemical Structure

I. *Ester group*
   1. Cocaine
   2. Benzocaine
   3. Procaine
   4. Tetracaine

II. *Amide (Nonester group)*
   1. Lidocaine
   2. Mepivacaine
   3. Prilocaine
   4. Etidocaine
   5. Bupivacaine

### B. Based on Duration of Action

1. Short acting
   - Procaine
2. Intermediate acting
   - Lidocaine
3. Long acting
   - Bupivacaine

The primary action of the local anesthetics agent in producing a nerve conduction block is to decrease the nerve permeability to sodium ($Na^+$) ions, thus preventing the inflow of $Na^+$ ions into the nerve. Therefore local anesthetics interfere with sodium conductance and inhibit the propagation of impulse along the nerve fibers (Fig. 11.1).

In tissues with lower pH, local anesthetics show slower onset of anesthesia while in tissues with higher pH, local anesthetic solution speeds the onset of anesthesia. This happens because at alkaline pH, local anesthetic is present in undissociated base form and it is this form penetrates the axon (Fig. 11.2).

### Composition of a Local Anesthetic Agent

- Local anesthetic—salt form of lidocaine hydrochloride.
- Vasoconstrictor—epinephrine
- Preservative for vasoconstrictor—sodium bisulfite
- Isotonic solution—sodium chloride
- Preservative—methyl paraben
- Sterile water to make the rest of the volume

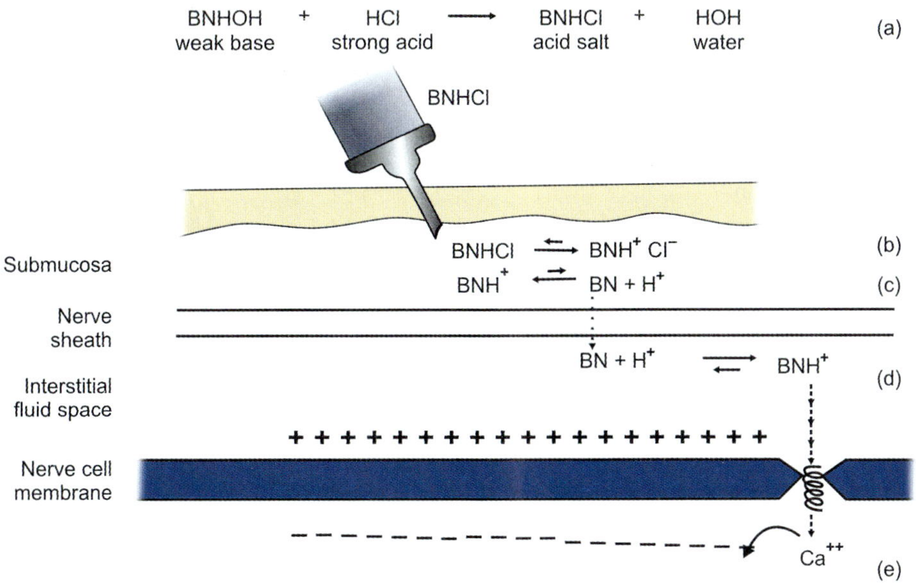


**Fig. 11.1:** Action of local anesthetic at normal pH

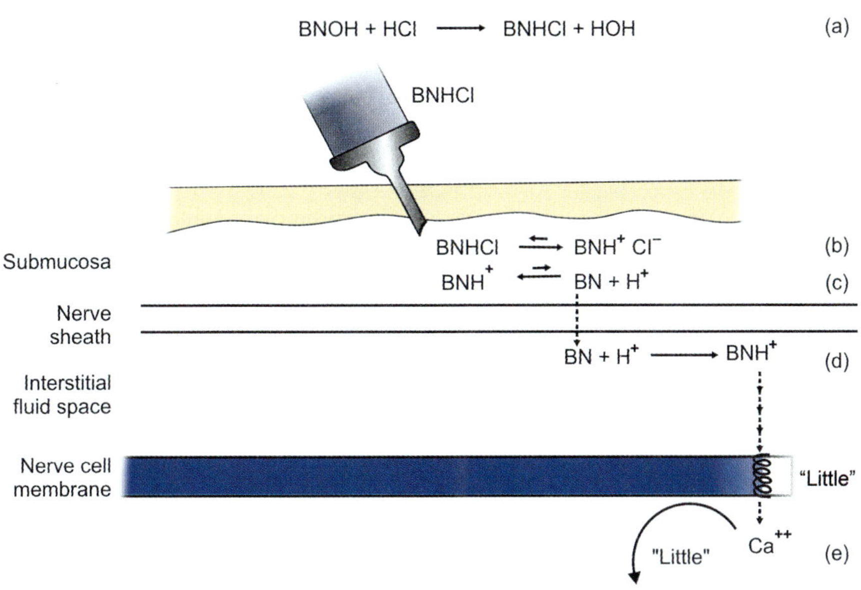


**Fig. 11.2:** Action of local anesthetic at low pH

### Following Factors should be kept in Mind Prior to Administration of Local Anesthesia

*Age:* In very young and extremely old persons, less than the normal therapeutic dose should be given.

*Allergy*: Since, it is life threatening in most of the cases, proper history about allergy should be taken before administering local anesthesia.

*Pregnancy*: It is better to use minimum amount of local anesthetic drugs especially during pregnancy.

*Thyroid disease*: Since patients with uncontrolled hyperthyroidism show increased response to the vasoconstrictor present in local anesthetics. Therefore, in such cases, local anesthesia solutions without adrenaline should be used.

*Hepatic dysfunction*: In hepatic dysfunction, the biotransformation cannot take place properly, resulting in higher levels of local anesthetic in the blood. So, in such cases low doses of local anesthetic should be administered.

### Precautions to be taken before Administration of Local Anesthesia

- Patient should be in supine position as it favors good blood supply and pressure to brain.
- Before injecting local anesthesia, aspirate a little amount in the syringe to avoid chances of injecting solution in the blood vessels.
- Do not inject local anesthesia into the inflamed and infected tissues as local anesthesia does not work properly due to acidic medium of inflamed tissues.
- Always use disposable needle and syringe in every patient. Needle should remain covered with cap till its use.
- To make injection a painless procedure, temperature of the local anesthesia solution should be brought to body temperature.
- Clean the site of injection with a sterile cotton pellet before injecting the local anesthesia.

- Insert the needle at the junction of alveolar mucosa and vestibular mucosa. If angle of needle is parallel to long axis, it causes more pain.
- Inject local anesthesia solution slowly not more than 1 ml per minute and in small increments to provide enough time for tissue diffusion of the solution.
- Needle should be continuously inserted inside till the periosteum or bone is felt by way of slight increase in resistance of the needle movement. The needle is slightly withdrawn and here the remaining solution is injected.
- Check the effect of anesthesia two minutes after injection.
- Patient should be carefully watched during and after local anesthesia for about half an hour for delayed reactions, if any.
- Discard needle and syringe in a leak-proof and hard-walled container after use.

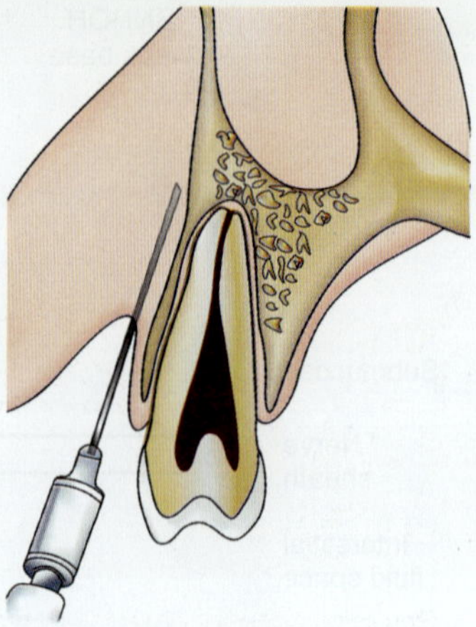

Fig. 11.3: Supraperiosteal technique of local anesthesia

## Various Techniques of Local Anesthesia

- Local infiltration technique
- Supraperiosteal technique
- Field block technique
- Nerve block technique

## Techniques Used for Maxillary Tissues

1. Supraperiosteal technique
*2. Anterior and middle superior alveolar nerve block
3. Posterior superior alveolar nerve block
4. Greater palatine nerve block (anterior palatine nerve block)
5. Nasopalatine nerve block
*6. Maxillary nerve block
7. Periodontal ligament injection

*Both can be given intraorally and extraorally while all other are given intraorally only.

## Techniques for Anesthetizing Maxillary Teeth

1. *Supraperiosteal technique:* It is also known as local infiltration and is most frequently used technique for obtaining anesthesia in maxillary teeth.

### *Technique*

The needle is inserted through the mucosa and the solution is slowly deposited in close proximity to the periosteum, in the vicinity of the apex of the tooth to be treated (Fig. 11.3).

### *Advantage*

It is simple to learn.

### *Disadvantage*

Multiple injections are required for large area.

2. *(a) Anterior superior alveolar nerve block:* Nerve anesthesized with this block are anterior, and middle superior alveolar nerve and infraorbital nerve; inferior palpebral, lateral nasal, superior labial nerves. It is given for anesthesizing the maxillary incisors, canines, premolars and mesiobuccal root of first molar (in 70% of cases). In this the target area is infraorbital foramen.

### *Technique*

Needle is inserted in the mucobuccal fold over the maxillary first premolar and directed towards the infraorbital foramen, once you have palpated. After aspirating, slowly deposit the solution 0.9 to 1.2 ml in the vicinity of the nerve (Fig. 11.4).

*(b) Middle superior alveolar nerve block:* It is used for anesthesizing the middle superior alveolar nerve and its terminal branches. It is given for anesthesizing the maxillary first and second premolars and mesiobuccal root of the first molar.

### *Technique*

Needle is inserted into the mucobuccal fold above the second premolar. After aspirating, slowly deposit local anesthetic solution (i.e. 0.9 to 1.2 ml).

3. *Posterior superior alveolar nerve block:* It is used for posterior superior alveolar nerves. It is given for anesthesizing the maxillary third, second and first molar (sometimes mesiobuccal root is not anesthesized) (Fig. 11.5) and overlying structures (buccal mucosa and bone).

### *Technique*

Needle is inserted distal to the zygomatic process in the mucobuccal fold over the maxillary molar teeth. After aspirating slowly deposit local anesthetic solution.

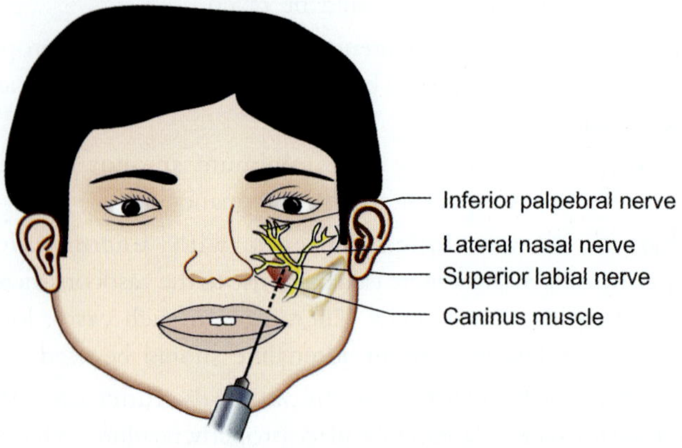


Fig. 11.4: Anterior superior alveolar nerve block

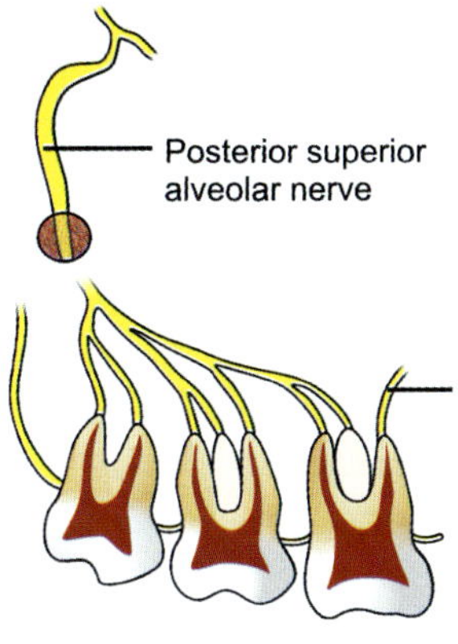


**Fig. 11.5:** Posterior superior alveolar nerve block

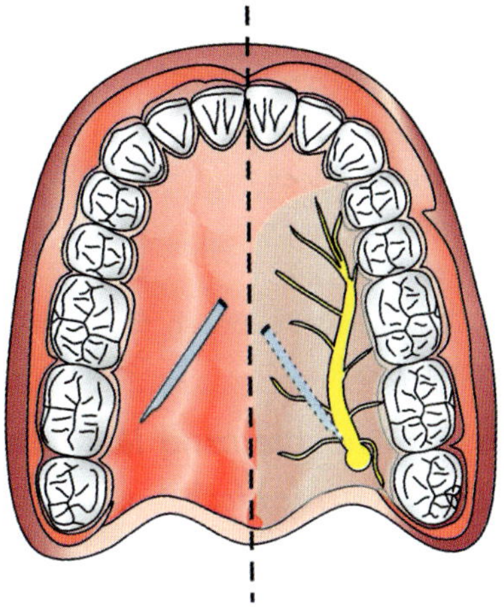

**Fig. 11.6:** Greater palatine nerve block

4. *Greater palatine nerve block:* It is used for anesthesizing greater palatine nerve. It is given for anesthesizing posterior portion of hard palate and its overlying soft tissue, up to the first bicuspid.

### Technique

In this target area is greater palatine foramen. The needle is inserted from the opposite side of mouth at a right angle to the foramen which lies 1 cm from palatal gingival margin towards midline (Fig. 11.6). After aspirating, deposit the solution slowly.

5. *Nasopalatine nerve block:* It is used for anesthesizing anterior portion of the hard palate (soft and hard tissues), extending from one side premolar to other side of first premolar.

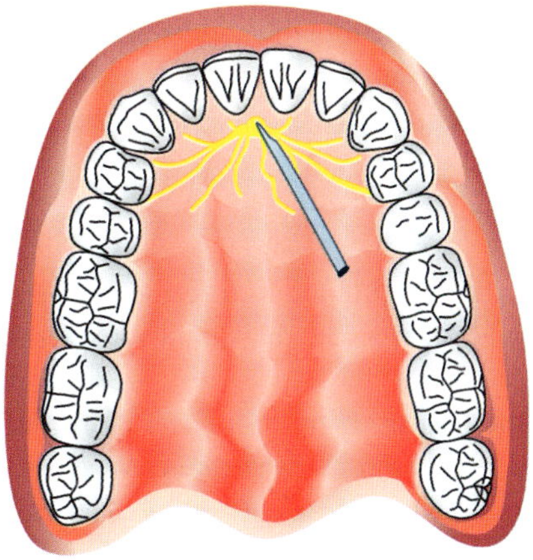

**Fig. 11.7:** Nasopalatine nerve block

### Technique

Needle is inserted in intraseptal tissue between the maxillary central incisors. Deposit slowly the local anesthetic solution in the tissue (Fig. 11.7).

6. *Maxillary nerve block:* It is used for anesthesizing the maxillary nerve of trigeminal nerve. In this, different techniques which can be used are:
   i. High tuberosity approach
   ii. Greater palatine canal approach
   iii. Extraoral technique

7. *Periodontal ligament injection:* It is used for anesthesizing terminal nerve endings in vicinity of the injection. The local anesthetic solution is deposited into the periodontal ligament or membrane.

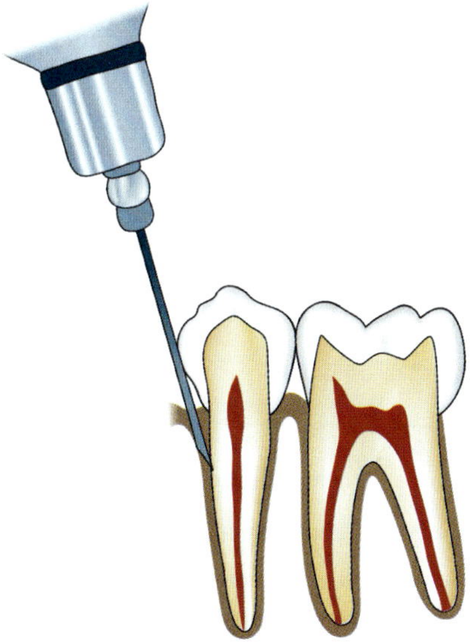

**Fig. 11.8:** Periodontal ligament injection

### Technique

Needle is inserted along the long axis of the tooth either on mesial or distal of the root (Fig. 11.8). Deposit local anesthetic solution (0.1-0.2 ml) slowly.

### Advantages

- Rapid onset of action
- It is a useful adjunct to normal local anesthesia
- Provides specific analgesia to isolated tooth.

### Disadvantage

Post injection discomfort due to temporary extrusion.

## Various Mandibular Anesthesia Techniques

1. Inferior alveolar nerve block
2. Long buccal nerve block
3. Mandibular nerve block
   - Gow-gates technique
   - Extraoral approach
4. Vazirani-Akinosi closed mouth technique
5. Mental nerve block

## Techniques of Anesthetizing Mandibular Teeth

1. ***Inferior alveolar nerve block:*** It is used for anesthesizing inferior alveolar nerve, lingual nerve and its terminal branches, i.e. mental and incisive.

*The areas anesthesized are*:

i. Mandibular teeth
ii. Body of the mandible and inferior portion of the ramus
iii. Buccal mucous membrane and its underlying tissues only up to first molar
iv. Anterior two third of tongue, lingual soft tissues, floor of the oral cavity.

### *Technique*

The target in this technique is inferior alveolar nerve. The operator should first palpate the anterior border of the ramus. Its deepest concavity is known as coronoid notch which determines the height of injection. The thumb is placed over the coronoid notch and also in contact with internal oblique ridge. The thumb is moved towards the buccal side, along with buccal sucking pad. This gives better exposure to pterygo-mandibular raphe (Fig. 11.9). Insert the needle parallel to occlusion of mandibular teeth from opposite side of mouth. Needle is finally inserted lateral to pterygomandibular raphe in pterygomandibular space.

Bone must be contacted as it determines the penetration depth. Solution required in this block vary from 1.5-1.8 ml.

2. ***Long buccal nerve block:*** It is used for anesthesizing buccal mucosa of mandibular molar teeth.

### *Technique*

In this, target is buccal nerve. Insert needle in the mucosa distal and buccal to last lower molar tooth in the oral cavity (Fig. 11.10).

3. ***Mandibular nerve block:*** For complete anesthesizing the mandibular nerve, following techniques may be used

i. Gow-gates technique
ii. Extraoral approach

4. ***Vazirani-Akinosi closed mouth technique:*** It is usually preferred in patients who have limited/restricted mouth opening. The areas anesthesized by this technique is very much similar to the area anesthesized by inferior alveolar nerve block. Target area is pterygomandibular space.

### *Technique*

In this technique first patient is asked to bring teeth in the occlusion. Needle is positioned at the level of mucogingival junction of maxillary molars. Needle is penetrated through the mucosa in the embrasure just medial to the ramus (Fig. 11.11). When tip of the needle reaches the target area, approximate 2 ml of solution is deposited slowly.

5. ***Mental nerve block:*** It is used for anesthesizing the buccal soft tissues anterior to the mental foramen and up to the midline.

### *Technique*

Insert the needle in the mucobuccal fold just anterior to mental foramen (Fig. 11.12). Slowly deposit the solution into the tissue.

## Intrapulpal Injection

Adequate pulpal anesthesia is required for treatment of pulpally involved tooth. Mandibular teeth usually offers some problems in obtaining profound anesthesia. This injection control spain, both by applying pressure and utilizing the pharmacologic action of local anesthetic agent.

### *Indication*

Lack of obtaining profound anesthesia in pulpally involved teeth by other techniques (mentioned above).

### *Nerves Anesthesized*

Terminal nerve endings at the site of injection.

### *Technique*

1. Insert 25 or 27 gauge needle firmly into the pulp chamber (Fig. 11.13).

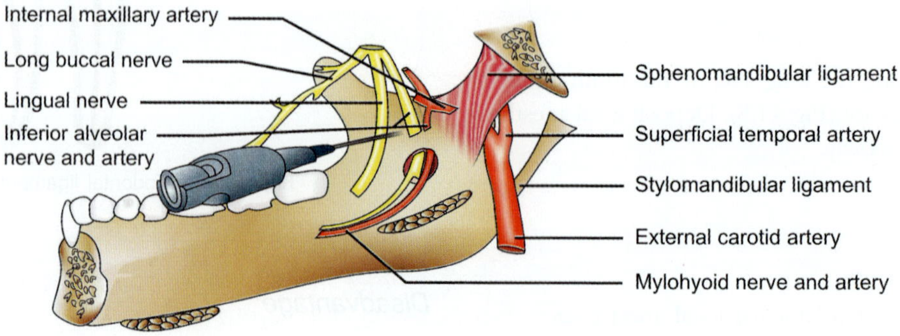


**Fig. 11.9:** Inferior alveolar nerve block

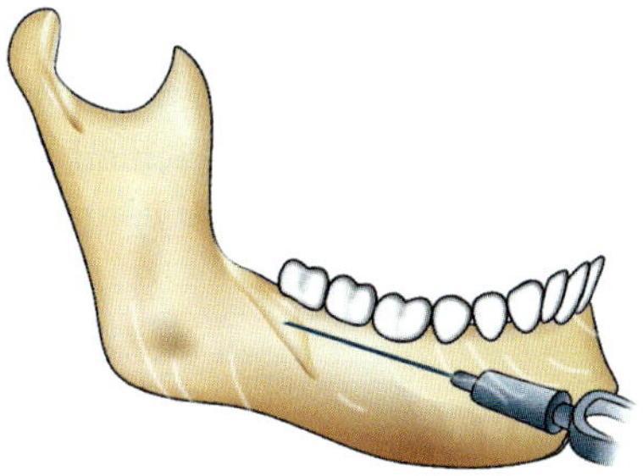

Fig. 11.10: Long buccal nerve block

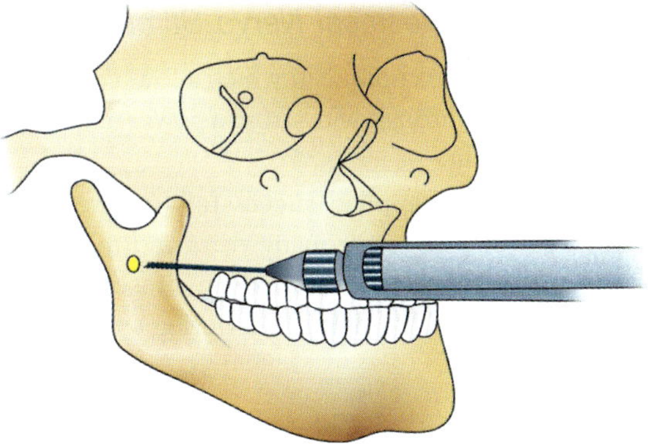

Fig. 11.11: Closed mouth technique

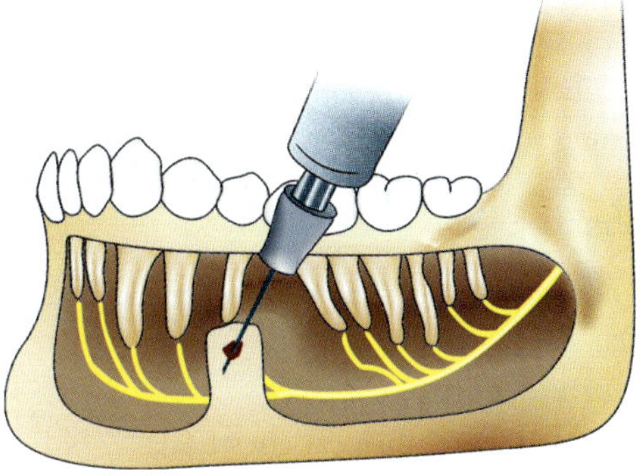

Fig. 11.12: Mental nerve block

2. Before inserting the needle, patient must be informed that he/she may experience a brief period of sensitivity (mild to very painful) after giving the injection.
3. Always deposit local anesthetic solution under pressure as back pressure is shown to be the major factor is producing anesthesia (Fig. 11.14).
   - For creating back-pressure, block the access with stoppers (cotton pellet). To prevent back-flow, other stoppers which can be used are gutta-percha, waxes or pieces of rubber.
   - Deposit a very small amount of solution (0.2-0.3 ml) under pressure (5-10 seconds).
   - Sometimes, bending of needle is done for gaining access to the canal.

### *Advantages*

1. Requires less volume
2. Early onset
3. Easy to learn

### *Disadvantages*

1. Results are not predictable as it may vary (it should always be given under pressure).
2. Taste of local anesthetic drug is not accepted by patients as it may spill during administration of intrapulpal injection.
3. Brief pain during or after insertion of solution (not tolerated by some patients).

## Recent Advances in Local Anesthesia

Many advances have been tried for making the experience of local anesthesia more comfortable and less traumatic. These advances are:

1. WAND system of local anesthesia
2. Comfort control syringe
3. TENS local anesthesia
4. Electronic Dental Anesthesia (EDA)
5. Needle-less syringes.

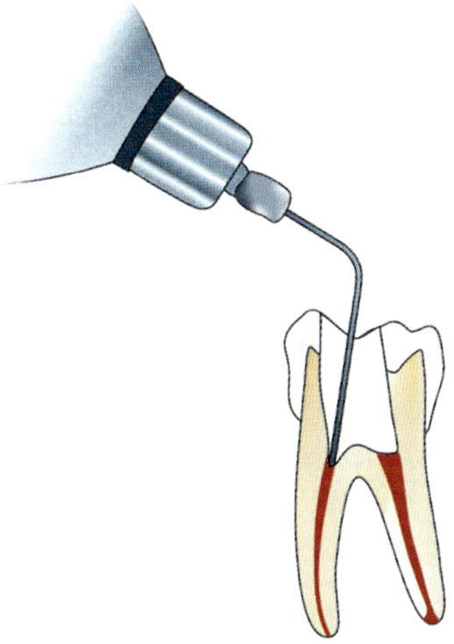

Fig. 11.13: Intrapulpal injection

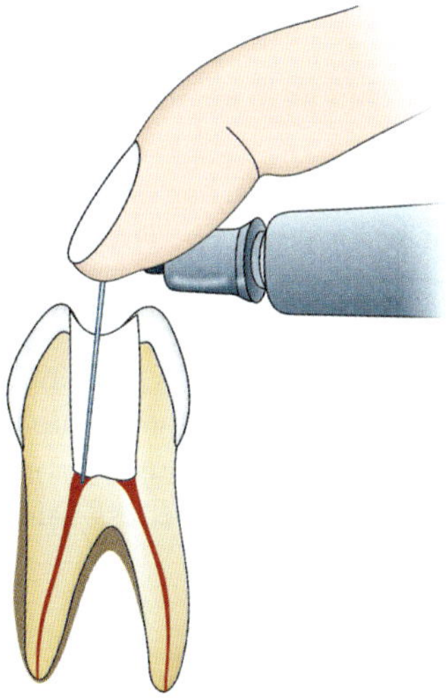

Fig. 11.14: During intrapulpal injection deposit the solution under pressure

### WAND System of Local Anesthesia

WAND local anesthesia system is considered as the significant advancement in the delivery of local anesthetic system. This is computer-automated injection system which allows precise delivery of anesthesia at a constant flow rate despite varying tissue resistance.

It has been renamed CompuDent—featuring the WAND handpiece. This has been approved by US Food and Drug Administration (FDA) as local anesthesia delivery device.

CompuDent system consists of two main elements:

1. CompuDent computer
2. WAND handpiece.

***Method:*** Topical anesthetic is first applied to freeze the mucosa and then a tiny needle is introduced through the already numb tissue to anesthetize the surrounding area. In this system, a disposable anesthetic cartridge is placed in a disposable plastic sleeve, which docks with the pump that delivers anesthetic solution through a microintravenous tubing attached to handpiece.

*Uses:* Considered as effective for all injections that can be performed using a standard aspirating syringe.

#### Advantages

1. Reduced pain and anxiety
2. More rapid onset of anesthesia
3. Considered as more accurate than standard aspirating syringe
4. Enables the operator to use pen grasp while injecting.

#### Disadvantages

1. Initial cost of the unit is expensive
2. Longer injection time
3. Due to longer tubing attached to handpiece, only 1.4 ml of anesthetic solution is injected from cartridge.
4. System does require sometime to get accustomed too.
5. System is operated by foot-pedal control and anesthetic cartridge is not directly visible.

### Comfort Control Syringe (CCS)

It is an electronic, pre-programmed delivery system for local anesthesia that dispenses the anesthetic in a slower, more controlled and more consistent manner than traditional manual syringe.

The comfort control syringe has two-stage delivery system in which injection begins at a very slow rate to decrease the discomfort associated with rapid injection. After ten seconds, CCS automatically increases injection rate for the technique which has been selected. There are five different injection rates to choose from that are pre-programmed into CCS system. As a result, CCS can be adapted for any intraoral injection and still deliver an injection that can be less painful than with a manual syringe.

#### Advantages

1. During the first-phase of injection, anesthetic is delivered at very slow rate. This minimizes pressure, tissue trauma and patient discomfort.
2. More rapid onset of anesthesia.
3. Enables the operator to use pen grasp while injecting.
4. It has anesthetic cartridge directly behind the needle, that as in traditional syringe and injection controls are on finger tip rather than on foot-pedal.

#### Disadvantages

1. Longer injection time
2. Cost of the unit is expensive
3. Handpiece is bulkier than WAND system.

### Transcutaneous Electrical Nerve Stimulation (TENS)

This is non-invasive technique in which a low-voltage electrical current is delivered through wires from a power unit to electrodes located on the skin.

TENS, has been applied successfully to treat acute and chronic pain in medicine for many years and more recently in dentistry. Its use for treatment of myofascial pain is well documented and has also been tried during simple restoration and electroanalgesia.

#### Mechanism of Action

1. Release of endogenous opiates
2. Based on Gate's control theory, which states that stimulating input from large pain conducting nerve fibers closes the gate on nociceptive sensory phenomena from the A-delta and C-fibers. This prevents descendent motor activity (tightening up).

#### Indications

- Most commonly used in temporomandibular disorders (TMDs)
- Restorative dentistry
- In patients, allergic to local anesthesia
- In patients having needle phobia.

#### Contraindications

- Patients having cardiac pacemakers
- Patients having neurological disorders such as epilepsy, stroke, etc.
- Pregnant patients.

#### Technique

1. Clean the surface by alcohol swab over the coronoid notch area
2. Dry the area with gauze piece
3. Apply electrode patches
4. Make sure that TENS unit is off
5. Attach electrode leads from patch to TENS unit
6. Adjust the timer
7. Adjust the controls to high bandwidth and high frequency.
8. Slowly adjust the amplitude so that patient feels a gentle pulsing sensation

9. Adjust pulse width and pulse rate
10. Proceed with dental procedure in usual manner
11. At the completion of the procedure, disconnect the leads and remove the electrode patches from the patient.

### *Electronic Dental Anesthesia (EDA)*

Electronic dental anesthesia developed in mid-1960s for management of acute pain, but the use of electricity as therapeutic modality is not new in the field of medical and dental sciences.

### *Indications*

1. Most common use is in temporomandibular disorders (TMDs)
2. Restorative dentistry
3. Patients with allergic to local anesthesia
4. Patient having needle phobia.

### *Contraindications*

1. In patients with cardiac pacemakers
2. Pregnant patients
3. In patients with neurological disorders such as epilepsy, stroke, etc.
4. Young pediatric patient
5. Dental phobics individuals afraid of every dental treatment
6. Very old patients with senile dementia.

### *Mechanism of EDA*

This is explained on the basis of Gate controls theory. In this, higher frequency is used which causes the patient to experience a sensation described as throbbing or pulsing. It also causes stimulation of larger diameter nerve fibers (A-fibers) which is usually responsible of touch, pressure and temperature.

These large diameter fibers (A-fibers) are said to inhibit the central transmission of effects of smaller nerve fibers (A-delta and C-fibers) which in turn are stimulated during drilling at high speed and curettage. So, when no impulse reaches the central nervous system, there would be no pain.

**Mechanism of EDA**

1. Based on Gate Controls theory
2. Uses higher frequency to experience a sensation
3. Causes the patient to experience a sensation described as throbbing or pulsing
4. Causes stimulation of large diameter nerves (A-fibers) which inhibit central transmission of effects of smaller nerve fibers.

### *EDA Advantages*

1. No fear of needle
2. No fear for injection of drugs
3. No residual anesthetic effect after the completion of procedure
4. Residual analgesic effects persists after completion of procedure

### *Disadvantages*

1. Expensive
2. Technique sensitive—requires training.

### *Needle-less Syringes*

Needle-less syringe are especially designed syringes to administer anesthetic drugs which shoot a pinpoint jet of fluid through the skin at high speed.

## INFECTION CONTROL

In the usual picture, pulpal invasion begins with the mixed infection of aerobes and anaerobes. As the infection increases, flora changes to obligate anaerobes and facultative organisms because of oxygen depletion. One of the primary goals of endodontic therapy is to eliminate a habitat of microorganisms in canal space. Thus thorough sterilization is needed starting from the pulpal debridement up to the step of obturation. It has been seen many times that chronic infection persists in periapical area, following root canal therapy. Studies have shown presence of bacteria in chronic asymptomatic periapical radiolucent lesions. Though antibiotics are considered as tool for fighting infection, endodontic therapy mainly emphasizes the importance of thorough debridement of canal apace.

When drainage from root canal system becomes difficult to obtain or when host resistance is low or when virulence of attacker is high, antibiotics are needed.

## ANTIBIOTICS

These drugs attack cell structure and metabolic paths, unique to bacteria and not shared with the human cells. Since ***Flemming*** produced the first antibiotic over 60 years ago, dealing with infection, has changed.

### Definition

These are substances which are produced by micro-organisms, suppress or kill other microorganisms at very low concentrations.

These drugs attack cell structure and metabolic pathways of bacteria but not the human cells. Nowadays, oral and systemic antibiotics are most frequently used so, the thorough understanding about their pharmacologic profile is necessary. In this topic, we will discuss the indications, uses and side effects of most commonly antibiotics.

### Classification of Antibiotics

**Classification**

I. Based on spectrum of activity
   a. Narrow spectrum
      i. Penicillin G
      ii. Streptomycin
      iii. Erythromycin
   b. Broad spectrum
      i. Tetracyclines
      ii. Chloramphenicol
II. Type of action
   1. Bactericidal
      a. Penicillin and cephalosporins
      b. Metronidazole

| | |
|---|---|
| c. Fluoroquinolone | i. Nalidixic acid |
| | ii. Ciprofloxacin |
| | iii. Ofloxacin |
| | iv. Sparfloxacin |
| | v. Gatifloxacin |
| d. Aminoglycosides | i. Streptomycin |
| | ii. Amikacin |

2. Primarily bacteriostatic
   a. Sulfonamides
   b. Tetracycline
   c. Clindamycin
   d. Erythromycin

III. On the basis of family
   Pencillins
   Cephalosporins
   Sulfonamides
   Tetracyclines
   Aminoglycosides
   Macrolides

**Factors determining the efficiency of antimicrobial agents**
- Host defense
- Source of infection
- Tissue affected
- Margin of safety
- Bacterial susceptibility/resistance to agent being used.

**Mechanism of action of antimicrobial agents**

| *Action* | *Antimicrobial agents* |
|---|---|
| 1. Inhibition of cell wall synthesis | Pencillins, cephalosporins vancomycin |
| 2. Inhibition of protein synthesis | Aminoglycosides, tetra-cycline chloramphenicol, lincomycin |
| 3. Interference in transcription/ translation of genetic information | Ciprofloxacin, ofloxacin gatifloxacin, metronidazole |
| 4. Antimetabolite actions | Sulfonamides, trimethoprim |

## FACTORS AFFECTING SELECTION OF ANTIBIOTICS

**Selection of antibiotic**
Selection of antibiotic depends upon several factors like:
- Clinical diagnosis
- Identification of causative organism
- Age
- Severity of the disease
- Drug resistance and toxicity
- Drug allergic reactions
- Cost of the therapy

- *Clinical diagnosis*: A clinical diagnosis should be made before initiating antimicrobial therapy.
- *Age of the patient*: Drug should be given according to age of the patient for example-Chloramphenicol is not given to infants.
- *Severity of the disease*: In general, antimicrobial therapy should be considered for patients with established orofacial infections. In mixed infections, a combination of antimicrobial should be used.
- *Pregnancy*: Many antimicrobial agents should be used with caution as these drugs cross placental barrier.

*Drugs which can be given in these conditions are*:
1. Pencillins
2. Cephalosporins
3. Erythromycin
4. Lincomycin
5. Clindamycin
6. Azithromycin.

### Drug Resistance and Toxicity

Drug resistance should also be kept in mind while prescribing antibiotic as some microorganisms are resistant to some antibiotics.

***For example***: Some strains of staphylococci are resistant to penicillin, then an alternative should be prescribed. Drug toxicity usually occurs when there is defect in excretion of drug. It is usually seen in hepatic and renal damage. Usually, the drugs are cleared by two mechanisms.
1. By renal excretion
2. Non-renal mechanism.

The mechanism of clearance of some commonly prescribed antibiotics is described in tabulated form as follows:

**Mechanism of clearance**

| *Renal excretion* | *Non-renal* |
|---|---|
| 1. Penicillins | 1. Erythromycin |
| 2. Fluoroquinolones | 2. Doxycycline |
| 3. *Cephalosporins | 3. Chloramphenicol |
| 4. Aminoglycosides | |

(* *Cephalosporin excluding cefoparazole*)

### Drug Allergic Reactions

Previous allergic reactions if any, to antimicrobials should be noted and alternative should be prescribed.

***For example***: If a person is allergic to penicillin and its products, he/she should be prescribed erythromycin.

### Cost Therapy

Presently many drugs are available in the market. Newer drugs are added from time-to-time which are usually more expensive but not necessarily more effective so proper selection of antibiotic is necessary.

## COMMONLY USED ANTIBIOTICS

### Beta-lactam Antibiotics

1. Penicillins
2. Cephalosporins.

#### Mechanism of Action

- Inhibition of cell wall synthesis.
- Bacteria possess a cell wall, which is absent in mammalian cells

- Bacterial cell contents are usually under high osmotic pressure and the viability of the bacteria depends upon the integrity of this peptidoglycan lattice in the cell wall
- These drugs bind to bacterial cell surface receptors which are actually enzymes involved in the transpeptidation reaction
- They also cause the inactivation of the cell wall inhibitor of autolytic enzymes in the cell wall which results in the enzymatic cell lysis.

## Classification of Penicillins

- Benzyl penicillin (penicillin G), penicillin V
- Penicillinase resistant penicillins: Methicillin, cloxacillin
- Broadspectrum penicillins: Ampicillin, amoxycillin
- Antipseudomonal penicillin: Carbencillin

### *Benzyl Penicillin (Penicillin G)*

- Not very effective orally, therefore used IM or IV.
- Easily destroyed by gastric acids
- Bactericidal active against gram-positive organisms. *(Available in different form-crystalline penicillin, procaine penicillin, benzathine penicillin)*
- Adverse reaction: Anaphylaxis.

### *Penicillin V (Phenoxymethyl penicillin)*

- This is not destroyed by gastric acid.
- Well absorbed orally.
- Antimicrobial spectrum-similar to penicillin G.

## Penicillinase Resistant Penicillins

Penicillinase can inactivate beta-lactam antibiotics. Chemical modifications in the beta-lactamase ring has led to the development of penicillinase resistant penicillins such as methicillin and cloxacillin.

## Broad-spectrum Penicillins (Ampicillin, Amoxycillin)

- Effective against gram-positive and gram-negative bacteria.
- They are destroyed by beta-lactamase enzyme but are acid stable
- Can be given orally
- Amoxycillin is better absorbed orally than ampicillin, has lower incidence of diarrhea and has a similar antibacterial spectrum.

## Cephalosporins

- Broad-spectrum of activity, effective against gram-positive and gram-negative organisms
- Adverse reaction – allergy.
  *(Usually patients sensitive to penicillins are allergic to cephalosporins also)*
- These drugs are classified according to their antibacterial spectrum into first, second, third and fourth generation cephalosporins.

| *Generation* | *Examples* | *Spectrum of activity* |
|---|---|---|
| First generation cephalosporins | Cephalexin<br>Cefadroxil | Effective against Gram+ve organisms |
| Second generation Cephalosporins | Cefuroxime<br>Cefaclor | Greater activity against Gram +ve organisms *Klebsiella, H. influenzae, E.coli* |
| Third generation cephalosporins | Cefotaxime<br>Ceftriaxone<br>Ceftazidime | Less activity against Gram +ve organisms *Pseudomonas, Enterobacteria Gonococci* |
| Fourth generation cephalosporins | Cefepime | *Enterococci, Gonococci* |

## Erythromycin

- Can be used in treating patients who are allergic to penicillin
- Effective against gram-positive cocci, streptococci, staphylococci
- Bacteriostatic in nature
- This drug is penicillinase resistant and thus can be used against staphylococcal infections
- Well absorbed orally.

## Tetracycline

### *Mechanism of Action*

- Inhibit bacterial protein synthesis
- Bacteriostatic in nature
- Broad-spectrum antibiotics
- Effective against gram-positive, gram-negative organisms, Mycoplasma and Rickettsia
- Problem of bacterial resistance
- Absorption of tetracycline is inhibited by chelation with milk
- Deposited into growing teeth and bones causing hypoplasia and staining. It should be avoided in children under 12 years of age and in pregnancy.

## Metronidazole

- Main indication is for anaerobic infections.
- Bactericidal
- Effective in orofacial infections
- Can be given orally or parentrally
- Adverse reactions: nausea and metallic taste.

## Ciprofloxacin

- Inhibition of DNA replication
- It inhibitis the enzyme DNA gyrase which prevents the supercoiling of the bacterial chromosome
- Bactericidal in nature
- Effective in treating gram-negative and gram-positive infections.

CHAPTER 12

# Endodontic Instruments



## INTRODUCTION

Although variety of instruments used in general dentistry, are applicable in endodontics, yet some special instruments are unique to endodontic purpose.

In early 1900s, there was availability of variety of tools like path finders, barbed broaches, reamers, files, etc. In that time, every clinical picture presented was tackled with unique formulae utilizing permutations and combinations of tools, medicaments and sealants available. In other words there was little uniformity in quality control, taper of canal or instrument and filling materials in terms of size and shape.

The year 1958 was hallmark year in the history of endodontic instrumentation. The manufacturers came together and a consensus was reached on instruments and obturation materials for root canal therapy. Then in 1959, standardized instruments and filling materials were introduced. In this standardization:

a. For each instruments and filling materials a formula for diameter and taper was made.
b. Formulae for graduated increment in size from one instrument to another were given.
c. Based on instrument diameter, numbering system for instruments was developed.

In 1968, Jack Jacklich of Loyola University formed a group with other dentists and performed endodontic therapy. The tedium of hand instrumentation and its ineffectiveness soon resulted in what he called *"the scourge of digital hyperkeratosis"*. Also the time and patience required for handling of gutta-percha points for lateral condensation technique led him on the path of discovery, which led to many innovations in techniques and tools. The result was a huge paradigm shift in the logic and technique.

Then in 1989, "American National Standards Institute (ANSI)" granted the approval of "ADA Specification No. 28" for endodontic files and reamers. It established the requirements for diameter length, resistance to fracture, stiffness, etc.

Latter on, in 1996, the specification No. 28 was again modified. Initially manufactures of endodontic instruments adhered closely to these specification but nowadays several variations regarding diameter, taper, tip feature, stiffness and metal type used have been noted.

## CLASSIFICATION OF ENDODONTIC INSTRUMENTS

ISO - FDI (Federation Dentaire International) grouped root canal instruments according to their method of use:

Group I : *Hand use only* for example, K and H-files, reamers, broaches, etc.

Group II : *Latch type Engine driven*: Same design as group I but can be attached to handpiece.

Group III : *Drills or reamers latch type engine driven* for example, Gates-Glidden, Peeso reamers.

Group IV : *Root canal points* like gutta-percha, silver point, paper point.

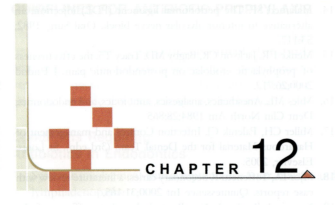

## Grossman's Classification

| *Function* | *Instruments* |
|---|---|
| Exploring | Smooth broaches and endodontic explorers. (To locate canal orifices and determine patency of root canal) |
| Dibriding or extirpating | Barbed broaches (To extirpate the pulp and other foreign materials from the root canal) |
| Cleaning and shaping | Reamers and files (used to shape the canal space) |
| Obturating | Pluggers, spreaders and lentulospirals (To pack gutta-percha points into the root canal space). |

# HAND OPERATED INSTRUMENTS

## Alloys Used for Manufacturing Endodontic Instruments

a. Carbon steel
b. Stainless steel
c. Nickle-titanium .

a. **Carbon steel:** These alloys contain less-than 2.1 percent of carbon.
   **Advantage:** They have high hardness than stainless steel instruments.
   **Disadvantages**
   - Prone to corrosion, so cannot be resterilized
   - Prone to rust.

   Example: Barbed broach.

b. Stainless steel instruments
   These are corrosion resistant instruments. They contain 18 percent chromium, 8-10 percent nickel and 0.12 percent carbon.
   **Advantage:** Corrosion resistant
   **Disadvantages**
   - Stiff in nature
   - Prone to fracture
   - Prone to distortion

   Example: K-file, H-file, reamer

c. **Nickel titanium**
   These instruments contain 55 percent nickel and 45 percent titanium. These alloys show stress induced martensitic transformation from parent austenitic structure. On releasing stresses, the material returns to austenitic and its original shape.
   **Advantages:**
   - Shape memory
   - Super elasticity
   - Low modulus of elasticity
   - Corrosion resistant
   - Softer
   - Good resiliency
   - Biocompatibility

**Disadvantages of NiTi files**
- Poor cutting efficiency.
- NiTi files do not show signs of fatigue before they fracture.
- Poor resistance to fracture as compared to stainless steel.
  Example: NiTi Hand files, profiles, protapers.

## Manufacturing of Hand Instruments

A hand operated instrument reamer or file begins as a round wire which is modified to form a tapered instrument with cutting edges. Several shapes and forms of such instruments are available. These are manufactured by two techniques

a. By machining the instrument directly on the lathe for example H-file and NiTi instruments are machined.
b. By first grinding and then twisting. Here the raw wire is ground into tapered geometric blanks, i.e. square, triangular or rhomboid. These blanks are then twisted counterclockwise to produce cutting edges.

## Standardization of Instruments given by Ingle and Levine

Ingle and Levine using and electronic microcomparator found variation in the diameter and taper for same size of instrument. They suggested few guidelines for instruments for having uniformity in instrument diameter and taper (Fig. 12.1). The guidelines were:

- Instruments are numbered from 10-100. There is increase in 5 units up to size 60 and in 10 units till they are size 100.
- Each number should represent diameter of instrument in 100th of millimeter at the tip.
- Working blade shall begin at tip ($D_1$) and extend 16 mm up the shaft ($D_2$). $D_2$ should be 0.32 mm greater than $D_1$, ensuring that there is constant increase in taper, i.e 0.02 mm per mm of instrument.
- Instruments handles should be color coded for their easier recognition (Pink, grey, purple, white, yellow, red, blue, green, black............)
- Instruments are available in following lengths: 21 mm, 25 mm, 28 mm, 30 mm and 40 mm. 21 mm length is commonly used for molars, 25 mm for interiors, 28 and 30 mm for canines and 40 mm for endodontic implants.

## Modifications from Ingle's Standardization (Fig. 12.2)

- An additional diameter measurement point at $D_3$ is 3 mm from the tip of the cutting end of the instrument at $D_0$ (Earlier it was $D_1$).

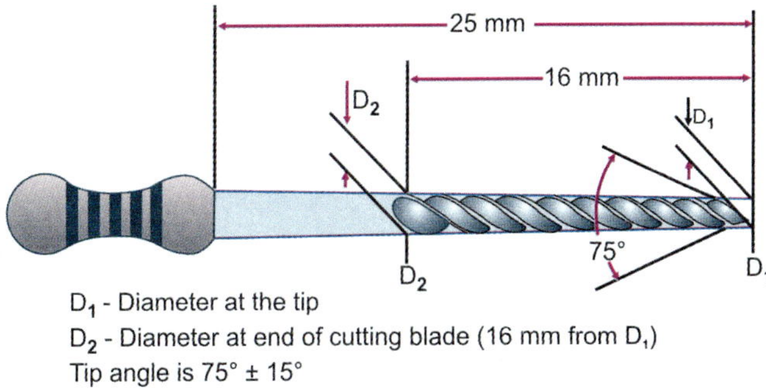


**Fig. 12.1:** Diagrammatic representation of an endodontic instrument in accordance with ANSI specification No. 57

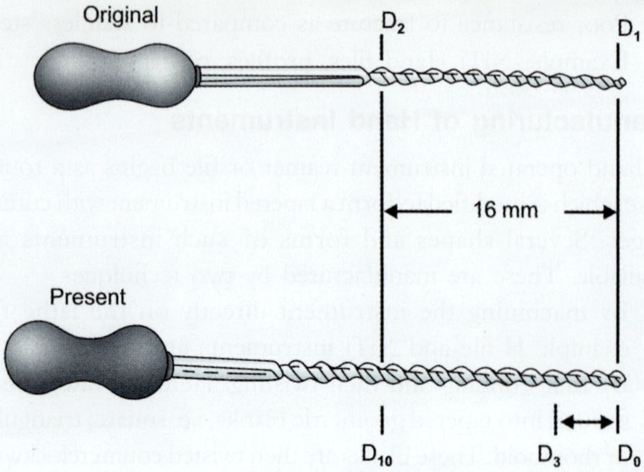


**Fig. 12.2:** Modification from Ingle's standardization

- Tip angle of an instrument should be 75° ± 15°.
- Greater taper instruments (0.04, 0.06, 0.08—) have also been made available.

**Color coding of endodontic instruments (Fig. 12.3)**

| *Color code* | *Instrument number* |
|---|---|
| Pink | 06 |
| Gray | 08 |
| Purple | 10 |
| White | 15 |
| Yellow | 20 |
| Red | 25 |
| Blue | 30 |
| Green | 35 |
| Black | 40 |
| White | 45 |
| Yellow | 50 |
| Red | 55 |
| Blue | 60 |
| Green | 70 |
| Black | 80 |

- Instruments available in length 21, 25, 28 and 30 mm are used for root canal therapy, and those of 40 mm size are used in preparing root canals for the endodontic implants.

## Broaches and Rasps

### *Broaches*

Broaches are of two types:

**a. Smooth broaches:** These are free of barbs. Previously they were used as pathfinder, but at present flexible files are used for this.

**b. Barbed broach (Fig. 12.4)**

- They are one of the oldest intracanal instruments with specifications by ANSI No. 63 and ISO No. 3630-1.
- They have ADA specification No.6
- Broaches are short handled instruments meant for single use only.
- They are made from round steel wires. The smooth surface of wire is notched to from barbs bent at an angle from the long axis

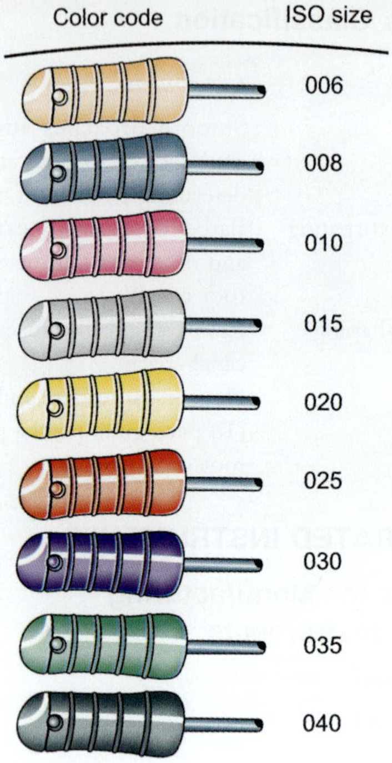


**Fig. 12.3:** Color coding of endodontic instruments

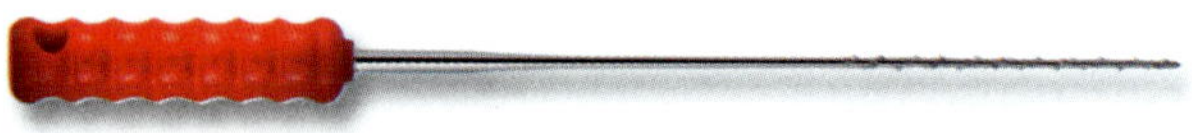

**Fig. 12.4:** Barbed broach

- Broach does not cut the dentin but can effectively be used to remove cotton or paper points which might have lodged in the canal
- Broach should not be forced apically into the canal, as its barbs get compressed by the canal wall. While removing this embedded instrument, barbs get embedded into dentin and broach may break on applying pressure.

## Uses of Broach

- Extirpation of pulp tissues
- Removal of cotton or paper points lodged in the canal.
- Loosen the necrotic debris from canal.

## Rasps

- They have ADA specification No. 63.
- Rasps have similar design to barbed broach except in taper and barb size. Barb size is larger in broach then rasp (Fig. 12.5).
- They are used to extirpate pulp tissue.

| *Broach* | *Rasp* |
|---|---|
| • Barb extends to half of its core diameter, making it a weaker instrument. | Barbs extend to one third of the core, so it is not as weak as barbed broach |
| • Less taper (0.007-0.010 taper/mm) | • More taper (0.015-0.020 taper/mm) |
| • Barbs are very fine and longer | • Barbs are blunt, shorter and shallower |

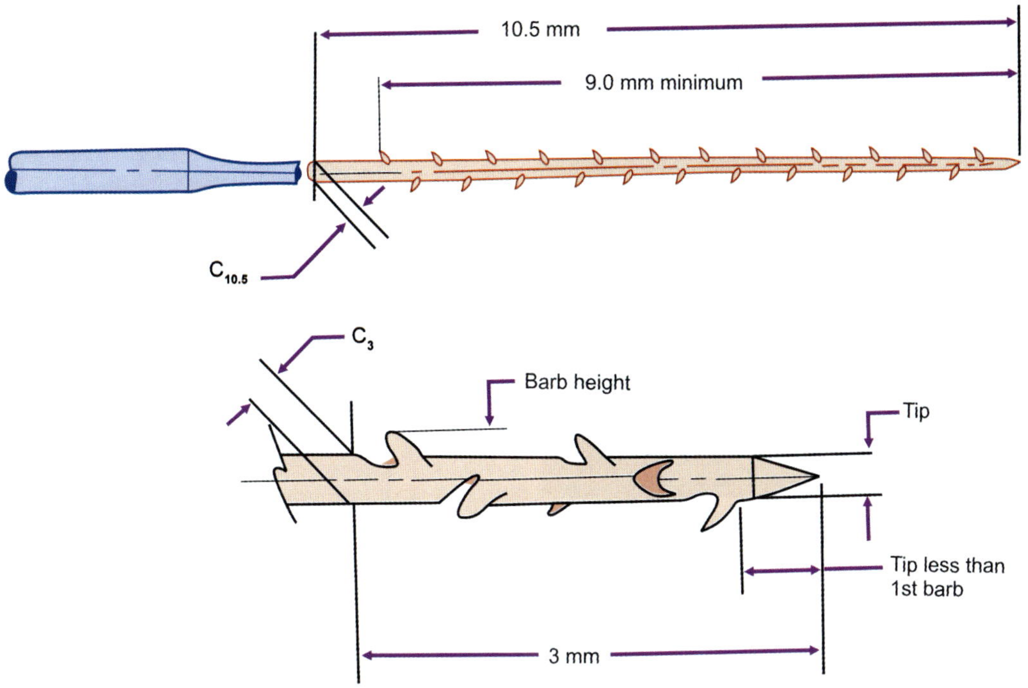


**Fig. 12.5:** Diagrammatic picture of a broach and rasp

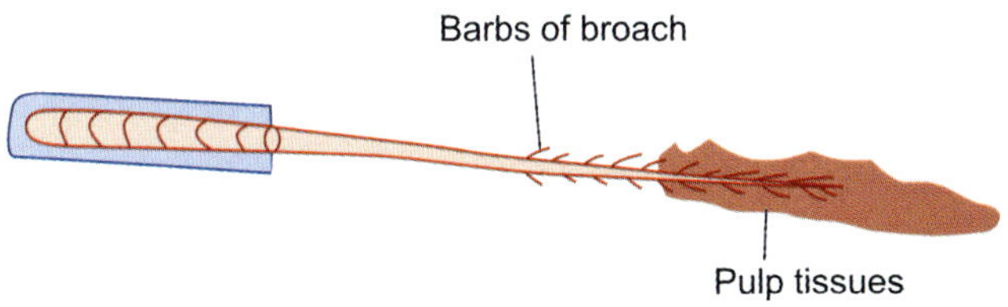


**Fig. 12.6:** Pulp extirpation using broach

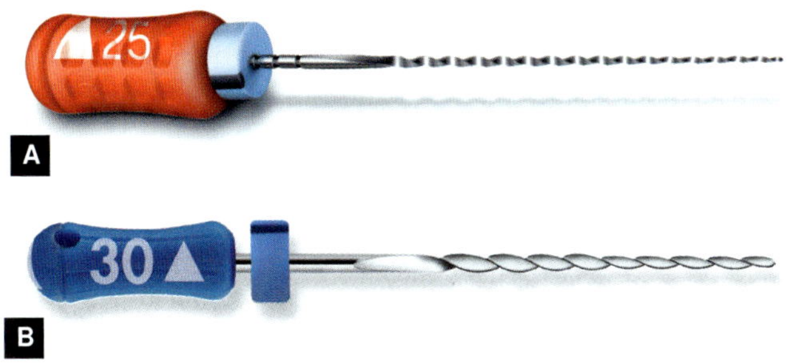


**Figs 12.7A and B:** Reamers

**Technique of pulp extirpation (Healey, 1984)**

Penetrate the barbed broach along the canal wall towards the apex

↓

As it reaches to the apical constriction, move it into the center of mass of pulp tissue

↓

Rotate the broach several times in a watch winding manner to entrap the pulp which is then withdrawn from the canal (Fig. 12.6)

## Reamers (Fig. 12.7)

1. Reamers are K-type instruments (manufactured by Kerr company), which are used to ream the canals. They cut by inserting into the canal, twisting clockwise one quarter to half turn and then withdrawing, i.e. penetration, rotation and retraction.
2. Reamers have triangular blank and lesser number of flutes than files (Fig. 12.8). Numbers of flutes in reamer are ½-1/mm, while in files the flutes are 1½-2½/mm (Fig. 12.9).
3. Though reamer has fewer numbers of flutes than file, cutting efficiency is same as that of files because more space between flutes causes better removal of debris.
4. Reamer tends to remain self centered in the canal resulting in less chances of canal transportation.

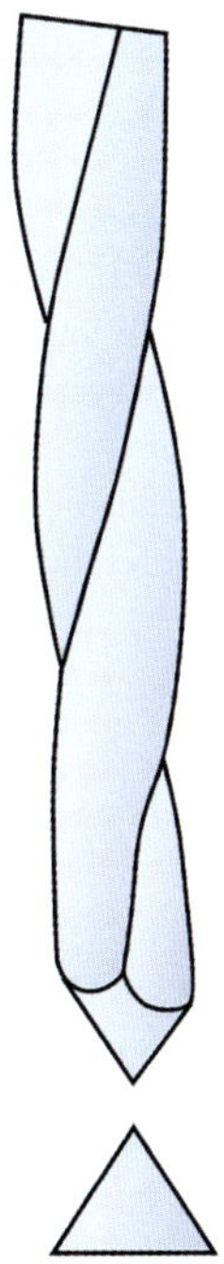

**Fig. 12.8:** Triangular blank and lesser number of flutes in reamer

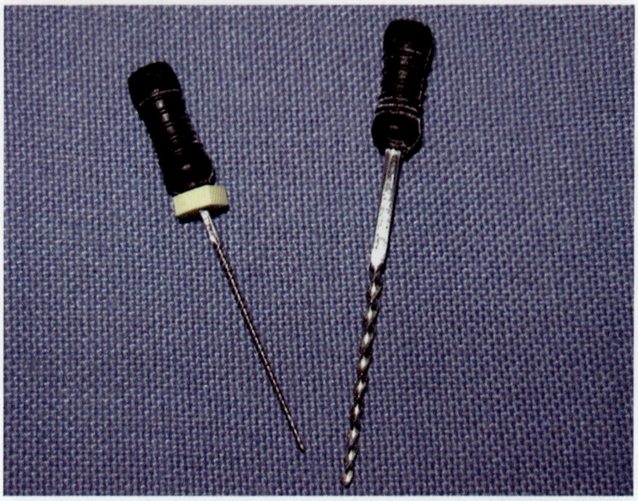

Fig. 12.9: Reamer has lesser number of flutes than file

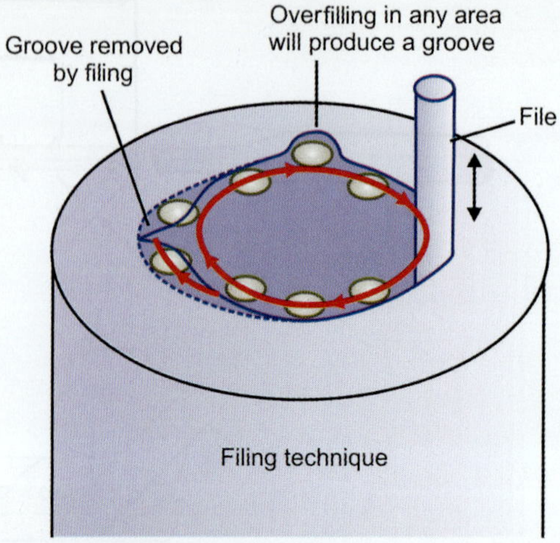


Fig. 12.10: Filing/Rasping action

## Files

Files are the instruments used during cleaning and shaping of the root canals for machining of the dentin. Since Kerr manufacturing company was first to produce them, the files were also called K-files.

Files are predominantly used with filing or rasping action in which there is little or no rotation in the root canals. It is placed in root canal and pressure is exerted against the canal wall and instrument is withdrawn while maintaining the pressure (Fig. 12.10).

**Difference between files and reamers**

| | *Files* | *Reamers* |
|---|---|---|
| 1. Cross-section | Square | Triangular |
| 2. Area of cross-section | More | less |
| 3. Flutes | more (1½-2/mm) | less (½-1/mm) |
| 4. Flexibility | Less | More (because of less work hardening) |
| 5. Cutting motion | Rasping penetration, (Push and pull) | Rotation and retraction. |
| 6. Preparation shape | Usually avoid | Round |
| 7. Transport of debris | Poor because of tighter flutes | Better because of space present in flutes |

**Commonly used files**

1. K-file
2. K-flex file
3. Flexo-file
4. Flex-R file
5. Hedstrom file
6. Safety H-file
7. S-file

## K-files (Fig. 12.11)

- They are triangular, square or rhomboidal in cross-section, manufactured from stainless steel wire, which is grounded into desired shape (Fig. 12.12).

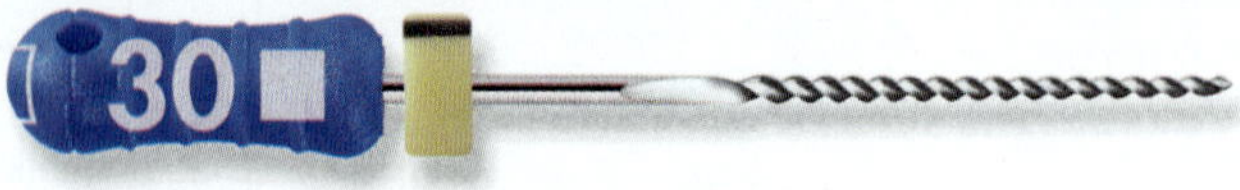


Fig. 12.11: K-file

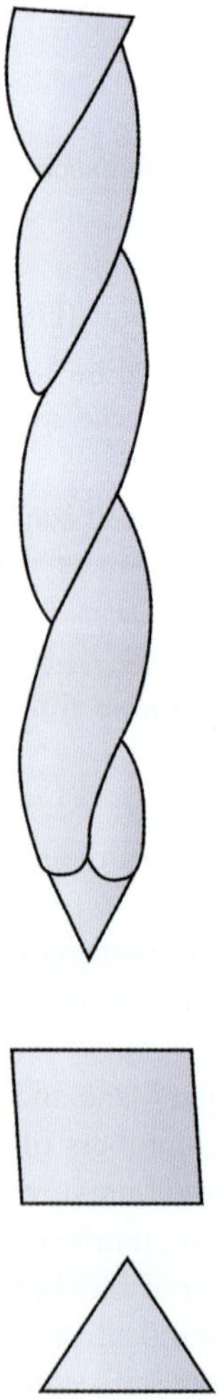

Fig. 12.12: Square or triangular cross-section of a K-file

- K-files have 1½ to 2½ cutting blades per mm of their working end
- Tighter twisting of the file spirals increases the number of flutes in files (more than reamer).
- Triangular cross-sectioned files show superior cutting and increased flexibility than the file or reamers with square blank (Fig. 12.13).

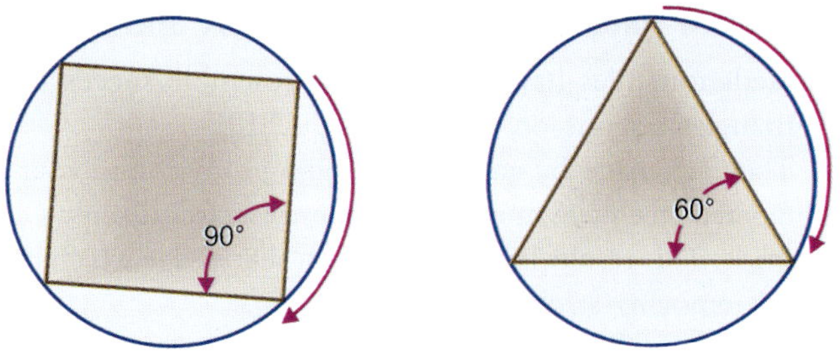


**Fig. 12.13:** Triangular cross-sectioned file shows better flexibility and cutting efficiency than square cross-sectioned file are reamer

## Disadvantage of K-files

1. Less cutting efficiency
2. Extrusion of debris periapically.

## K-flex Files (Fig. 12.14)

- They were introduced by Kerr manufacturing company in 1982. It was realized that square blank of file results in total decrease in the instrument flexibility. To maintain shape and flexibility of these files, K-flex files were introduced.
- K-flex files are rhombus in cross section having two acute angles and two obtuse angles (Fig. 12.15).
- Two acute angles increase sharpness and cutting efficiency of the instrument.
- Two obtuse angles provide more space for debris removal. Also the decrease in contact of instrument with canal walls provide more space for irrigation.
- They are used in filing and rasping motion.

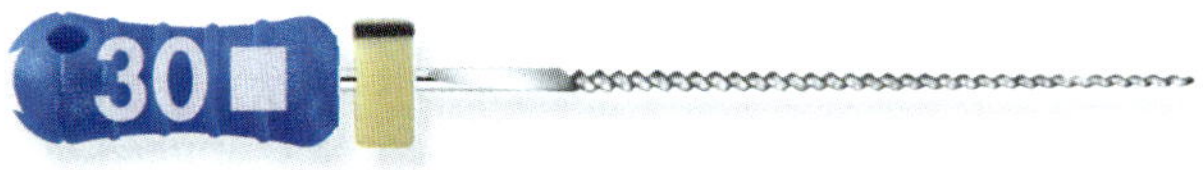


**Fig. 12.14:** K-flex file

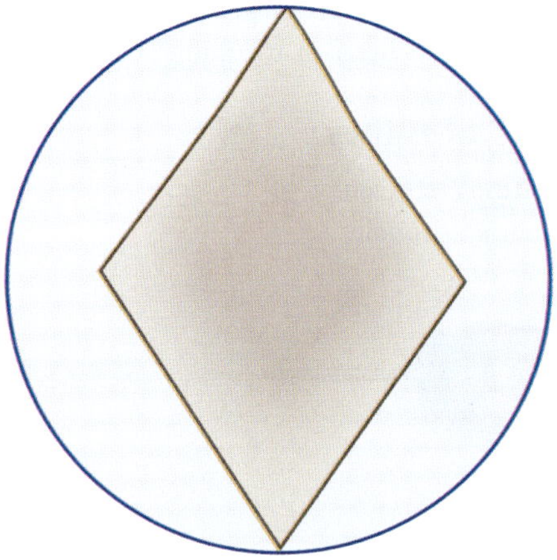

**Fig. 12.15:** Rhombus cross-section of K-flex file

## Flexo Files (Fig. 12.16)

- These are similar to the K-Flex files *except* that they have triangular cross section. This feature provides them more flexibility and thus ability to resist fracture.
- The tip of file is modified to non-cutting type.
- They are made up to NiTi.
- Flexo files have more flexibility but less of cutting efficiency.

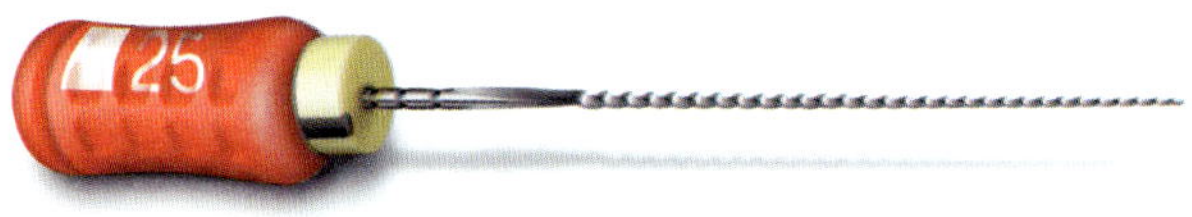


**Fig. 12.16:** Flexo-file

## Triple Flex Files

- They are made up of stainless steel and are triangular in cross section.
- They have more flutes than reamers but lesser than k-files.

## Flex-R-files/Roane Files

- Flex-R-files are made by removing the sharp cutting edges from the tip of instrument (Figs 12.17A and B). The noncutting tip enables the instrument to traverse along the canal rather than gouge into it.
- This design reduces the ledge formation, canal transportation and other procedural accidents when used with balanced force technique.
- Another feature of flex-R file is presence of triangular cross-section which provides it flexibility to be used in curved canals.
- They are made up of NiTi and cut during anticlock wise rotary motion.

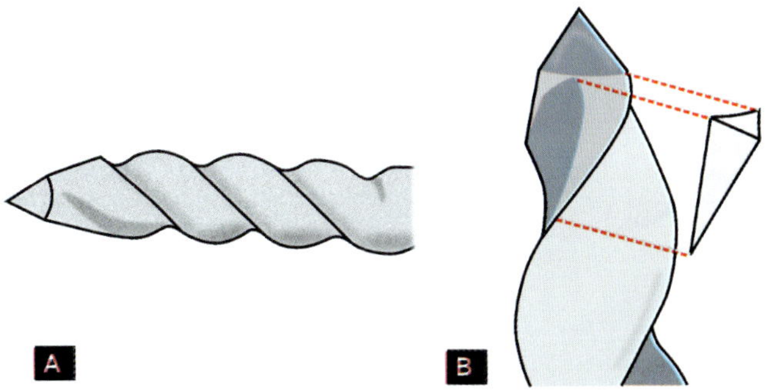


**Figs 12.17A and B:** Flex-R-file

## Hedstrom Files (H-files) (Figs 12.18A and B)

- Hedstrom files have flutes which resemble successively triangles set one on another (Fig. 12.19).
- They are made by cutting the spiral grooves into round, tapered steel wire in the same manner as wood screws are made. This results in formation of a sharp edge which cuts on removing strokes only (Fig. 12.20).
- Hedstrom files cut only when instrument is withdrawn because its edges face the handle of the instrument.
- When used in torquing motion, their edges can engage in the dentin of root canal wall and causing H - files to fracture.
- Rake angle and distance between the flutes are two main features which determine working of the file.
- H-files have positive rake angle, i.e. its cutting edge is turned in the same direction in which the force is applied which makes it dig into the dentin making it more aggressive in cutting.
- Hedstrom files should be used to machine straight canals because they are strong and aggressive cutters. Since they lack the flexibility and are fragile in nature, the H-files tend to fracture when used in torquing action.

### Advantages of H-files

1. Better cutting efficiency
2. Push debris coronally

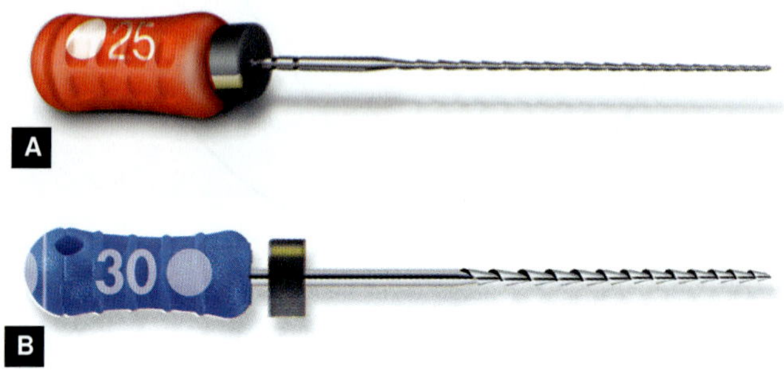


**Figs 12.18A and B:** Hedstrom file

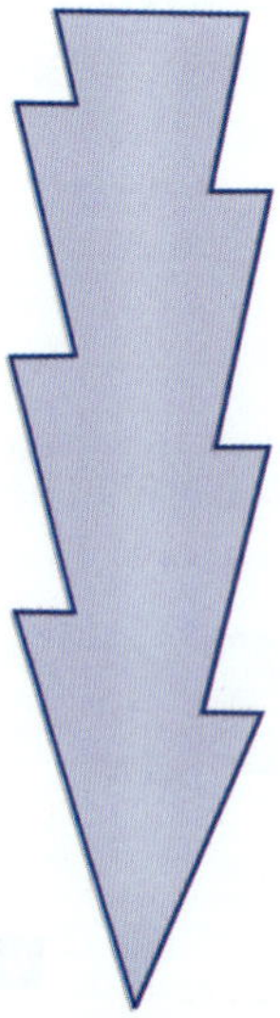

**Fig. 12.19:** Diagrammatic view of Hedstrom file

### Disadvantages of H-files

1. Lack flexibility
2. Tend to fracture
3. Aggressive cutter

### Safety Hedstrom File

- This file has non-cutting safety side along the length of the blade which reduces the chances of perforations. The non-cutting side is directed to the side of canal where cutting is not required. The non-cutting side of safety file prevents lodging of the canals (Fig. 12.21).

### S-file

- It is called 'S' file because of its cross-sectional shape.
- S-File is produced by grinding, which makes it stiffer than Hedstrom file. This file is designed with two spirals for cutting blades, forming double helix design (Fig. 12.22).

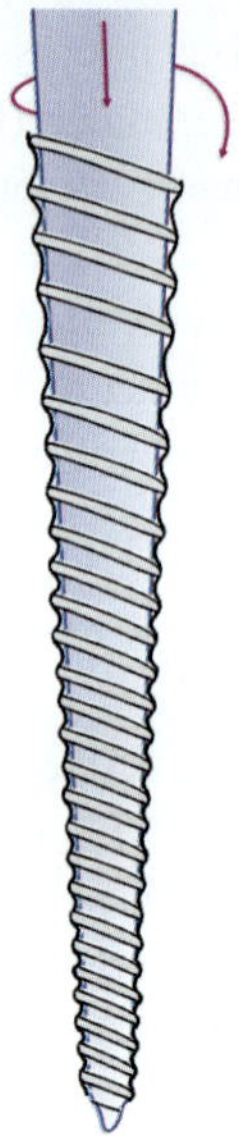

**Fig. 12.20:** Screw entering a piece of wood

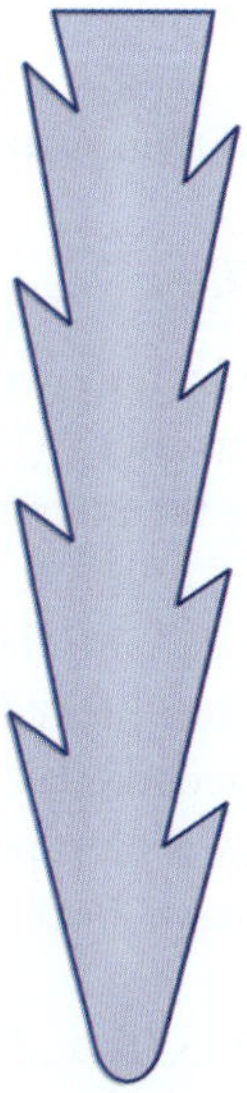

**Fig. 12.21:** Safety Hedstrom file

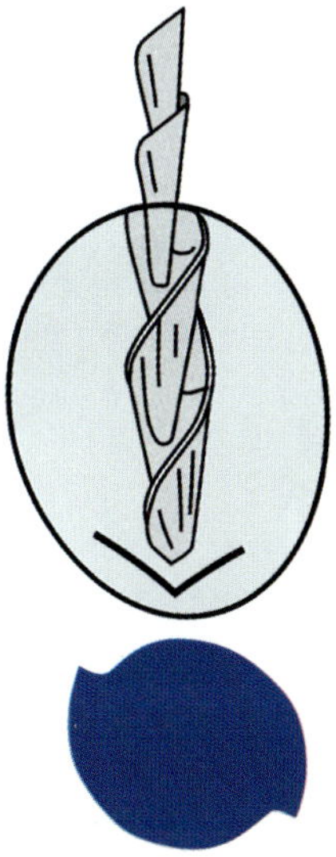

Fig. 12.22: S-file

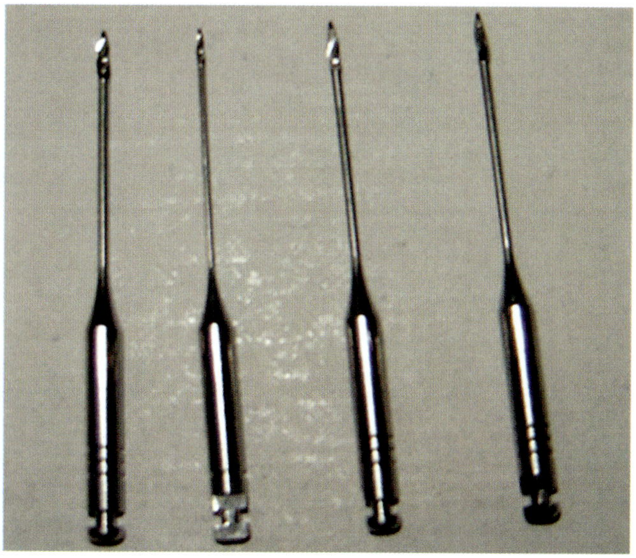

Fig. 12.23: Gates-Glidden drills

- S-file has good cutting efficiency in either filling or reaming action, thus this file can also be classified as a hybrid design.

### C+Files

- C+ files are used for difficult and calcified canals. They have better buckling resistance than K-files.
- They are available in size 8, 10 and 15 of length 18, 21 and 25 mm.

### Golden Medium Files

1. These files were described by Weine. They come under intermediate files provided with half sizes between conventional instruments.
2. They are available in sizes from 12-37 like 12, 17, 22, 27, 32 and 37.
3. They are used for narrow canals.
4. They are formed by cutting 1 mm from the tip of instrument. In this way No. 10 file can be converted to no. 12, and 15 to No. 17 and so on.

## ENGINE DRIVEN INSTRUMENTS

### Gates-Glidden Burs (Fig. 12.23)

- Traditional engine driven instruments include Gates-Glidden drills which have flame-shaped cutting point mounted on long thin shaft attached to a latch type shank (Fig. 12.24).
- Gates-Gliddens are available in a set from 1 to 6 with the diameters from 0.5 to 1.5 mm.
- Due to their design Gates-Glidden drills are side cutting instruments with safety tips (Fig. 12.25).
- They should be used at the speed of 750-1500 rpm. In brushing strokes.
- Safety design of Gates-Gliddens is that its weakest part lies at the junction of shank and shaft of the instrument. If its cutting tip jams against the canal wall, fracture occurs at the junction of shank and the shaft but not at the tip of the instrument. This makes the easy removal of fractured drill from the canal.
- They can be used both in crown down as well as step back fashion (Fig. 12.26).

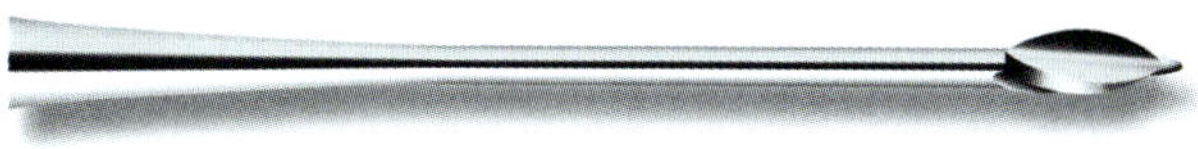

Fig. 12.24: Flame shaped head mounted on long thin shaft in Gates-Glidden drill

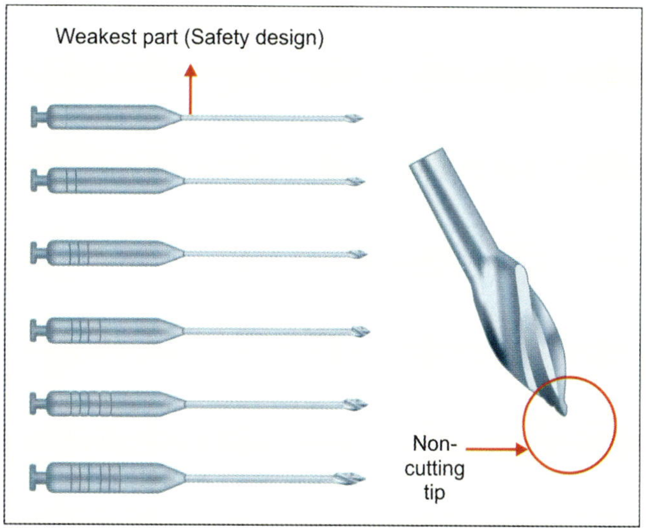


Fig. 12.25: Due to safety design, if cutting tip of instrument jams against canal wall, the fracture occurs at junction of shaft and shank and not at tip

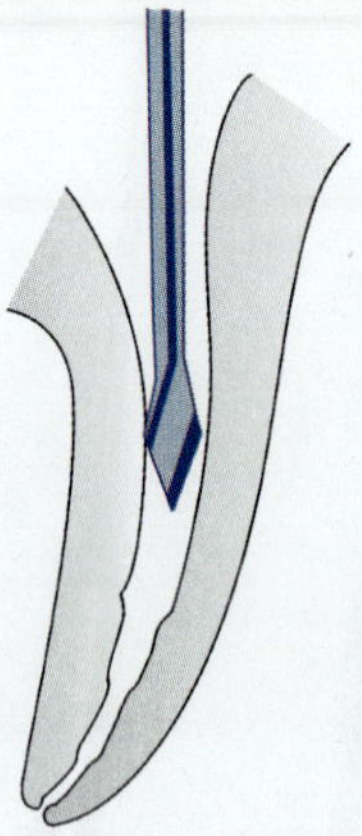

**Fig. 12.26:** Use of Gates-Glidden drill in canal

| *Number* | *Diameter at cutting tip* |
|---|---|
| 1. | 0.50 mm |
| 2. | 0.70 mm |
| 3. | 0.90 mm |
| 4. | 1.1 mm |
| 5. | 1.3 mm |
| 6. | 1.5 mm |

### Uses of Gates-Glidden Drills

1. For coronal flaring during root canal preparation (Figs 12.27A and B).
2. During retreatment cases or post space preparation for removal of gutta-percha.
3. During instrument removal, if used incorrectly for example using at high rpm, incorrect angle of insertion, forceful drilling, the use of Gates-Glidden can result in procedural accidents like perforations, instrument separation, etc.

### Flexogates (Fig. 12.28)

- Flexogates are modified Gates-Gliddens. They are made up of NiTi and have non-cutting tip.
- They are more flexible and used for apical preparation.
- Flexogates can be rotated continuously in a handpiece through 360°.
- These instruments have many advantages over the traditional instruments in that they allow increased debris removal because of continuous rotation, smoother and faster canal preparation with less clinician fatigue.

### Advantages of Flexogates

1. Safe non-cutting guiding tip.
2. Safety design, i.e its breakage point is 16 mm from the tip, so once fractured, it can be easily retrieved.
3. Flexible, so used in curved canals.

## PEESO REAMERS

- They are rotary instruments used mainly for post space preparations.
- They have safe ended non-cutting tip.

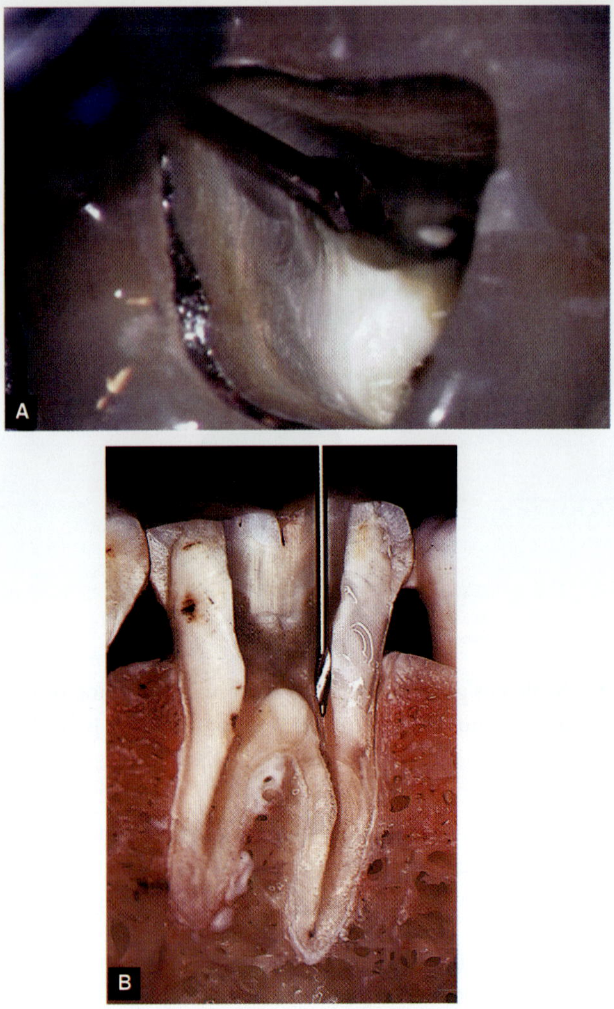


**Figs 12.27A and B:** Use of Gates-Glidden drill for coronal flaring

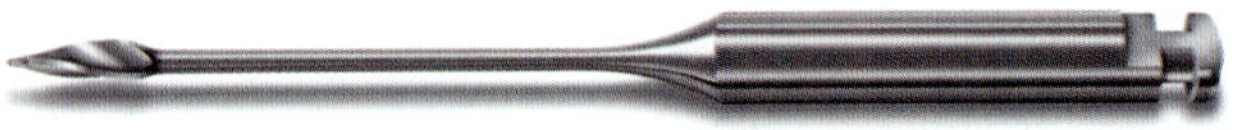

**Fig. 12.28:** Flexogates

- Their tip diameter varies from 0.7 to 1.7 mm.
- They should be used in brushing motion.

| *Number* | *Diameter at cutting tip* |
|---|---|
| 1. | 0.70 mm |
| 2. | 0.90 mm |
| 3. | 1.1 mm |
| 4. | 1.3 mm |
| 5. | 1.5 mm |
| 6. | 1.7 mm |

Disadvantages of using peeso reamers are:

1. They do not follow the canal curvature and may cause perforation by cutting laterally.
2. They are stiff instruments.
3. They have to be used very carefully to avoid iatrogenic errors.

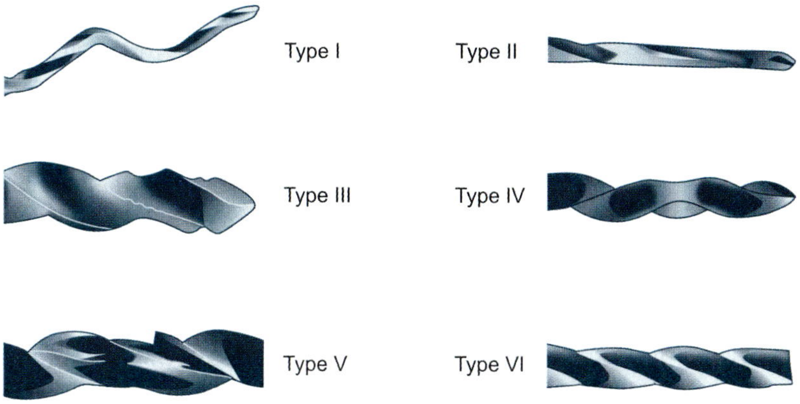


**Fig. 12.29:** Sotokowa's classification of instrument damage

**Sotokowa's classification of instrument damage (Fig. 12.29)**

| | |
|---|---|
| Type I | Bent instrument |
| Type II | Straightening of twisted flutes |
| Type III | Peeling of metal at blade edges |
| Type IV | Clockwise twist (Partial) |
| Type V | Cracking of instrument along its long axis |
| Type VI | Full fracture of instrument |

## NICKEL TITANIUM (NiTi) ENDODONTIC INSTRUMENTS

When using the stainless steel files, occurrence of procedural errors cannot be avoided specially in case of curved canals. Deviation from the original shape, ledge formation, zipping, stripping and perforations are the common problems which are seen in curved canals. But the superelasticity of NiTi alloy allows these instruments to flex more than the stainless steel instruments before exceeding their elastic limit, thereby allowing canal preparation with minimal procedural errors.

NiTi was developed by Buchler 40 years ago. NiTi is also known as the NiTinol (NiTi Navol Ordinance Laboratory in US). In endodontics commonly used NiTi alloys are called 55 NiTi nol (55% weight Ni and 45% Ti) and 60 NiTi nol (60% weight of Ni, 40% Ti).

First use of NiTi in endodontics was reported in 1988, by Walia et al when a 15 No. NiTi file was made from orthodontic wire and it showed superior flexibility and resistance to torsional fracture. This suggested the use of NiTi files in curved canals.

### Advantages of NiTi Alloys

1. Shape memory
2. Superelasticity
3. Low modulus of elasticity
4. Good resiliency
5. Corrosion resistance
6. Softer than stainless steel

Superelasticity and shape memory of NiTi alloys is because of phase transformation in their crystal structures when cooled from the stronger, high temperature form (Austenite) to the weaker low temperature form (Martensite). This phase transformation is mainly responsible for the above mentioned qualities of NiTi alloys.

### Disadvantages of NiTi Files

1. Poor cutting efficiency.
2. NiTi files do not show signs of fatigue before they fracture.
3. Poor resistance to fracture as compared to stainless steel.

### Manufacturing of NiTi Files

Because of the presence of superelasticity and shape memory, the NiTi files cannot be manufactured by twisting as done with K-files. Infact the NiTi files have to be grounded for their manufacturing.

Earlier there used to be NiTi hand files but later automated use of NiTi files was developed to increase the efficiency of clinical treatment.

## INSTRUMENT DEFORMATION AND BREAKAGE

An unfortunate thing about NiTi instruments is that their breakage can occur without any visible sign of unwinding or permanent deformation. In other words visual examination is not a reliable method for evaluation of any NiTi instrument.

Basically there are two modes of rotary instrument separation viz. Torsional fracture and flexural fracture.

### Torsional Fracture

Torsional fracture occurs when torque limit is exceeded. The term torque is used for the forces which act in the rotational manner. The amount of torque is related to mass of the instrument, canal radius and apical force when worked in the canal. As the instrument moves apically, the torque increases because of increased contact area between the file and the canal wall.

Theoretically an instrument used with high torque is very active but chances of deformation and separation increase with

2. Proper glide path must be established before using rotary files, i.e. getting the canal to at least size 15 before using them (Fig. 12.35).
3. Use crown down method for canal preparation. By this apical curves can be negotiated safely (Fig. 12.36).
4. Frequent cleaning of flutes should be done as it can lessen the chances that debris will enter the microfractures and resulting in propagation of original fracture and finally the separation (Fig. 12.37).
5. Do not force the file apically against resistance. Motion of file going into canal should be smooth, deliberate with 1-2 mm deep increments relative to the previous instrument.
6. Remove the maximum possible pulp tissue with broach before using rotary files.
7. Canals should be well lubricated and irrigated. This reduces the friction between instrument and the dentinal walls.
8. Dentin mud collected in the canal increases the risk of fracture, it should be cleared off by frequent irrigation.
9. Discard a file if it is bent, stretched or has a shiny spot.
10. Do not use rotary nickel titanium files to true working length specially in teeth with S- shaped canals, canals with multiple and sharp curves and if there is difficult access of orifice because it can place stresses on the instrument which will cross the breaking torque value. In such cases apical portion of canal should be prepared by hand files.
11. A file should be considered disposable when:
    a. It has been used in curved canals.
    b. Despite of existence of excellent glide path, if it does not cut dentin properly.

### Three Different Handing Protocols are followed for Rotary Instruments (Figs 12.38A to C)

a. Brushing technique: In this file is moved laterally so as to avoid threading in. This motion is done most effectively with stiffer instruments with positive rake angle like protaper instruments.
b. Up-and down motion: In this a rotary file is moved in an up and down motion with a very light touch so as to dissipate the forces. This motion is given to an instrument until desired working length is reached or resistance is met.
c. Third movement is feeding the rotary file into root canal with gentle apical pressure till the instrument meets resistance and then immediately withdraw the file. The file is then again inserted and similar motion is given, this motion is usually given for Race files.

## VARIOUS ROTARY NICKEL TITANIUM (RNT) SYSTEM

Since last many years innumerable amount of RNT file system have been made available. Though no system is perfect, but if used in proper way, they can result in desired canal shape. Various rotary nickel titanium systems available in the market are Profile, Greater Taper files, ProTaper, Quantec, Light Speed

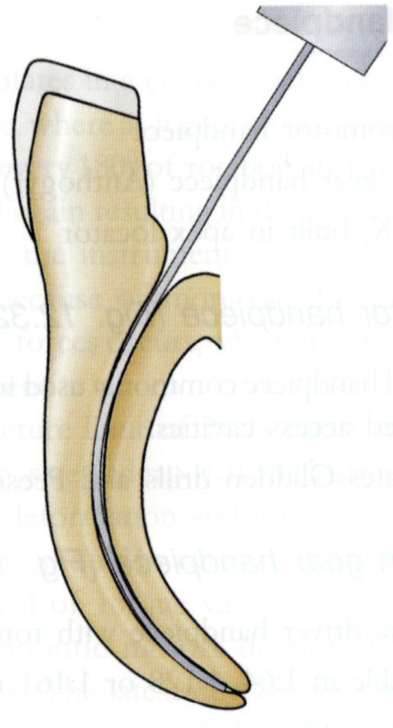

Fig. 12.35: Establish glide path before using rotary instrument

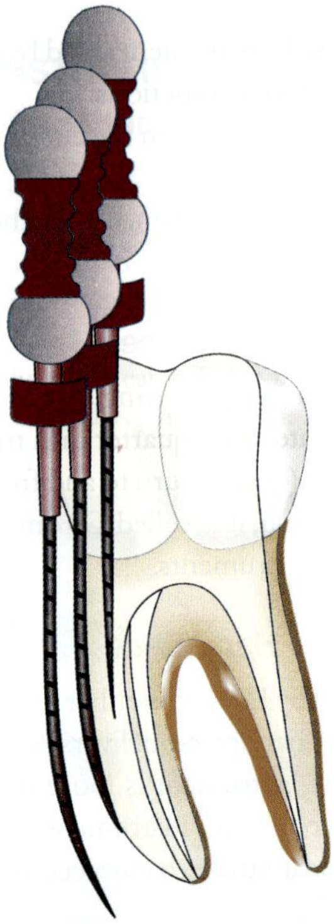

Fig. 12.36: Crown down method for canal preparation

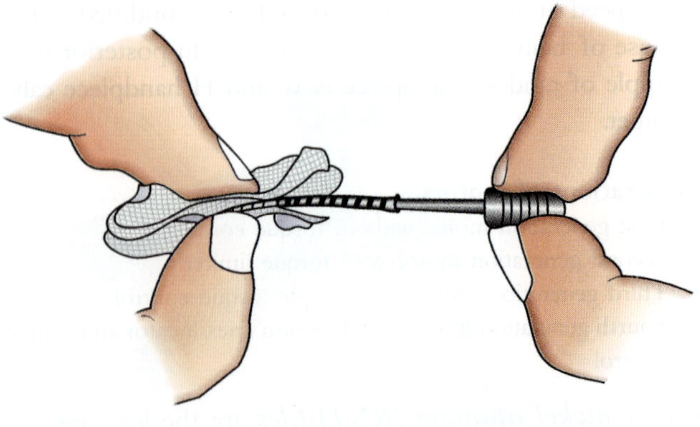

Fig. 12.37: Frequent cleaning of file decreases the chances of instrument fracture

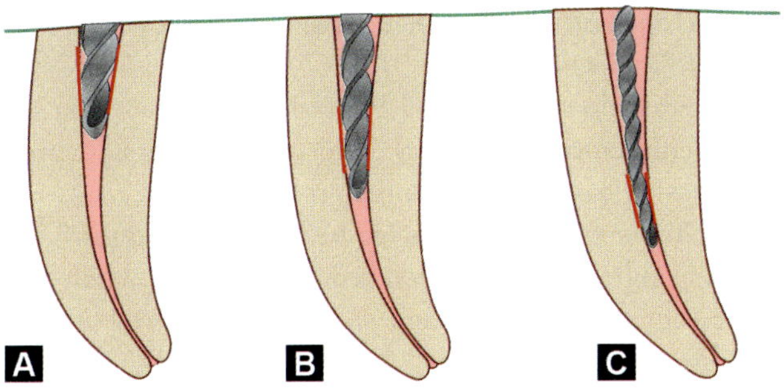


**Figs 12.38A to C:** Different types of handling protocols for rotary instruments: (A) Brushing technique; (B) Up and down motion; (C) Taking file in the canal till it meets resistance

System, $K_3$ system and HERO 642, RACE and Real World Endo Sequence file system.

**Generations of rotary instruments**

| | |
|---|---|
| • First generation: | Profiles, Quantec |
| • Second generation: | Profile GT |
| • Third generation: | $K_3$, RACE ProTaper |
| • Fourth generation: | V-taper |

## PROFILE SYSTEM

- Profile instruments made by Tulsa Dental were one of the first NiTi instruments available commercially. This system was introduced by Dr Johnson in 1944.
- Earlier Profile system was sold as series 29 instruments. In series 29, at the constant rate of 29 percent, there has been advantage of smooth transition among the smaller files but in larger files, the greater gap may create difficulties during cleaning and shaping of the root canals. After this profile series were introduced with greater tapers of 19 mm lengths and ISO sized tips (Fig. 12.39).
- Recommended rotational speed for profiles is 150-300 rpm.
- Cross-section of profiles show three equally shaped U-shaped grooves with radial lands (Fig. 12.40).
- Central parallel core present in profiles increase their flexibility (Fig. 12.41).
- They have negative rake angle (– 20°) which makes them to cut dentin in planning motion. Profile instruments tend to pull debris out of the canal because of presence of 20° helical angle (Fig. 12.42).

## GREATER TAPER FILES (GT FILES)

1. The GT rotary instruments possess a U-shaped file design with ISO tip sizes of 20, 30 and 40 and tapers of 0.04, 0.06, 0.08, .010 and 0.12.
2. Accessory GT files for use as orifice openers of 0.12 taper in ISO sizes of 35, 50, 70 and 90 are also available.
3. The maximum diameter of these instruments is 1.50 mm.
4. Recommended rotational speed for GT files is 350 rpm.
5. Negative rake angle of these files makes them to scrape the dentin rather than cutting it.

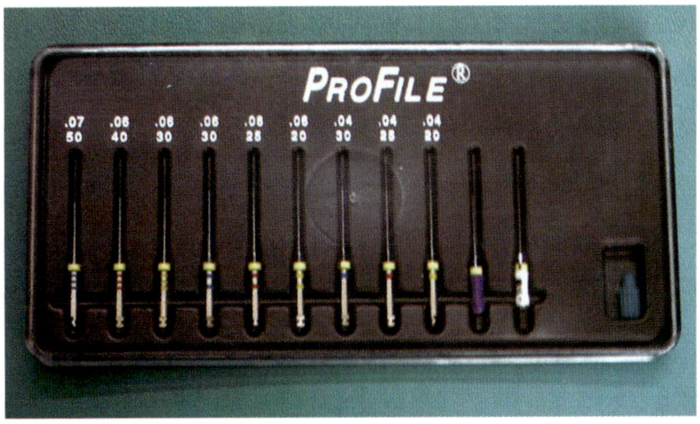


**Fig. 12.39:** Profile series

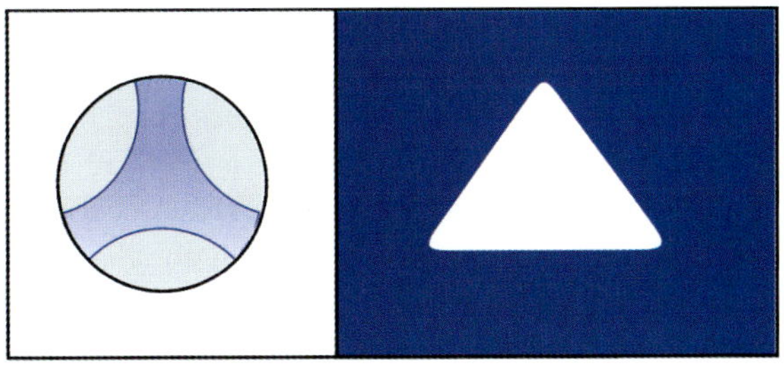

**Fig. 12.40:** U-shaped grooves with radial lands of profile

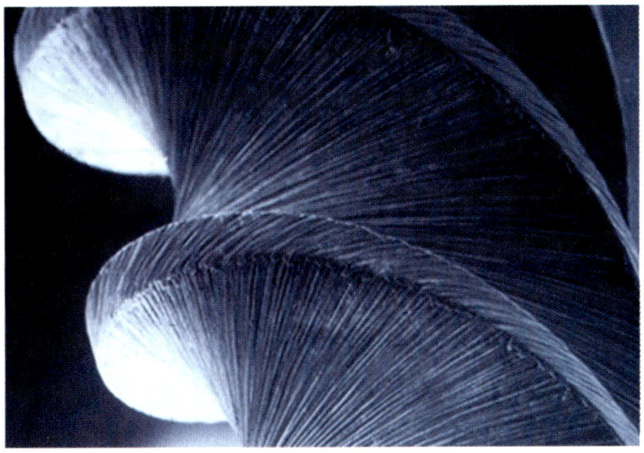

**Fig. 12.41:** Central parallel core in profile increases their flexibility

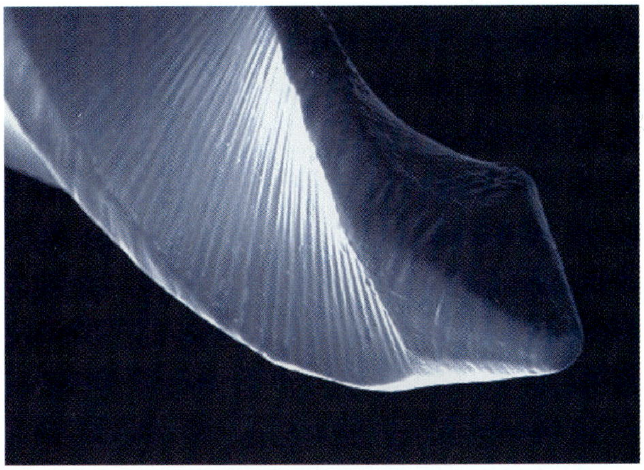

**Fig. 12.42:** Negative rake angle of profile cuts dentin in planning motion

**Difference between profile and ProTaper GT**

| | *Profile* | *ProTaper GT* |
|---|---|---|
| Working length | 16 mm | Depends upon the taper |
| Number of spirals | Same throughout its length | More at the tip than near handle |
| Taper | 0.02, 0.04, 0.06 0.08 and 0.10 | 0.04, 0.06, 0.08, 0.10, 0.12 with three primary sizes 20, 30 and 40 |

## PROTAPER FILES (FIG. 12.43)

1. It was introduced by D Cliff ruddle, Dr Johan West, Ben John and Dr Pierre.
2. ProTaper means progressively taper. A unique feature of the ProTaper files is each instrument has changing percentage tapers over the length of cutting blades. This progressively tapered design improves flexibility, cutting efficiency and the safety of these files (Fig. 12.44).
3. Recommended speed for their use is 150-350 rpm.
4. The ProTaper file has a triangular cross-section and is variably tapered across its cutting length (Fig. 12.45).
5. Convex triangular cross-section of these instrument decrease the friction between the blade of file and the canal wall and it increases its cutting efficiency.
6. ProTaper file has modified guiding tip which allows one to follow canal better.
7. Variable tip diameters of ProTaper file allows it to have specific cutting action in defined area of canal without stressing instrument in other sections.
8. ProTaper file has a changing helical angle and pitch over their cutting blades which reduces the instrument from screwing into the canal and allows better removal of debris (Fig. 12.46).
9. ProTaper file acts in active motion, this further increases its efficiency and reduces torsional strain.
10. Length of file handle is reduced from 15 to 12.5 mm which allows better access in posterior areas.
11. The ProTaper system consists of just three shaping and three finishing files.

### Shaping Files (Fig. 12.47)

These are termed as $S_x$, $S_1$ and $S_2$.

#### *$S_x$ (Fig. 12.48)*

- No identification ring on its gold colored handle
- Shorter length of 19 mm

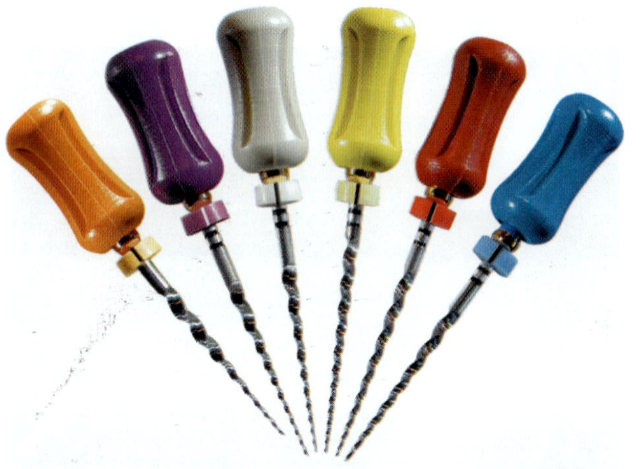

**Fig. 12.43:** ProTaper files

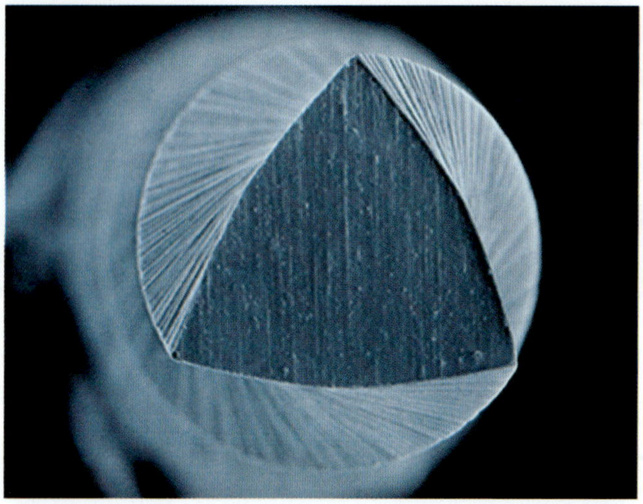

**Fig. 12.45:** Triangular cross-section of ProTaper

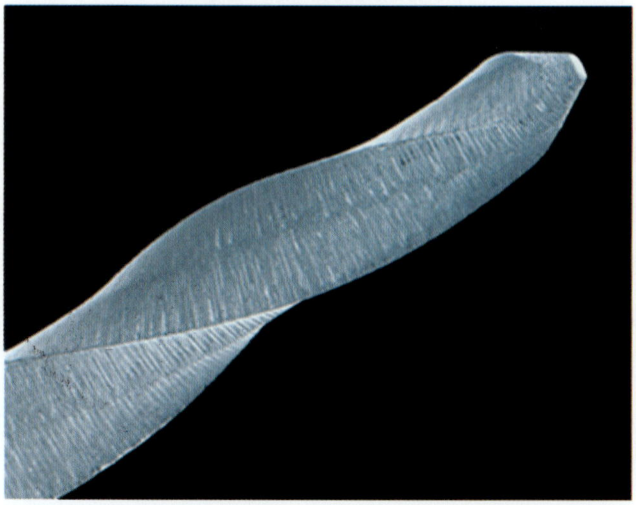

**Fig. 12.44:** Progressively taper design of ProTaper improves flexibility and its cutting efficiency

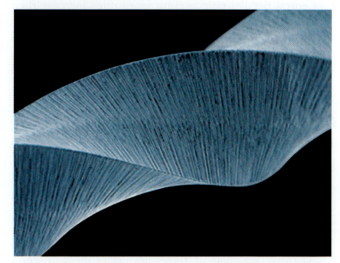

**Fig. 12.46:** Changing helical angle and pitch over their cutting blades decreases the chances of its screwing into the canal

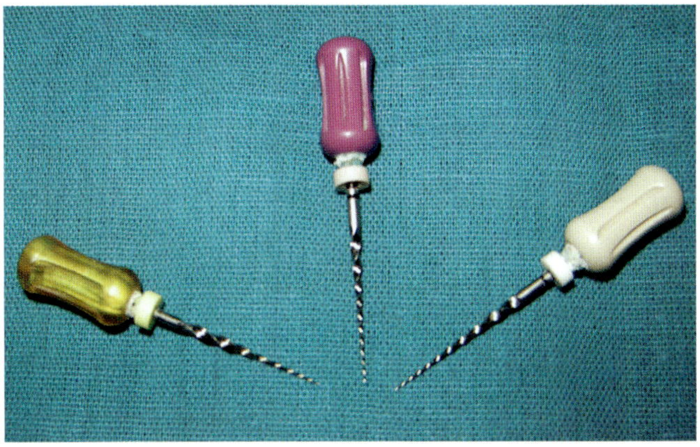

**Fig. 12.47:** Shaping files

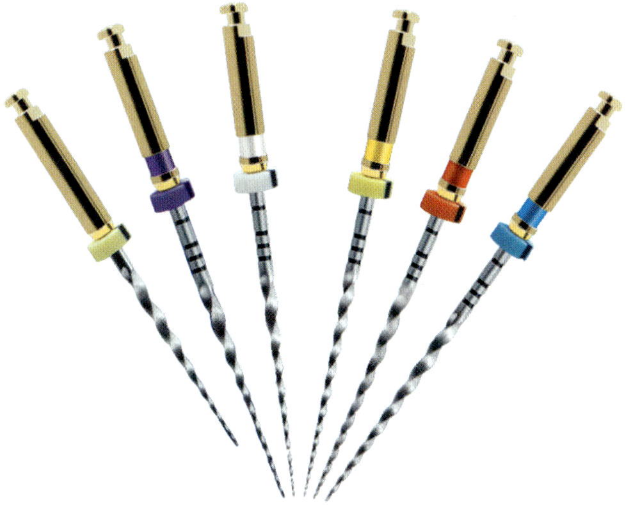

**Fig. 12.48:** Shaping and finishing files

- $D_0$ diameter is 0.19 mm
- $D_{14}$ diameter is 1.20 mm
- There is increase in taper up to $D_9$ and then taper drops off up to $D_{14}$ which increases its flexibility
- Use is similar to Gates-Glidden drills or orifice shapers.

*$S_1$ (Fig. 12.48)*

- Has purple identification ring on its handle
- $D_0$ diameter is 0.17 mm and $D_{14}$ is 1.20 mm
- Used to prepare coronal part of the root.

*$S_2$ (Fig. 12.48)*

- Has white identification ring on its handle
- $D_0$ diameter is 0.20 mm and $D_{14}$ is 1.20 mm
- Used to prepare middle third of the canal.

## Finishing Files

Three finishing files $F_1$, $F_2$, $F_3$ are used to prepare and finish apical part of the root canal (Fig. 12.49).

*$F_1$*

- Yellow identification ring
- $D_0$ diameter and apical taper is 20 and 0.07.

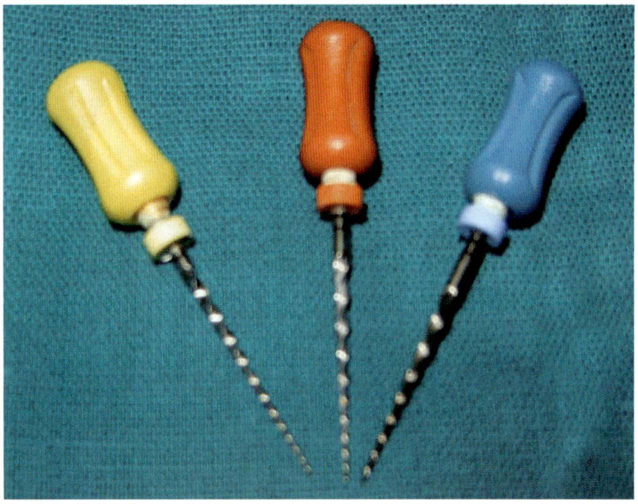

**Fig. 12.49:** Finishing files

*$F_2$*

- Red identification ring on handle
- D0 diameter and taper is 25 and 0.08.

*$F_3$*

- Blue colored ring on handle
- $D_0$ diameter and taper is 30 and 0.09.

Each instrument has decreasing percentage of taper from $D_4$ to $D_{14}$. This improves flexibility and decrease the potential for taper lock.

## QUANTEC FILE SYSTEM

1. Quantec file series are available in both cutting and noncutting tips with standard size of 25 No. in 0.12, 0.10, 0.08, 0.06, 0.05, 0.04, 0.03 and 0.02 tapers. 0.02 tapered Quantec file are also available in size 15-60 No.
2. Quantec system has a positive blade angle with two wide radial lands and relief behind the lands (Fig. 12.50).
3. This unique design minimizes its contact with the canal, thereby reducing the torque, also this design increases the strength of the instrument.
4. Quantec system utilizes the "graduated taper technique" to prepare a canal. It is thought that using a series of files of single taper results in decreases in efficiency as the larger instruments are used. This happens because more of file comes in contact with the dentinal wall which makes it more difficult to remove dentin, thereby retarding the proper cleaning and shaping of the canal. But in graduated taper technique, restricted contact of area increases the efficiency of the instrument because now forces are concentrated on smaller area.

## LIGHT SPEED SYSTEM

- This system was introduced by Steve and Willian Wildely in 1990.
- Light speed system is engine driven endodontic instrument manufactured from nickel-titanium. These are so named

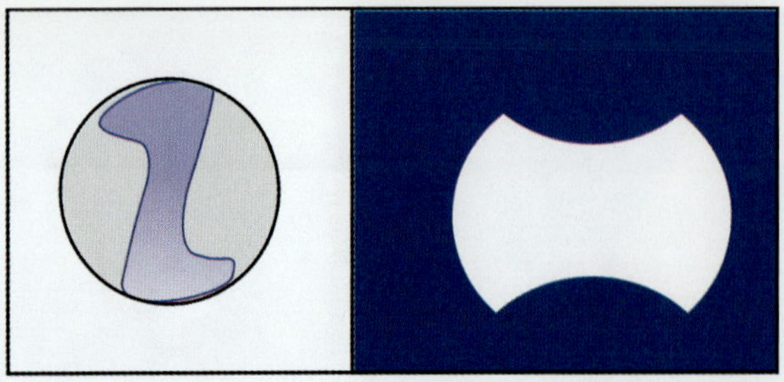

**Fig. 12.50:** Cross-section of quantec files

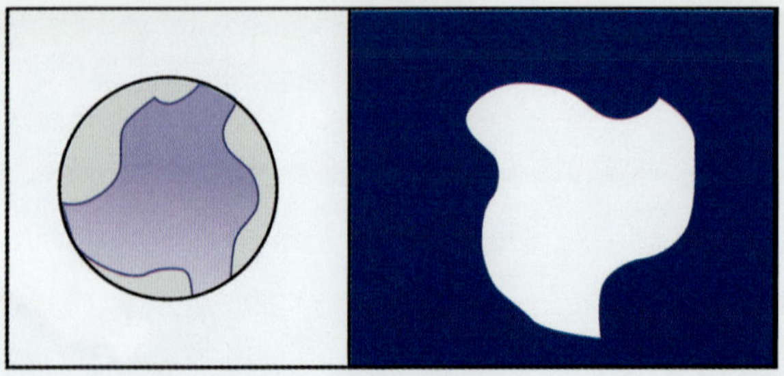

**Fig. 12.51:** Cross-section of $K_3$ rotary file

because a "light" touch is needed as "speed" of instrumentation is increased.

- Light speed instrument are slender with thin parallel shaft and have non-cutting tip with Gates-Glidden in configuration.
- Recommended speed for their use is 1000-2000 rpm.
- They are available in 21, 25, 31 and 50 mm length and ISO No. 20-140.
- Half sizes of light speed instrument are also available viz. 22.5, 27.5, 32.5. The half sizes are also color coded as full ones with only difference in that half size instruments have white or black rings on their handles.
- Cutting heads of light speed system has three different geometric shapes
    - i. Size 20-30-short, non-cutting tips at 75° cutting angle.
    - ii. Size 32.5 - longer non-cutting tip at 33° cutting angle.
    - iii. Size 35-140-longer non-cutting tip with 21° cutting angle.
- Cutting heads basically have three radial lands with spiral shaped grooves in between.

## $K_3$ ROTARY FILE SYSTEM

Dr John Mc Spadden in 2002 in North America introduced $K_3$ system.

1. $K_3$ files are available in taper of 0.02, 0.04 or 0.06 with ISO tip sizes. An Axxess handle design shortens the file by 5 mm without affecting its working length.
2. They are flexible because of presence of variable core diameter.
3. Cutting head of $K_3$ system show three radial lands with relief behind two radial lands. Asymmetrically placed flutes make the $K_3$ system with superior canal tracking ability, add peripheral strength to $K_3$ system, and prevent screwing into the canal (Fig. 12.51).
4. $K_3$ files have positive rake angle providing them an effective cutting surface.
5. They are color coded to differentiate various tip sizes and tapers.
6. Body shapers available in taper 0.08, 0.10, and 0.12 all with tip size 25, are used to prepare the coronal third of the canal.

## HERO 642

| | | |
|---|---|---|
| HERO | - | High elasticity in rotation |
| 642 | - | 0.06., 0.04 and 0.02 tapers |

- It was introduced by Daryl-Green.
- HERO 642 (High Elasticity in Rotation, 0.06, 0.04 and 0.02 tapers) is used in "Crown down" technique, between 300 and 600 rotations per minute (rpm) in a standard slow speed contra-angle air driven or electric motors.

### Features

1. It has trihelical Hedstorm design with sharp flutes (Fig. 12.52).
2. HERO instrument has positive rake angle.
3. Due to progressively increasing distance between the flutes, there is reduced risk for binding of the instrument in root canal.
4. Larger central core provides extra strength and hence resistance to fracture.
5. Used at speed of 300-600 rpm.
6. Available in size of 0.20-0.45.

## RACE (Reamers with Alternating Cutting Edges) FILES

- RACE has safety tip and triangular cross-section. This file has two cutting edges, first alternates with a second which has been placed at different angle (Fig. 12.53)

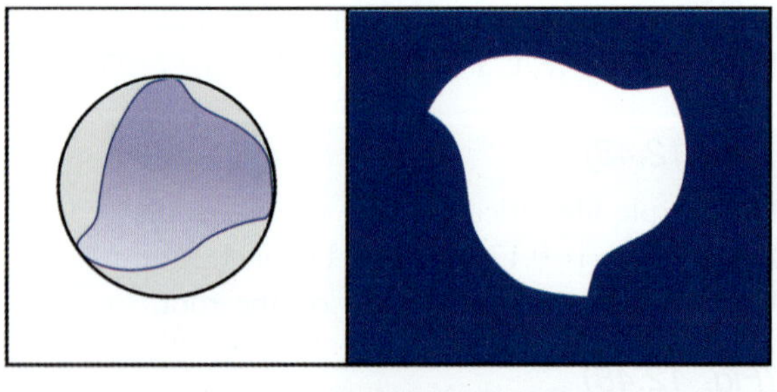

**Fig. 12.52:** Cross-section of HERO 642

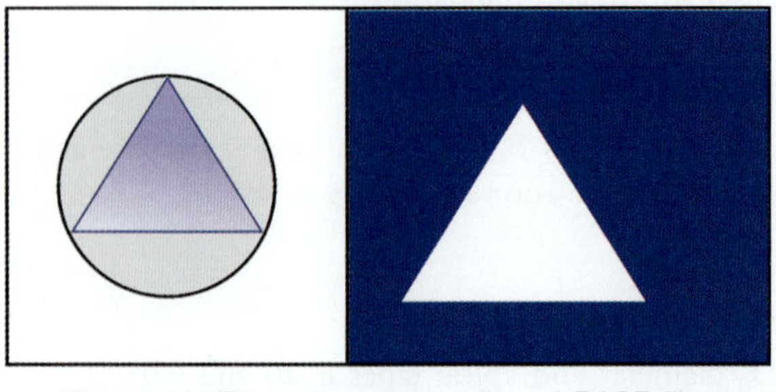

**Fig. 12.53:** Triangular cross-section of RACE files

- This file has an alternating spiral and has a cutting shank giving variable pitch and helical angles
- Variable helical angle and pitch prevents the file from screwing into the canal during its working
- Electrochemical treatment of these files provides better resistance to corrosion and metal fatigue.

### Advantages of RACE Files

1. Non-cutting safety tip helps in:
   a. Perfect control of the instrument.
   b. Steers clear of lateral canals.
2. Alternating cutting edges
   a. Reduced working time.
   b. Lowest operation torque.
   c. Non-threading or blocking effect
3. Sharp cutting edges
   a. Improved efficiency.
   b. Better debris evacuation.
4. Electrochemical treatment
   a. Better resistance to torsion and metal fatigue.

## REAL WORLD ENDO SEQUENCE FILE

1. Real World Endo sequence file system is recently introduced in NiTi rotary system. During manufacturing, these files are subjected to electropolishing for metal treatment. Electropolishing reduces the tendency of NiTi files for crack propagation by removing the surface imperfections.
2. Real World Endo sequence file system has a blank design in such a way that alternating contact points (ACPs) exist along the shank of the instrument. Because of presence of ACPs, there is no need of radial lands, which further make the instrument active shaper and thus more effective.
3. These files are available in 0.04 and 0.06 taper having the precision tip. Precision tip is defined as a non-cutting tip which becomes active at $D_1$. This results in both safety as well as efficiency.
4. Sequence files have variable pitch and helical angle which further increase its efficiency by moving the debris out of canal and thus decreasing the torque caused by debris accumulation.
5. They are worked at the speed of 450-600 rpm. Sequence files come in package of four files each, i.e. Expeditor file, 0.06 taper files in extra small, small, medium and large sizes.

## SONICS AND ULTRASONICS IN ENDODONTICS

The concept of using ultrasonics in endodontics was suggested by Richman in 1957. The pioneer research on endosonics was done by Cunningham and Martin in early 1980. But these machines showed lots of problems like tip design of instrument was such that it could not be used along with sodium hypochlorite as an irrigant because machines used to get blocked due to crystallization of NaOCl in irrigation lines. Since then a lot of changes have been made in endosonics for example tip design has been specifically turned for endodontic use, etc (Fig. 12.54).

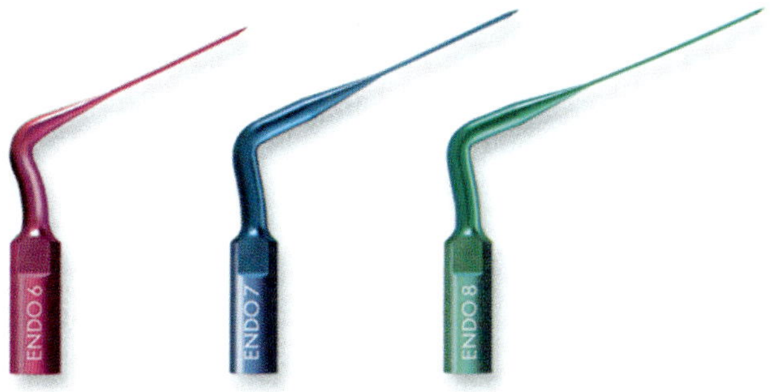


**Fig. 12.54:** Endosonic files

### Sonic Handpiece

1. It is attached to normal air line. In other words sonic instrument uses compressed air line at a pressure of 0.4 MPa, which is already available in the dental unit setup, as its source of power.
2. It has an adjustable ring to give oscillating range of 1500-3000 cycles/sec. Examples of sonic handpiece are sonic air 1500, Endo mm 1500.
3. There are two options for irrigating the root canal while using sonic handpieces. Either the water line of the dental units can be attached to the sonic handpiece, or the water can be cut off and the dental assistant can introduce sodium hypochlorite from a syringe.
4. Sonic handpiece uses three types of files:
   i. Heliosonic
   ii. Shaper sonic
   iii. Rispi sonic
3. All these instruments have safe ended non-cutting tip 1.5-2 mm in length. Also sizes for these instruments range from 15-40.
5. Instruments oscillate outside the canal which is converted into vibrational up and down movement in root canal. Sonic instruments are used in step down technique.
6. To permit the insertion of No. 15 sonic file, canal should be initially prepared with conventional hand files (no.20). Sonic file begins its rasping action 1.5-2.0 mm from the apical stop. This length is called as sonic length.

### Advantages of Sonic Instruments

- Better shaping of canal when compared to ultrasonic preparation
- Due to constant irrigation, amount of debris extruding beyond apex is less
- Produces clean canals free of smear layer and debris

### Disadvantages

- Walls of prepared canals are rough.
- Chances of transportation are more in curved canals.

### Ultrasonic Handpiece

1. Ultrasonics used in endodontics is called as endosonics. They were introduced by Richaman.

2. Ultrasonic endodontics is based on a system on which sound as an energy source (at 20 to 42 kHz), activates an endodontic file resulting in three-dimensional activation of the file in the surrounding medium.
3. The ultrasonic systems involve a power source to which an endodontic file is attached with a holder and an adapter.
4. Ultrasonic handpiece uses K-file as a canal instrument (Fig. 12.55). Before a size 15 can fully function, the canal must be enlarged with hand instruments to a size 20.
5. The irrigants are emitted from cords on the power source and travel down the file into the canal to be energized by the vibrations (Fig. 12.56).

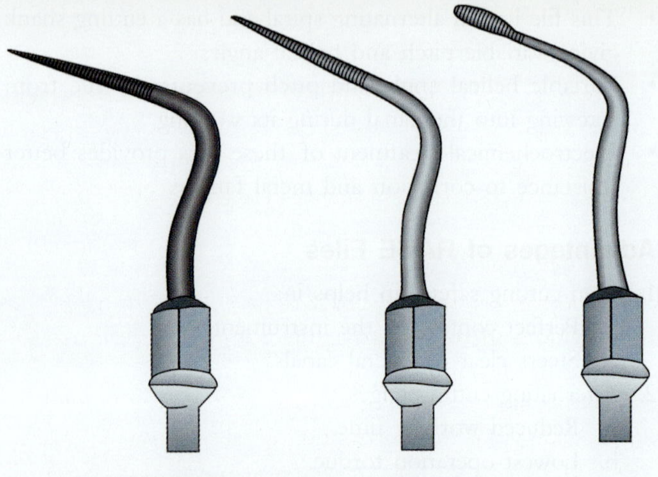

Fig. 12.55: Diagrammatic representation of endosonic files

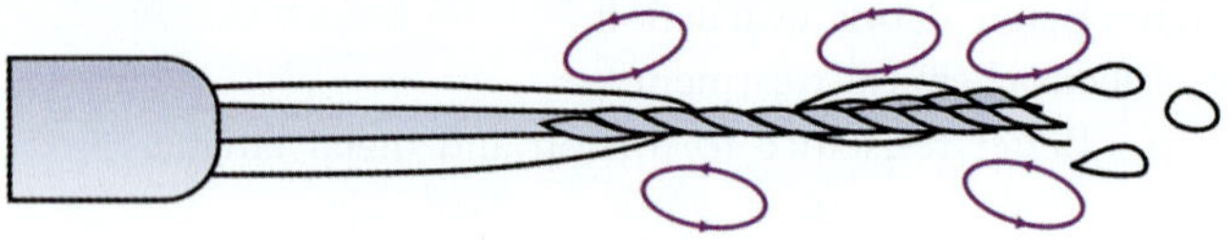

Fig. 12.56: Irrigants get energized with ultrasonic vibrations

## Advantages of Ultrasonics

- Clean canals free of smear layer and debris
- Enhanced action of NaOCl because of increased temperature and ultrasonic energy.

## Type of Ultrasonics

They are two types:

**Magnetostrictive:** It needs water coolant because it generates more heat. It is expensive, more clumpsy and less powerful.

**Piezoelectric:** Since, it generates less heat, it does not require water as coolant. It is used for location of calcified canals, retrieval of broken instrument and root-end preparation.

## Mechanism of Action

### *Cavitation and Acoustic Streaming*

Cavitation is defined as the growth and subsequent violent collapse of a small gas filled pre-existing inhomogeneity in the bulk fluid. This motion results in development of shock wave, increased temperature and pressure and free radical formation in the fluid (Fig. 12.57). Cavitation has been shown useful in removal of tooth deposits in scaling procedure but during its use in root canal regarding cavitation phenomenon, following points are to be considered:

- Threshold power setting at which this phenomenon occurs is beyond the range that is normally used for endodontic purpose.
- Cavitation depends on free displacement amplitude of the file. During root canal therapy, when file movement is restricted, this phenomenon is impossible to achieve.

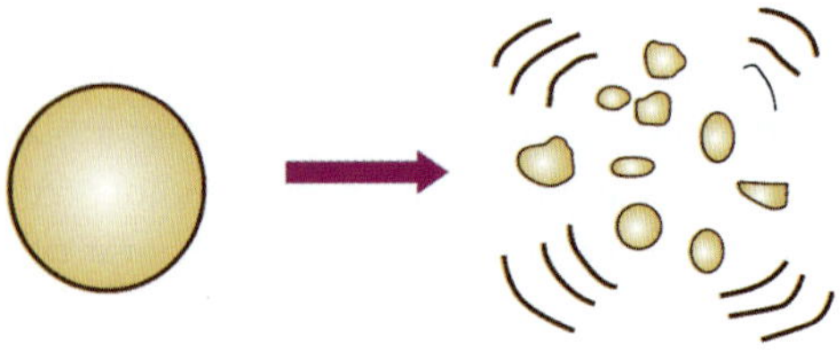

Fig. 12.57: Cavitation

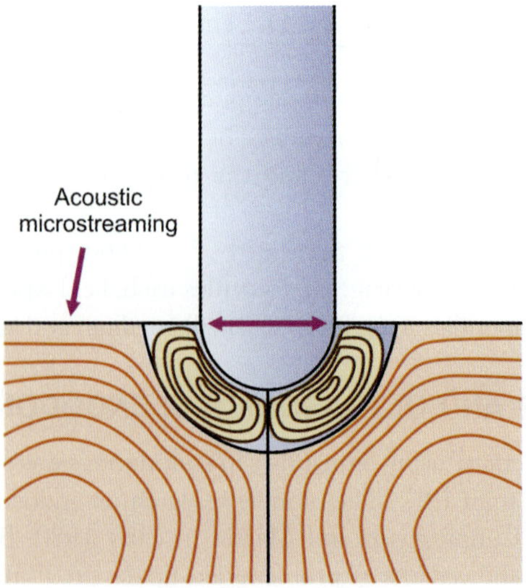


Fig. 12.58: Acoustic streaming

## Acoustic Streaming

Acoustic streaming is defined as the generation of time independent, steady unidirectional circulation of fluid in the vicinity of a small vibrating object (Fig. 12.58). This flow of liquid has a small velocity, of the order of a few centimeters per second, but because of the small dimensions involved the rate of change of velocity is high. This results in the production of large hydrodynamic shear stresses around the file, which are more than capable of disrupting most biological material. In endodontic file the greatest shear stresses around the points of maximum displacement, such as the tip of file and the antinodes along its length in the canal, therefore it may be of benefit to preheat the irrigant in the reservoir within the endosonic unit.

## Uses of Endosonics

### Access Enhancement

Performing access preparation with burs can lead to gauging of the pulpal floor and sides of the chamber. But use of round or tapered ultrasonically activated diamond coated tips has shown to produce smooth shapes of access cavity (Fig. 12.59).

### Orifice Location

Ultrasonic instruments are very useful in removal of the chamber calcifications as well as troughing for canals in isthmus and locating the canal orifices.

The troughing concept involves using an endodontic tip in back and forth brushing motion along a groove in the pulpal floor. By troughing there is better removal of tissue in the isthmus between the canals, and conservation of the tooth structure.

### Irrigation

Studies have shown that use of endosonics have resulted in cleaner canals. There is a synergetic action of the physical action of the tip along with the chemical action of the sodium irrigant.

Acoustic streaming forces within the irrigant together with the oscillation of the instrument are useful for dislodging out the debris out of the canal.

### Sealer Placement

One of the method of sealer placement is by using an ultrasonic file which runs without fluid coolant. A recent study found ultrasonic endodontic sealer placement significantly superior to hand reamer placement. A common problem encountered with this technique is the "whipping up" of the cement in the canal and causing it to set prematurely. This problem can be solved to an extent by replacing the ZnO-Eugenol sealer with a resin sealer like AH-26.

### Gutta-percha Obturation

Moreno first suggested the technique of plasticizing gutta-percha in the canal with an ultrasonic instrument. His technique advocated the placement of gutta-percha points to virtually fill the canal. The attached endodontic instrument is then inserted into the mass and the ultrasonic instrument is then activated. The gutta-percha gets plasticized by the friction being generated. Final vertical compaction is done with hand or finger pluggers.

### MTA Placement

MTA is a wonderful material with many uses. But its placement is difficult because of its sandy consistency. Low powered ultrasonics can be used to vibrate the material into position with no voids.

### Endodontic Retreatment (Fig. 12.60)

i. ***Intraradicular post removal***

   Teeth that present with intraradicular posts and periapical infections can be difficult to retreat from a coronal approach. Many techniques have been devised to aid in removal of posts from root canal spaces, of which ultrasonics are highly efficient as post removal can be achieved with minimal loss of tooth structure and decreased risk of other root damage. Ultrasonic instrumentation for post removal typically involves removing coronal cement and buildup material from around the post, then activating the tip of the ultrasonic instrument against the metal post. The ultrasound energy transfers to the post and breaks down the surrounding cement until the post loosens and is easily removed.

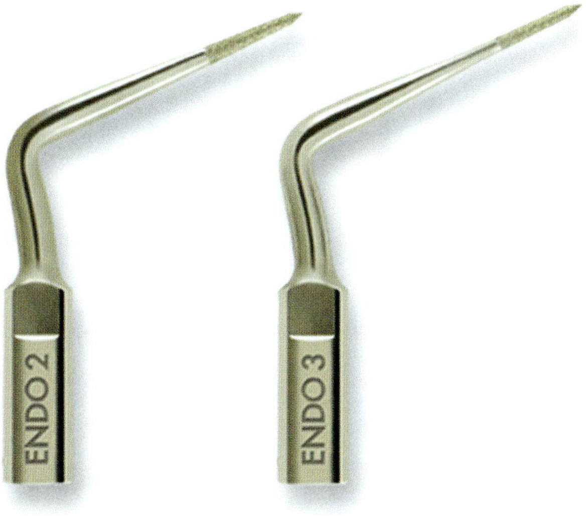


**Fig. 12.59:** Diamond coated ultrasonic tips

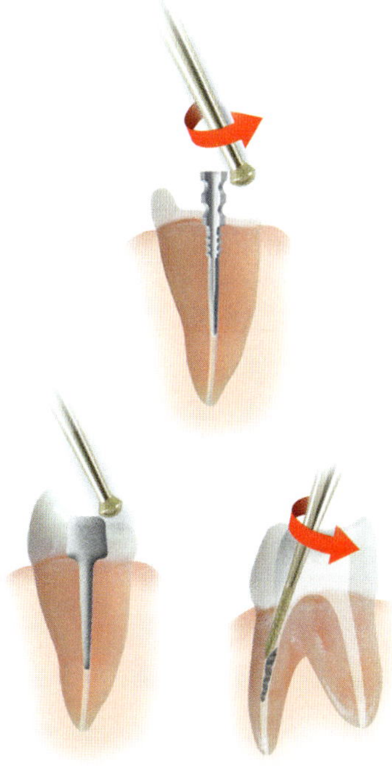

**Fig. 12.60:** Removal of post using ultrasonics

ii. ***Gutta-percha removal***

Studies have shown that ultrasonic instrumentation alone or with a solvent is as effective as hand instrumentation in removing gutta-percha from root canals. Although ultrasonic instrumentation requires less time than hand instrumentation to attain the working length, it uses significantly more solvent (chloroform or halothane) because the solvent not only acts as an irrigant but also gets volatilized.

iii. ***Silver point removal***

A conservative approach for removing defective silver points has been suggested by Krell. In this technique, a fine Hedstrom file is placed down into the canal alongside the silver point. The file is then enervated by the ultrasonic tip and slowly withdrawn. Ultrasonics with copious water irrigation along with gentle up and down strokes is quite effective in not only removing silver points and broken files, but spreader and burs tips as well.

It is apparent that no automated device will answer all needs in cleaning and shaping. Hand instrumentation is essential to prepare and cleanse the apical canal, no matter which device, sonic and ultrasonic is used later. Both ultrasonics and sonics will be a useful adjunct in endodontics if their limitations and characteristics are fully understood.

## INSTRUMENTS USED FOR FILLING ROOT CANALS

*Spreaders and pluggers* are the instruments used to compact the gutta-percha into root canal during obturation (Fig. 12.61). The use of instrument depends on the technique employed for obturation.

Earlier there used to occur the discrepancy in spreader size and shape with the gutta-percha points but in 1990, ISO/ADA endodontic standardization committee recommended the size of 15-45 for spreaders and 15-140 for pluggers (Figs 12.62A and B).

### Hand Spreaders

- They are made from stainless steel and are designed to facilitate the placement of accessory gutta-percha points around the master cone during lateral compaction technique (Fig. 12.63).
- These spreaders do not have standardized size and shape.
- They are not used routinely because excessive pressure on the root may cause fracture of root.

### Finger Spreaders (Fig. 12.64)

- They are shorter in length which allows them to afford a great degree of tactile sense and allow them to rotate freely around their axis.
- They are standardized and color coded to match the size of gutta-percha points.
- They can be manufactured from stainless steel or nickel titanium.

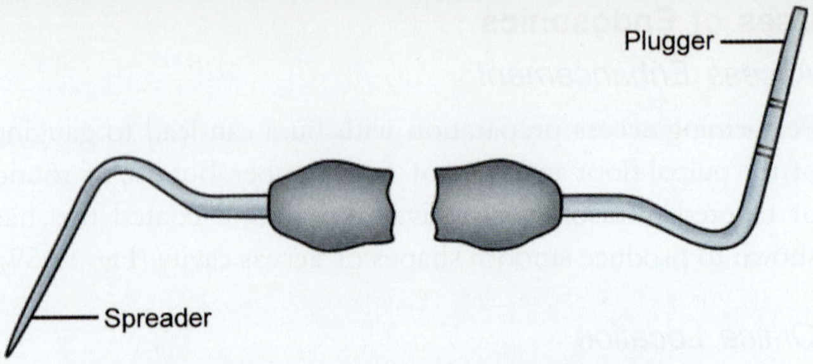


**Fig. 12.61:** Spreader and plugger tips

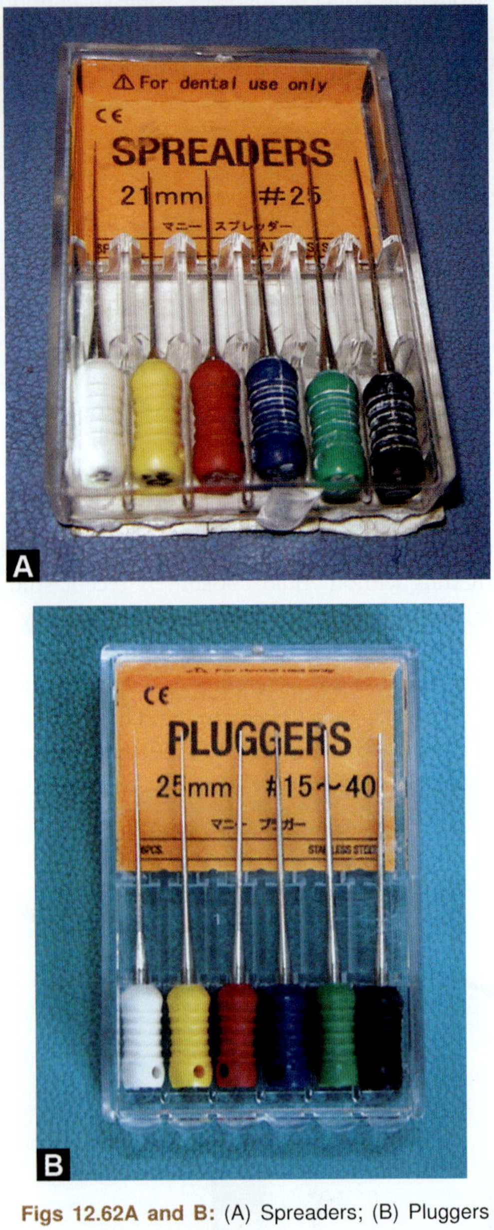


**Figs 12.62A and B:** (A) Spreaders; (B) Pluggers

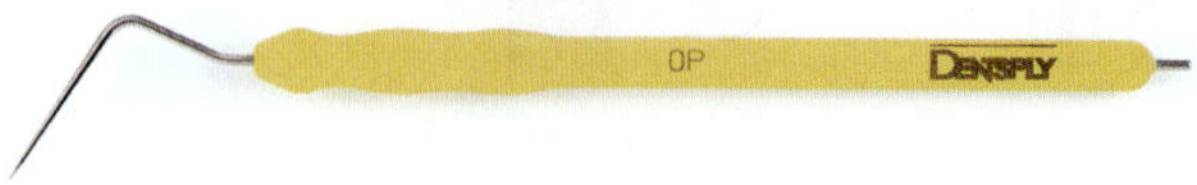


**Fig. 12.63:** Hand spreader

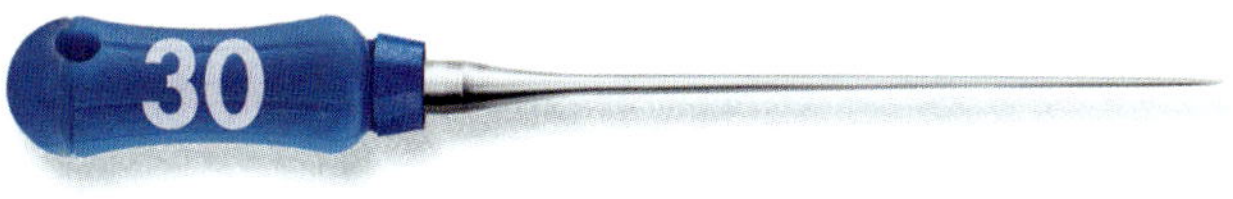


Fig. 12.64: Finger spreader

- Stainless steel spreaders may pose difficulty in penetration in curved canals, may cause wedging and root fracture if forced during compaction. They also produce great stresses while compaction.
- NiTi spreaders are recently introduced spreaders which can penetrate the curved canals and produce less stresses during compaction (Fig. 12.65). But they may bend under pressure during compaction. So, we can say that combination of both types of spreaders, i.e. stainless steel and NiTi is recommended for compaction of gutta-percha, NiTi spreaders in apical area and stainless steel in coronal part of the root canal.

## Hand Pluggers

- They consist of diameter larger than spreader and have blunt end (Figs 12.66A and B).
- They are used to compact the warm gutta-percha vertically and laterally into the root canal.
- They may also be used to carry small segments of gutta-percha into the canal during sectional filling technique (Fig. 12.67).
- Calcium hydroxide or MTA like materials may also be packed into the canals using pluggers.

## Finger Pluggers (Fig. 12.68)

- They are used for vertical compaction of gutta-percha. They apply controlled pressure while compaction, and have more tactile sensitivity than hand plugger.

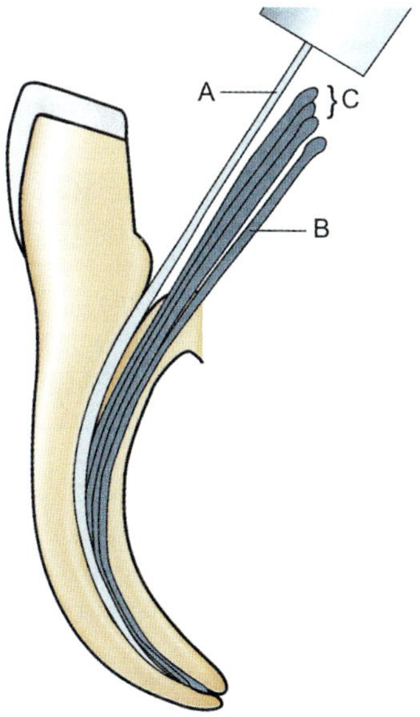


Fig. 12.65: Use of spreader during lateral compaction technique

Care should be taken with spreaders and pluggers while compacting the gutta-percha in canals. They should be cleaned prior to their insertion into the canal; otherwise the set sealer from previous insertion may roughen their surface and may pull the cone outside the canal rather than packing it. Also one should discard the instrument when it has become bent or screwed to avoid instrument separation while compaction.

## Lentulo Spirals (Fig. 12.69)

- They are used for applying sealer cement to the root canal walls before obturation.
- They can be used as hand or rotary instruments.

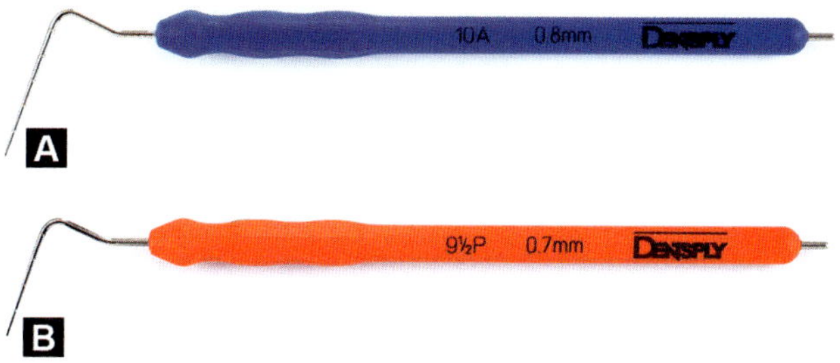


Figs 12.66A and B: Hand pluggers

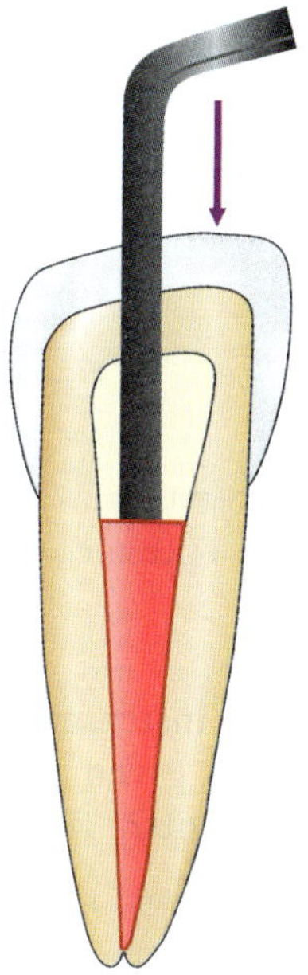

Fig. 12.67: Vertical compaction of gutta-percha using plugger

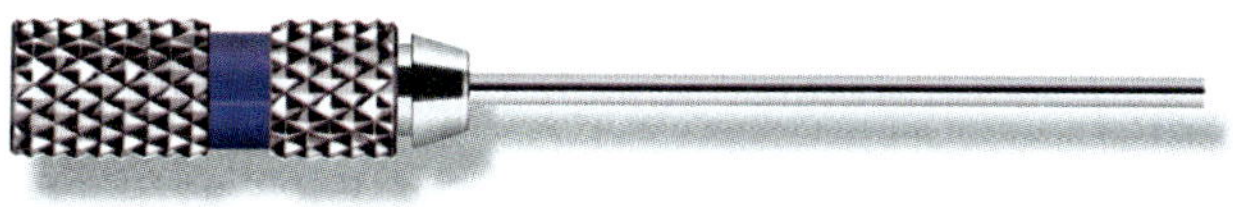

Fig. 12.68: Finger plugger

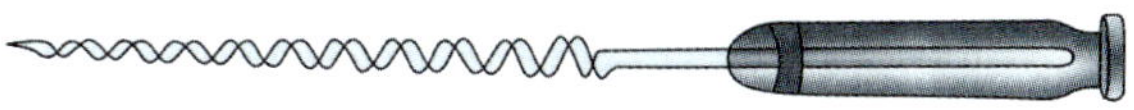

Fig. 12.69: Lentulo spiral

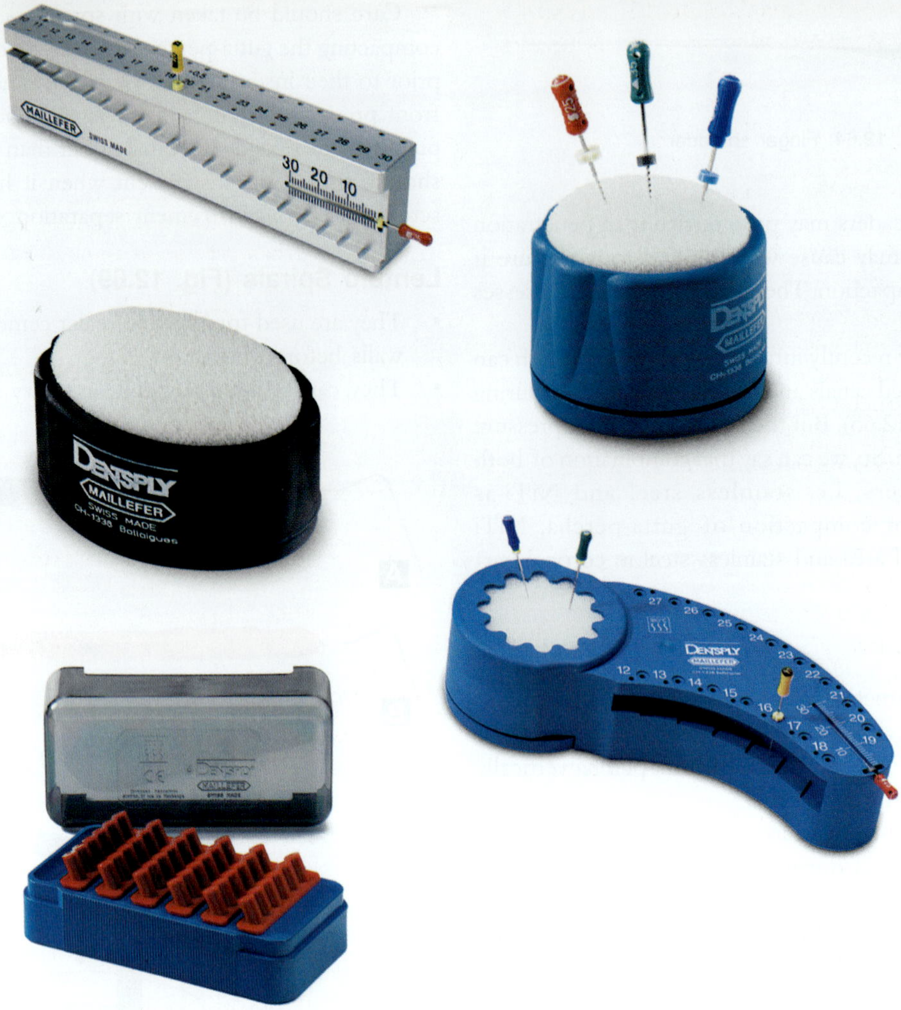


**Fig. 12.70:** Commercially available instrument holders and gauzes

Various design of instrument holders and gauzes are available commercially for operator's convenience (Fig. 12.70).

## QUESTIONS

**Q. Classify endodontic instruments**

**Q. What are guidelines given for standardization of endodontic instruments?**

**Q. Write short notes on:**

a. Broaches
b. Difference between files and reamers
c. K-files
d. H-files
e. ProTaper files
f. Profiles

**Q. Role of ultrasonics in endodontics.**

## BIBLIOGRAPHY

1. Ahmad M, Pitt Ford TR, Crum LA, Walton AJ. Ultrasonic debridement of root canals: Acoustic cavitation and its relevance. J Endod 1988;14:486-93.
2. Ahmad M, Pitt Ford TR, Crum LA. Ultrasonic debridement of root canals: An insight into the mechanisms involved. J Endod 1987;13:93-101.
3. Ahmad M, Pitt Ford TR, Crum LA. Ultrasonic debridement of root canals: Acoustic streaming and its possible role. J Endod 1987;13:490-9.
4. Ahmad M, Pitt Ford TR. Comparison of two ultrasonic units in shaping curved canals. J Endod 1989;15:457-62.
5. Ahmad M. Shape of the root canal after ultrasonic instrumentation with K-Flex files. Endod Dent Traumatol 1990;6:104-8.
6. Alapati SB, Brantley WA, Nusstein JM, et al. Vickers hardness investigation of work-hardening in used NiTi rotary instruments. J Endod 2006;32:1191-3.
7. Alapati SB, Brantley WA, Svec TA, et al. Proposed role of embedded dentin chips for the clinical failure of nickel-titanium rotary instruments. J Endod 2004;30:339-41.
8. Alapati SB, Brantley WA, Svec TA, et al. Scanning electron microscope observation of new and used nickel-titanium rotary files. J Endod 2003;29:667-9.
9. Alexandrou G, Chrissafis K, Vasiliadis L, et al. Effect of heat sterilization on surface characteristics and microstructure of Mani NRT rotary nickel-titanium instruments. Int Endod J 2006;39:770-8.
10. Alexandrou GB, Chrissafits K, Vasiliadis LP, et al. SEM observations and differential scanning calorimetric studies of new and sterilized nickel-titanium rotary endodontic instruments. J Endod 2006;32:675-9.

11. Andreasen GF, Hileman TB. An evaluation of 55 cobalt substitute nitinol wire for use in orthodontics. J Am Dent Assoc 1971;82:1373-5.
12. Andreasen GF, Morrow RE. Laboratory and clinical analyses of nitinol wire. Am J Orthod 1978;73:142-51.
13. Arens FC, Hoen MM, Steiman HR, Dietz GC. Evaluation of single-use rotary nickel-titanium instruments. J Endod 2003;29:664-6.
14. Ayar LR, Love RM. Shaping ability of profile and $K_3$ Rotary NiTi instruments when used in a variable tip sequence in simulated curved root canals. Int Endo J 2004;37:593-601.
15. Bahia MGA, Melo MCC, Buono VTL. Influence of simulated clinical use on the torsional behavior of nickel-titanium rotary endodontic instruments. Oral Surg Oral Med Oral Pathol Oral Radiol Endod 2006;101:675-80.
16. Baker MC, Ashrafi SH, Van Cura JE, Remeikis NA. Ultrasonic compared with hand instrumentation a scanning electron microscope study. J Endod 1988;14:435-40.
17. Barrieshi-Nusair KM. Gutta-percha retreatment: Effectiveness of nickel-titanium rotary instruments versus stainless steel hand files. J Endod 2002;28:454-6.
18. Barthel C, Gruber S, Rouler J. A new method to assess the results of instrumentation techniques in the root canal. J Endod 1999;25:535-8.
19. Berry KA, Loushine RJ, Primack PD, Runyan DA. Nickel-titanium versus stainless steel finger spreaders in curved canals. J Endod 1998;24:752-4.
20. Berutti E, Chiandussi G, Gaviglio I, Ibba A. Comparative analysis of torsional and bending stresses in two mathematical model of nickel-titanium rotary instruments. ProTaper versus Profile. J Endod 2003;29:15-19.
21. Best S, Watson P, Pillier R, et al. Torsional fatigue and endurance limit of a size 30.06 Profile rotary instrument. Int Endod J 2004;37:370-3.
22. Blum IY, Cohen A, Machtou P, Micallef IP. Analysis of forces developed during mechanical preparation of extracted teeth using profile NiTi instruments. Int Endod J 1999;32:32-46.
23. Blum J, Machton P, Micallef J. Location of contact areas on rotatry profile instruments in relationship to the forces developed during mechanical preparation on extracted teeth. Int Endod J 1999;32:108-14.
24. Blum J-Y Machtou P, Ruddle C, Micallef JP. Analysis of mechanical preparations in extracted teeth using ProTaper rotary instruments: Value of the Safety Quotient. J Endod 2003;29:567-75.
25. Bolanos OR, Sinai, IH, Gonsky MR, Srinivasan R. A comparison of engine and air-driven instrumentation methods with hand instrumentation. J Endod 1988;14:392-6.
26. Booth IR, Scheetz JP, Lemons JE, Eleazer PD. A comparison of torque required to fracture three different nickel-titanium rotary instruments around curves of the same angle but of different radius when bound at the tip. J Endod 2003;29:55-7.
27. Bortnick Kl, Steiman HR, Ruskin A. Comparison of nickel-titanium file distortion using electric and air-driven handpieces. J Endod 2001;27:57-9.
28. Bradley TG, Brantley WA, Culbertson BM. Differential scanning nickel-titanium orthodontic wire. Am J Orthod Dentofacial Orthop 1996;109:589-97.
29. Brantley WA, Svec TA, Iijima M, et al. Differential scanning calorimetric studies of nickel-titanium rotary endodontic instruments after simulated clinical use. J Endod 2002;28: 774-8.
30. Brantley WA, Iijima M, Grentzer TH. Temperature-modulated DSC provides new insight about nickel-titanium wire transformations. Am J Orthod Dentofacial Orthop 2003; 124:387-94.
31. Brantley WA, Svec TA, Iijima M, et al. Differential scanning calorimetric studies of nickel titanium rotary endodontic instruments. J Endod 2002;28:567-72.
32. Briggs PFA, Gulabivala K, Stock GJR, Setchell DJ. The Dentine-removing characteristics of an ultrasonically, energized K-file. Int Endod J 1989;22:259-68.
33. Briseno BM, Kremers L, Hamm G, Nitsch C. Comparison by means of a computer-supported device of the enlarging characteristics of two different instruments. J Endod 1993;19:281-7.
34. Briseno BM, Sonnabend E. The influence of different root canal instruments on root canal preparation: an in vitro study. Int Endod J 1991;24:15-23.
35. Brockhurst PJ, Denholm I. Hardness and strength of endodontic files and reamers. J Endod 1996;22(2):68-70.
36. Bryant ST, Dummer PMH, Pitoni C, Bourba M, Moghal S. Shaping ability of .04 and .046 taper profile rotary nickel-titanium instruments in simulated root canals. Int Endod I 1999;32:155-64.
37. Buchanan LS. The standardized-taper root canal preparation-part II GT file selection and safe handpiece-driven file use. Int Endod J 2001;34(1):63-71.
38. Cameron JA. The effect of ultrasonic endodontics on the temperature of the root canal wall. J Endod 1988;14:554-9.
39. Cameron JA. The use of ultrasonics in the removal of the smear layer: a scanning electron microscope study. J Endod 1983;9:289-92.
40. Canalda-Sahli C, Brau-Aguade E, Berastegui-Jimeno E. Torsional and bending properties of stainless steel and nickel-titanium Canal Master U and Flexogate instruments. Endod Dent Traumatol 1996;12:141-5.
41. Canalda-Sahli C, Brau-Aguade E, Berastequi-Jimeno E. A Comparison of bending and torsional properties of K files manufactured with different metallic alloys. Int Endod J 1996;29:185-9.
42. Canalda-Sahli C, Brau-Aguade E, Sentis-Vilalta J. The effect of sterilization on bending and torsional properties of K-files manufactured with different metallic alloys. Int Endod J 1998;31:48-52.
43. Cheung GSP, Peng B, Bian Z, et al. Defects in ProTaper SI instruments after clinical use: fractographic examination. Int Endod J 2005;38:802-9.
44. Cirnis GJ, Boyer TJ, Pelleu GB. Effect of three file type on the apical preparation of moderately curved canals. J Endod 1988;14:441-4.
45. Cunningham WT, Martin H, Pelleu GB, Stoops DE. A comparison of antimicrobial effectiveness of endosonic and hand root canal therapy. Oral Surg Oral Med Oral Pathol Oral Radiol Endod 1982;54:238-41.
46. Cunningham WT, Martin H. A scanning electron microscope evaluation of root canal debridement with the endosonic ultrasonic system. Oral Surg Oral Med Oral Pathol Oral Radiol Endod 1982;53:527-31.
47. Da Silva FM, Kobayashi C, Suda H. Analysis of forces developed during mechanical preparation of extracted teeth using RACE rotary instruments and Profiles. Int Endod J 2005;381:17-21.
48. Dalton BC, Orstavik D Phillips C, et al. Bacterial reduction with nickel-titanium rotary instrumentation. J Endod 1998;24:763-7.

49. Darabara M, Bourithis L, Zinelis S, Papadimitriou GD. Assessment of elemental composition, microstructure, and hardness of stainless steel endodontic files and reamers. J Endod 2004;30(7):523-6.
50. Darabara M, Bourithis L, Zinelis S, Papadimitriou GD. Susceptibility to localized corrosion of stainless steel and NiTi endodontics instruments in irrigating solutions. Int Endod 2004;37:705-10.
51. Daugherty DW, Gound TG, Comer TL, Comparison of fracture rate, deformation rate, and efficiency between rotary endodontic instruments driven at 150 rpm and 350 rpm. J Endod 2001:27:93-5.
52. Dautel-Morazin A, Vulcain JM, Guigand M, Bonnaure-Mallet M. An ultrastructural study of debris retention by endodontic reamers. J Endod 1995;21(7):358-61.
53. David Sonntag. Flex Master: a universal system. Endodontic Topics 2005;10:183-86.
54. Deplazes P, Peters O, Barbakow F. Comparing apical preparations of root canals shaped by nickel-titanium rotary instruments and nickel-titanium and instruments. J Endod 2001;27:196-202.
55. Di Fiore PM, Genov KA, Komaroff E, et al. Nickel-titianium rotary instrument fracture: A clinical practice assessment. Int Endod J 2006;39:700-8.
56. Dietz D, Di Fiore P, Bahcall J, Lautenschlager E. Effect of rotational speed on the breakage of nikel-titanium rotary files. J Endod 2000;26:68-71.
57. Dr Joseph Dovgan. Non-surgical endodontics in the new millennium. Endodontic Practice May, 2000.
58. Dummer PMH, Alodeh MHA, Doller R. Shaping of simulated root canals in resin blocks using files activated by a sonic handpiece. Int Endod J 1989;22:211-25.
59. Eggert C, Peters O, Barbakow F. Wear of nickel-titanium lightspeed instruments evaluated by scanning electron microscopy. J Endod 1999;25:494-7.
60. Ehrlich AD, Boyer TJ, Hicks ML, Pelleu GB. Effect of sonic instrumentation on the apical preparation of curved canals. J Endod 1989;15:200-3.
61. El Deeb ME, Boraas JC. The effect of different files on the preparation shape of curved canal. Int Endod J 1985;18:1-7.
62. Elliot LM, Curtis RV, Pitt Ford TR. Cutting patterns of nickel titanium files using two preparation techniques. Endod Dent Traumatol 1998;14:10-5.
63. Fairbourn DR, McWalter GM, Montgomery S. The effect of four preparation techniques on the amount of apically extruded debris. J Endod 1987;13:102-8.
64. Felt RA, Moser JB, Heuer MA. Flute design of endodontics instruments: Its influence on cutting efficiency. J Endod 1982;8:253-9.
65. Ferreira JJ, Rhodes JS, Pitt Ford TR. The efficacy of gutta-percha removal using Profiles. Int Endod J 2001;34:267-74.
66. Gambarini G. Shaping and cleaning the root canal system: A scanning electron microscopic evaluation of a new instrumentation and irrigation technique. J Endod 1999;25:800-3.
67. Gambarini G. Cyclic fatigue of profile rotary instruments after prolonged clinical use. Int. Endod J 2001;34:386-9.
68. Gambill JM, Alder M, del Rio CE. Comparison of nickel-titanium and stainless steel hand file instrumentation using computed tomography. J Endod 1996;22:369-75.
69. Gharai Sr, Thorpe JR, Strother JM, McClanahan SB. Comparison of generated forces and apical microleakage using nickel-titanium and stainless steel finger spreaders in curved canals. J Endod 2005;31:198-200.
70. Gianluca Gambarini. The K3 rotary nickel titanium instrument system. Endodontic Topics 2005;10:179-82.
71. Goldman M, Sakurai-Fuse E, Turco J, White RR. A silicone model method to compare three methods of preparing the root canal. Oral Med Oral Pathol Oral Radiol Endod 1989;68:457-61.
72. Haidet J, Reader A, Beck M, Meyers W. An in vivo comparison of the step-back technique versus a step-back/ultrasonic technique in human mandibular molars. J Endod 1989;15: 195-9.
73. Hilt BR, Cunningham CJ, Shen C, Richards N. Torsional properties of stainless steel and nickel-titanium files after multiple autoclave sterilizations. J Endod 2000;26:76-80.
74. Hulsman M, Stryga F. Comparison of root canal preparation using different automated devices and hand instrumentation. J Endod 1993;19:141-5.
75. Hulsmann M, Schade, Schafers F. A comparative study of root canal preparation with HERO 642 and Quantec SC rotary Ni-Ti instruments. Int Endod 2001;34:538-46.
76. Iqbal MK, Piric S, Tulcan J, et al. Comparison of apical transportation between Profile and ProTaper NiTi rotary instruments. Int Endod J 2004;37:359-64.
77. Kielt LW, Montgomery S. The effect of endosonic instrumentation in simulated root canals. J Endod 1987;13:215-19.
78. Kim JW, Griggs JA, Regan JD, et al. Effect of cryogenic treatments. Int Endod J 2005;38:364-71.
79. Klayman S, Brillant J. A comparison of the efficacy of serial preparation versus Giromatic preparation. J Endod 1975;1:334-7.
80. Knowles KI, Hammond NB, Biggs SG, Ibarrola JL. Incidence of instruments separation using Lightspeed rotary instruments. J Endod 2006;32:14-16.
81. Kosa D, Marshall G, Baumgartner J. An analysis of canal centering using mechanical instrumentation techniques. J Endod 1999;25:441-5.
82. Krell KV, Johnson RJ. Irrigation patterns of ultrasonic files. Part II. Diamond coated files. J Endod 1988;14:535-7.
83. Krell KV, Johnson RJ, Madison S. Irrigation patterns during ultrasonic canal instrumentation. Part I. K-type files. J Endod 1988;14:65-8.
84. Kuhn G, Jordan L. Fatigue and mechanical properties of nickel-titanium endodontic instruments. J Endod 2002;28: 716-20.
85. Kuhn G, Tavernier B, Jordan L. Influence of structure on nickel-titanium endodontic instruments failure. J Endod 2001;27:516-20.
86. Kum K-Y, Kazemi RB, Cha By, ZHU Q. Smear layer production of K3 and Profile NiTi Rotary instruments in curve root canals: A comparative SEM study. Oral Surg Oral Med Oral Pathol Oral Radiol Endod 2006;101:536-41.
87. Lev R, Reader A, Beck M, Meyers W. An in vitro comparison of the step-back technique versus a step-back/ultrasonic technique for 1 and 3 minutes. J Endod 1987;13:523-30.
88. Li U-M, Lee B-S, Shih C-T, et al. Cyclic fatigue of endodontic nickel titanium rotary instruments: Static and dynamic tests. J Endod 2002;28:448-51.
89. Linsuwanont P, Parashos P, Messer H. Cleaning of rotary nickel-titanium endodontics instruments. Int Endod J 2004;34:19-28.
90. Luebke NH, Brantley WA, Alapati SB, et al. Bending fatigue study of nickel-titanium Gates-Glidden drills. J Endod 2005;31:523-5.
91. Luebke NH, Brantley WA. Torsional and metallurgical properties of rotary endodontics instruments. II Stainless steel Gates-Glidden drill. J Endod 1991;17:319-23.

92. Luebke NH. Performance of Gates-Glidden drill with an applied deflection load. J Endod 1989;15:175.
93. Lumkey PJ, Walmsley AD, Walton Re, Rippin JW. Cleaning of oval canals using ultrasonic or sonic instrumentation. J Endod 1993;19:453-7.
94. Lumley PJ. Cleaning efficacy of two apical preparation regiments following shaping with hand files of greater taper. Int Endod J 2000;33:262-5.
95. Lumley PJ, Walmsley AD. Effect of precurving on the performance of endosonic K-files. J Endod 1992;18:232-6.
96. Machian GR, Peters DD, Lorton L. The comparative efficiency of four types of endodontic instruments. J Endod 1982;8:398-402.
97. Martin B, Zelada G, Varela P, et al. Factors influencing the fracture of nickel-titanium rotary instruments. Int Endod J 2003;36:262-6.
98. Martin H, Cunningham WT. An evaluation of postoperative pain incidence following endosonic and conventional root canal therapy. Oral Surg Oral Med Oral Pathol Oral Radiol Endod 1982;54:74-6.
99. Martin H, Cunningham WT, Norris JP. A quantitative comparison of the ability of diamond and K-type files to remove dentin. Oral Surg Oral Med Oral Pathol Oral Radiol Endod 1980;50:566-8.
100. Martin H. Ultrasonic disinfection of the root canal. Oral Surg Oral Med Oral Pathol Oral Radiol Endod 1976;42:92-9.
101. Masiero AV, Barletta FB. Effectiveness of different techniques for removing gutta-percha during retreatment. Int Endo J 2005;38:2-7.
102. McGurkin-Smith R, Trope M, Caplan D, Sigurdsson A. Reduction of intracanal bacteria using GT rotary instrumentation, 5.25 NaOCl. EDTA, and $Ca(OH)_2$. J Endod 2005;31:359-63.
103. Miyai K, Ebihara A, Hayashi Y, et al. Influence of phase transformation on the torsional and bending properties of nickel-titanium rotary endodontic instruments. Int Endod J 2006;39:119-26.
104. Mize SB, Clement DJ, Pruett JP, Carnes DL Jr. Effect of sterilization on cyclic fatigue of rotary nickel-titianium endodontic instruments. J Endod 1998;24:843-7.
105. Ottosen S, Nicholls J Steiner J. A comparison of instrumentation using naviflex and profile nickel-titanium engine-driven rotary instruments. J Endod 1999;25:457-60.
106. Paque F, Musch U, Hulsmann M. Comparison of root canal preparation using RACE and ProTaper rotary NiTi instruments. Int Endod J 2005;38:8-16.
107. Parashos P, Gordon I, Messer HH. Factors influencing defects of rotary nickel-titanium endodontics instruments after clinical use. Endod 2004;30:722-5.
108. Park H. A comparison of Greater Taper files. Profiles and stainless steel files to shape curved root canals. Oral Surg Oral Med Oral Pathol Oral Radiol Endod 2001;91:715-18.
109. Pedicord D, El Deeb ME, Messer HH. Hand versus ultrasonic instrumentation: Its effect on canal shape and instrumentation time. J Endod 1986;12:375-81.
110. Peters OA, Laib A, Gohring TN, Barbakow F. Changes in root canal geometry after preparation assessed by high-resolution computed tomography. J Endod 2001;27:1-6.
111. Peters OA, Peters CI, Schonenberger, K, Barbakow F. PròTaper rotary root canal preparation: Assessment of torque and force in relation to canal anatomy. Int Endod J 2003;36:93-9.
112. Peters OA, Schonenberger K, Laib A. Effects of four NiTi Preparation techniques on root canal geometry assessed by microcomputed tomography. Int Endod J 2001;34:221-30.
113. Pettiette M , Metzger S, Phillips C, Trope M. Endodontics Complications of root canal therapy performed by dental students-steel K-files and nickel-titanium hand files. J Endod 1999;25:230-4.
114. Pruett JP, Clement DJ, Carnes DL. Cyclic fatigue testing of nickel-titanium endodontic instruments. J Endod 1997;23:77-85.
115. Richman MJ. The use of ultrasonics in root canal therapy and root resection. J Dent Med 1957;12:12-18.
116. Rueggenberg FA, Powers JM. Mechanical properties of endodontic broaches and effects of bead sterilization. J Endod 1988;14:133-7.
117. Sae-Lim V, Rajamanickam I, Lim B, Lee H. Effectiveness of Profile. 04 taper rotary instruments in endodontics retreatment. J Endod 2000;26:100-4.
118. Sahafer E, Vlassis M. Comparative Investigation of two rotary nickel-titanium instruments: ProTaper Versus RaCe. Part 2. Cleaning effectiveness and shaping ability in severely curved root canals of extracted teeth. Int Endod J 2004;37:239-48.
119. Sattapan B, Palamara J, Messer H. Torque during canal instrumentation using rotary nickel-titanium files. J Endod 2000;26:156-60.
120. Sattapan B, Nervo GI, Palamara IEA, Messer HH. Defects in rotary nickel-titanium files after clinical use. J Endod 2000;26:161-3.
121. Schafer E, Dzepina A, Danesh G. Bending properties of rotary nickel-titanium instruments. Oral Surg Oral Med Oral Pathol Oral Radiol Endod 2003;96:757-63.
122. Schafer E, Schlingemann R. Efficiency of rotary nickel-titanium K3 instruments compared with stainless steel hand K-Flexofile, Part 2. Cleaning effectiveness and shaping ability in severely curved root canals of extracted teeth. Int Endod J 2003;36:208-17.
123. Schafer E. Shaping ability of HERO 642 rotary nicked- titanium instruments and stainless steel hand K-Flexofiles in simulated curved root canals. Oral Sung Oral Med Oral Pathol Oral Radiol Endod 2001;92:215-20.
124. Schäfer E. Effect of sterilization on the cutting efficiency of PVD-coated nickel-titanium endodontic instruments. Int Endod J 2002;35:867-72.
125. Schirrmesiter JF, Wrbas K-T, Meyer KM, et al. Efficacy of different rotary instruments for gutta-percha removal in root canal retreatment. J Endod 2006;32:469-72.
126. Schmidt K, Walker T, Johnson J, Nicoli B. Comparison of nickel-titanium and spreader penetration and accessory cone fit in curved canals. J Endod 2000;26:42-4.
127. Schrader C, Peters OA. Analysis of torque and force with differently tapered rotary endodontics instruments in vitro. J Endod 2005;31:120-3.
128. Scott GL, Walton RE. Ultrasonic endodontics: The wear of instruments with usage. J Endod 1986;12:279-83.
129. Sepic AO, Pantera EA, Neaverth EJ, Anderson RW. A comparison of flex-R files and K-type file for enlargement of severely curved molar root canals. J Endod 1989;15:240-5.
130. Shadid DB, Nicholls JI, Steiner JC. A comparison of curved canal transportation with balanced force versus Lightspeed. J Endod 1998;24:651-4.
131. Shen Y, Cheung GSP, Bian Z, Peng B. Comparison of defects in Profile and ProTaper Systems after clinical use. J Endod 2006;32:61-5.
132. Silvaggio J, Hicks ML. Effect of heat sterilization on the torsional properties of rotary nickel-titanium endodontic files. J Endod 1997;23:731-4.

133. Siqueria J, Lima K Magalhaes F, et al, Mechanical reduction of the bacterial population in the root canal by three instrumentation techniques. J Endod 1999;25:332-5.
134. Song YL, Bian Z, Fan B, et al. A Comparison of instrument-centering ability within the root canal for three contemporary instrumentation techniques. Int Endod J 2004;34:265-71.
135. Spyropoulos S, El Deeb ME, Messer HH. The effect of Giromatic files on the preparation shape of severely curved canals. Int Endod J 1987;20:133-42.
136. Stenman E, Spångberg LSW. Machining efficiency of Flex-R, K-Flex, Trio-Cut and S-Files. J Endod 1990;16:575-9.
137. Stenman E, Spangberg LSW. Matching efficiency of endodontic files: a new methodology. J Endod 1990;16:151-7.
138. Stokes OW, Di Flore PM, Barse JT, et al. Corrosion in Stainless-steel and nickel-titanium files. J Endod 1999;25:17-20.
139. Tasdemir T, Aydemir H Inan U, Unal O. Canal preparation with HERO 642 rotary NiTi instruments compared with stainless steel hand K-file assessed using computed tomography. Int Endod J 2005;38:402-8.
140. Thompson SA. An overview of nickel-titanium alloys used in dentistry. Int Endod J 2000;33:297-310.
141. Tripi TR, Bonaccorso A, Condorelli GG. Fabrication of hard coatings on NiTi instruments. J Endod 2003;29:132-4.
142. Tripi TR, Bonaccorso A, Condorelli GG. Cyclic fatigue of different nickel-titanium endodontic roratory instruments. Oral Surg Oral Med Oral Pathol Oral Radiol Endod 2006;102:E106-14.
143. Tripi TR, Bonaccorso A, Rapisarda E, et al. Depositions of nitrogen on NiTi instruments. J Endod 2002;28:197-500.
144. Tripi TR, Bonaccorso A, Tripi V, et al. Defects in GT rotary instruments after use, an SEM study. J Endod 2001;27:782-5.
145. Tronstad L, Niemczyk SP. Efficacy and safety tests of six automated devices for root canal instrumentation. Endod Dent Traumatol 1986;2:270-6.
146. Turpin Y, Chagneau E, Vulcain J. Impact of two theoretical cross-sections ontorsional and bending stresses of nickel-titanium root canal instrument models. J Endod 2000;26:414-17.
147. Turpin YL, Chargneau F, Bartier O, et al. Impact of torsional and bending inertia on root canal instruments. J Endod 2001;27:333-6.
148. Tygesen YA, Steiman HR, Ciavarro C. Comparison of distortion and separation utilizing Profile and Pow-R nickel-titanium rotary files. J Endod 2001;27:762-4.
149. Usman N, Baumgartner JC, Marshall JG. Influence of Instrument Size on root canal debridement. J Endod 2004:30:110-12.
150. Viana ACD, Gonzalez BM, Buono VTL, Bahia MGA. Influence of sterilization on mechanical properties and fatigue resistance of nickel-titanium rotary endodontic instruments. Int Endod J 2006;39:709-15.
151. Walia H, Brantley WA, Gerstein H. An initial investigation of the bending and torsional properties of Nitinol root canal files. J Endod 1988;14:346-51.
152. Walker TL, del Rio CE. Histological evaluation of ultrasonic and sonic instrumentation of curved root canals. J Endod 1989;18:49-59.
153. Walmsley AD, Lumley PJ, Laird WR. The oscillatory pattern of sonically powered endodontics files. Int Endod J 1989;22: 125-32.
154. Walmsley AD, Williams AR. Effects of constraint on the oscillatory pattern of endosonic files. J Endod 1989;15:189-94.
155. Walsh CL, Messer HH, El Deeb ME. The effect of varying the ultrasonic power setting on canal preparation. I Endod 1990;16:273-8.
156. Weine FS, Kelly RF, Bray KE. Effect of preparation with endodontic handpieces on original canal shape. J Endod 1976;2:298-303.
157. Wildey WL, Senia S. A new root canal instrument and instrumentation technique: a preliminary report. Oral Surg Oral Med Pathol Oral Radiol Endod 1989;67:198-207.
158. Yao JH, Sachwartz SA, Beeson TJ. Cyclic fatigue of three types of rotary nickel-titanium files in a dynamic model. J Endod 2006;32:55-7.
159. Yared G, Bou Dgher F, Kulkarni K. Influence of torque control motors and the operator's proficiency on ProTaper failures. Oral Surg Med Oral Pathol Radiol Endod 2003;96:229-33.
160. Yared G, Sleiman P. Failure of Profile instruments used with air, high torque contro, and low torque control motors. Oral Surg Oral Med Oral Pathol Oral Radiol Endod 2002;93:92-6.
161. Yared GM, Bou Dagher FE, Machtou P. Cyclic fatigue of Profile rotary instruments after clinical use. Int Endo J 2000; 33:204-7.
162. Yoneyama T, Doi H, Hamanaka H, et al. Super-elasticity and thermal behavior of NiTi alloy orthodontic arch wires. Dent Mater J 1992;11:1-10.
163. Yoshimine Y, Ono M, Akamine A. The Shaping effects of three nickel-titanium rotary instruments in simulated S-Shaped Canals. J Endod 2005;31:373-5.
164. Zakariasen KA, Zakariasen KL. Comaprison of hand, hand/ sonic and hand/ mechanical instrumentation methods. J Dent Res 1994;73:215
165. Zakariasen KL, Zakariasen KA, McMinn M. Today's Sonics; using the combined hand/sonic endodontic technique. I Am Dent Assoc 1992;123:67-78.
166. Zelada G, Varela P, Martin B, et al. The effect of rotational speed and the curvature of root canals on the breakage of rotary endodontic instruments. J Endod 2002;28:540-2.

# Internal Anatomy

CHAPTER 13



## INTRODUCTION

For the success of endodontic therapy, the knowledge of pulp anatomy cannot be ruled out. It is essential to have the knowledge of normal and usual configuration of the pulp cavity and its variations from the normal.

Before starting the endodontic therapy after correct diagnosis and treatment planning, one must have thorough knowledge of pulp anatomy. The pulp cavity must be mentally visualized three dimensionally. In addition to general morphology, variations in canal system must be kept in mind while performing the root canal therapy.

## PULP CAVITY

Various studies have been conducted regarding the anatomy of pulp cavity of teeth. The pulp cavity lies within the tooth and is enclosed by dentin all around except at the apical foramen. It is divided into two—a coronal and a radicular portion. The coronal portion, i.e. pulp chamber (Fig. 13.1) reflects the external from of crown. The roof of pulp chamber consists of dentin covering the pulp chamber occlusally or incisally. The floor of pulp chamber merges into the root canal at the orifices. Thus canal orifices are the openings in the floor of pulp chamber leading into the root canals (Fig. 13.2).

### Pulp Horns

Pulp horns are landmarks present occlusal to pulp chamber. They may vary in height and location. Pulp horn tends to be single horn associated with each cusp of posterior teeth and mesial and distal in anterior teeth. The occlusal extent of pulp horn corresponds to height of contour in young permanent teeth and cervical margin in older teeth and cervical margin in older teeth.

### Pulp Chamber

It occupies the coronal portion of pulp cavity. It acquires shape according to shape and size of crown of the tooth, age of person, and irritation, if any.

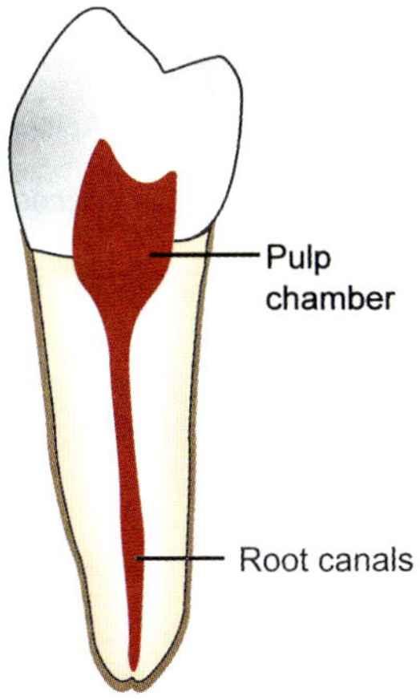


Fig. 13.1: Pulp cavity showing pulp chamber and root canals

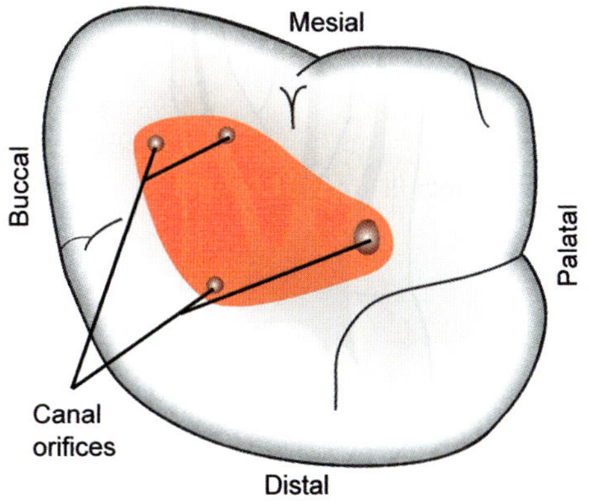


Fig. 13.2: Canal orifices

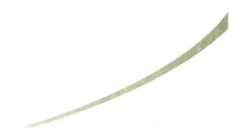

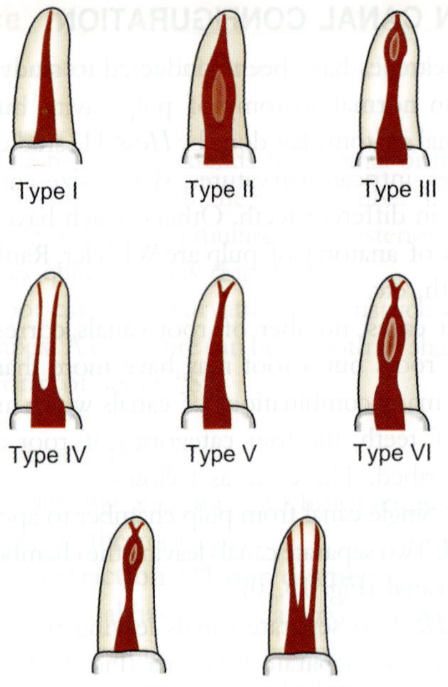


**Fig. 13.13:** Vertucci's is classification of root canal anatomy

**Type I:** A single canal extends from the pulp chamber to the apex (1).

**Type II:** Two separate canals leave the pulp chamber and join short of the apex to form one canal (2-1).

**Type III:** One canal leaves the pulp chamber and divides into two in the root; the two then merge to exit as one canal (1-2-1).

**Type IV:** Two separate, distinct canals extend from the pulp chamber to the apex (2).

**Type V:** One canal leaves the pulp chamber and divides short of the apex into two separate, distinct canals with separate apical foramina (1-2).

**Type VI:** Two separate canals leave the pulp chamber, merge in the body of the root, and redivide short of the apex to exit as two distinct canals (2-1-2).

**Type VII:** One canal leaves the pulp chamber, divides and then rejoins in the body of the root, and finally redivides into two distinct canals short of the apex (1-2-1-2).

**Type VIII:** Three separate, distinct canals extend from the pulp chamber to the apex (3).

**Vertucci classification**

| | | |
|---|---|---|
| One canal at apex | Type I | 1 → 1 |
| | Type II | 2 → 1 |
| | Type III | 1 → 2 → 1 |
| Two canals at apex | Type IV | 2 → 2 |
| | Type V | 1 → 2 |
| | Type VI | 2 → 1→2 |
| | Type VII | 1 → 2 → 1 → 2 |
| Three canals at apex | Type VIII | 3 → 3 |

This classification does not consider possible positions of auxiliary canals or portion at which apical foramen exit the root.

## METHODS OF DETERMINING PULP ANATOMY

Basically there are two ways of determining pulp anatomy of teeth. These are:

1. Clinical methods
   a. Anatomy studies
   b. Radiographs
   c. Exploration
   d. High resolution computed tomography
   e. Visualization endogram
   f. Fiberoptic endoscope
   g. Magnetic resonance imaging
2. *In vitro* methods
   a. Sectioning of teeth
   b. Use of dyes
   c. Clearing of teeth
   d. Contrasting media
   e. Scanning electron microscopic analysis

a. **Anatomic studies:** The knowledge of anatomy gained from various studies and textbooks is commonly used method.

b. **Radiographs:** Radiographs are also useful in assessing the root canal anatomy (Figs 13.14 to 13.17). But very good quality of radiographs is needed for this purpose. Since radiographs are two-dimensional picture of a three-dimensional object, one has to analyze the radiograph carefully.

c. **Exploration:** On reaching pulpal floor one finds the grooves and anatomic dark lines which connect the canal orifices, this is called dentinal map. Map should be examined and explored using an endodontic explorer.

d. **High resolution computed tomography:** It shows three-dimensional picture of root canal system using computer image processing.

e. **Visualization endogram:** In this technique, an irrigant is used which helps in visualization of the canals on radiograph. This solution is called Ruddle's solution. It consists of:

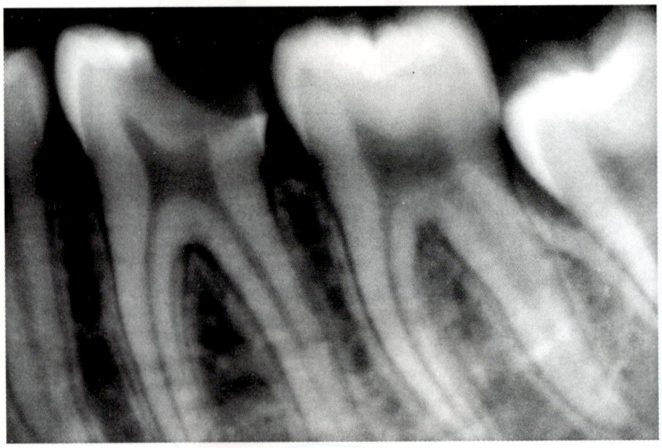

**Fig. 13.14:** Radiograph showing root canal anatomy of molars

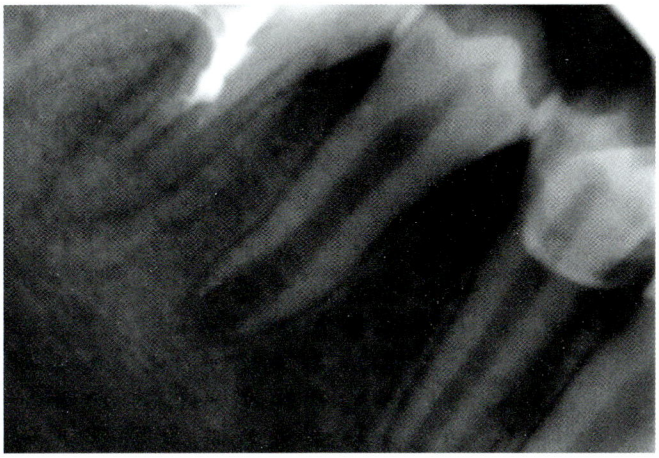

Fig. 13.15: Radiograph showing root canal anatomy of premolars

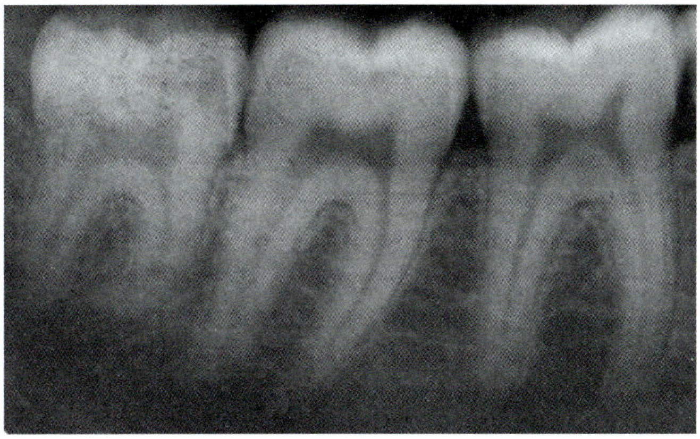

Fig. 13.16: Radiograph showing root canal anatomy of molars

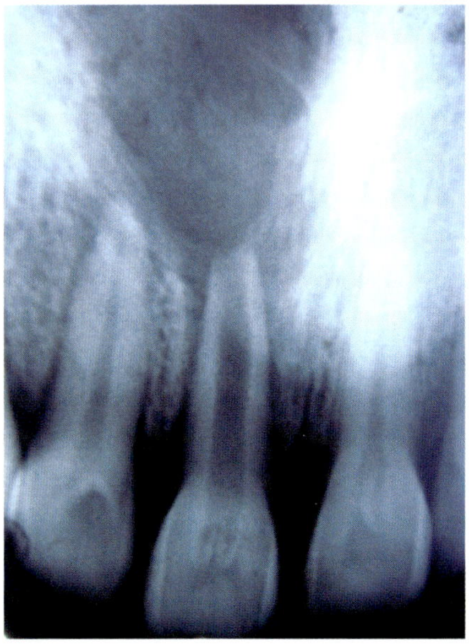

Fig. 13.17: Root canals of anterior teeth

a. Sodium hypochlorite-to dissolve organic tissues
b. 17% EDTA → to dissolve inorganic tissue
c. Hypaque: It is an iodine containing radiopaque contrast media.

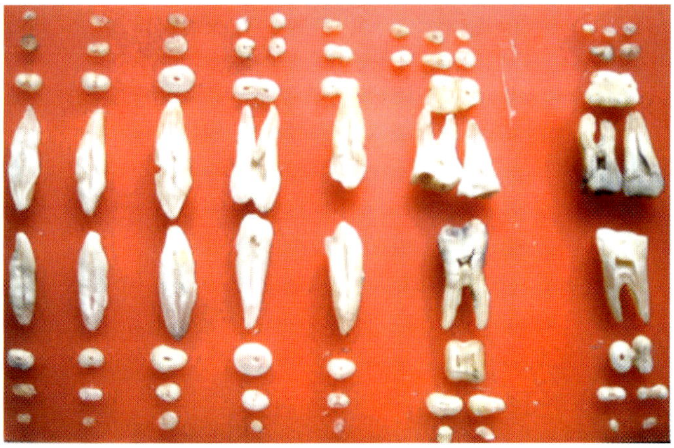

Fig. 13.18: Sectioning of teeth showing canal anatomy

After injecting Ruddle's solution into canal system, radiograph is taken to visualize the canal anatomy.

f. **Fiberoptic endoscope:** It is used to visualize canal anatomy.
g. **Magnetic resonance imaging:** It produces data on computer which helps in knowing canal morphology.

### *In vitro* Methods

a. **Sectioning:** In this teeth are sectioned longitudinally for visualization of root canal system (Fig. 13.18).
b. **Use of dyes:** Methylene blue or fluorescein sodium dyes (commonly used) help in locating pulp tissue preset in pulp chamber because dyes stain any vital tissue present in pulp chamber or root canals.
c. **Clearing of roots:** In this roots are initially decalcified using either 5 percent nitric acid or 10 percent hydrochloric acid and then dehydrated using different concentrations of alcohols and immersed in different clearing agents like methyl salicylate or xylene. By this treatment, tooth becomes transparent, then a dye is injected and anatomy is visualized (Fig. 13.19).
d. **Hypaque/contrasting media:** It is iodine containing media which as injected into root canal space and visualized on radiograph.
e. **Scanning electron microscopic (SEM) analysis:** It also helps in evaluating root canal anatomy.

## VARIATIONS IN THE INTERNAL ANATOMY OF TEETH

The canal configuration can vary in some cases because of numerous reasons like development anomalies, hereditary factors, trauma, etc. Usually the variations in root morphologies tend to be bilateral.

1. **Variations in development**
   i. Gemination
   ii. Fusion
   iii. Concrescence
   iv. Taurodontism
   v. Talon's cusp
   vi. Dilacerations
   vii. Dentinogenesis imperfecta

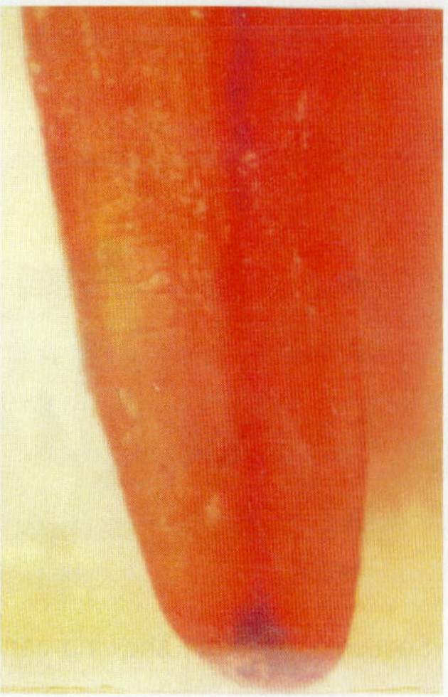

**Fig. 13.19:** Photograph showing transparent root made by use of chemicals and dye penetration in root canal

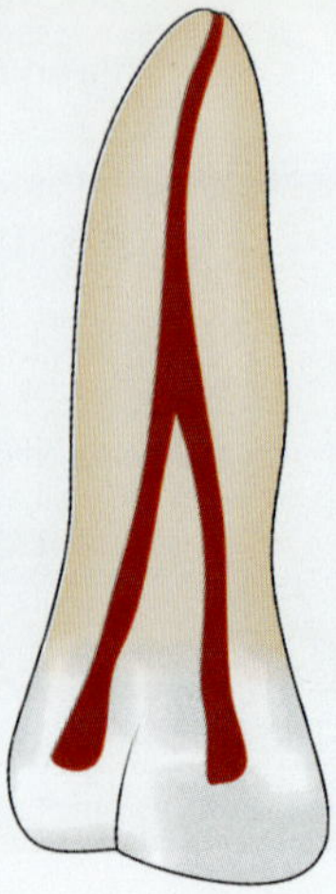

**Fig. 13.20:** Gemination

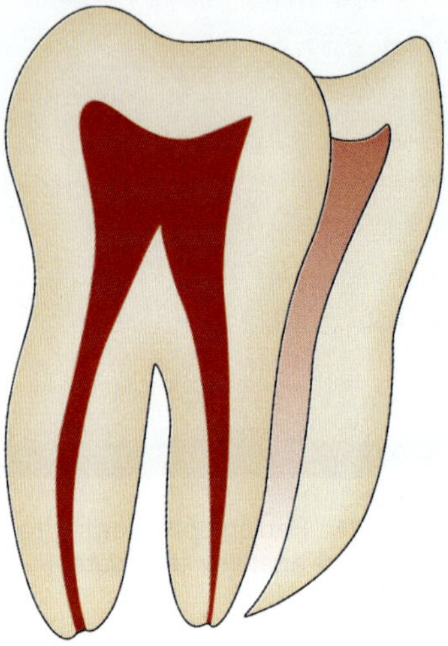

**Fig. 13.21:** Fusion

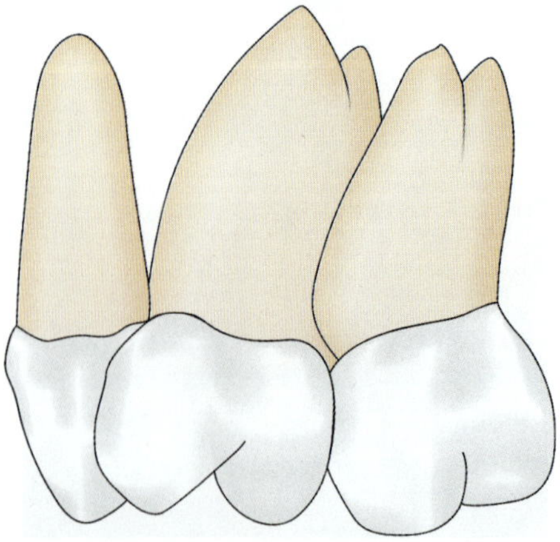

**Fig. 13.22:** Concrescence

viii. Dentin dysplasia
ix. Lingual groove
x. Extra root canal
xi. Missing root
xii. Dens evaginatus
xiii. Dens invaginatus

2. **Variations in shape of pulp cavity**
   i. Gradual curve
   ii. Apical curve
   iii. C-shaped
   iv. Bayonet shaped
   v. Dilaceration
   vi. Sickle shaped
3. **Variations in pulp cavity due to pathology**
   i. Pulp stones
   ii. Calcifications
   iii. Internal resorption
   iv. External resorption
4. **Variations in apical third**
   i. Different locations of apex
   ii Accessory and lateral canals
   iii. Open apex
5. **Variations in size of tooth**
   i. Macrodontia
   ii. Microdontia

1. **Variations in development**
   i. **Gemination:** It arises from an attempt at division of a single tooth germ by an imagination resulting in incomplete formation of two teeth (Fig. 13.20).
   ii. **Fusion:** Fusion results in union of two normally separated tooth germ. Fused teeth may show separate or fused pulp space (Fig. 13.21).
   iii. **Concrescence:** In this fusion occurs after the root formation has completed. Teeth are joined by cementum only (Fig. 13.22).
   iv. **Taurodontism:** In this body of tooth is enlarged at the expense of roots (also called bull like teeth). Pulp chamber in these teeth is extremely large with a greater apico-occlusal height (Fig. 13.23). Bifurcations/trifurcations may be present only few millimeters above the root apices. Pulp lacks the normal constriction at cervical level of

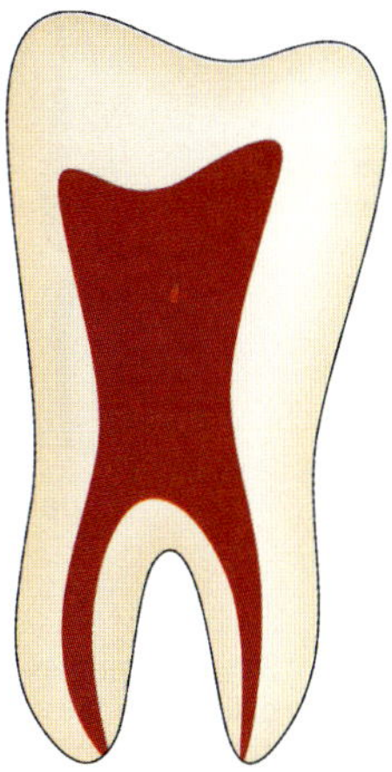

Fig. 13.23: Taurodontism

tooth. This condition is commonly seen associated with syndromes like ***Klinefelter's syndrome*** and ***Down syndrome***.

v. **Talon's cusp:** It resembles eagle's talon. In this, anomalous structure projects lingually from the cingulum area of maxillary or mandibular incisor. This structure blends smoothly with the tooth except that there is a deep developmental groove where that structure blends with lingual surface of the tooth.

vi. **Dilacerations:** Dilacerations is an extraordinary curving of the roots of the teeth. Etiology of dilacerations is usually related to trauma during the root development in which movement of the crown and a part of root may result in sharp angulation after tooth completes development (Figs 13.24).

vii. **Dentinogenesis imperfecta:** It results in defective formation of dentin. It shows partial or total precocious obliteration of pulp chamber and root canals because of continued formation of dentin.

viii. **Dentin dysplasia:** It is characterized by formation of normal enamel, atypical dentin and abnormal pulpal morphology. In this root canals are usually obliterated so need special care while instrumentation.

ix. **Lingual groove:** It is a surface infolding of dentin directed from the cervical portion towards apical direction. It is frequently seen in maxillary lateral incisors.

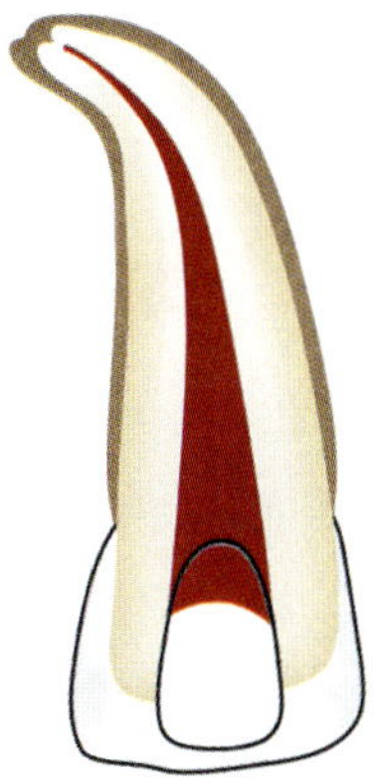

Figs 13.24: Dilacerated root

Deep lingual groove is usually associated with deep narrow periodontal pocket which often communicates with pulp causing endodontic-periodontal relationship. Prognosis of such teeth is poor and treatment is difficult.

x. **Presence of extracanals:** More than 70 percent of maxillary first molar have shown the occurrence of second mesiobuccal canal, and this is found to be most common reason for retreatment of maxillary molars. Location of orifice can be made by visualizing a point at the intersection between a line running from mesiobuccal to palatal canal and a perpendicular from the distobuccal canal.

In mandibular molars extracanals are found in 38 percent of the cases. A second distal canal is suspected when distal canal does not lie in midline of the tooth.

Two canals in mandibular incisors are reported in 41 percent of the cases. And among mandibular premolars more than 11 percent of teeth have shown the presence of two canals. In most of the cases no separate orifices are located for two different canals. Usually the lingual canal projects from the wall of main buccal canal at an acute angle.

xi. **Extra root or the missing root:** It is a rare condition which affects less than 2 percent of permanent teeth (Figs 13.25A to C).

xii. **Dens in dente or dens invaginatus:** This condition represents an exaggeration of the lingual pit (Fig. 13.26). Most commonly involved teeth are permanent maxillary lateral incisors. This condition may range from being superficial that is involving only crown part to pit in which both crown and root are involved. Tooth with dens invaginatus has tendency for plaque accumulation which predisposes it to early decay and thus pulpitis.

Types of dens invaginatus (According to Oehlers) (Fig. 13.27):

*Type I:* Minor type imagination occurring with in crown and not extending beyond CEJ.

*Type II:* Here invagination invades the root as a blind sac and may connect pulp.

*Type III:* Severe type invagination extending to root and opening in apical region without connection with pulp.

xiii. **Dens evaginatus:** In this condition an anomalous tubercle or cusp is located on the occlusal surface (Fig. 13.28). Because of occlusal abrasion, this tubercle wears off fast causing early exposure of accessory pulp horn that extends into the tubercle. This may further result in periradicular pathology in otherwise caries free teeth even before completion of the apical root development. This condition is commonly seen in premolar teeth.

2. **Variations in shape of pulp cavity**

i. **Gradual curve:** It is most common condition in which root canal gradually curves from orifice to the apical foramen (Fig. 13.29).

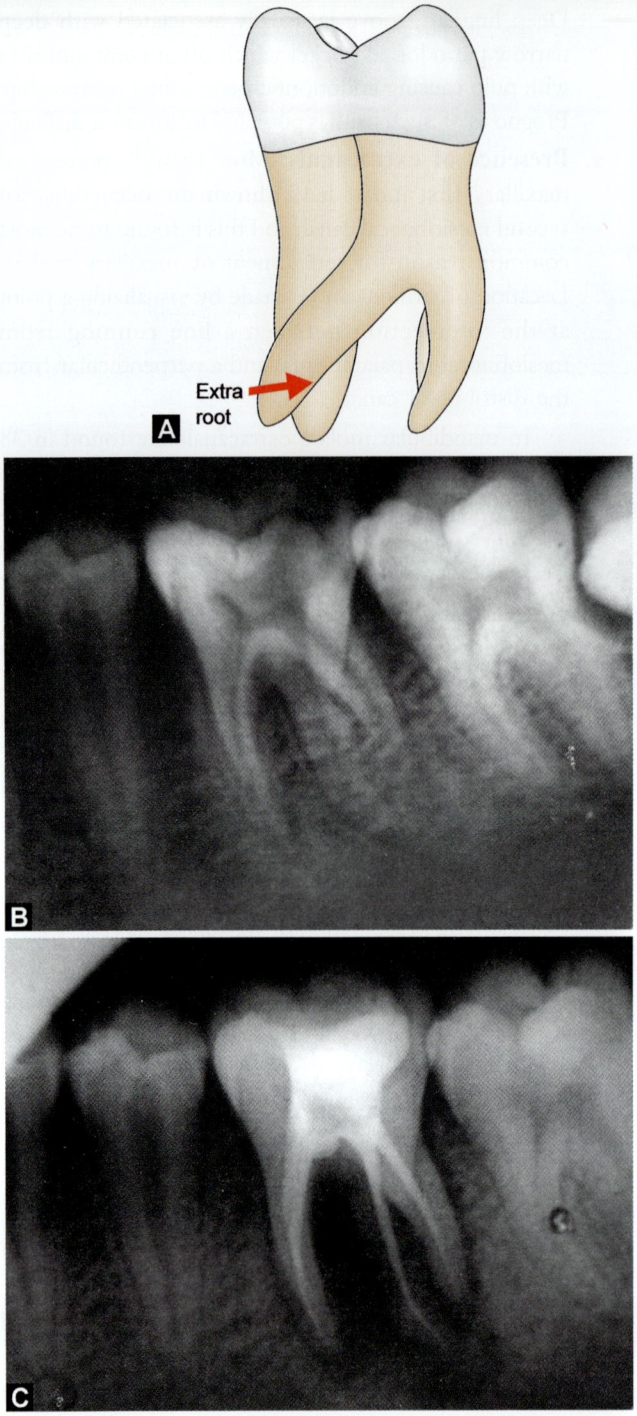


Figs 13.25 A to C: Extra root in mandibular molar

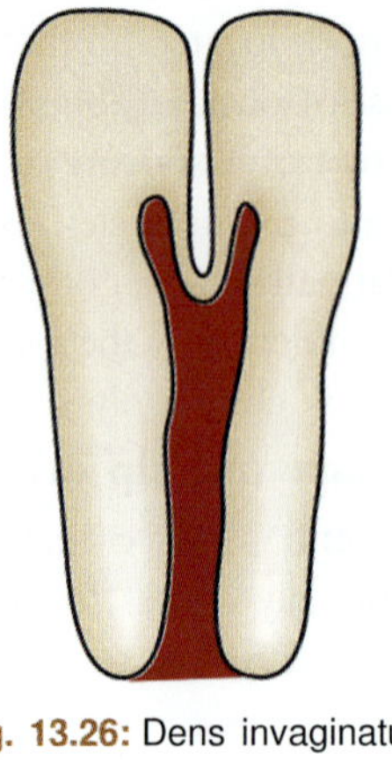

Fig. 13.26: Dens invaginatus

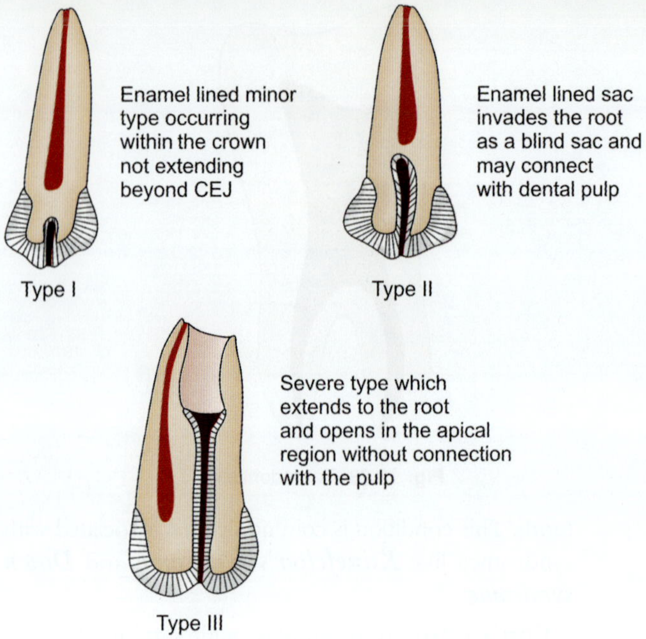


Fig. 13.27: Oehlers classification of Dens invaginatus

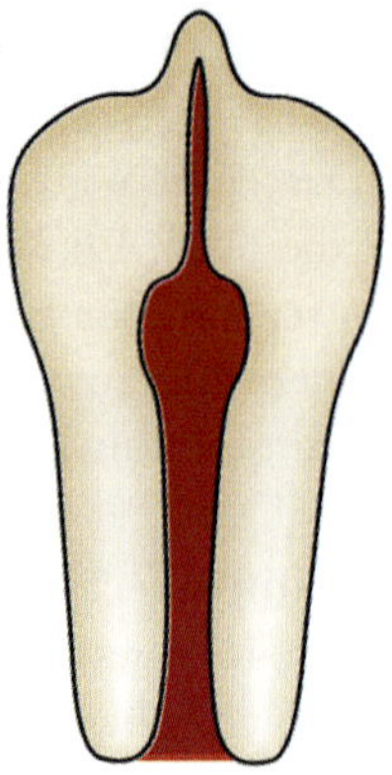

Fig. 13.28: Dens evaginatus

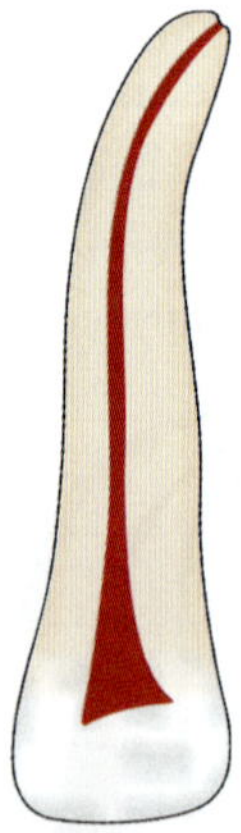

Fig. 13.29: Gradual curve in root canal

ii. **Apical curve:** In this root canal is generally straight but at apex it shows curve. It is commonly seen in maxillary lateral incisors and mesiobuccal root of maxillary molars (Fig. 13.30).

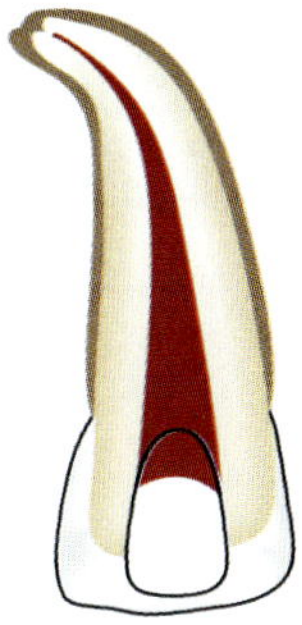

**Fig. 13.30:** Apical curve

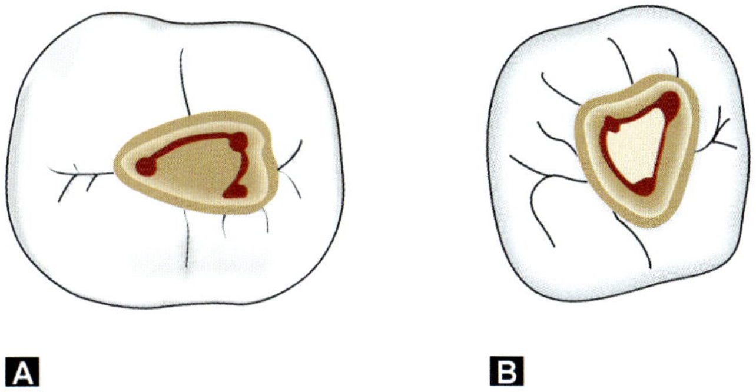


**Figs 13.31 A and B:** C-shaped canal

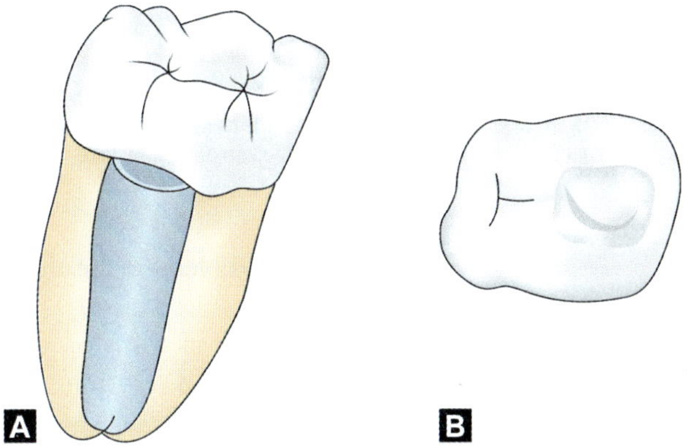


**Figs 13.32 A and B:** C-shaped canal forming 180° arc

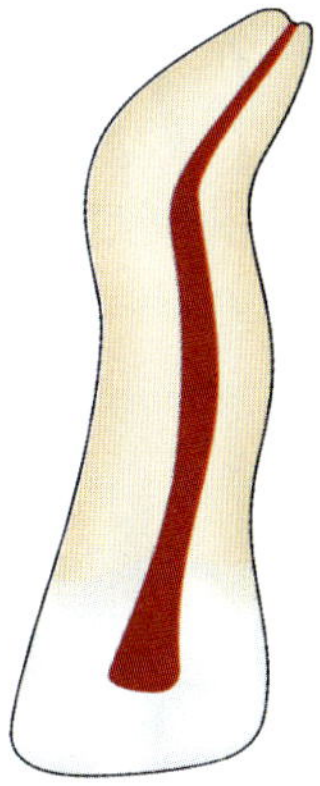

**Fig. 13.33:** Bayonet shaped canal

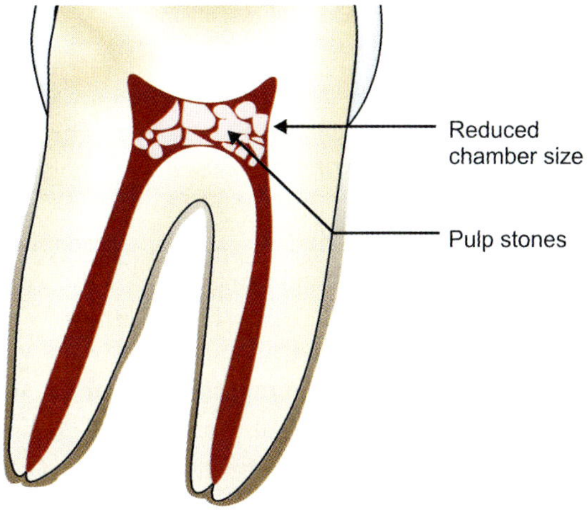


**Fig. 13.34:** Pulp stones and calcification

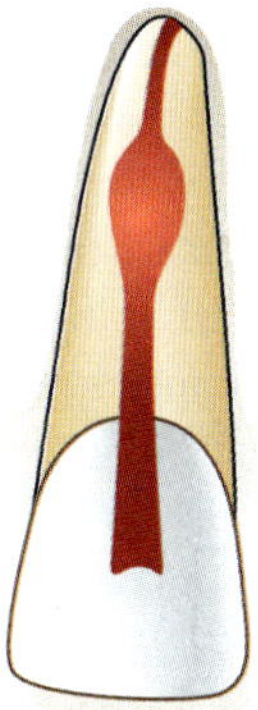

**Fig. 13.35:** Internal resorption

iii. **C-shaped canal:** This type of canal is usually found in mandibular molars. They are named so because of its morphology. Pulp chamber in C-shaped molar is single ribbon shaped with 180 degree arc or more (Figs 13.31 and 13.32). Root structure of C-shaped molar has various anatomic variations below the orifice level.

iv. **Bayonet shaped canal:** It is commonly seen in premolars (Fig. 13.33).

v. **Sickle shaped canals:** In this, canal is sickle shaped. It is commonly seen in mandibular molars. Cross-section of this canal shows ribbon shape.

3. **Variations in pulp cavity because of pathology**

i. **Pulp stones and calcifications:** Pulp stones are nodular calcified masses present in either coronal and radicular pulp or both of these. They are present in atleast 50 percent of teeth. Pulp stones may form either due to some injury or a natural phenomenon (Fig. 13.34). Presence of pulp stones may alter the internal anatomy of the pulp cavity. Thus, making the access opening of the tooth difficult. Sometimes calcifications become extremely large, almost obliterating the pulp chamber or the root canal.

ii. **Internal resorption:** "Internal resorption is an unusual form of tooth resorption that begins centrally within the tooth, apparently initiated in most cases by a peculiar inflammation of the pulp." It is characterized by oval shaped enlargement of root canal space (Fig. 13.35).

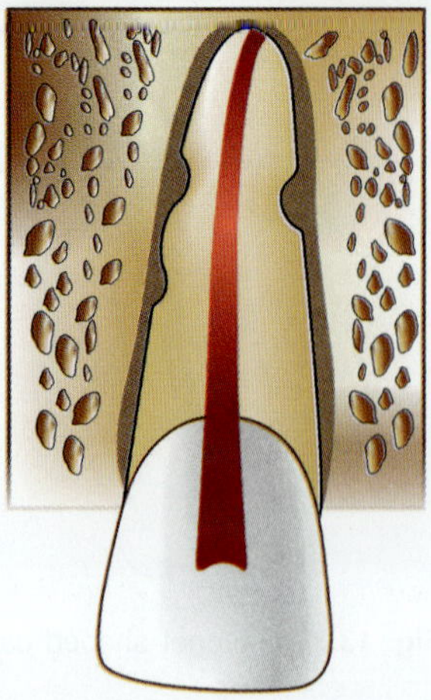

Fig. 13.36: External resorption

It is commonly seen in maxillary central incisors, but any tooth of the each can be affected. The typical ***radiographic appearance*** is smooth widening of root canal wall.

iii. **External resorption:** External root resorption is initiated in the periodontium and it affects the external or lateral surface of the root (Fig. 13.36).

4. **Variations in apical third**
   i. **Different locations of apical foramen:** Apical foramen may exit on mesial, distal, buccal or lingual surface of the root. It may also line 2-3 mm away from anatomic apex.
   ii. **Accessory and lateral canals:** They are lateral branches of the main canal that form a communication between the pulp and periodontium. They can be seen anywhere from furcation to apex but tend to more common in apical third and in posterior teeth.
   iii. **Open apex:** It occurs when there is periapical pathology before completion of root development or as a result of trauma or injury causing pulpal exposure. In this canal is wider at apex than at cervical area. It as also referred as Blunderbuss canal (Fig. 13.37). In vital teeth with open apex, treatment should be apexogenesis and in nonvital teeth, it is apexification.
5. **Variations in size of tooth**
   i. **Macrodontia:** In this condition pulp space and teeth are enlarged throughout the dentition. Commonly seen in gigantism.
   ii. **Microdontia:** In this condition, pulp space and teeth appear smaller in size. It is commonly seen in cases of dwarfism.

## FACTORS AFFECTING INTERNAL ANATOMY

Internal anatomy of teeth, i.e. pulp cavity though reflects the tooth form, yet various environmental factors whether physiological or pathological affect its shape and size because of pulpal and dentinal reaction to them. These factors can be enlisted as:

1. ***Age:*** With advancing age, there is continued dentin formation causing regression in shape and size of pulp cavity (Fig. 13.38). Clinically it may pose problems in locating the pulp chamber and canals.

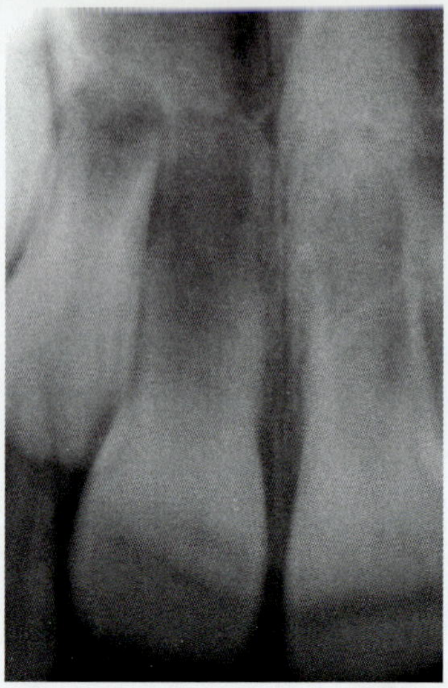

Fig. 13.37: Radiograph showing open apex of maxillary incisor tooth

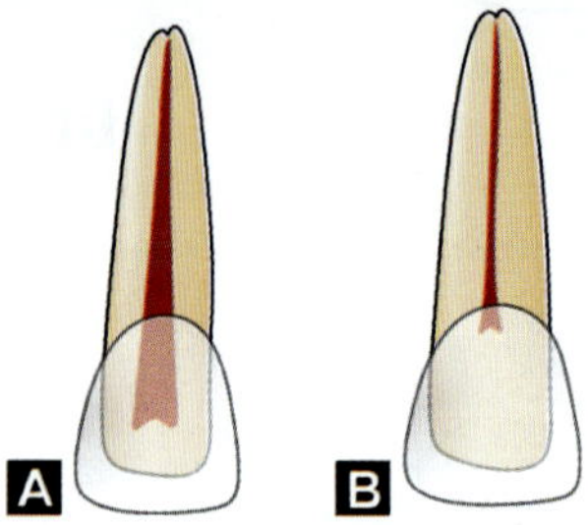



Figs 13.38 A and B: (A) Root canal anatomy of young patient (B) In older patient, pulp cavity decreases in size

2. ***Irritants:*** Various irritants whether in form of caries, periodontal disease, attrition, abrasion, erosion, cavity preparation and other operative procedures may stimulate dentin formation at the base of tubules in the underlying pulp leading to alteration in internal anatomy.
3. ***Calcific metamorphosis:*** It commonly occurs because of trauma to a recently erupted tooth.
4. ***Calcifications:*** In form of pulp stones or diffuse calcifications are usually present in chamber and the radicular pulp. These are either normal or may form as a result of irritation. These alter the internal anatomy of teeth and may make the process of canal location difficult.
5. ***Resorption:*** Chronic inflammation or for unknown cause internal resorption may result in change of shape of pulp cavity making the treatment of such teeth challenging.

**Factors affecting internal anatomy**
- Age
- Irritants
- Calcific metamorphosis
- Canal calcifications
- Resorption

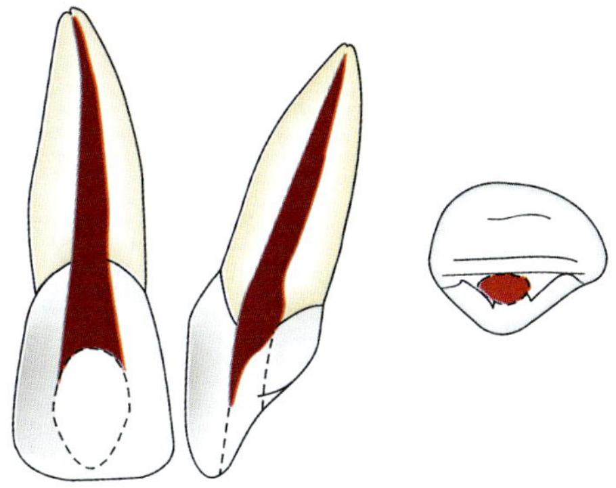

Fig. 13.39: Root canal anatomy of maxillary central incisor

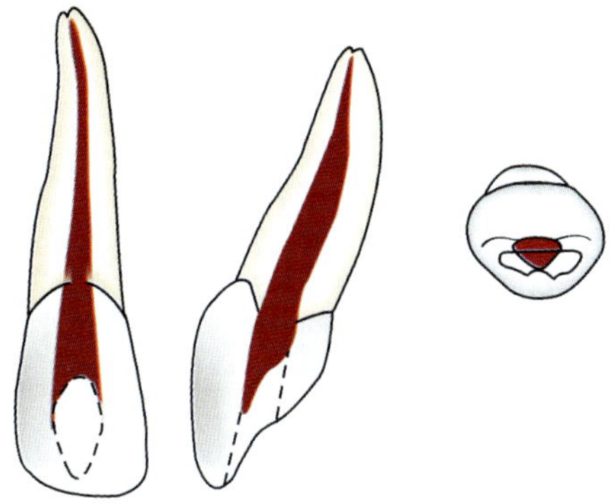

Fig. 13.40: Root canal anatomy of maxillary lateral incisor

## INDIVIDUAL TOOTH ANATOMY

### Maxillary Central Incisor (Fig. 13.39)

#### *Average Tooth Length*

The average length of the maxillary central incisor is 22.5 mm. The average pulp volume of this tooth is 12.4 mm$^3$.

#### *Pulp Chamber*

- It is located in the center of the crown, equal distance from the dentinal walls.
- Mesiodistally, pulp chamber follows the outline of the crown and it is ovoid in shape.
- Buccopalatally the pulp chamber is narrow as it transforms into the root canal with a constriction just apical to the cervix.
- In young patients, central incisors usually have three pulp horns that correspond to enamel mammelons on the incisal edge.

#### *Root Canal*

- Usually central incisor has one root with one root canal.
- Coronally, the root canal is wider buccopalatally.
- Coronally or cervically, the canal shape is ovoid in cross-section but in apical region, the canal is round.
- The root canal differs greatly in outline in mesiodistal and labiopalatal view.
  a. Mesiodistal view shows a fine straight canal.
  b. In labiopalatal view the canal is very much wider and often shows a constriction just apical to the cervix.
- Usually lateral canals are found in apical third.
- Most of the time, the root of central incisor is found to be straight.

#### *Clinical Considerations*

- A pulp horn can be exposed following a relatively small fracture of an incisal corner in the young patient.
- Placing the access cavity too far palatally makes straight line access difficult.
- In order to clean a ribbon shaped canal effectively, the operator relies on the effectiveness of irrigant solutions.

### Maxillary Lateral Incisor (Fig. 13.40)

#### *Average Length*

The average length of maxillary lateral incisor is 21 mm with average pulp volume of 11.4 mm$^3$.

#### *Pulp Chamber*

The shape of pulp chamber of maxillary lateral incisor is similar to that of maxillary central incisor but there are few differences.

I. The incisal outline of the pulp chamber tends to be more rounded.
II. Lateral incisors usually have two pulp horns, corresponding to the development mammelons.

#### *Root Canal*

- Root canal has finer diameter than that of central incisor though shape is similar to that.
- Labiopalatally, the canal is wider and usually shows constriction just apical to the cervix.
- Canal is ovoid labiopalatally in cervical third, ovoid in middle third and round in apical third.
- Apical region of the canal is usually curved in a palatal direction.

#### *Clinical Considerations*

- Cervical constriction may need to be removed during coronal preparation to produce a smooth progression from pulp chamber to root canal.
- Since palatal curvature of apical region is rarely seen radiographically, during cleaning and shaping ledge formation may occur at this curve. This may result in root canal filling short of apex and other problems.
- Apical curvature can also complicate surgical procedures like root end cavity preparation and root resection.

### Maxillary Canine (Fig. 13.41)

#### *Average Tooth Length*

It is the longest tooth with an average length of 26.5 mm with average pulp space volume of 14.7 mm$^3$.

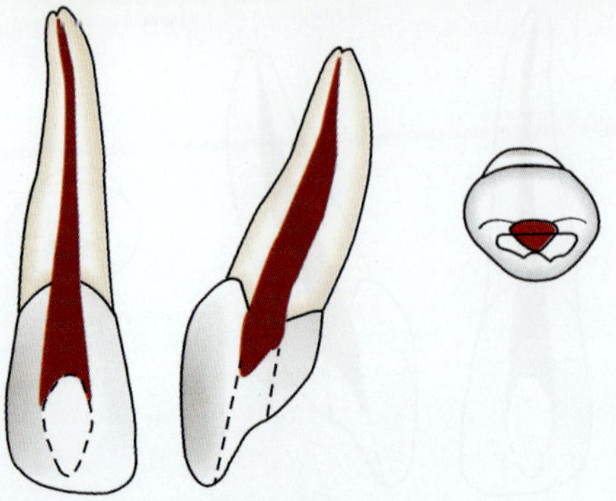

Fig. 13.41: Maxillary canine

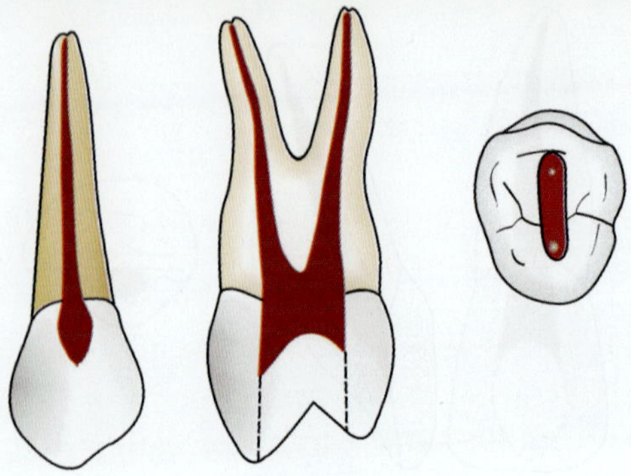

Fig. 13.42: Maxillary first premolar

### Pulp Chamber

- Labiopalatally, the pulp chamber is almost triangular shape with apex pointed incisally.
- Mesiodistally it is narrow, sometimes resembling a flame. At cervix, there can be constrictions sometimes.
- In cross-section it is ovoid in shape with larger diameter labiopalatally.
- Usually one pulp horn is present corresponding to one cusp.

### Root Canal

- Normally there is single root canal which is wider labiopalatally than in mesiodistal aspect.
- Cross-section at cervical and middle third show its oval shape, at apex it becomes circular.
- Canal is usually straight but may show a distal apical curvature.

### Clinical Considerations

- Cervical constriction needs to be shaped during coronal flaring to produce uniformly tapered preparation.
- When long, sclerosed canal is being present, care must be taken to avoid blockage of the root canal.
- Surgical access sometimes becomes difficult because of their long length.

## Maxillary First Premolar (Fig. 13.42)

### Average Tooth Length

This tooth has generally two roots with two canals and average length of 21 mm. The pulp space volume of maxillary first premolar is 18.2 $mm^3$.

### Pulp Chamber

- Pulp chamber is wider buccopalatally with two pulp horns, corresponding to buccal and palatal cusps.
- Roof of pulp chamber is coronal to the cervical line.
- Floor is convex generally with two canal orifices.

### Root Canal

- Maxillary first premolar has two roots in most (>60%) of the cases but cases with single root or three roots have also been reported.
- Buccal canal is directly under the buccal cusp and palatal canal is directly under the palatal cusp.
- Cross-section of root canals shows ovoid shape in cervical third with larger dimensions buccopalatally.

  At middle and apical third, they show circular shape in cross-section.
- The root canals are usually straight and divergent.

### Clinical Considerations

- To locate both the canals properly, a good quality of radiograph should be taken from an angle so as to avoid superimposition of canals.
- Avoid over flaring of the coronal part of the buccal root to avoid perforation of palatal groove present on it.
- Surgical procedures on first premolar should be given more consideration since palatal root may be difficult to reach.
- In maxillary first premolar, failure to observe the distal—axial inclination of the tooth may lead to perforation.

## Maxillary Second Premolar (Fig. 13.43)

Average length of maxillary second premolar is 21.5 mm. Average pulp volume is 16.5 $mm^3$.

### Pulp Chamber

- Maxillary second premolar usually has one root with a single canal, but shape of canal system is variable
- Pulp chamber is wider buccopalatally and narrower in mesiodistal direction
- In cross-section, pulp chamber has narrow and ovoid shape.

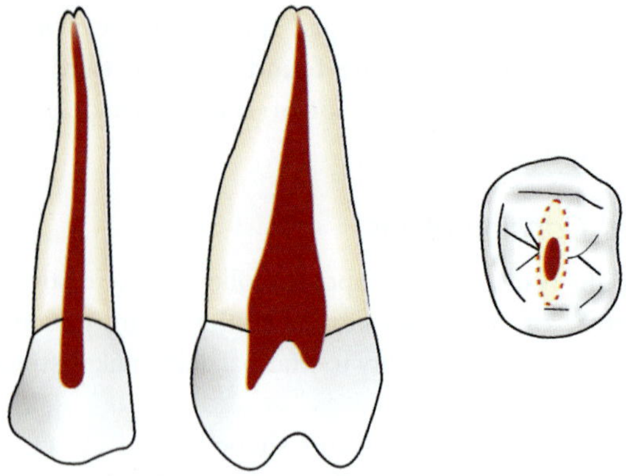

Fig. 13.43: Maxillary second premolar

### Root Canals

- In more than 60 percent of cases single root with single canal is found. There may be a single canal along the entire length of the root.
- If there are two canals, they may be separated or distinct along the entire length of the root or they may merge to form a single canal as they approach apically
- Canal is wider buccopalatally forming a ribbon like shape
- At cervix, cross-section shows ovoid and narrow shape, at middle third it is ovoid which becomes circular in apical third.

### Clinical Considerations

- Narrow ribbon like canal is often difficult to clean and obturate effectively
- Care should be taken to explore, clean and obturate the second canal of maxillary second premolar (40% of the cases).

## Maxillary First Molar (Fig. 13.44)

### Average Tooth Length

The average tooth length of this tooth is 21 mm and average pulpal volume is 68.2 $mm^3$.

### Pulp Chamber

- Maxillary first molar has the largest pulp chamber with four pulp horns, viz. mesiobuccal, mesiopalatal, distobuccal and distopalatal
- Bulk of pulp chamber lies mesial to the oblique ridge across the surface of the tooth
- The four pulp horns are arranged in such a fashion which gives it rhomboidal shape in the cross-section. The four walls forming roof converge towards the floor, where palatal wall almost disappears making a triangular form in cross-section
- Orifices of root canals are located in the three angles of the floor; Palatal orifice is largest and easiest to locate and appears funnel like in the floor of pulp chamber
- Distobuccal canal orifice is located more palatally than mesiobuccal canal orifice

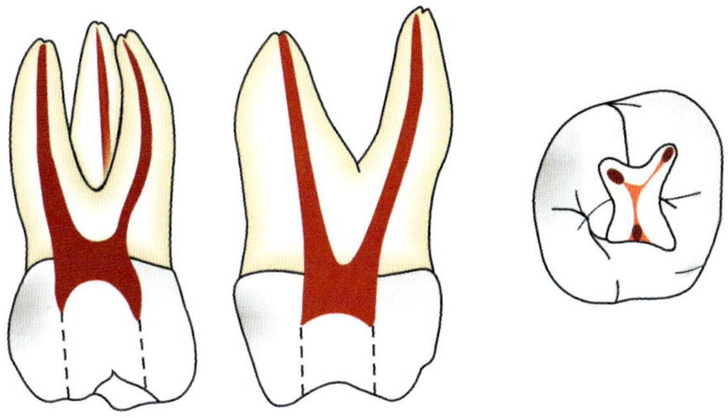

**Fig. 13.44:** Maxillary first molar

- More than 60 percent of maxillary first molars have shown the presence of two canals in mesiobuccal root. The minor mesiobuccal canal (MB2) is located on a line between palatal canal orifice and the main mesiobuccal canal orifice.

### Root Canals

- Maxillary is generally three rooted with three or four canals
- Two canals in mesiobuccal root are usually closely interconnected and sometimes merge into one canal
- Mesiobuccal canal is the narrowest of the three canals, flattened in mesiodistal direction at cervix but becomes round as it reaches apically
- Distobuccal canal is narrow, tapering canal, sometimes flattened in mesiodistal direction but generally it is round in cross-section
- The palatal root canal has largest diameter which has rounded triangular cross-section coronally and becomes round apically
- Palatal canal can curve buccally in the apically one-third
- Lateral canals are found in 40 percent of three canals at apical third and at trifurcation area.

### Clinical Considerations

- Buccal curvature of palatal canal may not be visible on radiographs, leading to procedural errors
- MB2 should be approached from distopalatal angle since the initial canal curvature is mesial
- Sometimes isthmus is present between mesiobuccal canals, it should be cleaned properly for success of the treatment
- Mesiobuccal canals show curvature sometimes which is not visible radiographically. So, care should be taken while doing endodontic therapy
- Since pulp chamber lies mesial to oblique ridge, pulp cavity is cut usually mesial to oblique ridge
- Caries, previous restorative procedures, attrition, etc. can lead to formation of secondary dentin causing alteration in pulp cavity. So careful study of preoperative radiographs is mandatory to avoid any procedural errors
- Perforation of a palatal root is commonly caused by assuming canal to be straight.

## Maxillary Second Molar (Fig. 13.45)

### Average Tooth Length

The average tooth length of this tooth is 20 mm and average pulp volume is 44.3 $mm^3$.

### Pulp Chamber

- It is similar to maxillary first molar except that it is narrower mesiodistally
- Roof of pulp chamber is more rhomboidal in cross-section and floor is an obtuse triangle
- Mesiobuccal and distobuccal canal orifices lie very close to each other, sometimes all the three canal orifices lie in a straight line.

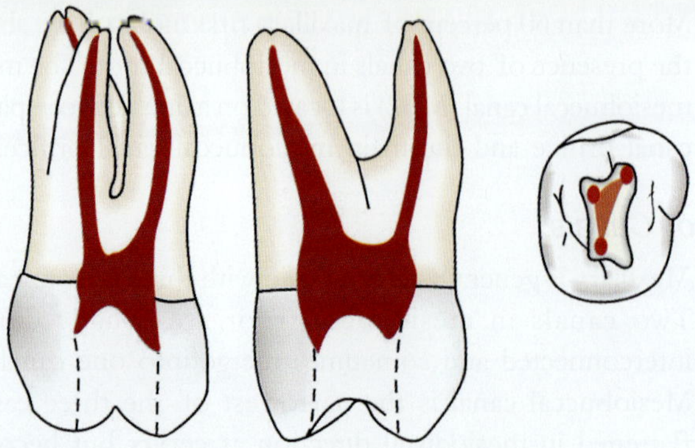

Fig. 13.45: Maxillary second molar

#### Root Canals

- Similar to first molar except that in maxillary second molar roots tend to be less divergent and may be fused
- Fewer lateral canals are present in roots and furcation area than in first molar.

#### Clinical Considerations

- Similar to maxillary first molar.

### Maxillary Third Molar

#### Average Tooth Length

Average length of tooth is 16.5 mm.

#### Pulp Chamber and Root Canal

It is similar to second molar but displays great variations in shape, size, and form of both pulp chamber as well as root canal.

There may be presence of one, two, three or more canals sometimes.

### Mandibular Teeth Central Incisor (Fig. 13.46)

#### Average Tooth Length

Average length of this tooth is 21 mm.
Average pulp volume is 6.1 $mm^3$.

#### Pulp Chamber

Mandibular central incisor is the smallest tooth in the arch.

- Pulp chamber is similar to maxillary central incisor being wider labiolingually pointed incisally with three pulp horns
- Cross-section of pulp chamber shows its ovoid shape.

#### Root Canals

- Various root canal formations have been seen in mandibular incisors. There can be a single canal from orifice to apex or a single canal by bifurcate into two canals or sometimes two separate canals are also found. Incidence of two canals can be as high as 41 percent
- Cross-section of root canals show wider dimension in labiolingual direction making it ovoid shape whereas round in the apical third

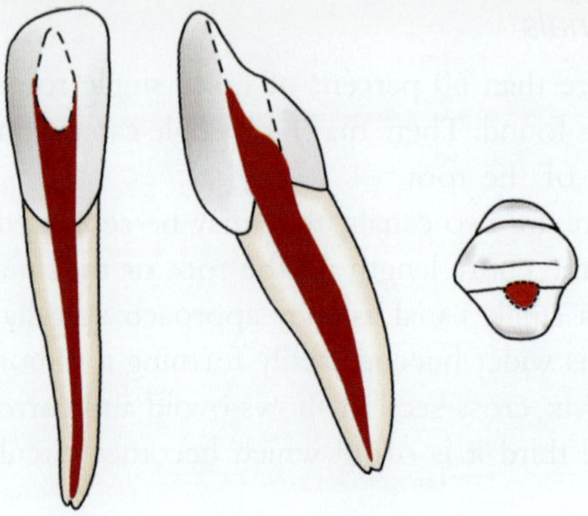

Fig. 13.46: Mandibular central incisor

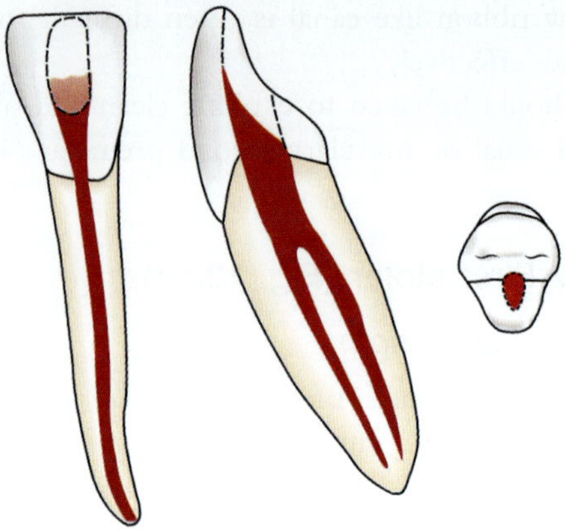

Fig. 13.47: Mandibular lateral incisor

- Since canal is flat and narrow mesiodistally and wide buccopalatally, ribbon shaped configuration is formed.

#### Clinical Considerations

- If root canals are overprepared, because of presence of groove along the length of root and narrow canals, weakening of the tooth structure or chances of strip perforations are increased
- It is common to miss presence of two canals on preoperative radiograph if they are superimposed
- Since apex of mandibular central incisor is inclined lingually, the surgical access may become difficult to achieve.

### Mandibular Lateral Incisor (Fig. 13.47)

#### Average Tooth Length

- Average length of mandibular lateral incisor is 21 mm.
- Average pulp volume is 7.1 $mm^3$.

#### Pulp Chamber

The configuration of pulp chamber is similar to that of mandibular central incisor except that it has larger dimensions.

#### Root Canal

- It has features similar to those of mandibular central incisor
- Usually the roots are straight or curved distally or labially, but distal curve is sharper than those of mandibular central incisors.

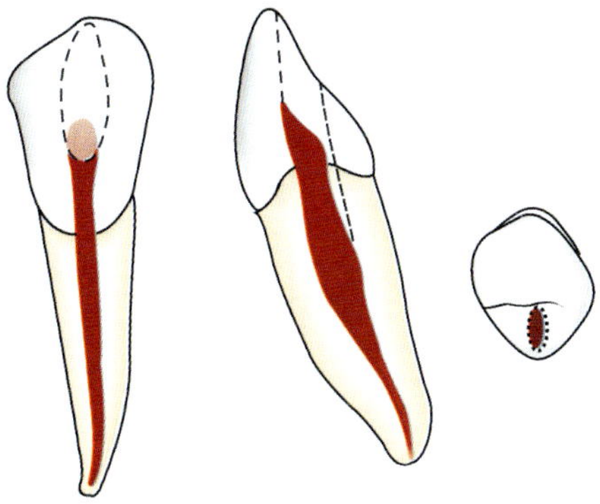

Fig. 13.48: Mandibular canine

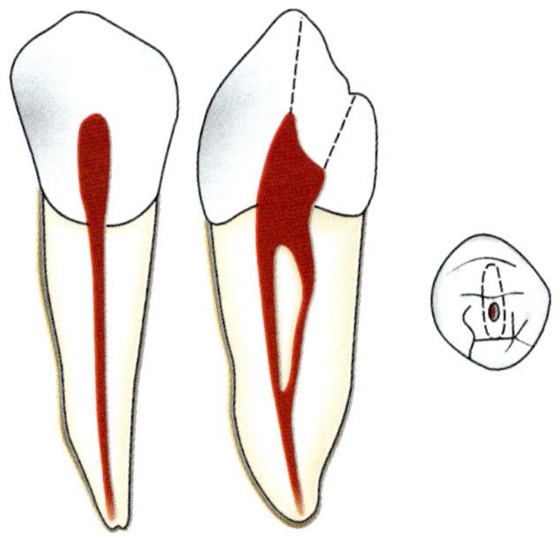

Fig. 13.49: Mandibular first premolar

### Clinical Consideration

They are similar to central incisor.

## Mandibular Canine (Fig. 13.48)

- ***Average tooth length:*** Average length of the tooth is 22.5 mm
- Average pulp volume is 14.2 $mm^3$.

### Pulp Chamber

- On viewing labiolingually, the pulp chamber tapers to a point in the incisal third of the crown
- In cervical third of tooth, it is wider in dimensions and ovoid in cross-section at this level
- Pulp chamber appears to narrower mesiodistally
- Cervical constriction is also present.

### Root Canals

- Mandibular canine usually has one root and one canal but can occasionally have two (14% cases)
- Coronally, the root canal is oval in cross-section, becomes round in the apical region
- Lateral canals are present in 30 percent of cases.

### Clinical Consideration

In older patients, where there is deposition of secondary dentine, it is necessary to incorporate the incisal edge into the access cavity for straight line access.

## Mandibular First Premolar (Fig. 13.49)

### Average Tooth Length

Average length of the tooth is 21.5 mm and average mature pulp volume is 14.9 $mm^3$.

### Pulp Chamber

- Mesiodistally, the pulp chamber is narrow in dimension
- Pulp chamber has two pulp horns, the buccal horn being most prominent
- Buccolingually, the pulp chamber is wide and ovoid in cross-section.

### Root Canal

- Mandibular first premolars usually have one root and one canal. Sometimes teeth have shown presence of second canal
- Mesiodistally, the canal is narrower in dimension
- Buccolingually, root canal cross-sections tend to be oval until the most apical extents, where they become round
- Lateral canals are present in 44 percent of the cases.

### Clinical Considerations

- The access cavity in these teeth should have extended on to the cusp tip, in order to gain straight line access
- Surgical access to the apex of the mandibular first premolar is often complicated by the proximity of the mental nerve
- The lingual canal when present, is difficult to instrument. Access can usually be gained by running a fine instrument down the lingual wall of the main buccal canal until the orifice is located
- Perforation at the distogingival is caused by failure to recognize the distal tilt of premolar
- Apical perforation should be avoided by taking care of buccal curvature of the canal at the apex.

## Mandibular Second Premolar (Fig. 13.50)

### Average Tooth Length

The average length of this tooth is 22.5 mm and average mature pulp volume is 14.9 $mm^3$.

### Pulp Chamber

- It is similar to that of mandibular first premolar except that lingual pulp horn is more prominent
- Cross-section of pulp chamber shows oval shape with greatest dimensions buccolingually.

### Root Canal

- Usually has one root and one canal and in 11 percent of the teeth, has a second canal
- Buccolingually, it is wider than that of mandibular first premolar
- Root canal cross-sections tend to be oval coronally and round apically.

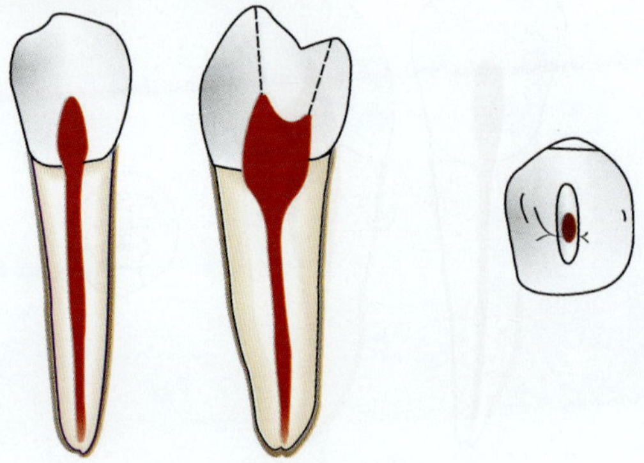

Fig. 13.50: Mandibular second premolar

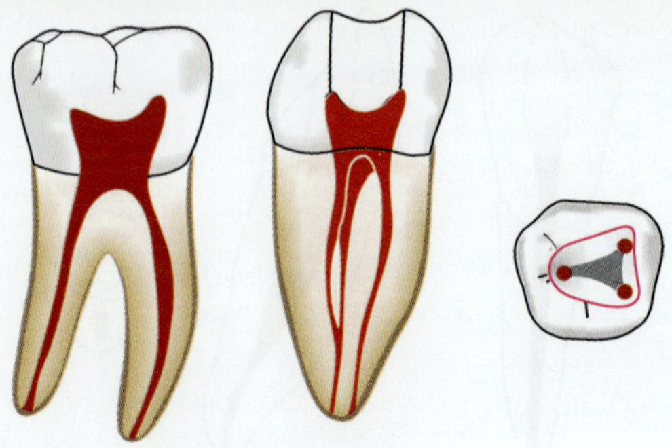

Fig. 13.51: Mandibular first molar

### Clinical Consideration

They are similar to mandibular first premolar.

## Mandibular First Molar (Fig. 13.51)

***Average tooth length:*** The average length of this tooth is 21 mm and an average pulp volume is 52.4 $mm^3$.

### Pulp Chamber

- It is quadrilateral in cross-section at the level of the pulp floor and is wider mesially than distally
- The roof of the pulp chamber is rectangular in shape with straight mesial wall and rounded distal wall
- There may be presence of four or five pulp horns
- Mesiobuccal orifice is present under the mesiobuccal cusp
- The mesiolingual orifice is located in a depression formed by mesial and the lingual walls. Usually a connecting groove is present between mesiobuccal and mesiolingual orifices
- Distal orifice is the widest of all three canals. It is oval in shape with greater diameter in buccolingual direction.

### Root Canals

Mandibular first molar usually has two roots with three canals. But teeth with three roots and four or five canals have also been reported.

- Mesial root has two canals, viz. mesiobuccal and mesiolingual which may exit in two foramina (>41% cases), exit in single foramen (30%) and may also exit in different pattern
- Mesiobuccal canal is usually curved and often exit in pulp chamber in a mesial direction
- Distal root generally has one canal (> 70% cases). But two canals are also seen in some cases (Fig. 13.52)
  A single distal canal is ribbon shaped and has largest diameter buccolingually. But when two canals are present in distal root, they tend to be round in the cross-section.

### Clinical Considerations

- Over-enlargement of mesial canals should be avoided to prevent procedural errors
- To avoid superimposition of the mesial canals, radiograph should be taken at an angle.

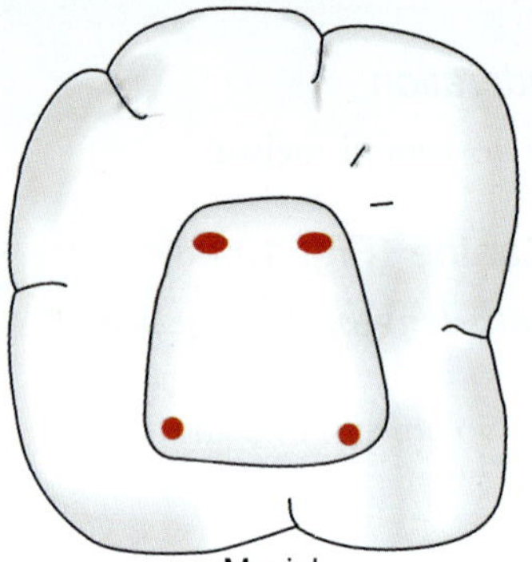


Fig. 13.52: Four canal in mandibular first molar

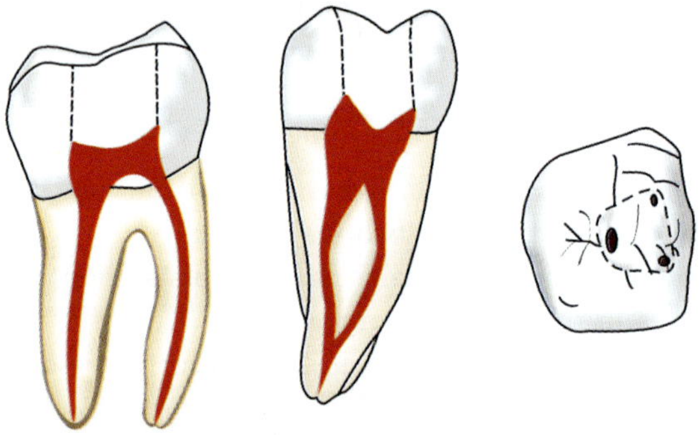

Fig. 13.53: Mandibular second molar

## Mandibular Second Molar (Fig. 13.53)

### Average Tooth Length

The average tooth length of this tooth is 20 mm and average pulp volume is 32.9 $mm^3$.

### Pulp Chamber

- It is similar to that of mandibular first molar except that it is smaller in size
- Root canal orifices are smaller and closer together.

### Root Canals

- Usually it contains two roots with three canals but variation in their presence (one or three roots, 2 canals) is also seen

- C-shaped canals are also seen, i.e. mesial and distal canals become fused into a fin.

### *Clinical Considerations*

- C-shaped canals make the endodontic procedures difficult so care should be taken while treating them
- There may be only one mesial canal. The mesial and distal canals may lie in midline of the tooth
- Perforation can occur at mesial cervical region if one fails to recognize the mesially tipped molar.

## Mandibular Third Molar

- Average tooth length
- Average length of this tooth is 17.5 mm.

### Pulp Chamber and Root Canals

It resembles to that of mandibular first and second molar but with enormous variations, i.e. there may be presence of one, two or three canals. Anomalous configurations such as "C-shaped" root canal orifices are also seen commonly.

## CLASSIFICATION OF C-SHAPED ROOT CANALS

### I. Melton's Classification

It was based on cross-sectional shape

1. **Category I:** Continuous C-shaped canal running from the pulp chamber to the apex defines a C-shaped outline without any separation (C1 in Fig. 13.54).
2. **Category II:** The semicolon shaped (;) in which dentin separates a main C-shaped canal from one mesial distinct canal (C2 in Fig. 13.54).
3. **Category III:** Refers to those with two or more discrete and separate canals (C3 in Fig 13.54).
   1. **Subdivision I:** C-shaped orifice in the coronal third that divides into two or more discrete and separate canals that join apically.
   2. **Subdivision II:** C-shaped orifice in the coronal third that divides into two or more discrete and separate canals in the midroot to the apex.
   3. **Subdivision III:** C-shaped orifice that divides into two or more discrete and separate canals in the coronal third to apex.

### II. Fan's Classification (anatomic classification)

Fan et al in 2004 modified Melton's method into the following categories:

1. **Category I (C1):** The shape was an interrupted "C" with no separation or division.
2. **Category II (C2):** The canal shape resembled a semicolon resulting from a discontinuation of the "C" outline but either angle $\alpha$ or $\beta$ (Fig. 13.55) should not be less than 60°.
3. **Category III (C3):** 2 or 3 separate canals and both angles $\alpha$ and $\beta$, were less than 60° (Fig. 13.56).
4. **Category IV (C4):** Only one round or oval canal in that cross-section (C4 in Fig. 13.54).

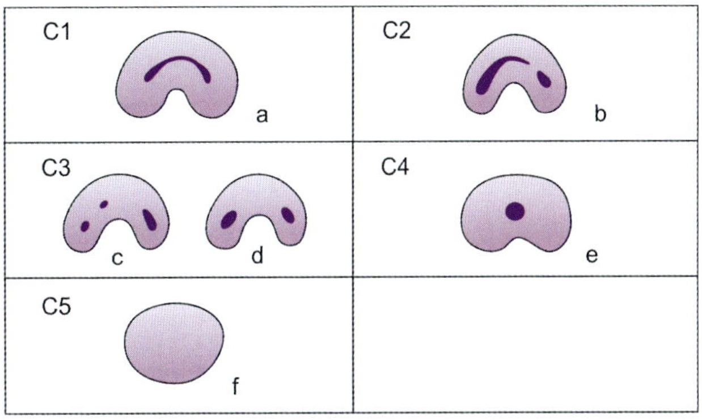


**Fig. 13.54:** Melton's classification of C canals

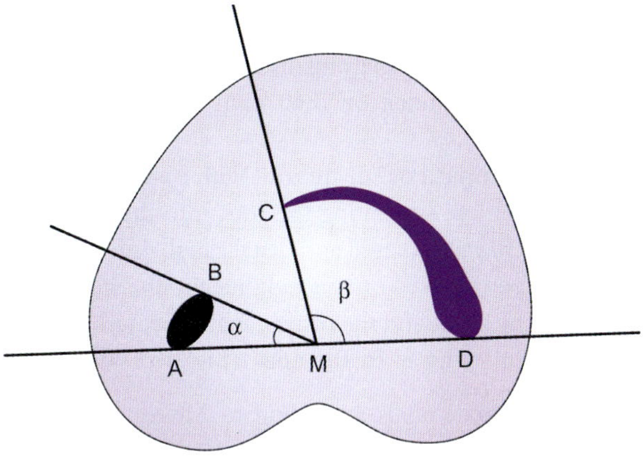


**Fig. 13.55:** In this $C_2$ category of Fan's classification, canal resembles a semicolon due to discontinuation of "C" outline, but either angle $\alpha$ of $\beta$ are not less than 60°

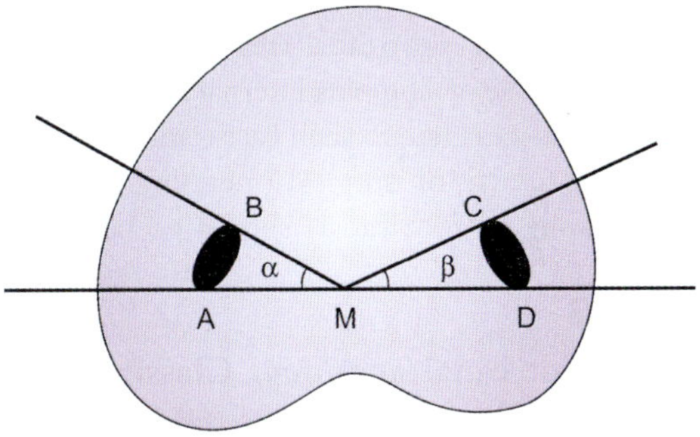


**Fig. 13.56:** In this $C_3$ category of Fan's classification, 2-3 separate canals are there with angle $\alpha$ and $\beta$ less than 60°

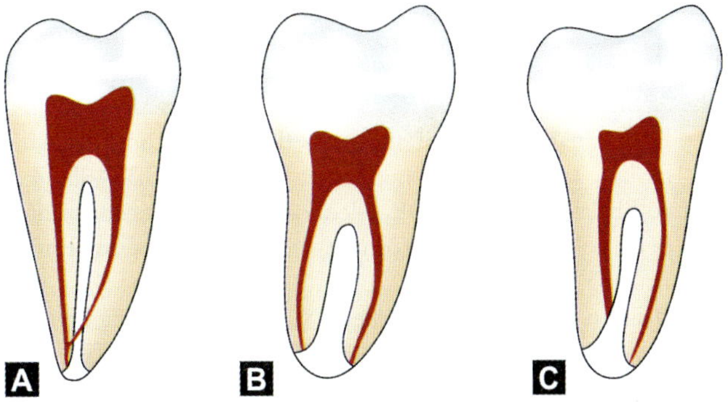


**Figs 13.57A to C:** Fan's radiographic classification

5. **Category V (C5):** No canal lumen could be observed (which is usually near the apex only) (C5 in Fig. 13.54).

### III. Fan's Classification (radiographic classification)

Fan et al classified C-shaped roots according to their radiographic appearance into three types:

1. **Type I:** Conical or square root with a vague, radiolucent longitudinal line separating the root into distal and mesial parts. There was a mesial and distal canal that merged into one before exiting at the apical foramen (foramina) (Fig. 13.57A).
2. **Type II:** Conical or square root with a vague, radiolucent longitudinal line separating the root into distal and mesial parts. There was a mesial and distal canal, and the two canals appeared to continue on their own pathway to the apex (Fig. 13.57B).
3. **Type III:** Conical or square root with a vague, radiolucent longitudinal line separating the root into distal and mesial parts. There was a mesial and distal canal, one canal curved to and superimposed on this radiolucent line when running towards the apex, and the other canal appeared to continue on its own pathway to the apex (Fig. 13.57C).

Type of C-shaped canals according to Melton:

**Type I :** Continuous C-shaped canal outline without any break.

**Type II :** C-shaped canal in semicolon shape in which dentin separates one distinct canal from a buccal or a lingual C-shaped canal in the same direction.

**Type III :** Two or more distinct canals below C-shaped orifice.

The prognosis of root canal treatment in such teeth is questionable because of complex internal anatomy. Therefore, to increase the success rate in such cases, additional treatment measures such as use of surgical operating microscope or microtomography of root canals should be taken.

## QUESTIONS

**Q. Define root canal anatomy. Classify root canal configuration?**

**Q. What are different factors affecting root anatomy?**

**Q. Write short notes on:**

a. Root canal anatomy of maxillary first molar
b. C-shaped canals

## BIBLIOGRAPHY


1. Al Shalabi RM, Omer OE, Glennon J, Jennings M, Claffey NM. Root canal anatomy of maxillary first and second permanent molars. International Endodontic Journal 2000;33:405-14.
2. Al-Shalabi Rm, Omer OE, Glennon J, et al. Root canal anatomy of maxillary first and second permanent molars. Int Endod J 2000;33.
3. Baisden MK, Kulild Jc, Weller RN. Root canal configuration of the mandibular first premolar. J Endod 1992;18:505.
4. Baldassari-Cruz LA, Lilly Jp, Rivera Em. The influence of dental operating microscope in locating the mesiolingual canal orifice. Oral Surg Oral Med Oral Pathol Oral Radiol Endod 2002;93:190.
5. Baugh D, Wallace J. Middle mesial canal of the mandibular first molar: A case report and literature review. J Endod 2004;30:185-86.
6. Buhrley LJ, Barrows MJ, BeGole E, Wenckus CS. Effect of magnification on locating the mb2 canal in maxillary molars. J Endod 2002;28:324.
7. Caliskan MK, Pehlivan Y, Sepetcioglu F, et al. Root canal morphology of human permanent teeth in a Turkish population. J Endod 1995;21:200.
8. Christie WH, Peikoff MD, Acheson DW. Endodontics treatment of two maxillary lateral incisors with anomalous root formation. J Endod 1981;7:528.
9. Coldero LG, McHugh S, Mackenzie D, Saunders WP. Reduction in intracanal bacteria during root canal preparation with and without apical enlargement. Int Endod J 2002;35:437.
10. Cooke HG, Cox FL. C-shaped canal configurations in mandibular molars. J Am Dent Assoc 1979;99:836-39.
11. Cunningham CJ, Senia ES. A three-dimensional study of canal curvatures in the mesial roots of mandibular molars. J Endod 1992;18:294.
12. De Moor RJ, Deroose CA, Calberon FL. The radix entomolaris in mandibular first molars: An endodontic challenge int. Endod J 2004;37:789-99.
13. Dempster WT, Adams WJ, Duddles RA. Arrangement in the jaws of the roots of the teeth. J Am Dent Assoc 1963;67:779.
14. Eskoz N, Weine FS. Canal configuration of the mesiobuccal root of the maxillary second molar. J Endod 1995;21:38.
15. Fabra- Campos H. Three canals in the mesial root of mandibular first permanent molars: A clinical study. Int Endod J 1989;22:39.
16. Genovese FR, Marsico Em. Maxillary central incisor with two roots; a case report. J Endod 2003;29:220.
17. Gorduysus MO, Gorduysus M, Friedman S. Operating microscope improves negotiation of second mesiobuccal canals in maxillary molars. J Endod 2001;27:683-86.
18. Green D. Double canals in single roots. Oral Surg Oral Med Oral Pathol Oral Radiol Endod 1973;35:689.
19. Gulabivala K, Aung TH, Alavi A, Mg Y-L. Root and canal morphology of Burmese mandibular molars. Int Endod J 2001;34:359-70.
20. Gutierrez JH, Aguayo P. Apical foraminal openings in human teeth-number and loction. Oral Surg Oral Med Oral Pathol Oral Radiol Endod 1995;79:769-77.
21. Hatton JF, Ferrillo PJ Jr. Successful treatment of a two canaled maxillary lateral incisor. J Endod 1989;15:216.
22. Helfer AR, Melnick S, Schilder H. Determination of the moisture content of vital and pulpless teeth. Oral Surg Oral Med Oral Pathol Oral Radiol Endod 1972;34:661.
23. Heling I, Gottlieb-Dadon I, Chandler NP. Mandibular canine with two roots canals. Endod Dent Traumatol 1995;11:301.
24. Howe CA, McKendry DJ. Effect of endodontics access preparation on resistance to crown-root fracture. J Am Dent Assoc 1990;121:712.
25. Imura N, Hata GI, Toda T, et al. Two canals in mesiobuccal roots of maxillary molars. Int Endod J 1998;31:410.
26. Janik JM. Access cavity preparation. Dent Clin North Am 1984;28:806.
27. Kartal N, Ozeelilk B, Cimilli H. Root canal morphology of maxillary premolars. J Endod 1998;24:417.
28. Kartal N, Yanikoglu FC. Root canal morphology of mandibular incisors. J Endod 1992;18:562.
29. Kasahara E, Yasuda E, Yamamoto A, Anzai M. Root canal system of the maxillary central incisor. J Endod 1990;16:158.

30. Krasner P, Rankow HJ. Anatomy of the pulp chamber floor. J Endod 2004;30:5-16.
31. LaTurno SA, Zillich RM. Straight-line endodontics access to anterior teeth. Oral Surg Oral Med Oral Pathol Oral Radiol Endod 1985;59:418.
32. Macri E, Zmener O. Five canals in a mandibular second premolar. J Endod 2000;26:304.
33. Mandibular second molars in Chinese population. Dent Traumatol 1988;4:160-63.
34. Mannocci F, Peru M, Sheriff M, et al. The isthmuses of the mesial root of mandibular molars: A microcomputed tomographic study. Int Endod J 2005;38:558.
35. Mauger Mj, Waite RM, Alexander JB, Schindler WG. Ideal endodntics access in mandibular incisors. J Endod 1999;25;206.
36. Melton DC, Krell KV, Fuller MW. Anatomical and histological features of C-shaped canals in mandibular second molars. J Endod 1991;17:384.
37. Min KS. Clinical management of a manidbular first molar with Multiple Mesial Canals. A case report J. Contemp Dent Pract 2004;(5).
38. Nallapati S. Three canal mandibular first and second premolars: a treatment approach. A case report. Int Endod 2005;31:474.
39. Orguneser A, Kartal N. Mandibular canine with two roots and three canals. Endod Dent Traumatol 1998;11:301.
40. Panitvisai P, Messer HH. Cuspal deflection in molars in relation to endodontics and restorative procedures. J Endod 1995;21:57.
41. Pecora JD, Saqury PC, Sousa Neto MD, Woelfel JB. Root form and canal anatomy of maxillary first premolar. Braz Dent J 1991;2:87.
42. Peikoff MD, Christie WH, Fogal HM. The maxillary second molar: variations in the number of roots and canals. Int Endod J 1996;29:365.
43. Peters OA. Current challenges and concepts in the preparation of root canal systems a review. J Endod 2004;30:559.
44. Peters OA, Gohring TN, Lutz F, Effect of a eugenol-containing sealer on marginal adaptation of dentine-bonded resin fillings. Int Endod J 2000;33:53.
45. Peters OA, Peters CI, Schonenberger K, Barbakow F. ProTaper rotary root canal preparation: effect of canal anatomyon final shape analysed by micro CT. Int Endod J 2003;36:86.
46. Pineda F, Kuttler Y. Mesiodistal and buccolingual roentgeno-graphic investigation of 7,275 root canals. Oral Surg Oral Med Oral Pathol Oral Radiol Endod 1972;33:101.
47. Pomeranz HH, Fishelberg G. The secondary mesiobuccal canal of maxillary molars. J Am Dent Assoc 1974;88:119.
48. Rankine-Wilson RW, Henry PJ. The bifurcated root canal in lower anterior teeth. J Am Dent Assoc 1965;70:1162.
49. Rhodes IS. A case of unusual anatomy: a mandibular second premolar with four canals. Int Endod J 2001;34:645.
50. Rice Rt, Gilbert BO Jr. A usual canal configuration in a mandibular first molar. J Endod 1987;13:515.
51. Rosen H. Operative procedures on mutilated endodontically treated teeth. J Prosthet Dent 1961;11:972.
52. Schwarze T, Baethge C, Stecher T, Geurtsen W. Identification of second canal in the mesiobuccal root of maxillary first and second molar using magnifying loupes or an operating microscope. Aust Endod J 2002;28:57-60.
53. Skidmore AE, Bjorndal AM. Root canal morphology of the human mandibular first molar. Oral Surg Oral Med Oral Pathol Oral Radiol Endod 1971;32:778.
54. Slowey RE. Root canal anatomy: Road map to successful endodontics. Dent Clin N Am 1979;23:555-73.
55. Sorensen JA, Engelman MJ. Ferrule design and fracture resistance of endodontically treated teeth. J Prosthet Dent 1990;63:529.
56. Sorensen JA, Martinoff JT. Intracoronal reinforcement and cornal coverage: A study of endodontically treated teeth. J Prosthet Dent 1984;51:780.
57. Stropko JJ. Canal morphology of maxillary molar, clinical observations of canal configurations. J Endod 1990;25:446-50.
58. Teplitsky PE, Surtherland JK. Endodontic access of cerestore crowns. J Endod 1985;11:555.
59. Thomas RP, Moule AJ, Bryant R. Root canal morphology of maxillary permanent first molar teeth at various ages. Int Endod J 1993;26:257.
60. Vertucci FJ, Gegauff A. Root canal morphology of the maxillary first premolar. J Am Dent Assoc 1979;99:194.
61. Vertucci FJ. Root canal morphology of madibular premolars. J Am Dent Assoc 1978;97:47.
62. Vertucci FJ. Root canal anatomy of the human permanent teeth. Oral Surg Oral Med Oral Pathol Oral Radiol Endod 1984;58:589-99.
63. Vertucci FJ. Root canal anatomy of the mandibular anterior teeth. J Am Dent Assoc 1974;89:369-71.
64. Walker RT. Root form and canal anatomy of maxillary first premolars in a Southern Chinese population. Endod Dent Traumatol 1987;3:130.
65. Weine FS, Harami S, Hata G, Toda T. Canal configuration of the mesiobuccal root of the maxillary first molar of a Japanese subpopulation. Int Endod J 1999;32:79-87.
66. Weine FS. Case report: Three canals in the mesial root of a mandibular first molar (?) J Endod 1982;8:517-20.
67. Zillich R, Dowson J. Root canal morphology of mandibular first and second premolars. Oral Surg Oral Med Oral Pathol Oral Radiol Endod 1973;36:738.
68. Zillich RM, Jerome JK. Endodontic access to maxillary lateral incisors. Oral Surg Oral Med Oral Pathol Oral Radiol Endod 1981;52:443.

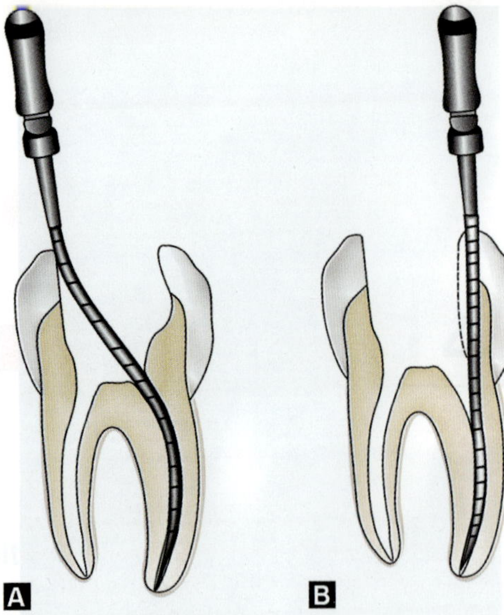


**Figs 14.7A and B:** (A) Not removing dentin from mesial wall causes bending of instrument while inserting in canal leading to instrumental errors; (B) Removal of extra-dentin from access opening gives straight line access to the canal without any undue bending

3. Conserve sound tooth structure as much as possible so as to avoid weakening of remaining tooth structure.

## INSTRUMENTS FOR ACCESS CAVITY PREPARATION (FIG. 14.8)

### Instruments for Access Opening

#### *Access Opening Burs*

They are round burs with 16 mm bur shank (3 mm longer than standard burs) (Fig. 14.9).

#### *Access Refining Burs (Fig. 14.10)*

These are coarse grit flame-shaped, tapered round and diamonds for refining the walls of access cavity preparation.

#### *Surgical Length Burs*

These are long 32 mm burs. They are useful in teeth which present problems with access and visibility. With there burs, visibility of cutting tip of instrument is increased because of displacement of handpiece away from incisal or occlusal surface of tooth.

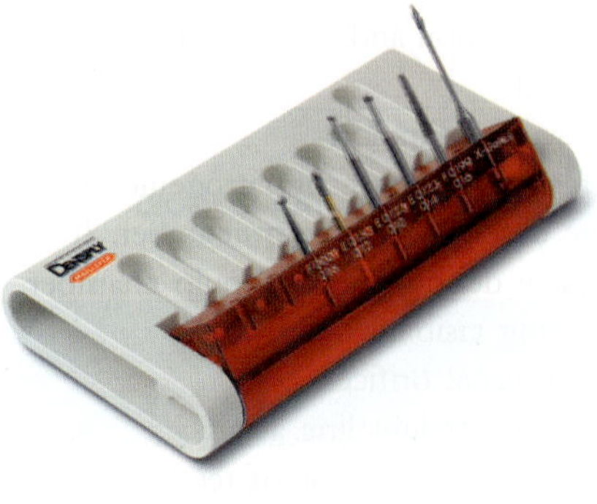

**Fig. 14.8:** Instruments for access preparation

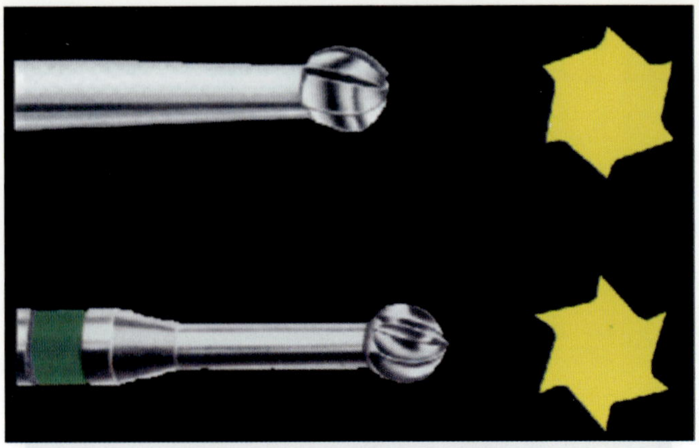

**Fig. 14.9:** Access opening burs

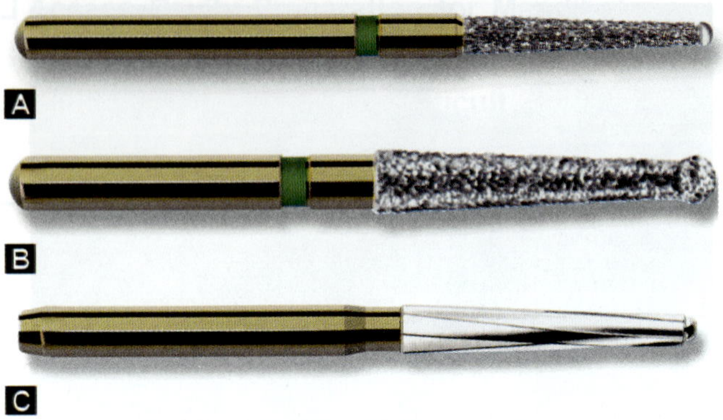


**Figs 14.10A to C:** Access refining burs

#### *Munce Discovery (MD) Burs*

They are 34 mm long round carbide tipped troughing burs with stiff shafts that are 1 mm in diameter. These burs are available in four sizes: #1/2, #1, #2 and #4. All sizes have the same shaft diameter.

This contrasts with Mueller burs which have variable shaft diameters, the smallest of which is a very flexible 0.5 mm. Additionally, the smallest Mueller bur tip size is 0.85 mm in diameter, compared to the #1 and #1/2 MD bur tip sizes of 0.77 mm and 0.58 mm in diameter, respectively. While the LN Burs do offer a #1/2 round tip size and a stiff narrow shift, they are only 28 mm in length and thus provide inadequate reach for deep troughing procedures.

### Uses

They are often required for safely locating calcified canals and exposing separated instruments deep within radicular structures.

*Comparison with ultrasonics*

1. They are much more efficient than ultrasonic tips for bulk troughing.
2. The effectiveness of ultrasonic tips is directly related to the amount of energy delivered to the tip—energy which generates heat. This heat can be dangerous to the delicate periodontal ligament, often only a fraction of a millimeter away from the tip. To reduce the risk of damage to the PDL, the level of energy can be decreased, making the tip less efficient, or water can be introduced into the deep cavity

to dissipate the heat. The use of water as a coolant requires the introduction of an evacuation device into an already-crowded field.
3. Of course, it goes without saying that, at $60-120 each, seemingly spontaneous—and frequently reported—ultrasonic tip breakage is more than a nuisance.

*Comparison with 30 mm long and 34 mm long standard shaft diameter round burs*

The fact that 30 mm long round burs with standard shaft diameters of 2.4 mm are useful on the chamber floor, but once troughing progresses beyond the level of the floor, two primary impediments will occur:
1. The view corridor beyond the handpiece head will become ineffective as the gap between coronal structure and the handpiece diminishes.
2. The large shaft diameter will impinge on the ever deepening cavity wall, forcing the tip of the bur toward ledging and perforation.

## Muler Burs (Fig. 14.11)

These are long shaft, round carbide tipped burs which are used in low speed handpiece. Their long shaft increases visibility of cutting tip. They are often used for safely locating calcified canals because their long shaft is useful for working deep in the radicular portion. But since they are made up of carbide, they do not tolerate sterilization cycles and become dull quickly.

## Guidelines for Access Cavity Preparation (Fig. 14.12)

1. Before starting the access cavity preparation one should check the depth of preparation by aligning the bur and handpiece against the radiograph. This is done so as to note the position and depth of the pulp chamber (Fig. 14.13).
2. Place a safe-ended bur in handpiece to complete the outline form. The bur is penetrated into the crown until the roof of pulp chamber is penetrated (Fig. 14.14).

   Commonly recommended access opening bur is round bur, that is to penetrate the pulp chamber (Fig. 14.15). It prevents the overpreparation. Once the "drop in" into the pulp chamber is obtained, round bur is replaced by tapered fissured bur (Figs 14.16 to 14.20).

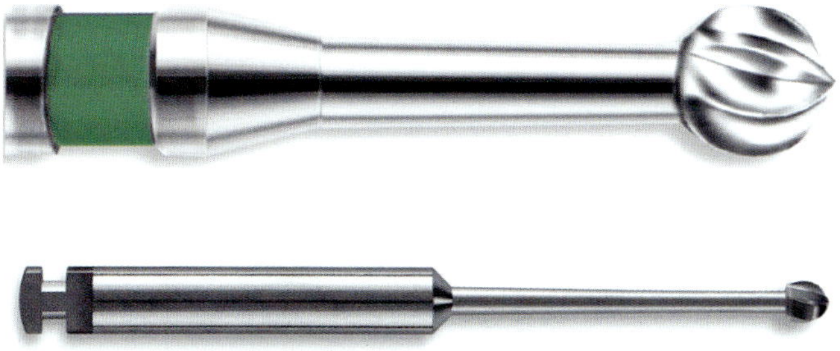

Fig. 14.11: Muler burs

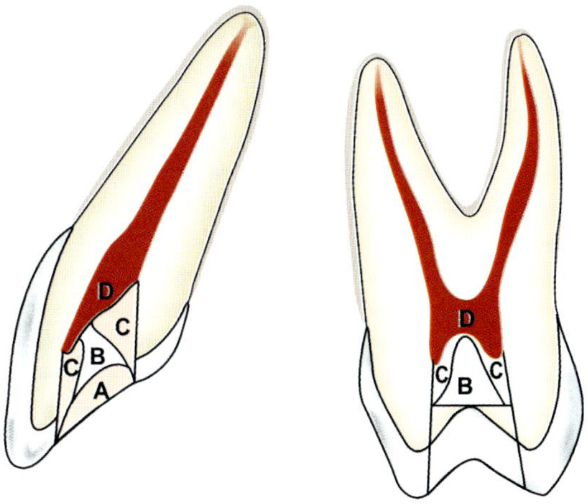


Fig. 14.12: Guidelines for access cavity preparation

A. Penetration into enamel with No. 2 or No. 4 high speed round bur;
B. Exposure of pulp chamber with tapered fissure bur;
C. Refinement of the pulp chamber and removal of pulp chamber roof using round bur from inside to outside;
D. Complete debridement of pulp chamber space

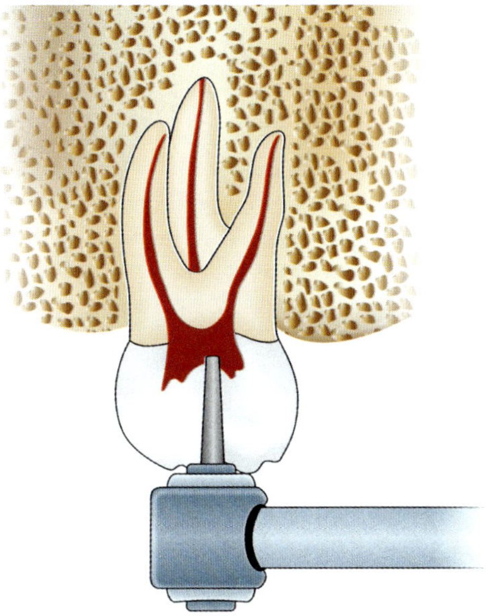

Fig. 14.13: Preoperative radiograph can help to note the position and depth of pulp chamber

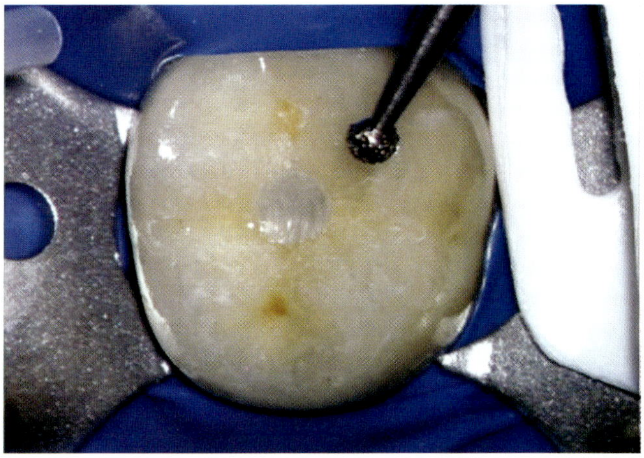

Fig. 14.14: Gain entry to pulp chamber with round bur

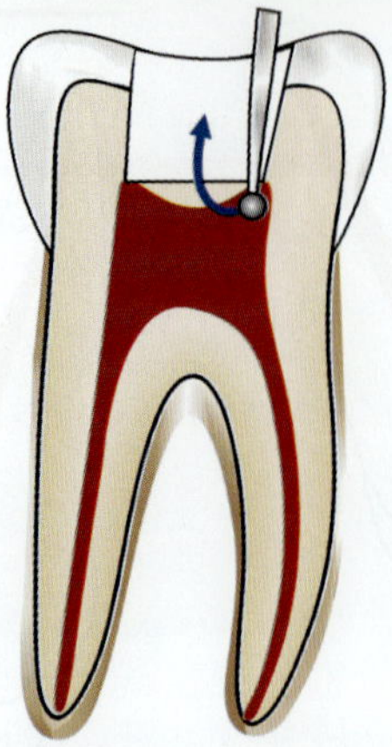

**Fig. 14.15:** Once "drop in" into pulp chamber is obtained bur is moved inside to outside

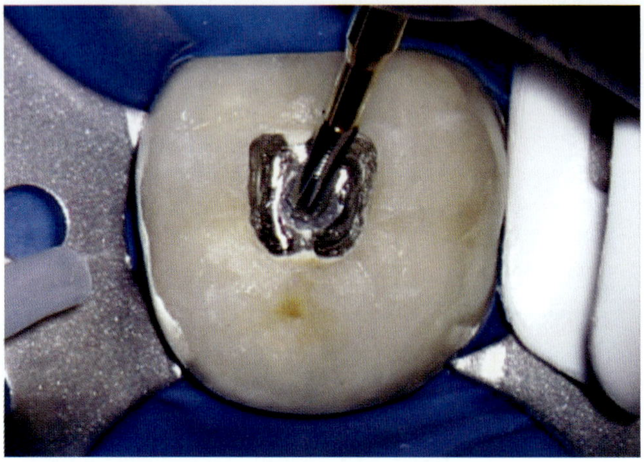

**Fig. 14.16:** Access preparation using tapered fissure burs

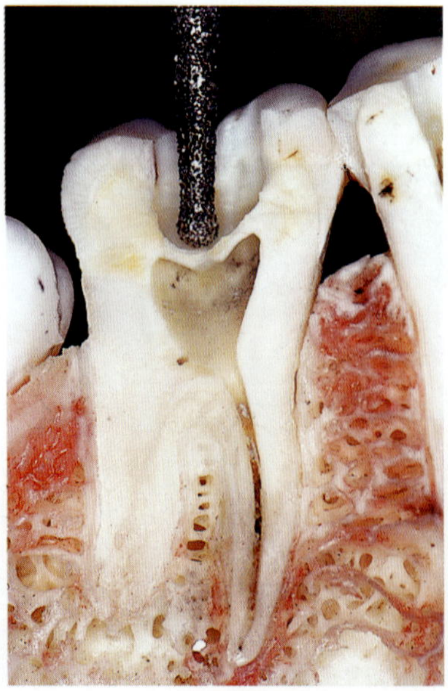

**Fig. 14.17:** Access preparation

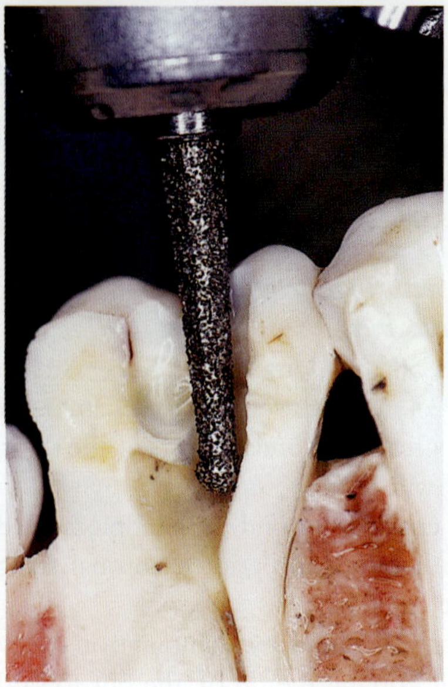

**Fig. 14.18:** Access preparation continues

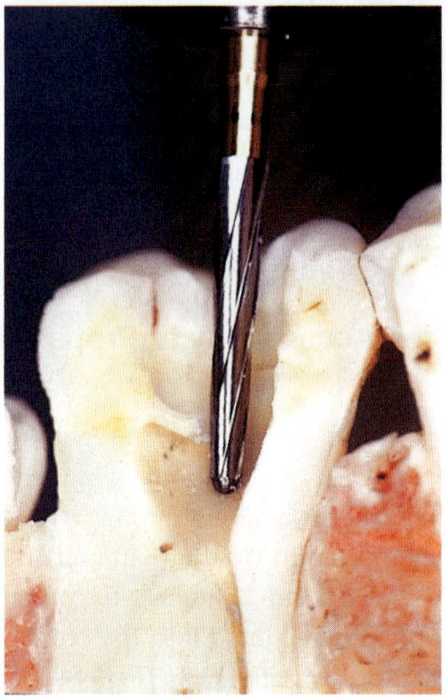

**Fig. 14.19:** Access refining

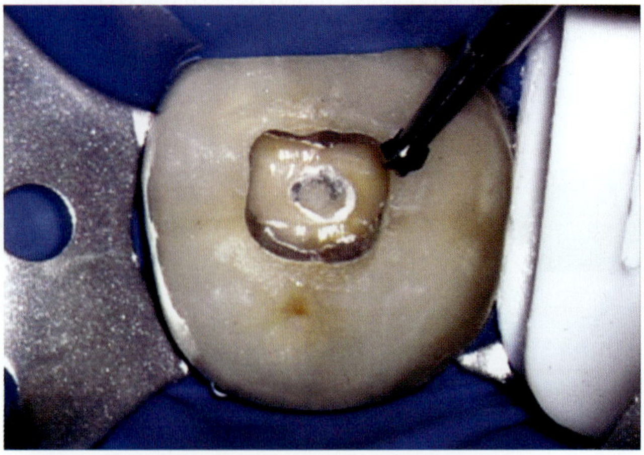

**Fig. 14.20:** Final access preparation

One should avoid using flat-ended burs which make highly irregular access walls, causing multiple ledges.

Round-ended carbide burs are used for access opening into cast restorations because they have distinct tactile sense when dropping into the pulp chamber.

Access finishing is best carried out by using burs with safe non-cutting ends (Fig. 14.21). ***Advantage*** of using these burs is that they are less likely to damage or perforate the pulp chamber floor. ***Disadvantages*** of using these burs are that they can cut laterally and they cannot drop into small orifices to funnel the point of transition between the access cavity and walls.

3. When locating the canal orifices is difficult, one should not apply rubber dam until correct location has been confirmed.
4. Remove all the unsupported tooth structure to prevent tooth fracture during treatment.
5. Remove the chamber roof completely as this will allow the removal of all the pulp tissue, calcifications, caries or any residuals of previous fillings. If pulp chamber is not completely deroofed, it can result in:
   a. Contamination of the pulp space.
   b. Discoloration of endodontically treated tooth.
6. The walls of pulp chamber are flared and tapered to form a gentle funnel shape with larger diameter towards occlusal surface (Fig. 14.22).
7. Endodontic access cavity is prepared through the occlusal or lingual surface, never through proximal or gingival surface. If access cavity is made through wrong entry, it will cause inadequate canal instrumentation resulting in iatrogenic errors (Figs 14.23).
8. Inspect the pulp chamber for determining the location of canals, curvatures, calcifications using well magnification and illumination.

***Shape of pulp chamber is determined by:***

***Size of pulp chamber:*** Access preparation in young patients is broader than the older patients, in which pulp cavity is shrunken.

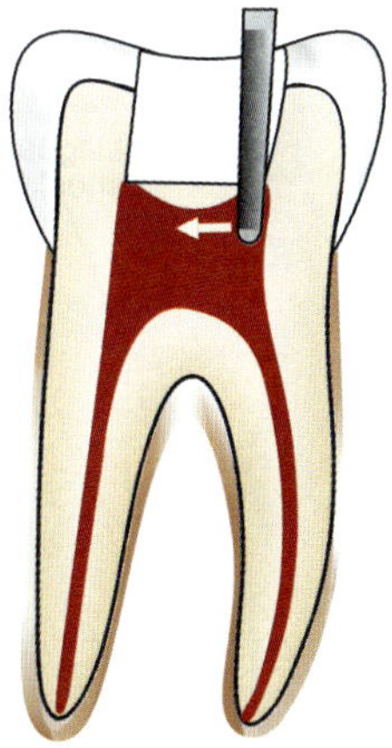

**Fig. 14.21:** Completely deroof the pulp chamber

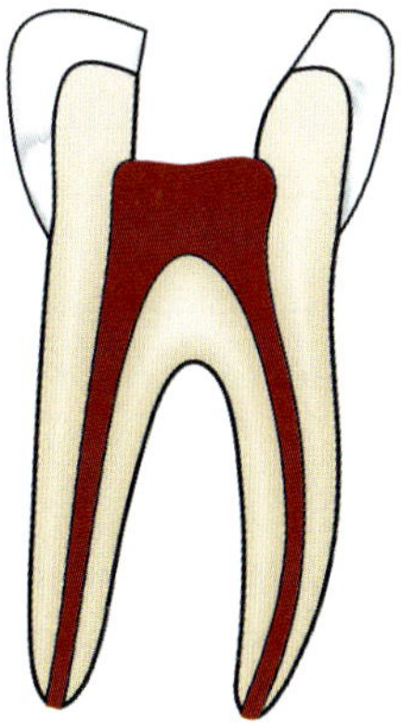

**Fig. 14.22:** Complete access cavity preparation

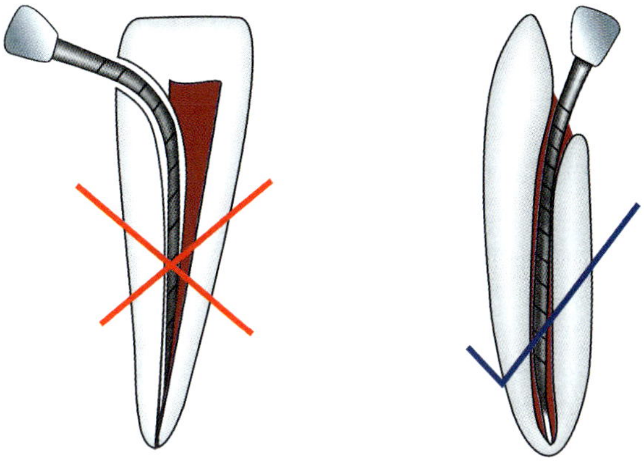

**Fig. 14.23:** Correct position for entering into the pulp cavity

***Shape of pulp chamber:*** The final outline form should reflect the shape of pulp chamber. It is triangular in anteriors, ovoid buccolingually in premolars and trapezoidal or triangular in molars.

***Number, position and curvature of the canal:*** It can lead to modified access preparation, like Shamrock preparation in maxillary molar because of presence of distally curved mesial root.

## Laws of Access Cavity Preparation for Locating Canal Orifices

### *Law of Centrality*

Floor of pulp chamber is always located in the center of tooth at the level of cementoenamel junction.

### *Law of Cementoenamel Junction*

Distance from external surface of clinical crown to the wall of pulp chamber is same throughout the tooth circumference at the level of CEJ.

### *Law of Concentricity*

Walls of pulp chamber are always concentric to external surface of tooth at the level of CEJ. This indicates anatomy of external tooth surface reflects the anatomy of pulp chamber.

*Law of Color Change*

Color of pulp chamber floor is darker than the cavity walls.

*Law of Symmetry*

Usually canal orifices are equidistant from a line drawn in mesial and distal direction through the floor of pulp chamber.

*Law of Orifice Location*

Canal orifices are located at the junction of floor and walls, and at the terminus of root development fusion lines.

## ACCESS CAVITY OF ANTERIOR TEETH

- Remove all the caries and any defective restorations so as to prevent contamination of pulp space as well as to have a straight line access into the canals.
- Access opening is started at center of the lingual surface (Fig. 14.24). If it is made too small and too close to the cingulum the instrument tends to bind the canal walls and thus may not work optimally.
- Direct a round bur perpendicular to the lingual surface at its center to penetrate the enamel. Once enamel is penetrated, bur is directed parallel to the long axis of the tooth, until 'a drop' in effect is felt (Fig. 14.25).
- Now when pulp chamber has been penetrated, the remainder of chamber roof is removed by working a round bur from inside to outside. This is done to remove all the obstructions of enamel and dentin overhangs that would entrap debris, tissues and other materials.
- Now locate the canal orifices using endodontic explorer. Sharp explorer tip is used to locate the canal orifices, to penetrate the calcific deposits if present, and also to evaluate the straight line access.
- Once the canal orifices are located, the lingual shoulder is removed using Gates-Glidden drills or safe tipped diamond or carbide burs. Lingual shoulder is basically a prominence of dentin formed by removal of lingual roof which extends from the cingulum to approximately 2 mm apical to the orifice (Fig. 14.26).

  During the removal of lingual shoulder, the orifice should also be flared so that it becomes confluent with all the walls of access cavity preparation. By this a straight line access to the apical foramen is attained, i.e. an endodontic file can reach up to apical foramen without bending or binding to the root canal wall. Any deflection of file occurring should be corrected because it can lead to instrumental errors (Fig. 14.27). The deflected instruments work under more stress, more chance of instrument separation is there. Deflected instruments also result in procedural accidents like canal transportations, perforations, ledging and zipping.
- After the straight line access of the canal is confirmed by passing a file passively into the canal, one should evaluate the access cavity using magnification and illumination.
- Finally smoothening of the cavosurface margins of access cavity is done because rough or irregular cavity margins can

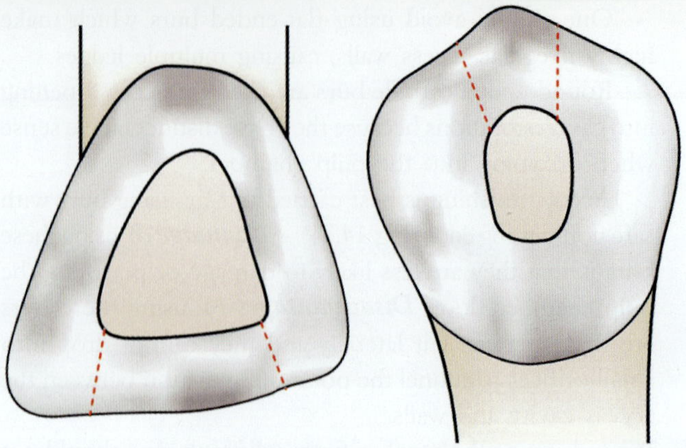

**Fig. 14.24:** Access opening is initiated at center of lingual surface

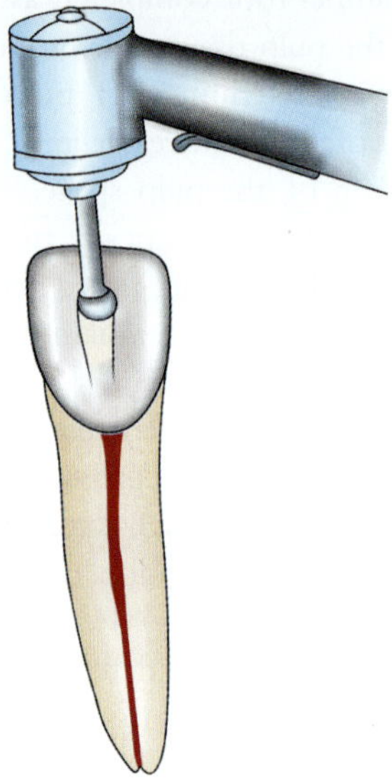

**Fig. 14.25:** Once enamel is penetrated, bur is directed parallel to long axis of tooth

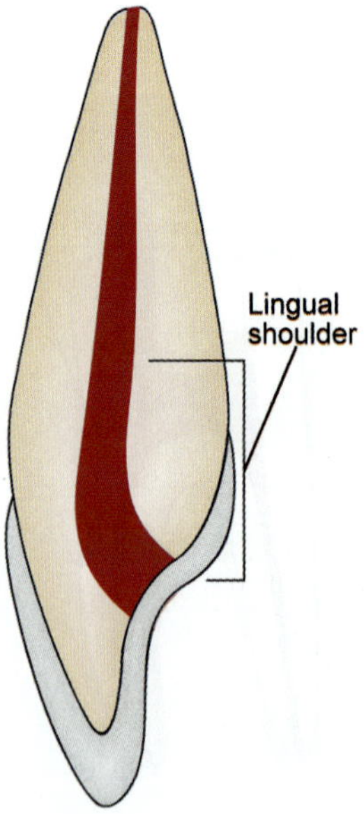


**Fig. 14.26:** Lingual shoulder is prominence of dentin formed by lingual roof. It extends from cingulum to 2 mm apical to the canal orifice

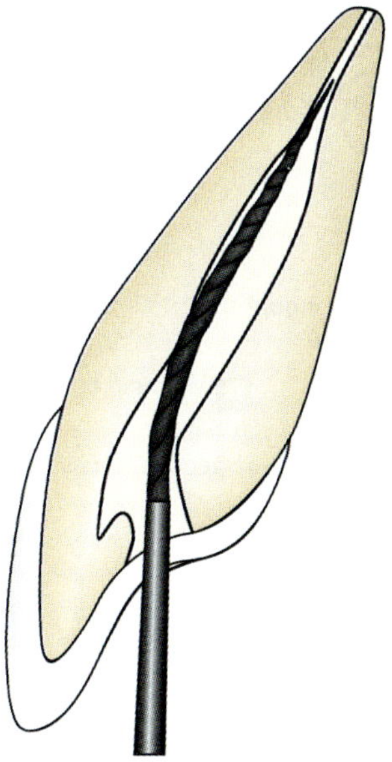

Fig. 14.27: Improper access cavity preparation causing deflection of instrument

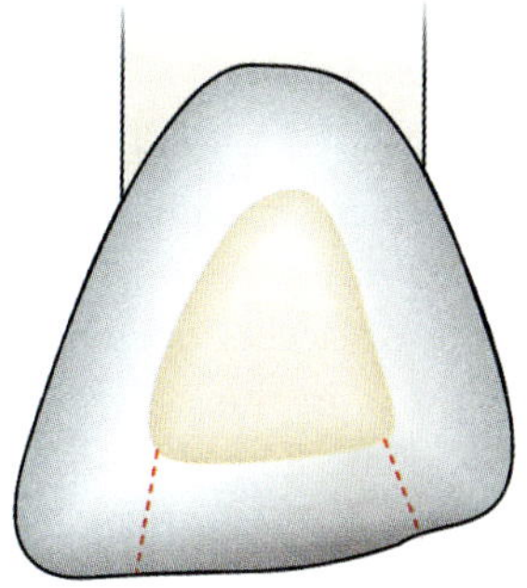

Fig. 14.28: Outline of access cavity of maxillary incisor

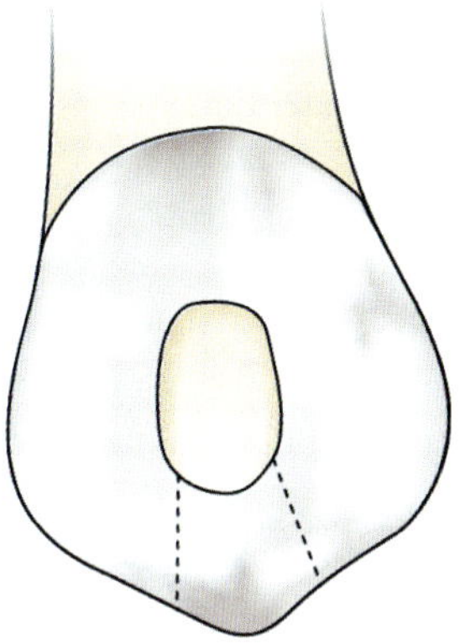

Fig. 14.29: Outline of access cavity of maxillary canine

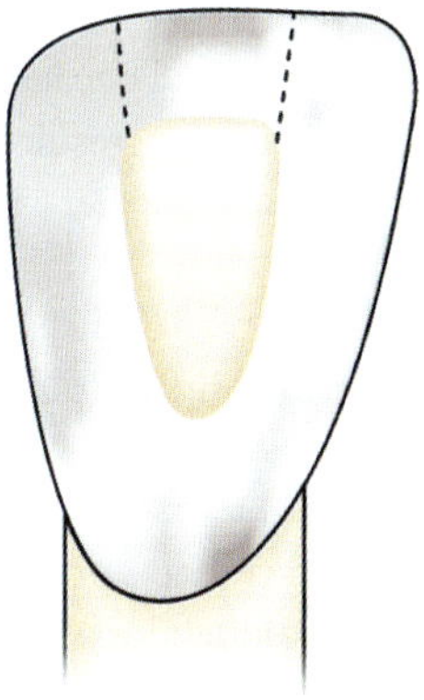

Fig. 14.30: Outline of access cavity of mandibular incisor

cause coronal leakage through restorations. Also smooth cavity margins allow better and précised placement of final composite restoration with minimal coronal leakage.

Since the outline form of access cavity reflects the internal anatomy of the pulp space, though technique of the access opening of anterior teeth is the same, the shape may vary according to internal anatomy of each tooth.

## Maxillary Central Incisor

The outline form of access cavity of maxillary central incisor is a rounded triangular shape with base facing the incisal aspect (Fig. 14.28). The width of base depends upon the distance between mesial and distal pulp horns. Shape may change from triangular to slightly oval in mature tooth because of less prominence of mesial and distal pulp horns.

## Maxillary Lateral Incisor

The shape of access cavity is almost similar to that of maxillary central incisor except that:

i. It is smaller in size.
ii. When pulp horns are present, shape of access cavity is rounded triangle.
iii. Generally the pulp horns are missing so shape of access cavity which results is oval.

## Maxillary Canine

Shape of access cavity of canine though is quite similar to incisors with following differences:

i. Canine does not have pulp horns
ii. Access cavity is oval in shape with greater diameter labiopalatally (Fig. 14.29).

## Mandibular Incisors

Mandibular central and lateral incisors are similar in shape of access cavity and the root canal system. Shape of access cavity of mandibular incisors is different from maxillary incisors in following aspects (Fig. 14.30):

i. It is smaller in shape.
ii. Shape is long oval with greatest dimensions directed incisogingivally.

## Mandibular Canine

The shape of access opening of mandibular canine is similar to that maxillary of canine except that:

i. It is smaller in size.
ii. Root canal outline is narrower in mesiodistal dimension.
iii. Generally two canals are present in mandibular canine.

## ACCESS CAVITY PREPARATION FOR PREMOLARS

- The basic step of access cavity preparation is removal of the caries and any other permanent restoration material if present.
- Determine the site of access opening on the tooth.

  In premolars, it is in the center of occlusal surface between buccal and the lingual cusp tips (Fig. 14.31).
- Slight variations exist between mandibular and maxillary premolars because of the lingual tilt of mandibular premolars.
- Penetrate the enamel with No. 4 round bur in high speed contra angle handpiece. The bur should be directed parallel to the long axis of tooth and perpendicular to the occlusal table. Generally the external outline form for premolars is oval in shape with greater dimensions of buccolingual side (Fig. 14.32).
- Once the clinician feels "drop" into the pulp chamber, penetrate deep enough to remove the roof of pulp chamber without cutting the floor of pulp chamber. To remove the roof of pulp chamber and pulp horns, place the bur alongside the walls of pulp chamber and work from inside to outside.

  For removal of pulp chamber roof, round bur, a tapered fissure or a safety tip bur can be used.
- After removal of roof of pulp chamber, locate the canal orifices with the help of sharp endodontic explorer. Ideally the canal orifices should be located at the corners of final preparation. Extension of orifices to the axial walls results in **Mouse Hole Effect**.

  Mouse hole effect is caused because of under extension of the access cavity. This may result in hindrance to the straight line access which may further cause procedural errors (Fig. 14.33).
- Remove any remaining cervical bulges or obstructions using safety tip burs or Gates-Glidden drills and obtain a straight line access to the canals.

  It can be confirmed by passing a file passively into the canal which should reach the apex or the first point of curvature without any deflection.
- The walls of access cavity are then smoothened and sloped slightly towards the occlusal surface. The divergence of access cavity walls creates a positive seat for temporary restorations.

  Access cavity preparation for all premolars is same except for some differences.

### Maxillary First Premolar

Shape of access cavity is ovoid in first premolar in which boundaries should not exceed beyond half the lingual incline of buccal cusp and half the buccal incline of lingual cusp.

### Maxillary Second Premolar

It is similar to that of maxillary first premolar and varies only by anatomic structure of the pulp chamber.

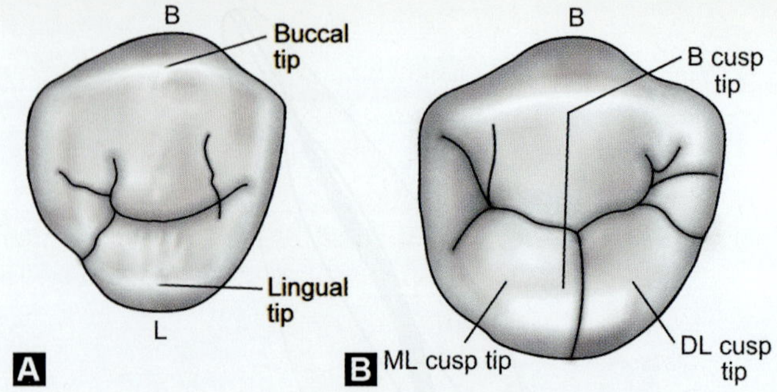


Fig. 14.31: Outline of access cavity of premolars

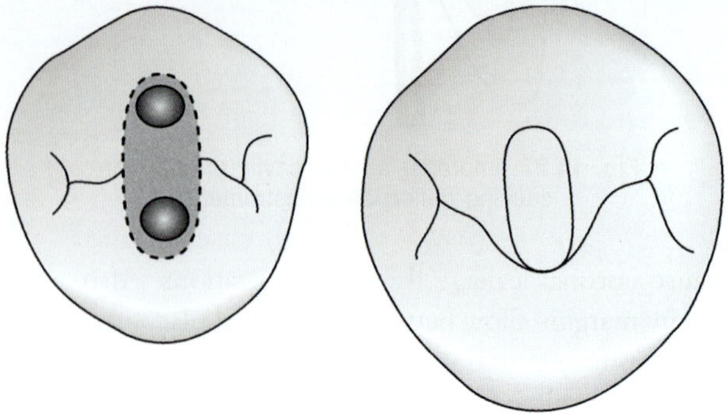

Fig. 14.32: Oval-shaped access cavity of premolars

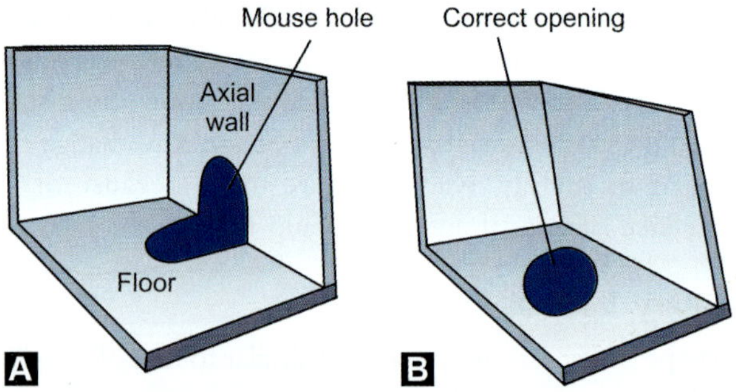


Fig. 14.33: Mouse hole effect: (A) Mouse hole effect—Due to under extension of axial wall, orifice opening appears partly in axial wall and partly in floor, (B) Correct opening

### Mandibular First Premolar

Following differences are seen in case of mandibular first premolar from the maxillary premolars:

i. There is presence of 30° lingual inclination of the crown to the root, hence the starting point of bur penetration should be halfway up the lingual incline of the buccal cusp on a line connecting the cusp tips (Fig. 14.38).
ii. Shape of access cavity is oval which is wider mesiodistally when compared with its maxillary counterpart.

### Mandibular Second Premolar

The access cavity preparation is similar to mandibular first premolar except that in mandibular second premolar:

i. Enamel penetration is initiated in the central groove because its crown has smaller lingual tilt.
ii. Because of better developed lingual half, the lingual boundary of access opening extends halfway upto the lingual cusp incline, i.e. pulp chamber is wider buccolingually.
iii. Root canals are more often oval than round.
iv. Ovoid access opening is wider mesiodistally.

## ACCESS CAVITY PREPARATION FOR MAXILLARY MOLARS

Though the technique of access cavity preparation of molar is similar to that of anterior teeth and premolar but because of anatomic differences, they are discussed separately.

- Remove all the carious portion or any restoration if present.
- Determine the shape and size of access opening by measuring the boundaries of pulp chamber mesially and distally and coronally on the radiograph.
- Determine the starting point of bur into the enamel. It is determined by mesial and distal boundary. Mesial boundary is a line joining the mesial cusps and the distal boundary is the oblique ridge. The starting point of bur penetration is on the central groove midway between mesial and distal boundaries (Fig. 14.34).
- Now penetrate the enamel with No. 4 round bur in the central groove directed palatally and prepare an external outline form.
- Penetrate the bur deep into the dentin until the clinician feels "drop" into the pulp chamber. Now remove the complete roof of pulp chamber using tapered fissure, round bur or safety tip diamond or the carbide bur working from inside to outside. The shape and size of the internal anatomy of pulp chamber guides the cutting.
- Explore the canal orifices with sharp endodontic explorer. All the canal orifices should be positioned entirely on the pulp floor and should not extend to the axial walls.
- After the canal orifices have been located, remove any cervical bulges, ledges or obstruction if present.
- Smoothen and finish the access cavity walls so as to make them confluent within the wall of pulp chamber and slightly divergent towards the occlusal surface.

### Maxillary First Molar

- The shape of pulp chamber is rhomboid with acute mesiobuccal angle, obtuse distobuccal angle and palatal right angles (Fig. 14.35).
- Palatal canal orifice is located palatally. Mesiobuccal canal orifice is located under the mesiobuccal cusp. Distobuccal canal orifice is located slightly distal and palatal to the mesiobuccal orifice.

  A line drawn to connect all three orifices (i.e. MB, DB and palatal) forms a triangle, termed as ***molar triangle***.

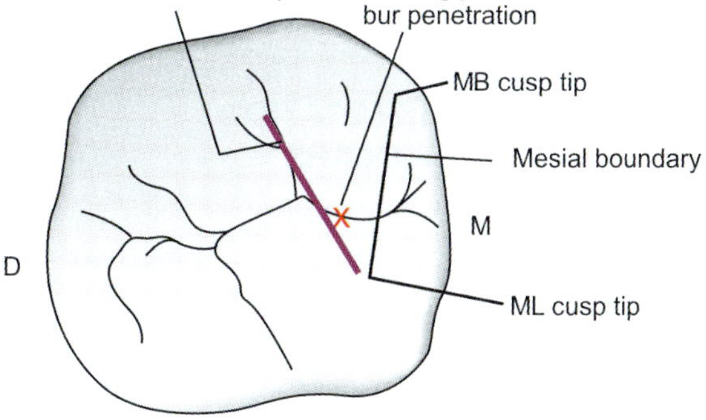


**Fig. 14.34:** Outline of access cavity of maxillary molars is determined by mesial and distal boundary. Mesial boundary is a line joining the mesial cusps and the distal boundary is the oblique ridge. The starting point of bur penetration is on the central groove midway between mesial and distal boundaries

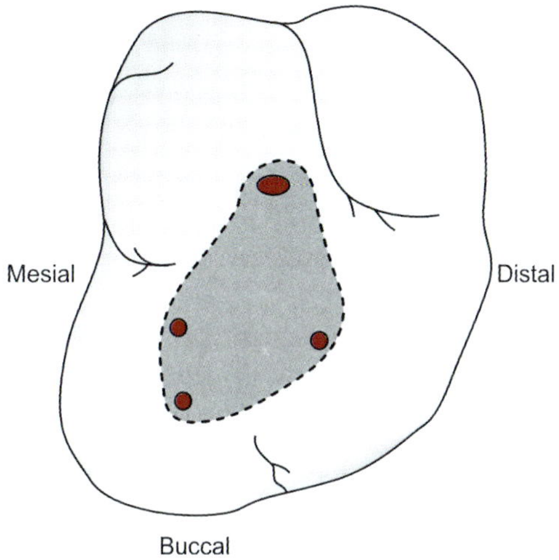


**Fig. 14.35:** Position of root canal orifices of maxillary first molar

- Almost always a second mesiobuccal canal, i.e. MB2 is present in first maxillary molars, which is located palatal and mesial to the MB1. Though its position can vary sometimes it can lie a line between MB1 and palatal orifices.
- Because of presence of MB2, the access cavity acquires a rhomboid shape with corners corresponding to all the canal orifices, i.e. MB1, MB2, DB and palatal.

***Luebke*** has shown that an entire wall is not extended to search and facilitate cleaning, shaping and obturation of extracanal. He recommended extension of only that portion of the wall where extracanal is present, and this may result in "***cloverleaf appearance***" in the outline form. Luebke referred this to as a ***Shamrock preparation***.

### Maxillary Second Molar

***Basic technique is similar to that of first molar but with following differences:***

i. Three roots are found closer which may even fuse to form a single root.
ii. MB2 is less likely to be present in second molar.
iii. The three canals form a rounded triangle with base to buccal.

iv. Mesiobuccal orifice is located more towards mesial and buccal than in first molar.

## ACCESS CAVITY PREPARATION FOR MANDIBULAR MOLARS

- It is similar to that of any other access cavity preparation in removal of caries and any restorative material if present.
- The enamel is penetrated with No. 4 round bur on the central fossa midway between the mesial and distal boundaries. The mesial boundary is a line joining the mesial cusp tips and the distal boundary is the line joining buccal and the lingual grooves (Fig. 14.36).
- Bur is penetrated in the central fossa directed towards the distal root. Once the "drop" into pulp chamber is felt, remove whole of the roof of pulp chamber working from inside to outside with the help of round bur, tapered fissure bur or the safety tip diamond or the carbide bur as it was done in maxillary molars.
- Explore the canal orifices with sharp endodontic explorer and finally finish and smoothen the cavity with slight divergence towards the occlusal surface.
- Second molars with fused roots usually have two canals, buccal and palatal though the number, type, shape and form of canals may vary.
- When four canals are present, the shape of access cavity is rhomboid but when two canals are present, access cavity is oval in shape with wider dimensions buccolingually.
- Shape and size of the access cavity may vary according to the size, shape and location of the canal orifices.

### Mandibular First Molar

Mesiobuccal orifice is under the mesiobuccal cusp. Mesiolingual orifice is located in a depression formed by mesial and the lingual walls. The distal orifice is oval in shape with largest diameter buccolingually, located distal to the buccal groove.

Orifices of all the canals are usually located in the mesial two-thirds of the crown (Fig. 14.37).

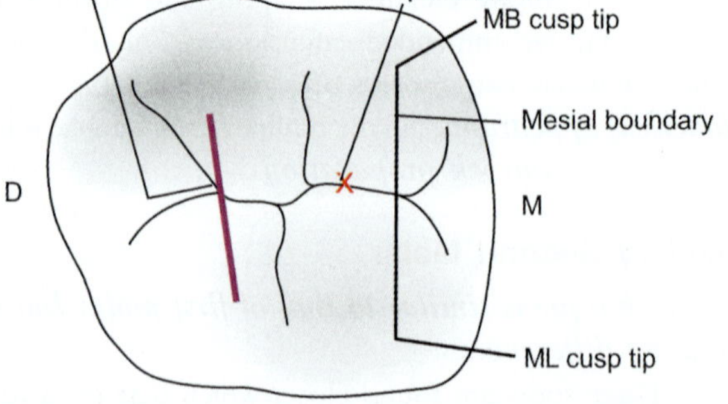


Fig. 14.36: Outline of access preparation of mandibular molars. The enamel is penetrated with No. 4 round bur on the central fossa midway between the mesial and distal boundaries. The mesial boundary is a line joining the mesial cusp tips and the distal boundary is the line joining buccal and the lingual grooves

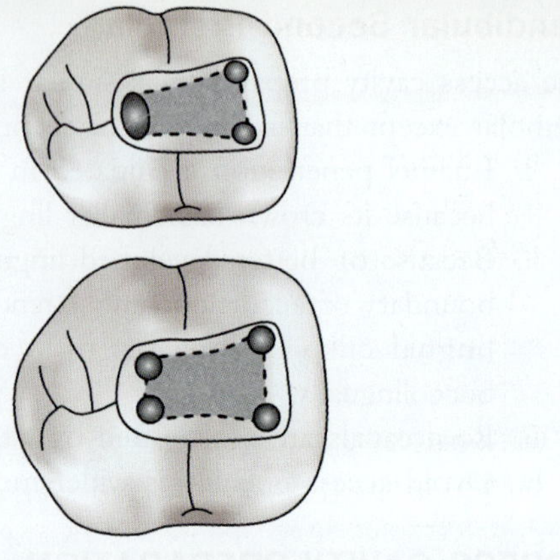

Fig. 14.37: Outline of access cavity of mandibular molars

Cases have also been reported with an extramesial canal, i.e. middle mesial canal (1-15%) lying in the developmental groove between mesiobuccal and mesiolingual canals. Distal root has also shown to have more than one orifices, i.e. distobuccal, distolingual and middle distal. These orifices are usually joined by the developmental grooves.

- The shape of access cavity is usually trapezoidal or rhomboid irrespective of number of canals present.

  The mesial wall is straight, the distal wall is round. The buccal and lingual walls converge to meet the mesial and distal walls.

### Mandibular Second Molar

Access opening of mandibular second molar is similar to that of first molar except for a few differences. In mandibular second molar:

i. Pulp chamber is smaller in size.
ii. One, two or more canals may be present.
iii. Mesiobuccal and mesiolingual canal orifices are usually located closer together.
iv. When three canals are present, shape of access cavity is almost similar to mandibular first molar, but it is more triangular and less of rhomboid shape.
v. When two canal orifices are present, access cavity is rectangular, wide mesiodistally and narrow buccolingually.
vi. Because of buccoaxial inclination, sometimes it is necessary to reduce a large portion of the mesiobuccal cusp to gain convenience form for mesiobuccal canal.

## CLINICAL MANAGEMENT OF DIFFICULT CASES FOR ACCESS OPENING

For optimal treatment of teeth with abnormal pulpal anatomy, following are required:

a. **Good quality radiographs:** Good quality radiographs with angled views, good contrast are preferred for better assessment of root canals anatomy. If a canal disappears midway from orifice to roof apex, one should always suspect bifurcation, if there is an asymmetry, one should suspect abnormal anatomy of pulp space.
b. **Magnification:** Use of surgical operating microscope is recommended for endodontic treatment. It magnifies the pulpal anatomy in great detail.

c. **Clinical anatomy:** One should evaluate gingival contour for abnormal anatomy of tooth. For example, broad labial gingival in maxillary premolar may suggest a broad buccal root and thus two root canals. Teeth with extra cusp may indicate aberrant pulp chamber.

d. **Pulpal floor:** In general pulpal floor is dark grey in color, whereas axial dentin is light in color. This color difference helps the clinician to be very accurate in removing axial dentin so as to expose pulpal floor.

e. **Extensions of access cavity:** Extensions of access cavity help in locating the canal orifices. The initial access shape is determined by shape of the pulpal floor but later it is extended to gain straight line access to the canals. Sometimes modified access cavity is prepared to locate MB2 in maxillary molars or second buccal canal in maxillary premolars.

## Management of Cases with Extensive Restorations

If extensive restorations or full veneer crowns are marginally intact with no caries, then they can be retained with access cavity being cut through them (Fig. 14.38). Restorative materials often alter the anatomic landmarks making the access cavity preparation difficult (Fig. 14.39).

If possible, complete removal of extensive restoration allows the most favorable access to the root canals. When restoration is not removed, and access cavity is made through it, following can occur:

i. Coronal leakage because of loosening of fillings due to vibrations while access preparation.
ii. Poor visibility and accessibility.
iii. Blockage of canal, because broken filling pieces may struck into the canal system.
iv. Misdirection of bur penetration (because in some cases restorations are placed to change the crown to root angulations so as to correct occlusal discrepancies).

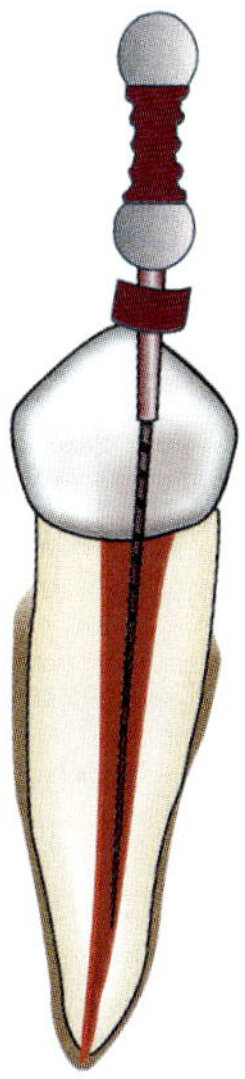

**Fig. 14.38:** When full veneer crown is marginally intact with no caries, access can be made through the crown

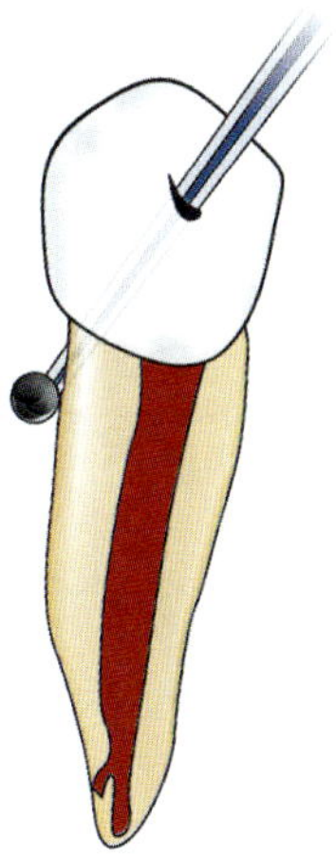

**Fig. 14.39:** Perforation caused during access cavity preparation while gaining entry through already placed crown

If the restorations show no defect, leaky margins, fractures or caries, access can be made through them. For cutting porcelain restorations diamond burs are effective and for cutting through metal crowns, a fine cross-cut tungsten carbide bur is very effective.

## Tilted and Angulated Crowns

If tooth is severely tilted, access cavity should be prepared with great care to avoid perforations. Preoperative radiographs are of great help in evaluating the relationship of crown to the root. Sometimes it becomes necessary to open up the pulp chamber without applying the rubber dam so that bur can be placed at the correct angulation.

If not taken care, the access cavity preparation in tilted crowns can result in:

i. Failure to locate canals
ii. Gouging of the tooth structure
iii. Procedural accidents such as
   a. Instrument separation
   b. Perforation
   c. Improper debridement of pulp space

## Calcified Canals

Calcifications in the pulp space are of common occurrence. Pulp space can be partially or completely obliterated by the pulp stones. Teeth with calcifications result in difficulty in locating and further treatment of the calcified canals.

Special tips for ultrasonic handpieces are best suited for treating such cases. They allow the précised removal of dentin from the pulp floor while locating calcified canals (Fig. 14.40). But magnification and illumination are the main requirements before negotiating a calcified canal.

If special tips are not available then a pointed ultrasonic scaler tip can be used for removal of calcifications from the pulp space. One should avoid over cutting of the dentin in order to locate the canals, this will further result in loss of landmarks and the tooth weakening. At the first indication that

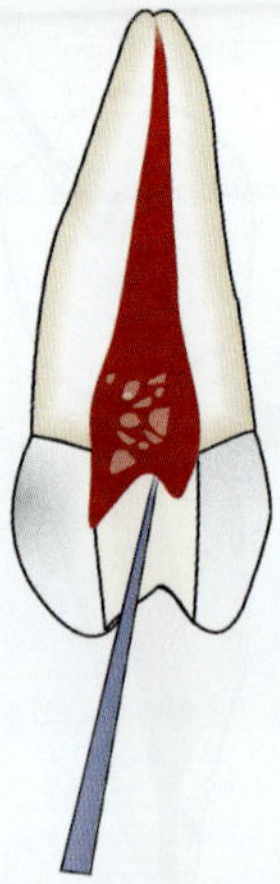

**Fig. 14.40:** Use of ultrasonic tip to remove dentin while locating calcified canals

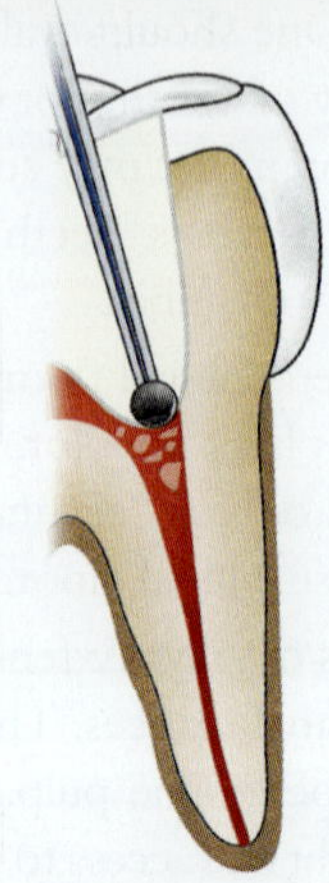

**Fig. 14.42:** Use of long shanked round bur to negotiate the sclerosed canal

canal is found, introduce the smallest instrument with gentle passive motion both rotational and apical in the canal to negotiate it (Fig. 14.41). Use of chelating agents is also of great help while negotiating the calcified canals.

## Sclerosed Canals

Sometimes sclerosed canals are found in teeth which make the endodontic treatment a challenge. For visualization, magnification and illumination are the main requirements. Dyes can be used to locate the sclerotic canals. While negotiating, the précised amount of dentin should be removed with the help of ultrasonic tips to avoid over cutting. Long shanked low speed No. 2 round burs can also be used (Fig. 14.42). Use of chelating agents in these cases is not of much help because it softens the dentin indiscriminately, resulting in procedural errors such as perforations.

## Teeth with No or Minimal Crown

Though it seems to be quite simple to prepare access cavity in such teeth, some precautions are needed while dealing with such cases:

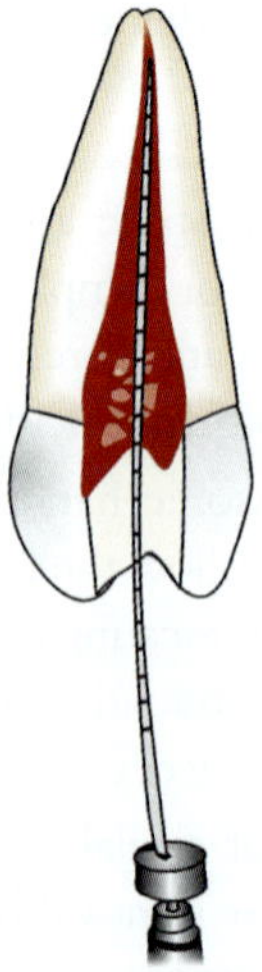

**Fig. 14.41:** Introduce the smallest instrument into the canal at first indication of canal orifice

a. Evaluate the preoperative radiograph to assess the root angulation.
b. Start the cavity preparation without applying rubber dam.
c. Evaluate the depth of penetration from preoperative radiograph.
d. Apply rubber dam as soon as the canals have been located.

If precautions are not taken in case of missing crown, there are chances of occurrence of iatrogenic errors like perforations due to misdirection of the bur. In such cases, sometimes it becomes imperative to rebuild the tooth previous to endodontic treatment. In teeth with weakened walls, it is necessary to reinforce the walls before initiating endodontic treatment. In other words, it is necessary to restore the natural form of a crown of the tooth to achieve following goals:

a. Return the tooth to its normal form and function.
b. Prevent coronal leakage during treatment.
c. Allow use of rubber dam clamps.
d. Prevent fracture of walls which can complicate the endodontic procedure.

## QUESTIONS

**Q. Define access cavity preparation. What are objectives of access cavity preparation?**

**Q. How will you do access preparation for mandibular molar?**

**Q. Write short notes on:**

a. Mouse-hole effect
b. Shamrock preparation

## BIBLIOGRAPHY

1. Cohen S, I lergreaves K. Pathways of pulp (9th edn), St Louis: Elsevier 2006;610-49.
2. Cooke HG, Cox FL. C-shaped canal configurations in mandibular molars. J Am Dent Assoc 1979;99:836-39.
3. De Moor RJ, Deroose CA, Calberon FL. The radix entomolaris in mandibular first molars: an endodontic challenge. Int Endod J 2004;37:789-99.
4. Ferreira CM, de Moraes IG, Bernardineli N. Three-rooted maxillary second premolar. J Endod 2000;26:105-06.

5. Kerekes K, Tronstad L. Long-term results of endodontic treatment performed with a standardized technique. J Endod 1979;5:83-90.
6. Manning SA. Root canal anatomy of mandibular second molars. Part II. C-shaped canals. Int Endod J 1990;23:40-45.
7. Soares JA, Leonardo RT. Root canal treatment of three-rooted maxillary first and second premolars: A case report. Int Endo J 2003;36:705-10.
8. Vertucci FJ, Seelig A, Gills R. Root canal morphology of the human maxillary second premolar. Oral Surg Oral Med Oral Pathol Oral Radiol Endod 1974;38:456-64.
9. Vertucci FJ. Root canal anatomy of the human permanent teeth. Oral Surg Med Oral Pathol Oral Radiol Endod 1984;58: 589-99.
10. Walton RE, Torabinejad M, Principles and Practice of endodontics (3rd edn). Philadelphia: Saunders 1996;213-15.
11. Weine FS, Hayami S, Hata G, Toda T. Canal configuration of the mesiobuccal root of the maxillary first molar of a Japanese subpopulations. Int Endod J 1999;32:79-87.
12. Weine FS. Endodontic Therapy (5th edn). St. Louis: Mosby-Yearbook Inc. 1996;243.

# Working Length Determination

CHAPTER 15



## INTRODUCTION AND HISTORY

Determination of an accurate working length is one of the most critical steps of endodontic therapy. The cleaning, shaping and obturation of root canal system cannot be accomplished accurately unless working length is determined precisely. Prognosis and microbiologic studies as well as histologic experiments involving healing after obturation show that it is preferable to confine instruments, irrigating solutions and obturating materials to the canal space. Thus we can say that predictable endodontic success demands an accurate determination of working length of root canal and strict adherence to it, in order to create a small wound site and good healing conditions.

**Historical perspectives**

| | | | |
|---|---|---|---|
| At the end of nineteenth century | | - | Working length was usually calculated when file was placed in the canal and patient experienced pain. |
| 1899 | Kells | - | Introduced X-rays in dentistry |
| 1918 | Hatton | - | Microscopically studied the diseased periodontal tissues. |
| 1929 | Collidge | - | Studied the anatomy of root apex in relation to treatment problem. |
| 1955 | Kuttler | - | Microscopically investigated the root apices. |
| 1962 | Sunada | - | Found electrical resistance between periodontium and oral mucous membrane. |
| 1969 | Inove | - | Significant contribution in evolution of Electronic apex locator |

Before we discuss various methods of determination of working length, we need to understand the anatomic consideration regarding it.

## DEFINITIONS

According to endodontic glossary *working length* is defined as "the distance from a coronal reference point to a point at which canal preparation and obturation should terminate" (Fig. 15.1).

*Reference point*: Reference point is that site on occlusal or the incisal surface from which measurements are made. A reference point is chosen which is stable and easily visualized during preparation. Usually this is the highest point on incisal edge of anterior teeth and buccal cusp of posterior teeth (Fig. 15.2). Reference point should not change between the appointments.

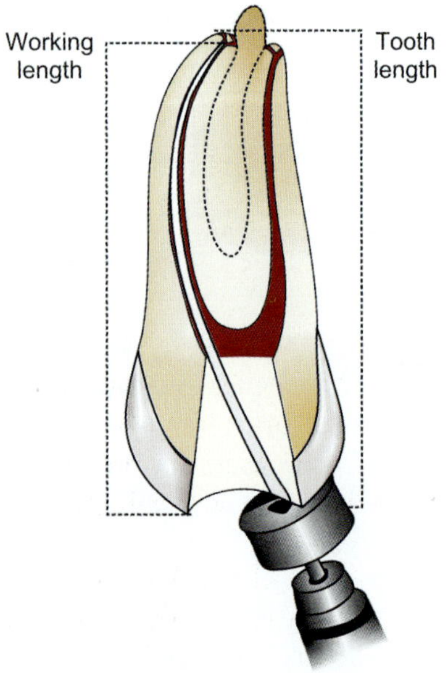


**Fig. 15.1:** Working length distance is defined as the distance from coronal referencer point to a point where canal preparation and obturation should terminate

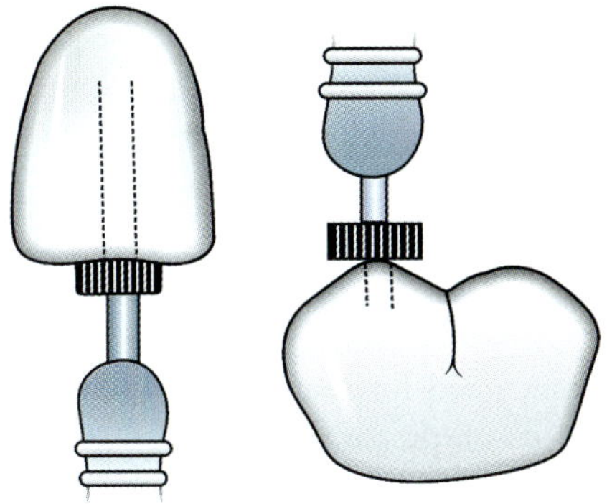

**Fig. 15.2:** Usually the reference point is highest point on incisal edge of anterior teeth and cusp tip of posterior teeth

Therefore in case of teeth with undermined cusps and fillings, they should be reduced considerably before access preparation.

***Anatomic apex*** is "tip or end of root determined morphologically".

***Radiographic apex*** is "tip or end of root determined radiographically".

***Apical foramen*** is main apical opening of the root canal which may be located away from anatomic or radiographic apex.

***Apical constriction*** (minor apical diameter) is apical portion of root canal having narrowest diameter. It is usually 0.5 -1 mm short of apical foramen (Fig. 15.3). The minor diameter widens apically to foramen, i.e. major diameter (Fig. 15.4).

***Cementodentinal junction*** is the region where cementum and dentin are united, the point at which cemental surface terminates at or near the apex of tooth. It is not always necessary that CDJ always coincide with apical constriction. Location of CDJ ranges from 0.5 - 3 mm short of anatomic apex (Fig. 15.5).

## SIGNIFICANCE OF WORKING LENGTH

- Working length determines how far into canal, instruments can be placed and worked.
- It affects degree of pain and discomfort which patient will experience following appointment by virtue of over and under instrumentation.
- If placed within correct limits, it plays an important role in determining the success of treatment.
- Before determining a definite working length, there should be straight line access for the canal orifice for unobstructed penetration of instrument into apical constriction.
- Once apical stop is calculated, monitor the working length periodically because working length may change as curved canal is straightened.
- Failure to accurately determine and maintain working length may result in length being over than normal which will lead to postoperative pain, prolonged healing time and lower success rate because of incomplete regeneration of cementum, periodontal ligament and alveolar bone.
- When working length is made short of apical constriction it may cause persistent discomfort because of incomplete cleaning and underfilling. Apical leakage may occur into uncleaned and unfilled space short of apical constriction. It may support continued existence of viable bacteria and contributes to the periradicular lesion and thus poor success rate.

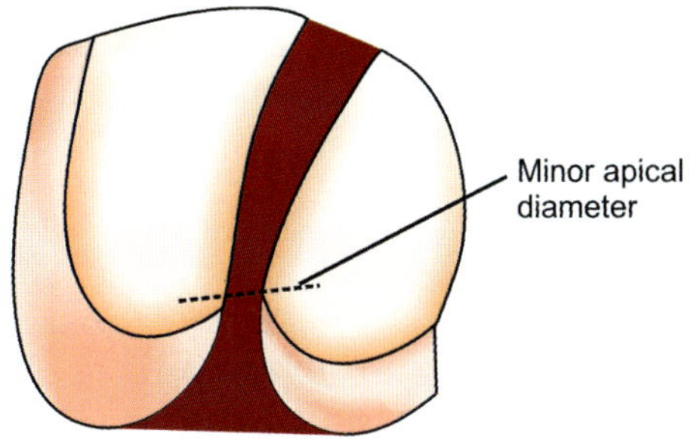


**Fig. 15.3:** Minor apical diameter

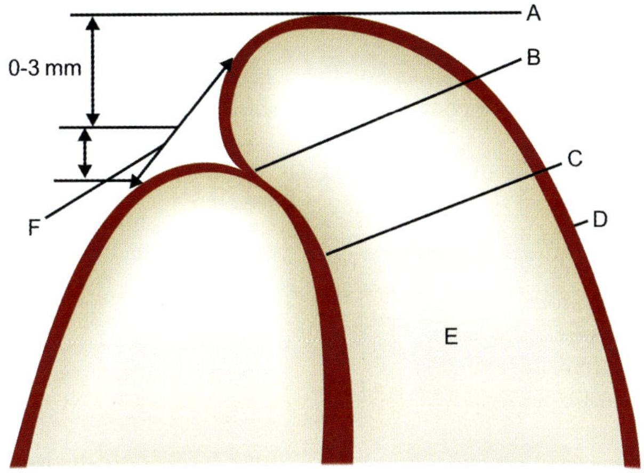

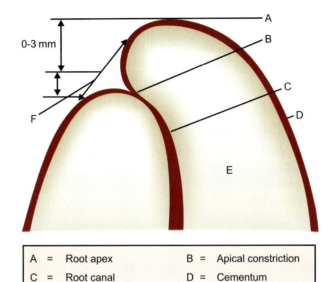

| | | | | | |
|---|---|---|---|---|---|
| A | = | Root apex | B | = | Apical constriction |
| C | = | Root canal | D | = | Cementum |
| E | = | Dentin | F | = | Apical foramen |

**Fig. 15.4:** Anatomy of root apex

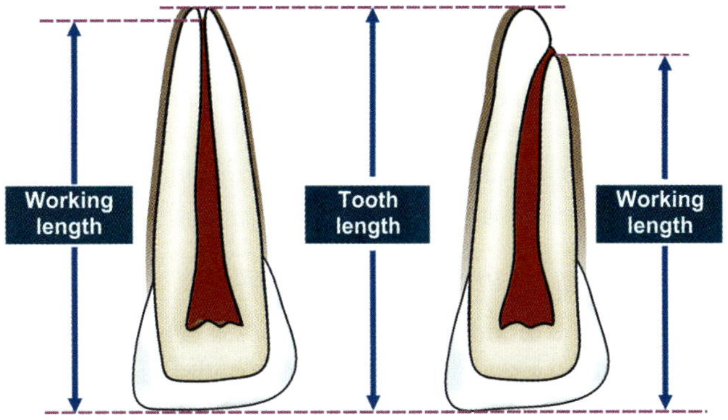


**Fig. 15.5:** CDJ needs not to terminate at apical constriction. It can be 0.5-3 mm short of the apex

### Working Width

Working width is defined as "initial and post instrumentation horizontal dimensions of the root canal system at working length and other levels".

**Consequences of over-extended working length**
- Perforation through apical construction
- Over instrumentation
- Overfilling of root canal
- Increased incidence of postoperative pain
- Prolonged healing period
- Lower success rate due to incomplete regeneration of cementum, periodontal ligament and alveolar bone.

**Consequences of working short of actual working length**
- Incomplete cleaning and instrumentation of the canal
- Persistent discomfort due to presence of pulpal remnants
- Underfilling of the root canal
- Incomplete apical seal
- Apical leakage which supports existence of viable bacteria, this further leads to poor healing and periradicular lesion.

**Causes of loss of working length**
- Presence of debris in apical 2-3 of canal
- Failure to maintain apical patency
- Skipping instrument sizes
- Ledge formation
- Inadequate irrigation
- Instrument separation
- Canal blockage.

The minimum initial working width corresponds the initial apical file size which binds at working length. The maximum final working width corresponds to the master apical file size, this master apical file size is usually three times than minimum initial working width.

### Determination of Minimum Initial Working Width

It depends upon following factors:

***Canal shape:*** It is easier to determine working width in round canals but variations occur in roots with oval, irregular or flattened ribbon like canals. It is difficult to calculate width in such canals thus resulting in discrepancy in value. This can further lead to incomplete cleaning and shaping and keyhole or dumbbell root canal preparation.

### Significance of Working Width

- To attain a round apical stop so as to achieve a three-dimensional impermeable seal. This round shape conforms to the round cross-sectional tip of gutta-percha
- Large working width of apical area removes more bacteria, and let the irrigants to reach apical area, more easily then in canals with small working width.

#### *Advantages of Narrow Apex*

- Decreases risk of canal transportation
- Avoids extrusion of debris and obturating material.

#### *Disadvantages*

- Incomplete removal of infected dentin
- Not ideal for lateral compaction
- Irrigants may not reach the apical-third of canal.

#### *Advantages of Wide Apex*

- Complete removal of infected dentin
- Better disinfection of canal at apical third.

#### *Disadvantages*

- Increased chances of extrusion of irrigants and obturating material
- Not recommended for thermoplastic obturation
- More chances of preparation errors.

## DIFFERENT METHODS OF WORKING LENGTH DETERMINATION

Various methods for determining working length include using average root lengths from anatomic studies, preoperative radiographs, tactile sensation, etc. Other common methods include use of paper point, working length radiograph, electronic apex locators or any combination of the above.

In this era of improved illumination and magnification, working length determination should be to the nearest 1.5 mm. So to achieve the highest degree of accuracy a combination of several methods should be used.

**Methods of determining working length**

| *Radiographic methods* | *Non-radiographic methods* |
|---|---|
| • Grossman formula | • Digital tactile sense |
| • Ingle's method | • Apical periodontal sensitivity |
| • Weine's method | • Paper point method |
| • Kuttler's method | • Electronic apex locators |
| • Radiographic grid | |
| • Endometric probe | |
| • Direct digital radiography | |
| • Xeroradiography | |
| • Subtraction radiography | |

### Directional Stop Attachments

Most commonly used stoppers for endodontic instruments are silicon rubber stops, though stop attachments can be made up of metal, plastic or silicon rubber. Stop attachments can be available in two shapes tear drop or round.

Irrespective of shape, the stop should be placed perpendicular to the instrument not at any other direction (oblique) so as to avoid variation in working length. Advantage of using tear shaped stopper is that in curved canal, it can be used to indicate the canal curvature by placing its tear shape towards the direction of curve.

## RADIOGRAPHIC METHOD OF WORKING LENGTH DETERMINATION

Radiographic apex has been used as termination point in working length determination since many years and it has showed promising results. But there are two school of thoughts regarding this:

Those who follow this concept say cementodentinal junction is impossible to locate clinically and the radiographic apex is the only reproducible site available for length determination.

According to it, a patent root tip and larger files kept with in the tooth may result in excellent prognosis.

Those who don't follow this concept say that position of radiographic apex is not reproducible. Its position depends on number of factors like angulation of tooth, position of film, film holder, length of X-ray cone and presence of adjacent anatomic structures, etc.

When radiographs are used in determining working length the quality of the image is important for accurate interpretations.

Among the two commonly used techniques, paralleling techniques have been demonstrated as superior to bisecting angle technique in determination and reproduction of apical anatomy.

As the angle increases away from parallel, the quality of image decreases. This occurs because as the angle increases, the tissue that X-rays must pass through includes a greater percentage of bone mass, therefore the root anatomy becomes less apparent.

Parallel working length radiographs can be difficult to attain because of disorientation, shallow palatal vault and tori, etc. But good film holders like Endo Ray II film holder may help in improving the results.

Before studying the X-rays for endodontics, under-standing of buccal object rule is essential. The basic concept of the rule is that as the vertical or horizontal angulation of X-ray tube changes, the object buccal or closest to tube head moves to opposite side of radiograph compared to the lingual object. To separate buccal and lingual roots (for example in maxillary first premolar) to visualize the working length, tube head should be moved from a 20° mesial angulation. This captures the buccal root to the opposite or distal side of radiograph and lingual root on mesial side of the radiograph. It is also known as SLOB rule that is same lingual opposite buccal.

When two superimposed canals are present (for example buccal and palatal canals of maxillary premolar, mesial canals of mandibular molar) one should take following steps:

a. Take two individual radiographs with instrument placed in each canal.
b. Take radiograph at different angulations, usually 20° to 40° at horizontal angulation.
c. Insert two different instrument, e.g. K file in one canal, H file/reamer in other canal and take radiograph at different angulations.
d. Apply SLOB rule, that is expose tooth from mesial or distal horizontal angle, canal which moves to same direction, is lingual where as canal which moves to opposite direction is buccal.

## A. Radiographic Methods

Before access opening, fractured cusps, cusps weakened by caries or restorations are reduced to avoid fracture of weakened enamel during the treatment. This will avoid the loss of initial reference point and thus the working length (Figs 15.6A and B).

In this method, preoperative periapical radiograph is used to calculate the working length for endodontic treatment. OrthoPantograph (OPG) radiographs are not advocated for calculating tentative working length because of gross magnification of 13-28 percent employed in OPG which will lead to errors in calculation of accurate readings.

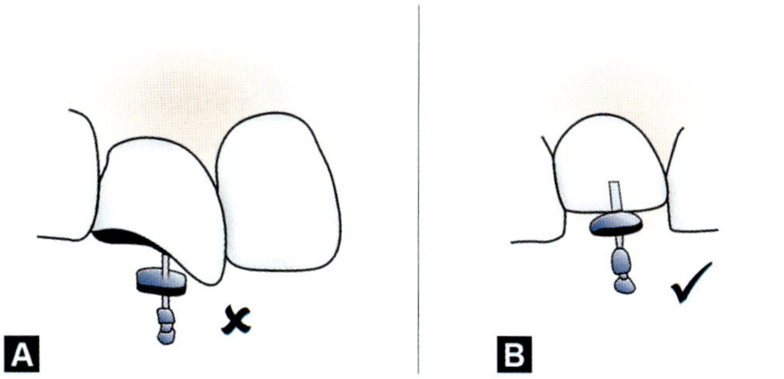


**Figs 15.6A and B:** Reference point should not be made of fractured tooth surface or carious tooth structure. These should be first removed for avoiding loss in working length

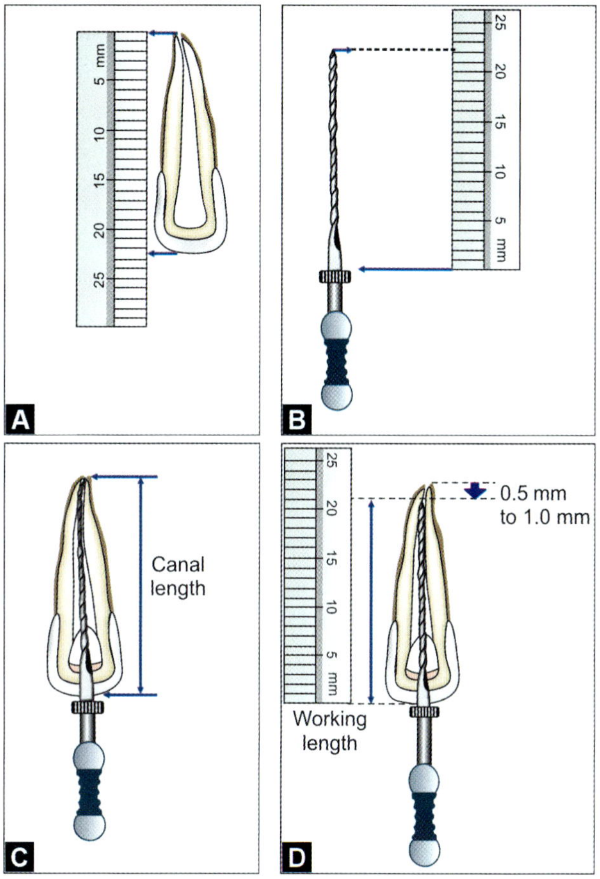


**Figs 15.7A to D:** Radiographic method of working length determination

This measurement is used as estimated working length which can then be confirmed by placing an endodontic instrument into the canal and taking a second radiograph (Figs 15.7A to D).

The instrument inserted in the canal should be large enough not to be loose in the canal because it can move while taking the radiograph and thus may result in errors in determining the working length.

Fine instruments are often difficult to be seen in a radiograph. The new working length is calculated by adding or subtracting the distance between the instrument tip and desired apical termination of the root.

The correct working length is finally calculated by subtracting 1 mm as safety factor from this new length. This technique was first introduced by John Ingle. Weine modified this subtraction rule (Figs 15.8A to C) as follows:

a. If radiograph shows absence of any resorption, i.e. bone or root apex, shorten the length by 1 mm (Fig. 15.8A).
b. If periapical bone resorption is present, shorten it by 1.5 mm (Fig. 15.8B).
c. If both bone and root resorption is seen, shorten length by 2 mm. This is done because if there is root resorption, loss of apical constriction may occur in such cases (Fig. 15.8C).

In curved canals, canal length is reconfirmed because final working length may shorten up to 1 mm as canal is straightened out by instrumentation. If root contains two canals, the cone should be positioned at 20 to 30° horizontal deviation from the standard facial projection.

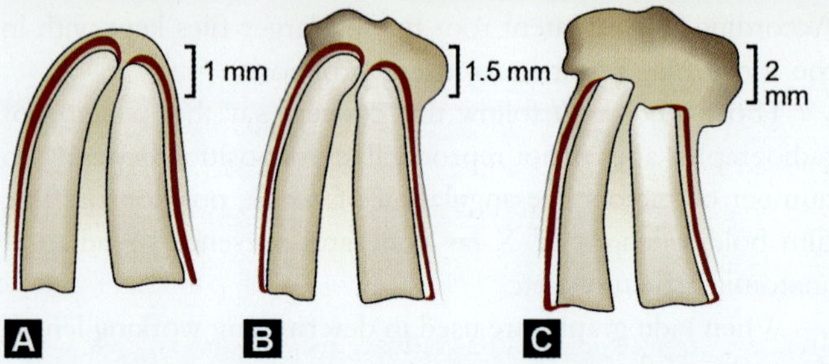

**Figs 15.8A to C:** Modification in length by substraction in case of root resorption

**Radiographic method of length determination**

1. Measure the estimated working length from preoperative periapical radiograph.
2. Adjust stopper of instrument to this estimated working length and place it in the canal up to the adjusted stopper.
3. Take the radiograph.
4. On the radiograph measure the difference between the tip of the instrument and root apex. Add or subtract this length to the estimated working length to get the new working length.
5. Correct working length is finally calculated by subtracting 1 mm from this new length.

**Modification in the length subtraction (Fig. 15.8)**

| | |
|---|---|
| 1. No resorption | - subtract 1 mm |
| 2. Periapical bone resorption | - subtract 1.5 mm |
| 3. Periapical bone + root apex resorption | - subtract 2 mm |

**Advantages of radiographic methods of working length determination**

1. One can see the anatomy of the tooth
2. One can find out curvature of the root canal
3. We can see the relationship between the adjacent teeth and anatomic structures.

**Disadvantages of radiographic methods of working length determination**

1. Varies with different observers
2. Superimposition of anatomical structures
3. Two-dimensional view of three-dimensional object
4. Cannot interpret if apical foramen has buccal or lingual exit
5. Risk of radiation exposure
6. Time consuming
7. Limited accuracy

## Grossman Method/Mathematic Method of Working Length Determination

It is based on simple mathematical formulations to calculate the working length. In this, an instrument is inserted into the canal, stopper is fixed to the reference point and radiograph is taken. The formula to calculate actual length of the tooth is as follows:

$$\frac{\text{Actual length of the tooth}}{\text{Actual length of the instrument}} = \frac{\text{Apparent length of tooth in radiograph}}{\text{Apparent length of instrument in radiograph}}$$

By above, as we see those three variables are known and by applying the formula, 4th variable, i.e. actual length of tooth can be calculated.

$$\text{Actual length of tooth} = \frac{\text{Actual length of the instrument} \times \text{Apparent length of tooth in radiograph}}{\text{Apparent length of instrument in radiograph}}$$

### *Disadvantages*

1. Wrong readings can occur because of:
   a. Variations in angles of radiograph
   b. Curved roots
   c. S-shaped, double curvature roots.

## Kuttler's Method

According to Kuttler, canal preparation should terminate at apical constriction, i.e. minor diameter. In young patients, average distance between minor and major diameter is 0.524 mm where as in older patients it 0.66 mm.

### *Technique*

- Locate minor and major diameter on preoperative radiograph
- Estimate length of roots from preoperative radiograph.
- Estimate canal width on radiograph. If canal is narrow, use 10 or 15 size instrument. If it is of average width, use 20 or 25 size instruments. If canal is wide, use 30 or 35 size instrument.
- Insert the selected file in the canal up to the estimated canal length and take a radiograph.
- If file is too long or short by more than 1 mm from minor diameter, readjust the file and take second radiograph.
- If file reaches major diameter, subtract 0.5 mm from it for younger patients and 0.67 for older patients.

### *Advantages*

- Minimal errors
- Has shown many successful cases
- Rapid development of increases the chances of retaining obturating material.

### *Disadvantages*

- Time consuming and complicated
- Requires excellent quality radiographs.

### Radiographic Grid

It was designed by Everett and Fixott in 1963. It is a simple method in which a millimeter grid is superimposed on the radiograph. This over comes the need for calculation. But it is not good method if radiograph is bent during exposure.

### Endometric Probe

In this method, one uses the graduations on diagnostic file which are visible on radiograph. But its main disadvantage is that the smallest file size to be used is number 25.

### Direct Digital Radiography

In this digital image is formed which is represented by spatially distributed set of discrete sensors and pixels.

Two types of digital radiography:

a. Radiovisiography
b. Phosphor imaging system.

#### *Xeroradiography*

It is new method for recording images without film in which the imaging is recorded on an aluminium plate coated with selenium particles.

The plate is removed from the cassette and subjected to relaxation which removes old images, then these are electrostatically charged and inserted into the cassette. Radiations are projected on film which cause selective discharge of the particles. This forms the latent image and is converted to a positive image by a process called 'development' in the processor unit.

#### *Advantages*

- This technique offers 'edge enhancement' and good detail.
- The ability to have both positive and negative prints together.
- Improves visualization of files and canals.
- It is two times more sensitive than conventional D-speed films.

#### *Disadvantages*

- Since saliva may act as a medium for flow of current, the electric charge over the film may cause discomfort to the patient.
- Exposure time varies according to thickness of the plate.
- The process of development cannot be delayed beyond 15 min.

### B. Non-radiographic Methods

1. *Digital tactile sense:* In this clinician may see an increase in resistance as file reaches the apical 2-3 mm.
   *Advantages*
   - Time saving
   - No radiation exposure.

   *Disadvantages*
   - Does not always provide the accurate readings
   - In case of narrow canals, one may feel increased resistance as file approaches apical 2-3 mm.
   - In case of teeth with immature apex instrument can go periapically.
2. *Periodontal sensitivity test:* This method is based on patient's response to pain. But this method does not always provide the accurate readings, for example in case of narrow canals, instrument may feel increased resistance as file approaches apical 2-3 mm and in case of teeth with immature apex instrument can go beyond apex. In cases of canal with necrotic pulp, instrument can pass beyond apical constriction and in case of vital or inflamed pulp, pain may occur several mm before periapex is crossed by the instrument.
3. *Paper point measurement method:* In this method, paper point is gently passed in the root canal to estimate the working length. It is most reliable in cases of open apex where apical constriction is lost because of perforation or resorption. Moisture of blood present on apical part of paper point indicates that paper point has passed beyond estimated working length. It is used as supplementary method.

## ELECTRONIC APEX LOCATORS

Radiographs are often misinterpreted because of difficulty in distinguishing the radicular anatomy and pathosis from normal structures. Electronic apex locators (EAL) are used for determining working length as an adjunct to radiography. They are basically used to locate the apical constriction or cementodentinal junction or the apical foramen, and not the radiographic apex. Hence the term apex locator is a misnomer one.

The ability to distinguish between minor diameter and major diameter of apical terminus is most important for the creation of apical control zone (Fig. 15.9). ***The apical control zone*** is the mechanical alteration of the apical terminus of root canal space which provides resistance and retention form to the obturating material against the condensation pressure of obturation. Various studies have shown that electronic apex locators have provided more accurate results when compared to conventional radiographs.

History of EALs goes back to 1918, when Custer first reported the use of electronic current to determine working length. In 1960's, Gordon reported the use of a clinical device for electrical measurement of root canals.

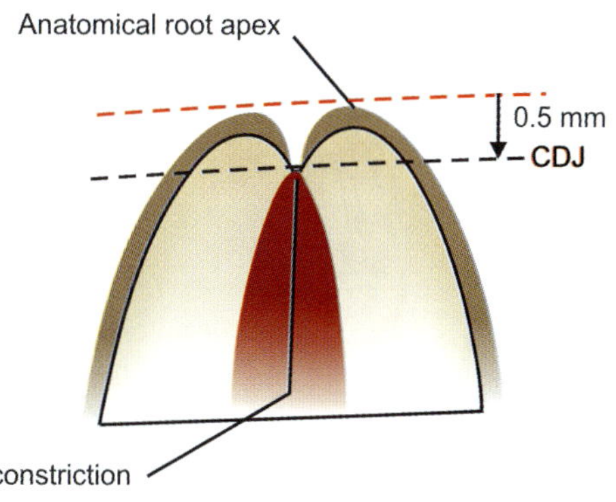


**Fig. 15.9:** Location of CDJ

In 1942, Suzuki's discovered that electrical resistance between an instrument inserted into root canal and an electrode attached to oral mucosa registered a constant value.

In 1962, Sunada using a direct current device with simple circuit demonstrated that consistent electrical resistance between periodontium and mucous membrane was 6.5 K ohms (Fig. 15.10).

In 1970s, frequency measurements were taken through the feedback of an oscillator loop by calibration at periodontal pocket depth of each tooth.

In mid 80's, there occurred the development of a relative value of frequency response method where apical constriction was picked by filtering the difference between two direct potentials after 1 KHz wave was applied to canal space.

A third generation electronic apex locator was developed in late 80's by Kobayashi. He used multiple channel impedance ratios based technology to simultaneously measure the impedance of two different frequencies; calculate the quotient of impedance and express it in terms of the position of electrode, i.e. file in the canal.

**Historical review of EALs**

| | | |
|---|---|---|
| 1918 | - Custer | - Use of electric current for working length |
| 1942 | - Suzuki | - Conducted scientific study of apex locator |
| 1960's | - Gordon | - Use of clinical device for measurement of length |
| 1962 | - Sunada | - Found electrical resistance between periodontium and oral mucous membranes |
| 1969 | - Inove | - Significant contribution in evolution of EAL |
| 1996 | - Pratten and McDonald | - Compared the efficacy of three parallel radiographs and Endex apex locators in cadaver. |

Thus, we can say that all of these apex locators function by using human body to complete an electrical circuit. One side of apex locator circuit is connected to endodontic instrument and other side is connected to patient's body. Circuit is completed when endodontic instrument is advanced into root canal until it touches the periodontal tissue.

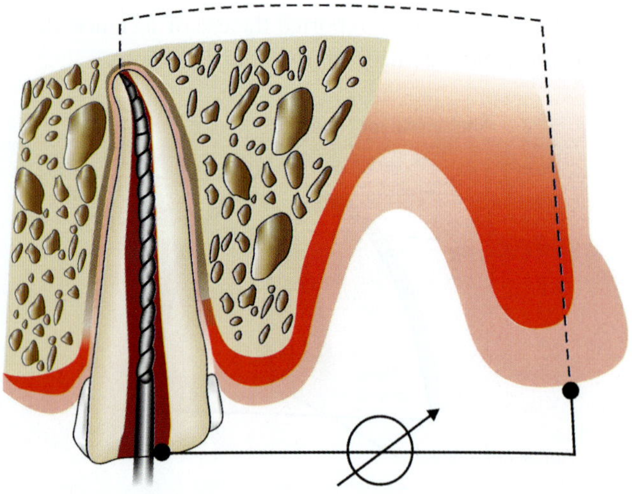

**Fig. 15.10:** Diagrammatic representation of working of resistance type of apex locator

## Components of Electronic Apex Locators

- Lip clip
- File clip
- Electronic device
- Cord which connects above three parts.

## Advantages of Apex Locators

- Provide objective information with high degree of accuracy.
- Accurate in reading (90-98% accuracy)
- Some apex locators are also available in combination with pulp tester, so can be used to test pulp vitality.

### *Disadvantages*

a. Can provide inaccurate readings in following cases:-
   i. Presence of pulp tissue in canal
   ii. Too wet or too dry canal
   iii. Use of narrow file
   iv. Blockage of canal
   v. Incomplete circuit
   vi. Low battery
b. Chances of over estimation
c. May pose problem in teeth with immature apex.

## Uses of Apex Locators

1. Provide objective information with high degree of accuracy.
2. Useful in conditions where apical portion of canal system is obstructed by:
   a. Impacted teeth
   b. Zygomatic arch
   c. Tori
   d. Excessive bone density
   e. Overlapping roots
   f. Shallow palatal vault.

   In such cases, they can provide information which radiographs cannot.
3. Useful in patient who cannot tolerate X-ray film placement because of gag reflex.
4. In case of pregnant patients, to reduce the radiation exposure, they can be valuable tool.
5. Useful in children who may not tolerate taking radiographs, disabled patients and patients who are heavily sedated.
6. Valuable tool for:
   a. Detecting site of root perforations (Fig. 15.13)
   b. Diagnosis of external and internal resorption which have penetrated root surface
   c. Detection of horizontal and vertical root fracture
   d. Determination of perforations caused during post preparation
   e. Testing pulp vitality
7. Helpful in root canal treatment of teeth with incomplete root formation, requiring apexification and to determine working length in primary teeth.

## Contraindications to the Use of Apex Locator

Older apex locators were contraindicated in the patients who have cardiac pacemaker functions. Electrical stimulation to such patients could interfere with pacemaker function. But this problem has been overcome in newer generation of apex locators.

It has been shown that in teeth with periapical radiolucencies, and necrotic pulps associated with root resorption, etc. the use of apex locators is not much beneficial. In such cases there is alteration of apical constriction and lack of viable periodontal ligament tissue to respond to EAL which may cause abnormally long readings.

### Classification of EALs

This classification is based on type of the current flow and opposition to current flow as well as number of frequencies involved. Following classification is modification of classification given by McDonald [DCNA 1992;36:293].

### First Generation Apex Locators (Resistance Apex Locators)

They are also known as resistance apex locators which measure opposition to flow of direct current, i.e. resistance. It is based on the ***principle*** that resistance offered by periodontal ligament and oral mucous membrane is the same, i.e. 6.5 K ohms. Initially ***Sonoexplorer*** was imported from ***Japan*** by ***Amadent***, but nowadays first generation apex locators are off the practice. Blood, pus, chelating agents, irrigants and other materials used within the canal can give false readings.

### Technique for Using Resistance Based EAL

1. Turn on the device and attach the lip clip near the arch being treated. Hold a 15 number file and insert it approximately 0.5 mm into sulcus of tooth (like PD probe). Adjust the control knob until the reference needle is centered on the meter scale and produces audible beeps. Note this reading.
2. Prepare the access cavity and apply rubber dam and remove pulp, debris, etc.
3. Using preoperative radiograph estimate the working canal width. Clean the canal if bleeding form vital pulp is excessive, dry it with paper points.
4. Insert the file into canal unless the reference needle moves from extreme left to center of scale and alarm beeps sound. Reset the stop at reference point and record the lengths (Figs 15.11A to D).
5. Take the radiograph with file in place at the length indicated by apex locator. If length is longer/shorter, it is possible that preoperative film can be elongated or apex locator is inaccurate.

#### *Advantages*

1. Easily operated
2. Digital read out
3. Audible indication
4. Detect perforation
5. Can be used with K-file.
6. May incorporate pulp tester.

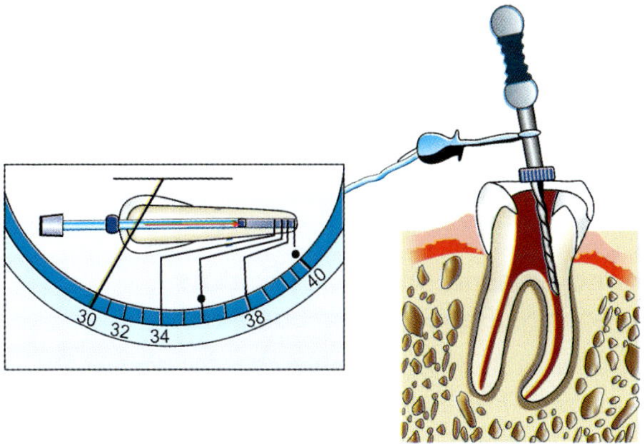


**Fig. 15.11A:** File being introduced in the canal

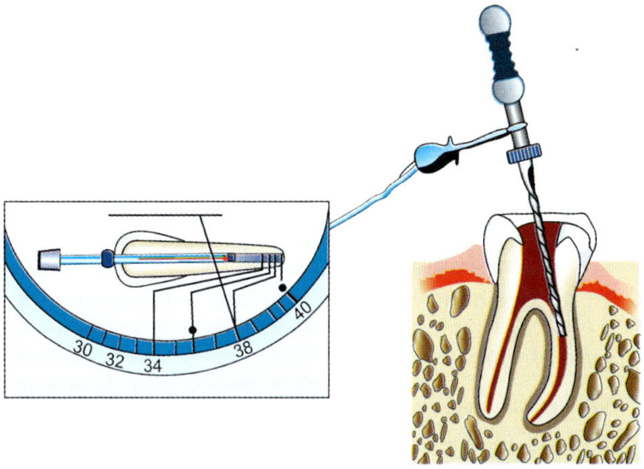


**Fig. 15.11B:** Steady increase in the reading as file approaches apex

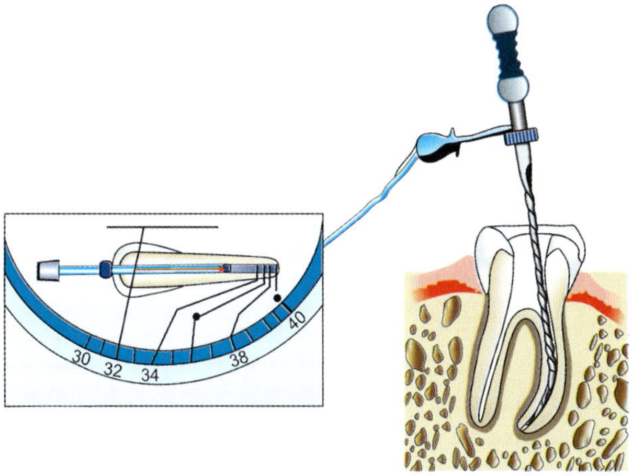


**Fig. 15.11C:** Reading showing that file has reached at apex

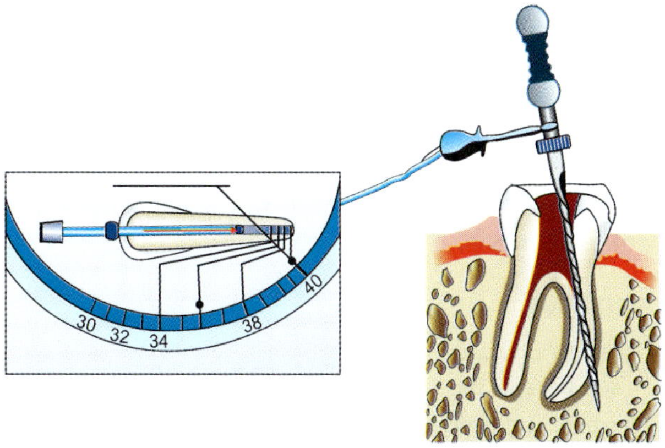


**Fig. 15.11D:** Sudden increase in reading indicates perforation

### Disadvantages

1. Requires a day field
2. Patient sensitivity
3. Requires calibration
4. Requires good contact with lip clip
5. Cannot estimate beyond 2 mm.

## Second Generation Apex Locators (Impedance Based Apex Locators)

They are also called as ***impedance apex locator*** which measure opposition to flow of alternating current or impedance. A major ***disadvantage*** of second generation apex locators is that root canal has to be free of electroconductive materials to obtain accurate readings. Presence of electroconductive irrigants changes the electric characteristics and lead to inaccurate readings. Various second generation apex locators are given below.

### Advantages

1. Does not require lip clip
2. No patient sensitivity
3. Analog method.

### Disadvantages

1. No digital read out
2. Difficult to operate
3. Canal should be free of electroconductive irrigants and tissue fluids.

**Various second generation apex locators**

- Sonoexplorer
- The apex finder (has digital LED indicator and is self calibrating)
- Endoanalyzer (combination of apex locator and pulp tester)
- Digipex (has digital LED indicator but requires calibration)
- Digipex II (combination of apex locators and pulp tester)
- Formation IV (digital LED light and display, self calibrating).

## Third Generation Apex Locators (Fig. 15.12)

They are also called ***frequency dependent apex locator***. They are based on the fact that different sites in canal give difference in impedance between high (8 KHz) and low (400 Hz) frequencies. The difference in impedance is least in the coronal part of canal. As the probe goes deeper into canal, difference increases. It is the greatest at cementodentinal junction.

Since impedance of a given circuit may be substantially influenced by the frequency of current flow, these are also known as frequency dependent. More appropriately, they should be termed as "Comparative Impedance" because they measure relative magnitudes of impedance which are converted into length information.

### Advantages

1. Easy to operate
2. Uses K-type file
3. Audible indication
4. Can operate in presence of fluids
5. Analog read out.

### Disadvantages

1. Requires lip clip
2. Chances of short circuit.

***Endex*** is original third generation apex locator which was described by Yamaoka et al. It uses two frequencies 5 and 1 KHz. As the instrument is moved apically, difference in impedance is noted. Commonly available third generation apex locators are mentioned in below:

**Various third generation apex locators**

| | |
|---|---|
| Endex | Original 3rd generation apex locator |
| Neosomo Ultimo | Apex locator with pulp tester |
| EZ apex locator | |
| Mark V plus | Apex locator with pulp tester |
| Root Zx | Shaping and cleaning of root canals with simultaneous monitoring of working length |
| *Combination of Apex Locator and Endodontic Handpiece* | |
| Tri Auto Zx | Cordless electrical handpiece with three safety mechanism |
| Endy 7000 | Reverses the rotation when tip reaches apical constriction |
| Sofy Zx | Monitor the location of file during instrumentation |

## Fourth Generation Apex Locators

Recently fourth generation electronic apex locators have been developed which measure resistance and capacitance separately rather than the resultant impedance value. There can be different combination of values of capacitance and resistance that provides the same impedance, thus the same foraminal reading. But by using fourth generation apex locator, this can be broken down into primary components and measures separately for better accuracy and thus less chances of occurrence of errors.

Though it is claimed to provide high accuracy but more studies are required for its confirmation.

## Combination Apex Locators and Endodontic Handpiece

***Tri Auto Zx*** (J Morita Calif) is cordless electric endodontic handpiece with built in root ZX apex locator. It has three safety mechanisms (Fig. 15.13).

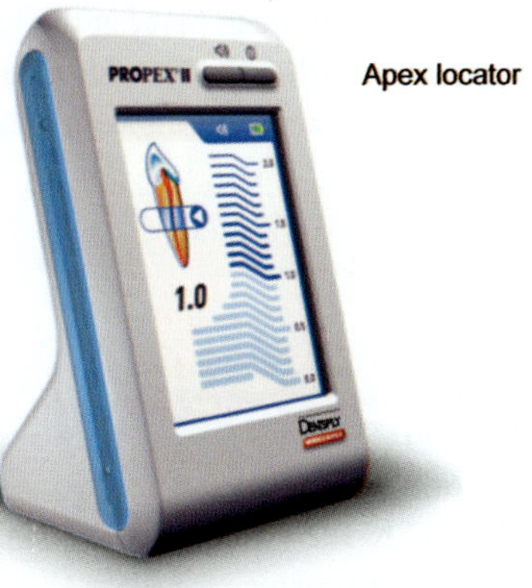


**Fig. 15.12:** Propex II apex locator

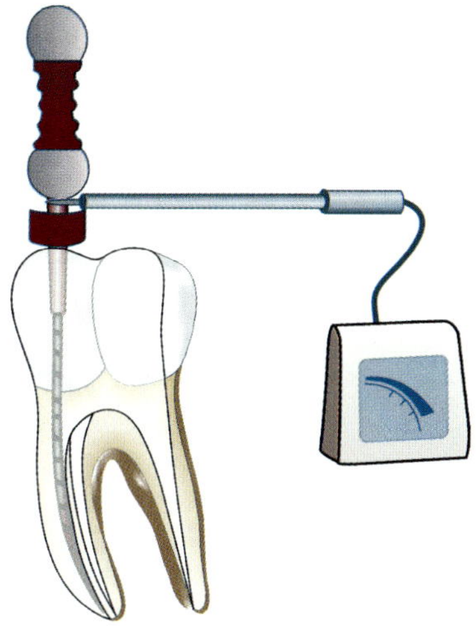

Fig. 15.13: Combination of apex locator and endodontic handpiece

*Autostart stop mechanism*: Handpiece starts rotation when instrument enters the canal and stops when it is removed.

*Autotorque reverse mechanism*: Handpiece automatically stops and reverses rotation when torque threshold (30 gm/cm) is exceed. It prevents instrument breakage.

*Autoapical-reverse mechanism*: It stops and reverses rotation when instrument tip reaches a distance from apical constriction taken for working length. It prevents apical perforation. Endy 7000 reverse the rotation when tip reaches the apical constriction. Sofy Zx (J Morita Calif) uses Root Zx to electronically monitor the location of file tip during whole of the instrumentation procedure.

## Basic Conditions for Accuracy of EALs

Whatever is the generation of apex locator; there are some basic conditions, which ensure accuracy of their usage.

1. Canal should be free from most of the tissue and debris.
2. The apex locator works best in a relatively dry environment. But extremely dry canals may result in low readings, i.e. long working length.
3. Cervical leakage must be eliminated and excess fluid must be removed from the chamber as this may cause inaccurate readings.
4. If residual fluid is present in the canal, it should be of low conductivity value, so that it does not interfere the functioning of apex locator.

   The descending order of conductivity of various irrigating solutions is 5.25 percent NaOCl > 17 percent EDTA > Saline.
5. Since EALs work on the basis of contact with canal walls and periapex. The better the adaptation of file to the canal walls, the more accurate as the reading.
6. Canals should be free from any type of blockage, calcifications, etc.
7. Battery of apex locator and other connections should be proper.

**Basic conditions for accuracy of EAL**
- Canal should be free from debris
- Canal should be relatively dry
- No cervical leakage
- Proper contact of file with canal walls and periapex
- No blockages or calcifications in canal

## SUMMARY

The most important thing to understand when determining working length is morphology of apical one-third of the canal. The consideration should be given to adopt the parameters of 0.5 - 0.0 mm (from the apical constriction) as most ideal terminating point in canal. One should use as many of techniques as possible during the course of treatment. First of all there should be a stable coronal reference point. Next step is to estimate working length from average anatomical length and preoperative radiograph. Finally calculate the correct working length using combination of various mentioned techniques, i.e. tactile sense, radiography, electronic apex locators, etc. Multiple measurements should be taken to determine accurate readings of working length. With so many advances coming up in the branch of endodontics we expect the future of apex locators to provide accurate readings in all the conditions of root canal without the need of calibrations.

## QUESTIONS

**Q. Define working length. What is significance of working length?**

**Q. Enumerate different methods of working length determination. Write in detail Ingle's method of working length determination.**

**Q. Classify apex locators. What are third generation apex locators.**

**Q. Write short notes on:**

a. Paper point sensitivity test

b. Advantages of apex locators

## BIBLIOGRAPHY

1. Bramante CM, Berbert A. Critical evaluation of methods of determining working length. Oral Surg 1974;37:463.
2. Cluster LE. Exact methods of locating the apical foramen. J Nat Dent Assoc 1918;5:815.
3. Ingle JI, Bakland LK. Endodontic cavity preparation. Textbook of endodontics (5th edn). Philadelphia: BC Decker, 2002.
4. Kim E, Lee SJ. Electronic apex locator. Dent Clin North Am 2004;48(1):35-54. (Review).
5. Krithika AC, Jandaswamy D, Velmurugan N, Krishna VG. Non-metallic grid for radiographic measurement. Aust Endod J 2008;34(1):36-38.
6. Kuttler Y. Microscopic investigation of root apexes. J Am Dent Assoc 1955;50:544-52.
7. McDonald NJ. The electronic determination of working length. Dent Clin North Am 1992;36:293.
8. Sunada I. New method for measuring the length of root canals. J Dent Res 1962;41(2):375-87.

# Irrigation and Intracanal Medicaments

CHAPTER 16



## INTRODUCTION

During the past 20 years, endodontics has begun to appreciate critically the important role of irrigation in successful endodontic treatment. The objective of endodontic treatment is to prevent or eliminate infection within the root canal. Over the years, research and clinical practices have concentrated on instrumentation, irrigation and medication of root canal system followed by obturation and the placement of coronal seal. It's truly said, "Instruments shape, irrigants clean". Every root canal system has spaces that cannot be cleaned mechanically. The only way we can clean webs, fins and anastomoses is through the effective use of an irrigation solution (Fig. 16.1). In order to get maximum efficiency from the irrigant, irrigant must reach the apical portion of the canal. Irrigation is an important part of root canal treatment because it assists us in (a) removing bacteria and debris (b) configuring the system so that it can be obturated to eliminate dead space. It has been found that use of saline as an irrigant before and after instrumentation, markedly resulted in a 100 to 1,000 fold reduction in bacterial counts (Bystrom, et al 1981).

### Ideal Requirements for an Irrigant

An ideal irrigant solution must fulfill the some criteria. It should

1. Have broadspectrum antimicrobial properties.
2. Aid in the debridement of the canal system.
3. Have the ability to dissolve necrotic tissue or debris.
4. Have low toxicity level.
5. Be a good lubricant.
6. Have low surface tension so that it can easily flow into inaccessible areas.
7. Be able to effectively sterilize the root canal (or at least disinfect them).
8. Be able to prevent formation of smear layer during instrumentation or dissolve the latter once it is formed.
9. Inactivate endotoxin.

Other desirable properties of ideal irrigants include availability, cost, ease of use, convenience, adequate shelf life and ease of storage. In addition to these properties, if endodontic irrigants come in contact with vital tissue, these should be systemically nontoxic, noncaustic to the periodontal tissue and have little potential to cause an anaphylactic reaction.

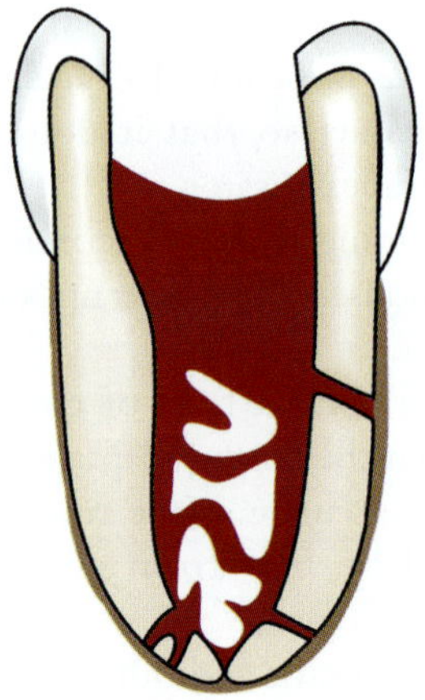

**Fig. 16.1:** Complicated root canal anatomy

**Properties of ideal irrigant solution**

1. Broad spectrum antimicrobial properties.
2. Aid in debridement of the root canal system.
3. Ability to dissolve necrotic tissue or debris.
4. Low toxicity level.
5. Good lubricant.
6. Low surface tension to flow into inaccessible area.
7. Ability to sterilize the canal.
8. Prevent/dissolve smear layer.
9. Inactivate endotoxin.

## FUNCTIONS OF IRRIGANTS

1. Irrigants perform physical and biologic functions. Dentin shavings get removed from canals by irrigation (Fig. 16.2). Thus, they do not get packed at the apex of root canal (Fig. 16.3).
2. Instruments do not work properly in dry canals. Their efficiency increases by use in wet canals. Instruments are less likely to break when canal walls are lubricated with irrigation.
3. Irrigants act as solvent of necrotic tissue, so they loosen debris, pulp tissue and microorganisms from irregular dentinal walls (Fig. 16.4).
4. Irrigants help in removing the debris from accessory and lateral canals where instruments cannot reach.
5. Most irrigants are germicidal but they also have antibacterial action.
6. Irrigants also have bleaching action to lighten teeth discolored by trauma or extensive silver restorations.
7. Though presence of irrigants in canal facilitate instrumentation but simultaneous use of some lubricating agents (RC prep, REDTAC, Glyde, etc.) make the instrumentation easier and smoother.

**Functions of irrigants**

1. Remove dentinal shavings by physical flushing.
2. Increase the efficiency of instruments.
3. Dissolve necrotic tissue.
4. Remove debris from lateral and accessory canals.
5. Germicidal as well as antibacterial properties.
6. Bleaching action.
7. Irrigants with lubricating agent further increase the efficiency.
8. Opening of dentinal tubules by removal of smear layer.

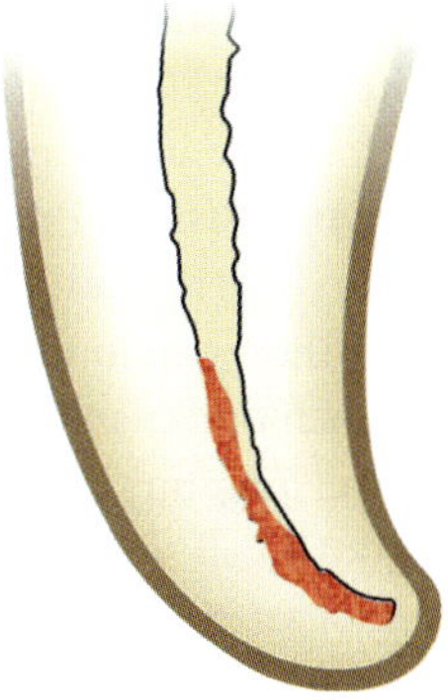

**Fig. 16.2:** Dentin shavings packed at apical third

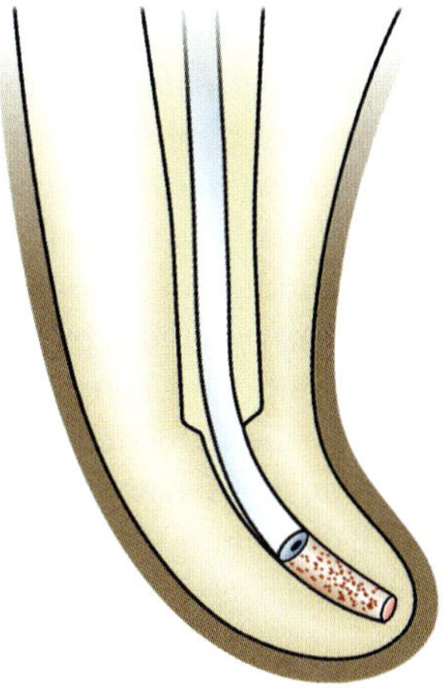

**Fig. 16.3:** Use of irrigating syringe to remove debris

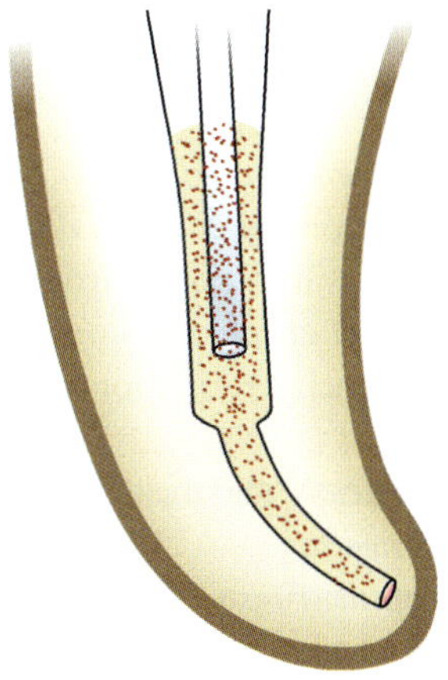

**Fig. 16.4:** Irrigation helps in loosening of debris

## FACTORS THAT MODIFY ACTIVITY OF INTRACANAL IRRIGATING SOLUTIONS

It is clear that there are several factors associated with the efficacy of the agents used. Some modifying factor such as host resistance, bacterial virulence, microbial resistance or susceptibility, etc. are beyond our control.

Other factors which can be controlled or at least predicted, such factors are:

1. ***Concentration:*** Several studies have revealed that the tissue dissolving ability of sodium hypochlorite is greater at a concentration of 5.2 percent than at 2.5 percent and 0.5 percent. But it has also been clearly demonstrated that higher concentrations are more cytotoxic than lower concentrations. This direct relationship of effectiveness and toxicity to concentration is generally true for all intracanal agents.
2. ***Contact:*** To be effective, the intracanal agent must contact the substrate (i.e. organic tissue or microbes). In case if it is not in contact with the substrate, it won't be able to dissolve or flushe out the debris. So, it is critical that the canals should be mechanically enlarged to carry the solution to the apical extent of canal preparation.

When the canals are sufficiently enlarged, the solution can be deposited directly in the apical area of the preparation with a fine irrigating needle (Fig. 16.3).

3. ***Presence of organic tissue:*** Presence of the organic tissues decreases the effectiveness of intracanal medicaments, so the organic tissue must be removed mechanically or chemomechanically by simultaneous use of instruments and irrigating solutions. If organic debris are present in root canal space, its protein content will coagulate as a result of its reaction with the medicament. This coagulation serves as a barrier to prevent further penetration of medicament, thus limiting its effectiveness.
4. ***Quantity of the irrigant used:*** Baber, et al proved that ability of solution to debride is directly related to the quantity of irrigating solution. In case of medicament, increase in quantity results in increase in cytotoxicity.
5. ***Gauze of irrigating needle:*** Usually a 27 or 28 gauze needle is preferred as it can go deeper in canal for better delivery and debridement action.
6. ***Surface tension of irrigant:*** Lower the surface tension, better is wettability, and hence more penetration in narrow areas for better debridement.
7. ***Temperature of the irrigant:*** It has been shown in studies that if sodium hypochlorite is warmed before irrigation, it is much (60-70°C) more effective as a tissue solvent.
8. ***Frequency of irrigation:*** Frequency of irrigation depends upon amount of work that a particular instrument performs. In general, a canal should be copiously irrigated during instrumentation. In case of narrow and longer canals, frequency of irrigation further increases.

   *Increased frequency of irrigation has two advantages:*
   - More irrigation causes better debridement of tissues.
   - Each time a fresh potent irrigants plays an action.
9. ***Level of observation:*** Maximum actions of irrigant occurs on coronal part of root canal where as minimal on apical end.
10. ***Canal diameter:*** Wider the canal, better is debridement action of irrigant.
11. ***Age of irrigant:*** Freshly prepared solutions are more efficient then older ones.

**Factors modifying the activity of irrigating solutions**

1. *Concentration:* Tissue dissolving capability of NaOCl is higher at 5.2 percent.
2. *Contact:* To effective, irrigant must come in contact with the substrate.
3. *Presence of organic tissue:* Organic tissues must be removed for effective irrigation.
4. *Quantity of the irrigant used:* Increase in quantity increases the effectiveness.
5. *Gauze of irrigating needle:* 27 or 28 gauze is preferred for better penetration in the canal.
6. *Surface tension of irrigant:* Lower the surface tension, better is wettability.
7. *Temperature of irrigant:* Warming the NaOCl increases its efficacy.
8. Frequency of irrigation: More is frequency, better are the results.
9. *Level of observation.*
10. *Canal diameter:* Wider the canal, better is action of irrigant
11. *Age of irrigant*: Freshly prepared solutions are more efficient then older ones.

**Commonly used irrigating solutions**

*Chemically non-active solution*
- Water
- Saline
- Local anesthetic

*Chemically active materials:*
- Alkalis: Sodium hypochlorite 0.5-5.25 percent
- Chelating agents: Ethylene diamine tetra acetic acid (EDTA)
- Oxidizing agents: Hydrogen peroxide, carbamide peroxide
- Antibacterial agents: Chlorhexidine, Bisdequalinium acetate
- Acids: 30 percent hydrochloric acid
- Enzymes: Streptokinase, papain, trypsin
- Detergents: Sodium lauryl sulfate

## CHOICE OF MAIN IRRIGANT SOLUTION

Currently, there is no single irrigant that can fulfill all of these criteria and so we have to rely on different irrigating solutions and sometimes their combination. The main irrigants include sodium hypochlorite, chlorhexidine and ethylene diamine tetra-acetic acid. Unfortunately, this does not seem to be one clear regimen that should be followed to maximize the benefits of each of these materials.

### Normal Saline (Fig. 16.5)

Normal saline causes gross debridement and lubrication of root canals. Since it very mild in action, it can be used as an adjunct to chemical irrigant. Normal saline as 0.9% W/V is commonly

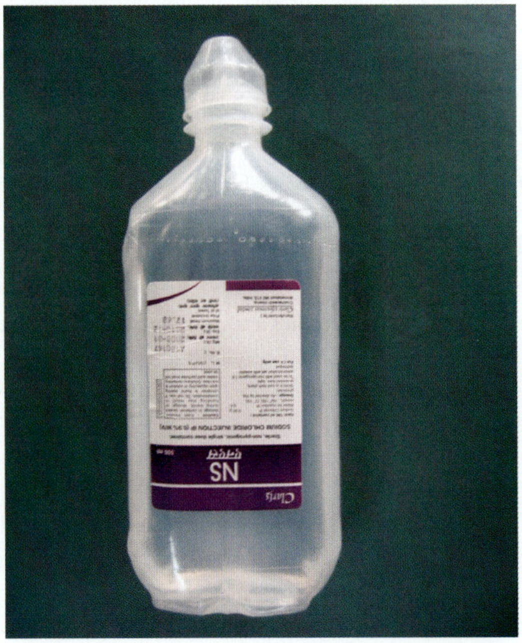

Fig. 16.5: Normal saline

used as irrigant in endodontics. It basically acts by flushing action. It can also be used as final rinse for root canals to remove any chemical irrigant left after root canal preparation.

### Advantage

It is biocompatible in nature. No adverse reaction even if extruded periapically because osmotic pressure of normal saline is same as that of the blood.

### Disadvantages

- Does not possess dissolution and disinfecting properties.
- Too mild to thoroughly clean the canals
- Cannot clear microbial flora from inaccessible areas like accessory canal
- Does not possess antimicrobial activity
- Does not remove smear layer.

## Sodium Hypochlorite

Sodium hypochlorite is a clear, pale, green-yellow liquid with strong odor of chlorine (Fig. 16.6). It is easily miscible with water and gets decomposed by light.

## Historical Review

1. Sodium hypochlorite was first introduced during the World War I by chemist **Henry Drysdale Dakin** for treating infected wounds. It is also known as **"Dakin's solution"**. The original concentration suggested by Dakin was 0.5 percent but concentration commonly used in practice is 5.25 percent.
2. Walker in 1936 first suggested its use in root canal therapy.
3. Grossman in 1941 demonstrated the tissue dissolving ability of Chlorinated soda when used double strength and recommend its use as intracanal medicament (Double strength chlorinated soda is same as 5 percent NaOCl).

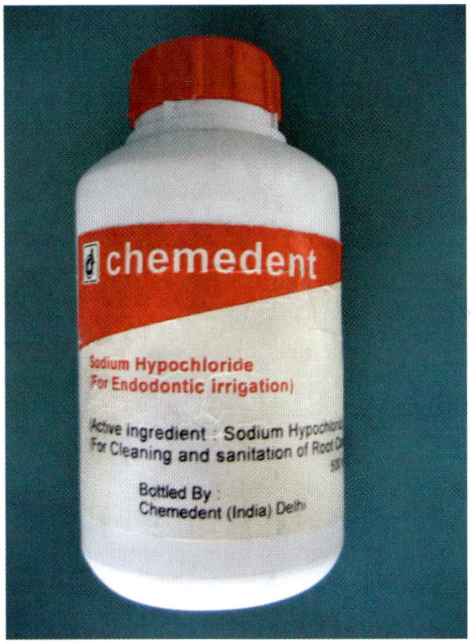


Fig. 16.6: Sodium hypochlorite

4. Spangberg in 1973 said that 0.5 percent NaOCl was sufficient to provide germicidal activity but was less toxic to tissue culture than 5 percent NaOCl.
5. Madden in 1977 compared 5, 2.5 and 0.5 percent NaOCl and found that 5 percent and 2.5 percent solution was better than 0.5 for tissue dissolving.
6. Foley, et al. in 1983 tested effectiveness of 0.5 percent NaOCl and Glyoxide and concluded that both can effectively kill bacteriod melaninogenicus and peptostreptococci.
7. Kozol, et al. concluded that sodium hypochlorite was detrimental to neutrophilic chemotaxis and toxic to fibroblasts and endothelial cells.

1. Introduced in World War Ist by Dakin.
2. Walker-1936—First suggested its use in root canal therapy.
3. Grossman-1941—Used it as an intracanal medicament.
4. Spangberg-1973-0.5 percent—NaOCl has good germicidal activity.
5. Madden-1977—Compared the different concentrations of Sodium hypochlorite.
6. Foley et al-1983—Compared effectiveness of 0.5 percent NaOCl and Glyoxide.

## Mechanism of Action of Sodium Hypochlorite

- At body temperature, reactive chlorine in aqueous solution exists in two forms-hypochlorite ($OCl^-$) and hypochlorous acid (HOCl). State of available chlorine depends on pH of solution, i.e. above pH of 7.6, it is mainly hypochlorite form and below this pH, it is hypochlorous acid
- Presence of 5 percent of free chlorine in sodium hypochlorite is responsible for breakdown of proteins into amino groups
- The pH of commonly used sodium hypochlorite is 12, at which the OCl form exits. Hypochlorite dissolves necrotic tissue because of its high alkaline nature (pH 12)
- To increase the efficacy of NaOCl solution, 1 percent sodium bicarbonate is added as buffering agent. Buffering makes the solution unstable, thus decreases its shelf life to even less than one week. Buffered and diluted sodium hypochlorite should be stored in dark and cool place.

**Methods by which we can increase the efficacy of sodium hypochlorite** are (Flow Chart 16.1):

1. *Time:* Since antimicrobial effectiveness of sodium hypochlorite is directly related to its contact time with the canal, greater the contact time, more effective it is. This is especially important in necrotic cases.
2. *Heat:* It has been shown that warming sodium hypochlorite to 60-70°, increases its tissue dissolving properties (Fig. 16.7). But one should be careful not to overheat the solution because this can cause breakdown of sodium hypochlorite constituents and thus may damage the solution.
3. *Specialized irrigating syringes:* Most researches have shown that unaided irrigation requires at least a size #25 apex for it to reach the more apical portions of canals. Newer specialized side venting endodontic syringes with narrower diameter (32 gauge) are available which aid in getting irrigant closer to apex and help the irrigant to move sideways (Fig. 16.8).

**Flow Chart 16.1:** Factors affecting the efficacy of sodium hypochlorite

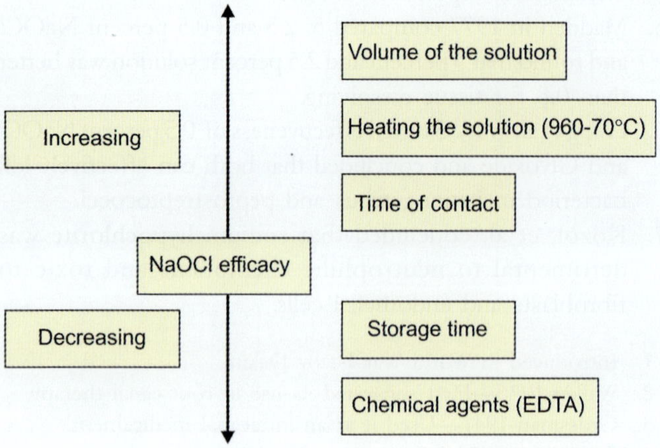


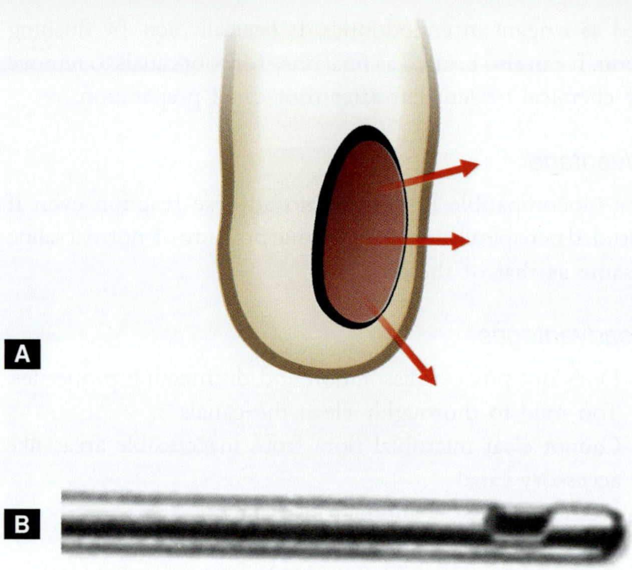


**Fig. 16.8:** Needle with side venting helps to move the irrigant sidways in whole canal

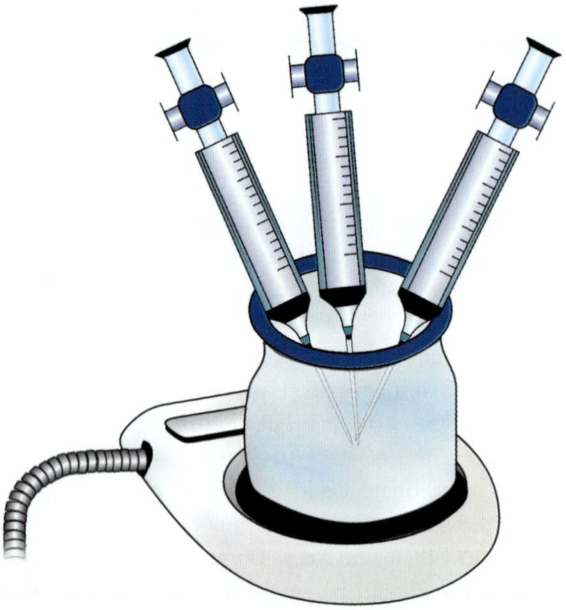

**Fig. 16.7:** To warm NaOCl, syringes filled with NaOCl are placed in 60-70°C (140°F) water bath

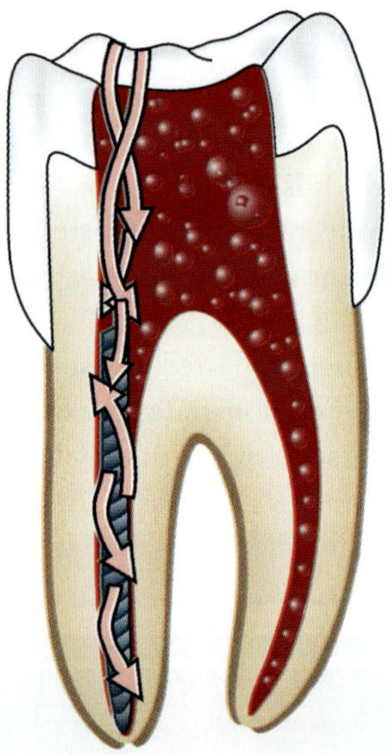

**Fig. 16.9:** Ultrasonic activation of irrigating solution

4. *Ultrasonic activation of:* Sodium hypochlorite has also shown to accelerate chemical reaction, create cavitational effect and thus achieve a superior cleansing action (Fig. 16.9). But it is seen that if ultrasonic activation of sodium hypochlorite is used, it is better to apply ultrasonic instrument after canal preparation. A freely oscillating instrument causes better effect than the instrument which binds to canal walls.

   Also the ultrasonic files cause more uncontrolled cutting of canal walls especially if used during preparation. Thus use of a noncutting instrument after canal preparation is best option for optimal effects.

## Precautions to be Taken While Using Sodium Hypochlorite Solution

It is important to remember that though sodium hypochlorite is nontoxic during intracanal use but 5.25 percent NaOCl can cause serious damage to tissue if injected periapically (Fig. 16.10).

If sodium hypochlorite gets extruded into periapical tissues, it causes excruciating pain, periapical bleeding and swelling. As potential for spread of infection is related to tissue destruction, medication like antibiotics, analgesics, antihistamine should be prescribed accordingly. In addition to these, reassurance to the patient is the prime consideration.

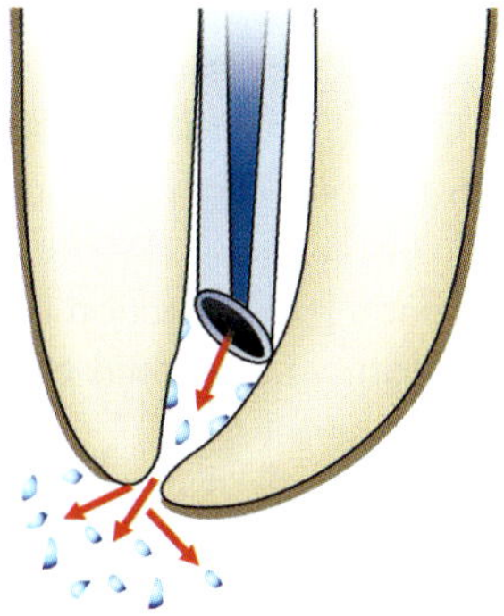

Fig. 16.10: Forceful irrigation can cause periapical extrusion of sodium hypochlorite solution

Thus irrigation with sodium hypochlorite solution should always be performed passively especially in cases with larger apical diameters and needles with very small diameter, also the syringe should never be locked in the canal.

### *Advantages of Sodium Hypochlorite*

1. It causes tissue dissolution.
2. It has antibacterial and bleaching action.
3. It causes lubrication of canals.
4. Economical.
5. Easily available.

### *Disadvantages*

1. Because of high surface tension, its ability to wet dentin is less.
2. Irritant to tissues, if extruded periapically, it can result in severe cellular damage.
3. If comes in contact, it cause inflammation of gingiva because of its caustic nature.
4. It can bleach the clothes if spilt.
5. It has bad odor and taste.
6. Vapors of sodium hypochlorite can irritate the eyes.
7. It can be corrosive to instruments.

### Use of Sodium Hypochlorite in Combination with other Medicaments

Many studies have shown that efficacy of sodium hypochlorite as antimicrobial agent is increased when it is used in combination with other solutions such as calcium hydroxide, EDTA or chlorhexidine.

The tissue dissolving capacity of sodium hypochlorite or chlorhexidine is found to be increased when tissue is pretreated with calcium hydroxide (Hasselgren, et al).

Wadachi, et al. in their study have shown that combination of calcium hydroxide and sodium hypochlorite was better than either of medicament alone. Various studies have shown that combination of sodium hypochlorite and EDTA has more bactericidal effect which is probably due to removal of contaminated smear layer by EDTA.

The alternate use of sodium hypochlorite and chlorhexidine results in greater reduction of microflora than the use of either alone as shown by ***Kuruvilla and Kamath***.

## UREA

It is a white, odorless, crystalline powder. It was used in World War first as a therapeutic agent for infected wounds. Urea solution (40% by weight) is mild solvent of necrotic tissue and pus and is mild antiseptic too. In 1951, Blechman and Cohen suggested that 30 percent urea solution can be used as root canal irrigant in patients with vital pulp as well as those with necrotic pulp.

### Mechanism of Action

1. *Denaturation of protein:* Urea denatures the protein by destroying bonds of the secondary structure resulting in loss of functional activity of protein. This mode of action is responsible for its antiseptic property.
2. It has the property of chemically debriding the wound by softening the underlying substrate of fibrin.

### Uses

1. It is excellent vehicle for antimicrobials such as sulfonamides.
2. It has low toxicity and so, it can be used in patients where vital uninfected pulp has been removed.
3. It can be used in open apex or in areas of resorptive defects.

## HYDROGEN PEROXIDE

It is clear, odorless liquid. It is mainly the 3 percent solution which is used as an irrigating agent (Fig. 16.11).

### Mechanism of Action

1. It is highly unstable and easily decomposed by heat and light. It rapidly dissociates into $H_2O$ + [O] (water and nascent oxygent). On coming in contact with tissue enzymes catalase and peroxidase, the liberated [O] produces bactericidal effect but this effect is transient and diminishes in presence of organic debris.
2. It causes oxidation of bacterial sulfhydryl group of enzymes and thus interferes with bacterial metabolism.

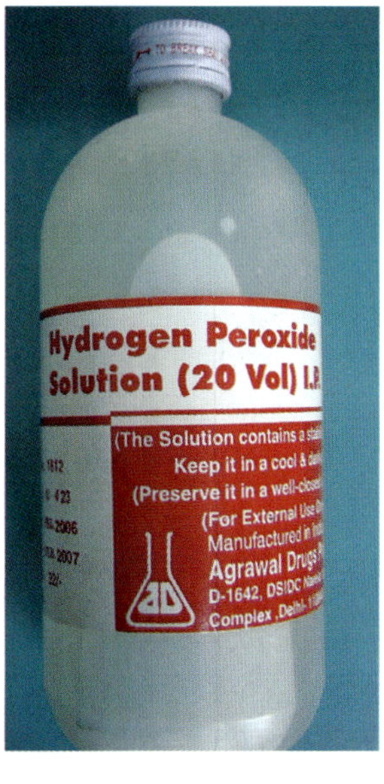


Fig. 16.11: Hydrogen peroxide

3. The rapid release of [O] nascent oxygen on contact with organic tissue results in effervescence or bubbling action which is thought to aid in mechanical debridement by dislodging particles of necrotic tissue and dentinal debris and floating them to the surface.

### Use

It is used as an irrigating solution either alone or alternatively with sodium hypochlorite. The advantage of using alternating solutions of 3 percent $H_2O_2$ and 5.2 percent NaOCl are:

1. Effervescent reaction by Hydrogen peroxide bubbles pushes debris mechanically out of root canal.
2. Solvent action of sodium hypochlorite on organic debris.
3. Disinfecting and bleaching action by both solutions.

While using in combination with sodium hypochlorite, always use sodium hypochlorite in the last because hydrogen peroxide can react with pulp debris and blood to produce gas (nascent oxygen) which builds up pressure on closing the tooth, this can result in severe pain.

## UREA PEROXIDE

It is white crystalline powder with slight odor. It is soluble in water, alcohol and glycerine.

### Mechanism of Action

It decomposes rapidly when exposed to heat, light or moisture. It dissociates into urea and hydrogen peroxide.

$$\text{Urea peroxide} \rightarrow \text{Urea} + H_2O_2$$

Its mechanism of action combines the effects of urea and hydrogen peroxide.

The anhydrous glycerol increases the stability of urea peroxide.

### Use

Ten percent solution of urea peroxide in anhydrous glycerol base is commonly available as (Glyoxide). The advantage of adding glycerol are:

i. It increases the stability of solution, thus increases shelf life.
ii. It acts as a good lubricant, so facilitates negotiation and instrumentation of thin, tortuous root canals.
iii. Glyoxide can be used along with EDTA to clean the walls of the canal.

#### *Disadvantages*

It dissociates more slowly than hydrogen peroxide ($H_2O_2$). So, its effervescence is prolonged but not as pronounced. This can be overcome by alternating irrigation with sodium hypochlorite.

## CHLORHEXIDINE

- Chlorhexidine was developed in the late 1940's in the research laborites
- Chlorhexidine was the most potent of the tested bisbiguanides
- It has strong base and is most stable in the form of its salts, i.e. chlorhexidine gluconate
- It is a potent antiseptic which is widely used for chemical plaque control in the oral cavity in concentrations of 0.2 percent
- It shows optimal antimicrobial action between pH 5.5-7.0
- For using it as an irrigant, it should be used as 2 percent in concentration.

### Combination of 0.2 percent Chlorhexidine and 2 percent Sodium Hypochlorite

This combination is commonly used as irrigant in root canals because:

- Chlorhexidine being a base forms salts of organic acids where as sodium hypochlorite being an oxidizing agent, oxidizing gluconate part chlorhexidine gluconate and forms gluconic acid
- There is an increase in ionizing capacity of chlorhexidine due to formation of chlorhexidine Cl. ($Cl^-$ group get attached to guanidine part chlorhexidine)
- Combination of chlorhexidine (PH 6.5) and sodium hypochlorite (PH 9-10) is more alkaline (pH 10) making it more effective.

### Mechanisms of Action

Chlorhexidine is broad spectrum antimicrobial agent. The antibacterial mechanism of chlorhexidine is related to its cationic bisbiguanide molecular structure. The cationic molecule is absorbed to the negatively charged inner cell membrane and causes leakage of intracellular components. At low concentration, it acts as a bacteriostatic, whereas at higher concentrations; it causes coagulation and precipitation of cytoplasm and therefore acts as bactericidal.

In addition, chlorhexidine has the property of substantivity (residual effect). Both 2 and 0.2 perent chlorhexidine can cause residual antimicrobial activity for 72 hours, if used as an endodontic irrigant.

#### *Advantages and Uses*

1. A 2 percent solution is used as root irrigant in canals.
2. A 0.2 percent solution can be used in controlling plaque activity.
3. It is more effective on gram-positive bacteria than gram-negative bacteria.

#### *Disadvantages*

1. It is not considered as the main irrigant in standard endodontic therapy.
2. It is unable to dissolve necrotic tissue remnants.
3. It is less effective on gram-negative than on gram-positive bacteria.

## CHELATING AGENTS

After canals are instrumented, an organic layer remains which covers the dentinal tubules. Controversies still exist whether

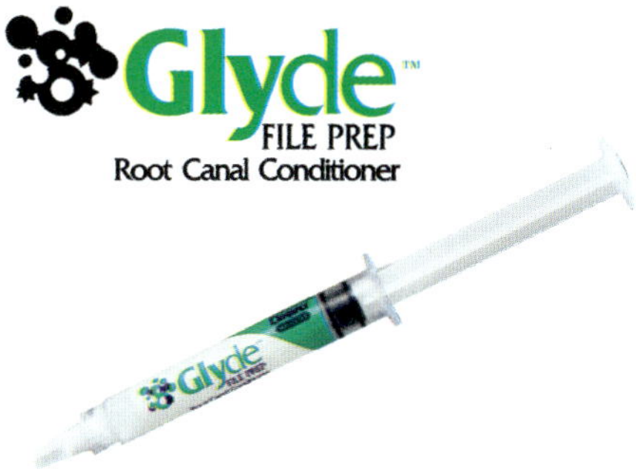


Fig. 16.12: Chelating agent

to keep or to remove smear layer as it relates to permeability of dentin. However most of studies have recommended removal of smear layer because it is the source of microorganisms and also the closest possible adaptation of endodontic filling is possible only after its removal.

Though sodium hypochlorite is thought to be almost ideal irrigating solution but it does not possess chelating properties. EDTA and other chelating agents like citric acid, polyacrylic acids are used for this purpose (Fig. 16.12).

**Chelating agent** is defined as a chemical which combines with a metal to form chelate.

EDTA is most commonly used chelating agent (Flow chart 16.2). It was introduced in dentistry by Nygaard Ostby for cleaning and shaping of the canals. It contains four acetic acid groups attached to ethylenediamine. EDTA is relatively nontoxic and slightly irritating in weak solutions. The effect of EDTA on dentin depends on the concentration of EDTA solution and length of time it is in contact with dentin. Serper and Calt in their study observed that EDTA was more effective at a neutral pH than at a pH 9.0. They showed that for optimal cleaning and shaping of canals EDTA should be used at neutral pH and with lower concentrations.

## Functions of EDTA

- Lubrication
- Emulsification
- Holding debris in suspension
- Smear layer removal (Figs 16.13A to C).

## Mechanism of Action

- It inhibits growth of bacteria and ultimately destroys them by starvation because EDTA chelates with the metallic ions in medium which are needed for growth of microorganisms.
- EDTA has self limiting action. It forms a stable bond with calcium and dissolve dentin, but when all chelating ions have reacted, an equilibrium reached which prevents further dissolution.

Flow Chart 16.2: Structural formula of EDTA

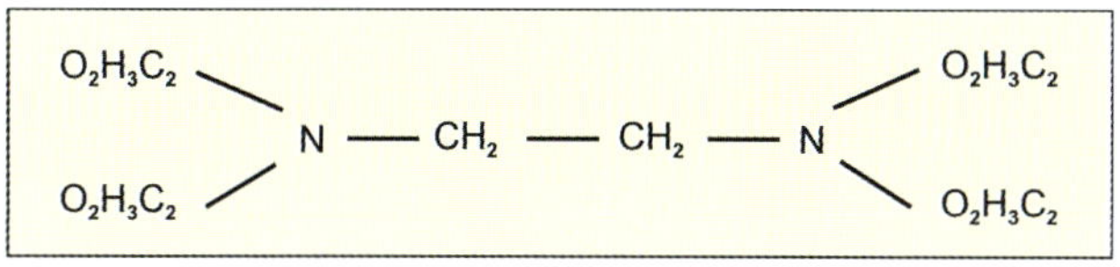


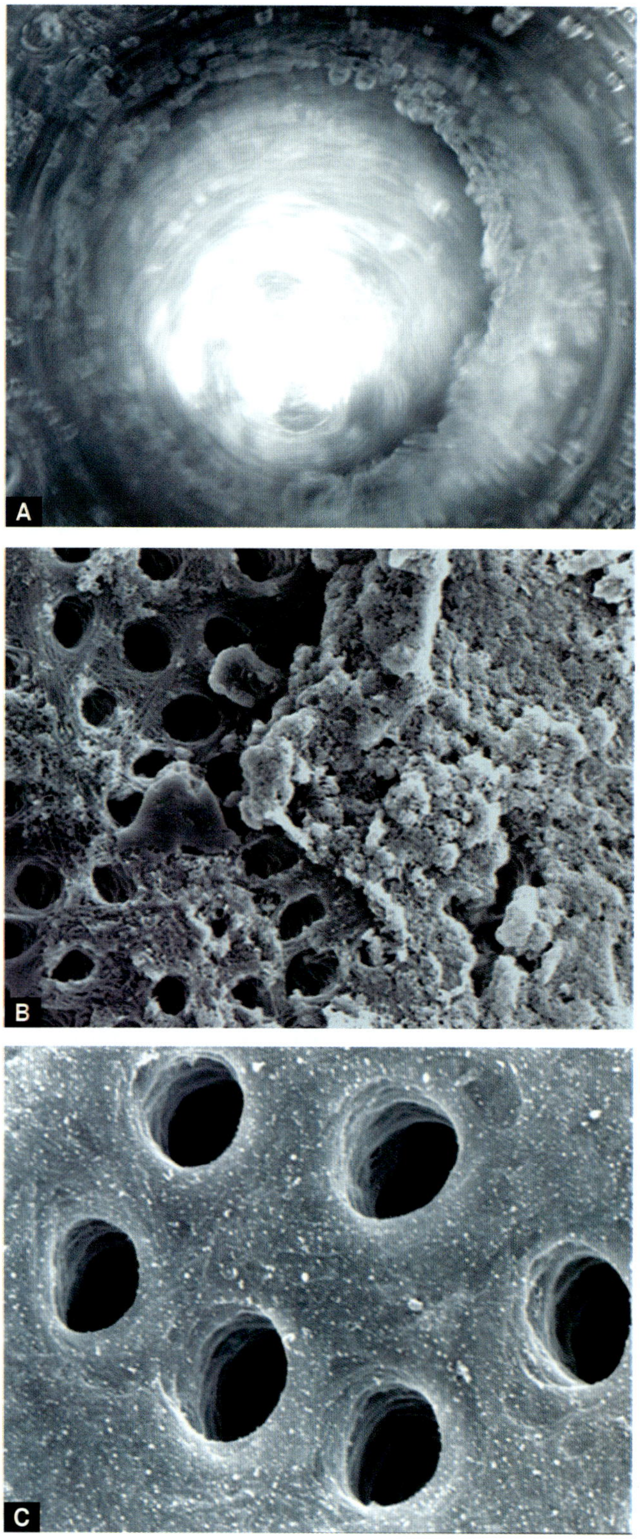


Figs 16.13A to C: (A) Dentin tubules blocked with smear lyear, (B) Application of chelating agent causes removal of smear layer, (C) Opening of dentinal tubules

## Uses of EDTA

- It has dentin dissolving properties
- It helps in enlarging narrow canals

- Makes easier manipulation of instruments
- Reduces time needed for debridement.

### Different Forms of EDTA

1. **R-EDTA:** In this EDTA is combined with cetrimide, i.e. cetyllrimethy 1 ammonium bromide. It helps in better cleaning of canals.
2. **EDTAT:** (EDTA + Texapon) here EDTA is combined with sodium lauryl sulfate which results in decreasing the surface tension.
3. **EDTA-C:** It is commercially available as 15 percent solution and pH of 7.3 under the name EDTAC because it contains cetavelon, a quaternary ammonium compound which has been added to it for its disinfecting properties. Also the introduction of surfactant reduces the contact angle of EDTA when placed on dentin surface and thus enhances its cleaning efficacy.

A chelating agent can be applied in liquid or paste form. The use of paste type preparation was first advocated by Stewart who devised a combination of urea peroxide with glycerol. Later this product was modified by combining EDTA, urea peroxide and water soluble carbowax, i.e. polyethylene glycol as vehicle. This product is commercially available as RC Prep. It is an effective lubricating and cleaning agent. Presence of glycol makes it a lubricant and coats the instrument which facilitates its movement in the canal.

A viscous suspension of chelator promotes the emulsification of organic debris and facilitates negotiation of the canal. Collagen is the major constituent of vital pulp which can be packed into glue like mass which contributes to iatrogenic blocks. Without the use of a chelator, vital tissue tends to collapse and readheres to itself but use of chelator does not allow this phenomenon to occur and accelerate emulsification of tissue.

Various studies have shown that combined use of sodium hypochlorite and RC Prep causes an efficient cleaning of canals. Their combination causes release of nascent oxygen which kills anaerobic bacteria and effervescence action which mechanically pushes the debris out of canal.

### Citric Acid

Other commonly used chelating agent for removal of smear layer as irrigating solution is citric acid.

It can be used alone or in combination with other irrigants but EDTA or citric acid should never be mixed with sodium hypochlorite because EDTA and citric acid strongly interact with sodium hypochlorite. This immediately reduces the available chlorine in solution and thus making it ineffective against bacteria.

### Polyacrylic Acid

Another chelating agent suggested as irrigant is polyacrylic acid, commercially available as Durelon and Fuji II liquid.

### Hydroxyethylidene Bisphosphonate (HEBP)

It is also known as Etidronate having chelating properties, suggested as an irrigating solution. The advantageous property of HEBP as chelating agent is that it shows only short term interference with sodium hypochlorite.

### Salvizol

It belongs to surface acting materials like quaternary ammonium group. It shows antibacterial property even in presence of

**Summary of Irrigants Used during Endodontic Therapy**

| *S.No.* | *Irrigant* | *Normal saline* | *Sodium hypochlorite* | *Hydrogen peroxide* | *EDTA* | *Chlorhexidine* |
|---|---|---|---|---|---|---|
| 1. | Concentration | 0.9% | 1%, 2.5%, 5.25% | 3% | 15%, 17% | 0.12%, .2%, 2% |
| 2. | pH | 7.3 | 10.8-12 | 6 | 7.3-8 | 5.5-7 |
| 3. | Mechanism of action | Physical flushing | Bactericidal | Bactericidal<br>i. Dissociates in $H_2O$ and [O][O] has bactericidal activity<br>ii. Causes oxidation of sulfhydryl groups of enzymes<br>iii. Effervescent reaction of $H_2O_2$ bubbles causes mechanical debridement | i. Lubrication, emulsification and holding debris in suspension<br>ii. Forms chelate with calcium ions of dentin making it more friable and easier to manipulate | i. At low concentration bacteriostatic<br>ii. At high concentration bactericidal by causing coagulation and precipitation of cytoplasm |
| 4. | Advantages | No side effects if extruded periapically | Has dissolution, disinfectant and antimicrobial properties | Has disinfectant and antimicrobial property | • Dentin dissolving property<br>• Makes easier manipulation of canals | i. Property of substantivity<br>ii. More effective against gram-positive bacteria |
| 5. | Disadvantages | • Too mild to be disinfectant | • Can cause tissue injury if extruded periapically | | | i. Unable to dissolve necrotic tissue remanants<br>ii. Less effective on gram-positive bacteria |

organic materials. It is most effective against gram-positive and gram-negative microorganisms and fungi.

## ULTRASONIC IRRIGATION

Ultrasonic irrigation has shown to clean the root canals or eliminates bacteria from the walls better than conventional methods (hand instrumentation alone).

Use of ultrasonics causes continuous flow of an irrigant in the canal, thus prevents accumulation of debris in the canal (Fig. 16.9).

### Mechanism of Action

When a small file is placed in canal and ultrasonic activation is given. The ultrasonic energy passes through irrigating solution and exerts its "acoustic streaming or scrubbing" effect on the canal wall (Fig. 16.14). This mechanical energy warms the irrigant solution (Sodium hypochlorite) and dislodges debris from canal. The combination of activating and heating the irrigating solution is adjunct in cleaning the root canal (Flow Chart 16.3).

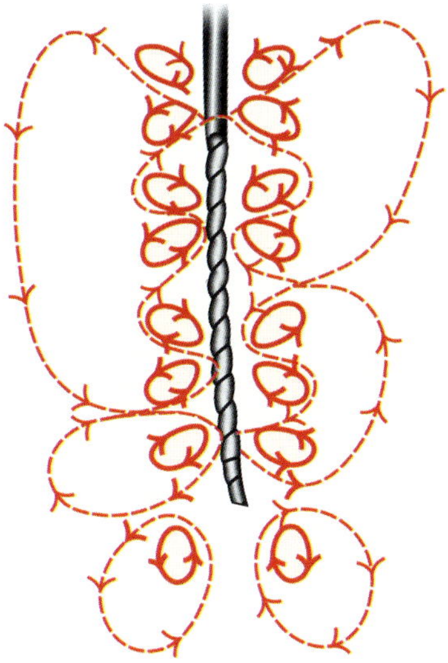

**Fig. 16.14:** Ultrasonic irrigation

**Flow Chart 16.3:** Ultrasonic irrigation

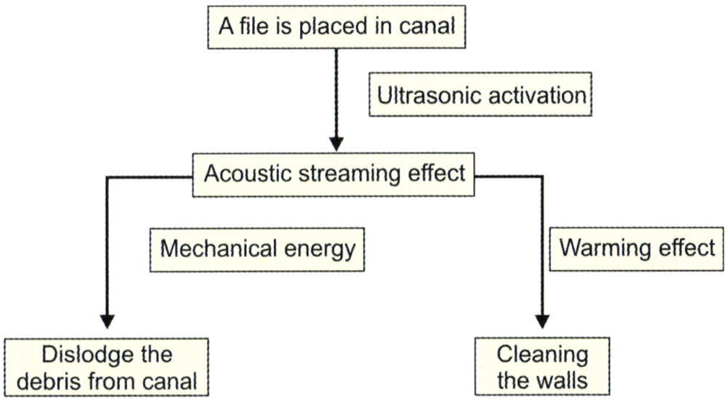


#### *Advantages*

1. It cleans the root canal walls better than conventional ones.
2. It removes the smear layer efficiently.
3. It dislodges the debris from the canal better due to acoustic effect.

#### *Disadvantages*

1. Ultrasonic preparation of the canal is found to be unpredictable.
2. It can lead to excessive cutting of canal walls and may damage the finished preparation.

## NEWER IRRIGATING SOLUTIONS

### Electrochemically Activated Solution

It is one of newer irrigant solution which is produced from the tap water and low concentrated salt solutions. Further, electrochemical treatment results in synthesis of two type of solutions, i.e. anolyte (produced in anode chamber) and catholyte (produced in cathode chamber) (Flow Chart 16.4).

Anolyte solution has also been termed as super oxidized water or oxidative potential water but now a days neutral and alkaline solutions has been recommended for clinical application.

Advantages of electrochemically activated solution:

1. Non-toxic to biological tissues.
2. Effective with wide range of microbial spectra.

**Flow Chart 16.4:** Electrochemically activated solution

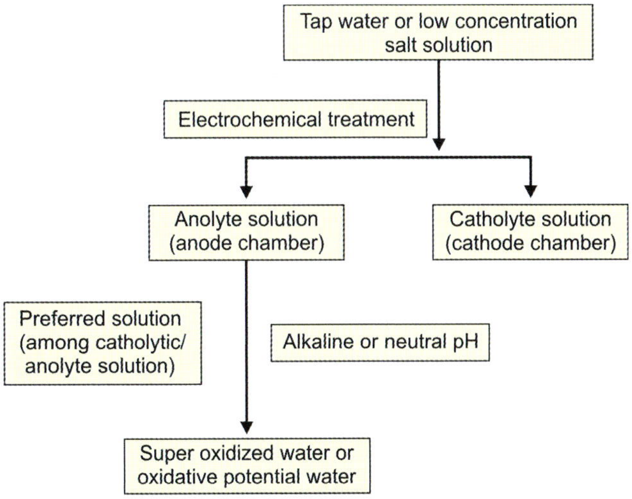


### Ozonated Water Irrigation

Ozonated water is newer irrigant solution which is shown to be powerful antimicrobial agent against bacteria, fungi, protozoa and viruses. It is suggested that ozonated water may prove to be useful in controlling oral infectious micro organism.

Its advantages include:

- Its potency
- Ease of handling
- Lack of mutagenicity
- Rapid microbial effects.

### Ruddle's Solution

It is a new experimental irrigating solution, introduce in the endodontics in an attempt to visualize the microanatomy of the canal system.

#### Composition

Ruddle's solution consists of:

a. Seventy percent EDTA
b. Five percent NaOCl
c. Hypaque which is an aqueous solution of iodide salts viz; Ditrizoate and sodium iodine.

#### Mechanism of Action

1. The solvent action of sodium hypochlorite, improved penetration due to EDTA and radiopacity because of hypaque helps to visualize the shape and microanatomy of canals and dentin thickness during endodontic therapy.
2. The solvent action of sodium hypochlorite clears the contents of root canal system and thus enables hypaque component to flow into every nook and corner of the canal system such as fracture, missed canals and defective restoration.

So Ruddle's solution can be helpful for improving diagnostic accuracy, treatment planning, management of procedural accidents, but further studies are needed to prove it as effective irrigating solution.

### Photo Activated Disinfection (PAD)

PAD is a breakthrough in the fight against pathogenic bacteria. It is a fast, effective and minimally invasive disinfection system which is considered to kill more than 99.99 percent of bacteria in the endodontic biofilm.

#### Mechanism of PAD

Here, low powered laser light is transmitted through the disposable fibro-optic tip to activate the PAD antibacterial solution. Within 1-3 minutes, the PAD system eliminates more than 99.99 percent bacteria found in root canals.

#### Advantages of PAD

1. It has shown to be the most effective antimicrobial agent. It can effectively kill gram-negative, gram-positive, aerobic and anaerobic bacteris, in other words it eliminates all types of bacteria.
2. It overcomes the problems of antibiotic resistance.
3. It can kill bacteria present in complex biofilm such as subgingival plaque which is typically resistant to action of antimicrobial agents.
4. PAD does not pose any thermal risk due to low power of PAD laser.
5. It does not cause any sensitization.
6. Neither the PAD solution nor its products are toxic to patients.

### MTAD (A Mixture of a Tetracycline Isomer, an Acid and a Detergent)

Recently MTAD has been introduced in 2000 as a final rinse for disinfection of root canal system. Torabinejad, et al have shown that MTAD is able to safely remove the smear layer and is effective against Enterococcus fecalis, a microorganism resistant to the action of antimicrobial medication.

#### Purpose of MTAD

The purpose of using MTAD is to:

a. Disinfect the dentin
b. Remove the smear layer
c. Open the dentinal tubules and allow the antimicrobial agents to penetrate the entire root canal system.

#### Composition

a. Tetracycline: It is bacteriostatic broad spectrum antibiotic.
   - It has low pH and acts as calcium chelator.
   - It removes smear layer
   - It has property of substanitivity
   - It promotes healing.
b. Citric acid: It is bactericidal in nature and removes smear layer.
c. Detergent (Tween 80): It decreases surface tension.

#### Advantages

1. It is an effective solution for removal of most of the smear layer.
2. It kills most significant bacterial stains, i.e. *E faecalis* which has been shown to resistant to many intracanal medicaments and irrigants
3. It is biocompatible
4. It has minimal effect on properties of teeth
5. MTAD has similar solubilizing effects on pulp and dentin to those of EDTA
6. The high binding affinity of doxycycline present in MTAD for dentin allows prolonged antibacterial effect (it's the main difference between MTAD and EDTA).

## METHOD OF IRRIGATION

Although the technique of irrigation is simple and easy, still, care should be taken while irrigating with different syringes or system. Following points should be in mind while irrigating the canal:

1. The solution must be introduced slowly and passively into the canal.
2. Needle should never be wedged into the canal and should allow an adequate back-flow (Fig. 16.15).
3. Blunted needle of 25 gauge or 27 gauge are preferred.
4. In case of small canals, deposit the solution in pulp chamber. Then file will carry the solution into the canal. Capillary action of narrow canal will stain the solution. To remove the excess fluid, either the aspirating syringe

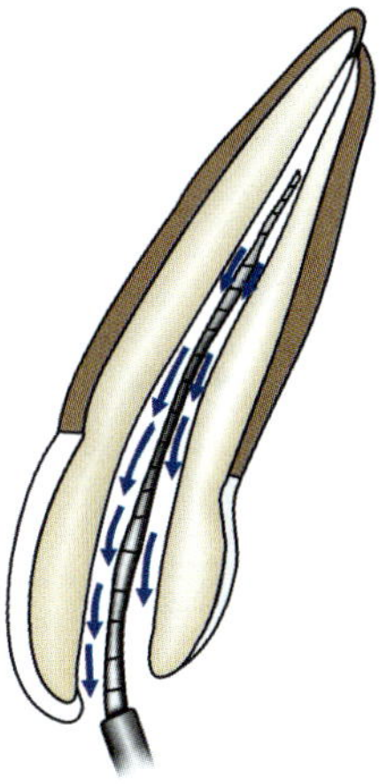

Fig. 16.15: Loose fitting needle providing space for optimal flow of irrigant

or 2 × 2 inches folded gauge pad is placed near the chamber (Fig. 16.16). To further dry the canal, remove the residual solution with paper point.

5. Canal size and shape are crucial for irrigation of the canal. For effective cleaning of apical area, the canals must be enlarged to size 30 and to larger size (Fig. 16.17).
6. Regardless of delivery system, irrigants must never be forcibly inserted into apical tissue rather gently placed into the canal.
7. For effective cleaning, the needle delivering the solution should be in close proximity to the material to be removed.
8. In case of large canals, the tip of needle should be introduced until resistance is felt, then withdraw the needle 2-3 mm away from that point and irrigate the canal passively. For removal of the solution sterile gauge pack or paper points should be used.
9. In order to clean effectively in both anterior and posterior teeth canals, a blunt bend of 30° in the center of needle can be given to reach the optimum length to the canal (Fig. 16.18).
10. Volume of irrigation solution is more important than concentration or type of irrigant.

**Various delivery systems for irrigation**

1. Stropko irrigator
2. 27 gauge needle with notched tip
3. Needle with bevel
4. Monojet endodontic needle
   a. 23 gauge
   b. 27 gauge
5. ProRinse—25, 28, 30 gauge probes
6. Ultrasonic handpiece.

**Ideal properties of irrigating needle**

1. Needle should be blunt.
2. It should allow back-flow.
3. It should be flexible.
4. Longer in length.
5. Easily available.
6. Cost-effective.

## Different Needle Designs

1. *Stropko irrigator*: In this system combination of delivery and recovery of irrigant is present in one probe. Here the needle delivers the solution and an aspirator held in same sheath retrieves the irrigant.
2. *27 gauge needle with Notched tip* (Fig 16.19): This needle is preferred as its notched tip allows backflow of the solution and does not create pressure in the periapical area. So, it ensures optimum cleaning without damage to periapical area (Figs 16.20A and B).

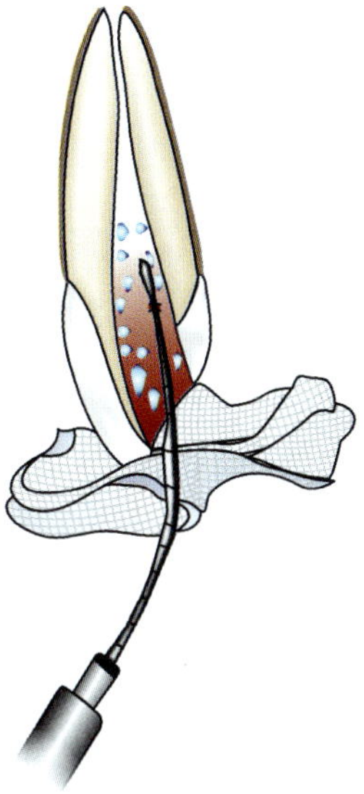

Fig. 16.16: A sterile gauge piece is placed near access opening to absorb excess irrigating solution and to check the debris from root canal

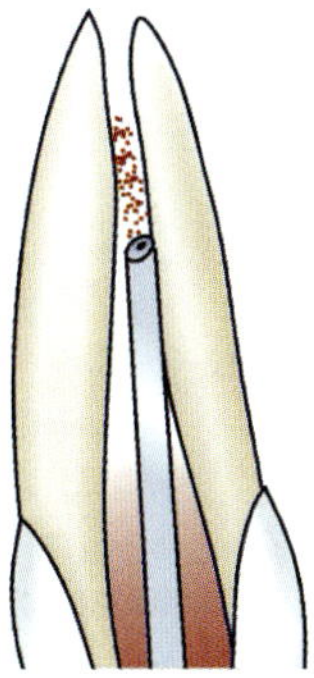

Fig. 16.17: A well-prepared canal allows better use of irrigant

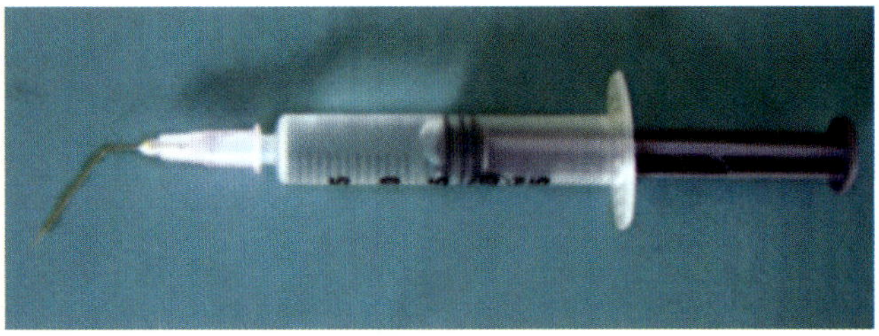

Fig. 16.18: 30° angle bend given in irrigation needle for efficient irrigation

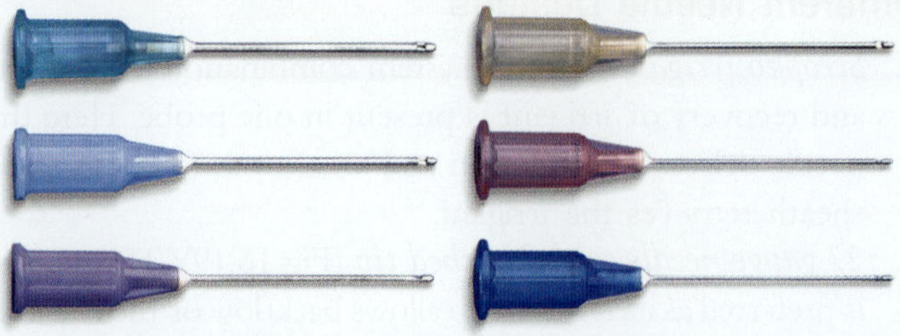

**Fig. 16.19:** Needle with notched tip

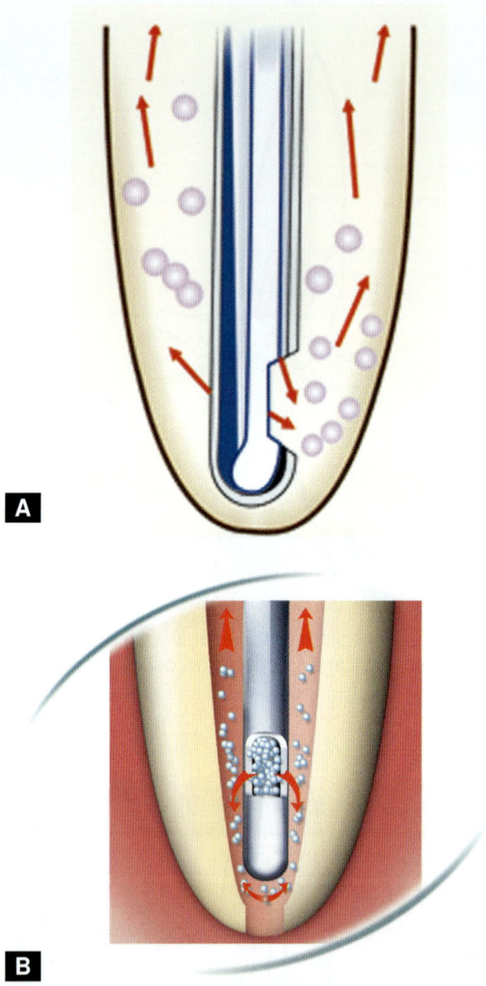

**Figs 16.20A and B:** Needle with notched tip allows back flow of solution and does not create pressure in periapical area

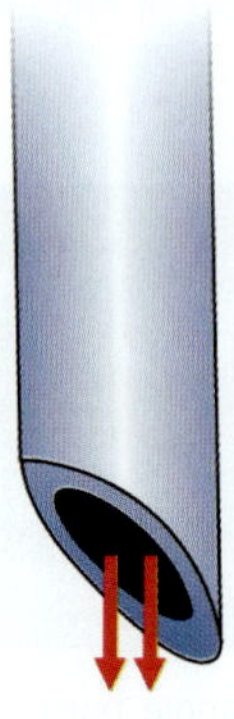

**Fig. 16.21:** Needle with bevel

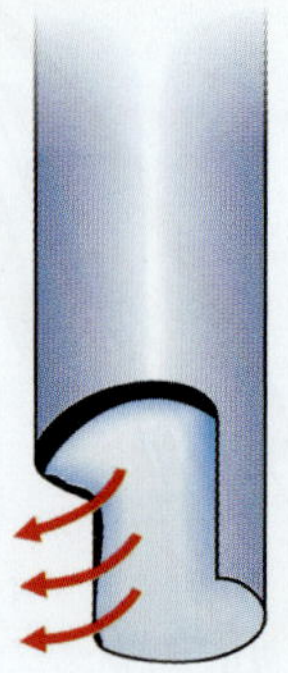

**Fig. 16.22:** Monojet endodontic needle

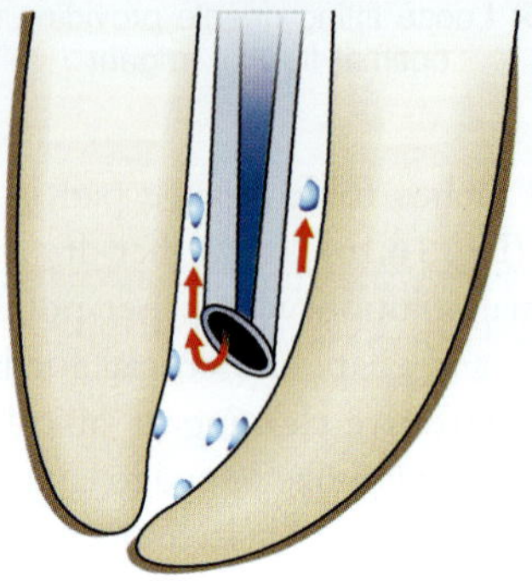

**Fig. 16.23:** Needle should not be wedged into the canal

3. *Needle with bevel*: Needle with bevel if gets lodged into the canal, there is risk of forcing irrigant past the apex (Fig. 16.21).
4. *Monojet endodontic needle*: This needle is also considered to be efficient one as the long blunt needles can be inserted to the full length of the canal to ensure optimum cleaning (Fig. 16.22). The only drawback observed is that if needles are placed near to the periapical area, it can cause damage.
5. *ProRinse probes*: This probe is proved to be highly effective in all gauges but 27gauge notch tip needle is proved to be highly effective as it can clean the periapical area without placing near the apical foramen. Its efficiency lie in its design as it has a blunt tip, with lumen 2 mm from the tip. Fluid from the lumen creates turbulence in all directions.
6. *Micro brushes and ultrasonic*: In this bristles are attached to braided wires or flexible plastic cores. These micro brushes can be used a rotary or ultrasonic end brushes. These micro brushes have tapers like non standardized gutta perchas cones. These are used in conjunction with sodium hypochlorite and EDTA to produce clean canals.

**Precautions to be taken while irrigation**

1. Avoid wedging the needle into the canal (Fig. 16.23).
2. Avoid forcing the solution into the canal.
3. Avoid placing the needle beyond the apical area or very near to apical area
4. Avoid using larger gauge needle.
5. Avoid using metallic, autoclavable syringe as they more prone to breakage.

## INTRACANAL MEDICAMENTS

Originally endodontics was mainly a therapeutic procedure in which drugs were used to destroy microorganisms, fix or mummify vital tissue and affect a sealing of the root canal space.

The drugs commonly used were caustics such as phenol and its derivatives which were shown to produce adverse effects on the periapical tissues. Gradually the reliance on drugs has been replaced by emphasis on thorough canal debridement. But drugs are still being used as intra-treatment dressings, although an ever increasing number of endodontists use them only for symptomatic cases.

### Functions

- Destroy the remaining bacteria and also limits the growth of new arrivals.
- Useful in treatment of apical periodontitis for example in cases of inflammation caused due to over instrumentation.

*A root canal disinfectant should have following properties:*

1. It should be effective germicide and fungicide.
2. It should be non-irritating to pulpal tissue.
3. It should remain stable in the solution.
4. It should have prolonged antimicrobial action.
5. It should remain active in presence of blood and pus, etc.
6. It should have low surface tension.
7. It should not interfere with repair of periapical tissue.
8. It should not stain tooth.
9. It should be capable of inactivation in the culture media.
10. It should not induce immune response.

**Various intracanal medicaments used are**

1. Essential oils — eugenol
2. Phenolic compounds —
   i. Phenol
   ii. Paramonochlor
   iii. Camphorated phenol
   iv. Cresatin
   v. Aldehydes
      a. Formocresol
      b. Paraformaldehyde
      c. Glutaraldehyde
3. Calcium hydroxide
4. Halogens
   i. Chlorine-sodium Hypochlorite
   ii. Iodine
      – 2% $I_2$ in 5% KI solution, i.e. iodophores.
      – 5 percent $I_2$ in tincture of alcohol
5. Chlorhexidine gluconate
6. Antibiotics
7. Corticosteroid-antibiotic combination

## CHARACTERISTICS OF INTRACANAL MEDICAMENTS

### Essential Oils

#### *Eugenol*

It has been used in endodontics for many years. It is a constituent of most root canal sealers and is used as a part of many

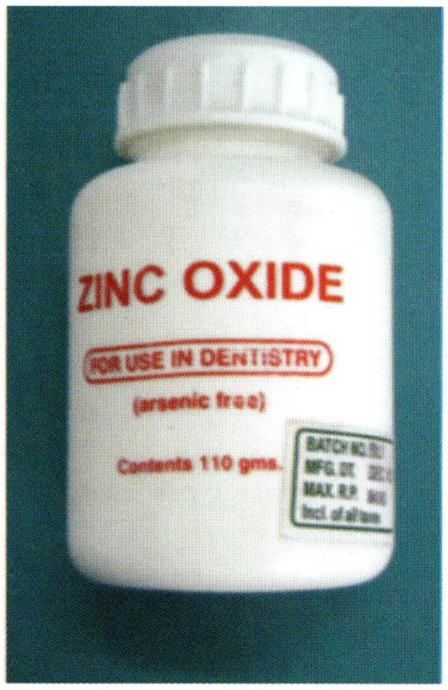


Fig. 16.24: Zinc oxide eugenol used as temporary restorative material

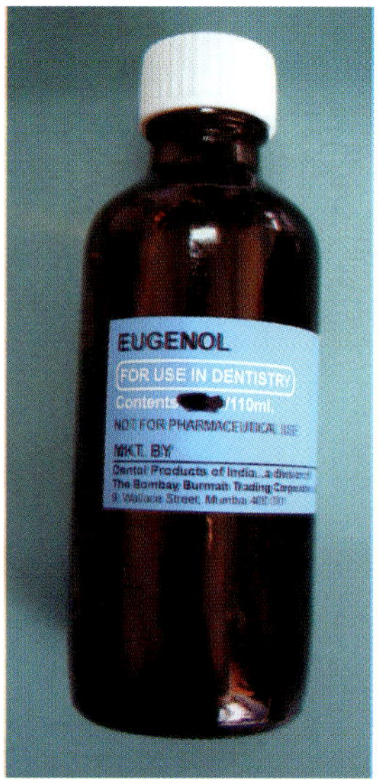


Fig. 16.25: Effects of eugenol depends on concentration of eugenol used

temporary sealing agents (Fig. 16.24). This substance is the chemical essence of oil of clove and is related to phenol. Effects of eugenol are dependent on tissue concentrations of the eugenol (Fig. 16.25). These are divided into low dose (beneficial effects) and high dose (toxic effects).

Low doses show anti-inflammatory activity while high doses exert cytotoxic effects.

**Eugenol**

| *Low dose (beneficial effects)* | *High dose (toxic effects)* |
|---|---|
| 1. Inhibits prostaglandins synthesis | 1. Induces cell death |
| 2. Inhibits nerve activity | 2. Inhibits cell respiration |
| 3. Inhibits white cell chemotaxis | |

#### *Uses of Eugenol*

1. Used as an intracanal medicament.
2. Used as a root canal sealers.
3. Part of temporary sealing agents.

## Phenolic Compounds

### Phenol

It was used for many years for its disinfectant and caustic action. However, it has strong inflammatory potential, so, at present, it is rarely used as an intracanal medicament.

Liquefied phenol (Carbolic acid) consists of 9 parts of phenol and 1 part of water.

### Uses

a. It is used for disinfection before periapical surgery.
b. It is also used for cauterizing tissue tags that resist removal with broaches or files.

### Parachlorophenol

Parachlorophenol has been a very popular component of dressing as phenol is no longer used in endodontics because of its high toxicity to efficacy ratio.

### Composition

This is substitution product of phenol in which chlorine replaces one of the hydrogen atoms ($C_6H_4OHCl$). On trituration with gum camphor, these products combine to form an oily liquid.

### Concentration

1 percent aqueous solution is preferred.

### Uses

Used as a dressing of choice for infected tooth.

## Camphorated Monoparachlorophenol (CMCP)

It is probably the most commonly used medicament in endodontics presently, even though its use has decreased considerably in the past few years (Fig. 16.26).

### Composition

2 parts of para-chlorophenol
\+
3 parts gum camphor
↓
Camphorated monochlorophenol (CMCP)

**Camphor is added to parachlorophenol (PCP) because it**
1. Has diluent action
2. Prolongs the antimicrobial effect
3. Reduces the irritating effect of PCP
4. Serves as a vehicle for the solution

### Uses

Used as a dressing of choice for infected teeth.

## Cresatin

As reported by Schilder and Amsterdam, Cresatin possesses the same desirable qualities and actions as that of CMCP, yet even less irritating to periapical tissues.

### Composition

This substance is clear, stable, oily liquid of low volatile nature known as Metacresyl acetate.

## Aldehydes

Formaldehyde, paraformaldehyde and glutaraldehyde are commonly used intracanal medicaments is root canal therapy. These are water soluble protein denaturing agents and are considered among the most potent disinfectants. They are mainly applied as disinfectants for surfaces and medical equipment which can not be sterilized, but they are quite toxic and allergic and some even may be carcinogenic.

### Formocresol

Formocresol contains formaldehyde as its main ingredient and is still widely used medicament for pulpotomy procedures in primary teeth but its toxic and mutagenic properties are of concern (Fig. 16.27).

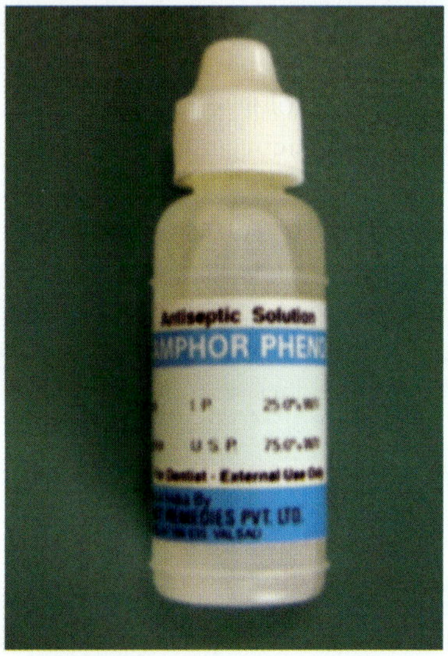


**Fig. 16.26:** Camphorphenol

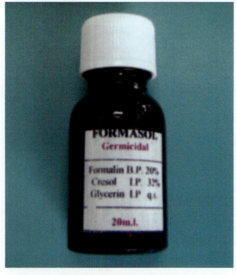


**Fig. 16.27:** Formocresol

| Composition of formocresol | | |
|---|---|---|
| Formaldehyde | — | 19 percent |
| Cresol | — | 35 percent |
| Water and glycerine | — | 46 percent |

### *Uses*

Used as dressing for pulpotomy to fix the retained pulpal tissue.

### *Paraformaldehyde*

It is polymeric form of formaldehyde and is commonly found as component of some root canal obturating materials like endomethasone. It slowly decomposes to give out formocresol, its monomer. Its properties are similar to formaldehyde that is toxic, allergenic and genotoxic in nature.

All phenolic and similar compounds are highly volatile with low surface tension. Therefore, if they are placed on a cotton pellet in the chamber of a tooth during treatment, the vapors will permeate the entire canal preparation, so, placement on a paper point is unnecessary. Only tiny quantity of medication is needed for effectiveness, otherwise, chances of periapical irritation are increased.

## Calcium Hydroxide

The use of calcium hydroxide in endodontics was introduced by Hermann in 1920. It has acquired a unique position in endodontics (Fig. 16.28). After its successful clinical applications for variety of indications, multiple biological functions have been attributed to calcium hydroxide.

## Effects of Calcium Hydroxide

### *Physical*

- Acts as a physical barrier for ingress of bacteria.
- Destroys the remaining bacteria by limiting space for multiplication and holding substrate for growth.

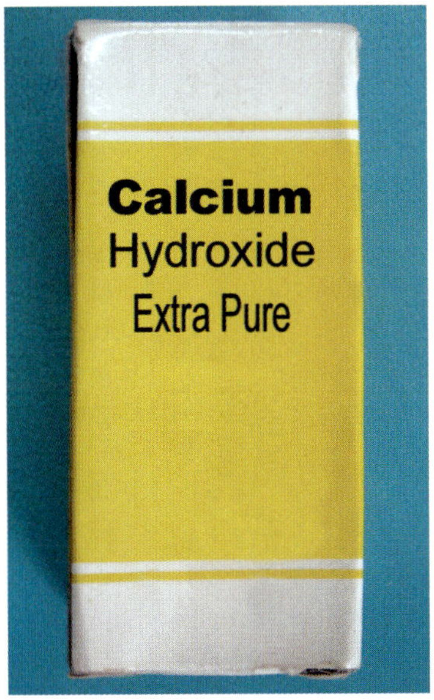


**Fig. 16.28:** Calcium hydroxide

### *Chemical*

- It shows antiseptic action probably because of its high pH and its leaching action on necrotic pulp tissues. It also increases the pH of circumpulpal dentin when placed into the root canal.
- Suppresses enzymatic activity and disrupts cell membrane
- Inhibits DNA replication by splitting it.
- It hydrolyses the lipid part of bacterial lipopolysaccharide (LPS) and thus inactivates the activity of LPS. This is a desirable effect because dead cell wall material remains after the killing of bacteria which may cause infection.

**Calcium hydroxide is available in**

a. *Paste form:* Single paste or in combination with iodoform.
b. *Powder form:* Powder form is mixed with saline and anesthetic solution. For placement in root canals it is coated with the help of paper points, spreaders or lentulo spirals.

## Indications of Calcium Hydroxide

- In weeping canals
- In treatment of phoenix abscess
- In resorption cases
- For apexification
- During pulpotomy
- For non surgical treatment of periapical lesion
- In cases of direct and indirect pulp capping
- As sealer for obturation
- To decrease postoperative pain after over instrumentation, it is used in combination with Ledermix (1:1)

## Disadvantages of Calcium Hydroxide as Intracanal Medicament

1. Difficult to remove from canals
2. Decreases setting time of zinc oxide eugenol based cements.

Studies have shown limited effectiveness of calcium hydroxide if used only for short time in root canals for disinfecting purposes. It is because of following reasons:

i. Low solubility and diffusibility of calcium hydroxide mater it difficult to attain rapid increases in pH.
ii. Different formulations having different alkaline potential
iii. Inability to reach in accessible areas like isthmus, ramification and canal irregularities.
iv. Bacterias loaded deeper in dentinal tubules are not affected by calcium hydroxide.
v. Inhibition of action of calcium hydroxide by dentinal protein buffering.

## Functions of $Ca(OH)_2$

1. Inhibits root resorption
2. Stimulates periapical healing
3. Encourage mineralization

## Use of Calcium Hydroxide in Weeping Canal Cases

Sometime a tooth undergoing root canal treatment shows constant clear or reddish exudation associated with periapical radiolucency. Tooth can be asymptomatic or tender on percussion. When opened in next appointment, exudates stops but it again reappears in next appointment. This is known as "Weeping Canal".

In these cases, tooth with exudates is not ready for filling, since culture reports normally show negative bacterial growth so, antibiotics are of no help in such cases. For such teeth, dry the canals with sterile absorbent paper points and place calcium hydroxide in the canal. By next appointment, one finds a dry canal, ready for obturation . It happens because pH of periapical tissues is acidic in weeping stage which gets converted into basic pH by Calcium hydroxide. Some say that caustic effect of calcium hydroxide burns the residual chronic inflamed tissue and also calcium hydroxide builds up the bone in the lesion due to its calcifying action.

## Halogens

Halogens include chlorine and iodine which are used in various formulations in endodontics. They are potent oxidizing agents with rapid bactericidal effects.

### Chlorine

*Sodium hypochlorite:* This compound is sometimes used as an intracanal medicament. In general, the disinfectant action of halogens is inversely proportional to their atomic weights. Chlorine (lowest atomic weight), has the greatest disinfectant action among the members of this group. Chlorine disinfectants are not stable compounds because they interact rapidly with organic matter. Mentz found sodium hypochlorite as effective intracanal medicament as well as irrigant. As the activity of sodium hypochlorite is intense but of short duration, the compound should preferably be applied to the root canal every other day.

*Iodides:* These compounds have been used as antiseptics for more than a century. Iodine is highly reactive, combining with proteins in a loosely bound manner so that its penetration is not impeded. It probably destroys micro-organisms by forming salts that are *inimical* to the life of the organism. Iodine is used as iodine potassium iodide and in Iodophors, which are organic iodine containing compounds that release iodine over time. It is also a very potent antibacterial agent of low toxicity, but may stain clothing if spilled. As Iodophors, it was used in a paste formulation to serve as a permanent root canal filling. Current applications of iodine compounds are as an irrigating solution and short-term dressing in a 2 percent solution of iodine in 4 percent aqueous potassium iodide and more recently, as a constituent in gutta-percha points for filling.

## Chlorhexidine Gluconate

Chlorhexidine gluconate has been widely used in periodontics because of its antibacterial activity. Its use as an irrigant solution has been compared with sodium hypochlorite.

Chlorhexidine exhibit substantivity (persistence in the area of interest), broadspectrum activity and low toxicity, these properties make it well suited for irrigation and dressing applications in endodontics. Effective concentrations commonly used are in range of 0.2-2 percent range. Innovative attempts are being made to utilize the disinfecting properties of chlorhexidine in gutta-percha points.

## PBSC Paste

As mentioned by Grossman, PBSC has enjoyed wide use among dentists. The constituents of the paste are as follows:
*Penicillin*—effective against gram-positive microorganisms
*Bacitracin*—effective against penicillin-resistant micro-organisms
*Streptomycin*—effective against the gram-negative micro-organisms
*Caprylate (sodium salt)*—effective against fungi.

Nystatin replaces sodium caprylate as the an antifungal agent and is available in form of PBSN. Both are available in a paste form that may be injected into root canals or impregnated on paper points. Because there is no volatility, the drug must be placed in the canal to have effect in that area.

PBSC may interfere with subsequent culturing procedures, therefore penicillinase may be added to culture media to inactivate penicillin. Reports of allergic reaction to the drug have been presented, if the patient reports history of allergy to any of the constituents, the drug should not be used. With the decline in popularity of intracanal drugs in general, and because of the potential for sensitivity due to topical use of antibiotics, PBSN largely has fallen into disuse.

### Sulfonamides

Sulfanilamide and Sulfathiazole are used as medicaments by mixing with sterile distilled water or by placing a moistened paper point into a fluffed jar containing the powder. Yellowish tooth discoloration has been reported after use. Sulfonamides are usually recommended while giving closed dressing in a tooth which had been left open after an acute periapical abscess.

### $N_2$ by Sargent

It is a compound consisting of paraformaldehyde as the main ingredient. It contains eugenol, phenyl mercuric borate and perfumes. Antibacterial effect of $N_2$ is short lived and dissipated in 7-10 days.

### Grossman Paste

It consists of

| | |
|---|---|
| Potassium penicillin G | 1,000 000 units |
| Bacitracin | 1, 00,00 |
| Streptomycin sulphate | 1.0 gm |
| Sodium caprylate | 1.0 gm |
| Silicon fluid | 3 ml |
| Nystatin | 1,00,00 units |

## Chloramines-T

It is a chlorine compound with good antimicrobial. It is used in the concentration of 5 percent. If remains stable for long period of time. It can be used to disinfect gutta-percha points, and can be used in patients allergic to iodine.

### Quaternary Ammonium Compounds

They are positively charged compounds which attract negatively charged microorganisms they have low surface tension for example Aminoacridine.

Aminoacridine is a mild antiseptic which is more effective than creation but less effective than CMCP. It is used more as an irritant than intracranial medicament.

### Corticosteroid-antibiotic Combinations

Medications that combine antibiotic and corticosteroid elements are highly effective in the treatment of over instrumentation; they must be placed into the inflamed periapical tissue by a paper point or reamer to be effective. Tetra-Cortril, Corti-sporin, Mycolog, and other combinations are available for their use in endodontics. Ledermix is one of best known corticosteroid-antibiotic combination. The corticosteroid constituent reduces the periapical inflammation and gives almost instant relief of pain to the patient who complains of extreme tenderness to percussion after canal instrumentation. While the antibiotic constituents present in the corticosteroid antibiotic combination prevent the overgrowth of microorganisms when the inflammation subsides.

**Root canal disinfectants**

**Halogens**

*Chlorine*

Irrigating solution: Sodium hypochlorite 0.5 to 5.25 percent in aqueous solution.

*Iodine*

Irrigating solution: 2 percent $I_2$ in 5 percent KI aqueous solution; iodophors.

Surface disinfection: 5 percent $I_2$ in tincture of alcohol.

**Chlorhexidine**

Chlorhexidine gluconate Irrigating solution: 0.12-2.0 percent aqueous solution.

**Calcium hydroxide**

*Dressing:* aqueous or viscous formulation with varying amounts of salts added. Antibacterials like iodine, chlorphenols, chlorhexidine may also be added.

**Aldehydes**

*Formocresol*

*Dressing:* 19 percent formaldehyde, 35 percent cresol, 46 percent water and glycerine.

**Phenols**

*Camphorated phenol*

*Paramonochlorphenol( PMCP)*

Irrigating solution; 2 percent aqueous solution .

*Dressing:* CMCP; 65 percent camphor, 35 percent PMCP.

**Eugenol**

Formation of electrochemically activated solution

## PLACEMENT OF INTRACANAL MEDICAMENT

1. Copiously irrigate the canal to remove debris present if any (Fig. 16.29).
2. Place the master apical file in the canal (Fig. 16.30).
3. Dry the canal using absorbent paper points (Fig. 16.31).

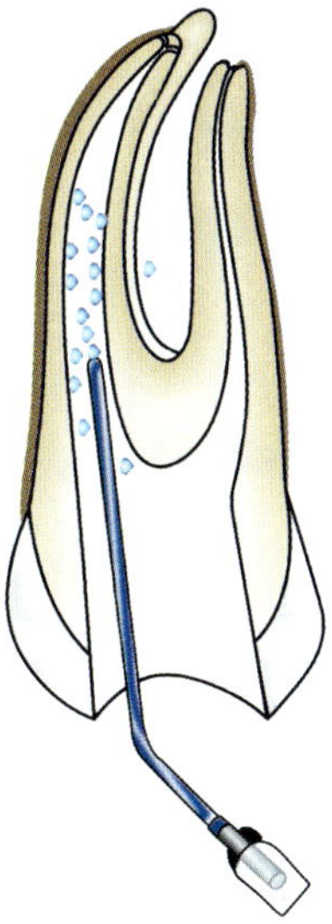

**Fig. 16.29:** Copiously irrigate the canal

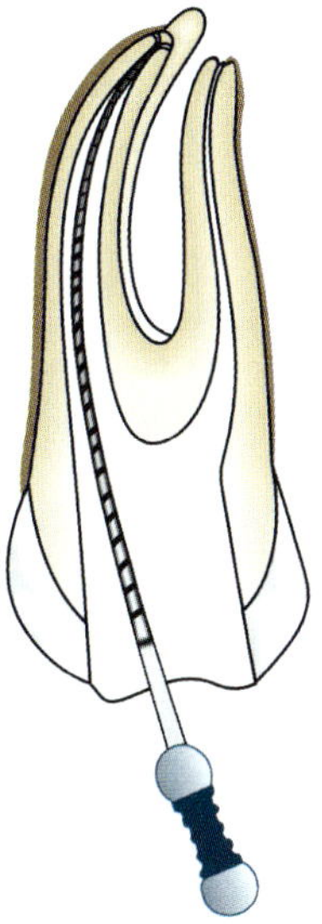

**Fig. 16.30:** Place the master apical file in the canal

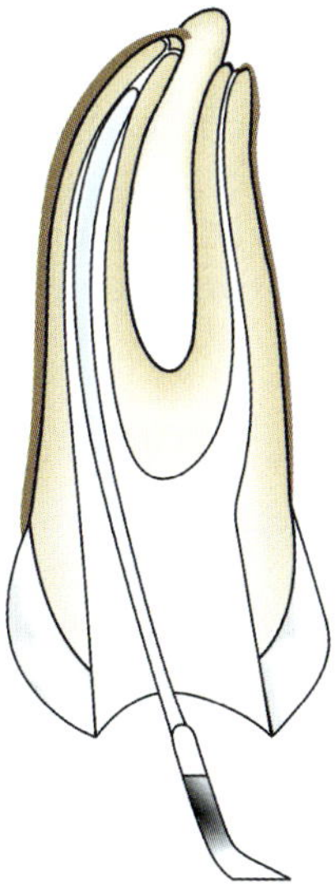

**Fig. 16.31:** Dry the canal using absorbent paper points

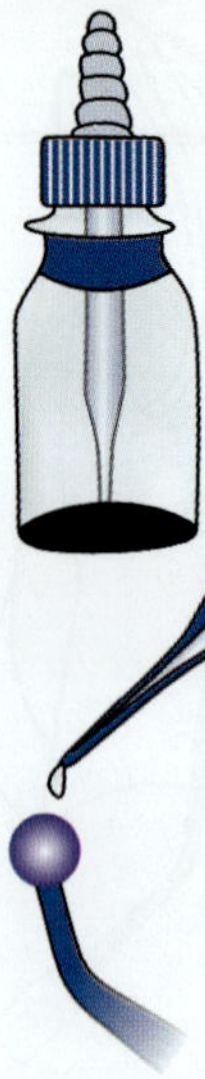

Fig. 16.32: Intracanal medicament

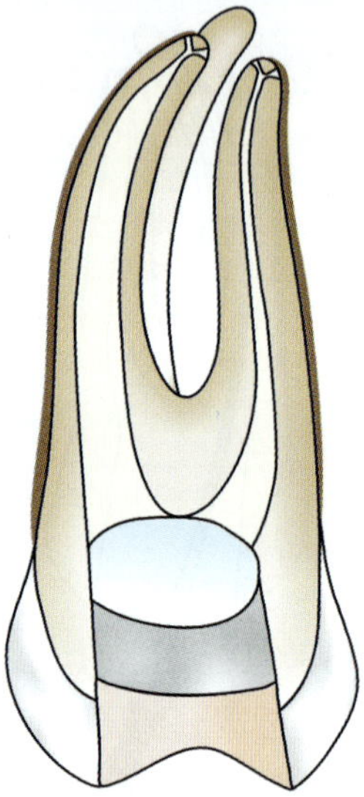

Fig. 16.33: Intracanal medicament on a cotton pellet is applied and placed in pulp chamber. Over it, a sterile dry cotton pellet is placed which is finally sealed with a temporary filling material

4. Place the intracanal medicament on a sterile cotton pellet and place it in the pulp chamber (Figs 16.32 and 16.33).
5. Over this another sterile cotton pellet is placed, which is finally sealed with a temporary restorative material (Fig. 16.33).

## Limitations of Intracanal Medicaments

1. For an intracanal, medicament to be effective, it should remain active during the time of inter appointment, which does not happen not in every case.
2. Clinical effectiveness of sustained release delivery systems is unknown.
3. Therapeutic action of medicaments depends upon its direct contact with tissues. But these substances may not reach all the areas where bacteria and tissues are present.

## QUESTIONS

**Q. What are properties of ideal irrigating solutions?**

**Q. What are functions of irrigating solution? Enumerate various irrigants used in endodontics.**

**Q. Write short notes on:**

a. Sodium hypochlorite
b. Hydrogen peroxide
c. MTAD
d. Ozonated water
e. Grossman paste

**Q. Define chelating agents. Write in detail about EDTA.**

**Q. Classify intracanal medicaments. What are ideal requirements for intracanal medicament?**

**Q. Explain role of calcium hydroxide in endodontics.**

## BIBLIOGRAPHY


1. Abbott PV. Medicaments: Aids to success in endodontics Part I. A review of literature. Aust Dent J 1990;35:438-48.
2. Basrani B, Ghanem A, Tjaderhane L. Physical and chemical properties of chlorhexidine and calcium hydroxide-containing medications. J of Endod 2004;30(6):413-17.
3. Basrani B, Lemonie C. Chlorhexidine gluconate. Aust Endod J. 2005;31(2):48-52. Review.
4. Baumgartner JC, Cuenin PR. Efficacy of several concentrations of sodium hypochlorite for root canal irrigation. J Endod 1992;18(12):605-12.
5. Baumgartner JC, Mader CL. A scanning electron microscopic evaluation of four root canal irrigation regimens. J Endod 1987;13:147-57.
6. Baumgartner JC, Watts CM, Xia T. Occurrence of Candida albicans in infections of endodontic origin. J Endod 2000;26:695-98.
7. Beltz RE, Torabinejad M, Pouresmail M. Quantitative analysis of the solubilizing action of MTAD, sodium hypochlorite, and EDTA on bovine pulp and dentin. J Endod 2003;29:334-7.
8. Bergenholtz G. Controversies in endodontics. Crit Rev Oral Biol Med 2004;15(2):99-114.
9. Busslinger A, Sener B, Barhakow F. Effect of sodium hypochlorite on nickel-titanium light speed instrument. Int Endod J 1998;31:290.
10. Byström A, Claesson R, Sundqvist G. The antibacterial effect of camphorated paramonochlorophenol, camphorated phenol and calcium hydroxide in the treatment of infected root canals. Endod Dent Traumatol 1985;1:170-75.
11. Byström A, Sundqvist G. Bacteriologic evaluation of the effect of 0.5 percent sodium hypochlorite in endodontic therapy. Oral Surg Oral Med Oral Surg Oral Med Oral Path 1983;55:307-12.
12. Caldero LG, McHugh SM, Mackenzie D. Reduction in intracanal bacteria during root canal bacteria during root canal preparation with and without apical enlargement. Int Endod J 2002;35:437.
13. Card SJ, Sigurdsson A, Ørstavik D, Trope M. The effectiveness of increased apical enlargement in reducing intracanal bacteria. J Endod 2002;28:779-83.
14. Carson KR, G Goodell, S Mc-Clanahan. Comparison of the antimicrobial Activity of Six Irrigants on Primary Endodontic Pathogens. J of Endod 2005;31(6):471-73.
15. Cheung GS, Stock CJ. In vitro cleaning ability of root canal irrigants with and without endosonics. Int Endod J 1993; 26:334.
16. Chong BS, Pitt Ford TR. The role of intracanal medication in root canal treatment. Int Endod J 1996;25:97-106.

17. Cunningham WT, Balekjian AY. Effect of temperature on collagen-dissolving ability of sodium hypochlorite endodontic irrigant. Oral Surg Oral Med Oral Patho 1980;49(2):175-77.
18. Curson I. Endodontic techniques. Part 8. The antibacterial treatment of root canals. Br Dent J 1996;121:381-83.
19. Ercan E, Ozekinci T, Atakul F, Gul K. Antibacteria activity of 2 percent chlorhexidine gluconate and 5.25 percent sodium hypochlorite in infected root canal. In vivo study. J Endod 2004;30:84.
20. Estrela C, et al. Mechanism of action of Sodium Hypochlorite. Braz Dent J 2002;13(2)113-17.
21. Estrela C, Pimenta F, Ito I, Bammann L. Antimicrobial Evaluation of Calcium hydroxide in infected Dentinal Tubules. J of Endod 1999;25(6):416-18.
22. Estrela C, Bammann L, F Pimenta, J Pecora. Control of microorganisms in vitro by calcium hydroxide pastes. Int. Endod J 2001;34:341-45.
23. Evan MD, Baumgartner JC, Khemaleelakul SU, Xia T. Efficacy of calcium hydroxide: Chlorhexidine paste as an intracanal medication in bovine dentin. J Endod 2003;29:338-39.
24. Evanov C, Liewehr FR, Buxton TB, Joyce AP. Antibacterial efficacy of calcium hydroxide and chlorhexidine at 37°C and 46°C. J Endod 2004;30:653.
25. Ferrari PH, S Cai, A Bombana. Effect of endodontic procedures on enterococci, enteric bacteria and yeasts in primary endodontic infections. Int Endod J 2005;38:372-80.
26. Ferreira FB, Torres SA, Rosa OP, Ferreira CM, Garcia RB, Marcucci MC, Gomes BP. Antimicrobial effect of propolis and other substances against selected endodontic pathogens. Oral Surg Oral Med Oral Pathol Oral Radiol Endod 2007; 104(5):709-16.
27. Foreman PC, Barnes IE. A review of calcium hydroxide. Int Endod J 1990;23:283-97.
28. Foster KH, Kulild JC, Weller RN. Effect of smear layer removal on the diffusion of calcium hydroxide through radicular dentin. J Endod 1993;19:136-40.
29. Goldberg F, Spielberg C. The effect of EDTAC and the variation of its working time analyzed with scanning electron microscopy. Oral Surg Oral Med Oral Pathol 1982;53(1):74-77.
30. Gomes B, et al. In vitro antimicrobial activity of several concentrations of sodium hypochlorite and chlorhexidine gluconate in the elimination of Enterococcus faecalis. Int Endod J 2001;34:424-28.
31. Gomes B, et al. Microbiological examination of infected root canals. Microbiological examination of infected root canals. Oral Microbiol Immunol 2004;19(2)71-76.
32. Grawehr M, Sener B, Waltimo T, Zehnder M. Interaction of ethylenediamine tetraacetic acid with sodium hypochlorite in aqueous solutions. Int Endod J 2003;36:411.
33. Grossman LI. Polyantibiotic treatment of pulpless teeth. J Am Dent Assoc 1951;43:265-78.
34. Haapasalo M, Ørstavik D. In vitro infection and disinfection of dentinal tubules. J Dent Res 1987;66:1375-79.
35. Haapasalo M, Qian W, Portenier I, Waltimo T. Effects of dentin on the teeth antimicrobial properties of endodontic medicaments. J Endod 2007;33:(8):917-25. Epub 2007;22. Review.
36. Haenni S, et al. Chemical and antimicrobial properties of calcium hydroxide mixed irrigating solutions. Int Endod J 2003:36:100-105.
37. Hand RE, Smith ML, Harrison JW. Analysis of the effect of dilution on the necrotic tissue dissolution property of sodium hypochlorite. J Endod 1978;4:60-64.
38. Hasselgren G, Olsson B, Cvek M. Effects of calcium hydroxide and sodium hypochlorite on the dissolution of necrotic porcine muscle tissue. J Endod 1988;14:125-27.
39. Hoshino E, Kurihara-Ando N, Sato I, Uematsu H, Sato M, Kota K, chong BS, Pitt ford TR. In vitro antibacterial susceptibility of bacteria take from infected root dentin to a mixture of ciprofloxacin, metronidazole and minocycline. Int Endod J 1996;29:125-30.
40. Hulsmann M, Hahn W. Complications during root canal irrigation. Literature review and case reports. Int Endod J 2000;33:186.
41. Ikhlas EI, Karim Kennedy J, Hussey D. The antimicrobial effects of root canal irrigation and medication. Oral Surg Oral Med Oral Pathol Oral Radiol Endod 2007;103(4):560-69.
42. Izu KH, Thomas SJ, Zheng P, Tzu AE. Effectiveness of sodium hypochlorite in preventing inoculation if periapical tissue with contaminated patency files. J Endod 2004;30:92.
43. Jeansonne MJ, White RR. A comparison of 2.0 percent chlorhexidine gluconate and 5.25 percent sodium hypochlorite as antimicrobial endodontic irrigants. J Endod 1997;20:276-78.
44. Kalaskar R, Damle SG, Tiku A. Nonsurgical treatment of periapical lesions using intracanal calcium hydroxide medicament- a report of cases. Quintessence Int 2007;28(5):e279-84.
45. Kaufman Ay, Greenberg I. Comparative study of the configuration and the cleanliness level of root canals prepared with the aid of sodium hypochlorite and bisdequalinium-acetate solutions. Oral Surg Oral Med Oral Pathol 1986; 62(2):191-97.
46. Krithikadatta J, Indira R, Dorothykalyani Al. Disinfection of dentinal tubules with 2 percent chlorhexidine, 2 percent metronidazole, bioactive glass when compared with calcium hydroxide as intracanal medicaments. J Endod 2007;33(12): 1473-76.
47. Kuruvilla JR, Kamath MP. Antimicrobial activity of 2.5 percent sodium hypochlorite and 0.2 percent chlorhexidine gluconate separately and combined, as endodontic irrigants. J Endod 1998;24:472-76.
48. Lee SJ, Wu MK, Wesslink PR. The effectiveness of syringe irrigation and ultrasonics to remove debris from simulated irregularities with in prepared root canals. Int Endod J 2004; 37:672.
49. Lin S, Levin L, Weiss EI, Peled M, Fuss Z. In vitro antibacterial efficacy of a new chlorhexidine slow-release device. Quintessence Int 2006;37(5):391-94.
50. Lin S, Zuckerman O, Weiss EI, Mazor Y, Fuss Z. Antibacterial efficacy of a new chlorhexidine slow release device to disinfect dentinal tubules. J Endod 2003;29:416-18.
51. Madison S, Krell KV. Comparison of ethylenediamine tetraacetic acid and sodium hypochlorite on the apical seal of endodontically treated teeth. J Endod 1984;10:499.
52. Marais JP. Cleaning efficacy of a new root canal irrigation solution. A preliminary evaluation. Int Endod J 2000;33:320.
53. Molander A, Reit C, Dahlen G, Kvist T. Microbiologial status of root filled teeth with apical periodontitis. Int Endod J 1998;31:1-7.
54. Molander A, Reit C, Dahlen G, Kvist T. Microbiological status of root filled teeth with apical periodontitis. Int Endod 1989;15:373-78.
55. Nair P, Sjögren U, Krey G, Kahnberg KE, Sundqvist G. Intraradicular bacteria and fungi in root-filled, asymptomatic human teeth with therapy-resistant periapical lesions: A long-term light and electron microscopic follow-up Study. J Endod 1990;16:580-88.

56. Nandini S, Velmurugan N, Kandaswamy D. Removal efficiency of calcium hydroxide intracanal medicament with two calcium chelators: volumetric analysis using spiral CT, an in vitro study. J Endod 2006;32(11):1097-1101.
57. Oliveira LD, Leão MV Carvalhi CA, Camargo CH, Valera MC, Jorge AO, Unterkircher CS. In vitro effects of calcium hydroxide and polymyxin B on endotoxins in root canals. J Dent. 2005;33(2):107-14. Epub 2004;10.
58. Ørstavik D, Kerekes K, Molven O. Effects of extensive apical reaming and calcium hydroxide dressing on bacterial infection during treatment of apical periodontitis: a pilot study. Int Endod J 1991;24:1-7.
59. Pallotta RC, Ribeiro MS, de Lima Machado ME. Determination of the minimum inhibitory concentration of four medicaments used as intracanal medication. Aust Endod J 2007;33(3):107-11.
60. Radcliff CE, et al. Antimicrobial activity of varying concentrations of sodium hypochlorite on the endodontic microorganisms Actinomyces Israeli, A. Naeslundi, Candida albicans and E faecalis. Int. Endod J 2004;37:438-46.
61. Schoeffel GJ. The EndoVac method of endodontic irrigation: safety first. Dent Today 2007;26(10):92,94,96 passim.
62. Sen BH, Piskin B, Demirci T. Observation of bacteria and fungi in infected root canal and dentinal tubules by SEM. Endod Dent Traumatol 1995;11:6-9.
63. Serper A, Çalt S. The demineralising effects of EDTA at different concentration and pH. J Endod 2002;28:501-02.
64. Silveira AM, Lopes HP, Siqueira JF Jr, Macedo SB, Consolaro A. Periradicular repair after two-visit endodontic treatment using two different intracanal medications compared to single-visit endodontic treatment. Braz Dent J 2007;18(4):299-304.
65. Siqueira J, et al. Chemomechanical reduction of the bacterial Population in the Root Canal after Instrumentation and Irrigation with 1 percent, 2.5 percent and 5.25 percent Sodium Hypochlorite. J of Endod 2000;26(6):331-34.
66. Siqueira J, Lopes H. Mechanisms of antimicrobial activity of calcium hydroxide: A critical review. Int Endod J 1999;32:361-69.
67. Sjögren U, Figdor D, Spångberg L, Sundqvist G. The antimicrobial effect of calcium hydroxide as a short-term intracanal dressing. Int Endod J 1991;24:119-25.
68. Squeira JF Jr, Lopes HP. Mechanisms of antimicrobial activity of calcium hydroxide: A critical review. Int Endod 1999; 132:361-69.
69. Stuart KG, Miller CH, Brown CE Jt, Newton CW. The comparative antimicrobial effect of calcium hydroxide. Oral Surg Oral Med Oral Pathol 1991;72:101-04.
70. Sundqvist G, Figdor D, Persson S, Sjögren U. Microbiologic analysis of teeth with failed endodontic treatment and the outcome of conservative re-treatment. Oral Surg Oral Med Oral Path Oral Radiol Endod 1998;85:86-93.
71. Torabinejad M, Ung B, Kettering J. In vitro bacterial penetration of coronally unsealed endodontically treated teeth. J Endod 1990;16:566-69.
72. Villegas JC, Yoshioka T, Kobayashi C, Suda H. Obturation of accessory canals after four different final irrigation regimens. J Endod 2002;28:534-36.
73. Virtej A, MacKenzie CR, Raab WH, Pfeffer K, Barthel CR. Determination of the performance of various root canal disinfection methods after in situ carriage. J Endod 2007; 33(8):926-29.
74. Waltimo TM, Siren EK, Torkko HL, Olsen I, Haapasalo MP. Fungi in therapy-resistant apical periodontitis. Int Endon J 1997;30:96-101.
75. Walton REm, Torabinejad M. Principles and practice of Endodontics (2nd edn). Philadelphia, Pa:WB saunders Company; 1996;201-32.
76. Wang CS, Debelian GJ, Teixeira FB. Effect of intracanal medicament on the sealing ability of root canals filled with Resilon. J Endod. 2006;32(6):532-6. Epub 2006 Apr 4.
77. Weston CH, Ito S, Wadgaonkar B, Pashley DH. Effects of time and concentration of sodium ascorbate on reversal of NaOCl-induced reduction in bond strengths. J Endod 2007; 33(7):879-81.
78. White RR, Hays GL, Janer LR. Residual antimicrobial activity after canal irrigation with chlorhexidine. J Endod 1997;23:229-31.
79. Wu MK, Wesselink PR. Efficacy of three techniques in cleaning the apical portion of curved root canals. Oral Surg Oral Med Oral Path Oral Radiol Endod 1995;79:492-96.
80. Wu MK, Dummer PMH, Wesselink PR. Consequences of and strategies to deal with residual post-treatment root canal infection. Int Endod J 2006;39:343-56.
81. Yesilsoy C, Whitaker E, Cleveland D, Phillips E, Trope M. Antimicrobial and toxic effects of established and potential root canal irrigants. J Endod 1995;21(10):513-15.
82. Yeung SY, Huang CS, Chan CP, Lin CP, Lin HN, Lee PH, Jia HW, Huang SK, Jeng JH, Chang MC. Antioxidant and pro-oxidant properties of chlorhexidine and its interaction with calcium hydroxide solutions. Int Endod J 2007;40(11):837-44.
83. Zamany A, Safavi K, Spångberg LS. The effect of chlorhexidine as an endodontic disinfectant. Oral Surg Oral Med Oral Pathol Oral Radiol Endod 2003;96(5):578-81.

# Cleaning and Shaping of Root Canal System

CHAPTER 17



## INTRODUCTION

Endodontic treatment mainly consists of **three steps:**

1. Cleaning and shaping of the root canal system
2. Disinfection
3. Obturation

Cleaning and shaping is one of the most important step in the root canal therapy for obtaining success in the root canal treatment.

### Cleaning

It comprises the removal of all potentially pathogenic contents from the root canal system.

### Shaping

The establishment of a specifically shaped cavity which performs the dual role of three-dimensional progressive access into the canal and creating an apical preparation which will permit the final obturation instruments and materials to fit easily (Fig. 17.1).

For the success of endodontic treatment one must remove all the contents of the root canal completely because any communication from root canal system to periodontal space acts as portal of exit which can lead to formation of lesions of endodontic origin (Fig. 17.2).

Cleaning and shaping, i.e. biomechanical preparation of the root canal system was a hit and trial method, before **Dr. Schilder** gave the concept of cleaning and shaping.

Initially the root canals were manipulated primarily to allow the placement of intracanal medicaments. But with the advent of role of radiographs in endodontics, one could see the lesion of bone and teeth and concept was changed to remove the pathogenic cause from the tooth. With the changing concepts of root canal treatment, the preparation is described as instrumentation, chemomechanical instrumentation, biomechanical preparation, etc. which describes the mode of root canal therapy, but the ultimate goal is of cleaning and shaping of the root canal system.

The two concepts, cleaning and shaping and the three-dimensional obturation are interdependent. Obturation of root canal cannot be achieved better if canals are not thoroughly cleaned and shaped (Fig. 17.3).

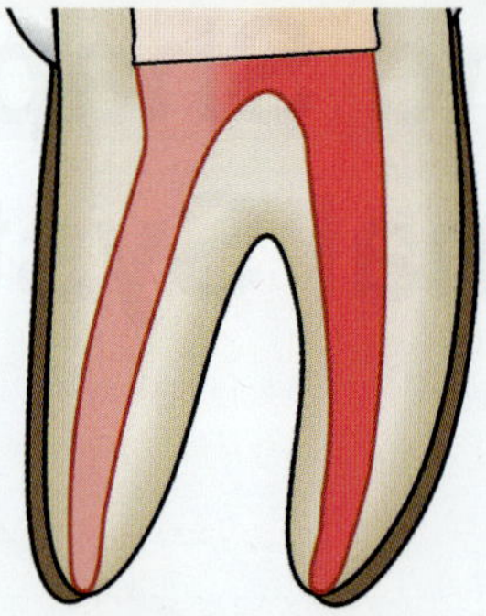

Fig. 17.1: Complete cleaning and shaping of root canal system

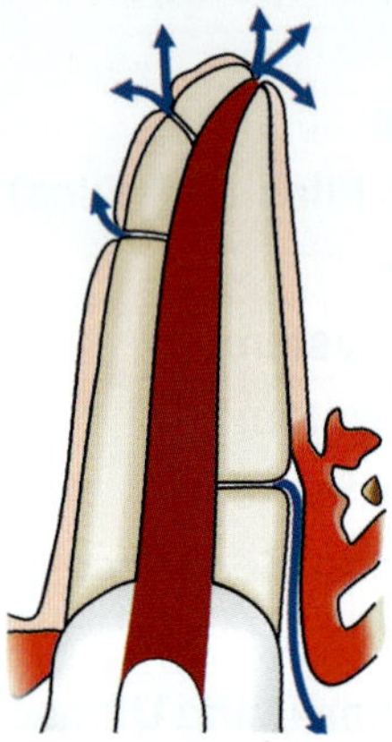

Fig. 17.2: Portals of communication of root canal system and periodontium

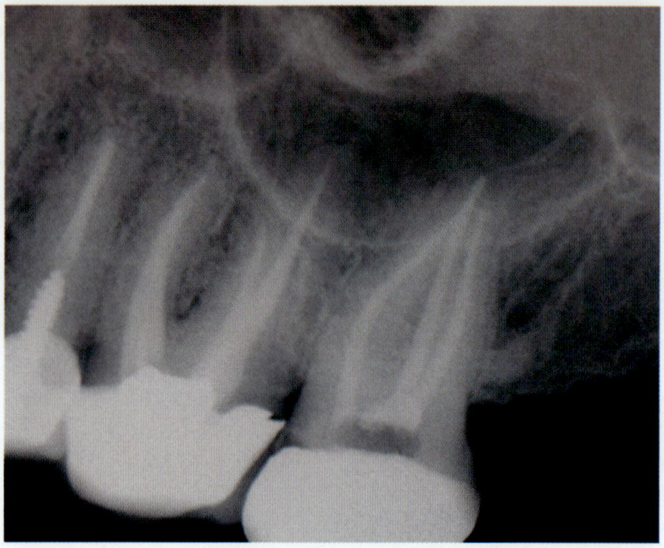

Fig. 17.3: Three-dimensional obturation of root canal system

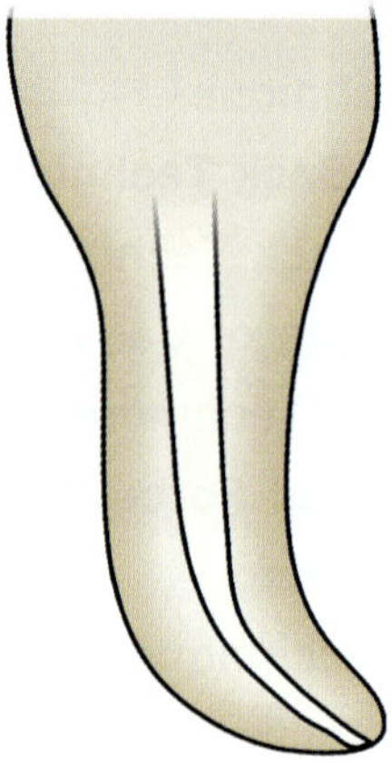

Fig. 17.4: Prepared root canal shape should be continuous tapered

The mechanics of cleaning and shaping may be viewed as an extension of the principles of coronal cavity preparation to the full length of the root canal system. **Schilder** gave five mechanical objectives for successful cleaning and shaping 30 years ago. The objectives taught the clinicians to think and operate in three dimensions.

The objectives given by **Schilder** are:

1. ***The root canal preparation should develop a continuously tapering cone (Fig. 17.4.) :*** This shape mimics the natural canal shape. Funnel shaped preparation of canal should merge with the access cavity so that instruments will slide into the canal. Thus access cavity and root canal preparation should form a continuous channel.
2. ***Making the preparation in multiple planes which introduces the concept of "flow":*** This objective preserves the natural curve of the canal.
3. ***Making the canal narrower apically and widest coronally:*** To create a continuous tapers up to apical third which creates the resistance form to hold gutta-percha in the canal (Fig. 17.5).
4. ***Avoid transportation of the foramen:*** There should be gentle and minute enlargement of the foramen while maintaining its position (Fig. 17.6).

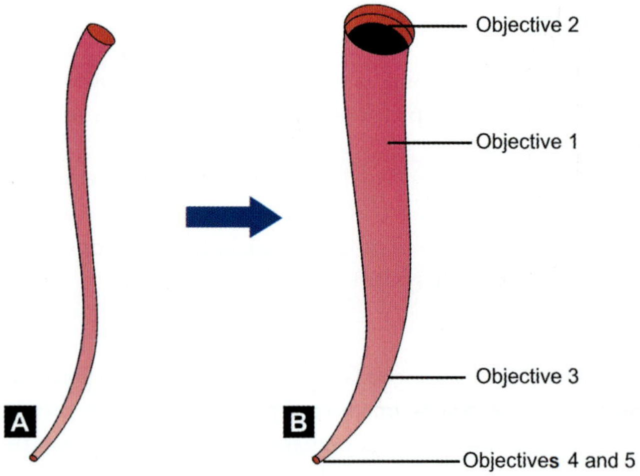


Fig. 17.5: Diagrammatic representation of objectives of canal preparation

5. ***Keep the apical opening as small as possible:*** The foramen size should be kept as small as possible as overlapping of foramen contributes to number of iatrogenic problems. Doubling the file size apically increases the surface area of foramen four folds ($\pi r^2$) (Fig. 17.7). This overlapping of apical foramen should be avoided.

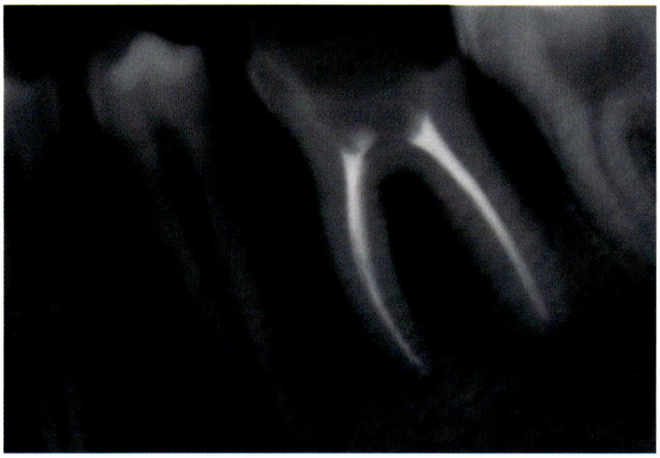

Fig. 17.6: Radiograph showing obturated first molar

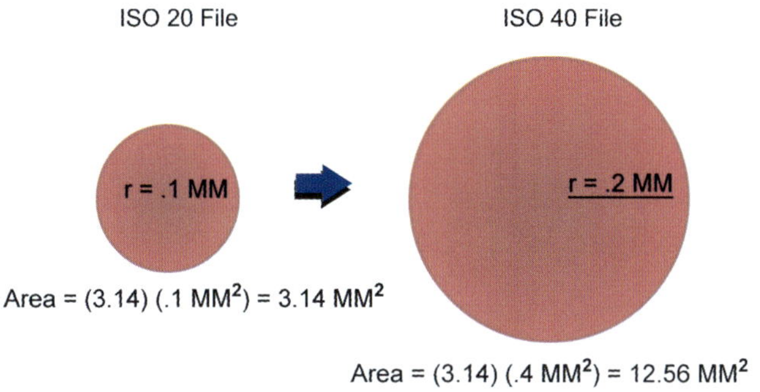


Fig. 17.7: Doubling the file size apically, increases the surface area of foramen four times

**Mechanical objectives of root canal preparation (given by Schilder)**

- The root canal preparation should develop a continuously tapering cone.
- Making the preparation in multiple plane which introduces the concept of "Flow".
- Making the canal narrower apically and widest coronally.
- Avoid transportation of foramen.
- Keep the apical opening as small as possible.

## Objectives of Biomechanical Preparation

### *Biologic Objectives of Root Canal Preparation*

Biologic objectives of biomechanical preparation are to remove the pulp tissue, bacteria and their by-products from the root canal space.

1. Procedure should be confined to the root canal space.
2. All infected pulp tissue, bacteria and their by products should be removed from the root canal.
3. Necrotic debris should not be forced periapically.
4. Sufficient space for intracanal medicaments and irrigants should be created.

## Clinical Objectives of Biomechanical Preparation

Before starting the endodontic therapy, the clinicians should plan the whole treatment so as to obtain the successful treatment results.

The clinician should evaluate the tooth to be treated to ensure that the particular tooth has favorable prognosis. Before performing cleaning and shaping, the straight line access to canal orifice should be obtained. All the overlying dentin should be removed and there should be flared and smooth internal walls to provide straight line access to root canals (Fig. 17.8). Since shaping facilitates cleaning, in properly shaped canals, instruments and irrigants can go deeper into the canals to remove all the debris and contents of root canal. This creates a smooth tapered opening to the apical terminus for obtaining three-dimension obturation of the root canal system.

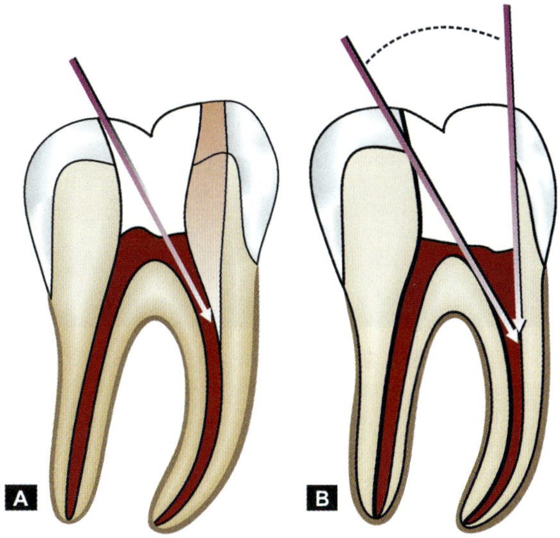


Fig. 17.8: Removal of overlying dentin causes smooth internal walls and provide straight line access to root canals

After obturation, there should be complete sealing of the pulp chamber and the access cavity so as to prevent microleakage into the canal system (Fig. 17.9). Tooth should be restored with permanent restoration to maintain its form, function and aesthetics and patient should be recalled on regular basis to evaluate the success of the treatment (Fig. 17.10). For past many years, there has been a gradual change in the ideal configuration of the prepared root canal. Earlier a round tapered and almost parallel shape was considered an ideal preparation but later when **Schilder** gave the concept of finished canal with gradually increasing the taper having the smallest diameter apically and widest diameter at the coronal orifice.

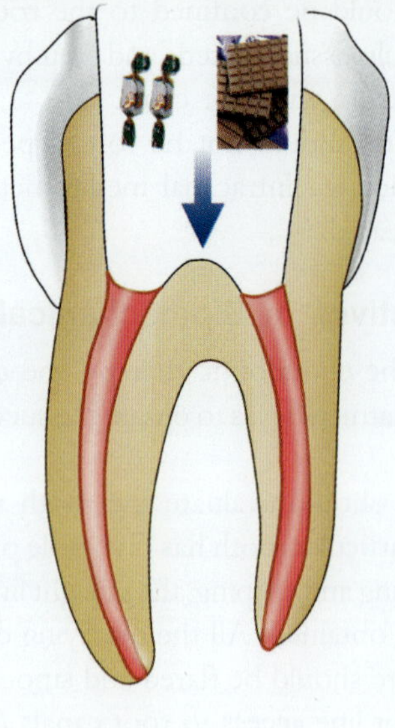

**Fig. 17.9:** Microleakage of root canal system in nonrestored tooth

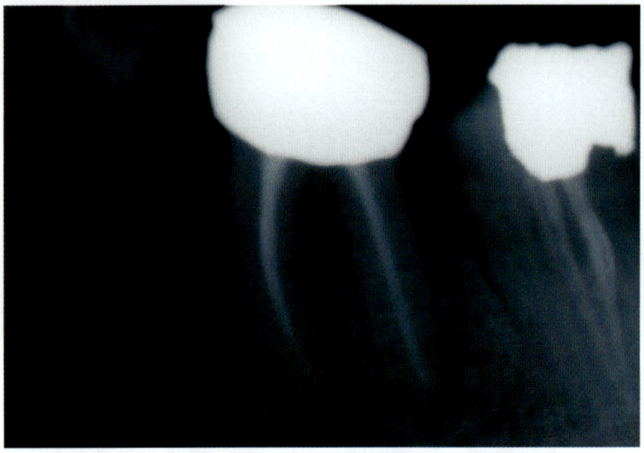

**Fig. 17.10:** Radiograph showing root canal treatment of first molar

**Instruments used for radicular preparation**

1. Hand instruments
   - i. Broaches
   - ii. Files
     - a. K files
     - b. Reamers
     - c. H-files
     - d. NiTi hand files
2. Rotary instruments
   - i. Gates glidden drills
   - ii ProTaper
   - iii. Profile
   - iv. Greater taper
   - v. Quantec file series
   - vi. Light speed
   - vii. RACE
   - viii. $K_3$ files
   - ix. Hero 642
3. Automated (ultrasonic/sonic)
4. Lasers

## DIFFERENT MOVEMENTS OF INSTRUMENTS

### Reaming

In Layman's terms, ream indicates use of sharp edged tool for enlarging holes. In endodontic practice, reaming is commonly done by use of reamers , though files can also be used. It involves clockwise rotation of an instrument. The instrument may be controlled from insertion to generate a cutting effect (Fig. 17.11).

### Filing

The term filing indicates push-pull motion with the instrument (Fig. 17.12). This method is commonly used for canal preparation.

But this active insertion of instrument with cutting force is a combination of both resistance to bending and apically directed hand pressure. This may lead to canal ledging, perforation and other procedural errors.

Nowadays, to avoid such errors, current modalities employ the technique of passive insertion of instrument, precurving of instruments and a quarter turn insertion.

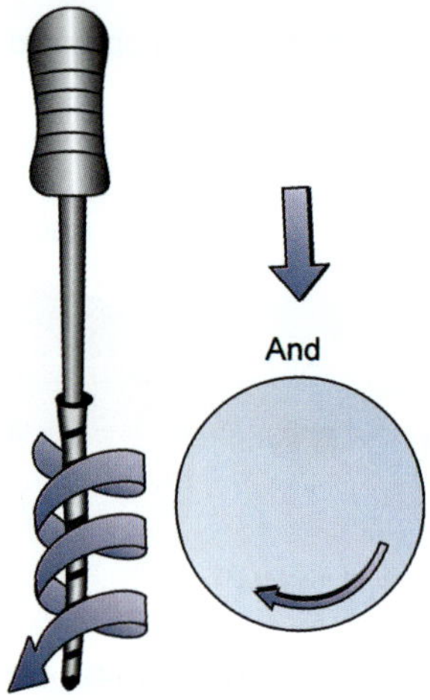


**Fig. 17.11:** Reaming motion involving clockwise rotation of instrument

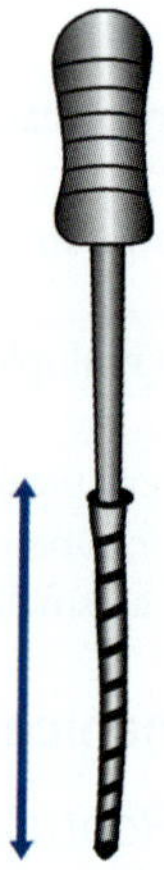

**Fig. 17.12:** Filing motion showing push and pull action of instrument

## Combination of Reaming and Filing (Fig. 17.13)

In this technique file is inserted with a quarter turn clockwise and apically directed pressure (i.e. reaming) and then is subsequently withdrawn (i.e. filing).

File edges get engaged into dentin while insertion and breaks the loose dentin during its withdrawal. By performing this combination of reaming and filing repeatedly, canal enlargement takes place. But this technique has also shown the occurrence of frequent ledge formation, perforation and other procedural errors.

To overcome these shortcomings, this technique was modified by Schilder. He suggested to give a clockwise rotation of half revolution followed by directing the instrument apically. In this method every time when a file is withdrawn, it is followed by next in the series. Though this method is effective in producing clean canals but it is very laborious and time consuming.

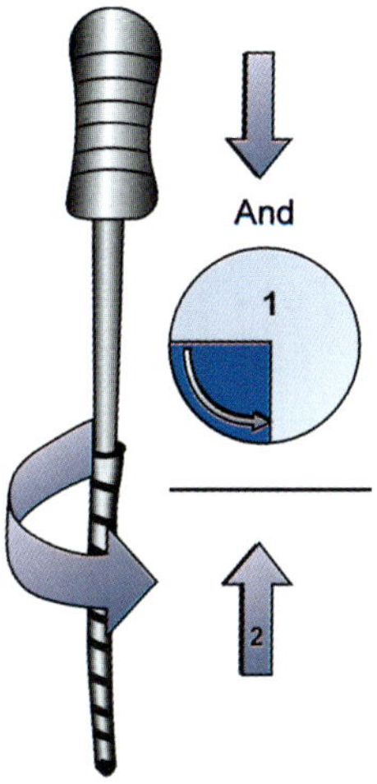


Fig. 17.13: Combination of reaming and filing

## Balanced Force Technique

This technique involves oscillation of instrument right and left with different arcs in either direction. Instrument is first inserted into the canal by moving it clockwise with one quarter turn. Then to cut dentin, file is rotated counter clockwise and simultaneously pushing apically to prevent it from backing out of the canal. Finally, the file is removed by rotating file clockwise simultaneously pulling the instrument out of the canal (Fig. 17.14).

This technique offers most efficient dentin cutting but care should be taken not to apply excessive force with this technique because it may lock the instrument into the canal (Fig. 17.15).

Since H-files and broaches do not possess left hand cutting efficiency, they are not used with this technique. Simultaneous apical pressure and anticlock-wise rotation of the file maintains the balance between tooth structure and the elastic memory of the instrument, this balance locates the instrument near the canal axis and thus avoids transportation of the canal.

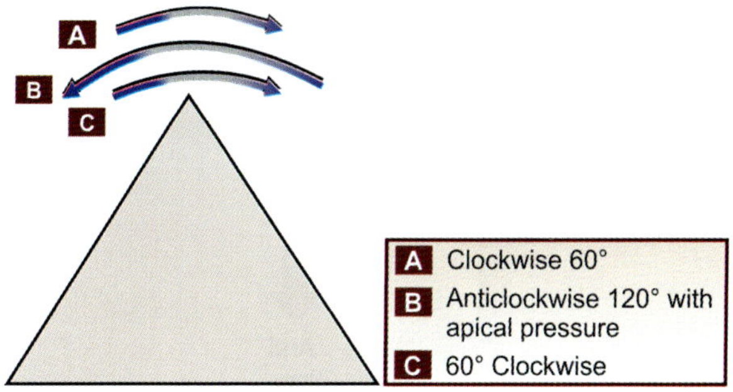


Fig. 17.14: Balanced force technique

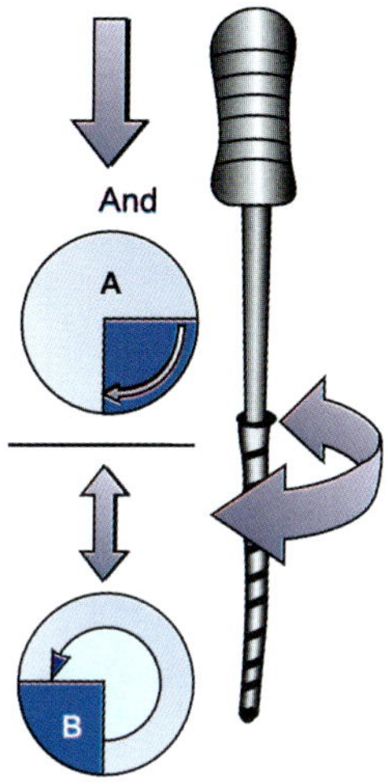


Fig. 17.15: If excessive force is applied, instrument may lock into the root canal system during rotation

## Watch Winding

It is back and forth oscillation of the endodontic instrument (file or reamer) right and left as it is advanced into the canal. The angle of rotation is usually 30 to 60 degrees (Figs 17.16 and 17.17).

This technique is efficient with K-type instruments. This motion is quite useful during biomechanical preparation of the canal. Watch winding motion is less aggressive than quarter turn and pull motion because in this motion, the instrument tip is not forced in to the apical area with each motion, thereby reducing the frequency of instrumental errors.

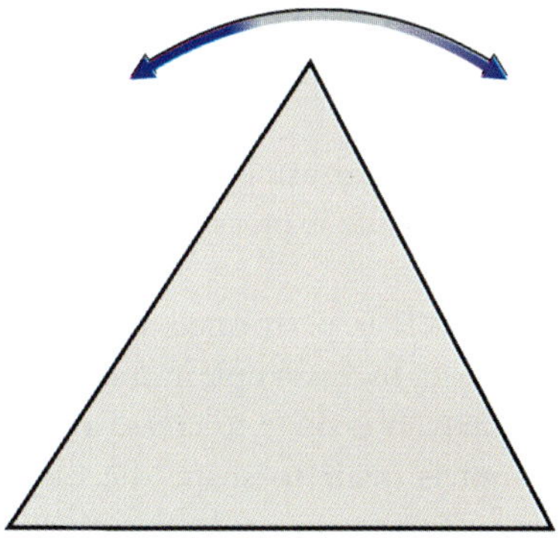


Fig. 17.16: Watch winding motion

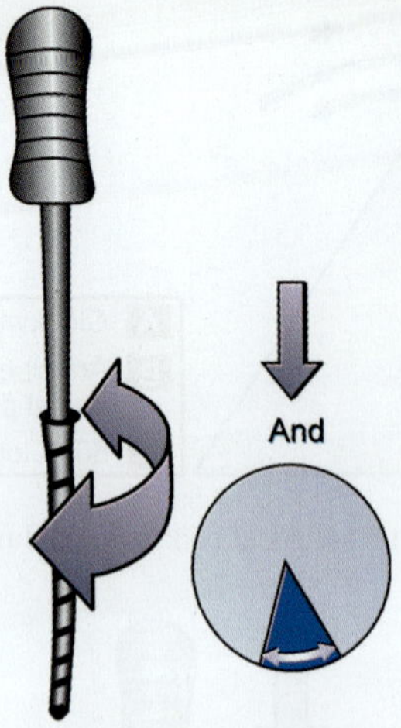


**Fig. 17.17:** Rotation of file in watch winding motion

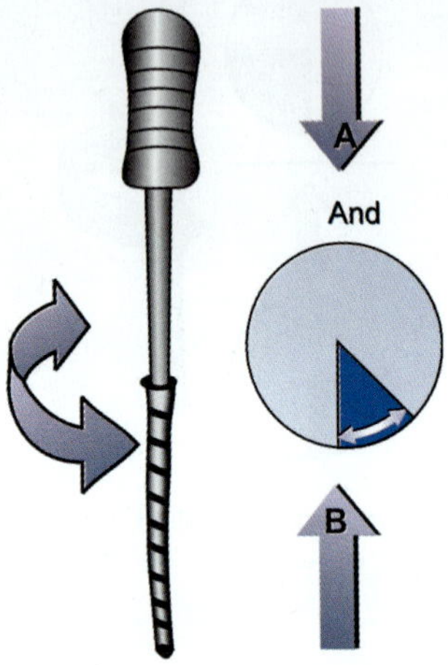


**Fig. 17.18:** Watch winding and pull motion

### Watch Winding and Pull Motion

In this, first instrument is moved apically by rotating it right and left through an arc. When the instrument feels any resistance, it is taken out of the canal by pull motion (Fig. 17.18). This technique is primarily used with Hedstroem files. When used with H-files, watch winding motion cannot cut dentin because H-files can cut only during pull motion.

### Motions of Instruments for Cleaning and Shaping

For effective use of reamers and files, following six different motions are given.

1. Follow: It is performed using files during initial cleaning and shaping. In this file is precurved so as to follow canal curvatures.
2. Follow withdraw: It is performed with files when apical foramen is reached. In this simple in and out motion is given to the instrument. It is done to create a path for foramen and no attempt is made to shape the canal.
3. Cart: Cart means transporting. In this precurved reamer is passed through the canal with gentle force and random touch with dentinal wall up to the apical foramen. It is done to transport pulp remnants and dentinal debris.
4. Carve: Carve is performed with reamers to do shaping of the canals. In this a precurved reamer as touched with dentinal wall and canal is shaped on withdrawal.
5. Smooth: It is performed with files. In this circumferential motion is given to smoothen the canal walls.
6. Patency: It is performed with files or reamers. Patency means that apical foramen has been cleared of any debris in its path.

## BASIC PRINCIPLES OF CANAL INSTRUMENTATION

1. There should be a straight line access to the canal orifices (Fig 17.19). Creation of a straight line access by removing overhang dentine influences the forces exerted by a file in apical third of the canal.
2. Files are always worked with in a canal filled with irrigant. Therefore, copious irrigation is done in between the instrumentation, i.e. canal must always be prepared in wet environment.
3. Preparation of canal should be completed while retaining its original form and the shape (Fig. 17.20).
4. Exploration of the orifice is always done with smaller file to gauge the canal size and the configuration.

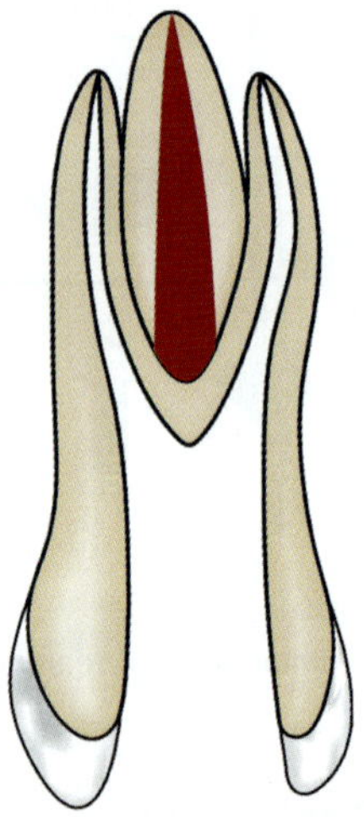

**Fig. 17.19:** Straight line access to root canal system

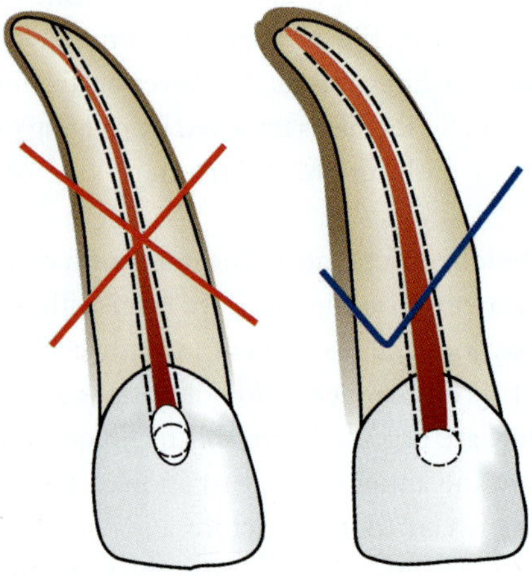

**Fig. 17.20:** Prepared canal should retain its original form and shape

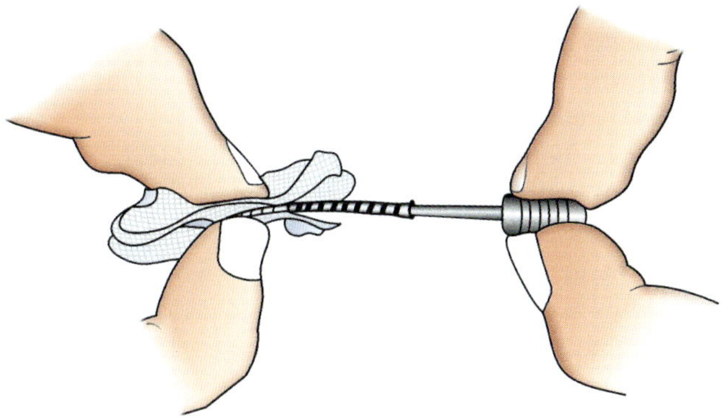

Fig. 17.21: Cleaning of flutes should be done after each instrumentation

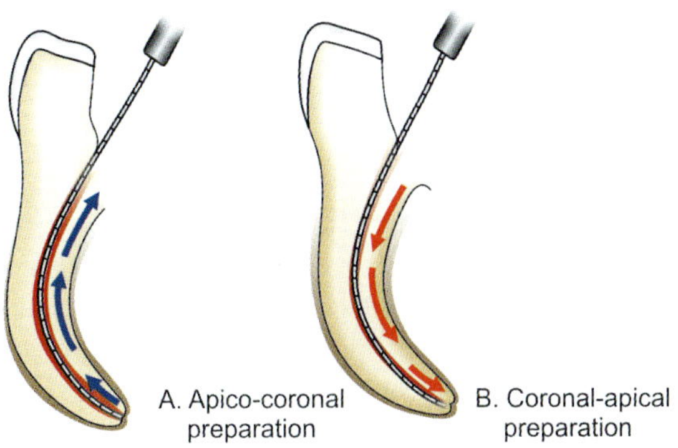


Fig. 17.22: Techniques of biomechanical preparation

5. Canal enlargement should be done by using instruments in the sequential order without skipping sizes.
6. All the working instruments should be kept in confines of the root canal to avoid any procedural accidents.
7. Instrument binding or dentin removal on insertion should be avoided.
8. After each insertion and removal of the file, its flutes should be cleaned and inspected (Fig. 17.21).
9. Smaller number instruments should be used extravagantly.
10. Recapitulation is regularly done to loosen debris by returning to working length. The canal walls should not be enlarged during recapitulation.
11. Over preparation and too aggressive over enlargement of the curved canals should be avoided.
12. Creation of an apical stop may be impossible if apical foramen is already very large. Overusing of larger files should be avoided in such cases as it may result in further enlargement of apical opening.
13. Never force the instrument in the canal. Forcing or continuing to rotate an instrument may break the instrument.
14. Establish the apical patency before starting the biomechanical preparation of tooth. Apical patency of the canal established and checked, by passing a smaller number file (No. 10) across the apex. The aim is to allow for creation of a preparation and filling extending fully to the periodontal ligament. Establishing the patency is believed to be non-harmful considering the blood supply and immune response present in the periapical area.

## TECHNIQUES OF ROOT CANAL PREPARATION

Basically, there are ***two approaches*** used for ***biomechanical preparation***, either starting at the apex with fine instruments and working up to the orifice with progressively larger instruments, this is ***Step back technique*** or starting at the orifice with larger instrument and working up to apex with larger instruments, this is ***Crown down technique (Fig. 17.22).***

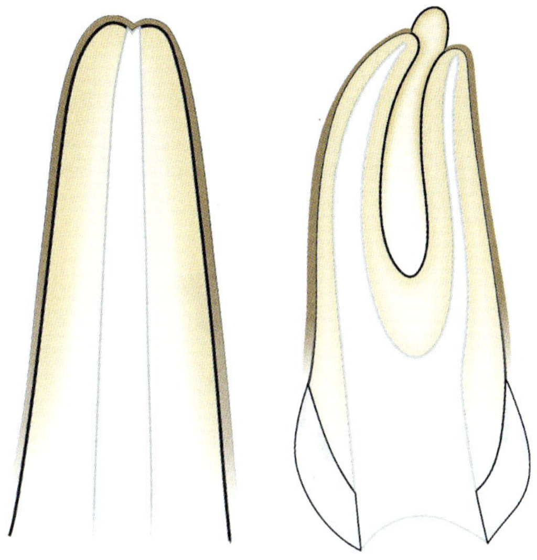

Fig. 17.23: Tapered canal preparation

Various other techniques have been modified out of these two basic techniques. Whichever the techniques is used for canal preparation one should ensure to stay within the confines of root canal and produce a continuous tapered preparation of the canal (Fig. 17.23).

## STANDARDIZED TECHNIQUE OF CANAL PREPARATION

It was introduced by Ingle. It was one of the first techniques to be used.

### Technique

1. Determine working length and select initial apical file.
2. Do circumferential filing to increase the apical construction 2-3 files sizes greater than initial apical file. In circumferential filing, file is inserted into the root canal to the desired length engaged into canal wall by applying lateral pressure and then withdrawn. This procedure is performed around all the canal walls.

## Disadvantages of Standardized Technique

- Chances of loss of working length due to accumulation of dentin debris.
- Increased incidences of ledging, zipping and perforation in curved canals.

## STEP BACK TECHNIQUE

Step back technique is also known as ***Telescopic canal preparation*** or ***serial root canal preparation.*** Step back technique emphasizes keeping the apical preparation small, in its original position and producing a gradual taper coronally. This technique was first described in 1960 by Mullaney.

Basically this technique involves the canal preparation into ***two phases; phase I*** involves the preparation of apical constriction and ***phase II*** involves the preparation of the remaining canal.

### *Phase I*

1. Evaluate the carious tooth before initiating endodontic treatment (Fig 17.24).
2. Initially prepare the access cavity, and locate the canal orifices (Figs 17.25).
3. Establish the working length of the tooth using pathfinder.
4. Now insert the first instrument into the canal with watch winding motion. In watch winding motion, a gentle clockwise and anticlockwise rotation of file with minimal apical pressure is given (Fig. 17.26).
5. Remove the instrument and irrigate the canal.
6. Don't forget to lubricate the instrument for use in apical area because it is shown that lubricant emulsifies the fibrous pulp tissue allowing the instrument to remove it whereas irrigants may not reach the apical area to dissolve the tissues.
7. Place the next larger size files to the working length in similar manner and again irrigate the canal (Fig. 17.27).
8. Don't forget to recapitulate the canal with previous smaller number instrument. This breaks up apical debris which are washed away with the irrigant.
9. Repeat the process until a size 25 K-file reaches the working length (Fig. 17.28). Recapitulate between the files by placing a small file to the working length (Fig. 17.29).

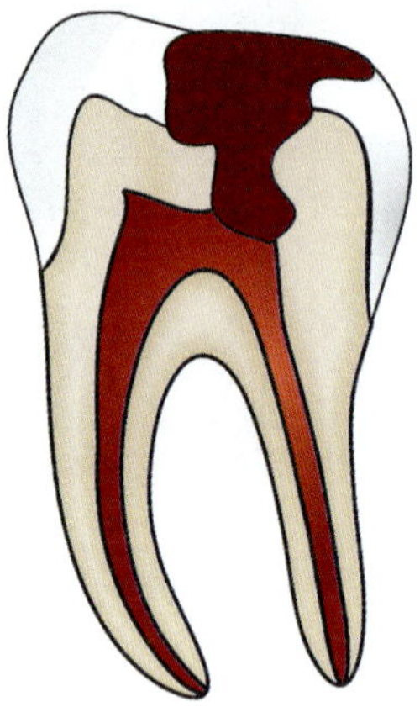

**Fig. 17.24:** Tooth decay causing pulp exposure

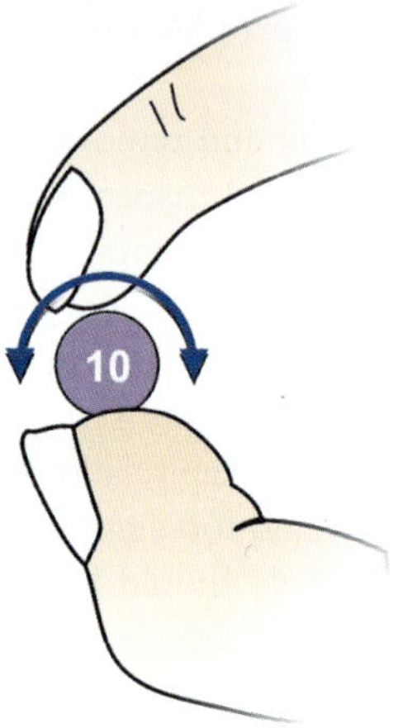


**Fig. 17.26:** Watch winding motion with gentle clockwise and anticlockwise motion of the file

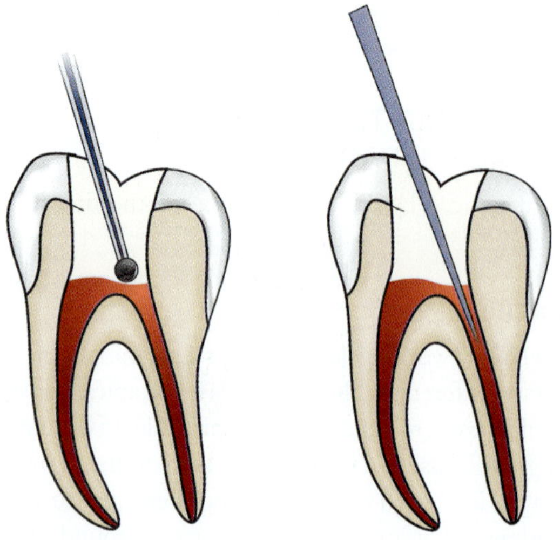

**Fig. 17.25:** Prepare the access cavity and locate the canal orifices

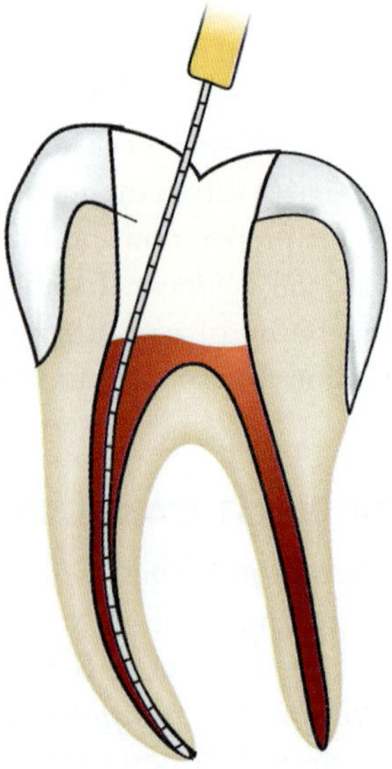

**Fig. 17.27:** Place file to working length

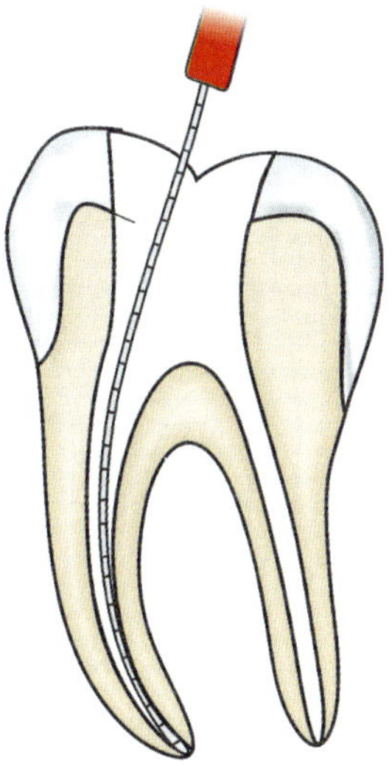

**Fig. 17.28:** 25 No. file at working length

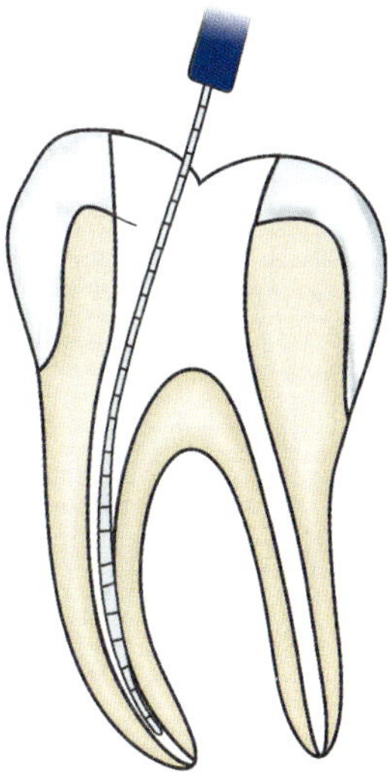

**Fig. 17.30:** 30 No. file 1 mm short of working length

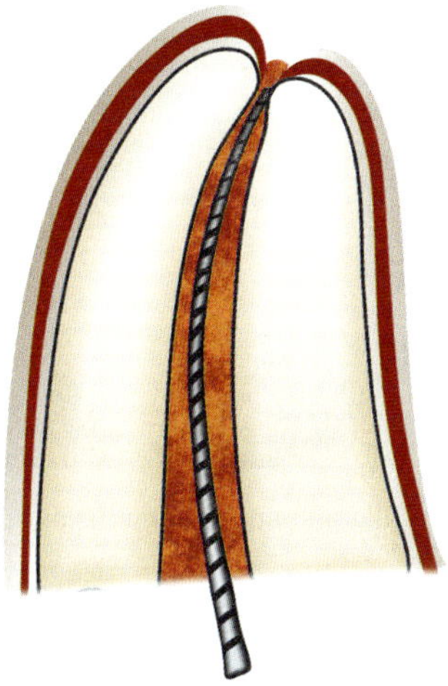

**Fig. 17.29:** Recapitulation using smaller file

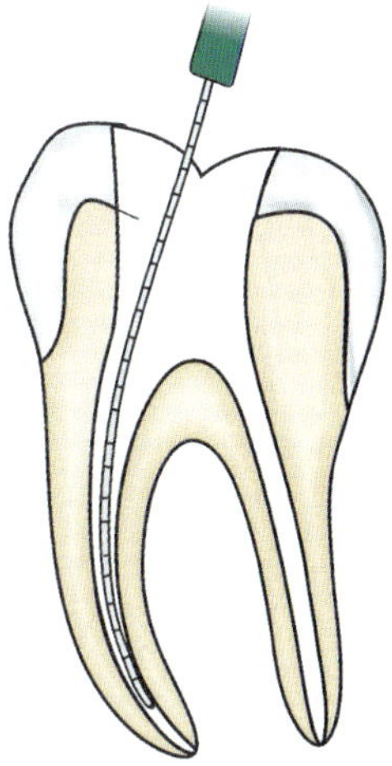

**Fig. 17.31:** 35 No. file 2 mm short of working length

### *Phase II*

1. Place next file in the series to a length 1 mm short of working length. Insert the instrument into the canal with watch winding motion, remove it after circumferential filing, irrigate and recapitulate (Fig. 17.30).
2. Repeat the same procedure with successively larger files at 1 mm increments from the previously used file (Fig. 17.31).
3. Similarly mid canal area and coronal part of the canal is prepared and shaped with larger number files (Figs 17.32 and 17.33).
4. Finally, refining of the root canal is done by master apical file with push-pull strokes to achieve a smooth taper form of the root canal (Fig. 17.34).

### *Variations in the Step Back Technique*

It involves following:

a. Use of Gates Glidden drills for initial enlargement of the coronal part of root canal (Figs 17.35A and B).

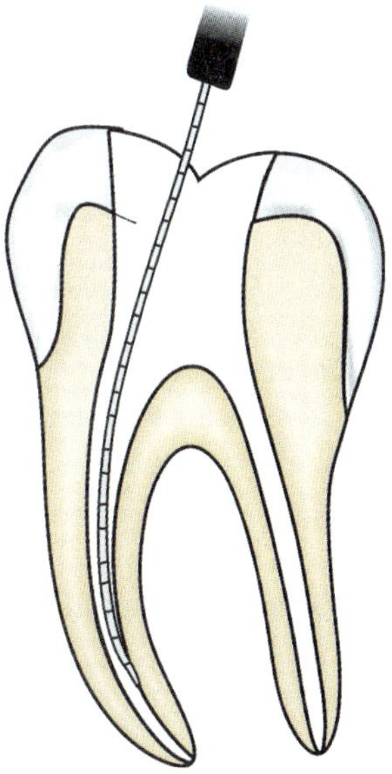

**Fig. 17.32:** 40 No. file 3 mm short of working length

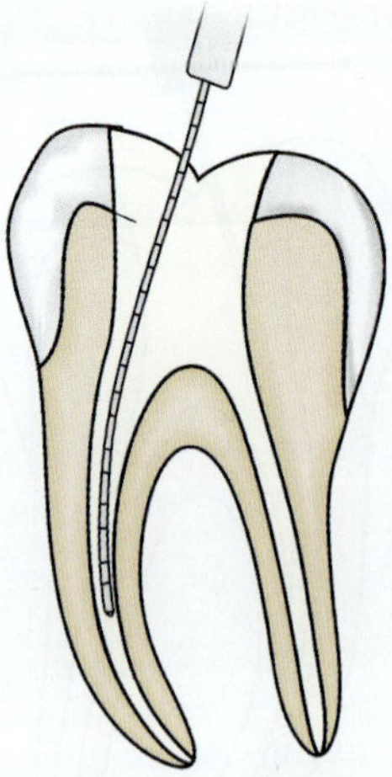

Fig. 17.33: 45 No. file 4 mm short of working length

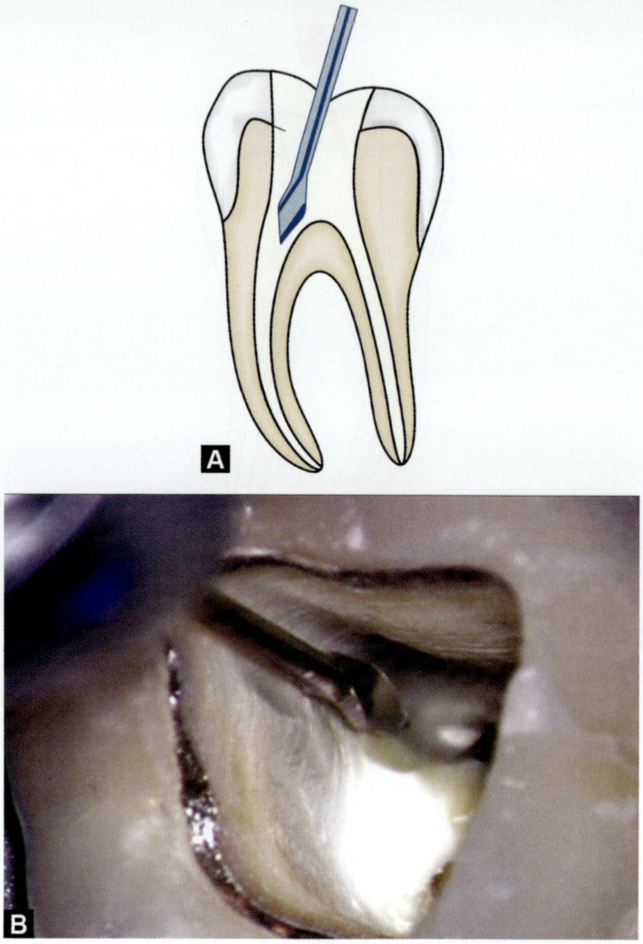


Figs 17.35A and B: Enlargement of canal using Gates-Glidden drill

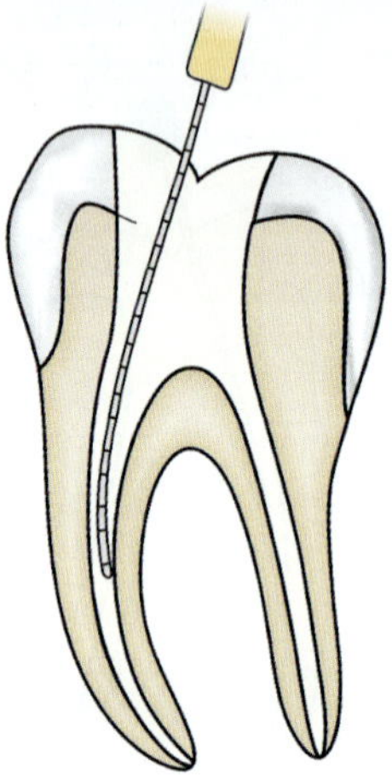

Fig. 17.34: 50 No. file for canal preparation

b. Use of smaller Gates-Glidden drills to prepare the mid root level (Figs 17.36A and B).
c. Use of Hedstorm files to flare the preparation.

Before using Gate-Glidden, one must gain access to the canal orifices by removing the overlying dentinal structure.

Thus we see that step back technique creates small apical preparation with larger instruments used at successively decreasing lengths to create a taper. The taper of canal preparation could be altered by changing the interval between the consecutive instruments for example taper of prepared canal could be increased by reducing the intervals between each successive file from 1 to 0.5 mm.

Though this technique has been used since long time, but various studies have shown that this apical to coronal preparation of root canals can cause deformation of the canal shape, instrument separation, zipping of the apical area, significant apical extrusion of debris, apical blockage, etc. (Figs 17.37A to C).

## Advantage of Step Back Technique

More flare at coronal part of root canal with proper apical stop.

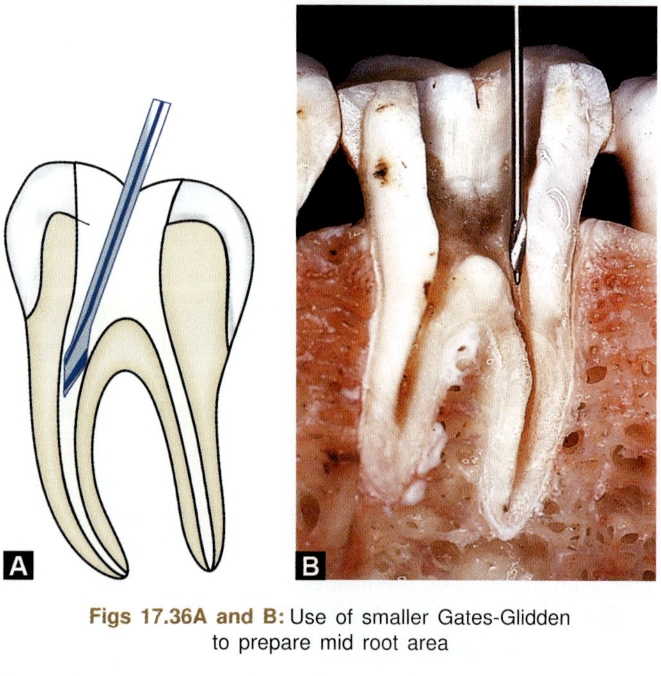


Figs 17.36A and B: Use of smaller Gates-Glidden to prepare mid root area

## Disadvantages of Step Back Technique

1. Difficult to irrigate apical region
2. More chances of pushing debris periapically.
3. Time consuming.
4. Increased chances of iatrogenic errors for example ledge formation in curved canals.

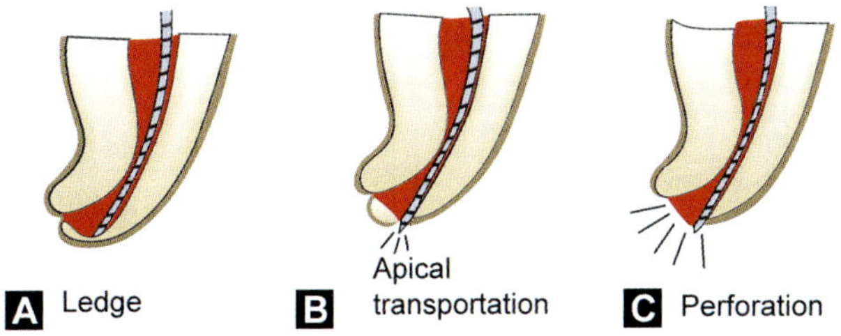


**Figs 17.37A to C:** Procedural errors

5. Difficult to penetrate instruments in canal.
6. More chances of instrument fracture.

## MODIFIED STEP BACK TECHNIQUE

In this technique, the preparation is completed in apical third of the canal. After this step back procedure is started 2-3 mm short of minor diameter/apical constriction so as to give an almost parallel retention form at the apical area. This receives the primary gutta-percha point which shows slight tug back, when the point is removed. This explains that cone fits snuggly into the last 2-3 mm of the prepared canal.

### Advantages

- Less chances of apical transportation
- Increases the chances of canal walls being planed.

### Disadvantages

- Less space for irrigants, leads to accumulation of debris in the canals.
- Chances of a change in working length because coronal constriction is removed at the end.
- Passing a precurved instrument in coronally tight canals, straightens the instrument. This may result in ledge formation.

## PASSIVE STEP BACK TECHNIQUE

Passive step back technique was developed by ***Torabinajed.*** This technique involves the combination of hand instruments (files) and the rotary instruments (Gates-Glidden drills and Pesso reamers) to attain an adequate coronal flare before apical root canal preparation.

It provides gradual enlargement of the root in an apical to coronal direction without applying force, thereby reducing the occurrence of procedural errors like transportation of the canal, ledge or zip formation and this is convenient to both patient as well as doctor.

### Technique

1. First of all, after preparation of the access cavity, locate the canal orifices and flare the walls of access cavity using tapered diamond burs.
2. Now establish the correct working length using a number 15 file. A number 15 file is inserted to the estimated working length using very light pressure with one eighth to one quarter turn with push-pull stroke to establish the apical patency.
3. After this additional files of number 20, 25, 30, 35 and 40 are inserted into the canal passively. This step removes the debris and creates a mildly flared preparation for insertion of Gates-Glidden drills.
4. Copious irrigation of the canal system is frequently done with sodium hypochlorite.
5. After this, number 2 Gate-Glidden drill is inserted into mildly flared canal to a point, where it binds slightly. It is pulled back 1 to 1.5 mm and then activated.
   With up and down motion and slight pressure, the canal walls are flared. In the similar fashion, numbers 3 and 4 Gates-Gliddens are then used coronally.
6. Since flaring and removal of curvatures reduces the working length, so reconfirmation of the working length should be done before apical preparation.
7. After this, a number 20 file is inserted into the canal upto working length. The canal is then prepared with sequential use of progressively larger instruments placed successively short of the working length. Narrow canal should not be enlarged beyond the size of number 25 or 30 files.

### Advantages of Passive Step Back Technique

- Removal of debris and minor canal obstructions.
- Knowledge of the canal morphology.
- Gradual passive enlargement of the canal in an apical to coronal direction.
- This technique can also be used with ultrasonic instruments.
- Decrease incidence of procedural errors like transportation of the canal, ledge or zip formation.

## HYBRID TECHNIQUE OF CANAL PREPARATION

In this technique a combination of step back and crown down preparation is used.

### Technique

In hybrid technique both rotary and hand instruments are used to prepare the canal.

1. Check the patency of canal using number 10 or 15 K flex files.
2. Prepare the coronal third of canal using hand or gates glidden drills till the point of curvature without applying excessive pressure.
3. Determine the working length.
4. Prepare the apical portion of canal using step back technique.
5. Recapitulate and irrigate the canal at every step so as to maintain patency of the canal.
6. Blend step back with step down procedure.

### Advantages

- Less chances of ledge formation.
- This technique maintains the integrity of dentin by avoiding excessive removal of radicular dentin.

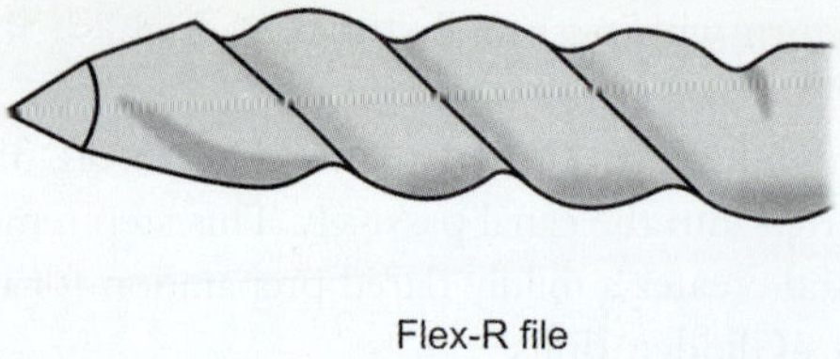


**Fig. 17.38:** Use of flex-R file for balanced force technique

## BALANCED FORCE TECHNIQUE

This technique was developed by ***Roane and Sabala in 1985***. It involves the use of instrument with noncutting tip. Since the K-type files have pyramidal tips with cutting angles which can be quite aggressive with clockwise rotation. For this technique, use of triangular cross sectioned instruments should be done. The decreased mass of the instrument and deeper cutting flutes improves the flexibility of instrument and decrease the restoring force of the instrument when placed in curved canals.

Use of Flex-R files is recommended for this technique. This file has "safe tip design" with a guiding land area behind the tip which allows the file to follow the canal curvature without binding in the outside wall of the curved canal (Fig. 17.38).

### Technique

1. In balanced force technique, first file which binds short of working length is inserted into the canal and rotated clockwise a quarter of a turn. This movement causes flutes to engage a small amount of dentin (Figs 17.39A and B).
2. Now file is rotated counterclockwise with apical pressure at least one third of a revolution (Fig. 17.40). It is the counterclockwise rotation with apical pressure which actually provides the cutting action by shearing off small amount of dentin engaged during clockwise rotation.
3. If there is little curvature or if instrument does not bind, only one or two counterclockwise motions are given. It should not be forced to give the counterclockwise rotation because it may lead to fracture of the instrument.
4. Then a final clockwise rotation is given to the instrument which loads the flutes of file with loosened debris and the file is withdrawn.

### Advantages of Balanced Force Technique

- With the help of this technique, there are lesser chances of canal transportation.
- One can manipulate the files at any point in the canal without creating a ledge or blockage.
- File cutting occurs only at apical extent of the file.

## REVERSE BALANCED FORCE PREPARATION

For reverse balanced force technique NiTi greater taper hand files are used because flutes of these files are machined in a reverse direction unlike other files. Also handle of these files is increased in size to make the manipulation of files easier for reverse balanced for technique.

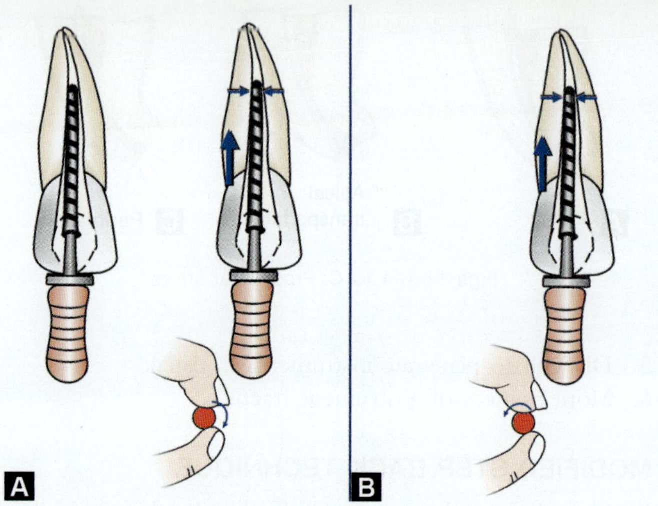


**Figs 17.39A and B:** (A) Engaging dentin with quarter clockwise turn, (B) Cutting action by anticlockwise motion with apical pressure

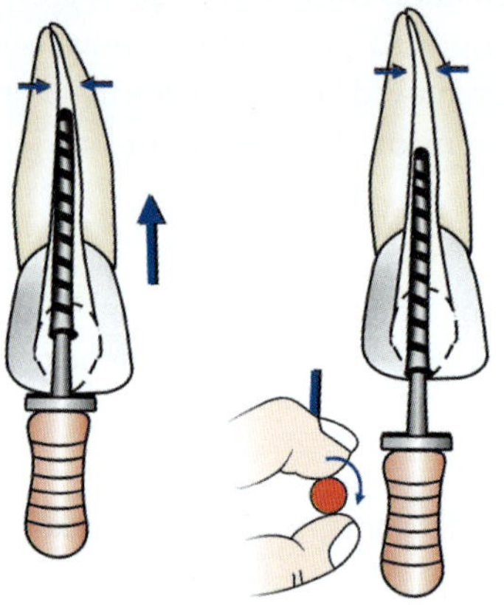

**Fig. 17.40:** Now file is turned quarter clockwise. It picks the debris and withdraws the instrument

### Technique

- Insert file in the canal and rotate it 60° in anticlockwise direction and then 120° in clockwise direction with apical pressure using GT files.
- These files are used in the sequence from largest to the smallest in crown down sequence progressively towards the apical direction till the estimated working length is achieved.
- Determine the working length.
- Prepare apical portion of canal using 2 percent tapered ISO files in balance force technique.

## ANTICURVATURE FILING

Concept of anticurvature filing was given by Lim and stock. Anticurvature filing was introduced to prevent excessive removal of dentin from thinner part of curved canals for example in mesial root of mandibular molar and mesiobuccal root of maxillary molar. If care is not taken while biomechanical preparation, strip formation can occur in danger zone area. It is seen that furcation side, i.e. danger zone has less dentin thickness than safety zone (for example on mesial side of mesial root of mandibular molar).

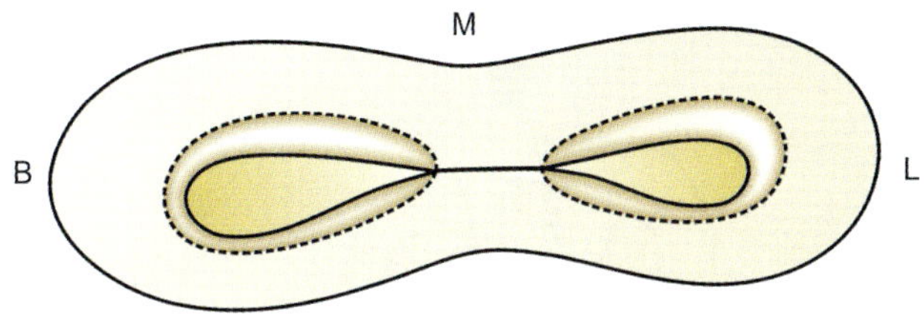


**Fig. 17.41:** Anticurvature filing

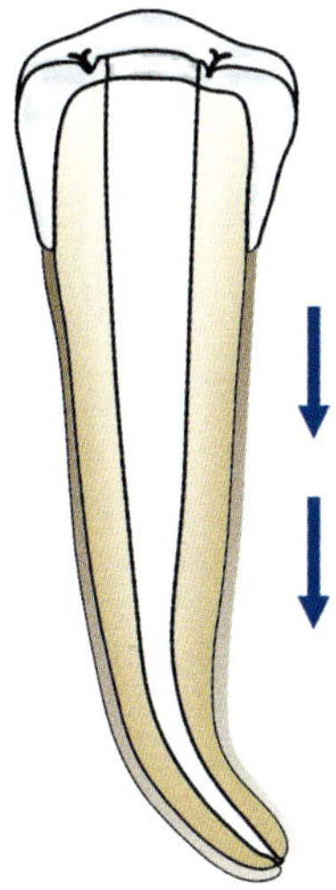

**Fig. 17.42:** Crown-down technique

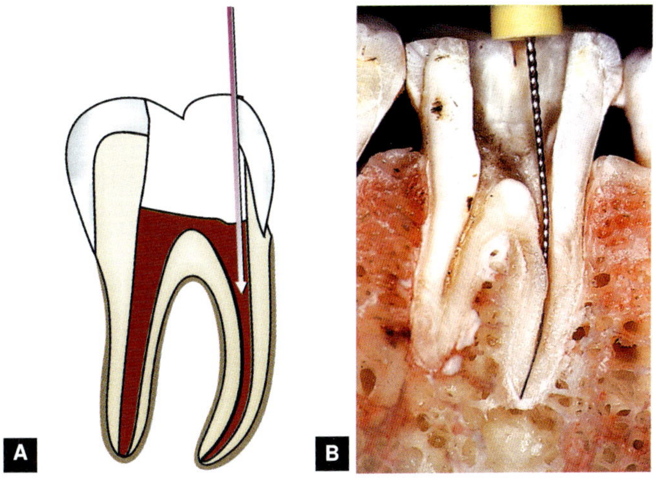


**Figs 17.43A and B:** Straight line access to root canal system

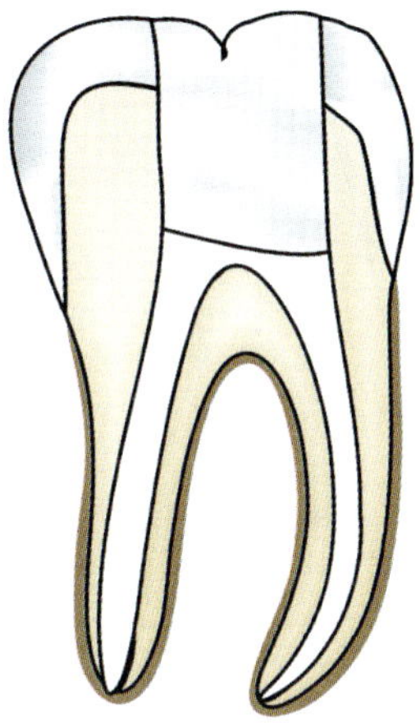

**Fig. 17.44:** Filling the chamber with irrigant solution

### Technique (Fig. 17.41)

Initial coronal flaring is done using rotary files. But for middle and apical third precurved hand instruments are used so as to avoid strip perforation.

Anticurvature filing involves lesser filing of the canal wall which is facing the curvature. For example in case of mesial root of mandibular molar, more filing is done on mesial side than on distal side.

## DOUBLE FLARE TECHNIQUE

It was introduced by Fava In this canal is explored using a small file. Then canal is prepared in crown down manner using K files in decreasing sizes. After this step back technique is followed in 1 mm increments with increasing file sizes. Frequent irrigation and recapitulation using master apical file is done during instrumentation.

## CROWN DOWN TECHNIQUE

In the crown down technique, the dentist prepares the canal from crown of the tooth, shaping the canal as he/she moves towards the apical portion of the canal (Fig. 17.42). Morgan and Montgomery found that this "crown down pressureless" techniques resulted in a rounder canal shape when compared to usual step back technique. Moreover, many studies have shown that greater apical enlargement without causing apical transportation can be achieved if coronal obstructions are eliminated.

### Technique of Crown Down Preparation

1. First step in the crown down technique is the access cavity preparation with no pulp chamber obstructions (Fig. 17.43). Locate the canal orifices with sharp explorer which shows binding in the pulp chamber.
2. Now fill the access cavity with an irrigant and start preflaring of the canal orifices (Fig. 17.44). Preflaring of the coronal third of the canal can be done by using hand instruments, Gates-Glidden drills or the nickle-titanium rotary instruments.
3. Gates-Glidden drills can be used after scouting the canal orifices with number 10 or 15 files. The crown down approach begins with larger Gates-Glidden first (Fig. 17.45). After using this subsequent, smaller diameter Gates-Glidden are worked into the canal with additional mm to complete coronal flaring. One should take care to avoid carrying all the Gates-Glidden drills to same level which may lead to excessive cutting of the dentin, weakening of the roots and thereby "Coke Bottle Appearance" in the radiographs (Fig. 17.46).
4. Frequent irrigation with sodium hypochlorite and recapitulation with a smaller file (usually No. 10 file) to prevent canal blockage.

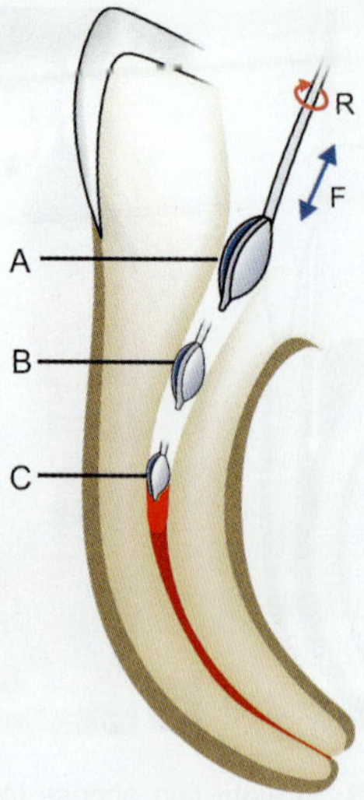


**Fig. 17.45:** Use of Gates-Glidden for preflaring

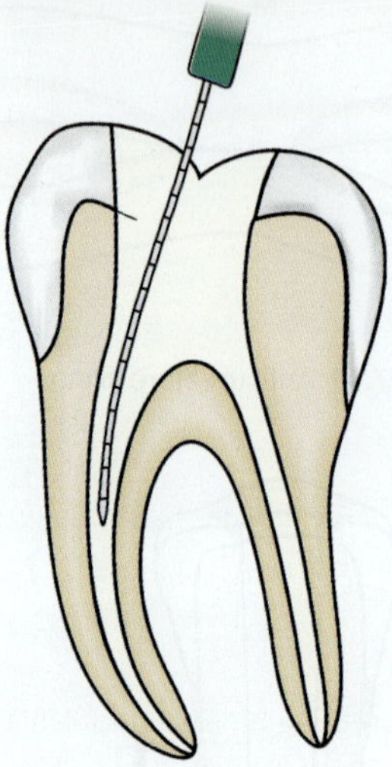

**Fig. 17.48:** Use of larger files to prepare coronal third

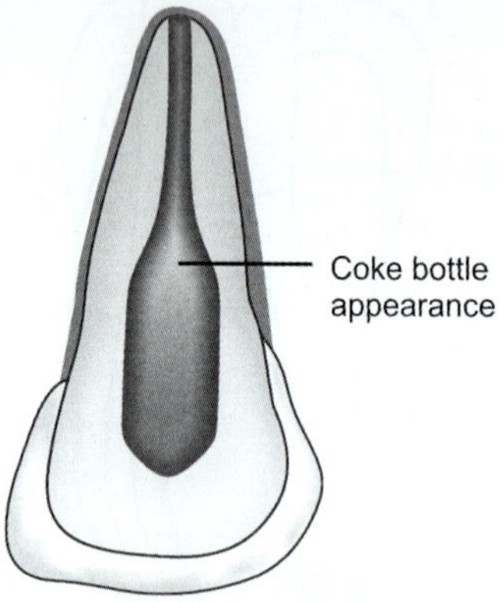


**Fig. 17.46:** "Coke-bottle appearance" caused by excessive use of Gates-Glidden drills

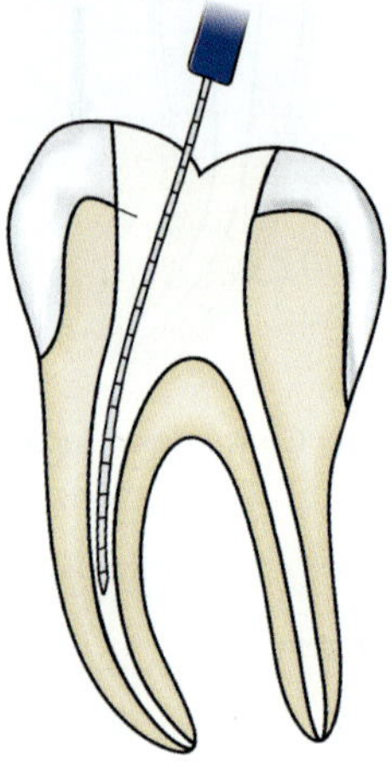

**Fig. 17.49:** Preparation of canal at middle third

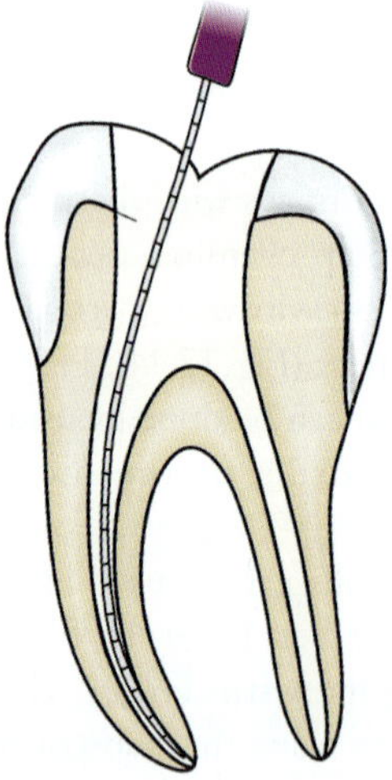

**Fig. 17.47:** Establishing working length using a small instrument

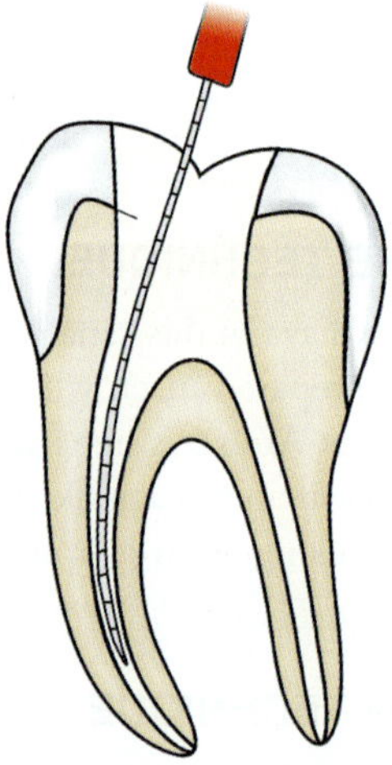

**Fig. 17.50:** Apical preparation of canal

5. After establishing coronal and mid root enlargement explore the canal and establish the working length with small instruments (Fig. 17.47).
6. Introduce larger files to coronal part of the canal and prepare it (Fig. 17.48). Subsequently introduce progressively smaller number files deeper into the canal in sequential order and prepare the apical part of the canal (Figs 17.49 and 17.50).
7. Final apical preparation is prepared and finished along with frequent irrigation of the canal system.

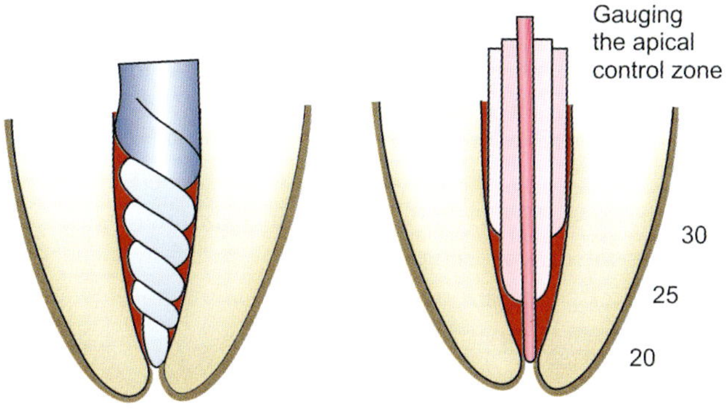


Fig. 17.51: Apical gauging of root canal

The classical apical third preparation should have a tapered shape which has been enlarged to at least size 20 at apex and each successive instrument should move away from the foramen by 1/2 mm increments.

## Apical Gauging

1. The function of apical gauging is to measure the apical diameter of the canal prior to cutting the final shape. This is necessary to insure that the final tapered preparation extends all the way to the terminus of the canal (Fig. 17.51).
2. Use NiTi K-files for gauging. The flexibility allows for much more accurate apical gauging in curved canals than with stainless steel, insuring the apical accuracy of obturation.
3. No effort is made to cut dentin during apical gauging. The gauging instruments are inserted straight in and are pulled straight out with no rotation.
4. Always use *17 percent aqueous EDTA* as an irrigant during gauging to remove the smear layer.

## Biological Benefits of Crown Down Technique

1. Removal of tissue debris coronally, thus minimizing the extrusion of debris periapically.
2. Reduction of postoperative sensitivity which could result from periapical extrusion of debris.
3. Greater volumes of irrigants can reach in canal irregularities in early stages of canal preparation because of coronal flaring.
4. Better dissolution of tissue with increased penetration of the irrigants.
5. Rapid removal of contaminated and infected tissues from the root canal system.

## Clinical Advantages of the Crown Down Technique

1. Enhanced tactile sensation with instruments because of removal of coronal interferences (Fig. 17.52).
2. Flexible (smaller) files are used in apical portion of the canal; where as larger (stiffer) files need not be forced but kept short of the apex.
3. In curved canals, after doing coronal flaring, files can go upto apex more effectively due to decrease deviation of instruments in the canal curvature.

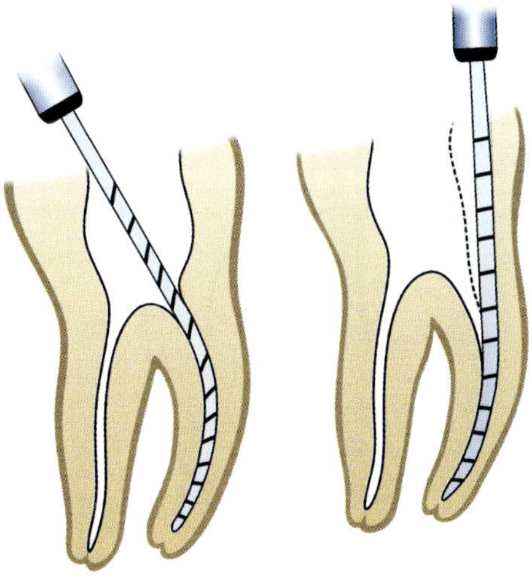

Fig. 17.52: Preflaring of canal causes removal of coronal interferences

4. Provides more space of irrigants.
5. Straight line access to root curves and canal junctions.
6. Enhanced movement of debris coronally.
7. Desired shape of canal can be obtained that is narrow at apex, wider at coronal (Figs 17.53 and 17.54).
8. Predictable quality of canal cleaning and shaping.
9. Decreased frequency of canal blockages.

The crown down is often suggested as a basic approach using nickel-titanium rotary instruments. Very few limitations exist in the application of the crown-down technique. Its application may be limited however to the use of hand instruments in specific situations. As with any technique, there will be a learning curve in its implementation, and the achievements with this technique of root canal cleaning and shaping may be affected by:

1. Operator desire to learn and skill level developed in application.
2. The use of end cutting rotary instruments in small or partially calcified canals may predispose to perforation as the instrument moves apically.
3. In canals that curve severely the rotary instruments cannot be precurved for placement and ease of penetration to enlarge the coronal third of the canal. In these cases, the

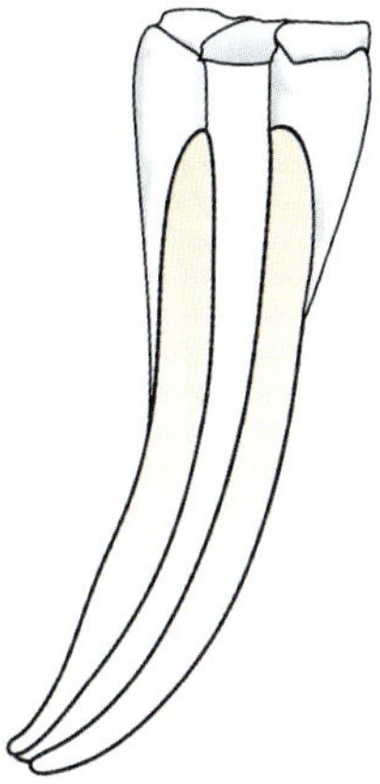

Fig. 17.53: A well-prepared canal mandibular premolar

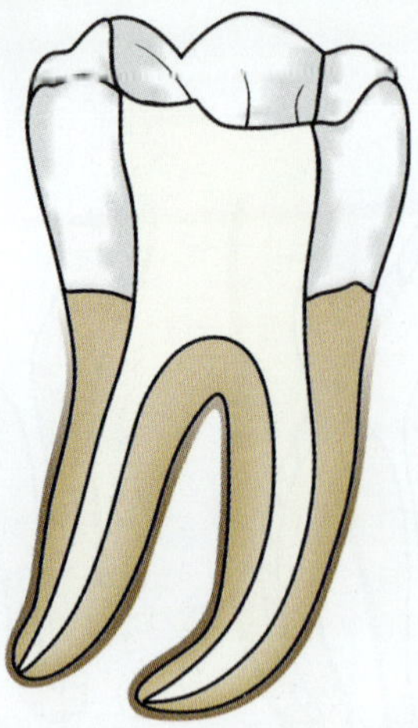

Fig. 17.54: A well prepared tapered preparation of mandibular molar

crown down technique can still be implemented by using hand instruments prior to rotary instruments.

4. If large, less flexible rotary instruments are used too rapidly and deeply in the root canal, a ledge may form (Fig. 17.55).

**Step back vs. crown down technique**

| *Step back technique* | *Crown down technique* |
|---|---|
| 1. Apico-coronal technique | 1. Corono-apical technique |
| 2. Has been used for past many year | 2. Introduced recently an gaining popularity. |
| 3. Starts with smallest instruments | 3. Starts with largest instruments. |
| 4. Shapes apical 1/3rd initially | 4. Shapes coronal 1/3rd initially. |
| 5. Commonly uses hand files | 5. Commonly uses rotary files. |

## ENGINE DRIVEN PREPARATION WITH NiTi INSTRUMENTS

These instruments were introduced in early 1990s, and since then they have become indispensable tools for canal enlargement. Before using these instruments one should take care to have a straight line access to the canal system. Canals should be thoroughly explored and passively enlarged before using rotary instrument. Instruments should be constantly moving and speed of rotation of each instrument should be known.

All of these NiTi rotary systems incorporate:

- Crown down preparation.
- Apical preparation as finale.
- Increasing taper instruments.

## PROFILE SYSTEM

Profile instruments system was introduced by Dr Johnson in 1944. Earlier profile system was sold as series 29 instruments. After this profile series were introduced with greater tapers of 19 mm lengths and ISO sized tips. Suggested rotational speed for profiles is 150-300 RPM. Cross section of profiles shows central parallel core with three equally shaped U-shaped grooves along with radial lands (Fig. 17.56). The negative rake angle of profiles makes them to cut dentin in planning motion.

### Clinical Technique for Use of Profiles

1. Make a straight line access to the canal orifice.
2. Estimate the working length of the canal from preoperative radiograph.
3. Create a glide path before using orifice shapers. Establish this path with a small, flexible, stainless steel number 15 or 20 file.
4. Use orifices shapers sizes 4, 3, 2, and 1 in the coronal third of the canal.
5. Perform crown down technique using the profile instruments of taper/size 0.06 /30,0.06/25,0.04/30 and 0.04/25 to the resistance. For larger canals use 0.06/35,0.06/30,0.04/35 and 0.04/30.
6. Now determine the exact working length by inserting conventional number 15 K-file (2% taper).
7. After establishing the exact working length complete the crown down procedure up until this length. Use profile 0.04/25, 0.04/30 for apical preparatio.

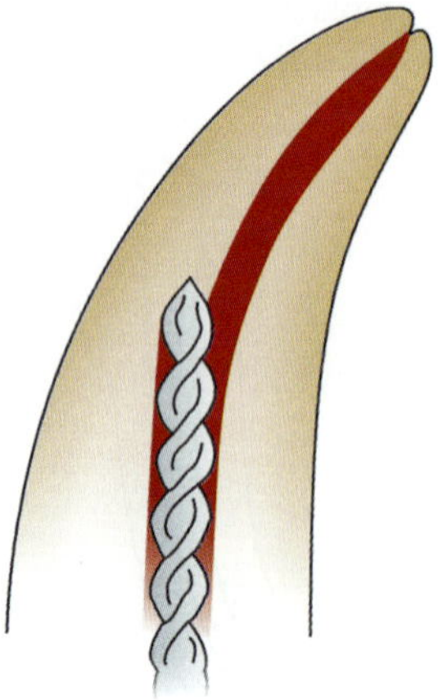

Fig. 17.55: Ledge formation caused by use of stiff instrument in curved canals

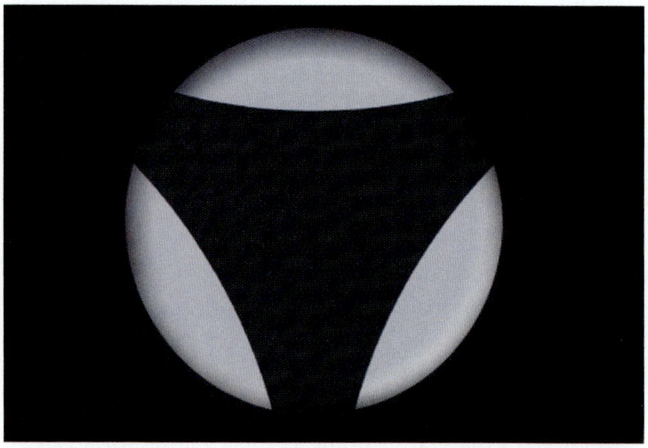

Fig. 17.56: U-shaped grooves with radial land

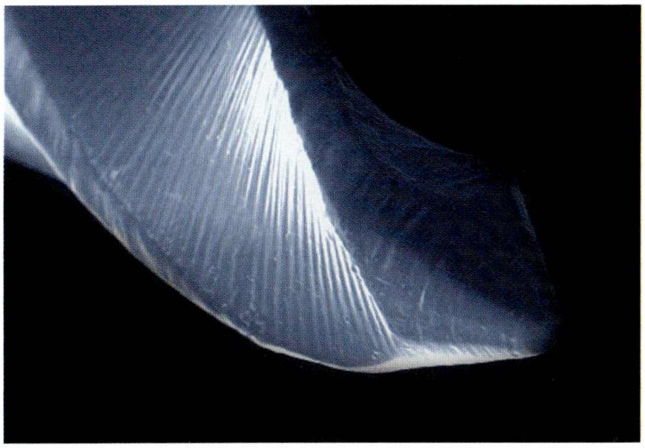

Fig. 17.57: Presence of radial land and non-cutting tip keeps profile self centered in root canals

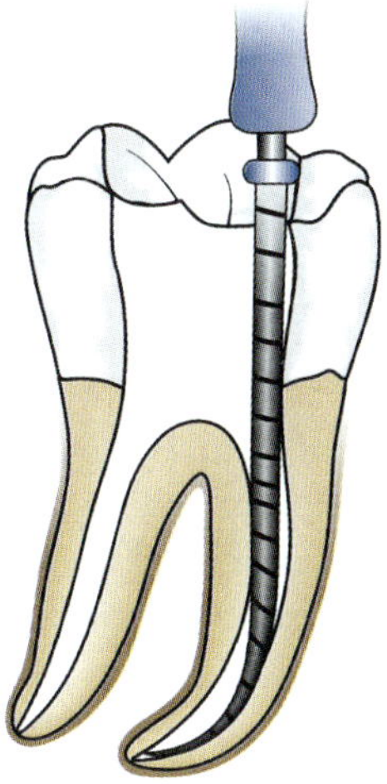

Fig. 17.58: Straight line access to canal orifices

8. Now final flaring is done using profile 0.06/25 short of working length to merge coronal and apical preparation.

In summary the profile instruments are used in both descending order of the diameter (i.e. for crown down from largest to the smallest) and in ascending order of diameter (for preparation to the exact working length and for final flaring from smallest to the largest).

### Advantages

1. Presence of radial land and non-cutting tip keep the Profiles self centered in root canal thus preserving the natural canal path (Fig. 17.57). It also avoids risk of zip or transportation of canal.
2. Presence of 20° helical angle allows effective removal of dentin debris, thus eliminating the risk of debris blocking the canal or being pushed into the periapical area.
3. Presence of radial land prevents its screwing into the canal and thus reduces the fracture risk.
4. Because of presence of modified tip without transition angle and negative rake angle, profiles work the dentin in planning motion.

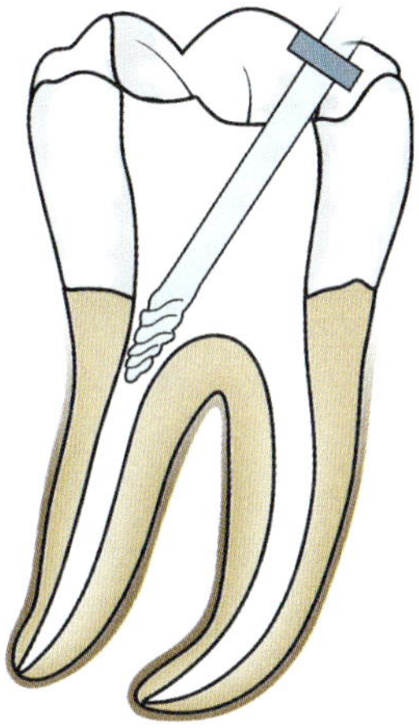

Fig. 17.59: Use of 0.12 GT files for coronal preparation

## GREATER TAPER FILES (GT FILES)

The GT rotary instruments possess a U-shaped file design with ISO tip sizes of 20, 30 and 40 and tapers of 0.04, 0.06, 0.08,.010 and 0.12. Accessory GT files for use as orifice openers are available in sizes of 0.12 taper in ISO sizes of 35, 50, 70 and 90.Negative rake angle of these files makes them to cut the dentin in planning motion.

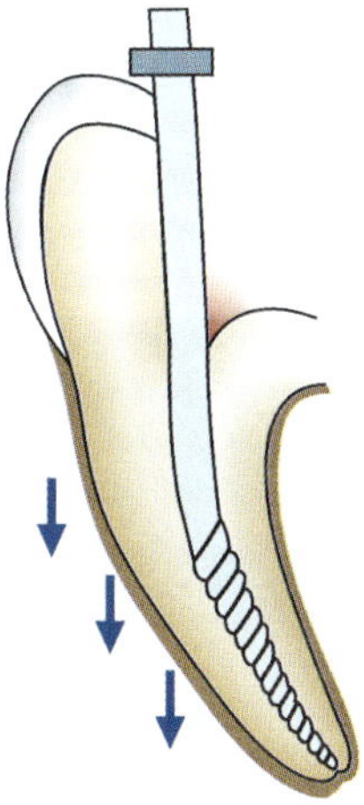

Fig. 17.60: Apical preparation using GT files

### Clinical Technique

1. Obtain a straight line access to the canal orifice and establish the glide path using No. 15 stainless steel file (Fig. 17.58).
2. Lubricate the canal and use GT files (0.12, 0.10, 0.08 and 0.06 taper) in crown down fashion at 150-300 rpm (Fig. 17.59).
3. When GT file reaches the two-thirds of estimated working length, establish the correct working length using 15 number stainless steel file.
4. Select the final shaping instrument and penetrate in canal steadily. Remove the instrument, irrigate the canal and reinsert it. Continue to progress apically until working length is achieved (Fig. 17.60).
5. Apical gauging is done thereafter to assure smooth apical taper.

## PROTAPER FILES

As we have seen that ProTaper files have a triangular cross-section and is variably tapered across its cutting length (Fig. 17.61). The progressively tapered design improves flexibility, cutting efficiency and the safety of these files (Fig. 17.62).

The ProTaper system consists of three shaping and three finishing files.

1. Shaping files are termed as $S_x$, $S_1$ and $S_2$.
   $S_x$ these are files of shorter length of 19 mm with $D_0$ diameter of 0.19 mm and $D_{14}$ diameter of 1.20 mm. The increase of taper up to $D_9$ and then taper decrease up to $D_{14}$ increases its flexibility.
   $S_1$ has $D_0$ diameter of 0.17 mm and $D_{14}$ of 1.20 mm. it is used to prepare coronal part of the root.
   $S_2$ has $D_0$ diameter of 0.20 mm and $D_{14}$ of 1.20 mm. it is used to prepare middle third of the canal.
2. Finishing files $F_1$, $F_2$, $F_3$ are used to prepare and finish apical part of the root canal.
   $F_1$ $D_0$ diameter and apical taper is 20 and 0.07.
   $F_2$ $D_0$ diameter and taper is 25 and 0.08.
   $F_3$ $D_0$ diameter and taper is 30 and 0.09.

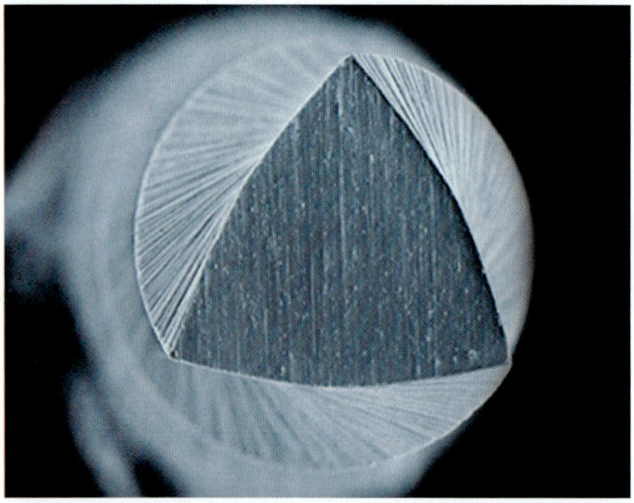

**Fig. 17.61:** Triangular cross-section of proTaper

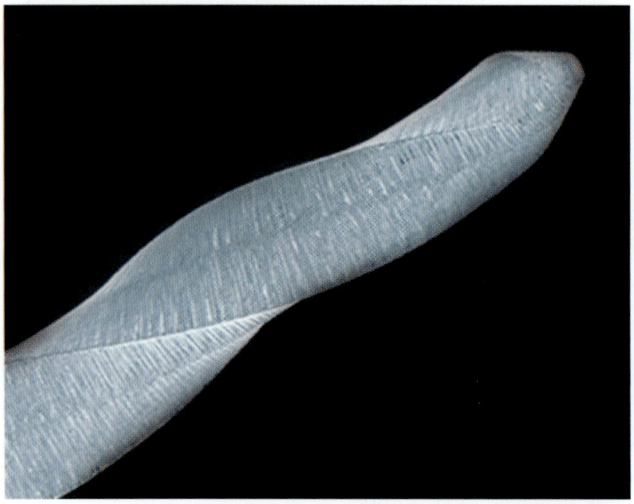

**Fig. 17.62:** Progressively tapered design improves flexibility and cutting efficiency of proTapers

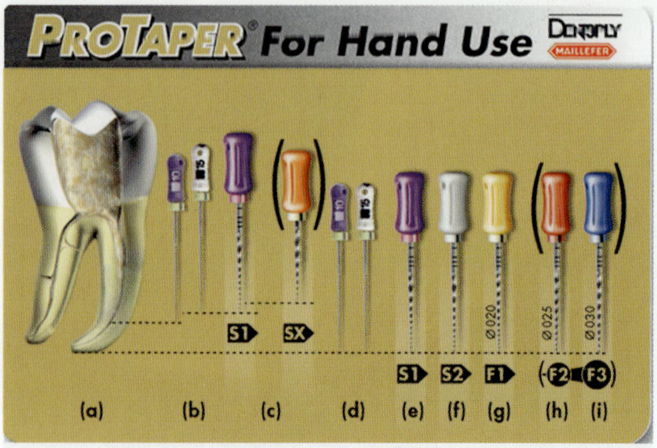


**Fig. 17.63:** ProTaper for hand use

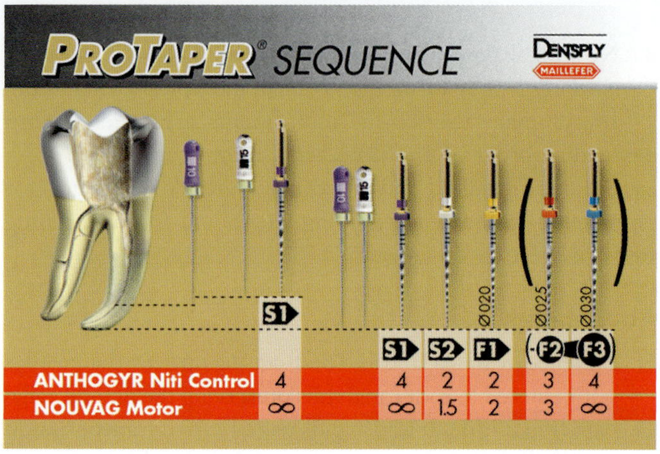


**Fig. 17.64:** ProTaper for rotary instrumentation

### Clinical Technique (Figs 17.63 and 17.64)

1. The foremost step is gaining straight line access to the canal orifices.
2. Establish a smooth glide path before doing any instrumentation with ProTaper system.
3. Now prepare the coronal third of the canal by inserting S1 into the canal using passive pressure. Don't go more than third fourth of the estimated canal length.
4. Irrigate and recapitulate the canal using number 10 file.
5. In shorter teeth, use of Sx is recommended.
6. After this $S_2$ is worked up to the estimated canal length.
7. Now confirm the working length using small stainless steel K- files up to size 15 by electronic apex locators and/or with radiographic confirmation.
8. Use $F_1$, $F_2$ and $F_3$ (if necessary) finishing files up to established working length and complete the apical preparation. Then refine the apical preparation using corresponding stainless steel file to gauge the apical foramen and to smoothen the canal walls.

### Advantages of ProTaper Files

- ProTaper files have modified guiding tip which allow them to follow canal better (Figs 17.65 and 17.66).

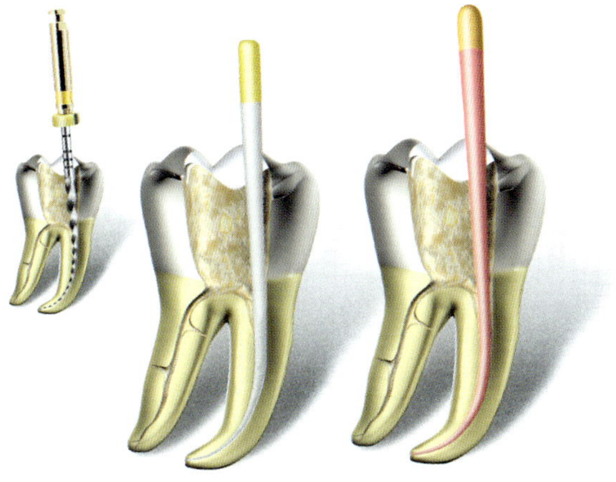

Fig. 17.65: Modified guiding tip of protaper allows them to follow canal better

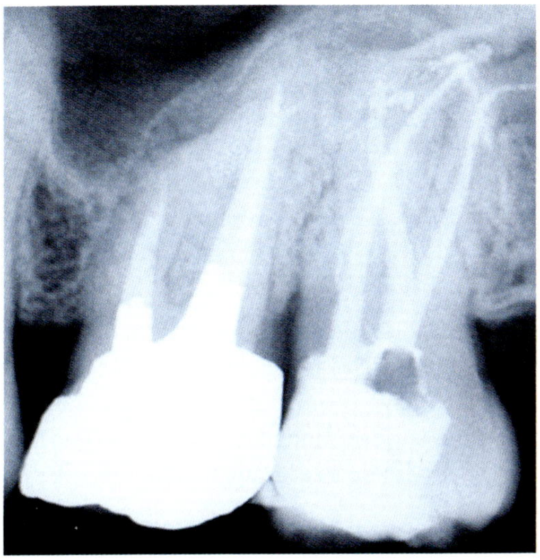

Fig. 17.66: Radiograph showing canals obturated after protaper instrumentation

- Variable tip diameters of ProTaper files allow them to have specific cutting action in defined area of canal without stressing instrument in other sections.
- Changing helical angle and pitch over the cutting blades of ProTaper files reduce the instruments from screwing into the canal and allow better removal of debris.
- ProTaper files act in active motion, this further increases its efficiency and reduces torsional strain.
- Length of file handle is reduced from 15 to 17.5 mm. which allows better access in posterior areas.

## QUANTEC FILE SYSTEM

Quantec file series are available in both cutting and non-cutting tips with standard size of 25 No. in 0.12, 0.10, 0.08, 0.06, 0.05, 0.04, 0.03 and 0.02 tapers.

This unique design of Quantec system that is a positive blade angle with two wide radial lands and relief behind the lands reduces its contact with the canal, thereby minimizing the torque. Quantec system utilizes the "graduated taper technique" to prepare a canal. It is thought that using a series of files of single taper result in the decreased efficiency as the larger instruments are used. This happens because more of file comes in contact with the dentinal wall which makes it more difficult to remove dentin, thereby retarding the proper cleaning and shaping of the canal. But in graduated taper technique, restricted contact of area increases the efficiency of the instrument because now forces are concentrated on smaller area.

### Clinical Technique

1. Obtain the straight line access to the canal orifices.
2. Establish the patency of canal using number 10 or 15 stainless steel files.
3. Insert the Quantec number 25, taper 0.06 file passively into the canal.
4. After negotiation of the canal using Quantec file, prepare the canal from 0.12 to 0.03 taper.
5. Finally complete the apical preparation of canal using 40 or 45 No., 0.02 taper hand or rotary files.

## LIGHT SPEED SYSTEM

These are so named because a "light" touch is needed as "speed" of instrumentation is increased.

Light speed instrument have non-cutting tip with Gates-Glidden in configuration and are available in 21, 25, 31 and 50 mm length and ISO numbers 20-140.

Half sizes of light speed instrument are available in numbers 22.5, 27.5, 32.5.

### Clinical Technique

While doing cleaning and shaping using the light speed system, three special instruments are used—

- Initial Apical Rotary (IAR) (Begins to cut canal walls at working length).
- Master Apical Rotary (MAR) (Last instrument to perform the apical preparation).
- Final Rotary (FR) (Last step back instrument which completes the step back procedure).

1. Obtain a straight line access to the canal orifice and establish a glide path using number 15 stainless steel file (Fig. 17.67).

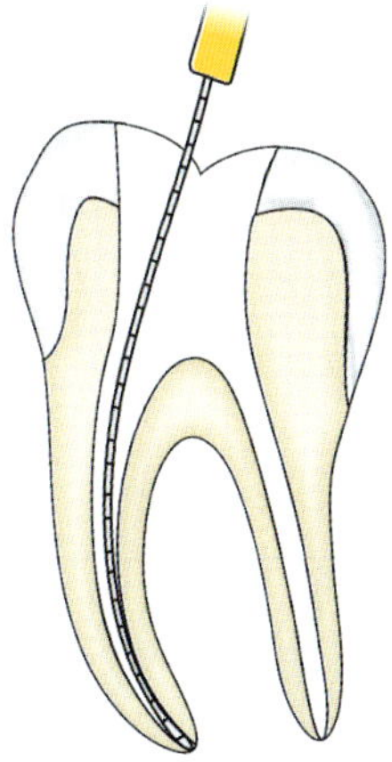

Fig. 17.67: Obtain straight line access

2. Slightly (1-2 mm) enlarge the canal orifice with the help of Gates-Glidden drills.
3. Determine the working length using number 15 stainless steel file.
4. Use initial apical rotary up to working length (Fig. 17.68).
5. Now prepare the canal using light speed instruments in forward and backward movement from smaller to larger number (Fig. 17.69).
6. Last instrument used in canal for canal preparation is master apical rotary which could be 5-12 size larger than the initial apical rotary instrument.
7. After using MAR, light speed instruments are used in step back procedure to complete the canal preparation (Fig. 17.70). Use the final rotary (FR) as the last back instrument.
8. Finally recapitulated with Master Apical Rotary (MAR) up to the working length.

## Advantages of Light Speed System

1. Short cutting blades provide more accurate tactile feedback of canal preparation.
2. Flexibility of light speed system keeps it centered, virtually eliminating ledging, perforation or zipping of canal.

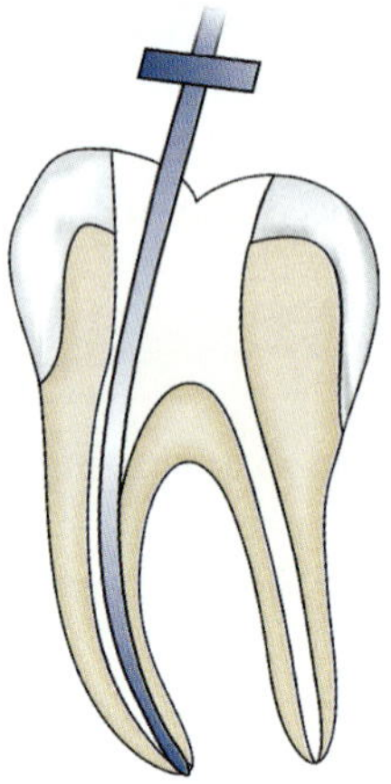

Fig. 17.68: Use of initial apical rotary in canal

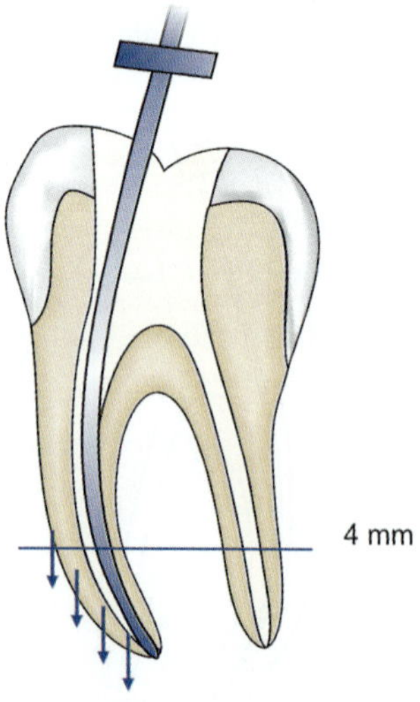


Fig. 17.69: Use of light speed instrument in forward and backward movement

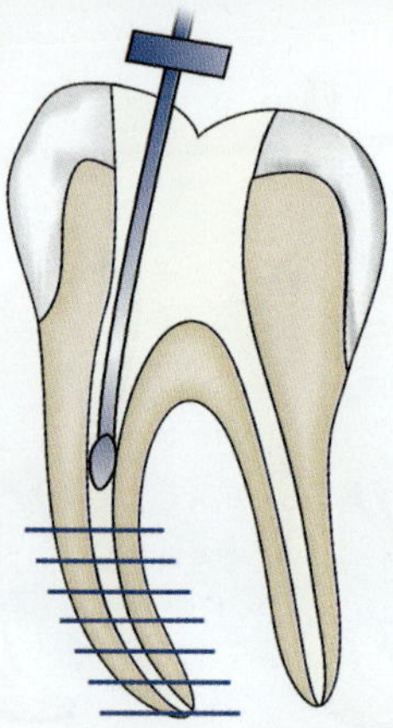

Fig. 17.70: Use of light speed instrument in step back procedure

3. Light speed instrumentation is conservative which prevents weakening of the root.
4. When used correctly, risk of instrument separation is low but if it does separate, it is designed to separate 18 mm from the tip which makes its removal fast.
5. Short cutting blades with non-cutting shaft minimize the torque and stress on the instrument.

## $K_3$ ROTARY FILE SYSTEM

$K_3$ files are available in taper of 0.02, 0.04 or 0.06 with ISO tip sizes. The presence of variable core diameter makes them flexible. $K_3$ files have positive rake angle providing them an effective cutting surface. Body shapers available in taper 0.08, 0.10, and 0.12 all with tip size 25, are used to prepare the coronal third of the canal.

### Clinical Technique

1. Obtain a straight line access to the canal orifices and enlarge them with $K_3$ shaper files. The shaper files are used to light resistance which is usually 3 to 4 mm apically.
2. After preparing coronal third of canal with shaper file, prepare the middle third of the canal.
   Obtain the glide path using number 15 stainless steel hand file before using $K_3$ system.
3. Then 0.06/40 $K_3$ can be inserted up to middle third of the canal. If it is difficult to use, switch over smaller files (0.06/35). On the whole 0.06/40 is used first followed by 0.06/35,0.06/30, etc. until the middle third and apical third is reached.
4. Don't forget to irrigate and recapitulate in between the files.
5. In narrow canals use 0.04 tapered files instead of 0.06 taper.
6. Now prepare the apical third of the canal using smaller $K_3$ files upto estimated working length.

## REAL WORLD ENDO SEQUENCE FILE

A recently introduced in NiTi world is Real World Endo Sequence File system. Electropolishing treatment of these files during manufacturing lessens the propensity of NiTi files for crack propagation. The blank design with alternating contact points (ACPs) and absence of radial lands, makes the instrument shaper and more efficient in cutting.

### Clinical Technique

1. Gain the straight line access to canal orifice and confirm the coronal patency with number 10 or 15 stainless steel hand file.
2. Use Expeditor file first into canal to determine the appropriate size of the canal.
3. Remove the Expeditor file from the canal, irrigate the canal and choose appropriate sequence file according to the canal size and perform crown down technique.
4. Now establish the working length of the canal, after using the second rotary file.
5. Complete the crown down technique up to the established working length.

### Advantages of Real World Endo Sequence File System

1. These files are available in 0.04 and 0.06 taper having the precision tip. Presence of precision tip results in both safety as well as efficiency.
2. These files keep themselves centered in the canal and produce minimal lateral resistance because of:
   i. Presence of ACPs
   ii. Electropolishing
   iii. Absence of radial lands.

Sequence files have variable pitch and helical angle which further increase its efficiency by moving the debris out of canal and thus decreasing the torque caused by debris accumulation.

## HERO 642

HERO 642 (High Elasticity in Rotation, 0.06. 0.04 and 0.02 tapers-) has trihelical hedstorm design with sharp flutes. It is used in "Crown down" technique, between 300 and 600 rotations per minute (rpm) in a standard slow speed contra-angle air driven or electric motors.

Due to progressively increasing distance between the flutes, there is reduced risk for binding of the instrument in root canal.

### Technique

In this crown down technique is achieved using variable size and taper. First and foremost step of canal preparation is to obtain straight line access to the canal orifices.

1. Start with size 30 of 0.06 taper, penetrate it in the canal with light up and down motion at the speed of 300-600 RPM and prepare the coronal part of the canal (Fig. 17.71).
2. Remove the file, irrigate the canal.
3. Now insert file size 30, 0.04 taper and continue the canal preparation up to the level of 2 mm of working length (Fig. 17.72).
4. Finally, complete the apical preparation using NiTi hand instruments or 0.02 taper rotary (Fig. 17.73).

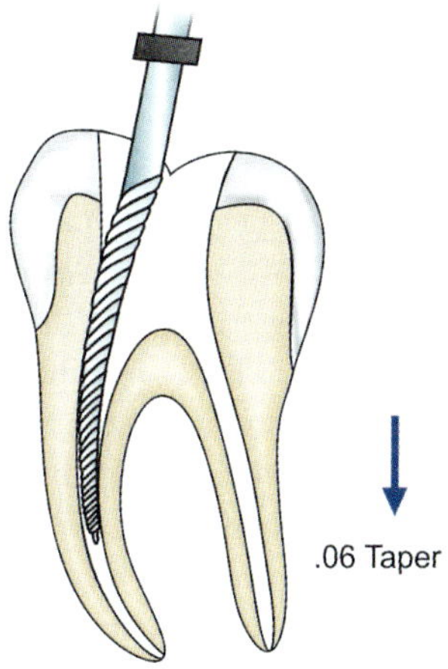


**Fig. 17.71:** 0.06 taper file to prepare coronal two-third of the canal

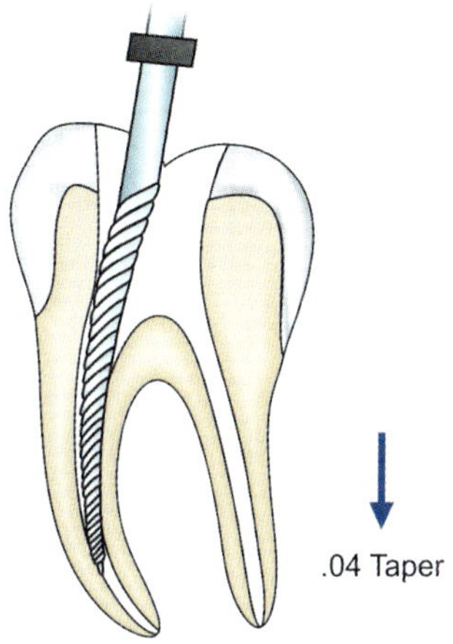


**Fig. 17.72:** Use of 0.04 taper file for mid root preparation

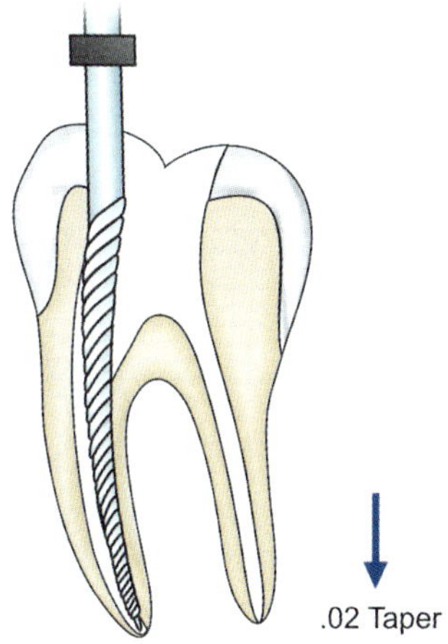


**Fig. 17.73:** Use of 0.02 tapered instrument for final apical preparation

## CANAL PREPARATION USING ULTRASONIC INSTRUMENTS

The concept of using ultrasound in endodontic therapy was suggested in 1957 by **Richman**. But it was the late 1970s, when ultrasonic scaling units became common for use in endodontics resulting in endosonics. Since that time a lot of research is being done on endosonics to make it an integral part of endodontics. The machines used for this purpose are designed to transmit low frequency ultrasonic vibration by conversion of electromagnetic energy to the mechanical energy to produce oscillation of file (Fig. 17.74). File oscillates at the frequency of 20,000-25, 000 vibrations/seconds. For free movement of file in the canal, it should not have any binding specially at the apical end (Fig. 17.75). During the oscillation of file, there is continuous flow of irrigants solutions from the handpiece along the file. This causes formation of cavitation. Cavitation is growth and subsequent violent collapse of the bubbles in the fluid which results in formation of a shock wave, increase temperature, pressure and the free radical formation in the fluid. Cavitation is considered as one of the primary beneficial effect in endosonics (Fig. 17.76).

Another effect is acoustic streaming which is produced around an object oscillating in a liquid. In this, there is production of shear forces which are capable of dislodging the lumps of material. Thus, acoustic streaming is be useful in reducing number of smear layer and loosening the aggregates of the bacteria.

## Technique

1. Before starting with ultrasonic instrumentation apical third of the canal should be prepared to at least size 15 file.

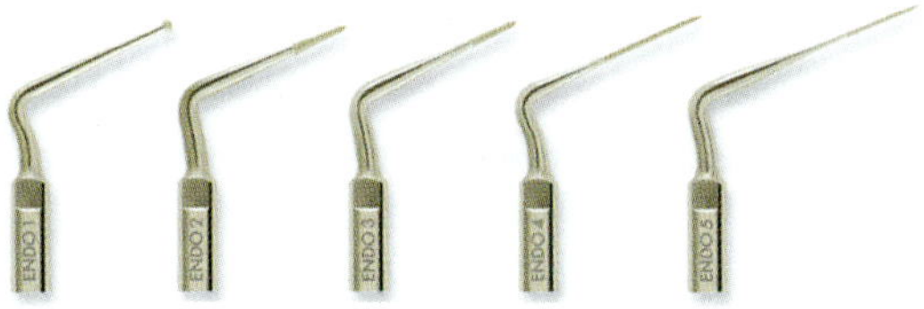


**Fig. 17.74:** Endosonic tips

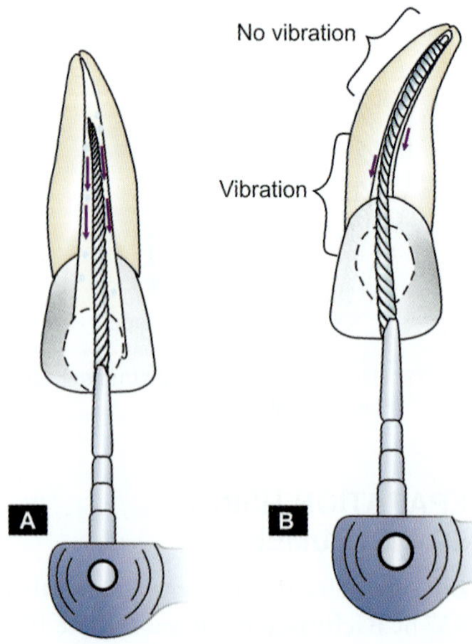


**Figs 17.75A and B:** (A) Ultrasonic instrument and irrigation work actively in straight canal. (B) Curvature in canal may impede vibration

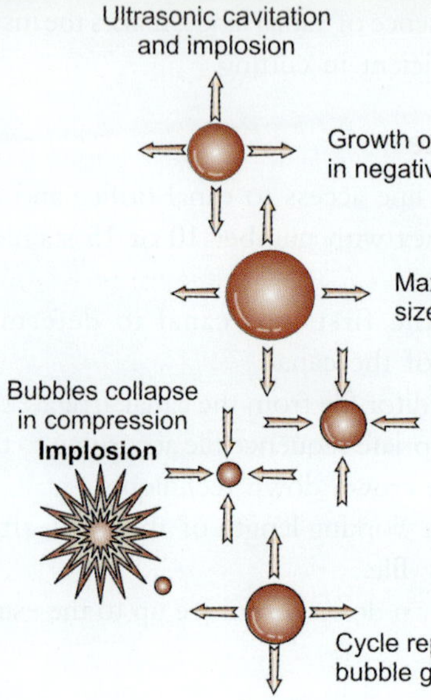


**Fig. 17.76:** Cavitation in ultrasonics

2. After activation, ultrasonic file is moved in the ***circumferential*** manner with push-pull stroke along the walls of canal.
3. File is activated for one minute. This procedure is repeated till the apex is prepared to at least size 25.

***The root canal debridement depends on:***

1. Choice of irrigant solution (sodium hypochlorite is irrigant of choice).
2. Oscillation of file.
3. The form of irrigation with ultrasonic irrigation being supplied.

## Advantages of Ultrasonic Canal Preparation

1. Less time consuming.
2. Produces cleaner canals because of synergetic relationship between the ultrasound and the sodium hypochlorite.
3. Heat produced by ultrasonic vibration increase the chemical effectiveness of the sodium hypochlorite.

### *Disadvantages*

1. Increased frequency of canal transportations.
2. Increased chances of overinstrumentation.

## Canal Preparation Using Sonic Instruments

Design of sonic instruments is similar to that of ultrasonics. They consist of a driver on to which an endosonic file is attached. The oscillatory pattern of driver determines the nature of movement of the attached file. In sonic instruments, there is longitudinal pattern of the vibration when activated in the root canal. This longitudinal file motion produces superior cleaning of the root canal walls.

Sonic system uses three types of file system for root canal preparation, viz. Heliosonic, Rispisonic and the Canal shaper instruments. These files have spiral blades protruding along their length and non-cutting tips.

### Technique

1. After gaining the straight line access to the canal orifices, penetrate small number file in the canal. Enlarge the canal upto 20 or 25 number file upto 3 mm of the apex to make some space for sonic file.
2. Now insert the sonic file 0.5-1 mm short of number 20 file, and do circumferential filling with up and down motion for 30-40 seconds.
3. after this use the larger number sonic file and do the coronal flaring.
4. After completion with this, determine the working length and prepare the apical third of the canal with hand files.
5. Finally blend the apical preparation with coronal flaring using smaller number sonic file.

Though sonic files have shown to enlarge and debride the canals effectively in lesser time but care should be taken not to force the file apically to prevent instrument separation, ledge formation or canal transportation.

**Apexum**

In nonsurgical endodontics, healing of apical periodontitis is achieved by complete cleaning and shaping of root canal system. The recently introduced Apexum procedure is used for enucleation of periapical tissue by minimally invasive technique through root canal access, thereby enhancing the healing kinetics of periapical lesions. For apexum procedure, after completing biomechanical preparation, apical foramen is enlarged with No. 35. rotary file about 1 to 2 mm periapically (Fig. 17.77). This is done for insertion of apexum device which is a nickel-titanium wire into periapical area This device rotates and minces the tissue. After this a biodegradable fiber is rotated at high speed so as to make this tissue into thin suspension. This can be latter removed with normal saline irrigation.

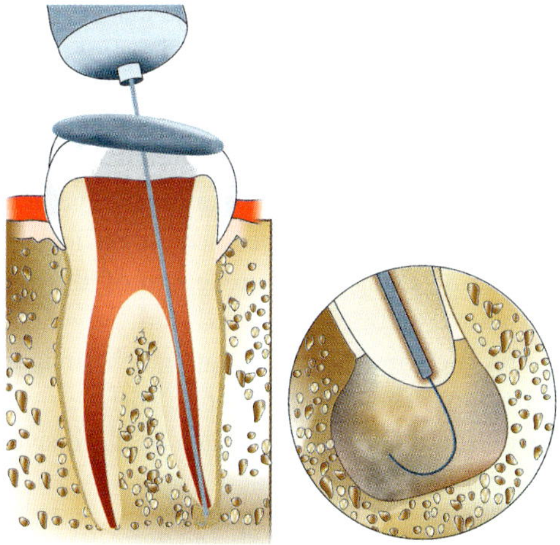

Fig. 17.77: Diagram showing working of apexum

## LASER ASSISTED ROOT CANAL THERAPY

Weichman and Johnson in 1971 were the first to suggest the use of lasers in endodontics. The most important benefits of this revolutionary technology for endodontic treatment is the ease of using it and great degree of patient comfort during and after the procedure.

Nd:YAG, Ar, Excimer, Holium, Ebrium laser beam are delivered through the optical fiber with the diameter of 200-400 mm equivalent to size 20-40 number file. Studies have shown different results with lasers.

Bahcall et al in 1992 found that though the use of Nd:YAG laser can produce cleaner canals, but heat produced by it may damage the surrounding supporting tissues, i.e. bone and PDL. Hibst et al showed that use of Er:YAG laser may pose less thermal damage to the tissues because it causes localized heating thereby minimizing the absorption depth.

Recently a new root canal treatment using the Er, Cr:YSGG (erbium, chromium: Yettruim scandium gallium garnet) has been introduced to help reduce the patient fear and provide better comfort to the patient. The device which provides such a treatment is the waterlase—Hydrokinetic Hard and Soft tissue laser, the only laser system to receive FDA clearance for complete endodontic therapy and other root canal procedures. This laser uses specialized fibers of various diameters and lengths to effectively clean the root canal walls and prepare the canal for obturation. By using hydrokinetic process in which water is energized by the YSGG laser photons to cause molecular excitation and localized microexpansion, hard tissues are removed precisely with no thermal side effects.

With this technique there is minimal patient discomfort, and postoperative complications such as inflammation, swelling and pain. Moreover, antibacterial action of YSGG laser has reduced the use of postoperative antibiotics therapy.

Thus we see that laser is one of the important revolution in endodontics. The intracanal irradiation with laser has shown to reduce the microbial reduction, inflammation, and other post-operative complications, simultaneously providing the comfort to patient. However performance of the equipment safety measures, temperature rise and level of microbial reduction should be well documented before it becomes a current method of choice for treatment.

## EVALUATION CRITERIA OF CANAL PREPARATION

1. Spreader should be able to reach within 1 mm of the working length. If spreader does not reach the estimated length, it indicates canal is not well prepared (Fig. 17.78).

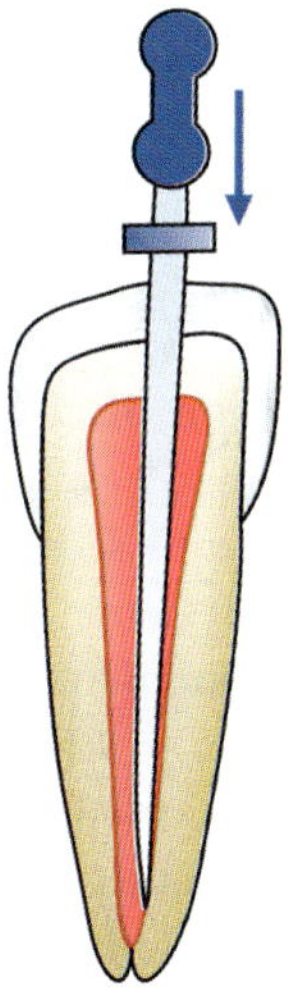

Fig. 17.78: Spreader should reach 1 mm short of apex in a well prepared canal

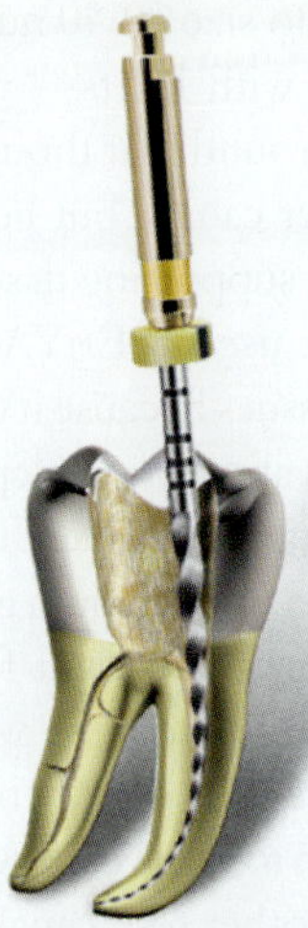

Fig. 17.79: Master apical file should feel smooth in a well-prepared canal

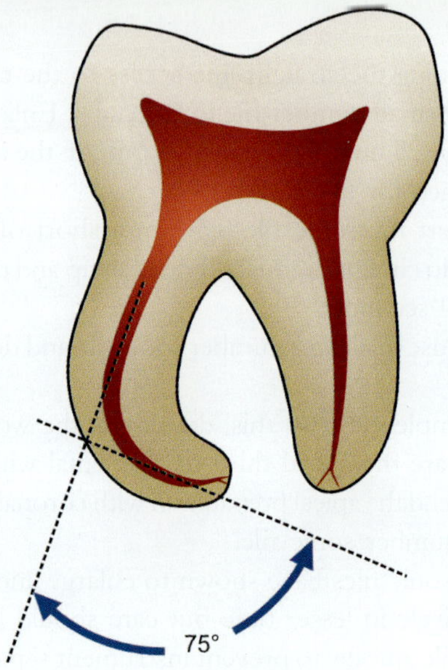


Fig. 17.80: Internal angle formed by interaction of lines is angle of curvature

2. After canal preparation, when master apical file is pressed firmly against each wall, it should feel smooth (Fig. 17.79).
3. Recently a three-dimensional, nondestructive technique has developed for detailed study of root canal geometry. A micro-computed tomography scanner is used to record the precise canal anatomy before and after the instrumentation. A three-dimensional analysis of root canal geometry by high resolution CT is then performed.

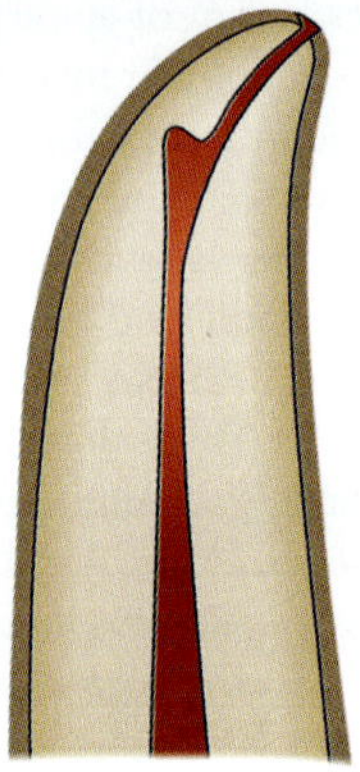

Fig. 17.81: Formation of ledge in a curved canal

## SPECIAL ANATOMIC PROBLEMS IN CANAL CLEANING AND SHAPING

1. Management of curved canals.
2. Management of calcified canals.
3. Management of C-shaped canals.
4. Management of S-shaped canals

### 1. Management of Curved Canals

The controlled, uniformly tapered radicular preparation is a great challenge in endodontics. But nowadays, introduction of flexible non-ISO taper NiTi instruments has brought a major change to overcome the problems of cleaning and shaping in curved canals earlier caused by use of stiff stainless steel files in push-pull motion.

In management of curved canals first of all estimate the angle of curvature. To calculate angle of curvature, imagine a straight line from orifice towards canal curvature and another line from apex towards apical portion of the curve. The internal angle formed by interaction of these lines is the angle of curvature (Fig. 17.80).

In curved canals, frequently seen problem is occurrence of uneven cutting. File can cut dentine evenly only if it engages dentine around its entire circumference. Once it becomes loose in a curved canal, it will tend to straighten up and will contact only at certain points along its length. These areas are usually outer portion of curve apical to the curve, on inner part of curve at the height of curve and outer or inner curve coronal to the curve. All this can lead to occurrence of procedural errors like formation of ledge, transportation of foramen, perforation or formation of elbow and zip in a curved canal (Fig. 17.81). To avoid occurrence of such errors there should be even contact of file to the canal dentine. But because file has tendency to straighten up to its original shape and it is difficult to control removal of dentine along the entire length of file in push-pull motion, the above errors can be reduced by:

- Decreasing the force by means of which straight files apt to bend against the curved dentine surface.
- Decreasing the length of file which is aggressively cutting at the given span.

***Decrease in the filing force can be done by:***

i. ***Precurving the file:*** A precurved file has shown to traverse the curve better than a straight file. Two types of precurving are done (Fig. 17.82):
   - Placing a gradual curve for the entire length of the file.
   - Placing a sharp curve of nearly 45 degrees near the apical end of the instrument. This type of curved file is used in cases when a sharp curve or an obstruction is present in the canal. Curve can be placed by grasping the flutes with gauze sponge and carefully bending the file until the preferred curvature is attained.

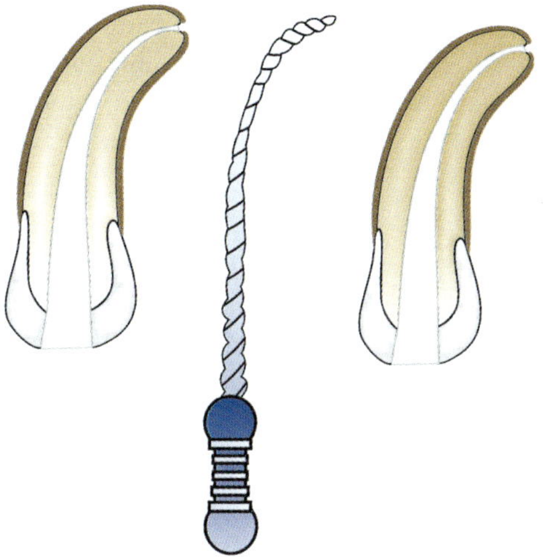

**Fig. 17.82:** Precurving of file

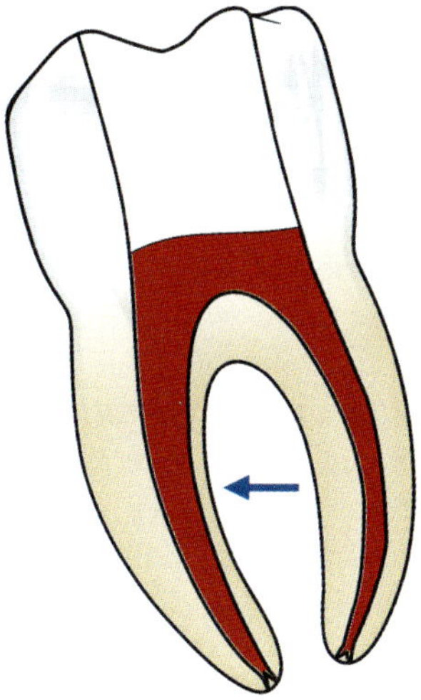

**Fig. 17.83:** Arrow showing area where chances of strip perforation are more

Once the precurved file is placed in the canal, there are chances of loosing the direction of curve. To avoid this problem teardrop shape rubber stopper is usually recommended with point showing the direction of the curve.

ii. ***Extravagant use of smaller number files:*** Since smaller sized instruments can follow the canal curvature because of their flexibility, they should be used until the larger files are able to negotiate the canal without force.

iii. ***Use of intermediate sizes of files:*** It has been seen that increment of 0.05 mm between the instruments is too large to reach the correct working length in curved canals. To solve this problem, by cutting off a portion of the file tip a new instrument size is created which has the size intermediate to two consecutive instruments. There is increase of 0.02 mm of diameter per millimeter of the length, cutting 1 mm of the tip of the instrument creates a new instrument size, for example cutting 1 mm of a number 15 file makes it number 17 file. In severely curved canals the clinician can cut 0.0 5 mm of the file to increase the instrument diameter by 0.01 mm. This allows the smoother transition of the instrument sizes to cause smoother cutting in curved canals.

iv. ***Use of flexible files:*** It has been seen that use of flexible files cause less alteration of the canal shape than the stiffer files. Flexible files help in maintaining the shape of the curve and avoid occurrence of procedural errors like formation of ledge, elbow or zipping of the canal.

Decrease in length of actively cutting file can be achieved by:

i. ***Anticurvature filing:*** In some roots like mesial root of mandibular molar and mesiobuccal root of maxillary molars, if care is not taken while preparing them, incidence of strip formation are seen. The canal wall facing the curve or furcation makes the danger zone because in this portion, less of the tooth structure is present as compared to the outer portion (safety zone) (Figs 17.83 and 17.84). In these teeth, to reduce the incidence of strip perforation, the concept of anticurvature filing is employed as given by Lim and Stock. It involves lesser filing of the canal wall which is facing the curvature (Fig. 17.85). For example, in case of filing of mesiobuccal canal of mandibular molars,

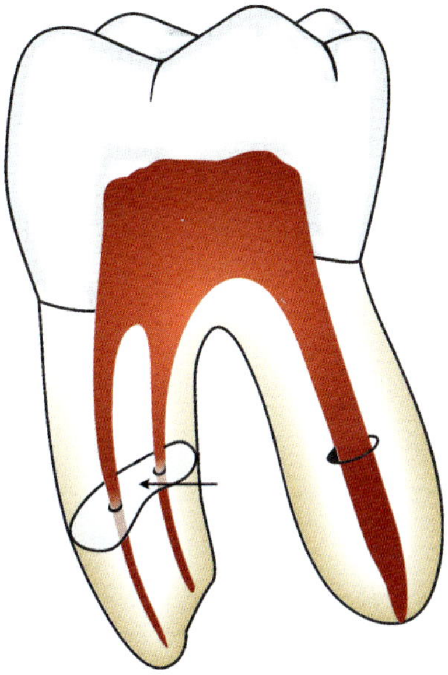

**Fig. 17.84:** Arrow showing danger zone

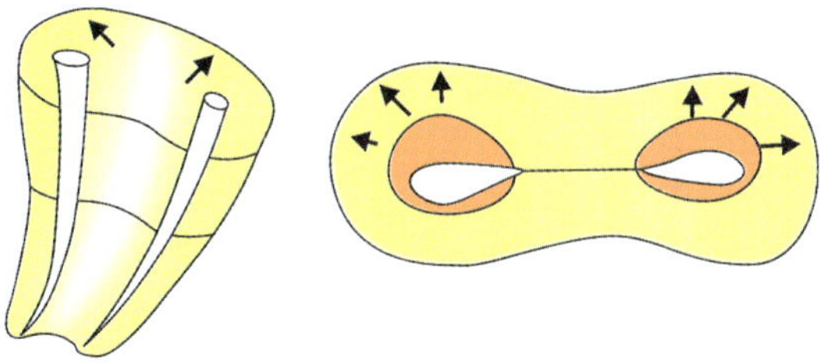

**Fig. 17.85:** Removal of dentin should be done more in shaded area to avoid perforation

more filing is done on mesial and buccal wall as compared to distal and lingual walls (Fig. 17.86).

ii. ***Modifying cutting edges of the instrument:*** The cutting edges of the curved instrument can be modified by dulling the flute of outer portion of the apical third and inner portion of the middle third. Dulling of the flutes can be done with the help of diamond file (Fig. 17.87).

iii. ***Changing the canal preparation techniques:*** crown down technique, i.e. preparation of coronal part of the canal before apical part removes the coronal interferences and allow the files to reach up to the apex more effectively (Fig. 17.88).

## 2. Management of Calcified Canals

Calcifications in the root canal system are commonly met problem in root canal treatment. The dentist must recognize that pulpal calcifications are signs of the pathosis, not the cause. Various etiological factors seem to be associated with calcifications are caries, trauma, drugs and aging.

### Steps

*Access Preparation*

1. Success in negotiating small or calcified canals is predicted on a proper access opening and identification of the canal orifice.
2. To locate the calcified orifice, first mentally visualize and plan the normal spatial relationship of the pulp space onto a radiograph of calcified tooth. In a tooth with a calcified pulp chamber, the distance from the occlusal surface to the pulp chamber is measured from the preoperative radiograph (Fig. 17.89). The geometric patterns of canal orifices and their variations have to be mentally projected on the calcified pulp chamber floor.
3. After this, access preparation is initiated, with the rotary instrument directed toward the assumed location of pulpal

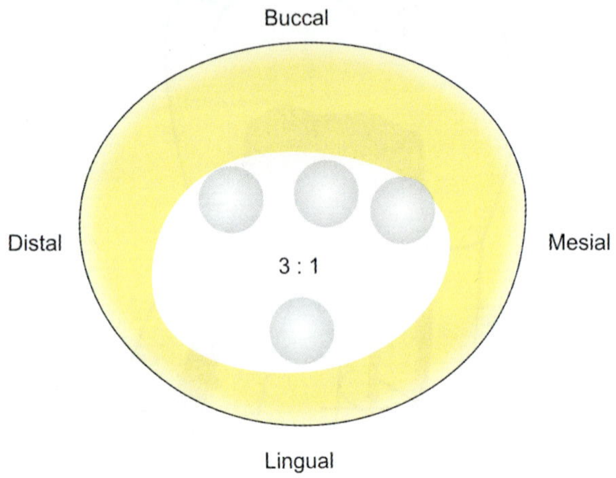


**Fig. 17.86:** In mesiobuccal canal of mandibular molars, more filing is done on mesial and buccal wall than on lingual and distal wall

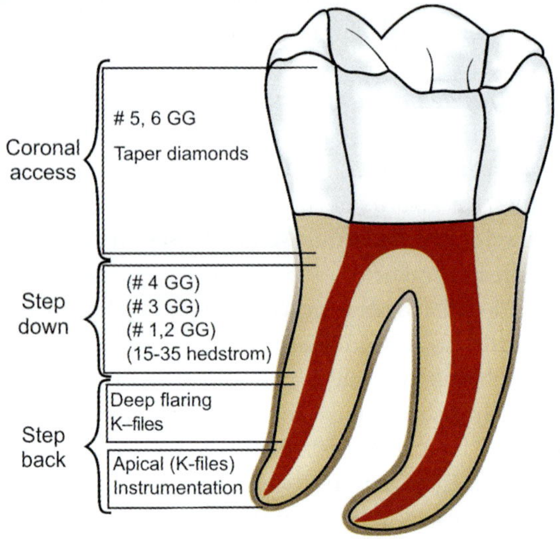


**Fig. 17.88:** Crown down technique for curved canals

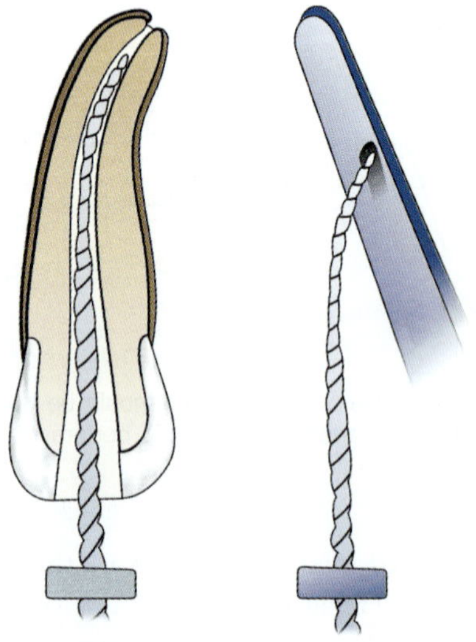

**Fig. 17.87:** Modifying the cutting edges of instrument

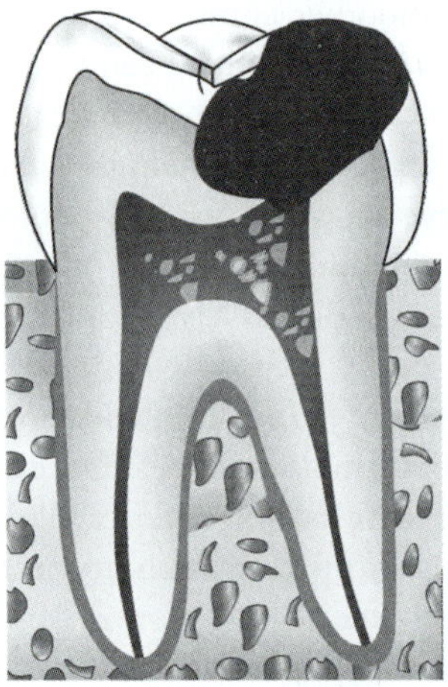

**Fig. 17.89:** Radiograph showing pulp stones and calcifications present in pulp cavity and also the location of pulp chamber

space (Fig. 17.90). Accurate radiographic visualization and intermittent evaluation of bur penetration and orientation helps recognize the calcified orifice.

*Location of the Canal Orifice*

1. The most significant instrument for orifice location is the DG – 16 explorer (Fig 17.91). If an orifice is present, firm pressure will force the instrument slightly into the orifice, and it will "stick" (Fig. 17.92). At this suspected point a fine instrument number 8 or 10 K-file, is placed into the orifice, and an effort is made to negotiate the canal. An alternative choice is to use instruments with reduced flutes, such as a canal pathfinder which can penetrate even highly calcified canals.
2. Although most of the attempts to locate canal orifices with calcifications are successful still there is a probability for perforation. Probing with the explorer yields a characteristic "stick" but if explorer lies too close to the root surface, it actually penetrates a thin area of remaining dentin. The most common sign of accidental perforation is bleeding, but bleeding may also indicate that the pulp in the calcified canal is vital. If there is any doubt as to whether the orifice has actually been found, place a small instrument in the opening and take a radiograph.

*Penetration and Negotiation of the Calcified Canal*

Once the orifice has been located, a No. 8 K-file is penetrated into the canal to negotiate the calcified canal (Fig. 17.93). A No. 10 K-file is too large, and a No. 6 K-file is too weak to apply any firm apical pressure. Also the use of Nickel- Titanium files is not recommended for this purpose because of lack of strength in the long axis of the file. Before the file is inserted into the canal, a small curve is placed in its apical 1 mm. In negotiating the fine-curved canal, the precurved instrument must be positioned along the pathway the canal is most likely to follow; as a result it is important to know in which direction the curve in the instrument is pointed. This is easily accomplished by observing the rubber stop on the instrument shaft.

Forceful probing of the canal with fine instruments and chelating agents results in formation of a false canal and continued instrumentation in a false canal results in perforation. In a calcified canal, it is necessary to confirm the position of the instrument with a radiograph. In cases of teeth with calcified canals, the prognosis of the root canal treatment depends on the continued health of the pulp or the periradicular tissues on the apical side of the blockage. In the absence of symptoms or evidence of apical pathosis, it is clinically practical and satisfactory to instrument and fill the canal to the level negotiated, followed by regular recall of the patient.

## Guidelines for Negotiating Calcified Canals (Figs 17.94A to C)

1. Copious irrigation all times with 2.5 to 5.25 percent NaOCl enhances dissolution of organic debris, lubricates the canal, and keeps dentin chips and pieces of calcified material in solution.
2. Always advance instruments slowly in calcified canals.

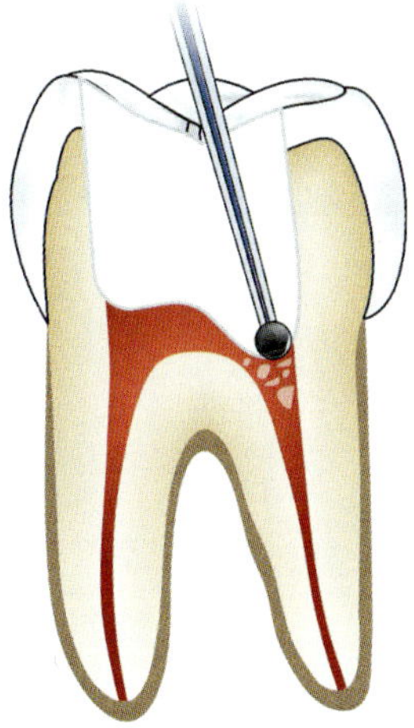

**Fig. 17.90:** Direct the rotary instrument to assumed pulp space

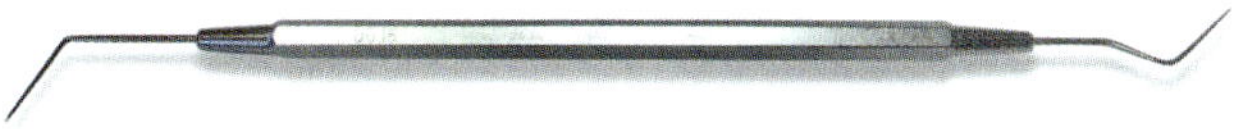

**Fig. 17.91:** DG-16 explorer

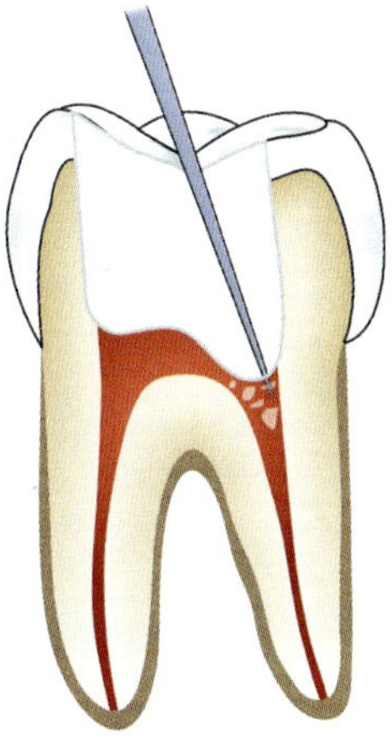

**Fig. 17.92:** Use of sharp endodontic explorer in tentative location of orifice

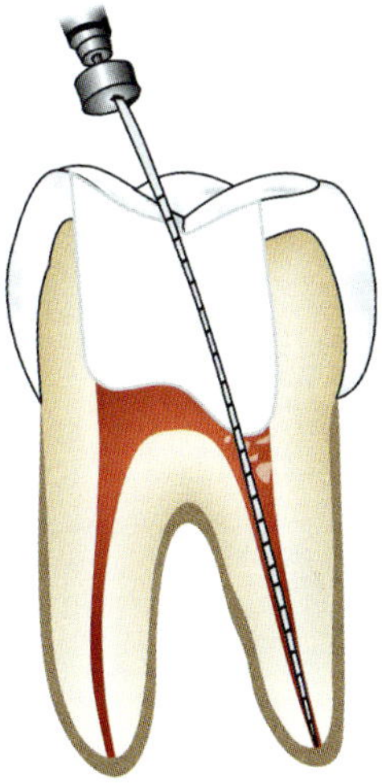

**Fig. 17.93:** Use of small instrument to negotiate calcified canal

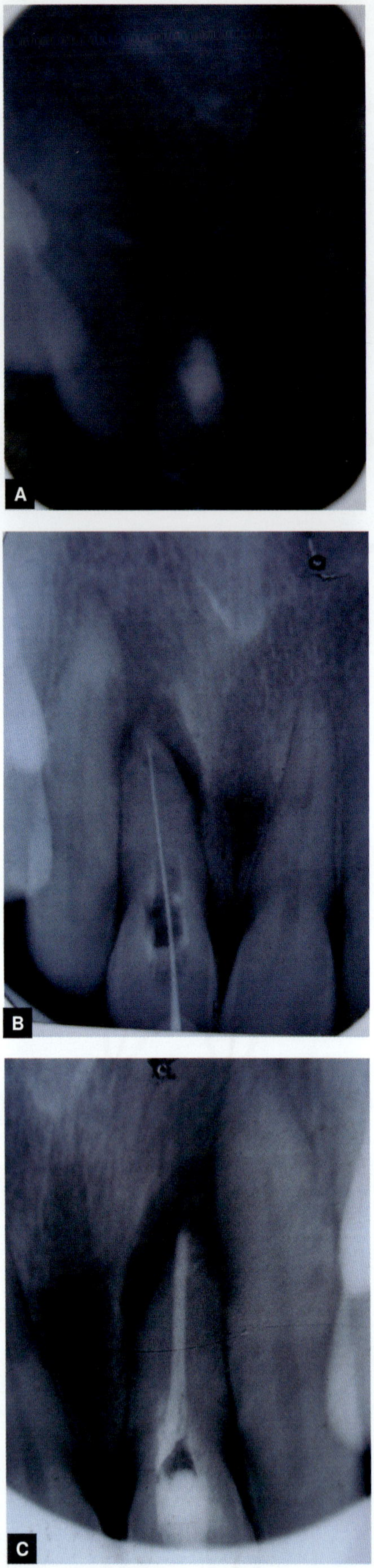

**Figs 17.94A to C:** A. Radiograph showing calcified central incisor, B. Straight line access gained and biomechanical preparation done, C. Obturation of central incisor

3. Always clean the instrument on withdrawal and inspect before reinserting it into the canal.
4. When a fine instrument reaches the approximate canal length, do not remove it; rather obtain a radiograph to ascertain the position of the file.
5. Use chelating agents to assist canal penetration.
6. Flaring of the canal orifice and enlargement of coronal third of canal space improves tactile perception.
7. The use of nickel-titanium rotary orifice penetrating instruments also helps in these cases.
8. Well angulated periapical and bite wing radiographs should be taken. They not only indicate the position of canals but also give important information about the relative position of canal orifice in calcified cases. Failure to recognize changes in the axis of the tooth that occurs during crown restoration, can lead to perforations. Proximal restorations can be used as guide to locate canals.
9. Not anesthetizing the patient while performing access opening can be useful in some cases. Patient should be told to indicate when he/she feels a sharp sensation during access with a bur. At that point a sharp DG 16 Endo explorer is used to locate the canal. It is easy to tell the difference between PDL and pulp with a small file. If file is inserted only a mm or two into the pulp, the reaction will be sharp. If it is in PDL, reaction is often less sharp.
10. Avoid removing large amount of dentin in the hope of finding a canal orifice. By doing this all the pulp floor landmarks are lost also the strength and dentinal thickness of tooth gets compromised.
11. Small round burs should be used to create a glide path to the orifice. This will further ease the instruments into the proper lane to allow effortless introduction of files into the canals.

## 3. Management of C-shaped Canals

Though the prevalence of C-shaped canals is low, but those requiring endodontic treatment present a diagnostic and treatment difficulties to the clinician. Some C-shaped canals are difficult to interpret on radiographs and often are not identified until an endodontic access is made. These are commonly seen in mandibular second molars and maxillary first molars especially when roots of these teeth appear very close or fused (Fig. 17.95).

In maxillary molars, the C-shaped canal includes mesiobuccal and palatal canals or the distobuccal and palatal canals. In the mandibular second molar, the C-shaped canal includes mesiobuccal and distal canals (Figs 17.96A and B).

In any of these cases, canal orifices may be found within the C-shaped trough or the C-shape may be continuous throughout the length of the canal.

Major problems come across during biomechanical preparation of C-shaped canals are difficulty in removing pulp tissue and necrotic debris, excessive hemorrhage, and persistent discomfort during instrumentation. Because of large volumetric

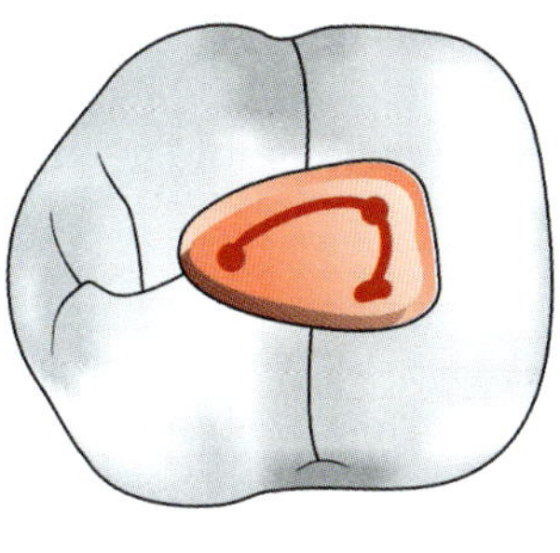
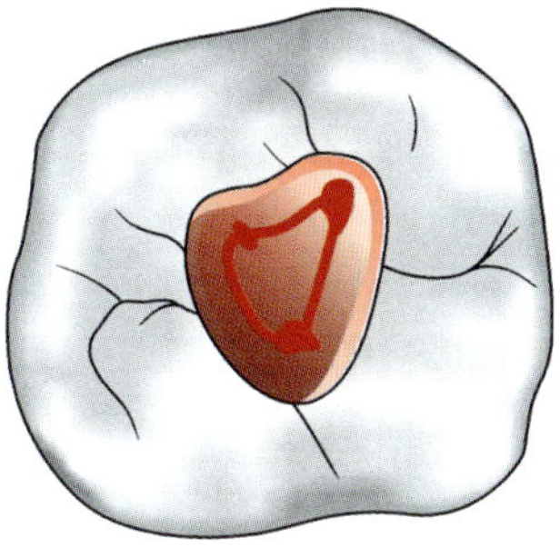

**Fig. 17.95:** Maxillary and mandibular molar showing C-shaped canal anatomy

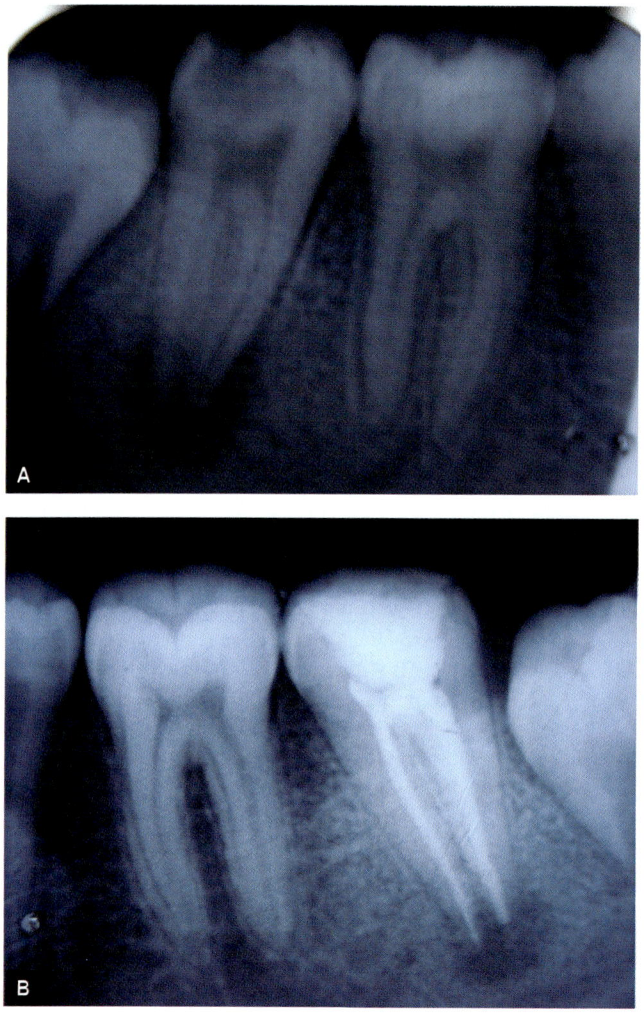


**Figs 17.96A and B:** (A) Carious second molar with C-shaped canals, (B) Obturation of molar

capacity of the C-shaped canal system, along with transverse anastomoses and irregularities, continuous circumferential filing along the periphery of the C with copious amounts of 5.25 percent NaOCl is necessary for maximum tissue removal and for control of bleeding. If hemorrhage continues, ultrasonic removal of tissue or placement of calcium hydroxide between appointments may be used to enhance tissue removal and control hemorrhage. Over preparation of C-shaped canals should be avoided, because of presence of only little dentin between the external root surface and the canal system in these teeth.

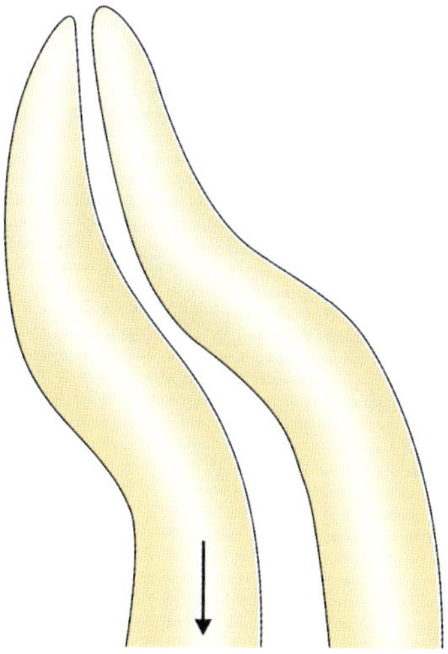

**Fig. 17.97:** Bayonet shaped canal

## 4. Management of S-shaped/ Bayonet shaped Canals

S-shaped or bayonet shaped canals pose great problems while endodontic therapy, since they involve at least two curves, with the apical curve having maximum deviations in anatomy (Fig. 17.97). These double curved canals are usually identified radiographically if they cross in mesiodistal direction. If they traverse in a buccolingual direction, they may be recognized with multi-angled radiographs, or when the initial apical file is removed from the canal and it simulates multiple curves. S-shaped canals are commonly found in maxillary lateral incisors, maxillary canines, maxillary premolars, and mandibular molars (Figs 17.98A to C).

For optimal cleaning and shaping of S-shaped canals, the three-dimensional nature of these canals must be visualized with special consideration and evaluation to the multiple concavities along the external surfaces of the root. Failure to know these may result in stripping of the canal along the inner surface of each curve. During initial canal penetration, it is essential that there be an unrestricted approach to the first curve. For this, the access preparation is flared to allow for a more direct entry. Once the entire canal is negotiated, passive shaping of the coronal curve is done first, to facilitate the cleaning and shaping of the apical curve. Constant recapitulation with small files and copious irrigation is necessary to prevent blockage and ledging in the apical curve. Over curving the apical 3 mm of the file aids in maintaining the curvature in the apical portion of the canal as the coronal curve becomes almost straight during the later stages of cleaning and shaping. Gradual use of small files with short amplitude strokes is essential to manage these canals effectively. To prevent stripping in the coronal curve, anticurvature or reverse filing is recommended, with primary pressure being placed away from curve of coronal curvature.

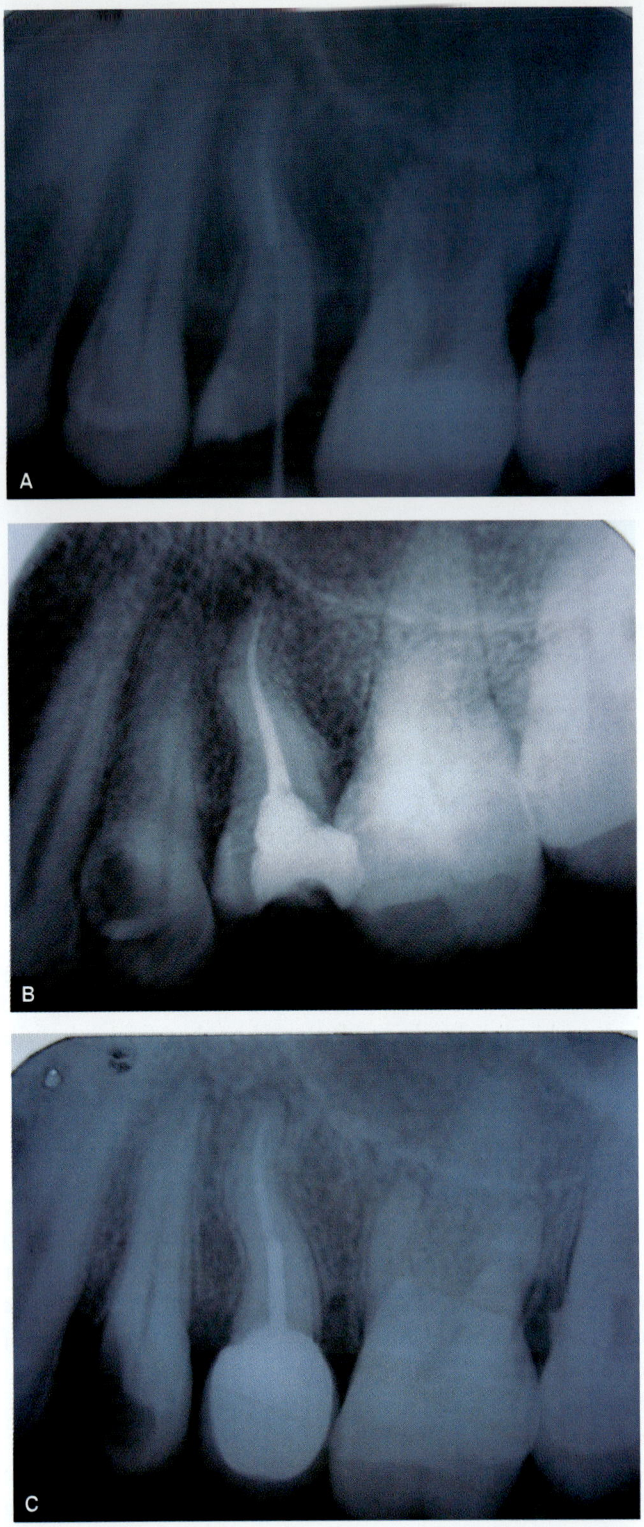

**Figs 17.98A to C:** A. 25 showing bayonet canal negotiated with 10 No. file, B. Obturation of bayonet shaped canal, C. Completed endodontic therapy of 25

## QUESTIONS

Q. What are Schilder's concept of root canal preparation?
Q. What are biologic and clinical objectives of root canal preparation?
Q. What are different movements of instruments?
Q. Write in detail about step-back technique of canal preparation with its advantages and disadvantages.
Q. What is crown down technique? What are its advantages over step-back technique?
Q. How will you manage a case of carious molar with curved canals?

## BIBLIOGRAPHY


1. Abou-Rass M, Frank AL, Glick DH. The anticurvature filing method to prepare the curved root canal. J Am Dent Assoc 1980;101:792.
2. Abou-Rass M, Jastrab RJ. The use of rotary instruments as auxillary aids to root canal preparation of molars. J Endod 1982;8(2):78-82.
3. Ahmad M, Ford TR, Crum LA, Walton AJ. Ultrasonic debridement of rot canals; acoustic cavitation and its relevance. J Endod 1988;14:486.
4. Ahmad M, Pitt Ford TR, Crum LA. Ultrasonic debridement of root canals; An insight into the mechanisms involved. J Endod 1987;13:93.
5. Ahmad M, Pitt Ford TR, Crum LA. Ultrasonic debridement of root canals; acoustic streaming and its possible role. J Endod 1987;13:490.
6. Allison DA, Weber CR, Walton RE. The influence of the method of canal preparation on the quality of apical and coronal obturation. J Endod 1979;5:298.
7. Al-Omari MA, Dummer PM. Canal blockage and debris extrusion with eight preparation techniques. J Endod 1995;21:154.
8. Anthony LP, Grossman LI. A brief history of root-canal therapy in the United States. I Am Med Assoc 1945;32:43.
9. Archer R, Reader A, Nist R, et al. An in vivo evaluation of the efficacy of ultrasound after step-back preparation in mandibular molars. J Endod 1992;18:549.
10. Arora RK, Gulabivala K. An in vivo evaluation of the ENDEX and RCM Mark II electronic apex locators in root canals with different contents. Oral Surg Oral Med Oral Pathol Oral Radiol Endod 1995;79:497-503.
11. Attin T, Buchalla W, Zirkel C, Lussi A. Clinical evaluation of the cleansing properties of the noninstrumental technique for cleaning root canals. Int Endod J 2002;35:929.
12. Balto KA. Modern electronic apex locators are reliable for determining root canal working length. Evid Based Dent 2006;7:31.
13. Barbakow F. The status of root canal therapy in Switzerland in 1993. J Dent Assoc S Afr 1996;51:819.
14. Barbakow. The LightSpeed system. Dent Clin North Am 2004;48:113.
15. Baugh D, Wallace J. The role of apical instrumentation in roof canal treatment: A review of the literature. J Endod 2005;31:333.
16. Baumgartner JC, Cuenin PR. Efficacy of several concentrations of sodium hypochlorite for root canal irrigation. J Endod 1992;18:605.
17. Beeson TJ, Hartwell GR, Thornton JD, Gunsolley JC. Comparison of debris extruded apically in straight canals; conventional filling versus ProFile. 04 taper series 29. J Endod 1998;24:18.
18. Berutti E, Angelini E, Rigolone M, et al. Influence of sodium hypochlorite on fracture properties and corrosion of ProTaper rotary instruments. Int Endod J 2006;39:693.
19. Blum JY, Machine P, Ruddle C, Micallef JP. Analysis of mechanical preparations in extracted teeth using ProTaper rotary instruments value of the safety quotient. J Endod 2003;29:567.

20. Boessler C, Peters OA, Zehnder. Impact of lubricant parameter on rotary instrument torque and force. J Endod 2007;33:280.
21. Borg E, Grondahl HG. Endodontics measurements in digital radiographs acquired by a photostimulable, storage phosphor system. Endod Dent Traumatol 1996;12:20.
22. Bortnick KL, Steiman HR, Ruskin A. Comparison of nickel-titanium file distortion using electric and air-driven handpieces. J Endod 2001;27:57.
23. Briseno BM, Sonnabend E. The influence of different root canal instruments on root canal preparation an in vitro study. Int Endod J 1991;24:15.
24. Brunton PA, Adbeen D, Macfarlane TV. The effect of an apex locator on exposure to radiation during endodontic therapy. J Endod 2002;28:524-6.
25. Buchanan LS. Paradigm shifts in cleaning and shaping. J Calif Dent Assoc 1991;19:23.
26. Buchanan LS. The standardized-taper root canal preparation-Part. Concepts for variably tapered shaping instruments. Int Endod J 2000;33;516.
27. Bystrom A, Sundqvist G. Bacteriologic evaluation of the effect of 0.5 percent sodium hypochlorite in endodontic therapy. Oral Surg Oral Med Oral Pathol Oral Radiol Endod 1983;55:307.
28. Bystrom A, Sundqvist G. The antibacterial action of sodium hypochlorite and EDTA in 60 cases of endodontics therapy. Int Endod J 1985;18:35.
29. Calhoun G, Montgomery S. The effects of four instrumentation techniques on root canal Shape. J Endod 1988;14:273.
30. Cameron JA. The use of ultrasonics in the removal of the smear layer: A scanning electron microscope study. J Endod 1983;9:289.
31. Cameron JA. The effect of ultrasonic endodontics on the temperature of the root canal wall. J Endod 1988;14:554.
32. Chenail BL, Teplitsky PE. Endosonics in curved root canals. Part II. J Endod 1988;14:214.
33. Clem WH. Endodontics: The adolescent patient. Dent Clin North Am 1969;13:482.
34. Cox VS, Brown CE Jr, Bricker SL, Newton CW. Radiographic interpretation of endodontic file length. Oral Surg Oral Med Oral Pathol Oral Radiol Endod 1991;72:340.
35. Crump MC, Natkin E. Relationship of broken root canal instruments to endodontic case prognosis; A clinical investigation. J Am Dent Assoc 1970;80:1341.
36. Cruse WP, Bellizzi R. A historic review of endodontics, 1689-1963, part 1. J Endod 1980;6:495.
37. Custer LE. Exact methods of locating the apical foramen. Natl Dent Assoc J 1918;5:815-19.
38. Dalton BC, Orstavik D, Phillips C, et al. Bacterial reduction with nickel-titanium rotary instruments. J Endod 1998;24:763.
39. Dietz DB, Di Fiore PM, Bahcall JK, Lautenschlager EP. Effect of rotational speed on the breakage of nickel-titanium rotary files. J Endod 2000;26:68.
40. El Ayouti A, Weiger R, Lost C. Frequency of overinstrumentation with an acceptable radiographic working length. J Endod 2001;27:49.
41. El Ayouti A, Weiger R, Lost C. The ability of root ZX apex locator to reduce the frequency of overestimated radiographic working length. J Endod 2002;28:116.
42. Fava LR. The double-flared technique: An alternative for biomechanical preparation. J Endod 1983;9:76-80.
43. Felt RA, Moser JB, Heuer MA. Flute design of endodontic instruments; its influence on cutting efficiency. J Endod 1982;8:253.
44. Forsberg J. Radiographic reproduction of endodontics "working length" comparing the paralleling and the bisecting angle techniques. Oral Surg Oral Med Oral Pathol Oral Radiol Endod 1987;64:353-60.
45. Forsberg J. A comparison of the paralleling and bisecting angle radiographic techniques in endodontics. Int Endod J 1987;20:177-82.
46. Fouad AF, Krell KV, Mc Kendry Dj, et al. Clinical evaluation of five electronic root canal length measuring instruments. J Endod 1990;16:446-9.
47. Frank AL, Torabinejad M. An in vivo evaluation of endex electronic apex locator. J Endod 1993;19:177-9.
48. Gabel WP, Hoen M, Steiman HR, et al. Effect of rotational speed on nickel-titanium file distortion. J Endod 1999;25:752.
49. Gambarini G. Shaping and cleaning the root canal system: A scanning electron microscopic evaluation of a new instrumentation and irrigation technique. J Endod 1999;25:800.
50. Goldberg F, Massone EJ. Patency file and apical transportation; an in vitro study. J Endod 2002;28:510.
51. Goldman M, Pearson AH, Darzenta N. Endodontics success-who's reading the radiograph? Oral Surg Oral Med Oral Pathol Oral Radiol Endod 1972;33:432-7.
52. Gordon MPJ, Chandler NP. Electronic apex locators. Int Endod J 2004;37:425-37.
53. Grawehr M, Sener B, Waltimo T, Zehnder M. Interactions of ethylenediaminetetra-acetic acid with sodium hypochlorite in aqueous solutions. Int Endod J 2003;36:411.
54. Green D. Double canals in single roots. Oral Surg Oral Med Oral Pathol Oral Radiol Endod 1973;35:689-96.
55. Green EN. Microscopic investigation of root canal diameters. J Am Dent Assoc 1958;57:636.
56. Green TL, Walton RE, Taylor JK, Merrell P. Radiographic and histologic periapical findings of root canal treated teeth in cadaver. Oral Surg Oral Med Oral Pathol Oral Radiol Endod 1997;83:707.
57. Grossman LI. Endodontics 1776-1976; A bicentennial history against the background of general dentistry. J Am Dent Assoc 1976;93:78.
58. Guiterrez Jh, Aguayo P. A apical foraminal openings in human teeth. Number and location. Oral Surg Oral Med Oral Path oral Radiol 1995;79:769.
59. Gutmann JL, Rakusin H. Perspectives on root canal obturation with thermoplasticized injectable gutta-percha. Int Endod J 1987;20:261.
60. Haapasalo M, Endal U, Zandi H, Coil JM. Eradication of endodontic infection by instrumentation and irrigation solutions. Endod Top 2005;10:77.
61. Harty FJ, Parkins BJ, Wengraf AM. Success rate in root canal therapy. A retrospective study of conventional cases. Br Dent J 1970;128:65-70.
62. Harty FJ, Stock C. The Giromatic system compared with hand instrumentation in endodontics. Br Dent J 1974;137:239.
63. Hoer D, Attin T. The accuracy of electronic working length determination. Int Endod J 2004;37:125.
64. Hommez GM, Braem M, De Moor RJ. Root canal treatment performed by Flemish dentists. Part 1. Cleaning and Shaping. Int Endod J 2003:36;166-73.
65. Hulsmann M, Peters OA, Dummer PMH. Mechanical preparation of root canals: Shaping goals, techniques and means. Endod Top 2005;10:30.
66. Hulsmann M, Rummelin C, Schafers F. Root canal cleanliness after preparation with different endodontic handpieces and

instruments: A comparative SEM investigation. J Endod. 1997;23(5):301-6.
67. Hulsmann M, Stryga F. Comparison of root canal preparation using different automated devices and hard instrumentation. J Endod 1993;19:141.
68. Ingle JI. A standardized endodontic technique using newly development instruments and filling materials. Oral Surg Oral Med Oral Pathol Oral Radiol Endod 1996;14:83.
69. Inoue N, Skinner DH. A simple and accurate way to measuring root canal length. J Endod 1985;11:421-7.
70. Izu KH, Thomas SJ, Zhang P, et al. Effectiveness of sodium hypochlorite in preventing inoculation of periapical tissue with contaminated patency files. J Endod 2004;30:92.
71. Jensen SA, Walker TL, Hutter JW, Nicoll BK. Comparison of the cleaning efficacy of passive sonic activation and passive ultrasonic activation after hand instrumentation in molar root canals. J Endod 1999;25:735.
72. Johnson TA, Zelikow R. Ultrasonic endodontics: a clinical review. J Am Dent Assoc 1987;114:655.
73. Kartal N, Cimilli HK. The degrees and configurations of mesial canal curvatures of mandibular first molars. J Endod 1997; 23(6):358-62.
74. Kast'akova A, Wu Mk, Wesselink PR. An in vitro experiment on the effect of an attempt to create an apical matrix during root canal preparation on coronal leakage and material extrusion. Oral Med Oral Pathol Oral Radiol Endod 2001;91:462.
75. Keller ME, Brown CE, Ir Newton CW. A clinical evaluation of the Endocater-an electronic apex locator. J Endod 1991;17: 271-4.
76. Kerekes K, Tronstad L. Long-term results of endodontic treatment performed with a standardized technique. J Endod 1979;5:83.
77. Kerekes K, Tronstad L. Morphometric observation on root canals of human anterior teeth. J Endod 1977;3:24.
78. Kerekes K. Radiographic assessment of an endodontics treatment method. J Endod 1978;4:210-13.
79. Khademi A, Yadzdizadeh M, Feizianfard M. Determination of minimum instrumentation size for the penetration of irrigants to the apical third of root canal systems. J Endod 2006;32:417.
80. Kim F, Lee SJ. Electronic apex locator. Dent Clin North Am 2004;48:35-54.
81. Kirkevang LL, Horsted-Bindslev P. Technical aspects of treatment in relation to treatment outcome. Endod Top 2002;2:89.
82. Klayman SM, Brilliant JD. A comparison of the efficacy of serial preparation versus Giromatic preparation. J Endod 1975;1:334.
83. Kobayashi C, Suda H. New electronic canal measuring device based on the ration method. J Endod 1994;20:111-14.
84. Kobayashi C. Electronic canal length measurement. Oral Surg Oral Med Oral Pathol Oral Radiol Endod 1995;79:226-31.
85. Kuttler Y. Microscopic investigation of root apexes. J Am Dent Assoc 1955;50:544.
86. Kyomen SM, Caputo AA, White SN. Critical analysis of the balanced force technique in endodontics. J Endod 1994;20:332.
87. Langeland K. The histopathologic basis in endodontics treatment. Dent Clin North Am 1967;491.
88. Leddy BJ, Miles DA, Newton CW, Brown CE Jr. Interpretation of endodontics file lengths using RadioVisiography. J Endod 1994;20:542.
89. Leeb J. Canal orifice enlargement as related to biomechanical preparation. J Endod 1983;9:463.
90. Li UM, Lee BS, Shih CT, et al. Cyclic fatigue of endodontic nickel titanium rotary instruments: static and dynamic tests. J Endod 2002;28:448.
91. Lilley JD. Endodontic instrumentation before 1800. J Br Endod Soc 1976;9:67.
92. Lim SS, Stock CJ. The risk of performation in the curved canal: anticurvature filing compared with the stepback technique. Int Endod J 1987;20:33.
93. Lin LM, Rosenberg PA, Lin J Do. Procedural errors cause endodontics treatment failure? J Am Dent Assoc 2005;136:187.
94. Lumley Pl. A comparison of dentine removal using safety or conventional Hedstrom files. Endod Dent Traumatol 1997;13:65.
95. Lussi A, Nussbacher U, Grosrey J. A novel noninstrumented technique for cleansing the root canal system. J Endod 1993;19:549.
96. MA Bauman NiTi. Options and challenges. Dent Clin N Am (48)55-67.
97. MA Bauman. Reamer with alternating cutting edges-concept and clinical application. Endodontic Topics 2005;10:176-8.
98. Martin H, Cunningham W. Endosonic endodontics: The ultrasonic synergistic system. Int Dent J 1984;34:198.
99. Martin H, Cunningham WT, Norris JP, cotton WR. Ultrasonic versus hand filing of dentin; a quantitative study. Oral Surg Oral Med Oral Radiol Endod 1980;49:79.
100. McDonald NJ. The electronic determination of working length. Dent Clin North Am 1992;36:293-307.
101. McGurkinn-Smith R, Trope M, Caplan D, Sigurdsson A. Reduction of intracanal bacterial using GT rotary instrumentation 5.25% NaOCl, EDTA and $Ca(OH)_2$. J Endod 2005;31:359.
102. Melius B, Jiang J, Zhu Q. Measurement of the distance between the minor foramen and the anatomic apex by digital and conventional radiography. J Endod 2002;28:125-6.
103. Meredith N, Gulabivala K. Electrical impedance measurements of root canal length. Endod Dent Traumatol 1997;13:126-31.
104. Michael Hu Ismann, Ove A. Peters, Paul MH. Dummer mechanical preparation of foot canals: Shaping goals, techniques and means. Endodontic Topics 2005;10:30-76.
105. Miserendino LJ, Miserendino CA, Moser JB, Heuer MA, Osetek EM. Cutting efficiency of endodontic instruments. Part III: comparison of sonic and ultrasonic instrument systems. J Endod 1988;14:24-30.
106. Miserendino LJ, Moser JB, Heuer MA, Osetek EM. Cutting efficiency of endodontic instruments. Part II: Analysis of tip design. J Endod 1986;12(1):8-12.
107. Morgan LF, Montgomery S. An Evaluation of the crow-down pressureless techniques. J Endod 1984;10:491.
108. Mullaney TP. Instrumentation of finely curved canals. Dent Clin North Am 1979;23:575.
109. Nagy CD, Bartha K, Bernath M, Verdes E, Szabo J. The effect of root canal morphology on canal shape following instrumentation using different techniques. Int Endod J 1997;30: 133-40.
110. Nair MK, Nair UP. Digital and advanced imaging in endodontics: a review. J Endod 2007;33:1.
111. Nair PMR. Apical periodontitis; a dynamic encounter between root canal infection and host response. Periodontology 2000 2000;13:121.
112. Nair PN. On the causes of persistent apical periodontitis: A review. Int Endod J 2006;39:249.
113. Nguyen HQ, Kaufman AY, Komorowski RC, Friedman S. Electronic length measurement using small and large files in enlarged canals. Int Endod J 1996;29:359.
114. O'Hoy PY Messe HH, Palamara JE. The effect of cleaning procedures on fracture properties and corrosion of NiTi files. Int Endod J 2003;36:724.

115. Olson AK, Goerig AC, Cavataio RE, Luciano J. The ability of the radiograph to determine the location of the apical foramen. Int Endod J 1991;24:28-35.
116. Ounsi HF, Haddad G. In Vitro evaluation of the reliability of the Endex electronics apex locator. J Endod 1998;24:120.
117. Palmer MJ, Weine FS, Healey HJ. Position of the apical foramen in relation to endodontic therapy. I Can Dent Assoc 1971;37:305-8.
118. Parashos P, Messer HH, Rotary NiTi. Instrument fracture and its consequences. J Endod 2006;32:1031.
119. Parris J, Wilcox L, Walton R. Effectiveness of apical clearing: histological and radiographical evaluation. J Endod 1994;20:219.
120. Pascon EA, Introcaso JH, Langeland K. Development of predictable peripical lesion monitored by subtraction radiography. Endod Dent Traumatol 1987;3:192.
121. Paul Calas HERO shapers. The adapted pitch Concept. Endodontic topics 2005;10:155-62.
122. Pecora JD, Capelli A, Guersoli DM, et al. Influence of cervical preflaring on apical size determination. Int Endod J 2005;38.
123. Pedicord D, elDeeb ME, Messer HH. Hand versus ultrasonic instrumentation: Its effect on canal shape and instrumentation time. J Endod 1986;12:375.
124. Pekruhn RB. The incidence of failure following single-visit endodontic therapy. J Endod 1986;12:68.
125. Peng B, Shen Y, Cheung GS, Xia TJ. Defects in ProTaper SI instruments after clinical use: longitudinal examination. Int Endod J 2005;38:550.
126. Peters IB, Wesselink Pr, Moorer WR. The fate and the role of bacteria left in root dentinal tubules. Int Endod J 1995;28:95.
127. Peters OA, Barbakow F, Peters CI. An analysis of endodontic treatment with three nickel-titanium rotary root canal preparation techniques. Int Endod 2004;37:849.
128. Peters OA, Barbakow F. Dynamic torque and apical forces of ProFile. 04 rotary instruments during preparation of curved canals. Int Endod J 2002;35:379.
129. Peters OA, Schönenberger K, Laib A. Effects of four NiTi preparation techniques on root canal geometry assessed by micro computed tomography. Int Endod J 2001;34:221-30.
130. Pettiette MT, Delano EO, Trope M. Evaluation of success rate of endodontic treatment performed by students with stainless-steel K-files and nickel-titanium hand files. J Endod 2001;27:124.
131. Pineda F, Kuttler Y. Mesiodistal and buccolingual roentgenographic investigation of 7,275 root canals. Oral Surg Oral Med Oral Pathol Oral Radiol Endod 1972;33:101-10.
132. Ponce de Leon Del Bello T, Wang N, Raone JB. Crown down tip design and shaping. J Endod 2003;29:513.
133. Radel RT, Goodell GG, McClanahan SB, Cohen ME. In vitro radiographic determination of distance from working length files to root ends comparing Kodak RVG 6000, Schick CDR, and Kodak insight film. J Endod 2006;32:566-8.
134. Ram Z. Effectiveness of root canal irrigation. Oral Surg Oral Med Oral Pathol Oral Radiol Endod 1977;44:306.
135. Ricucci D, Langeland K. Apical limit of root canal instrumentation and obturation, Part 2. A histological study. Int Endod J 1998;31:394.
136. Rig AC, Michelich RJ, Schultz IIII. Instrumentation of root canals in molar using the step-down techniques. J Endod 1982;8:550.
137. Roane JB, Powell SE. The optimal instrument design for canal preparation. J Am Dent Assoc 1986;113:596.
138. Roane JB, Sabala C. Clockwise or counterclockwise. J Endod 198;10:349.
139. Roane JB, Sabala CL, Duncanson MG Jr. The "balanced force" concept for instrumentation of curved canal. J Endod 1985;11:203.
140. Rowan MB, Nicholls JI, Steiner J. Torsional Properties of stainless steel and nickel-titanium endodontic files. J Endod 1996;22:341.
141. Ruddle C. The ProTaper technique. Endod Top 2005;10:187.
142. Ruddle C. Cleaning and shaping the root canal system. In Cohen S, Burns R, (Eds): Pathways of the Pulp, 8th edn. St Louis, MO:Mosby 2002;231-92.
143. Ruddle CJ. Cleaning and shaping the root canal system. In S Cohen and RC Burns (Eds): Pathways of the Pulp (8th edn). St Louis: Mosby, 2002.
144. Saad, Ay, al-Nazhan S. Radiation dose reduction during endodontic therapy a new technique combining an aped locator (Root ZX) and a digital imaging system (Radiovision Graphy) J Endod 2000;26:144-7.
145. Sabala CL, Roane JB, Sothard LZ. Instruments of curved canals using a modified tipped instrument: a comparison study. J Endod 1988;14:59.
146. Sabins RA, Johnson JD, Hellstein JW. A comparison of the cleaning ability of short-term sonic and ultrasonic passive irrigation after hand instrumentation in molar root canals. J Endod 2003;29:674.
147. Sattapan B, Nervo GJ, Palamara JEA, Messer HH. Defects in rotary nickel-titanium files after clinical use. J Endod 2000;26:161.
148. Saunders WP, Chestnutt IG, Saunders EM. Factors influencing the diagnosis and management of teeth with pulpal and periradicular disease by general practitioners. Part 2. By Dent J 1999;187:548-54.
149. Schäfer E, Schulz-Bongert U, Tulus G. Comparison of hand stainless steel and nickel titanium rotary instrumentation: A clinical study. J Endod 2004;30:432-35.
150. Schafer E, Zapke K. A comparative scanning electron microscopic investigation of the efficacy of manual and automated instrumentation of root canals. J Endod 2000;26:660.
151. Schafer E. Effects of four instrumentation techniques on curved canals: a comparison study. J Endod 1996;2:685.
152. Schrader C, Ackermann M, Barbakow F. Step-by-step description of a rotary root canal preparation technique. Int Endod J 1999;32:312.
153. Schrader C, Peters OA. Analysis of torque and force during step-back with differently taperd rotary endodontic instruments in vitro. J Endod 2005;31:120.
154. Schroeder KP, Walton RE, Rivera EM. Straight line access and coronal flaring effect on canal length. J Endod 2002;28:474.
155. Segall RO, del Rio CE, Brady JM, Ayer WA. Evaluation of debridement techniques for endodontic instruments. Oral Surg Oral Med Oral Pathol 1977;44(5):786-91.
156. Segall RO, del Rio CE, Brady JM, Ayer WA. Evaluation of endodontic instruments as received from the manufacturer: The demand for quality control. Oral Surg Oral Med Oral Pathol 1977;44(3):463-7.
157. Serota KS, Nahmias Y, Barnett F, et al. Predictable endodontic success. The apical control zone. Dentistry Today 2003;22:90.
158. Shearer AC, Horner K, Wilson NH. Radiovisiography for length estimation in root canal treatment: An in-vitro comparison with conventional radiography. Int Endod J 1991;24:233-9.
159. Simon JH. The apex: how critical is it? Gen dent 1994;42:330.
160. Siqueira JF Jr, Rjcas IN, Santos SR, et al. Efficacy of instrumentation techniques and irrigation regimens in reducing the bacterial population within root canals. J Endod 2002;28:181.

161. Siqueira JF. The etiology of root canal treatment failure: Why well-treatment teeth can fail. Int Endod J 2001;24:1.
162. SJ Jardine, K Gulabivala. An in vitro comparison of canal preparation using two automated rotary nickel-titanium instrumentation techniques. International Endodontic Journal 2000;381-91.
163. Sjogren U, Haglund B, Sundqvist G, Wing K. Factors affecting the long-term results of endodontics treatment. J Endod 1990;16:498-504.
164. Spångberg L. Endodontics in the era of evidence-based practice. Oral Surg Oral Med Oral Pathol Oral Radiol Endod 2003; 96(5):517-8.
165. Spangberg L. The wounderful world of rotary root canal preparation. Oral Surg Oral Med Oral Pathol Oral Radiol Endod 2001;92:479.
166. Sunada I. New method for measuring the length of the root canal. J Dent Res 1965;41:375-87.
167. Swartz DB, Skidmore AE, Griffin JA Jr. Twenty years of endodontics success and failure. J Endod 1983;9:198-202.
168. Swindle RB, Neaverth EJ, Pantera EA Jr, Ringle RD. Effect of coronal-radicular flaring on apical transportation. J Endod 1991;17:147.
169. Tan BT, Messer HH. The effect of instrument type and preflaring on apical file size determination. Int Endod J 2002;35:752.
170. Taylor GN. Advanced techniques for intracanal preparation and filling in routine endodontic therapy. Dent Clin North Am 1984;28:819.
171. Teixeira FB, Souza-Filho FL. Apical extrusion of debris and irrigants using two hand and three engine-driven instrumentation techniques. Int Endod J 2001;34:354-8.
172. Tepel J, Schafer E. Endodontic hand instruments: Cutting efficiency, instrumentation of curved canals, beding and torsional properties. Endod Dent Traumatol 1997;13(5):201-10.
173. Teresa Ponce de Leo Del Bello, Nancy Wang, James B. Roane, Crown-down Tip Design and Shaping. Journal of Endodontics 2003;29(8).
174. Thompson SA, Dummer PM. Shaping ability of ProFile. 04 Taper Series 29 rotary nickel-titanium Instruments in simulated root canals: Part I. Int Endod J 1997a;30:7.
175. Thompson SA, Dummer PMH. Shaping ability of HERO 642 rotary nickel-titanium in simulated root canal: Part 2. Int Endod J 2000 b;33:255-61.
176. Thompson SA. An overview of nickel-titanium alloys used in dentistry. Int Endod J 2000;33:297.
177. Tidmarsh BG. Radiograpic interpretation of endodontic lesions – a shadow of reality. Int Dent J 1987;37:10-15.
178. Tinaz AC, Alacam T, Uzun O, et al. The effect of disruption of the apical constriction on periapical extrusion. J Endod 2005;31:533.
179. Tinaz AC, Karadag LS, Alacam T, Mihcioglu T. Evaluation of the smear layer removal effectiveness of EDTA using two techniques: An SEM study. J Contem Dent Pract 2006;15:7(1): 9-16.
180. Torabinejad M. Passive step-back technique. Oral Surg Oral Med Oral Pathol Oral Rathol Endod 1994;77:398.
181. Ushiyama J. New Principle and method for measuring the root canal length. J Endod 1983;9:97-104.
182. Vande Voorde HE, Bjorndahl AM. Estimating endodontic "working length" with paralleling radiographs. Oral Surg Oral Med Oral Pathol Oral Radiol Endod 1969;27:106.
183. Velders XL, Sanderink GC, van der Stelt PF. Dose reduction of two digital sensor systems measuring file lengths. Oral Surg Oral Med Oral Pathol Oral Radiol Endod 1996;81:607-12.
184. Vertucci F. Root Canal Morphology and its relationship to endodontic procedures. Endod Top 2005;10:3.
185. Vertucci FJ. Root canal anatomy of the human permanent teeth. Oral Surg Oral Med Oral Pathol Oral Radiol Endod 1984;58:589-99.
186. Von der Lehr, WN Marsh RA. A radiographic study of the point of endodontic egress. Oral Surg Oral Med Oral Pathol Oral Radiol Endod 1973;35:705.
187. Walmsley AD, Lumley PJ, Laird WRE. The oscillatory pattern of sonically powered endodontic files. Int Endod J 1989;22:125.
188. Walmsley AD, Williams AR. Effects of constraint on the oscillatory pattern of endosonic files. J Endod 1989;15:189.
189. Walton RE. Current concepts of canal preparation. Dent Clin North Am 1992;36:309.
190. Walton RE. Histologic evaluation of different methods of enlarging the pulp canal shape. J Endod 1976;2:304.
191. Weiger R, John C, Geigle H, Lost C. An in vitro comparison of two modern apex locators. J Endod 1999;25:765-8.
192. Weiger R, El Ayouti A, Lost C. Efficiency of hand and rotary instruments in shaping oval root canals. J Endod 2002;28:580.
193. Weine FS, Healey HJ, Gerstein H, Evanson I. Pre-curved files and incremental instrumentation for root canal enlargement. J Can Dent Assoc 1970;36:155.
194. Weine FS, Kelly RF, Bray KE. Effect of preparation with endodontic handpieces on original canal shape. J Endod 1976;2:298.
195. Woolhiser GA, Brand JW, Hoen MM, et al. Accuracy of film-based, digital and enhanced digital images for endodontic length determination. Oral Surg Oral Med Oral Path Oral Radiol Endod 2005;99:499.
196. Wu MK, Dummer PM, Wesselink PR. Consequences of and stratergies to deal with residual post-treatment root canal infection. Int Endod J 2006;39:343.
197. Wu M-K, Van der Sluis LW, Wesselink PR. The risk of furcal perforation in mandibular molars using Gates-Glidden drills with anticurvature pressure. Oral Surg Oral Med Oral Pathol Oral Radiol Endod 2005;99:378.
198. Wu Mk, Wesselink PR, Walton RE. Apical terminus location of root canal treatment procedures. Oral Surg Oral Med Oral Pathol Oral Radiol Endod 2000;89:99.
199. Wu MK, Wesselink PR. A primary observation on the preparation and obturation of oval canals. Int Endod J 2001;34:137.
200. Yared G, Kulkarni GK. Accuracy of the DTC torque control motor for nickel-titanium rotary instruments. Int Endod J 2004;37:399.
201. Yared G, Kulkarni GK. Accuracy of the TCM Endo III torque-control motor for nickel-titanium rotary instruments. J Endod 2004;30:644.
202. Yared GM, Bou Daugher FE, Machtou P. Influence of rotational speed, torque and operator's proficiency on ProFile Failures. Int Endod J 2001;34:37.
203. Yeung-Yi Hsu, Syngcuk Kim. The profile system. Dent Clin N Am 2004;48(1):69-85.
204. Yusuf H. The significance of the presence of foreign material periapically as a cause of failure of root treatment. Oral Surg Oral Med Oral Pathol Oral Radiol Endod 1982;54:566.
205. Zehnder M. Root Canal Irrigants. J Endod 2006;32:389.
206. Zuolo MI, Walton RE. Instrument deterioration with usage; nickel-titanium versus stainless steel. Quintessence Int 1997; 28:397.

# Obturation of Root Canal System

CHAPTER 18



## INTRODUCTION

Root canal therapy may be defined as the complete removal of the irreversibly damaged dental pulp followed by thorough cleaning, shaping and filling of the root canal system that the tooth may remain as a functional unit within the dental arch (Fig. 18.1). The rationale of root canal treatment relies on the fact that the nonvital pulp, being avascular, has no defense mechanisms. The damaged tissue within the root canal undergoes autolysis and the resulting break down products diffuse into the surrounding tissues. They cause periapical irritation associated with the portals of exit even in the absence of bacterial contamination. It is essential therefore, that endodontic therapy must seal the root canal system three dimensionally so as to prevent tissue fluids from percolating in the root canal and toxic by-products from both necrotic tissue and microorganisms regressing into the periradicular tissues (Figs 18.2 and 18.3).

The current accepted method of obturation of prepared canals employs the use of solid or a semisolid core such as gutta-percha and a root canal sealer. Gutta-percha has no adhesive qualities to dentin regardless of the obturation technique used. Therefore, use of root canal sealer along with solid core plays a major role in achieving the hermetic seal by filling the accessory root canals, voids, spaces and irregularities and hence reducing the chances of failure of root canal treatment.

Not all teeth with positive bacterial cultures fail, nor do all teeth with negative cultures succeed. Thus, entombing residual microorganisms and irritants by sealing them within the root canal system may have a major influence on clinical outcome. Leakage of fluids through an obturated root canal can occur

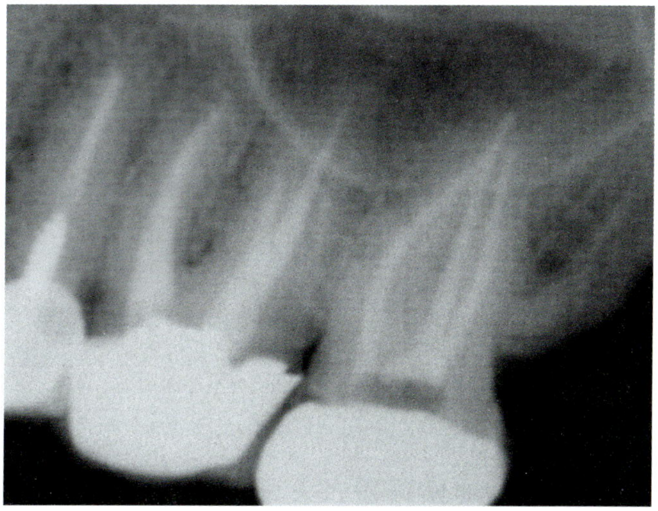

Fig. 18.1: Radiograph showing three-dimensional obturation

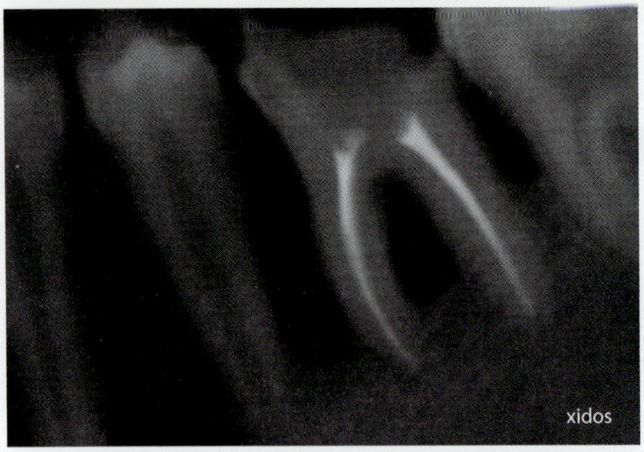


**Fig. 18.2:** Radiograph showing three-dimensional obturation of 36

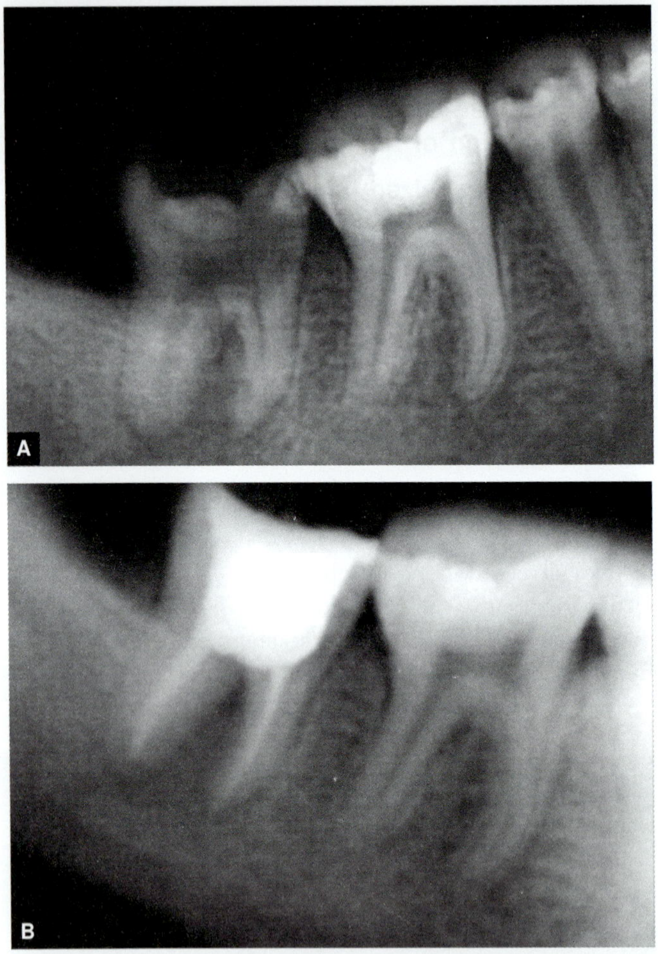


**Figs 18.3 A and B:** (A) Carious 47 with pulp exposure (B) Endodontic treatment done in 47

between the sealer and dentin, the sealer and gutta-percha, or through the voids within the sealer (Fig. 18.4). Although sealers enhance sealing ability by filling in any residual spaces and bonding to dentin, the optimal outcome of obturation is to maximize the volume of the core material and minimize the amount of sealer between the inert core and the canal wall.

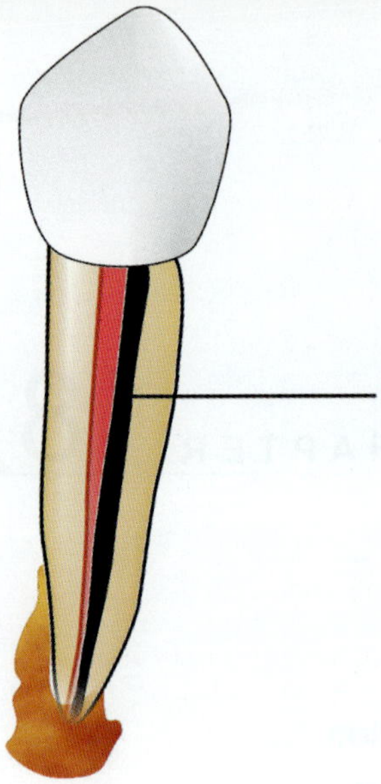


**Fig. 18.4:** Leakage in an obturated canal leading to root canal failure

Thus we can say that a three dimensional well fitted root canal with fluid tight seal is the **main objective of the root canal obturation.** ***Three-dimensional fluid tight seal of root canal system*** serves the following:

a. Prevents percolation and microleakage of periapical exudate into the root canal space.
b. Prevents infection by completely obliterating the apical foramen and other portals of communication.
c. Creates a favorable environment for process of healing to take place.

## PURPOSE OF OBTURATION

1. To achieve total obliteration of the root canal space so as to prevent ingress of bacterias and body fluids into root canal space as well as egress of bacterias which are left in canal.
2. To attain fluid tight seal so as to prevent bacterial micro-leakage.
3. To replace the empty root canal space with an inert filling material so as to prevent recurrent infection.
4. To seal the root canal space as well as to have coronal seal for long term success of root canal therapy.

**History**

1757 - Carious teeth were extracted, filled with Gold/lead and replanted again.
1847 - Hill's stopping was developed.
1867 - CA Bowman claimed to be the first to use gutta-percha for root canal filling.
1914 - Lateral condensation technique was developed by Callahan.
1953 - Acerbach advised filling of root canals with silver wires.
1961 - Use of stainless steel files in conjunction with root canal sealer as given by Sampeck.
1979 - Mc Spadden technique.

## TIMING OF OBTURATION

Various factors like patient symptoms, pulp and periradicular status and procedural difficulties affect the timings of obturation and number of appointment.

### Patient Symptoms

- If patient presents with sensitivity on percussion, it indicates inflammation in periodontal ligament space, canal should not be obturated before the inflammation has subsided.
- In case of irreversible pulpitis, obturation can be completed in single visit if the main source of pain, i.e. pulp has been removed.

### Pulp and Periradicular Status

- Teeth with vital pulp can be obturated in same visit.
- Teeth with necrotic pulp may be completed in single visit if tooth is asymptomatic.
- Presence of even a slight purulent exudate may indicate possibility of exacerbation. If canal is sealed, pressure and subsequent tissue destruction may proceed rapidly.

### Negative Culture

The reliance on negative cultures has decreased now since the researches have shown that false negative results can give inaccurate assessment on microbial flora, also the positive results do not indicate the potential pathogenicity of bacteria.

## EXTENT OF OBTURATION

Many studies have been conducted regarding the apical extent of obturation. It has been found that obturation should be done at the level of dentinocemental junction. Kutlur described DCJ as minor apical diameter which ends 0.5 mm short of apical foramen in young patients and 0.67 mm short in older patients. One should avoid overextension and overfilling of the root canal system.

**Overfilling** is complete obturation of root canal system with excess material extruding beyond apical foramen.

**Overextension** is extrusion of filling material beyond apical foramen but the canal may not have been filled completely.

**Features of an ideal root canal obturation**

- Three-dimensional obturation close to CDJ.
- Radiographically, filling should be seen 0.5-0.75 mm from radiographic apex.
- Minimal use of a root canal sealer which is confined to root canal.

## MATERIALS USED FOR OBTURATION

After the pulp space has been prepared appropriately, it must be obturated with a material which is capable of completely preventing communication between oral cavity and periapical tissue. The prepared apical connective tissue wound area cannot heal with epithelium, thus root canal filling material placed against this wound serves as an alloplastic implant. There are expectations which make the selection of a good obturation material. These materials may be introduced into the canals in different forms and may be manipulated by different ways. Grossman grouped acceptable filling materials into plastics solids, cements and pastes. He also delineated ***ten requirements for an ideal root canal filling materials.***

**Characteristics of an ideal root canal filling material**

1. Easily introduced in the canal.
2. Seal canal laterally and apically.
3. Dimensionally stable after being inserted.
4. Impervious to moisture.
5. Bacteriostatic or at least should not encourage bacterial growth.
6. Radiopaque.
7. Non staining to tooth structure.
8. Non irritating.
9. Sterile/easily sterilized.
10. Removed easily from canal if required.

**Materials used for obturation**

- Plastics: Gutta-percha, resilon
- Solids or metal cores: Silver points, Gold, stainless steel, titanium and irridio-platinum.
- Cements and pastes:
  - Hydron
  - MTA
  - Calcium phosphate
  - Gutta flow

### Gutta-percha

Gutta-percha was initially used as a restorative material and later developed into an indispensable endodontic filling material. Gutta-percha was earlier used as splints for holding fractured joints, to control hemorrhage in extracted sockets, in various skin diseases such as psoriasis, eczema and in manufacturing of golf balls (known as ***"Gutties"*** in past).

***Gutta-percha is derived from two words.***
"GETAH" - meaning gum
"PERTJA" - name of the tree

**Historical background**

- 1843 : ***Sir Jose d Almeida*** – First introduced gutta-percha to Royal Asiatic society of England
- In Dentistry : ***Edwin Truman*** – Introduced gutta-percha as temporary filling material.
- 1847 : ***Hill*** – Introduced Hill's stopping (a mixture of bleached gutta-percha and carbonate of lime and quartz).
- 1867 : ***Bowman*** – First to use gutta-percha as root canal filling material
- 1883 : ***Perry*** – Packed gold wire wrapped with gutta-percha in root canals
- 1887 : ***SS White company*** – First company to start the commercial manufacture of gutta-percha points.
- 1893 : ***Rollins*** – Used gutta-percha with pure oxide of mercury in root canals
- 1914 : ***Callahan*** – Did softening and dissolution of gutta-percha with use of rosins and then used for obturation of the canals.
- 1959 : ***Ingle and Levine*** – Proposed standardization of root canal instruments and filling materials.

### Sources

Gutta-percha is a dried coagulated extract which is derived from ***Brazillian trees (Palaquium)***. These trees belong to Sapotaceae family. In India, these are found in ***Assam and Western Ghats***.

### Chemistry

Its molecular structure is close to natural rubber, which is also a cis-isomer of polyisoprene.

## Chemical Structure

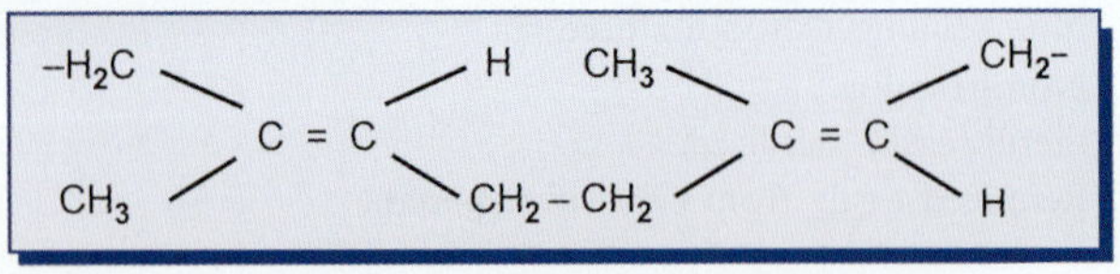


**In Crude form, the composition of gutta-percha is**

| | | |
|---|---|---|
| Gutta | - | 75-82 percent |
| Alban | - | 14-16 percent |
| Fluavil | - | 04-06 percent |

* Also contains tannins, salts and saccharine.

**Composition of commercially available gutta-percha (Given by Friedman, et al)**

| | | |
|---|---|---|
| • Matrix (Organic) | Gutta-percha | 20 percent |
| • Filler (Inorganic) | Zinc Oxide | 66 percent |
| • Radioopacifiers (Inorganic) | Heavy metal sulfates | 11 percent |
| • Plasticizers (Organic) | Waxes or resins | 3 percent |

***In other words,***

- Organic Content – Gutta-percha + Waxes = 23 percent
- Inorganic content – ZnO + Metal Sulfates = 77 percent

Chemically, pure gutta-percha exists in two different crystalline forms, i.e. $\alpha$ and $\beta$ which differ in molecular repeat distance and single bond form. Natural Gutta-percha coming directly from the tree is in $\alpha$–form while the most commercial available product is in $\beta$–form (Fig. 18.5).

**Different forms of gutta-percha**

*Alpha form*

- Pliable and tacky at 56°-64°.
- Available in form of bars or pellets.
- Used in thermoplasticized obturation technique.

*Beta form*

- Rigid and solid 42°-44°.
- Used for manufacturing gutta-percha points and sticks.

*Amorphous form*

- Exists in molten stage.

## Phases of Gutta-percha

These phases are interconvertible.

- $\alpha$ - runny, tacky and sticky (lower viscosity)
- $\beta$ - solid, compactable and elongatable (higher viscosity)
- $\gamma$ - unstable form
- On heating, gutta-percha expands which accounts for increased volume of material which can be compacted into the root canal. Gutta-percha shrinks as it returns to normal temperature. So, vertical pressure should be applied in all warm gutta-percha technique to compensate for volume change when cooling occurs (Schilder et al)
- Aging of gutta-percha causes brittleness because of the oxidation process (Fig. 18.6). Storage under artificial light also speeds up their deterioration. This brittle gutta-percha can be rejuvenated by a technique described by ***Sorien and Oliet***. In this, gutta-percha is immersed in hot water (55°C) for one or two seconds and then immediately immersed in cold water for few seconds.
- Gutta-percha cannot be heat sterilized. For disinfection of gutta-percha points, they should be immersed in 5.25 percent NaOCl for one minute (Fig. 18.7). Then, gutta-percha should be rinsed in hydrogen peroxide or ethyl alcohol. The aim of rinsing is to remove crystallized NaOCl before obturation, as these crystallized particles impair the obturation.
- Gutta-percha should always be used with sealer and cement to seal root canal space as gutta-percha lacks adhering qualities.
- Gutta-percha is soluble in certain solvents like chloroform, eucalyptus oil, etc. This property can be used to plasticize Gutta-percha by treating it with the solvent for better filling in the canal. But it has shown that gutta-percha shrinks (1-2%) when solidifies.

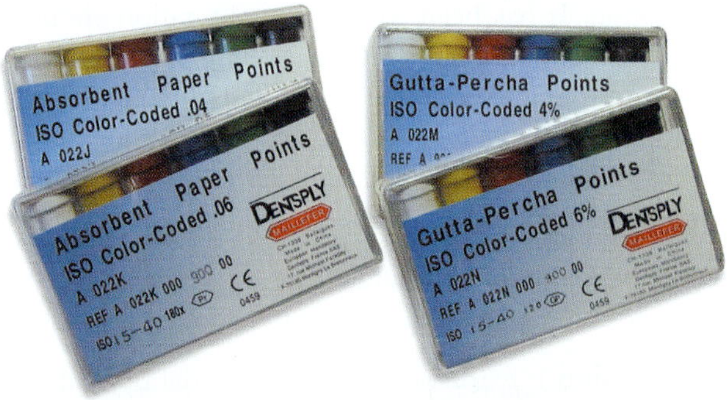


**Fig. 18.5:** Gutta-percha cones

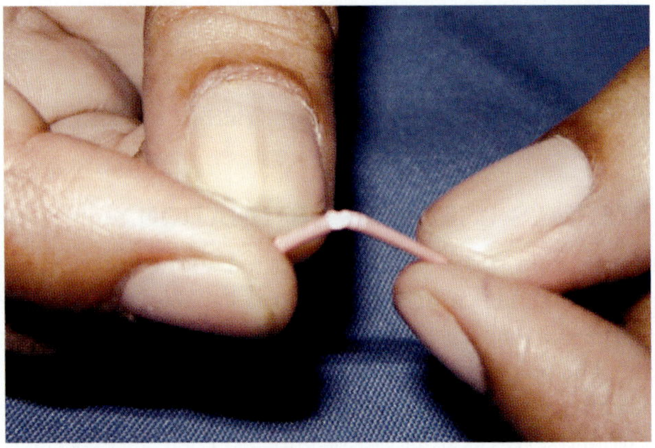

**Fig. 18.6:** Brittle gutta-percha point breaks on bending

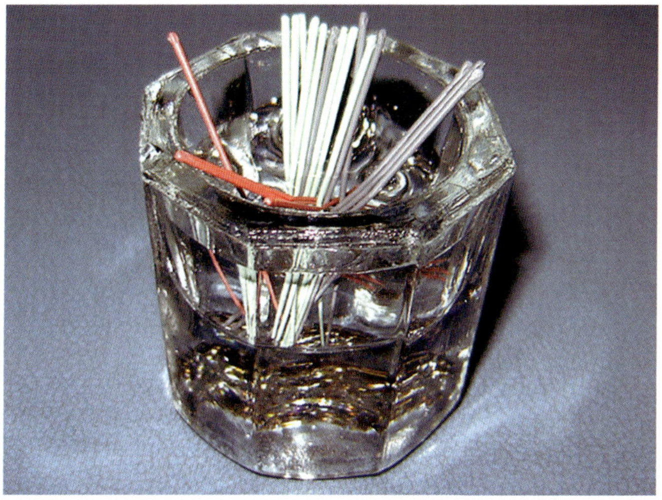

Fig. 18.7: Sterilization of gutta-percha by immersing them in 5.25 percent sodium hypochlorite for one minute

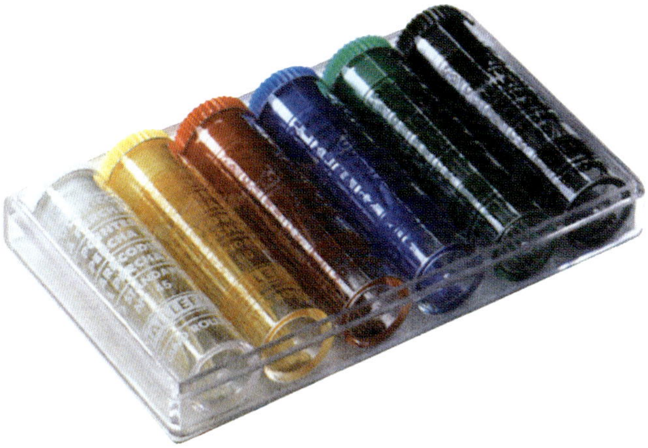

Fig. 18.8: Gutta-percha points

- Gutta-percha also shows some tissue irritation which is due to high content of zinc oxide.

## Current Available Forms of Gutta-percha

1. Gutta-percha points (Fig. 18.8): Standard cones are of same size and shape as that of ISO endodontic instruments.
2. Auxiliary points: Non-standardized cones; perceive form of root canal (Fig. 18.9).
3. Greater taper gutta-percha points: Available in 4 percent, 6 percent, 80 percent and 10 percent taper (Fig. 18.10).
4. Gutta-percha pellets/bars: They are used in thermoplastisized gutta-percha obturation e.g. obtura system.
5. Precoated core carrier gutta-percha: In these stainless steel, titanium or plastic carriers are precoated with alpha phase gutta-percha for use in canal. e.g. thermafil (Fig. 18.11).
6. Syringe systems: They use low viscosity gutta-percha. e.g. successful and alpha seal.
7. Gutta flow: In this gutta-percha powder is incorporated into resin based sealer.
8. Gutta-percha sealers like chloropercha and eucopercha:- In these gutta-percha is dissolved in chloroform/eucalyptol to be used in the canal.

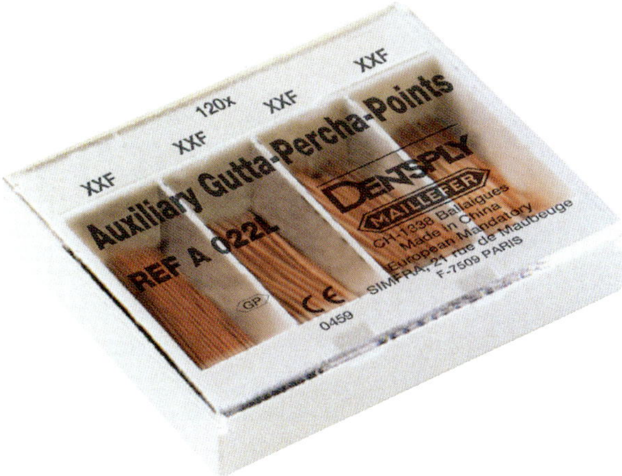


Fig. 18.9: Auxiliary points

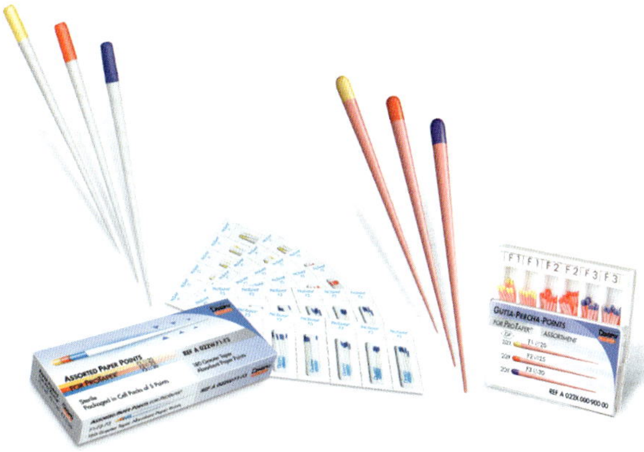

Fig. 18.10: Greater taper points

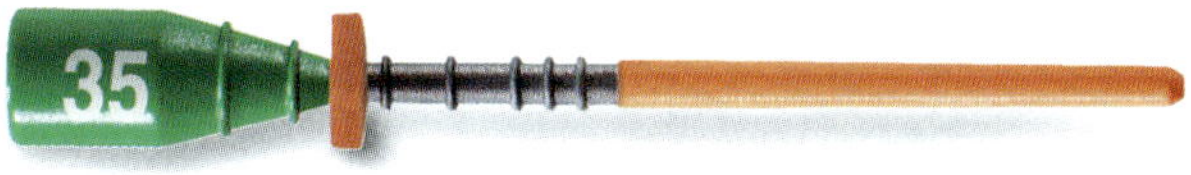


Fig. 18.11: Thermafil gutta-percha

9. Medicated gutta-percha: calcium hydroxide, iodoform or chlorhexidine diacetate containing gutta-percha points.

## Advantages of gutta-percha

- ***Compactiblity:*** adaptation to canal walls
- ***Inertness:*** makes it non-reactive material
- ***Dimensionally stable***
- ***Tissue tolerance***
- ***Radiopacity:*** easily recognizable on radiograph (Fig. 18.12)
- ***Plasticity:*** becomes plastic when heated
- ***Dissolve in some solvents*** like chloroform, eucalyptus oil, etc. This property makes it ***more versatile as canal filling material.***

## Disadvantages

- Lack of rigidity: Bending of gutta-percha is seen when lateral pressure is applied. So, difficult to use in smaller canals

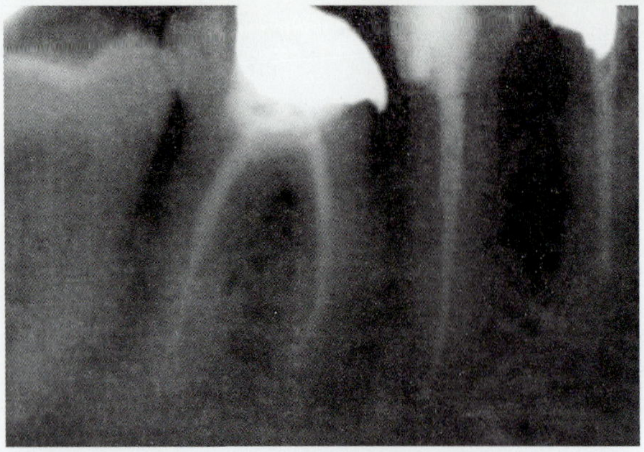

Fig. 18.12: Radiograph showing radiopaque Gutta-percha obturation

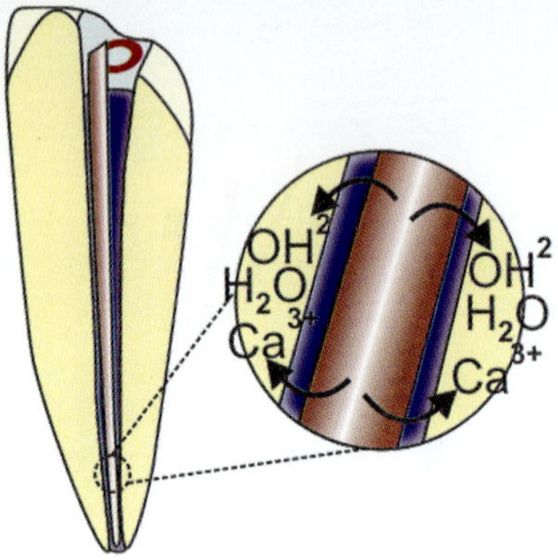


Fig. 18.13: Calcium hydroxide containing Gutta-percha

- Easily displaced by pressure
- Lacks adhesive quality.

## Medicated Gutta-percha

1. *Calcium hydroxide containing gutta-percha:* $Ca(OH)_2$ points (Fig. 18.13).
   They are made by combing 58 percent of calcium hydroxide in matrix of 42 percent gutta-percha. They are available in ISO size of 15-140. Action of $Ca(OH)_2$ is activated by moisture in canal.

### *Advantages of $Ca(OH)_2$ points*

- Ease of insertion and removal
- Minimal or no residue left
- Firm for easy insertion

### *Disadvantages*

- Short-lived action
- Radiolucent
- Lack of sustained release.

### *$Ca(OH)_2$ plus points*

Along with $Ca(OH)_2$ and gutta-percha they contain tenside which reduces the surface tension. Due to presence of water soluble components tenside and sodium chloride, they are 3 times more reactive then $Ca(OH)_2$ points.

They have superior pH and increases wettability of canal surface with increased antibacterial property. They have sustained alkaline pH for one week.

2. *Iodoform containing gutta-percha:* Iodoform containing gutta-percha remains inert till it comes in contact with the tissue fluids. On coming in contact with tissue fluids, free iodine is released which is antibacterial in nature.
3. *Chlorhexidine diacetate containing gutta-percha:* In this gutta-percha matrix embedded in 5 percent chlorhexidine diacetate. This material is used as an intracanal medicament.

## Silver Points

They have been used in dentistry since 1930's but now a days their use has been declined, because of corrosion caused by them.

Silver cones contain traces of metal like copper, nickel which add up the corrosion of the silver points. It has been seen that silver corrosion products are toxic in nature and thus may cause tissue injury.

Due to stiffness of silver cones, they are mainly indicated in round, tapered and narrow canals. They cannot conform with the shape of root canal because they lack plasticity; the use of silver points is not indicated in filling of large, triangular canals as in maxillary anterior teeth.

Silver cones do not possess adhering qualities, so a sealer is required to adequately seal the canal.

# ROOT CANAL SEALERS

The purpose of sealing root canals is to prevent periapical exudates from diffusing into the unfilled part of the canal, to avoid reentry and colonization of bacteria and to check residual bacteria from reaching the periapical tissues. Therefore, to accomplish a fluid tight seal, a root canal sealer is needed.

The sealer performs several functions during the obturation of a root canal system with gutta-percha; it lubricates and aids the seating of the master gutta-percha cone, acts as a binding agent between the gutta-percha and the canal wall and fills anatomical spaces where the primary filling material fails to reach. Root canal sealers, although used only as adjunctive materials in the obturation of root canal systems, have been shown to influence the outcome of root canal treatment.

The adequate combination of sealing ability and biocompatibility of root canal sealer is important for a favorable prognosis of the root canal treatment. Many studies have shown that most commercially available sealers can irritate the periapical tissues. Initially some type of cytotoxic reaction may even be partially beneficial with respect to eventual periapical healing. So, for a root canal filling material this toxicity should be minimal and clinically acceptable at the time of obturation. At a later time period, the material should become as inert as possible.

There are a variety of sealers that have been used with different physical and biological properties. The clinician must be careful to evaluate all characteristics of a sealer before selecting.

## Requirements of an Ideal Root Canal Sealer

Grossman listed eleven requirements and characteristics of a good root canal sealer:

1. It should be tacky when mixed so as to provide good adhesion between it and the canal wall when set. Only polycarboxylates, glass ionomers and resin sealers satisfy the requirement of good adhesion to dentin.
2. It should create hermetic seal.
3. It should be radiopaque so that it can be visualized in the radiograph. Radiopacity, is provided by salts of heavy metals such as silver, barium, bismuth.
4. The particles of powder should be very fine so that they can be mixed easily with the liquid.
5. It should not shrink upon setting. All of the sealers shrink slightly on setting, and gutta-percha also shrinks when returning from a warmed or plasticized state.
6. It should not stain tooth structure. Grossman's cement, zinc oxide-eugenol, Endomethasone, and N2 induce a moderate orange-red stain, Diaket and Tubli-Seal cause a mild pink discoloration, AH-26 gives a distinct color shift towards grey, Riebler's paste cause a severe dark red stain. Diaket causes the least discoloration. Leaving any sealers or staining cements in the tooth crown should be avoided.
7. It should be bacteriostatic or at least not encourage bacterial growth. All root canal sealers exert antimicrobial activity to a varying degree and those containing paraformaldehyde to a greater degree initially.
8. It should set slowly. The working and setting times of sealers are dependent on the constituent components, their particle size, temperature and relative humidity. There is no standard working time for sealers, but it must be long enough to allow placement and adjustment of root filling if necessary.
9. It should be insoluble in tissue fluids.
10. It should be tolerant, nonirritating to periradicular tissue.
11. It should be soluble in a common solvent if it is necessary to remove the root canal fitting.

*The following were added to Grossman's 11 basic requirements:*

12. It should not provoke an immune response in periradicular tissue.
13. It should be neither mutagenic nor carcinogenic.

**Requirements of an ideal root canal sealer**

- Should be tacky when mixed to provide good adhesion between it and the canal wall when set.
- Should create hermetic seal.
- Should be radiopaque.
- Powder particles size should be very fine, for easy mixing with liquid.
- Should not shrink upon setting.
- Should not stain tooth structure.
- Should be bacteriostatic.
- Should set slowly.
- Should be insoluble in tissue fluids.
- Should be non-irritating to periradicular tissue.
- Should be soluble in a common solvent.
- Should not provide immune response in periradicular tissue.
- Should not be mutagenic or carcinogenic.

## Functions of Root Canal Sealers

Root canal sealers are used in conjunction with filling materials for the following purposes:

1. ***Antimicrobial agent:*** All the popularly used sealers contain some antibacterial agent, and so a germicidal quality is excreted in the period of time immediately after its placement.
2. Sealers are needed to ***fill in the discrepancies*** between the filling material and the dentin walls (Fig. 18.14).
3. ***Binding agent:*** Sealers act as binding agent between the filling material and the dentin walls.
4. ***As lubricant:*** With the use of semisolid materials, the most important function for the sealer to perform is its action of lubrication.
5. ***Radiopacity:*** All sealers display some degree of radiopacity; thus they can be detected on a radiograph. This property can disclose the presence of auxiliary canals, resorptive areas, root fractures, and the shape of apical foramen.
6. ***Certain techniques dictate the use of particular sealer.*** The choropercha technique, for instance, uses the material as sealer as well as a solvent for the master cone. It allows the shape of normal gutta-percha cone to be altered according to shape of the prepared canal.

**Functions of root canal sealers**

- As antimicrobial agent
- Fill the discrepancies between the materials and dentin walls
- As binding agent
- As lubricant
- Give radiopacity
- As canal obturating material

## Classification

There are numerous classifications of root canal sealers. Classifications according to various authors are discussed below.

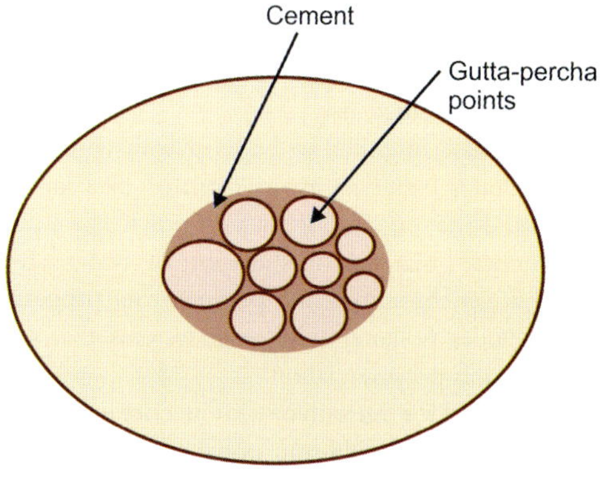


**Fig. 18.14:** Sealer fills the space between Gutta-percha points

**Sealers may be broadly classified according to their composition**

1. Eugenol
2. Non-eugenol
3. Medicated

*Amongst these, eugenol containing sealers are widely accepted.*

**1. Eugenol group may be divided into subgroups namely:**

a. *Silver containing cements:*
  - Kerr sealer (Rickert, 1931)
  - Procosol radiopaque silver cement (Grossman, 1936)

b. *Silver free cements:*
  - Procosol nonstaining cement (Grossman, 1958)
  - Grossman's sealer (Grossman, 1974)
  - Tubliseal (Kerr, 1961)
  - Wach's paste (Wach)

**2. Non-eugenol**

These sealers do not contain eugenol and consist of wide variety of chemicals.

**Examples:**
- Diaket
- AH-26
- Chloropercha and Eucapercha
- Nogenol
- Hydron
- Endofil
- Glass ionomer
- Polycarboxylate
- Calcium Phosphate cement

**3. Medicated**

These include the group of root canal sealers which have therapeutic properties. These materials are usually used without core materials.

**Examples:**
- Diaket-A
- $N_2$
- Endomethasone
- SPAD
- Iodoform paste
- Riebler's paste
- Mynol cement
- $Ca(OH)_2$ paste

**Classification of sealer according to Grossman**
- Zinc oxide resin cements
- Calcium hydroxide cements
- Paraformaldehyde cements
- Pastes

**According to Cohen (ADA and ANSI)**

According to the intended use:

**Type I** Material's intended to be used with core material.
- *Class I:* Includes materials in the form of powder and liquid that set through a non polymerizing process.
- *Class II:* Includes materials in the form of two pastes that set through a non polymerizing process.
- *Class III:* Includes polymers and resin systems that set through polymerization.

**Type II** Intended for use with or without core material or sealer.
- *Class I:* Powder and liquid-non polymerizing
- *Class II:* Paste and paste-non polymerizing
- *Class III:* Metal amalgams
- *Class IV:* Polymer and resin systems-polymerization

**According to Clark**
- Absorbable
- Non-absorbable

**According to Ingle**
- Cements
- Pastes
- Plastic
- Experimental sealers

## Zinc Oxide Eugenol Sealers (Fig. 18.15)

### Kerr Root Canal Sealer or Rickert's Formula

The original zinc oxide-eugenol sealer was developed by Rickert. This is based on the cement described by Dixon and Rickert in 1931. This was developed as an alternative to the gutta-percha based sealers (chloropercha and eucapercha sealers) as they lack dimensional stability after setting.

**Composition:**

| | |
|---|---|
| ***Powder*** | |
| Zinc oxide | 34-41.2 percent |
| Precipitated silver | 25-30.0 percent |
| Oleo resins | 30-16 percent |
| Thymol iodide | 11-12 percent |
| ***Liquid*** | |
| Oil of cloves | 78-80 percent |
| Canada balsam | 20-22 percent |

### *Advantages*

1. Excellent lubricating properties.
2. It allows a working time of more than 30 minutes, when mixed in 1:1 ratio.
3. Germicidal action and biocompatibility.
4. Greater bulk than any sealer and thus makes it ideal for condensation techniques to fill voids, auxilliary canals and irregularities present lateral to gutta-percha cones.

### *Disadvantage*

The major disadvantage is that the presence of silver makes the sealer extremely staining if any of the material enters the

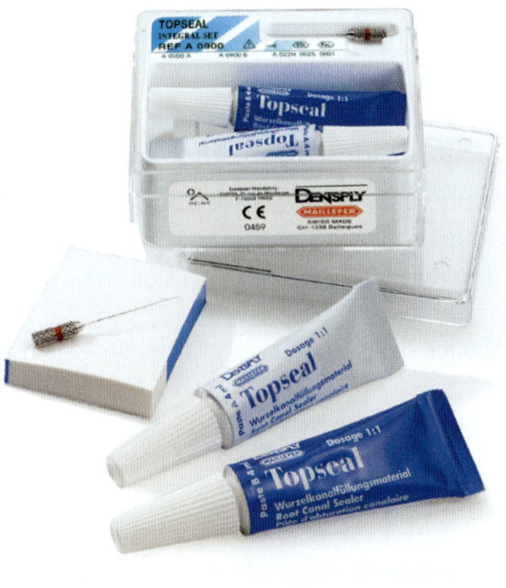


**Fig. 18.15:** Top seal sealer

dentinal tubuli. So sealers must be removed carefully from the pulp chamber with xylol.

## Manipulation

Powder is contained in a pellet and the liquid in a bottle. One drop of liquid is added to one pellet of powder and mixed with a heavy spatula until relative homogenicity is obtained.

Kerr pulp canal sealer completely sets and is inert within 15-30 minutes, thus reduces the inflammatory responses.

## Procosol Radiopaque-silver Cement (Grossman, 1936)

**Composition**

| | |
|---|---|
| ***Powder*** | |
| Zinc oxide | 45 percent |
| Precipitated Silver | 17 percent |
| Hydrogenated resins | 36 percent |
| Magnesium oxide | 2 percent |
| ***Liquid*** | |
| Eugenol | 90 percent |
| Canada balsam | 10 percent |

## Procosol Non Staining Cement (Grossman 1958)

**Composition**

| | |
|---|---|
| ***Powder*** | |
| Zinc oxide (reagent) | 40 percent |
| Staybelite resin | 27 percent |
| Bismuth Subcarbonate | 15 percent |
| Barium Sulfate | 15 percent |
| ***Liquid*** | |
| Eugenol | 80 percent |
| Sweet oil of almond | 20 percent |

## Grossman's Sealer

**Composition**

| | |
|---|---|
| ***Powder*** | |
| Zinc oxide (reagent) | 40 parts |
| Staybelite resin | 30 parts |
| Bismuth Subcarbonate | 15 parts |
| Barium Sulfate | 15 parts |
| Sodiumborate | 1 part |
| ***Liquid*** | |
| Eugenol | |

### Properties

1. It has plasticity and slow setting time due to the presence of sodiumborate anhydrate.
2. It has good sealing potential.
3. Zinc eugenolate is decomposed by water through continuous loss of eugenol, which makes zinc oxide eugenol a weak unstable compound.

### Disadvantage

Resin has coarse particle size, so the material is spatulated vigorously during mixing. If it is not done, a piece of resin may lodge on the canal walls.

### Setting Time

Cement hardens approximately in 2 hours at 37°C.

The setting time is influenced by:

1. Quality of the ZnO and pH of the resin used.
2. Technique used in mixing the cement.
3. Amount of humidity in the temperature.
4. Temperature and dryness of the mixing slab and spatula.

## Wach's Sealer

**Composition**

| | |
|---|---|
| ***Powder*** | |
| Zinc oxide | 10 g |
| Tricalcium phophate | 2 g |
| Bismuth subnitrate | 3.5 g |
| Bismuth subiodide | 0.3 g |
| Heavy magnesium oxide | 0.5 g |
| ***Liquid*** | |
| Canada balsam | 20 ml |
| Oil of clove | 6 ml |

### Properties

1. Medium working time.
2. Medium lubricating quality.
3. Minimal periapical irritation.
4. It is sticky due to the presence of Canada balsam
5. Increasing the thickness of the sealer lessens its lubricating effect. So this sealer is indicated when there is a possibility of over extension beyond the confines of the root canal.

### Advantages

1. It is germicidal
2. Less periapical irritation.

### Disadvantage

1. Odor of liquid

## Tubliseal (1961)

Slight modifications have been made in Rickert's formula to eliminate the staining property. It has marketed as 2 paste system containing base and catalyst.

**Composition**

| | |
|---|---|
| ***Base*** | |
| Zinc oxide | 57-59 percent |
| Oleo resins | 18.5-21.25 percent |
| Bismuth trioxide | 7.5 percent |
| Thymol iodide | 3.75-5 percent |
| Oil and waxes | 10 percent |
| ***Catalysts*** | |
| Eugenol | |
| Polymerized resin | |
| Annidalin | |

### Setting Time

- 20 minutes on the glass slab.
- 5 minutes in the root canal.

### Advantages

1. Easy to mix
2. Extremely lubricated.
3. Does not stain the tooth structure.
4. Expands after setting.

### Disadvantages

1. Irritant to periapical tissue.
2. Very low viscosity makes extrusion through apical foramen.
3. Short working time.

### Indications

1. When apical surgery is to be performed immediately after filling.
2. Because of good lubricating property, it is used in cases where it is difficult for a master cone to reach last apical third of root canal.

## Endoflas

It is zinc oxide based medicated sealer with setting time of 35-40 minutes.

**Composition**

***Powder***

Zinc oxide
Iodoform
Calcium hydroxide
Barium sulfate

***Liquid***

Eugenol
Parachlorophenol

### Setting Reaction of Zinc Oxide-Eugenol Cement

Zinc oxide and eugenol sets because of a combination of physical and chemical reaction, yielding a hardened mass of zinc oxide embedded in matrix of long sheath like crystals of zinc eugenolate. Hardening of the mixture is due to formation of zinc eugenolate. The presence of free eugenol tends to weaken the set. The significance of free eugenol is most apparent on increased cytotoxicity rather than alteration of the physical properties of dentin. Practically all ZOE sealer cements are cytotoxic and invoke an inflammatory response in connective tissue.

### Advantages of Zinc Oxide-Eugenol Cement

- Ease of manipulation.
- Shows only slight dimensional change.
- Radiopaque
- Germicidal properties.
- Minimal staining.
- Ample working time

### Disadvantages

- Irritant to periapex.
- Not easily absorbed from the apical tissues.

## Root Canal Sealers Without Eugenol

## Kloroperka N-Ø Sealers

This formula was given by Nyborg and Tullin in 1965.

**Composition**

***Powder***

| | |
|---|---|
| Canada balsam | 19.6 percent |
| Rosin | 11.8 percent |
| Gutta-percha | 19.6 percent |
| Zinc oxide | 49 percent |

***Liquid***

Chloroform

Kloroperka N-Ø was first introduced in 1939. The powder is mixed with liquid chloroform. After insertion the chloroform evaporates, leaving voids. It has been shown to be associated with a greater degree of leakage than other materials.

## Chloropercha

This is a mixture of gutta-percha and chloroform.

### Modified Chloropercha Methods

There are two modifications:

1. Johnston-Callahan
2. Nygaard-Ostby

1. ***Johnston-Callahan Method:*** In this method, the canal is repeatedly flooded with 95 percent alcohol and then dried. After this, it is flooded with Callahan resin chloroform solution for 2-3 minutes. A gutta-percha cone is inserted and compressed laterally and apically with a plugger until the gutta-percha is dissolved completely in the chloroform solution in the root canal. Additional points are added and dissolved in the same way.
2. ***Nygaard Ostby:*** It consists of Canada balsam; colophonium and zinc oxide powder mixed with chloroform. In this technique, the canal walls are coated with Kloroperka, the primary cone dipped in sealer is inserted apically pushing partially dissolved tip of the cone to its apical seal. Additional cones dipped in sealer are packed into the canal to obtain a good apical seal.

## Hydron

Hydron is a rapid setting hydrophilic, plastic material used as a root canal sealer without the use of a core. This was introduced by Wichterle and Lim in 1960. It is available as an injectable root canal filling material.

### Advantages

1. A biocompatible material.
2. Conforms to the shape of the root canal because of its plasticity.

### Disadvantages

1. Short working time.
2. Very low radiopacity.
3. Irritant to periapical tissues.
4. Difficult to remove from the canals.

## Nogenol

Nogenol was developed to overcome the irritating quality of eugenol. Base is ZnO with Barium sulfate as radiopacifier along with vegetable oil. Set is accelerated by hydrogenated rosin, chlorothymol and salicylic acid.

## Appetite Root Canal Sealer

Several root canal sealers composed of hydroxyapatite and tricalcium have been promoted.

*There are three types:*

**Type I:**

| | |
|---|---|
| *Powder* | |
| Tricalcium phosphate | 80 percent |
| Hydroxyapatite | 20 percent |
| *Liquid* | |
| Polyacrylic acid | 25 percent |
| Water | 75 percent |

***This is used for vital pulpectomy.***

**Type II:**

| | |
|---|---|
| *Powder* | |
| Tricalcium phosphate | 52 percent |
| Hydroxyapatite | 14 percent |
| Iodoform | 30 percent |
| *Liquid* | |
| Polyacrylic acid | 25 percent |
| Water | 75 percent |

**Type III:**

| | |
|---|---|
| *Powder* | |
| Tricalcium phosphate | 80 percent |
| Hydroxyapatite | 14 percent |
| Iodoform | 5 percent |
| Bismuth subcarbonate | 1 percent |
| *Liquid* | |
| Polyacrylic acid | 25 percent |
| Water | 75 percent |

## Resin Based Sealers

### *Diaket*

Diaket is a polyvinyl resin (Polyketone), a reinforced chelate formed between zinc oxide and diketone. It was introduced by Schmidt in 1951.

**Composition**

*Powder*
- Zinc oxide
- Bismuth phosphate

*Liquid*
- 2, 2, dihydroxy-5, 5 dichloro diphenyl methane.
- B-diketone
- Triethanolamine
- Caproic acid
- Copolymers of vinyl chloride, vinyl acetate and vinyl isobutyl ether.

### *Advantages*

- Good adhesion
- Fast setting
- Stable in nature
- Superior tensile strength

### *Disadvantages*

- Toxic in nature
- Tacky material so difficult to manipulate
- If extruded, can lead to fibrous encapsulation.
- Setting is adversely affected by presence of camphor or phenol (used as intracanal medicaments)

## AH-26

This is an epoxy resin recommended by Shroeder in 1957. Epoxy resin based sealers are characterized by the reactive epoxide ring and are polymerized by the breaking this ring. Feldman and Nyborg gave the following composition.

**Composition**

| | |
|---|---|
| *Powder* | |
| Bismuth oxide | 60 percent |
| Hexamethylene tetramine | 25 percent |
| Silver powder | 10 percent |
| Titanium oxide | 5 percent |
| *Liquid* | |
| Bisphenol diglycidyl ether | |

The formulation has been altered recently with the removal of silver as one of the constituent to prevent tooth discoloration.

### *Properties*

1. Good adhesive property.
2. Good flow
3. Antibacterial
4. Contracts slightly while hardening
5. Low toxicity and well tolerated by periapical tissue.
6. The addition of a hardener, hexamethylene tetramine, makes the cured resin inert chemically and biologically.

AH 26 consists of a yellow powder and viscous resin liquid and mixed to a thick creamy consistency. The setting time is 36 to 48 hours at body temperature and 5-7 days at room temperature.

AH 26 produces greater adhesion to dentin especially when smear layer is removed. Smear layer removal exposes the dentinal tubules creating an irritating surface thus enhancing adhesion.

## Thermaseal

Thermaseal has a formulation very similar to that of AH-26. It has been tested in several studies in the united states and is highly rated for both sealing ability and periapical tolerance. Thermaseal may be used with condensation techniques other than Thermafil.

## AH Plus (Fig. 18.16)

AH Plus is an Epoxide-Amine resin pulp canal sealer, developed from its predecessor AH26 because of color and shade stability,

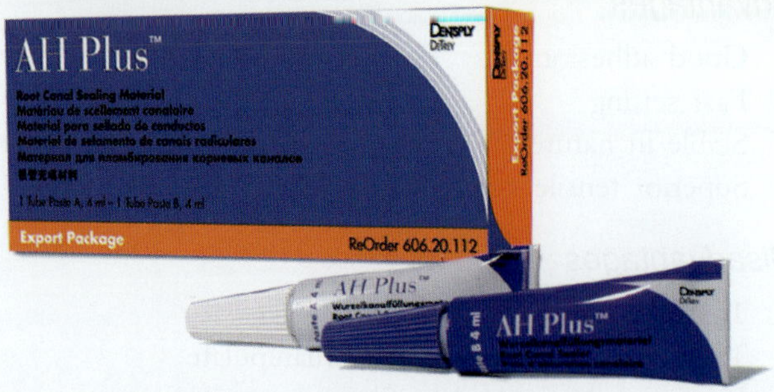


**Fig. 18.16:** AH plus root canal sealer

this is the material of choice where aesthetic demands are high. This easy-to-mix sealer adapts closely to the walls of the prepared root canal and provides minimal shrinkage upon setting as well as outstanding long-term dimensional stability and sealing properties.

**Composition**

***AH Plus Paste A***

Epoxy Resins
Calcium tungstate
Zirconium oxide
Silica
Iron oxide

***AH Plus Paste B***

Adamantianeamine
N, N-Dibenzyl-5-Oxanonane-diamine-1, 9, TCD-diamine
Calcium tungstate
Zirconium oxide
Silica
Silicone oil

Properties of AH plus sealer

| | |
|---|---|
| Radiopacity | 13.6 mm/ mm Al |
| Working time | 4 hours |
| Setting time | 8 hours |
| Flow | 36 mm |
| Film thickness | 26 μm |
| Shrinkage | 1.76% |
| Solubility | 0.31% |

Although pure AH plus contains calcium tungstate, but calcium release is absent from this material. Durarte et al in 2003 suggested addition of 5 percent calcium hydroxide makes it a low viscosity material, and increases its pH and calcium release. This higher alkalinity and enhanced calcium release leads to improved biological and antimicrobiological behavior, because more alkaline pH favors the deposition of mineralized tissue and exerts an antimicrobial action.

### *Dosage and Mixing*

Mix equal volume units (1:1) of Paste A and Paste B on a glass slab or mixing pad using a metal spatula. Mix to a homogeneous consistency.

**Difference between AH 26 and AH plus**

| | *AH 26* | *AH plus* |
|---|---|---|
| 1. | Available in powder and liquid systems | Available in two paste systems. |
| 2. | Releases small amount of formaldehyde on mixing, making it toxic in nature | Less toxic so biocompatible in nature. |
| 3. | Causes tooth staining | Does not cause staining |
| 4. | Film thickness is 39 μm. | It is 20 μm. |
| 5. | Setting time 24-36 hrs. | Setting time 8 hrs. |
| 6. | Good radiopacity | Better radiopacity. |
| 7. | Less soluble | Half solubility when compared to AH 26. |

### *Fiberfill*

Fiberfill is a new methacrylate resin-based endodontic sealer. Fiberfill root canal sealant is used in combination with a self-curing primer (Fiberfill primers A and B). Its composition resembles to that of dentin bonding agents.

**Composition**

***Fiberfill root canal sealant***

Mixture of UDMA, PEGDMA, HDDMA, Bis-GMA resins
Treated barium borosilicate glasses
Barium sulfate
Silica
Calcium hydroxide
Calcium phosphates
Initiators
Stabilizers
Pigments
Benzoyl peroxide

***Fiberfill primer A***

Mixture of acetone and dental surface active monomer NTG-GMA magnesium

***Fiberfill primer B***

Mixture of acetone and dental methacrylate resins of PMGDMA, HEMA Initiator

The bond between the adhesive systems and dentin depends on the penetration of monomers into the dentin surface, to create micromechanical interlocking between the dentin collagen and resin, thus to form a hybrid layer.

### *Manipulation*

Mix equal number of drops of Fiberfill primer A and B. Apply this mix into the root canal.

## Calcium Hydroxide Sealer

Calcium hydroxide has been used in endodontics as a root canal filling material, intra canal medicaments or as a sealer in combination with solid core materials. The pure calcium hydroxide powder can be used alone or it can be mixed with normal saline solution. The use of calcium hydroxide paste as a root canal filling material is based on the assumption that it results in formation of hard structures or tissues at the apical foramen (Fig. 18.17). The alkalinity of calcium hydroxide stimulates the formation of mineralized tissue.

***Calcium hydroxide sealers can:***
- Induce mineralization
- Induce apical closure via cementogenesis
- Inhibit root resorption subsequent to trauma
- Inhibit osteoclast activity via an alkaline pH
- Seal or prevent leakage as good as or better than ZOE sealers
- Less toxic than ZOE sealers

### *Disadvantages*

- Calcium hydroxide content may dissolve, leaving obturation voids.
- There is no objective proof that a calcium hydroxide sealer provides any added advantage of root canal obturation or has any of the its desirable biological effects.
- Although calcium hydroxide has dentin regenerating properties, the formation of secondary dentin along the canal wall is prevented by the absence of vital pulp tissue.

### *Seal Apex*

It is a non eugenol calcium hydroxide polymeric resin root canal sealer.

### *Advantage*

It has good therapeutic effect and biocompatible. The extruded material resorbs in 4-5 months.

### *Disadvantages*

- Poor cohesive strength
- Takes long time to set (three weeks)
- Absorbs water and expands on setting.

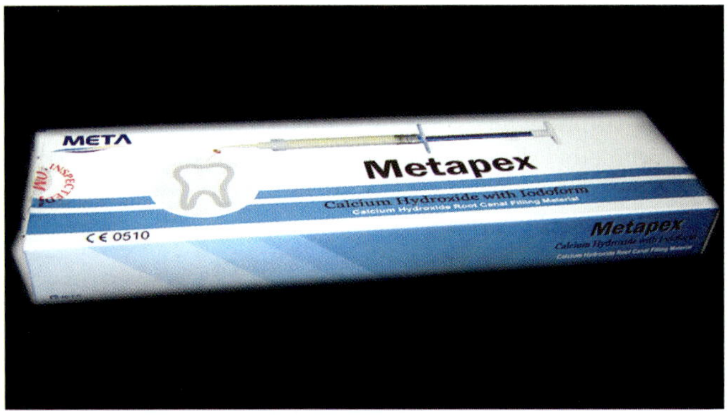


**Fig. 18.17:** Metapex sealer

**Composition**

***Base***

| | |
|---|---|
| Calcium hydroxide | 25 percent |
| Zinc oxide | 6.5 percent |
| Calcium oxide | |
| Butyl benzene | |
| Fumed silica (silicon dioxide) | |

***Catalyst***

| | |
|---|---|
| Barium sulfate | 18.6 percent |
| Titanium dioxide | 5.1 percent |
| Zinc stearate | 1.0 percent |
| Isobutyl salicylate | |
| Disalicylate | |
| Trisalicylate | |
| Bismuth trioxide | |

In 100 percent humidity it takes three weeks to reach a final set. It never sets in a dry atmosphere.

### *Calcibiotic Root Canal Sealer (CRCS)*

**Composition**

***Powder***

| | |
|---|---|
| Zinc oxide | Hydrogenated resin |
| Barium sulfate | Calcium hydroxide |
| Bismuth subcarbonate | |

***Liquid***

Eugenol
Eucalyptol

CRCS is a zinc oxide, eugenol-eucalyptol sealer to which calcium hydroxide has been added for its osteogenic effect. CRCS takes three days to set fully in either dry or humid environment. Because of little water resorption property, it is quite stable. Though sealing is improved, but since calcium hydroxide is not released from the cement, its main role (osteogenic effect) becomes questionable.

## CRCS

### *Advantages*

- Biocompatible
- Takes three days to set
- Stable in nature
- Shows little water resorption
- Easily disintegrates in tissues.

### *Disadvantages*

- Extruded sealer is resistant to resorption by tissue fluids.
- It shows minimal antibacterial activity.

## Apexit

Apexit is a calcium hydroxide based root canal sealer available in syringes.

**Composition**

| | |
|---|---|
| ***Base*** | |
| Calcium hydroxide | 31.9 percent |
| Hydrogenized colophony | 31.5 percent |
| Highly dispersed silicon dioxide | 8.1 percent |
| Calcium oxide | 5.6 percent |
| Zinc oxide | 5.5 percent |
| Tricalcium phosphate | 4.1 percent |
| Polydimethylsiloxane | 2.5 percent |
| Zinc stearate | 2.3 percent |
| Alkyl ester of phosphoric acid | |
| Paraffin oil | |
| Pigments | |
| ***Activator*** | |
| Trimethyl hexanedioldisalicylate | 25.0 percent |
| Bismuth carbonate | 18.2 percent |
| Bismuth oxide | 18.2 percent |
| Highly dispersed silicon dioxide | 15.0 percent |
| 1.3 Butanedioldisalicylate | 11.4 percent |
| Hydrogenized colophony | 5.4 percent |
| Tricalcium phosphate | 5.0 percent |
| Zinc stearate | 1.4 percent |
| Alkyl ester of phosphoric acid | |

### Advantages

- Biocompatible calcium hydroxide base.
- Easy to mix due to paste delivery form
- Radiopaque.
- Hard setting.

## Medicated Sealers

### $N_2$

$N_2$ was introduced by Sargenti and Ritcher (1961). N2 refers to the so called second nerve. ***(Pulp is referred to as first nerve)***

**Composition of $N_2$**

| | |
|---|---|
| ***Powder*** | |
| Zinc oxide | 68.51 g |
| Lead tetraoxide para | 12.00 g |
| Paraformaldehyde | 4.70 g |
| Bismuth subcarbonate | 2.60 g |
| Bismuth subnitrate | 3.70 g |
| Titanium dioxide | 8.40 g |
| Phenyl mercuric borate | 0.09 g |
| ***Liquid*** | |
| Eugenol | |
| Oleum rosae | |
| Oleum lavandulae | |

The corticosteroids are added to the cement separately as hydrocortisone powder or Terra-Cortril.

The object of introducing formaldehyde within the root-filling is to obtain a continued release of formaldehyde gas, which causes prolonged fixation and antiseptic action.

### Toxicity

Degree of irritation is severe with the overfilling when $N_2$ is forced into the maxillary sinus or mandibular canal, persisting paresthesia was observed.

### Endomethasone

The formation of this sealer is very similar to $N_2$ composition.

**Composition**

| | |
|---|---|
| ***Powder*** | |
| Zinc oxide | 100.00 g |
| Bismuth subnitrate | 100.00 g |
| Dexamethasone | 0.019 g |
| Hydrocortisone | 1.60 g |
| Thymol iodide | 25.0 g |
| Paraformaldehyde | 2.20 g |
| ***Liquid*** | |
| Eugenol | |

## Silicone-based Root Canal Sealers

### Endofill

Endofill is an injectable silicone resin endodontic sealant known as Lee Endofill. Endofill, a silicone elastomer, consists essentially of a silicone monomer and a silicone based catalyst plus bismuth subnitrate filler.

Active ingredients are hydroxyl terminated dimethyl polysiloxane, benzyl alcohol and hydrophobic amorphous silica. Catalysts are tetra ethylorthosilicate and polydimethyl siloxane.

Setting time can be controlled from 8 to 90 minutes by varying the amount of catalyst used. If more amount of catalyst is used, it decreases the setting time and increases the shrinkage of set mass.

### Advantages

1. Ease of penetration
2. Adjustable working time
3. Low working viscosity
4. Rubbery consistency
5. Non-resorbable.

### Disadvantages

1. Cannot be used in presence of hydrogen peroxide.
2. Canal must be absolutely dry.
3. Shrinks upon setting but has affinity for flowing into open tubuli.
4. Difficult to remove from the canals.

## Rocko Seal

It is silicon based root canal sealer with low film thickness, good flow, biocompatibility and low solubility. Its main constituent is poly dimethyl siloxane. Instead of showing shrinkage, Rocko seal shows 0.2 percent expansion on setting.

## Glass Ionomer Sealer (Ketac-Endo)

Recently glass ionomer cements has been introduced as endodontic sealer (Ketac-Endo). Glass ionomer cement is the reaction product of an ion-leachable glass powder and a polyanion in aqueous solution. On setting it forms a hard polysalt gel, which adheres tightly to enamel and dentin. Because of its adhesive qualities, it can be used as root canal sealer (Fig. 18.18).

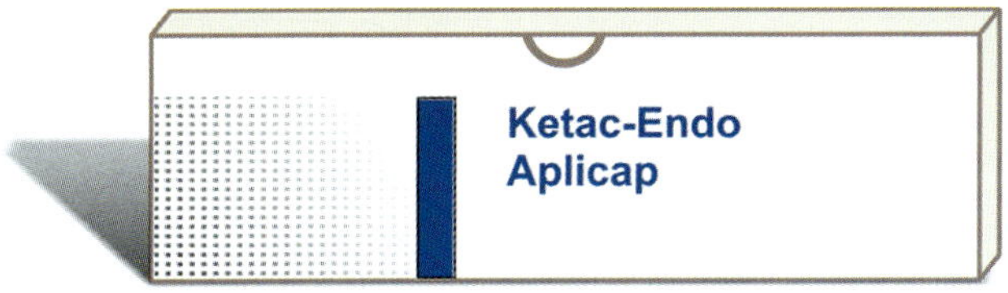


Fig. 18.18: Ketac-Endo sealer

**Composition**

***Powder***

Calcium aluminium lanthanum flurosilicate glass
Calcium volframate
Cilicic acid
Pigments

***Liquid***

Polyethylene polycarbonic acid/Maleic acid
Copolymer
Tartaric acid
Water

### *Advantages*

1. Optimal physical qualities.
2. Shows bonding to dentin
3. Shows minimum number of voids.
4. Low surface tension.
5. Optimal flow property.

### *Disadvantages*

It cannot be removed from the root canal in the event of retreatment as there is no known solvent for glass ionomer. However, Toronto/Osract group has reported that Ketac- endo sealer can be effectively removed by hand instruments or chloroform solvent followed by 1 minute with an ultrasonic No. 25 file.

## Resilon (Fig. 18.19)

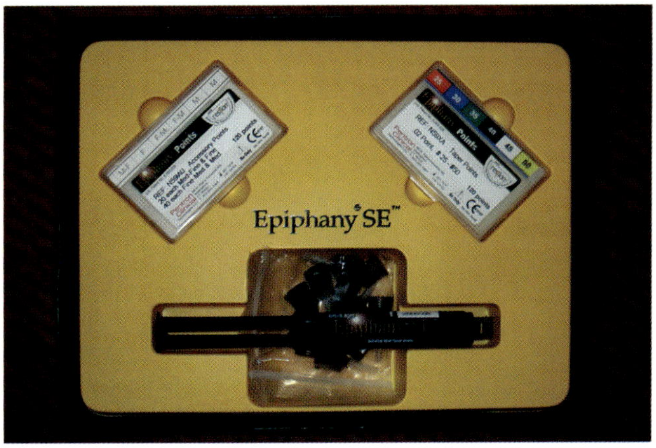


Fig. 18.19: Resilon

A new material, Resilon (Epiphany, Pentron Clinical Technologies; Wallingford, CT; RealSeal, SybronEndo; Orange, CA) has been developed to replace gutta-percha and traditional sealers for root canal obturation.

It offers solutions to the problems associated with gutta-percha:

1. Shrinkage of gutta-percha after application of heat.
2. Shrinkage of gutta-percha on cooling: since gutta-percha does not bind physically to the sealer, it results in gap formation between the sealer and the gutta-percha.

This resilon core material only shrinks 0.5 percent and is physically bonded to the sealer by polymerization. When it sets, no gaps are seen due to shrinkage.

*Resilon system is comprised of following components:*

1. ***Primer:*** It is a self etch primer, which contains a sulfonic acid terminated functional monomer, HEMA, water and a polymerization initiator.
2. ***Resilon sealer*** a dual-cured, resin-based composite sealer. The resin matrix is comprised of Bis-GMA, ethoxylated Bis-GMA, UDMA, and hydrophilic difunctional methacrylates. It contains fillers of calcium hydroxide, barium sulphate, bioactive glass, bismuth oxychloride and silica. The total filler content is approximately 70 percent by weight. The preparation of the dentin through these chemical agents may prevent shrinkage of the resin filling away form the dentin wall and aid in sealing the roots filled with resilon material.
3. ***Resilon core material:*** It is a thermoplastic synthetic polymer based (polyester) root canal core material that contains bioactive glass, bismuth oxychloride and barium sulphate. The filler content is approximately 65 percent by weight.

This new material has shown to be biocompatible, non-cytotoxic and non-mutagenic. The excellent sealing ability of the resilon system may be attributed to the "mono block" which is formed by the adhesion of the resilon cone to the Epiphany sealer, which adheres and penetrates into the dentin walls of the root canal system.

## The Monoblock Concept

An ideal endodontic filling material should create a "monoblock". This term refers to a continuous solid layer that consists of an etched layer of canal dentin impregnated with resin tags which are attached to a thin layer of resin cement that is bonded to a core layer of resilon which makes up the bulk of the filling material. ***In other words the monoblock concept means the creation of a solid, bonded, continuous material from one dentin wall of the canal to the other. One added benefit of the monoblock is that research has shown that it strengthens the root by approximately 20 percent.***

**Classification of Monoblock concept (Fig. 18.20)** based on number of interfaces present between corefilling material and bonding substrate:

**Primary:** In this obturation is completely done with core material, for example, use of MTA for obturation in cases of apexification.

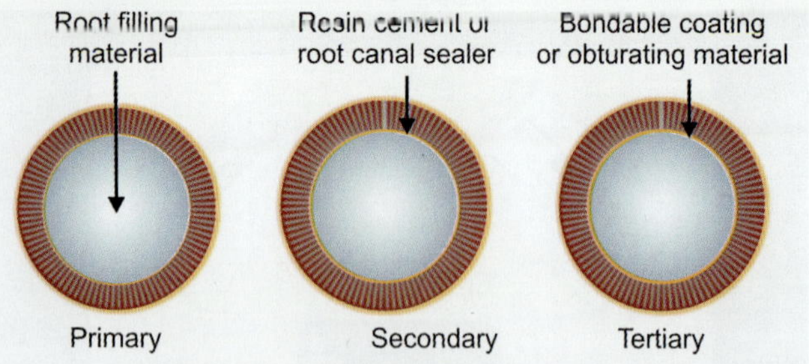


**Fig. 18.20:** Types of Monoblock concept

**Secondary:** In this bond is there between etched dentin of canal wall impregnated with resin tags which are attached to resin cement that is bonded to core layer, e.g. resilon based system.

**Tertiary:** In this conventional gutta-percha surface is coated with resin which bond with the sealer, which further bond to canal walls, e.g. Endo Rez and Activ GP system.

### Method of Use

1. Canal is prepared with normal preparation method.
2. ***Smear layer removal:*** Sodium hypochlorite should not be the last irrigant used within the root canal system due to compatibility issues with resins. Use 17 percent EDTA or 2 percent Chlorhexidine as a final rinse.
3. ***Placement of the primer:*** After the canal is dried with paper points, the primer is applied up to the apex. Dry paper points are then used to wick out the excess primer from the canal. The primer is very important because it creates a collagen matrix that increases the surface area for bonding. The low viscosity primer also draws the sealer into the dentinal tubules.
4. ***Placement of the sealer:*** The sealer can be placed into the root canal system using a lentulospiral at low rpm or by generously coating the master cone.
5. ***Obturation:*** The root canal system is then obturated by preferred method (lateral or warm vertical, etc.)
6. ***Immediate cure:*** The resilon root filling material can be immediately cured with a halogen curing light for 40 seconds.
7. ***Coronal restoration:*** A coronal temporary or permanent restoration should then be placed to properly seal the access cavity.

#### *Advantages of Epiphany*

1. Biocompatible
2. Good coronal seal so less microleakage
3. Non-toxic
4. Non-mutagenic
5. Forms monoblock
6. Increases resistance to fracture in endodontically treated teeth

#### *Disadvantage*

Does not retain its softness after heating.

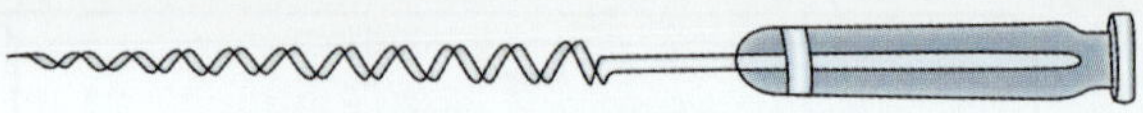

**Fig. 18.21:** Lentulo spiral for carrying sealer

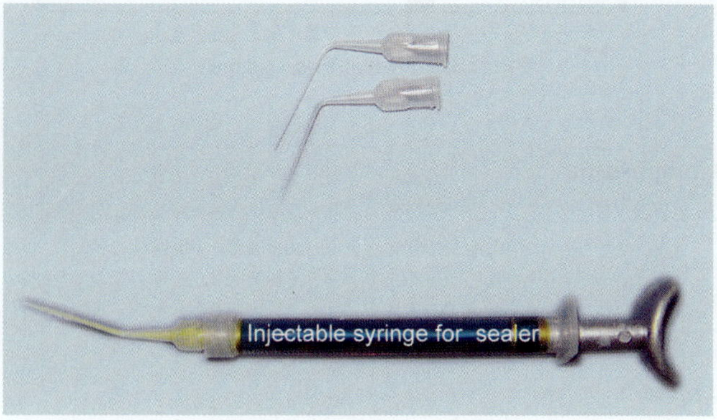


**Fig. 18.22:** Injectable syringe for carrying sealer

## METHODS OF SEALER PLACEMENT

Various methods are employed for placing sealer prior to inserting master cone. The common methods are:

1. Coating the master cone and placing the sealer in the canal with a pumping action.
2. Placing the sealer in the canal with a lentulo spiral (Fig. 18.21).
3. Placing the sealer on the final file used at the corrected working length and turning the file counterclockwise.
4. Injecting the sealer with special syringes (Fig. 18.22).

Sealer placement techniques vary with the status of apical foramen. If apex is open, only apical one third of master cone is coated with sealer to prevent its extrusion into periapical tissues. In closed apex root, any of above techniques can be used.

## OBTURATION TECHNIQUES

The main objective of root canal obturation is the three dimensional sealing of the complete root canal system. As we have seen that gutta-percha is the most common material used for root canal obturation, however, it must be stressed that a sealer is always required to lute the material to the root canal wall and to fill the canal wall irregularities.

Various root canal obturation techniques have been portrayed in the literature, each technique having its indications, contraindications, advantages and disadvantages (Fig. 18.23). Generally speaking the root canal obturation with gutta-percha as filling material, can be mainly divided in to following groups:

1. Use of cold gutta-percha
   - Lateral compaction technique
2. Use of chemically softened gutta-percha
   - Chloroform
   - Halothane
   - Eucalyptol
3. Use of heat softened gutta-percha
   - Vertical compaction technique
   - System B continuous wave condensation technique

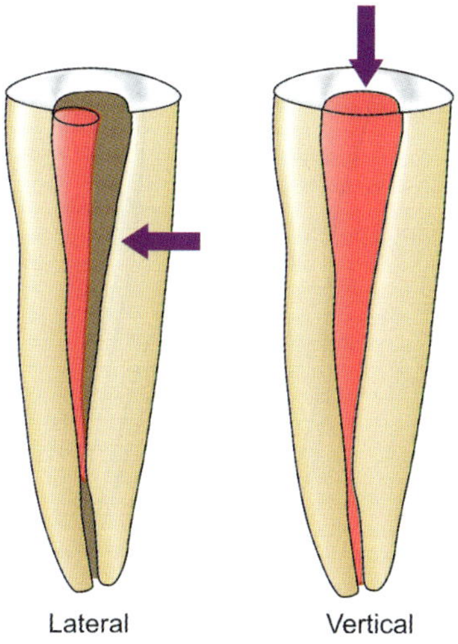


**Fig. 18.23:** Lateral and vertical compaction of gutta-percha

- Lateral/vertical compaction
- Sectional compaction technique
- McSpadden compaction of gutta-percha
- Thermoplasticized gutta-percha technique including
  - Obtura II
  - Ultrasonic plasticizing
  - Ultrafil system
- Solid core obturation technique including
  - Thermafil system
  - Silver point obturation

## ARMAMENTARIUM FOR OBTURATION (Fig. 18.24)

- primary and accessory gutta-percha points.
- Spreaders and pluggers for compaction of gutta-percha
- Absorbent paper points for drying the prepared root canal before applying sealer.

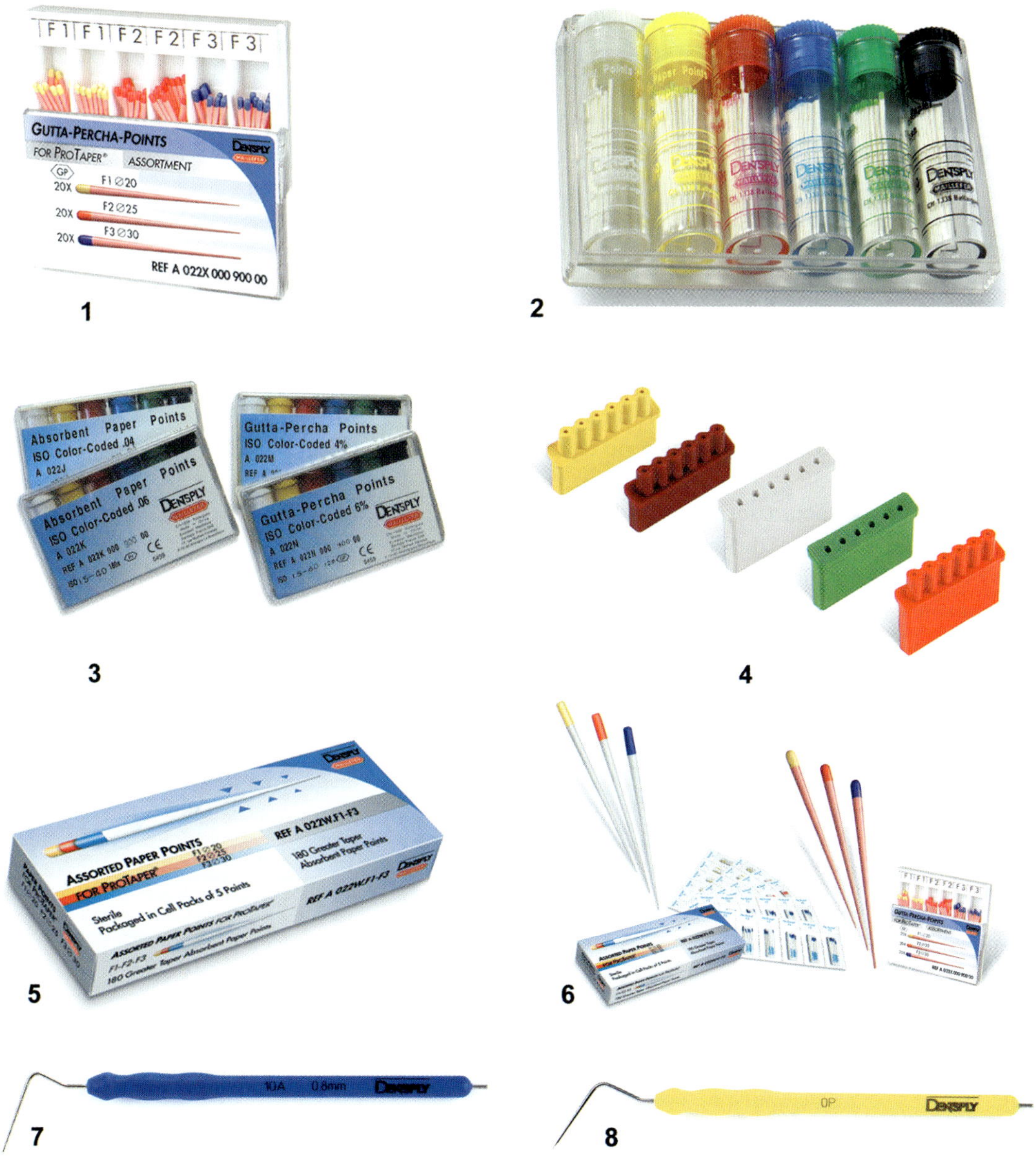


**Fig. 18.24:** Armamentarium for obturation

- Lentulospirals for placing sealer
- Scissors for cutting gutta-percha
- Endo gauge for measuring size of gutta-percha
- Endo block for measuring gutta-percha points
- Endo organizer for arranging gutta-percha and accessory points of various sizes.
- Heating device like spirit lamp or butane gas torch
- Heating instrument like ball burnisher, spoon excavator, etc.

## LATERAL COMPACTION TECHNIQUE

It is one of the most common methods used for root canal obturation. It involves placement of tapered gutta-percha cones in the canal and then compacting them under pressure against the canal walls using a spreader. A canal should have continuous tapered shape with a definite apical stop, before it is ready to be filled by this method (Fig. 18.25).

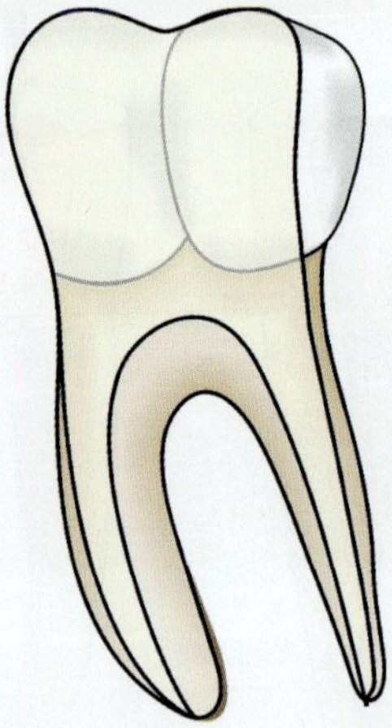

**Fig. 18.25:** Tapered preparation of root canal system

### Technique

1. Following the canal preparation, select the master gutta-percha cone whose diameter is consistent with largest file used in the canal up to the working length. One should feel the tugback with master gutta-percha point (Fig. 18.26). Master gutta-percha point is notched at the working distance analogous to the level of incisal or occlusal edge reference point (Fig. 18.27).
2. Check the fit of cone radiographically.
   - If found satisfactory, remove the cone from the canal and place it in sodium hypochlorite.
   - If cone fits short of the working length, check for dentin chip debris, any ledge or curve in the canal and treat them accordingly (Figs 18.28 and 18.29).
   - If cone selected is going beyond the foramen, either select the larger number cone or cut that cone to the working length (Fig. 18.30).
   - If cone shows "s" shaped appearance in the radiograph that means cone is too small for the canal. Here a larger cone must be selected to fit in the canal (Fig 18.31).
3. Select the size of spreader to be used for lateral compaction of that tooth. It should reach 1-2 mm of true working length (Fig. 18.32).
4. Dry the canal with paper points.
5. Apply sealer in the prepared root canal (Fig. 18.33).
6. Now premeasured cone is coated with sealer and placed into the canal. After master cone placement, spreader is placed into the canal alongside the cone (Fig. 18.34). Spreader helps in compaction of gutta-percha. It act as a wedge to squeeze the gutta-percha laterally under vertical pressure not by pushing it sideways (Fig. 18.35). It should reach 1-2 mm of the prepared root length.
7. After placement, spreader is removed from the canal by rotating it back and forth. This compacts the gutta-percha and a space gets created lateral to the master cone (Fig. 18.36).
8. An accessory cone is placed in this space and the above procedure is repeated until the spreader can no longer penetrate beyond the cervical line (Fig. 18.37).

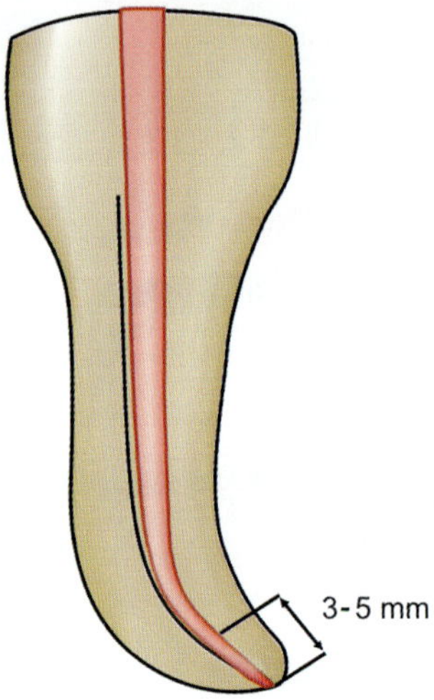


**Fig. 18.26:** Tugback with master gutta-percha cone

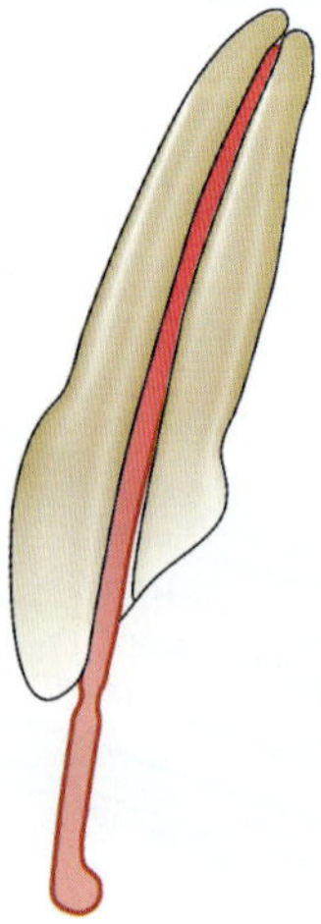

**Fig. 18.27:** Notching of gutta-percha at the level of reference point

9. Now sever the protruding gutta-percha points at canal orifice with hot instrument (Fig. 18.38).

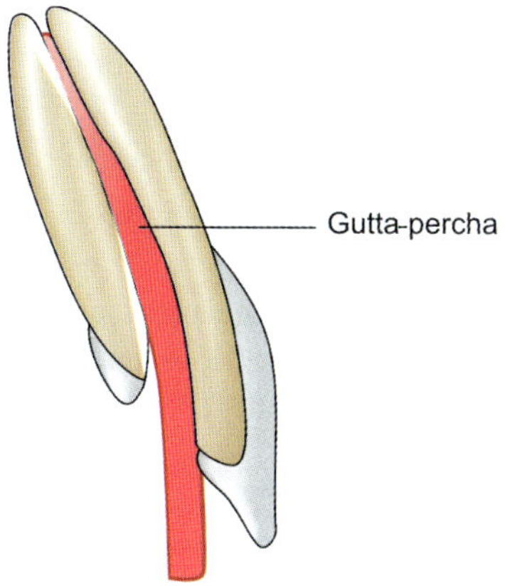


Fig. 18.28: Gutta-percha showing tight fit in middle and space in apical third

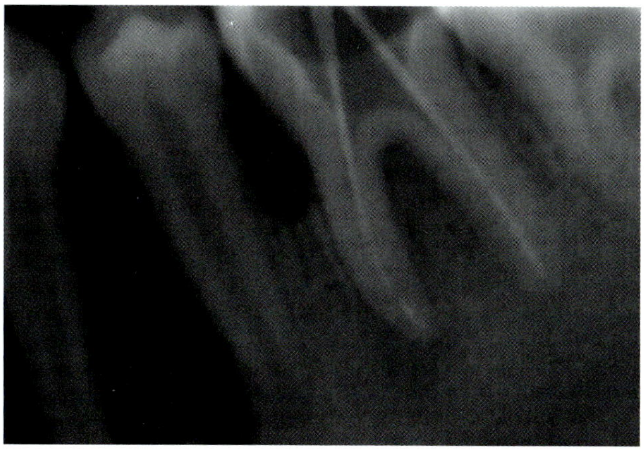

Fig. 18.31: S-shaped appearance of cone in mesial canal shows that cone is too small for the canal, replace it with bigger cone

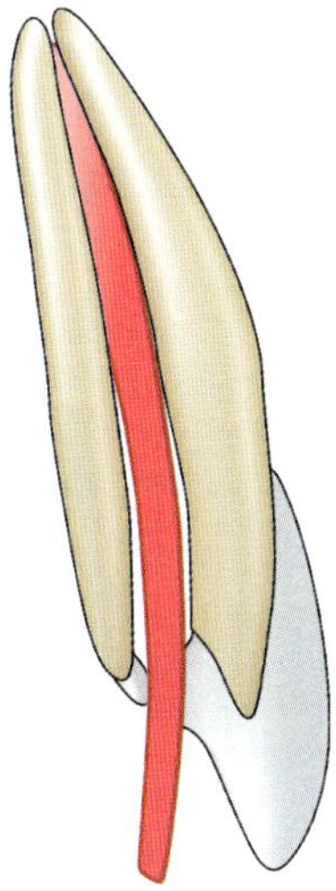

Fig. 18.29: Gutta-percha cone showing tight fit only on apical part of the canal

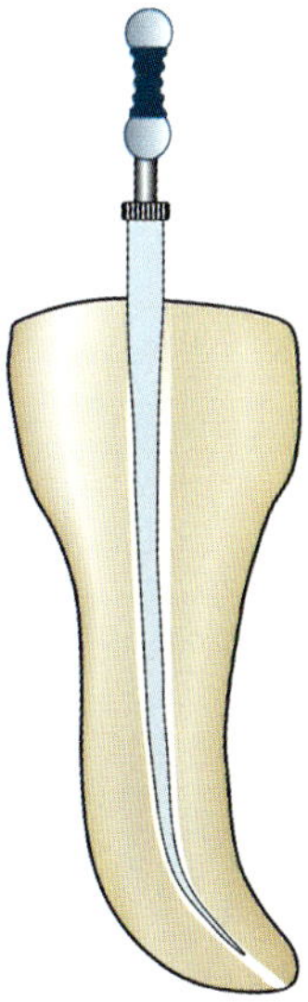

Fig. 18.32: Spreader should match the taper of canal

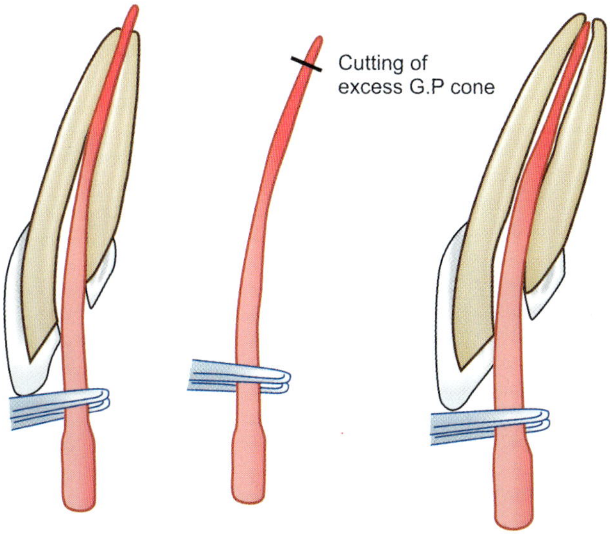


Fig. 18.30: If cone is going beyond apical foramen, cut the cone to working length or use larger number cone

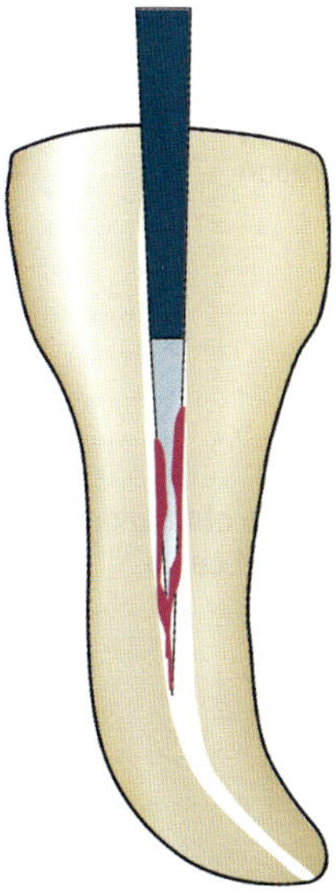

Fig. 18.33: Apply sealer in the prepared canal

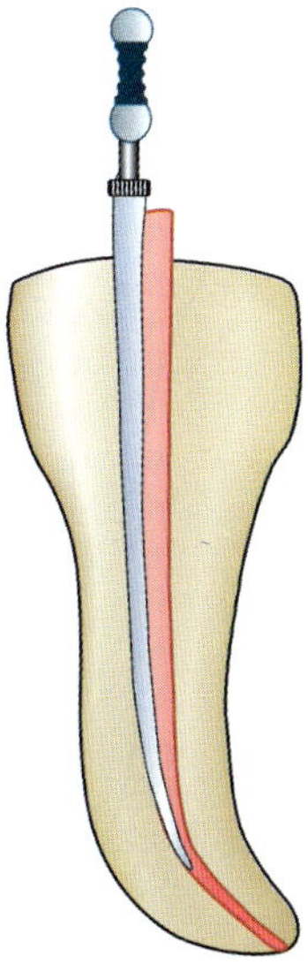

Fig. 18.34: Placing spreader along gutta-percha cone

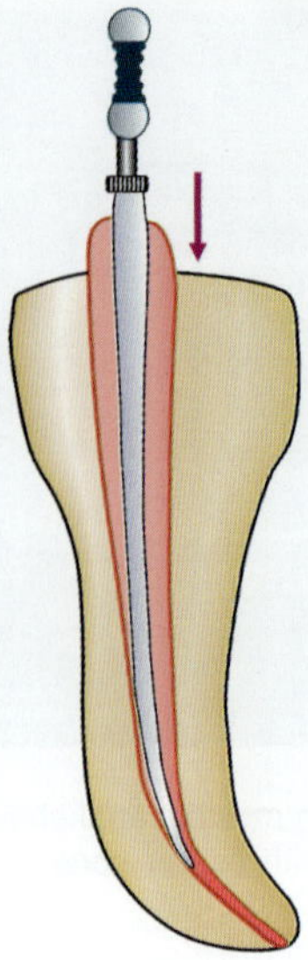

Fig. 18.35: Compaction of gutta-percha using spreader

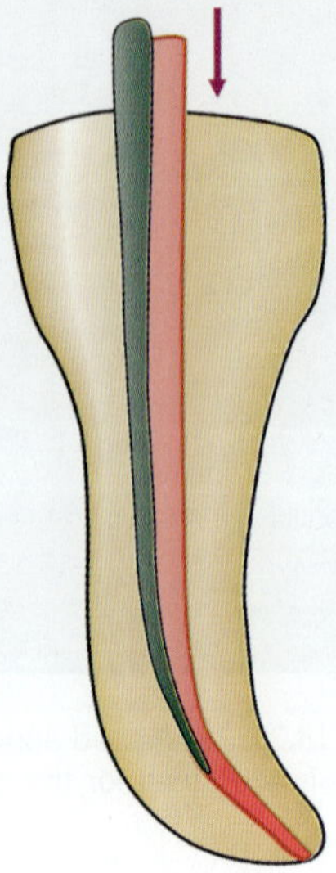

Fig. 18.36: Placing accessory cone along master cone

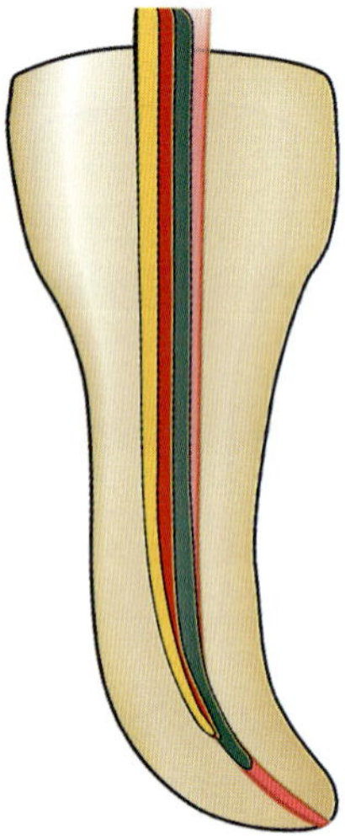

Fig. 18.37: Use of more accessory cones to complete obturation of the canal

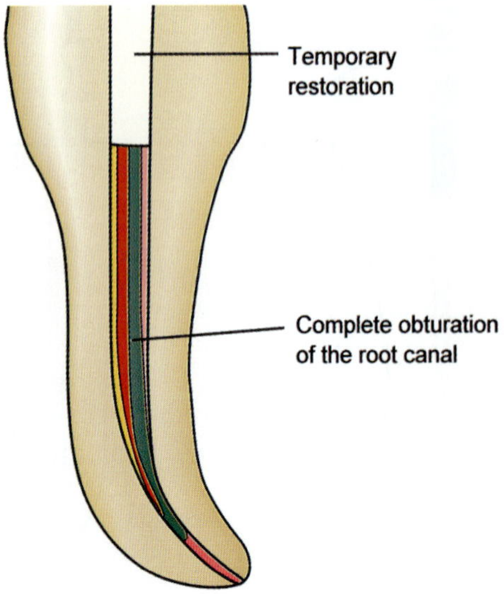


Fig. 18.38: Cut the protruding gutta-percha points at orifice with hot instrument and place temporary restoration over it

### *Advantages of Lateral Compaction Technique*

1. Can be used in most clinical situations.
2. During compaction of gutta-percha, it provides length control, thus decreases the chances of overfilling.

### *Disadvantages*

1. May not fill the canal irregularities efficiently.
2. Does not produce homogenous mass.
3. Space may exist between accessory and master cones (Fig. 18.39).

## VARIATION OF LATERAL COMPACTION TECHNIQUE

### For Tubular Canals (Figs 18.40A and B)

- Tubular canals are generally large canals with parallel walls.
- Since these canals don't have apical construction, the main criterion of obturation is to seal the apical foramen in order to permit the compaction of obturation material.
- These cases can be obturated by tailor made gutta-percha or with gutta-percha cone which has been made blunt by cutting at tip.

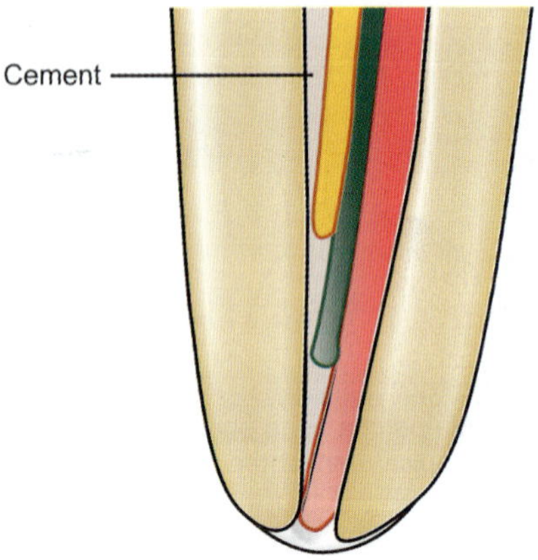


Fig. 18.39: In lateral compaction of gutta-percha, cones never fit as homogeneous mass, sealer occupies the space in between the cones

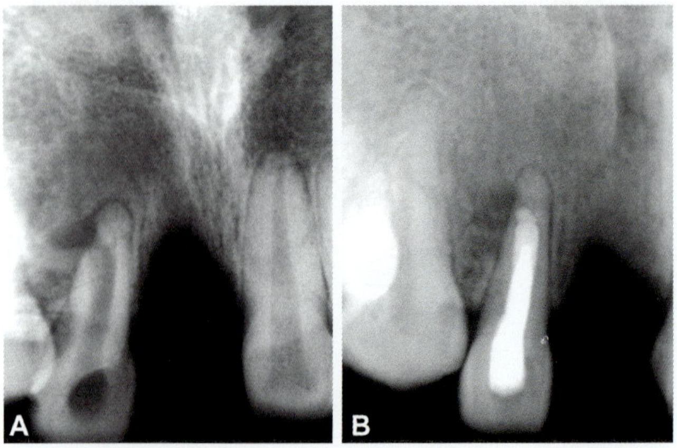


Figs 18.40A and B: (A) Carious 12 with tubular canal (B) Radiograph showing obturation of 12

## For Curved Canals (Fig. 18.41)

- Canals with gradual curvature are treated by same basic procedure which includes the use of more flexible (NiTi) spreader.
- For these canals, finger spreaders are preferred over hand spreaders.
- For canals with severe curvature like bayonet shaped or dilacerated canals, thermoplasticized gutta-percha technique is preferred (Fig. 18.42).

## Blunderbuss/Immature Canals (Figs 18.43A and B)

- Blunderbuss canals are characterized by flared out apical foramen. So a special procedure like apexification is required to ensure apical closure.
- For complete obturation of such canals, tailor made gutta-percha or warm gutta-percha techniques are preferred.

*Technique of preparing tailor made gutta-percha:*

- Tailor made gutta-percha is made by joining multiple gutta-percha cones from butt to tip until a roll is achieved.

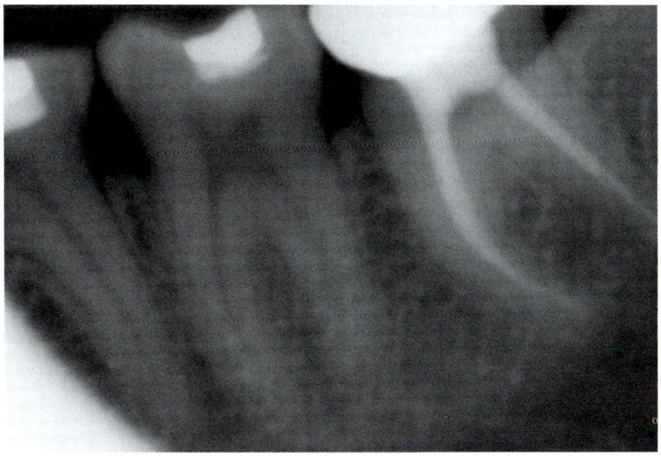

Fig. 18.41: Radiograph showing obturation of curved canals of 48

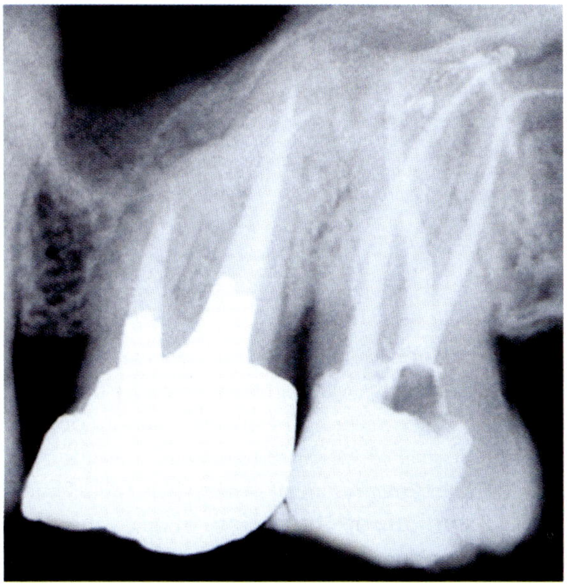

Fig. 18.42: Thermoplasticized gutta-percha technique should be used for severely curved canals

- This roll is then stiffened by using ice water or ethyl chloride spray.
- If this cone is loose fitting, more gutta-percha points are added to this.
- If this roll is large, it is heated over a flame and again rolled.
- For use in the canal, the outer surface of tailor made cone is dipped in chloroform, eucalyotol or halothane and then cone is placed in the canal. By this internal impression of canal is achieved.
- Finally, cone is dipped in alcohol to stop action of gutta-percha solvent.

## CHEMICAL ALTERATION OF GUTTA-PERCHA

Gutta-percha is soluble in number of solvents viz: chloroform, eucalyptol, xylol. This property of gutta-percha is used to adapt it in various canal shapes which are amenable to be filled by lateral compaction of gutta-percha technique. For example:

- In teeth with blunderbuss canals
- Root ends with resorptive defects, delta formation.
- In teeth with internal resorption.

In these cases an imprint of apical portion of the canal is obtained by following method:

- Root canal is cleaned and shaped properly (Fig. 18.44).
- The cone is held with a plier which has been adjusted to the working length (Fig. 18.45).
- The apical 2-3 mm of cone is dipped for a period of 3-5 seconds into a dappen dish containing solvent (Fig. 18.46).
- Softened cone is inserted in the canal with slight apical pressure until the beaks of plier touch the reference point (Fig. 18.47).
- Here take care to keep the canal moistened with irrigation, otherwise some of softened gutta-percha may stick to the desired canal walls, though this detached segment can be easily removed by use of H-file.
- Radiograph is taken to verify the fit and correct working length of the cone. When found satisfactory, cone is removed from the canal and canal is irrigated with sterile water or 99 percent isopropyl alcohol to remove the residual solvent.

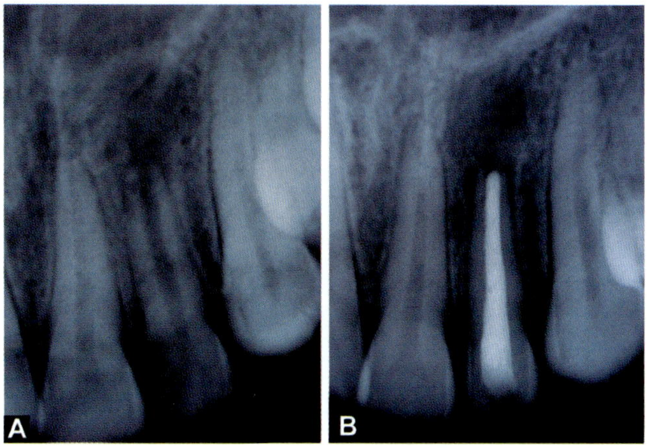


Figs 18.43A and B: (A) Carious 22 with blunderbass canals; (B) Obturation of 22 done

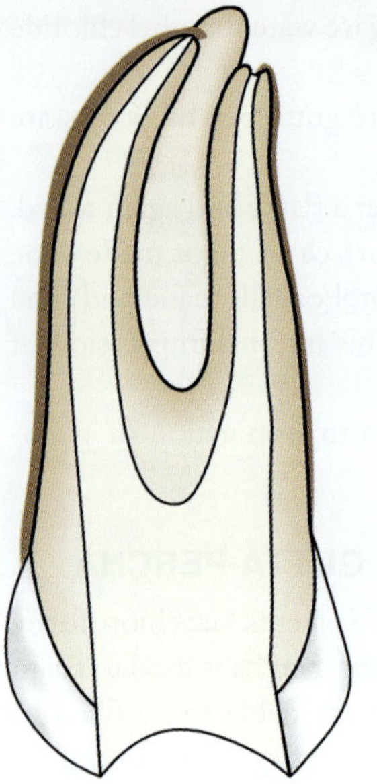

Fig. 18.44: Cleaned and shaped canal

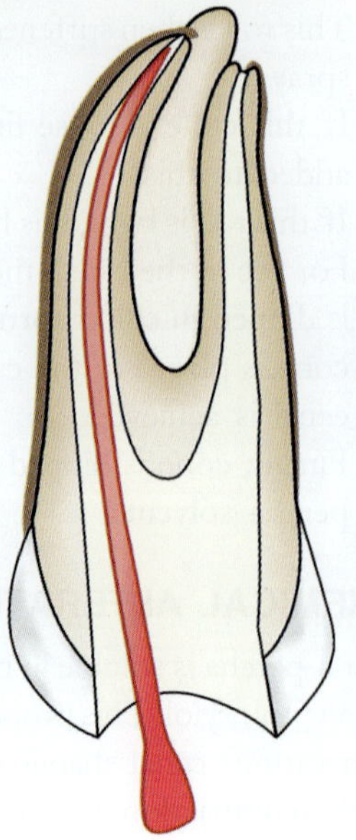

Fig. 18.45: Checking the fit of gutta-percha cone

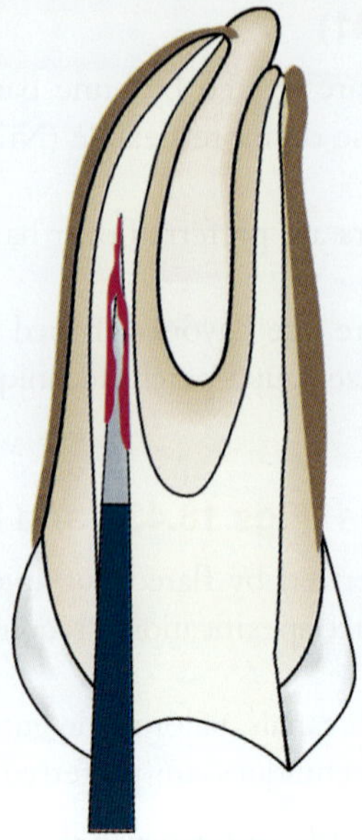

Fig. 18.47: Application of sealer in the canal

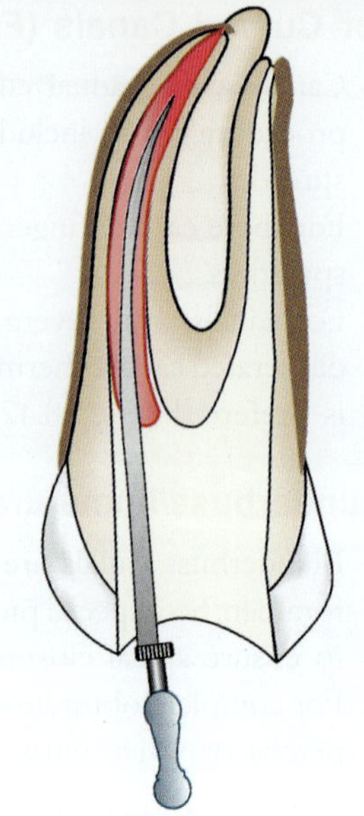

Fig. 18.48: Softened gutta-percha placed in the canal

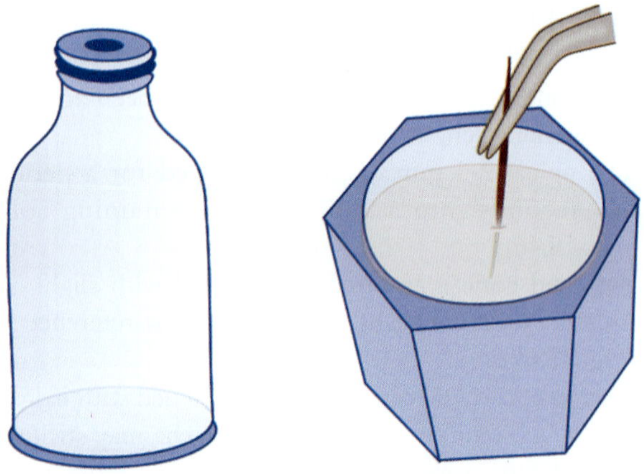

Fig. 18.46: Softening of gutta-percha cone by placing in chloroform

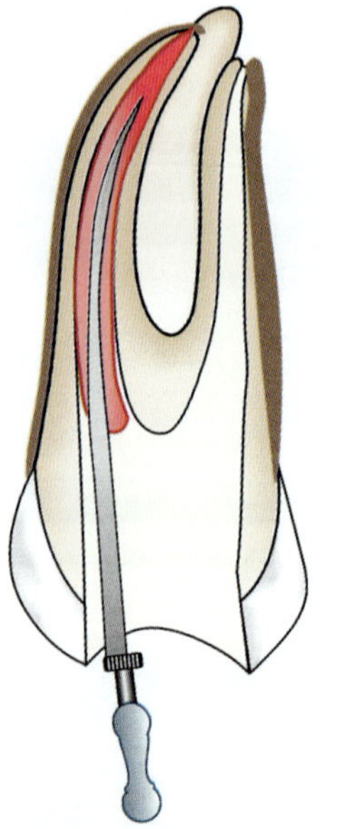

Fig. 18.49: Compaction of gutta-percha using spreader

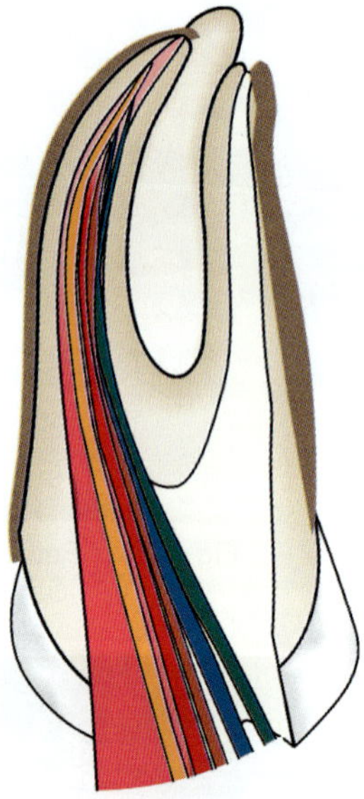

Fig. 18.50: Complete obturation of the canal using accessory cones

- After this canal is coated with sealer (Fig. 18.48), cone is dipped again for 2-3 seconds in the solvent and thereafter inserted into the canal with continuous apical pressure until the plier touches the reference point.
- A finger spreader is then placed in the canal to compact the gutta-percha laterally (Fig. 18.49).
- Accessory gutta-percha cones are then placed in the space created by spreader (Fig. 18.50).
- Protruding gutta-percha points are cut at canal orifice with hot instrument (Fig. 18.51).

Though this method is considered good for adapting gutta-percha to the canal walls but chloroform dip fillings have shown to produce volume shrinkage which may lead to poor apical seal.

## VERTICAL COMPACTION TECHNIQUE

It has been shown that root canal is not just a tubular structure present in the root. Infact presence of many lateral and accessory canals and anastomoses give it a complex shape (Fig. 18.52). Vertical compaction of warm gutta-percha method of filling the root canal was introduced by Schilder with an objective of filling all the portals of exit with maximum amount of gutta-percha and minimum amount of sealer. This is also known as **Schilder's technique of obturation**. In this technique using heated pluggers, pressure is applied in vertical direction to heat softened gutta-percha which causes it to flow and fill the canal space (Fig. 18.53).

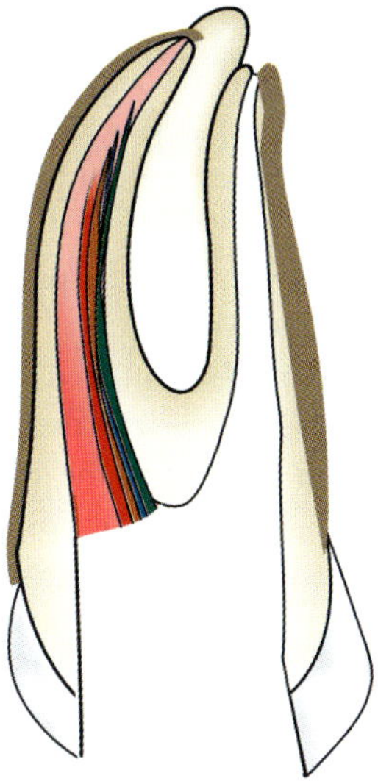

**Fig. 18.51:** Sever the protruding gutta-percha cones using hot burnisher

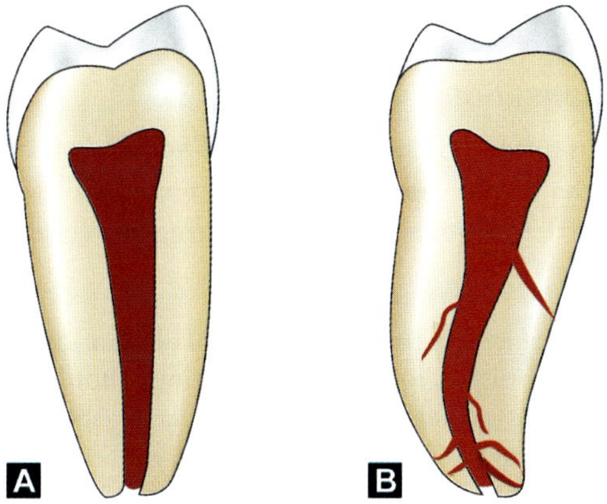


**Figs 18.52A and B:** (A) Theoretical canal formation (B) Actual root canal configuration with branches and ramifications

***Basic requirements of a prepared canal to be filled by this technique are:***

a. Continuous tapering funnel shape from orifice to apex (Fig. 18.54).
b. Apical opening kept as small as possible.
c. Decreasing the cross-sectional diameter at every point apically and increasing at each point as canal is approached coronally.

## Technique

- Select a master cone according to shape and size of the prepared canal. Cone should fit in 1-2 mm of apical stop because when softened material moves apically into prepared canal, it adapts more intimately to the canal walls (Fig. 18.55).
- Confirm the fit of cone radiographically, if found satisfactory, remove it from the canal and place in sodium hypochlorite.
- Irrigate the canal and then dry by rinsing it with alcohol and latter using the paper points.
- Select the heat transferring instrument and pluggers according to canal shape and size.
- Pluggers are prefitted at 5 mm intervals so as to capture maximum cross section area of the softened gutta-percha (Figs 18.56 to 18.58).
- Lightly coat the canal with sealer.
- Cut the coronal end of selected gutta-percha at incisal or occlusal reference point.
- Now use the heated plugger to force the gutta-percha into the canal. The blunted end of plugger creates a deep depression in the centre of master cone (Fig. 18.59). The outer walls of softened gutta-percha are then folded inward to fill the central void, at the same time mass of softened gutta-percha is moved apically and laterally. This procedure also removes 2-3 mm of coronal part of gutta-percha.

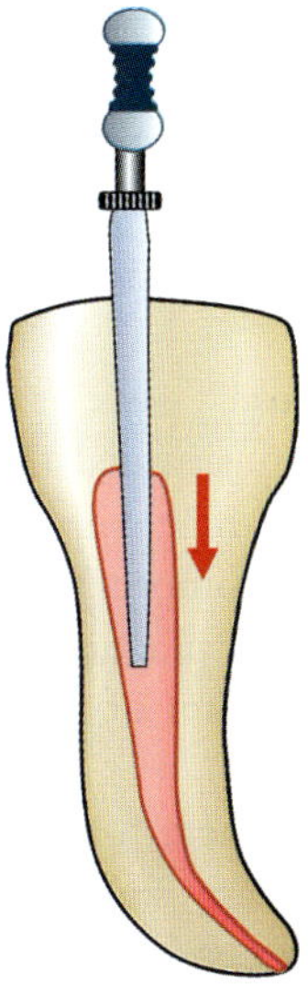

**Fig. 18.53:** Vertical compaction of gutta-percha using plugger

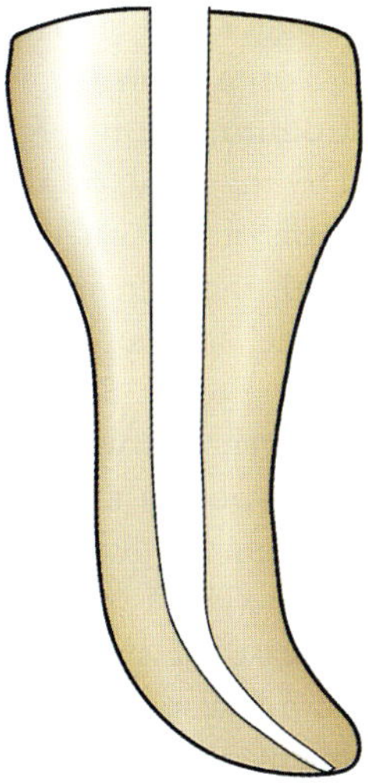

**Fig. 18.54:** Completely cleaned and shaped tapered preparation

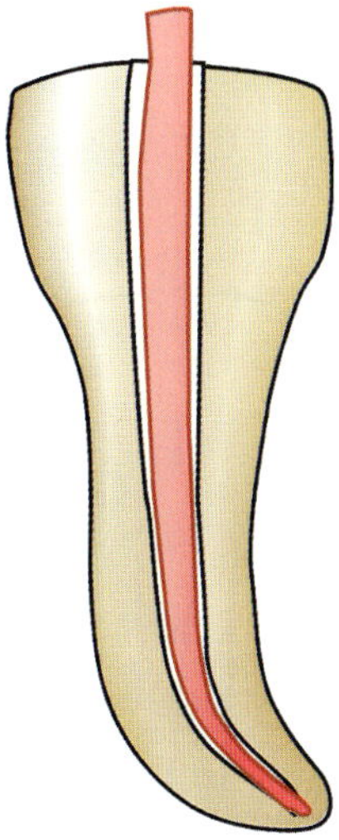

**Fig. 18.55:** Select the master gutta-percha cone

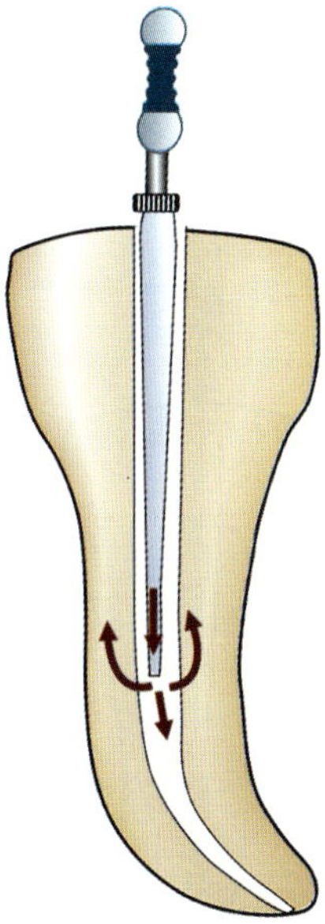

**Fig. 18.56:** Select the plugger according to canal shape and size

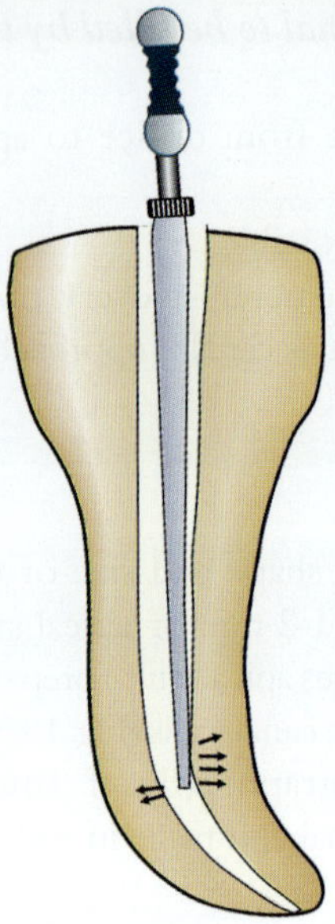

**Fig. 18.57:** Larger sized plugger may bind the canal and may split the root

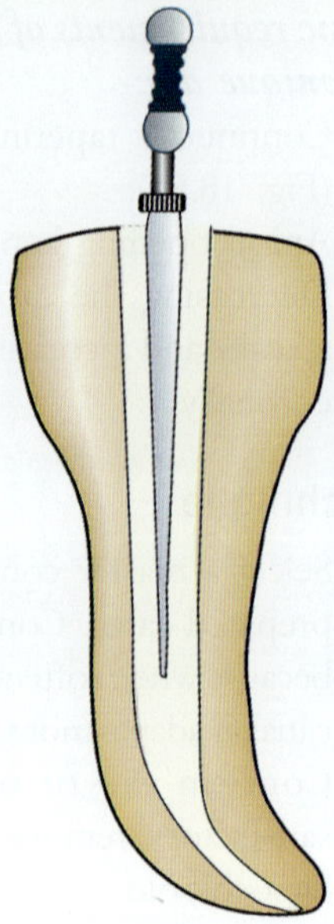

**Fig. 18.58:** Small plugger is ineffective for compaction

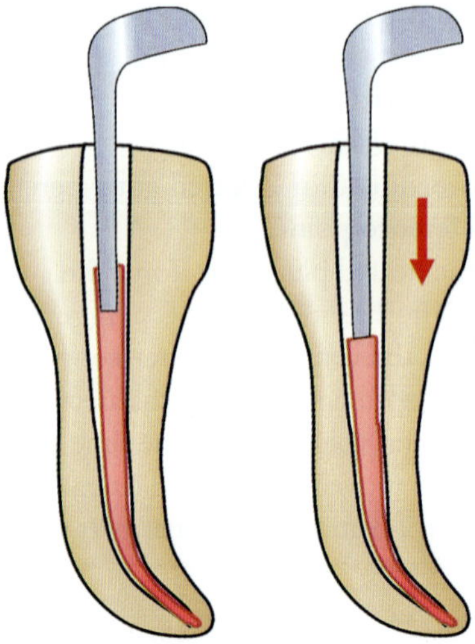

**Fig. 18.59:** Heated plugger used to compact gutta-percha

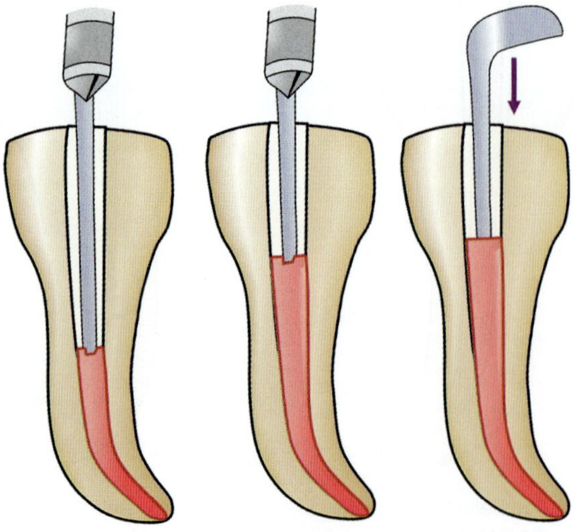

**Fig. 18.60:** Back filling of the canal

- Once apical filling is done, complete obturation by doing backfilling. Obturate the remaining canal by heating small segments of gutta-percha, carrying them into the canal and then compacting them using heated pluggers as described above (Fig. 18.60).
- Take care not to overheat the gutta-percha because it will become too soft to handle.
- Do not apply sealer on the softened segments of gutta-percha because sealer will prevent their adherence to the body of gutta-percha present in the canal.
- After completion of obturation, clean the pulp chamber with alcohol to remove remnants of sealer or gutta-percha.

### *Advantage of Vertical Compaction Technique*

Excellent sealing of canal apically, laterally and obturation of lateral as well as accessory canals.

### *Disadvantages of this Technique*

- Increased risk of vertical root fracture.
- Overfilling of canals with gutta-percha or sealer from apex.
- Time consuming.

## System B: Continuous Wave of Condensation Technique

System B is newly developed device by ***Buchanan*** for warming gutta-percha in the canal. It monitors temperature at the tip of heat carrier pluggers, thereby delivering a précised amount of heat.

**To have satisfactory, three-dimensional obturation by using system B technique, following precautions should be taken**

- Canal shape should be continuous perfectly tapered.
- Do not set the system B at high temperature because this may burn gutta-percha.
- While down packing, apply a constant firm pressure.

### Technique

1. Select the Buchanan plugger which matches the selected gutta-percha cone (Fig. 18.61). Place rubber stop on the plugger and adjust it to its binding point in the canal 5-7 mm short of working length.
2. Confirm the fit of the gutta-percha cone (Fig. 18.62).
3. Dry the canal, cut the gutta-percha ½ mm short and apply sealer in the canal.
4. With the system B turned on to "use", place it in touch mode, set the temperature to 200°C and dial the power setting to 10. Sever the cone at the orifice with preheated plugger. Afterwards plugger is used to compact the softened gutta-percha at the orifice. Push the plugger smoothly though the gutta-percha to with 3-4 mm of the binding point (Fig. 18.63).
5. Release the switch. Hold the plugger here for 10 seconds with a sustained pressure to take up any shrinkage which might occur upon cooling of gutta-percha (Fig. 18.64).
6. Maintaining the apical pressure, activate the heat switch for 1 second followed by 1 second pause, and then remove the plugger (Fig. 18.65).

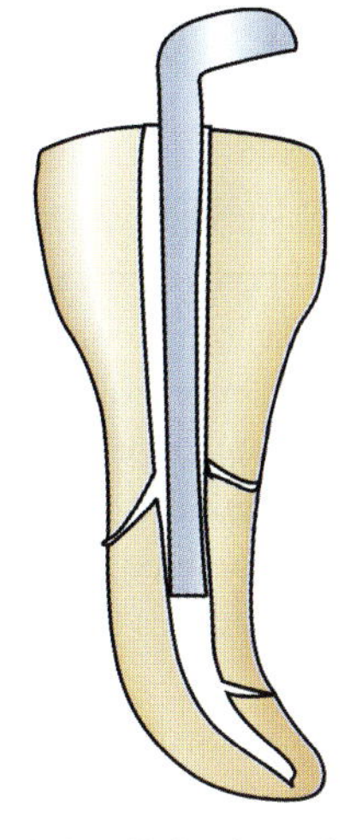

**Fig. 18.61:** Selection of plugger according to shape and size of the canal

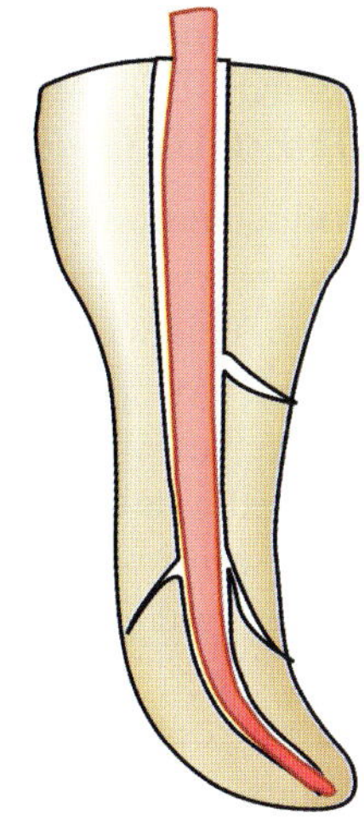

**Fig. 18.62:** Confirm fit of the cone

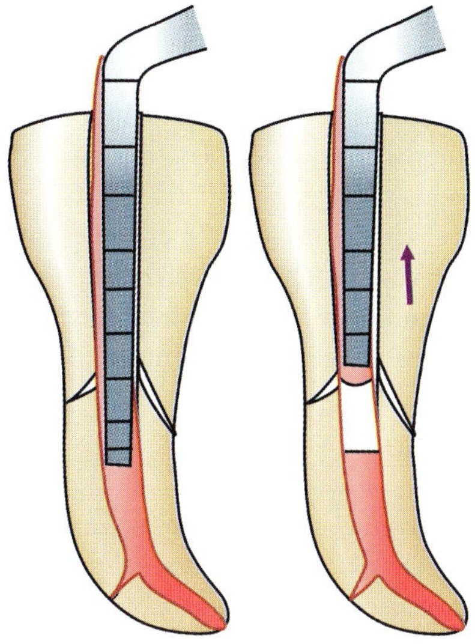

**Fig. 18.65:** Removal of plugger

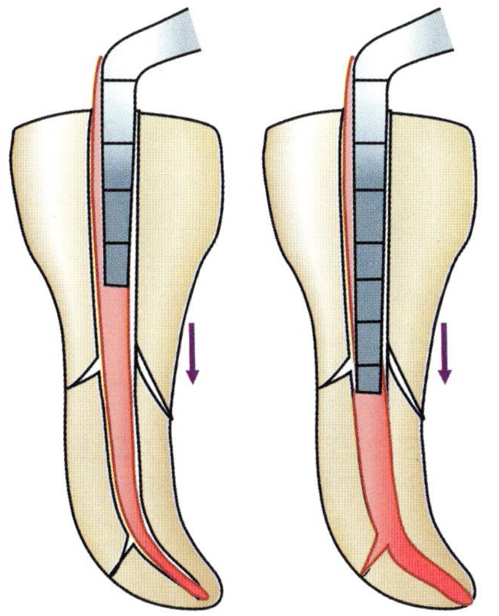

**Fig. 18.63:** Filling the canal by turning on system-B

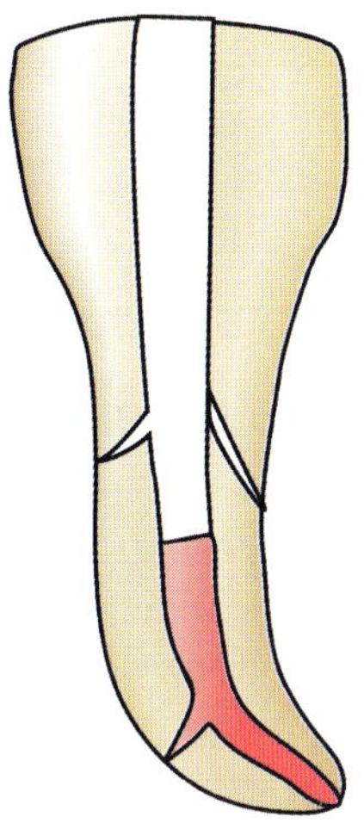

**Fig. 18.66:** Apical filling of root canal completed

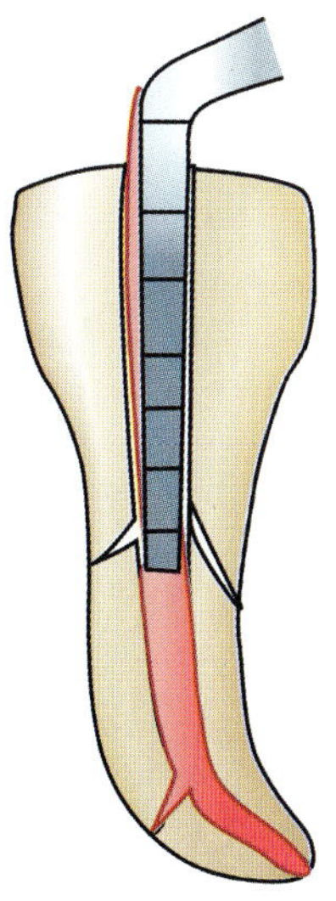

**Fig. 18.64:** Compaction of gutta-percha by keeping the plugger for 10 seconds with sustained pressure

7. After removal of plugger, introduce a small flexible end of another plugger with pressure to confirm that apical mass of gutta-percha has not dislodged, has cooled and set (Fig. 18.66).

Following radiographic confirmation canal is ready for the backfill by any means.

## Advantages of System B

- It creates single wave of heating and compacting thereby compaction of filling material can be done at same time when it has been heat softened.
- Excellent apical control.
- Less technique sensitive.
- Fast, easy, predictable.
- Thorough condensation of the main canal and lateral canals.
- Compaction of obturating materials occurs at all levels simultaneously throughout the momentum of heating and compacting instrument apically.

## LATERAL/VERTICAL COMPACTION OF WARM GUTTA-PERCHA

Vertical compaction causes dense obturation of the root canal, while lateral compaction provides length control and satisfactory ease and speed.

Advantages of both of these techniques are provided by a newer device viz ***Endotec II*** which helps the clinician to employ length control with warm gutta-percha technique. It comes with battery which provides energy to heat the attached plugger and spreader.

### Techniques

1. Adapt master gutta-percha cone in canal.
2. Select Endotec plugger and activate the device.
3. Insert the heated plugger in canal beside master cone to within 3-4 mm of the apex using light apical pressure.
4. Afterwards unheated spreader can be placed in the canal to create more space for accessory cones. This process is continued until canal is filled.

### Advantages

- Three-dimensional obturation of canal.
- Better sealing of accessory and lateral canals.
- ***Endotec*** can also be used to soften and remove the gutta-percha.

## SECTIONAL METHOD OF OBTURATION

In this technique, small pieces of gutta-percha cones are used to fill the sections of the canal. It is also known as ***Chicago technique*** because it was widely promoted by ***Coolidge, Lundquist, Blayney,*** all from ***Chicago***.

### Techniques

1. A gutta-percha cone of same size of the prepared root canal is selected and cut into sections of 3 to 4 mm long.
2. Select a plugger which loosely fits within 3 mm of working length.
3. Apply sealer in the canal.
4. One end of gutta-percha is mounted to heated plugger and is then carried into the canal and apical pressure is given. After this disengage the plugger from gutta-percha by rotating it.
5. Radiograph is taken to confirm its fit.

   If found satisfactory, fill the remainder of the canal in same manner.

### Advantages

- It seals the canals apically and laterally.
- In case of post and core cases, only apical section of canal is filled.

### Disadvantages

- Time consuming.
- If canal gets overfilled, difficult to remove sections of gutta-percha.

## McSPADDEN COMPACTION/ THERMOMECHANICAL COMPACTION OF THE GUTTA-PERCHA

McSpadden introduced a technique in which heat was used to low the viscosity of gutta-percha and thereby increasing its plasticity. This technique involves the use of a compacting instrument (McSpadden compacter) which resembles reverse Hedstorm file (Fig. 18.67). This is fitted into latch type handpiece and rotated at 8000-15000 rpm alongside gutta-percha cones inside the canal walls. At this speed, heat produced by friction softens the gutta-percha and designs of blade forces the material apically.

Because of its design, the blades of compaction break easily if it binds, so it should be used only in straight canals. But now days, its newer modification in form of Microseal condenser has come which is made up of nickel-titanium. Because of its flexibility, it can be used in curved canals.

### Advantages

- Requires less chair side time.
- Ease of selection and insertion of gutta-percha.
- Dense, three-dimensional obturation.

### Disadvantages

- Liability to use in narrow and curved canals.
- Frequent breakage of compactor blades.
- Overfilling of canals.
- Shrinkage of gutta-percha on cooling.

## THERMOPLASTICIZED INJECTABLE GUTTA-PERCHA OBTURATION

### Obtura II Heated Gutta-Percha System/High Heat System

This technique was ***introduced in 1977 at Harvard institute***. It consists of an electric control unit with pistol grip syringe and specially designed gutta-percha pellets which are heated to

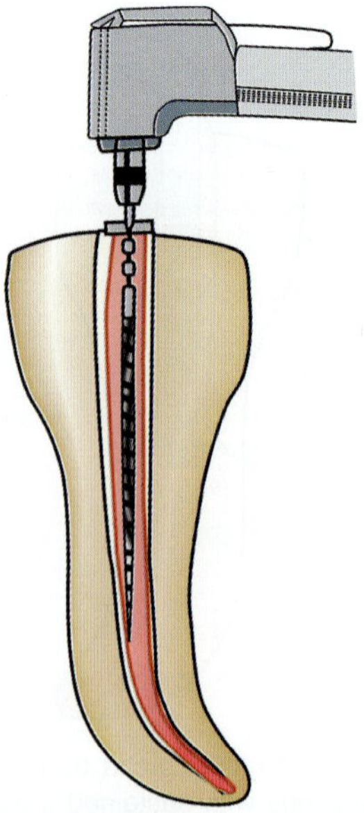

**Fig. 18.67:** Thermomechanical compaction of gutta-percha

approximately 365-390°F (185-200°C) for obturation. In this, regular Beta phase of gutta-percha is used. For canals to filled by Obtura II they need to have:

a. Continuous tapering funnel shape for unrestricted flow of softened gutta-percha (Fig. 18.68).
b. A definite apical stop to prevent overfilling.

### Indications

- Roots with straight or slightly curved canals.
- For backfilling of canals.
- For obturation of roots with internal resorption, perforations, etc.

### Techniques

a. Before starting the obturation, applicator needle and pluggers are selected. The needle tip should reach ideally 3-5 mm of the apical terminus passively (Fig. 18.69).
b. Apply sealer along the dentinal walls to fill the interface between gutta-percha and dentinal walls.
c. Place obtura needle loosely 3-5 mm short of apex, as warm gutta-percha flows and fills the canal, back pressure pushes the needle out of the canal (Fig. 18.70).
d. Now use pluggers to compact the gutta-percha, pluggers are dipped in isopropyl alcohol or sealer to prevent sticking of the gutta-percha.

Continuous compaction force should be applied throughout the obturation of whole canal to compensate shrinkage and to close any voids if formed.

### Variations in Thermoplasticizing Technique of Gutta-percha

#### *1. Ultrasonic Plasticizing of Gutta-Percha*

It has been seen that ultrasonics can be used to fill the canals by plasticizing the gutta-percha.

Earlier cavitron US scaler was used for this purpose but its design limited its use only in anterior teeth. Recently Enac Ultrasonic unit comes with an attached spreader which has shown to produce homogenous compaction of gutta-percha.

#### *2. Ultrafil System*

This system uses low temperature (i.e. 70°C) plasticized alpha phase gutta-percha. Here gutta-percha is available in three different viscosities for use in different situations.

Regular set and the firm set with highest flow properties primarily used for injection and need not be compacted manually. Endoset is more of viscous and can be condensed immediately after injection.

#### *Techniques*

1. Cannula needle is checked in canal for fitting. It should be 6-7 mm from apex (Fig. 18.71). After confirmation it is placed in heater (at 90°C) for minimum of 15 minutes before use.
2. Apply sealer in the canal and passively insert the needle into the canal. As the warm gutta-percha fills the canal, its backpressure pushes the needle out of the canal.
3. Once needle is removed, prefitted plugger dipped in alcohol is used for manual compaction of gutta-percha.

**Difference between obtura II and ultrafil**

| *Obtura II* | *Ultrafil* |
|---|---|
| 1. Uses high temperature | Uses low temperature |
| 2. Uses gun with heating element | There is no heating element |
| 3. Uses needles of 18, 20, 22 and 25 guage. | Uses needles of 22-gauge |
| 4. Digital display of temperature | No digital read out |
| 5. Working time is 3-10 minutes | Working time is less than one minute |

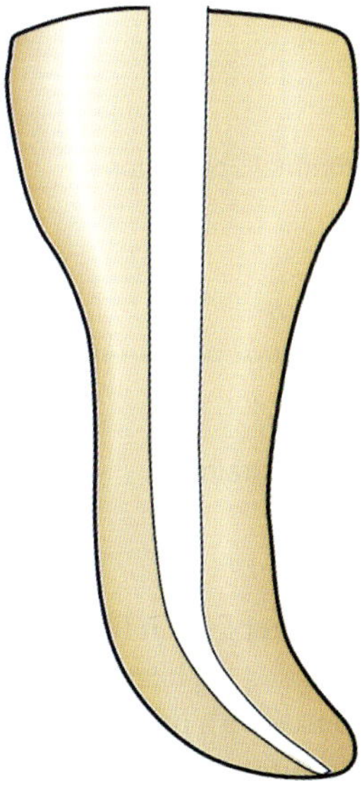

**Fig. 18.68:** Tapering funnel shaped of prepared canal is well suited for obturation using obtura II

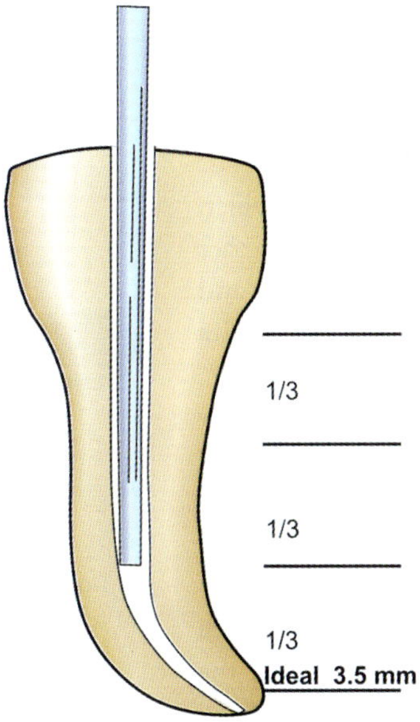


**Fig. 18.69:** Needle tip of obtura II should reach 3-5 mm of apical end

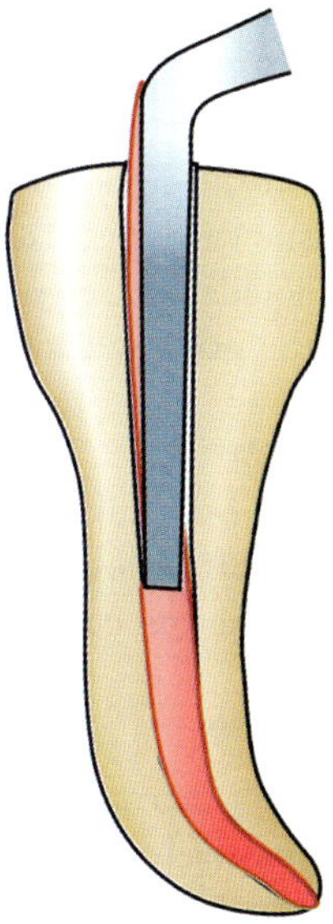

**Fig. 18.70:** Compaction of gutta-percha using plugger

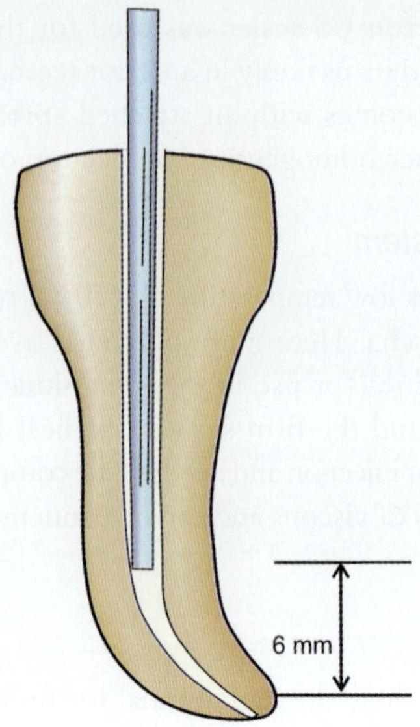


**Fig. 18.71:** Needle should reach 6-7 mm from the apical end

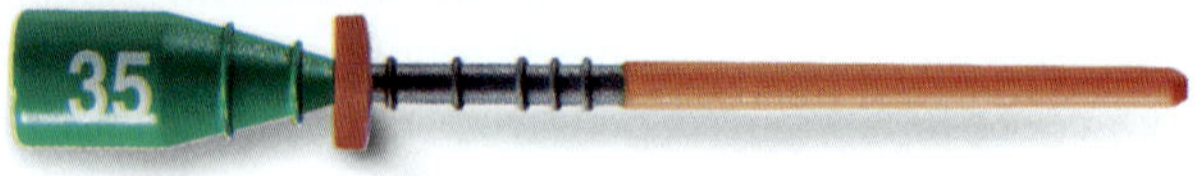


**Fig. 18.72:** Thermafil cones

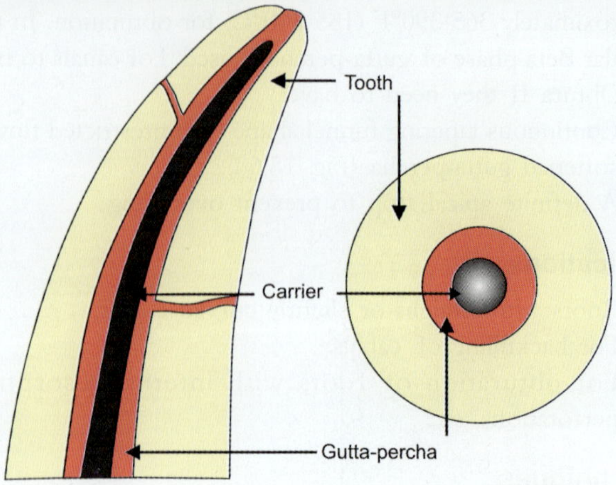


**Fig. 18.73:** The carrier is not primary cone for obturation. It acts as a carrier for carrying thermoplasticized gutta-percha

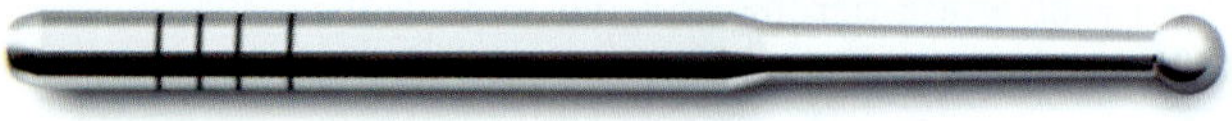

**Fig. 18.74:** Therma cut bur

## SOLID CORE CARRIER TECHNIQUE

### Thermafil Endodontic Obturators

Thermafil endodontic obturators are specially designed flexible steel, titanium or plastic carriers coated with alpha phase gutta-percha. Thermafil obturation was devised by W Ben Johnson in 1978. This technique became popular because of its simplicity and accuracy.

In this carriers are made up of stainless steel, titanium or plastic. They have ISO standard dimension with matching color coding in the sizes of 20-140 (Fig. 18.72).

Plastic carrier is made up of special synthetic resin which can be liquid plastic crystal or polysulphone polymer. The carrier is not the primary cone for obturation. It acts as carrier and condenser for thermally plasticized gutta-percha (Fig. 18.73).

Plastic cores allow post space to be made, easily and they can be cut off by heated instrument, stainless steel bur, diamond stone or therma cut bur (Fig. 18.74).

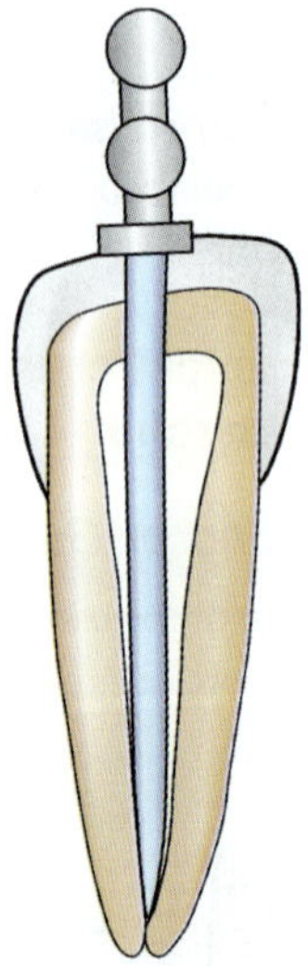

**Fig. 18.75:** Selection of thermafil obturator

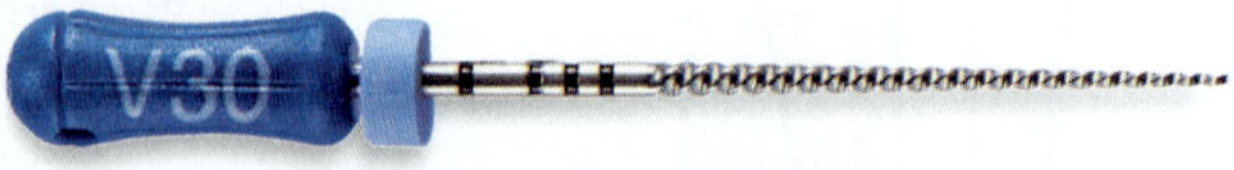


**Fig. 18.76:** Thermafil obturator

### Technique

1. Select a thermafil obturator of the size and shape which fits passively at the working length (Fig. 18.75). Verify the length of verifier by taking a radiograph (Figs 18.76 to 18.78).
2. Now disinfect the obturator in 5.25 percent sodium hypochlorite for one minute and then rinse it in 70 percent alcohol.
3. Preheat the obturator in "Therma Prep" oven for sometime (Fig. 18.79). This oven is recommended for heating obturator because it offers a stable heat source with more control and uniformity for plasticizing the gutta-percha.
4. Dry the canal and lightly coat it with sealer. Place the heated obturator into the canal with a firm apical pressure (Fig. 18.80) to the marked working length (Figs 18.81 and 18.82).

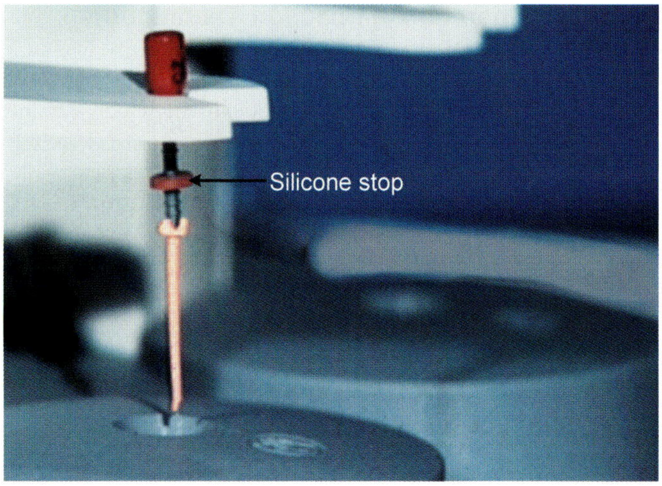


Fig. 18.77: Taking thermafil obturator for obturation

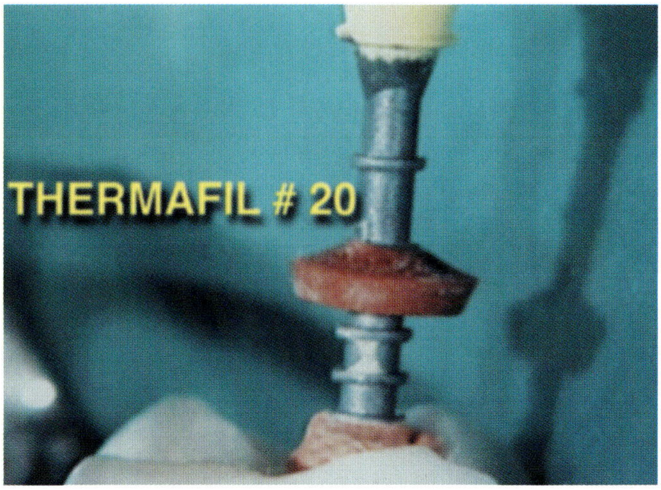


Fig. 18.78: Checking fit of cone up to marked working length

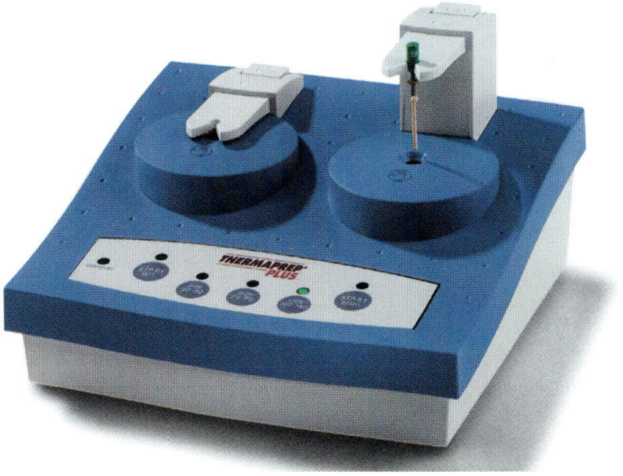


Fig. 18.79: Therma prep oven

5. Working time is 8-10 seconds after removal of obturator from oven. If more obturators are required, insert them immediately.

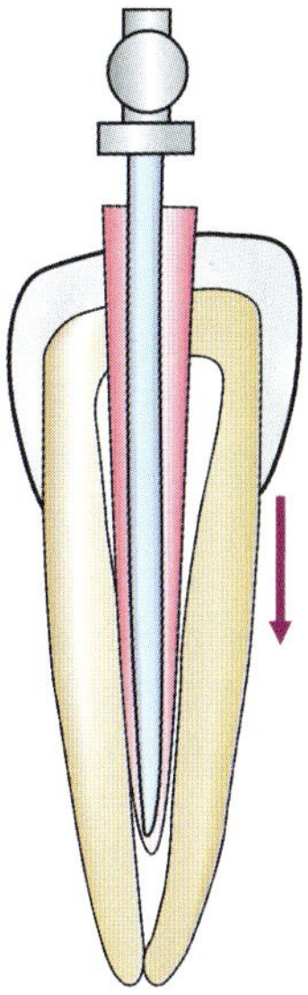

Fig. 18.80: Placing heated obturator in the canal with firm pressure

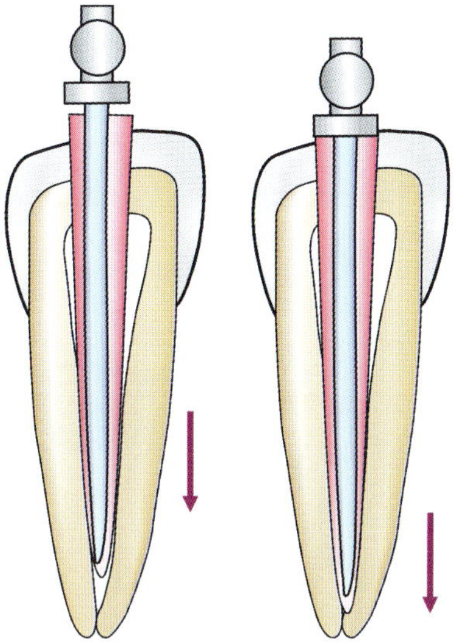

Fig. 18.81: It should reach up to the working length

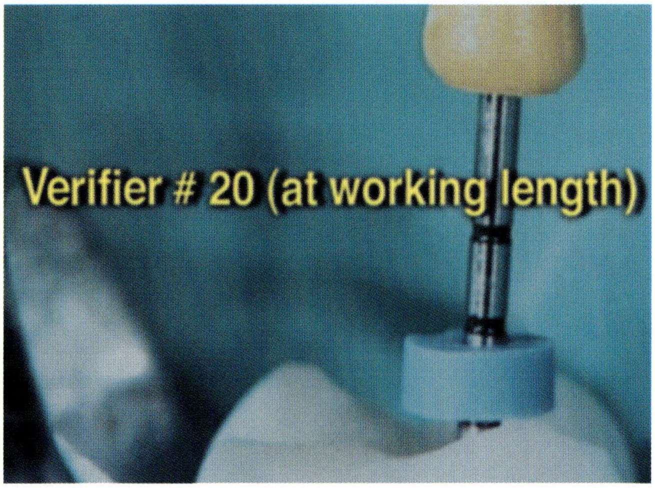


Fig. 18.82: Silicon stop should be used for confirming the length of cone

6. Verify the fit of obturation in radiograph. When found accurate, while stabilizing the carrier with index finger, sever the shaft level with the orifice using a prepi bur or an inverted cone bur in high speed handpiece (Figs 18.83 and 18.84).
7. Do not use flame heated instrument to sever the plastic shaft because instrument cools too rapidly and thus may cause inadvertent obturator displacement from the canal.
8. Now use a small condenser coated with vaseline or dipped in alcohol, to condense gutta-percha vertically around the shaft.
9. When the use of post is indicated, sever the obturator with the fissure bur at the selected length and give counter-clockwise rotation of shaft following insertion to disengage the instrument.

### Advantages

- Requires less chair side time.
- Provides dense three dimensional obturation as gutta-percha flows into canal irregularities such as fins, anastomoses, and lateral canals, etc.
- No need to precurve obturators because of flexible carriers.
- Since this technique requires minimum compaction so less strain while obturation with this technique.

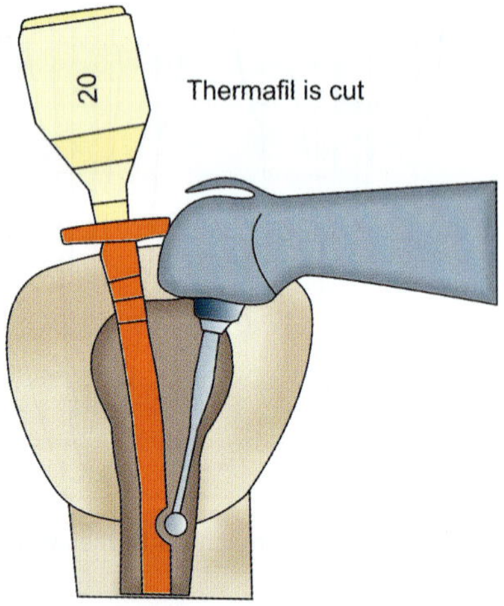


**Fig. 18.83:** Cut the thermafil using therma cut bur

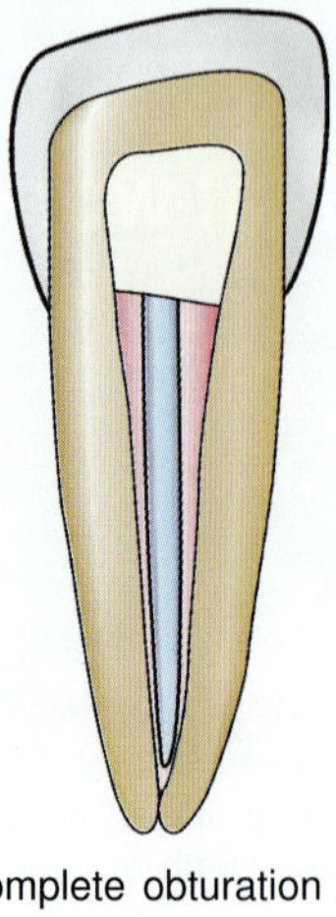

**Fig. 18.84:** Complete obturation using thermafil

## Cold Gutta-percha Compaction Technique

### *Gutta Flow*

Gutta flow is eugenol free radiopaque form which can be injected into root canals using an injectable system. It is self polymerizing filling system in which gutta-percha in powder form is combined with a resin sealer in one capsule.

### *Composition*

Gutta flow consists polydimethyl silloxan matrix filled with powdered gutta-percha, silicon oil, paraffin oil, palatinum, zirconium dioxide and nano silver.

### *Advantages*

- Easy to use
- Time saving
- Does not require compaction
- Does not require heating
- Biocompatible
- Can be easily removed for retreatment.

## OBTURATION WITH SILVER CONE

Silver cones are most usually preferred method of canal obturation mainly because of their corrosion. Their use is restricted to teeth with fine, tortuous, curved canals which make the use of gutta-percha difficult (Fig. 18.85).

### Indications

- In sound and straight canals
- In mature teeth with small calcified canals.

### Contraindications

- Teeth with open apex
- Large ovoid shaped canals

### Advantages

- Easy handling and placement.
- Negotiates extremely curved canals.
- Radiopaque in nature
- Mild antibacterial property.

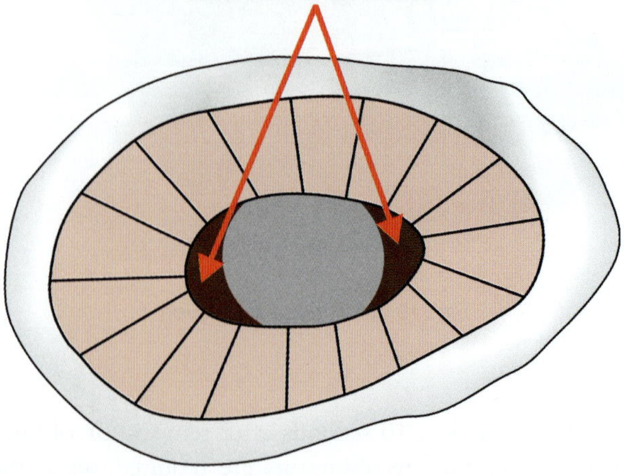


**Fig. 18.85:** Cross-section of canal obturated with silver cone showing poor adaptation of the cone in irregularly shaped canal

### Disadvantages

- Prone to corrosion resulting in loss of apical seal.
- Difficult to retrieve if it is snuggly fitting.
- Non-adaptable so does not seal accessory canals.

### Steps

1. Select a silver cone conforming the final shape and size of the prepared canal. Check its fitting radiographically. If found satisfactory, remove it from the canal and sterilize it over an alcohol flame.
2. Dry the canal and coat the canal walls with sealer.
3. Insert the cone into the canal with sterile cotton plier or Stieglitz forceps.
4. Take a radiograph to see the fitting of cone. If satisfactory, fill the remaining canal with accessory gutta-percha cones.
5. Remove excess of sealer with cotton pellet and place restoration in the pulp chamber.

#### *Stainless Steel*

They are more rigid than silver points and are used for fine and tortuous canals. They cannot seal the root canals completely without use of sealer.

#### *Apical Third Filling*

Sometimes apical barriers are needed to provide apical stop in cases of teeth with incomplete root development, over instrumentation and apical root resorption. Various materials can be used for this purpose. They are designed to allow the obturation without apical extrusion of the material in such cases.

**Apical third filling**

| | |
|---|---|
| A. Carrier based system: | 1. Simplifill obturator |
| | 2. Fiberfill obturator |
| B. Paste system: | 1. Dentin chip filling |
| | 2. Calcium hydroxide filling |
| | 3. MTA filling. |

### Simplifill Obturator

It was originally developed at light speed technology as to complement the canal shape formed by using light speed instruments. In this, the apical gutta-percha size is same ISO size as the light speed master apical rotary. Here a stainless steel carrier is used to place gutta-percha in apical portion of the canal.

### Steps

1. Try the size of apical GP plug so as to ensure an optimal apical fitting. This apical GP plug is of same size as the light speed master apical rotary.
2. Set the rubber stop 2 mm short of the working length and advance GP plug apically without rotating the handle.
3. Coat the apical third apical rotary.
4. Again set the rubber stop on carrier to working length and coat the GP plug with sealer.
5. Penetrate the GP plug to the working length without rotating the handle.
6. Once GP plug fits apically, rotate the carrier anticlockwise without pushing or pulling the handle of carrier.
7. Now backfilling of canal is done using syringe system.

### Fiberfill Obturator

This obturation technique combines a resin post and obturator forming a single until and apical 5 to 7 mm of gutta-percha. This apical gutta-percha is attached with a thin flexible filament to be used in moderately curved canals. Advantage of this technique is that due to presence of dure cure resin sealer, chances of coronal microleakage are less. But it poses difficulty in retreatment cases.

### Dentin Chip Filling

Dentin chip filling forms a ***Biologic seal***. In this technique, after thorough cleaning and shaping of canal, H-file is used to produce dentin powder in central portion of the canal, which is then packed apically with butt end of paper point.

#### *Technique*

- Clean and shape the canal
- Produce dentin powder using hedstroem file or gates glidden drill (Fig. 18.86)
- Use butt end of a paper point to push dentin chips apically (Fig. 18.87) and compact them apically (Fig. 18.88).
- 1-2 mm of chips should block the apical foramen. The density of pack is checked by resistance to perforation by no. 15 or 20 file.
- Backpacking is done using gutta-percha compacted against the plug (Fig. 18.89).

#### *Advantages*

- Biocompatible
- Promotes healing and decreases inflammation
- Prevent extrusion of filling material from the canal space.

#### *Disadvantage*

Infected dentin chips may cause harmful effects. Though it is biocompatible but care must be taken in this technique, because infected pulp tissue can be present in the dentinal mass.

### Calcium Hydroxide

It has also been used frequently as apical barrier. Calcium hydroxide has shown to stimulate cementogenesis. It can be used both in dry or moist state.

Moist calcium hydroxide is placed with the help of plugger and amalgam carrier, injectable syringes or by lentulospirals.

Dry form of $Ca(OH)_2$ is carried into canal by amalgam carrier which is then packed with pluggers (Fig. 18.90). Calcium hydroxide has shown to be a biocompatible material with potential to induce an apical barrier in apexification procedures.

### Mineral Trioxide Aggregate (MTA)

MTA was developed by Dr Torabinejad in 1993 (Fig. 18.91). It contains Tricalcium silicate, Dicalcium silicate, Tricalcium aluminate, Bismuth oxide, Calcium sulfate and Tetracalcium aluminoferrite.

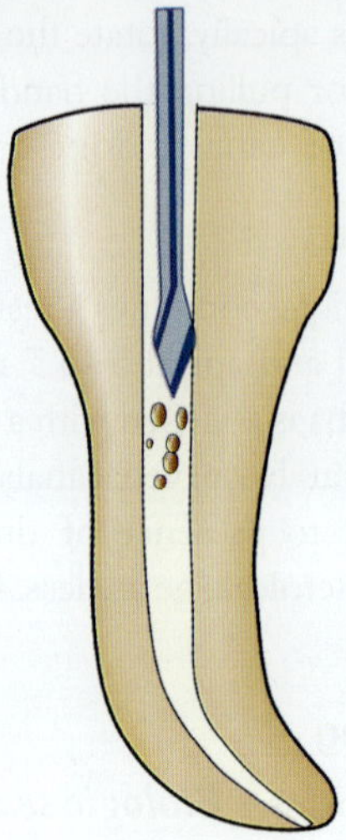

Fig. 18.86: Dentin chips produced by use of Gates-Glidden drills

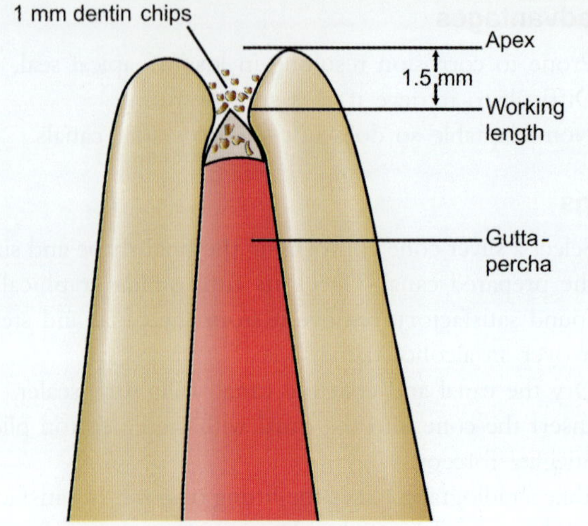


Fig. 18.89: Compaction of dentin chips in apical 2 mm from working length to stimulate hard tissue formation

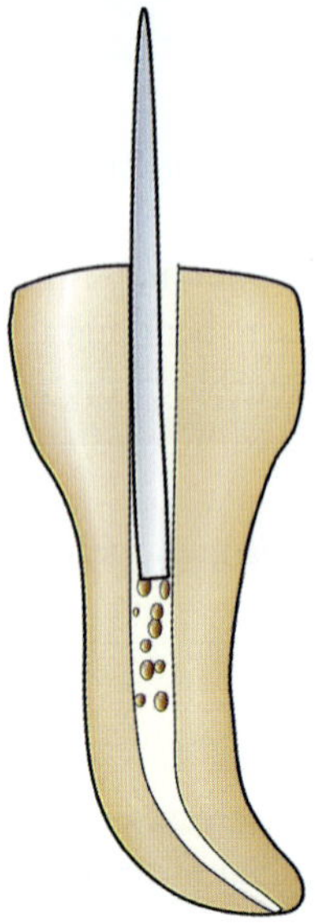

Fig. 18.87: Chips being compacted with blunt end of instrument/paper point

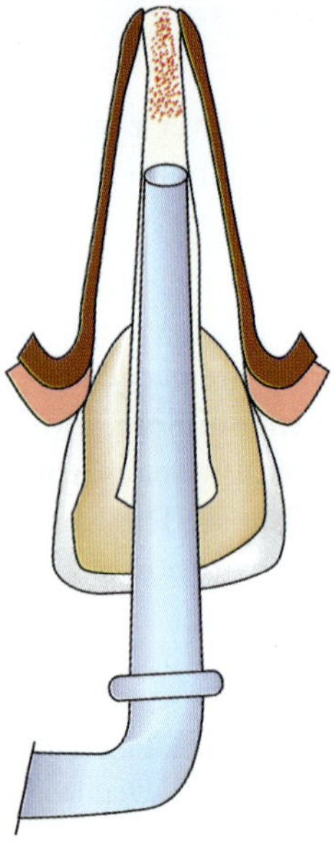

Fig. 18.90: Placement of $Ca(OH)_2$ in the canal

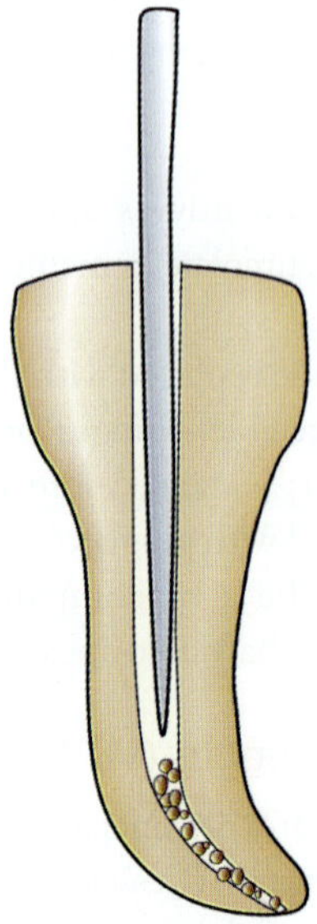

Fig. 18.88: Compaction of dentin chips apically

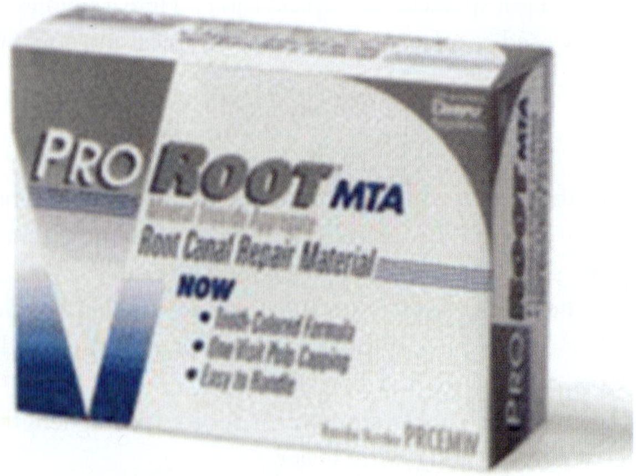


Fig. 18.91: Mineral trioxide aggregate

pH of MTA is 12.5, thus having its biological and histological properties similar to calcium hydroxide. Setting time is 2 hours and 45 minutes. In contrast to $Ca(OH)_2$, it produces hard setting nonresorbable surface.

Because of being hydrophilic in nature, it sets in a moist environment. It has low solubility and shows resistance to marginal leakage. It also exhibits excellent biocompatibility in relation with vital tissues.

To use MTA, mix a small amount of liquid and powder to putty consistency. Since, MTA mix is a loose granular aggregate, it can't be carried out in cavity with normal cement carrier and thus has to be carried in the canal with Messing gun, amalgam carrier or specially designed carrier (Fig. 18.92). After its placement, it is compacted with micropluggers.

Advantages of MTA include its excellent biocompatibility, least toxicity of all the filling materials, radiopaque nature, bacteriostatic nature and resistance to marginal leakage. However, it is difficult to manipulate with long setting time (3-4 hours).

## POSTOBTURATION INSTRUCTIONS

Sometimes patient should be advised that tooth may be slightly tender for a few days. It may be due to sensitivity to excess of filling material pushed into periapical tissues.

For relief of pain, NSAID and warm saline rinses are advised. Anti-inflammatory drugs such as corticosteroids and antibiotics should be prescribed in severe cases. Patient is advised not to chew unduly on the treated tooth until it is protected by permanent restoration.

### Patient Recall

Patient should be recalled regularity to evaluate tissue repair and healing progress.

In case of periapical radiolucency, radiographs should be taken at 3, 6 and 9 months internal period to see continued new bone formation.

The radiograph of a successful filling should show uniformly thickened periodontal ligament and continuous lamina dura along the lateral surfaces of root and around the apex. The tooth should be completely comfortable to patient.

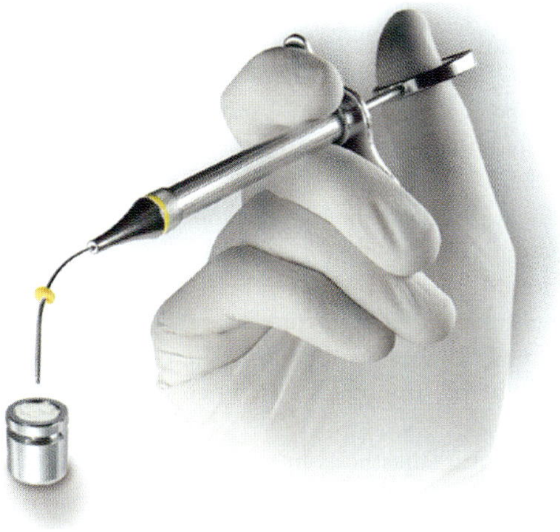

**Fig. 18.92:** Due to loose, granular nature of MTA, a special carrier like Messing Gun or amalgam carrier is used for carrying it

## QUESTIONS

**Q. What are different materials used for obturation? Write in detail about gutta-percha with its advantages and disadvantages?**

**Q. What are functions of root canal sealers? Classify different root canal sealers?**

**Q. How would you know that root canal is ready for obturation?**

**Q. Classify different obturation techniques. Explain in detail about lateral compaction technique?**

**Q. What are advantages and disadvantages of vertical compaction technique?**

**Q. Write short notes on:**

a. System B obturation system
b. Sectional method of obturation
c. Obtura II
d. Thermafil endodontic obturation

## BIBLIOGRAPHY


1. Abarca AM, Bustos A, Navia M. A comparison of apical sealing and extrusion between ThermaFil and lateral condensation techniques. J Endod 2001;27(11):670.
2. Adenubi JO, Rule DC. Success rated for root fillings in young patients. BR Dent J 1976;141:237.
3. Almeida JF, Gomes BP, Ferraz CC, Souza-Filho FJ, Zaua AA. Filling of artificial lateral canals and microleakage and flow of five endodontic sealers. Int Endod J 2007; 40(9):692-99.
4. Bailey GC NgYL, Cunnington SA, Barber P, Gulabivala K, Setchell DJ. Part II: an in vitro investigation of the quality of obturation. Int Endod J 2004;37:694-98.
5. Baksi Akdeniz BG, Eyuboglu TF, Sen BH, Erdilek N. The effect of three different sealers on the radiopacity of root fillings in simulated canals. Oral Pathol Oral Radiol Endod 2007;103(1):138-41.
6. Bal AS, Hicks ML, Barnett F. Comparison of lateral condensed .06 and .02 tapaered gutta-percha and sealer in vitro. J Endod 2001;27(12);786.
7. Baldissara P, Zicari F, Valandro LF, Scotti R. Effect of root canal treatments on quartz fiber posts bonding to root dentin. J Endod 2006;32(10):985-88.
8. Barbizam JV, Souza M, Cechin D, Dabbel J. Effectiveness of a silicon-based root canal sealer for filling of simulated lateral canal. Braz Dent J 2007;18(1):20-23.
9. Berg B. Endodontic management of multi rooted teeth. Oral Surg Oral Med Oral Pathol Oral Radio Endod 1953;3:399.
10. Berry KA, Louchine RJ, Primack PD, Runyan DA. Nickeltitanium versus stainless-steel finger spreadersin curved canals. J Endod 1998;24:752-54.
11. Biggs SG, Knowles KI, Ibarrola JL, Pashley DH. An in vitro assessment of the sealing ability of resilon/epiphany using fluid filtration. J Endod 2006;32(8):759-61.
12. Blayney JR. The medicinal treatment and filling of root canals. J Am Dent Assoc 1928;15:239.
13. Bodrumlu E, Semiz M. Antibacterial activity of new endodontic sealer against Enterococcus faecalis. J Can Dent Assoc 2006;72(7):637.

14. Bouillaguet S, Wataha JC Tay FR, Brackett MG, Lockwood PE. Initial in vitro biological response to contemporary endodontic sealers. J Endod 2006;32(10):989-92.
15. Bowman CJ, Baumgartner JC. Gutta-percha obturation of lateral grooves and depression. J Endod 2002;28:220-23.
16. Brady JM, del Rio CE. Corrosion of endodontic silver conesin bone: a scanning electron microscope and e-ray microprobe study. J Endod 1975;1:205.
17. Brothman P. A comparative study of the vertical and lateral condensation of gutta-percha. J Endod 1981;7:27.
18. Buchanan LS. Filling root canal system with centered condensation: concepts, instruments and techniques. Endod Prac 2005;8:9-15.
19. Caicedo R, von Fraunhofer JA. The properties of endodontic sealers. J Endod 1988;14:527.
20. Camps JJ, Pertot WJ, Escavy JY, et al. Young's modules of warm and cold gutta-percha. Endod Dent Traumatol 1996;12:50.
21. Canoglu H, Tekcicek MU, Cehreli ZC. Comparison of conventional, rotary, and ultrasonic preparation, different final irrigation regiments, and 2 sealers in primary molar root canal therapy. Pediatr Dent 2006;28(6):518-23.
22. Chogle S, Mickel AK, Huffaker SK, Neibaur B. An in vitro assessment of iodoform gutta-percha. J Endod 2005;31: 814-16.
23. Chohayeb AA, Chow LC, Tsaknis PJ, et al. Evaluation of calcium phosphate as a root canal sealer-filler material. J Endod 1987;13:384.
24. Chu CH, Lo ECM, Cheung GSP. Outcome of root canal treatment using ThermaFil and Cold lateral condensation filing techniques. Int Endod J 2005;38:179.
25. Clinton K, Van Himel T. Comparison of a warm gutta-percha obturation technique and lateral condensation. J Endod 2001;27:692-95.
26. Cobankara FK, Altinoz HC, Ergani O, et al. In vitro antibacterial activities of root canal sealers by using two different methods. J Endod 2004;30(1):57.
27. Cobankara FK, Orucoglu H, Sengun A, Belli S. The quantitative evaluation of apical sealing of four endodontic sealers.
28. Cohen BD, Combie ED, Lilley JD. Effect of thermal placement techniques on some physical properties of gutta-percha. Int Endod J 1992;25:292.
29. Collins J, Walkerm MP, Kulild J, et al. A comparison of three gutta-percha obturation techniques to replicate canal irregularities. J Endod 2006;32(8):399.
30. Combankara FK, Adair N, Belli S, et al. A quantitative evaluation of apical leakage of four root canal sealers. Int Endod J 2002;35(12):979.
31. Da saliva Neto UX, de Moraes IG, Westphalen VP, Menezes R, Carneiro E, Fariniuk LF. Leakage of 4 resin-based root-canal sealers used with a single-cone technique. Oral Surg Oral Med Oral Pathol Oral Radiol Endod 2007;104(2):e53-7.
32. Dalat DM, Onai B. Apical leakage of a new glass ionomer root canal sealer. J Endod 1998;24:161.
33. De Almeida WA, Leonardo MR, Tanomara FM, et al. Evaluation of apical sealing of three endodontic sealers. Int Endod J 2000;33(1):25.
34. De-Deus G, Coutingo-Filho T, Reis C, Murad C, Paciornik S. Polymicrobial leakage of four root canal sealers at two different thicknesses. J Endod 2006;32(10):998-1001.
35. Dow PR, Ingle JI. Isotope determination of root canal failure. Oral Surg Oral Med Oral Pathol Oral radiol Endod 1955;8:1100.
36. Dubrow H. Silver points and gutta-percha and the role of root canal fillings. J Am Dent Endod Assoc 1976;93(11);976-80.
37. Economides N, Panagiotis B, Kolokouris I, Gogos C, Kokorikos I. Comparative study of the sealing ability of a poly-dimethylsiloxane-based root canal sealer. Braz Dent J 2005;16(2):145-48.
38. Ehram EH. Treatment with $N_2$ root canal sealer. Br Dent J 1964;117:409.
39. El Deeb ME. The sealing ability of injection molded thermoplasticized gutta-percha. J Endod 1985;11:84.
40. Eldeniz AU, Erdemir A, Hadimli HH, Belli S, Erganis O. Assessment of antibacterial activity of EndoREZ. Oral Surg Oral Med Oral Pathol Oral Radiol Endod 2006;102(1):119-26.
41. Eldeniz AU, Erdemir A, Kurtoglu F, Esener T. Evaluation of pH and calcium ion release of acroseal sealer in comparison with Apexit and Sealapex sealers. Oral Surg Oral Med Oral Pathol Oral Radiol Endod 2007;103(3):e86-91.
42. Eldeniz AU, Mustafa K, Orstavik D, Dahl JE. Cytotoxicity of new resin-, calcium hydroxide –and silicone-based root canal sealers on fibroblasts derived from human gingiva and L929 cell lies. Int Endod J 2007;40(5):329-37.
43. Ewart A, Saunders EM. An investigation into the apical leakage of root filled teeth prepared for a post crown. Int Endod J 1990;23:239.
44. Fabra- Campos H. Experimental apical seal with a new canal obturation system. J Endod 1993;19:71.
45. Frank AL. Calcuim hydroxide: the ultimate medicament? Dent Clin North Am 1979;23:691.
46. Gambarini G, Testarelli L, Pongione G, Gerosa R, Gagliani M. Radiographic and rheological properties of a new endodontic sealer. Aust Endod J 2006;32(1):31-34.
47. Gencoglu N. Comparison of 6 different gutta-percha techniques (part II): Thermafil, JS Quick-Fill, Soft Core, Microseal, system B, and lateral condensation. Oral Surg Oral Med Oral Pathol Oral Radiol Endod 2003;96:91-95.
48. Gernjardt CR, Kruger T, Bekes K, Schaller HG. Apical sealing ability of 2 epoxy resin-based sealers used with root canal obturation techniques based on warm gutta-percha compared to cold lateral condensation. Quintessence Int 2007;38(3): 229-34.
49. Gesi A, Raffaelli O, Goracci C, Pashley DH, Tay FR, Ferraru M. Interfacial strength of resilon and gutta-percha to intraradicular dentin. J Endod 2005;31:809-13.
50. Ghoddusi J, Rohani A, Rashed T, Ghaziani P, Akbari M. An evaluation of microbial leakage after using MTAD as a final irrigation. J Endod 2007;33(2):173-76.
51. Gillespie WT, Loushine RJ, Weller RN, et al. Improving performance of endorez root canaa sealer with a dual-cured two step self etch adhensive. II Apical and Coronal seal. J endod 2006:32(8):771.
52. Glickman GN, Gutmann JL. Contemporary perspectives on canal obturation. Dent Clin North AM 1992;36(2);330.
53. Gordon MPJ, Love RM, Chandler NP. AN evaluation of .06. tapered gutta-percha cones for filling of .06 taper prepared curved root canal. Int Endod J 2005;38:87-96.
54. Grossman LI. Endodontic Practice. Philadelphia: Lea and Febiger, 1978.
55. Grossman LI. Paresthesia from $N_2$ or $N_2$ substitute. Oral Surg Oral Med Oral Pathol Oral Radiol Endod 1978;45:114.
56. Guess GM, Edwards KR, Yang ML, Iqbal MK, Kim S. Analysis of continuous-wave obturation using a singlecone and hybrid technique. J. Endod 1993;29:509-12.

57. Gutmann J, Witherspoon D. Chapter 9: Obturation of the cleaned and shaped Root Canal System. Pathways of the pulp, 7th edn. St Louis: Cohen and Burns 2002;293-364.
58. Gutmann JL, Saunders UP, Saunders EM. An assessment of the plastic ThermaFil obturation technique. Part 2 Material adaptation and sealability. Int Endod J. 1993:26:179.
59. Hiraishi N, Loushine RJ, Vano M, Chieffi N, Weller RN, Ferrari M, Pashley DH, Tay FR. Is an oxygen inhibited layer required for bonding of resin-coated gutta-percha to a methacrylate-based root canal sealer? J Endod 2006;32(5):429-33.
60. Holland R, de Sousa V, Nery MJ, et al. Tissue reaction following apical plugging of the root canal with infected dentine chips. Oral Surg Oral Med Oral Pathol Oral Radiol Endod 1980;49:366.
61. Hume WR. The pharmacologic and toxicological properties of zinc oxide eugenol. J Am Dent Assoc 1986;113:789.
62. Huumonen S, Lenander-Lumikari M, Sigurdsson A, Ørstavik D. Healing of apical periodontitis after endodontictreatment: a comparison between a siliconebased and a zinc oxide-eugenol-based sealer. Int. Endod J 2003;36:296-301.
63. Johnson WB. A new gutta-percha technique. J Endod 1978;4:184.
64. Juhasz A, Verdes E, Tokes L, Kobor A, Dobo-Nagy C. The influence of root canal shape on the sealing ability of two root canal sealers. Int Endod J 2006;39(4):282-86.
65. Kardon BP, Kuttler S, Hardigan P, Dorn SO. An in vitro evaluation of the sealing ability of a new root canal- obturation system. J Endod 2003;29:658-61.
66. Kardon BP, Kuttler S, Hardigan P, et al. An in vitro evaluation of sealing ability of a new root canal-obturation syste. J Endod 2003;29(10):658.
67. Kontakiotis EG, Tzanetakis GN, Loizides AL. A comparative study of contact angles of four different root canal sealers. J Endod 2007;33(3):299-302.
68. Kosti E, Lambrianidis T, Economides N, Neofitou C. Ex vivo study of the efficacy of H-files and rotary NiTi instruments to remove gutta-percha and four types of sealer. Int Endod J 2006;39(1):48-54.
69. Kuttler Y. Microscopic investigation of root apices. J Am dent Assoc 1955;50:544.
70. Lacey S, Pitt Ford TR, Yuan XF, Sherrif M, Watson T. The effect lf temperature on viscosity of root canal sealers. Int Endod J 2006;39(11):860-33.
71. Lea CS, Apicella MJ, Mines P, et al. Comparison of the obturation density of cold lateral compaction versus warm vertical compaction using the continuous wave of condensation technique. J Endod 2005;31(1):37.
72. Lee DH, Lim BS, Lee YK, Yang HC. Mechanisms of root ranal sealer cytotoxicity on esteoblastic cell line MC3T3-E1. Oral Surg Oral Med Oral Pathol Oral Radiol Endod 2007;104(5):717-21.
73. Lee K, Williams MC, Camp JJ, Pashley DH. Adhesion of endodontic sealers to dentin and gutta-percha. J Endod 2002;28(10):684.
74. Lee YY, Hung SL, Pai SF, Lee YH, Yang SF. Eugenol suppressed the expression of lipopolysaccharide-induced proinflammatory mediators in human macrophages. J Endod 2007;33(6):698-702.
75. Levitan ME, Himel VT, Luckey JB. The effect of insertion rate on fill length and adaptation of a thermoplasticized gutta-percha technique. J Endod 2003;29(8);505.
76. Lohbauer U, Gambarini G, Ebert J, Dasch W, Petschelt A. Calcium release and pH-characteristics of calcium hydroxide plus points. Int Endod J 2005;38:683-9.
77. Lucena –Martin C, Ferre-Luque CM, Gonzalez-Rodriguez MP, et al. A comparative study of apical leakage of endomethasone, top-seal and rocko-seal sealer cements. J Endod 2002;28(6):423.
78. Lui JN, Sae-Lim v, Song KP, Chen NN. In vitro antimicrobial effect of chlorhexidine-impregnated gutta-percha points on Enterococcus faecalis. Int Endod J 2004;37:105-13.
79. MC Michen FR, Pearson G, Rahbaren S, et al. A comparative study of selected physical properties of five root canal sealers. Int Endod J 2003;36(9):629.
80. Melegari KK, Botero TM, Holland GR. Prostaglandin E production and viability of cells cultured in contact with freshly mixed endodontic materials. Int Endod J 2006;39(5):357-62.
81. Merdad K, Pascon AE, Kulkarni G, Santerre P, Friedman S. Short–term cytotoxicity assessment of components of the epiphany resin-percha obturating system by indirect and direct contact millipore filter assays. J Endod 2007;33(1):24-27.
82. Molloy D, Goldman M, white RR, et al. Comparative tissue tolerance of a new endodontic sealer. Oral Surg Oral Med Oral Pathol Oral Radiol Endod 1992;73:490.
83. Moreno A. thermomechanically softened gutta-percha root canal filling. J Endod 1977;3:186.
84. Newton CW, Patterson SS, Kafrawy AH, et al. Studies of sargenti's technique of endodontic treatment six month and one year response. J Endod 1980;6:509.
85. Nielsen BA, Baumgartner JC. Spreader penetration during lateral compaction of Resilon and gutta-percha. J Endod 2006;32(1):52.
86. Oliver CM, Abbott PV. Correlation Between clinical success and apical dye penetration. Int Endod J 2001;34(8):637.
87. Orlay H. Overfilling in root canal treatment. Two accidents with $N_2$. Br Dent J 1966;120:376.
88. Ozata F, Onai B, Erdilek N, et al. A comparative study of apical leakage of apexit, Ketac-endo and diaket root canal sealers. J Endod 1999;25:603.
89. Partovi M, Al-Havvaz AH, Soleimani B. In vitro computer analysis of crown discolouration from commonly used endododntic sealers. Aust Endod J 2006;32(3);116-19.
90. Patel DV, Sherriff M, Ford TR, Watson TF, Mannocci F. The penetration of RealSeal primer and tibliseal into root canal dentinal tubules: a confocal microscopic study. Int. Endod J 2007;40(1):67-71.
91. Pommel L, About I, Pashley D, et al. Apical Leakae of four endodontic sea;ers. J Endod 2003;29(3):208.
92. Ramsey WD. Hermetic sealing of root canals. J Endod 1982;8(3):100.
93. Robert G, Liewehr FR, Buston TB, et al. Apical diffusion of Calcuim hydroxide in a in vitro model. J Endod 2005;31(1);57.
94. Saw LH, Messer HH. Root strains associated with different obturation techniques. J Endod 1995;21:314-20.
95. Schaeffer MA, White RR, Walton RE. Determining the optimal obturation length: a meta-analysis of the literature. J Endod 2005;31:271-74.
96. Schafer E, Zandbiglari T. Solubility of root canal sealers in water and artificial saliva. Int Endod J 2003;36(10):660.
97. Schumacher JW, Rutledge RE. An alternative to apexification. J Endod 1993;19:529.
98. Shipper G, Ørstavik D, Teixeira FB, Trope M. An evaluation of microbial leakage in root filled with a thermoplastic synthetic polymer-based root canal filling material (resilon), J Endod 2004;30:342-47.
99. Silver GK, Love RM, Purton DG. Comparison of two vertical condensation obturation techniques: touch 'n heat modified and system B. Int Endod J 1999;32:287-95.
100. Siskin, M. The obturation of the root canal. Dent Clin North Am 1957;November:855.
101. Sjogren U, Figdor D, Persson S, et al. Influence of infection at the time of root filling on the outcome of the endodontic

visit without compromising quality of the treatment. An inexperienced clinician should not attempt single visit endodontics.

- ***Positive patient acceptance:*** Patient should be cooperative to allow single visit treatment. Non-cooperative patients like patients with TMJ problems, limited mouth opening should be avoided for single visit endodontics.
- ***Absence of anatomical interferences:*** Anatomical problems like presence of fine, curved or calcified canals require more than usual time for the treatment (Figs 19.1 and 19.2). Teeth with such canals should be better treated in multiple visits rather than single visit.
- ***Accessibility:*** Teeth for single visit should have sufficient accessibility and visibility. For example, anterior teeth are more accessible than posterior teeth, so they should be treated before attempting treatment in posterior teeth.
- ***Availability of sufficient time to complete the case:*** Both clinician as well as patient should have sufficient time for single visit endodontics.
- ***Pulp status:*** Vital teeth are better candidate for single visit treatment than the nonvital teeth because of less flare-ups in teeth with vial pulp.
- ***Clinical symptoms:*** Teeth with acute alveolar abscess should not be treated by single visit. Whereas teeth with sinus tract are good candidate for single visit endodontics because presence of sinus acts as safety valve and prevents build up of pressure, so these teeth seldom show flare-ups.

**Criteria of case selection as given by Oliet include**
- Positive patient acceptance
- Absence of acute symptoms
- Absence of continuous hemorrhage or exudation
- Absence of anatomical interferences like presence of fine, curved or calcified canals
- Availability of sufficient time to complete the case
- Absence of procedural difficulties like canal blockage, ledge formation or perforations.

## Conditions where Single Visit Endodontics cannot be Performed

- Teeth with anatomic anomalies such as calcified and curved canals
- Asymptomatic nonvital teeth with periapical pathology and no sinus tract
- Acute alveolar abscess cases with frank pus discharge
- Patients with acute apical periodontitis
- Symptomatic nonvital teeth and no sinus tract
- Retreatment cases
- Patients with allergies or previous flare-ups
- Teeth with limited access
- Patients who are unable to keep mouth open for long durations such as patients with TMJ disorders.

## Indications of Single Visit Endodontics

- Vital teeth
- Fractured anteriors where esthetics is the concern (Fig. 19.3)

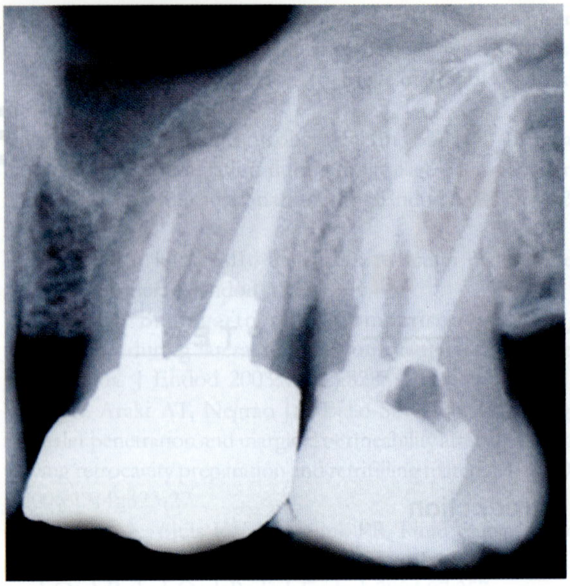

**Fig. 19.1:** Molars showing curved canals

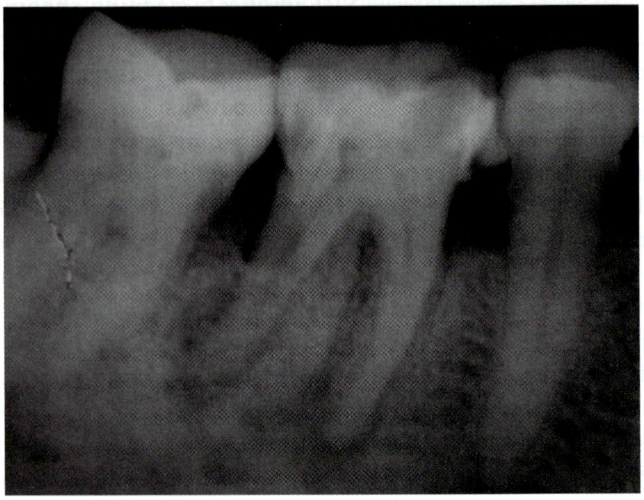

**Fig. 19.2:** Radiograph showing three rooted 46

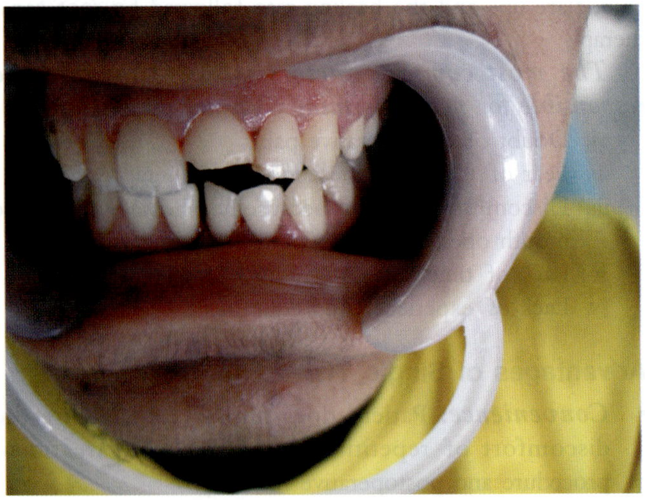

**Fig. 19.3:** In anterior teeth, single visit endodontic therapy is indicated because of esthetic reasons

- Patients who require sedation every time
- Nonvital teeth with sinus tract
- Teeth with limited access
- Nonsurgical retreatment cases
- Medically compromised patients who require antibiotics prophylaxis
- Physically compromised patients who cannot come to dental clinics frequently.

In conclusion, single-visit endodontics has been shown to be an effective treatment modality, which compared to multiple-visit therapy, is more beneficial to patients and dentists in many ways provided there is careful case selection and adherence to standard endodontic principles. The prevention and elimination of apical periodontitis are the goals of a successful endodontics therapy, once the way to accomplish these goals is determined, the decision to provide treatment in multiple visits or single visit will follow itself.

## QUESTION

**Q. What are indications and contraindications of single visit endodontics? Mention its advantages and disadvantages.**

## BIBLIOGRAPHY


1. Imura N, Zuolo ML. Factors associated with endodontic flare-ups: A prospective study. Int Endod J 1995;28(5):261-65.
2. Ng Y-L, Glennon JP, Setchell DJ, Gulabivala K. Prevalence of and factors affecting post-obturation pain in patients undergoing root canal treatment. Int Endod J 2004;37(6):381-91.
3. Ng Y-L, Mann V, Rahbaran S, Lewsey J, Gulabivala K. Outcome of primary root canal treatment: Systematic review of the literature—Part 1. Effects of study characteristics on probability of success. Int Endod J 2007;40(12):921-39.
4. Ng Y-L, Mann V, Rahbaran S, Lewsey J. Gulabivala review of the literature–Part 2. Influence of clinical factorts. Int Endod J 2008;41(1):6-31.
5. Peters LB, Wesselink PR. Periapical healing of endodontically treated teeth in one and two visits obturated in the presence or absence of detectable microorganisms. Int Endod J 2002;35(8):660-607.
6. Sathorn C, Parashos P, Messer H. Effectiveness of single-versus multiple-visit endodontic treatment of teeth with apical periodontitis: A systemic review and meta-analysis. Int Endod J 2005;38(6):347-55. (Review)
7. Sathorn C, Parashos P, Messer H. The prevalence of postoperative pain and flare-up in single-and multiple visit endodontic treatment: A systematic review. Int Endod J 2008;41(2):91-99.
8. Trope M, Bergenholtz G. Microbiological basis for endodontic treatment: Can a maximal outcome be achieved in one visit? Endod Topics 2002;1(1):40-53.

# Mid Treatment Flare-ups in Endodontics

CHAPTER 20



## INTRODUCTION

*Flare-up is described as the occurrence of pain, swelling or the combination of these during the course of root canal therapy, which results in unscheduled visits by patient.* Pain may occur soon after initiating endodontic treatment for an asymptomatic tooth or shortly after the initial emergency treatment or during the course of treatment.

*American Association of Endodontists (AAE) defines a flare-up "As an acute exacerbation of periradicular pathosis after initiation or in continuation of root canal treatment".* Mor C et al in 1992 have suggested that incidence of inter-appointment emergency with endodontic treatment is 4.2 percent and it is not related to patient's sex, age or tooth location.

The mid treatment flare-up is a true emergency and is so severe that an unscheduled patient visit and treatment are required. Despite judicious and careful treatment procedures, complications such as pain, swelling or both may occur. These inter-appointment emergencies are undesirable and disruptive events, so it should be resorted quickly. Occasionally flare-ups are unexpected; sometimes these are predicated due to patient presenting factors.

Flare-ups may even occur with the best of the therapy but these flare-ups usually happen due to improper treatment or when insufficient time is allowed for specific modalities in therapy (*Weine*).

Acute periapical inflammation is the most common cause of mid treatment pain and swelling. Mid treatment emergencies are usually due to irritants left within root canal system or iatrogenic factors such as operator's fault and host factors. The occurrence of mild pain is relatively common following root canal therapy; it should be expected and anticipated by patients, whereas severe pain and swelling associated with flare-up is a rare occurrence (1.4-16%) (Fig. 20.1).

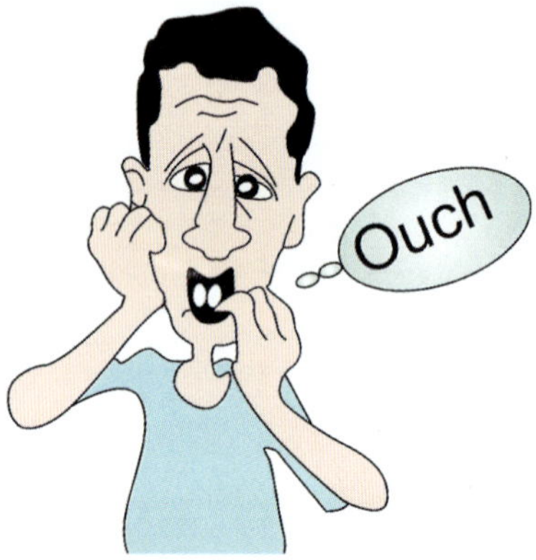


**Fig. 20.1:** Patient with endodontic flare-up presents lot of anxiety

## ETIOLOGY

Its etiology is multifactorial and can be categorized as related to the patient, to pulpal or periapical diagnosis or to treatment procedures done. Although many factors have been quoted for the etiology of mid flare-up but, if a patient comes with a history of preoperative swelling and pain, one can still think of inter-appointment emergencies.

A tooth with vital pulp is less likely to demonstrate the symptoms of inter-appointment emergencies; while on the other hand, a tooth with acute apical abscess along with pain shows severe emergency treatment in flare-ups.

## CLINICAL CONDITIONS OF FLARE-UP

1. ***Apical periodontitis secondary to treatment:*** An asymptomatic tooth before the initiation of endodontic treatment becomes sensitive to percussion during the course of treatment. In this condition, pain may become severe

causing a throbbing or gnawing pain. The cause of this pain may be:

- Overinstrumentation
- Over medication
- Forcing debris into periapical tissues

*Confirmatory test:* Apply the rubber clamp and use a sterile paper point. Access and mark the working length. Then, place the paper point in the canal. If over instrumentation has happened by fault, then the paper point will go beyond the working length without obstruction. On withdrawal, tip of the point will show a reddish or brownish color indicating inflamed tissue in the periapical region and absence of stop in apical preparation (Fig. 20.2).

2. ***Incomplete removal of pulp tissue:*** Whenever a pulpotomy or partial pulpectomy has been done, the patient may experience pain due to incomplete removal of inflamed pulp tissue (Fig. 20.3). In this condition, sensitivity to hot and cold or pain on percussion is usually seen.

   *Confirmatory test:* Apply rubber dam, place a sterile paper point, of course short of working length. When paper point is removed, it will display brownish discoloration indicative of inflamed seeping tissue.

3. ***Recrudescence of chronic apical periodontitis: (Phoenix Abscess):*** It is a condition that occurs in teeth with necrotic pulps and apical lesions that are asymptomatic. There is no exacerbation of previously symptomless periradicular lesion. The reason for this phenomenon is thought, to be due to the alteration of the internal environment of root canal space during instrumentation which activates the bacterial flora. Mobility, tenderness and swelling are usually the sign and symptoms found in phoenix abscess.

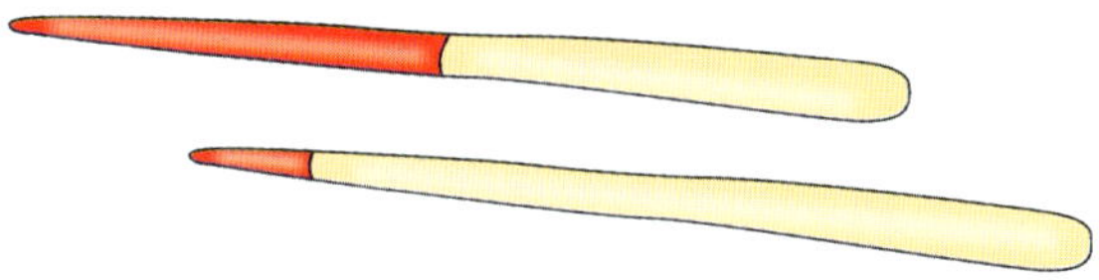

**Fig. 20.2:** Absorbent paper point showing reddish color indicating inflamed periapex

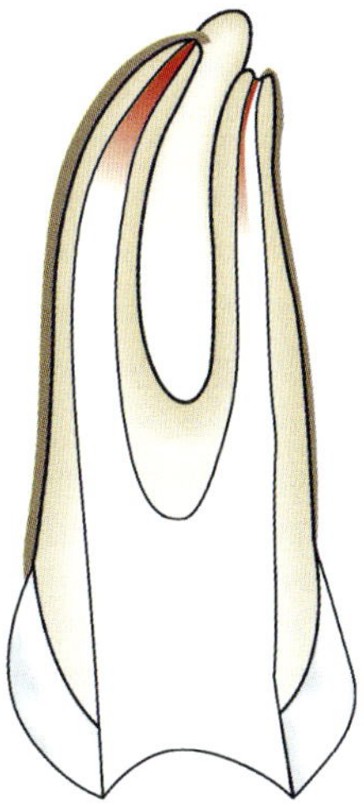

**Fig. 20.3:** Incomplete removal of pulp tissue

4. ***Recurrent periapical abscess:*** It is a condition where a tooth with an acute periapical abscess is relieved by emergency treatment after which the acute symptoms return (Fig. 20.4). In some cases, the abscess may recur more than once, due to microorganism of high virulence or poor host resistance.

**Clinical conditions of flare-up**

- Apical periodontitis secondary to treatment
- Incomplete removal of pulp tissue
- Recrudescence of chronic apical periodontitis
- Recurrent periapical abscess

## CONTRIBUTING FACTORS FOR FLARE-UPS

Factors Contributing for Flare-ups

- Overinstrumentation
- Inadequate debridement
- Periapical extrusion of debris
- Overfilling
- Periapical lesion
- Re-treatment
- Host factors

1. ***Overinstrumentation:*** It is most common cause for mid-treatment flare-ups (Fig. 20.5). Inter treatment pain is directly proportional to over instrumentation.
2. ***Inadequate debridement:*** Inadequate debridement or incomplete removal of pulp tissue may cause pain, and also the mid-treatment flare-ups (Fig. 20.6).
3. ***Periapical extrusion of debris:*** When pulp tissue fragments, necrotic tissues, microorganisms and dentinal filling are extruded beyond apical foramen, it leads to periapical inflammation and flare-ups (Fig. 20.7). The extrusion of irrigant solutions can also produce sudden reaction for example if sodium hypochlorite gets extruded beyond apex, it may result in violent tissue reaction and unbearable pain.

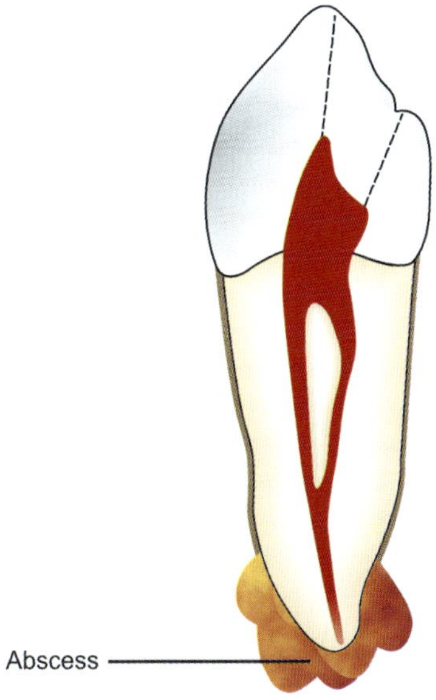


**Fig. 20.4:** Periapical abscess

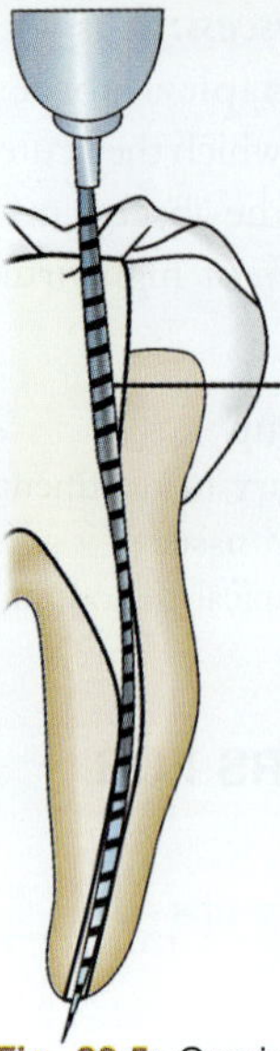


Fig. 20.5: Overinstrumentation

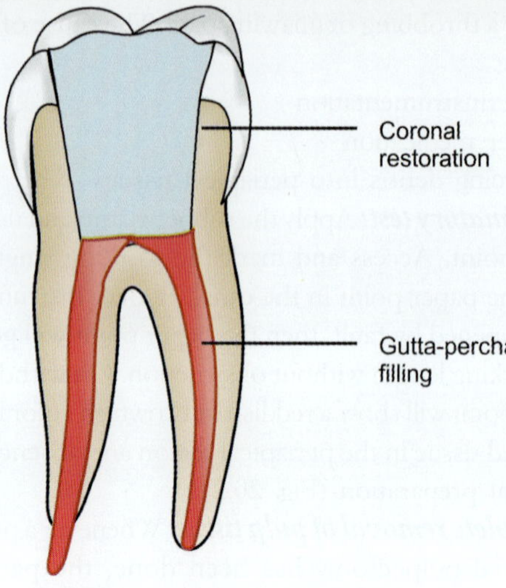


Fig. 20.8: Overfilling of obturating material causing inflammation of periapical area

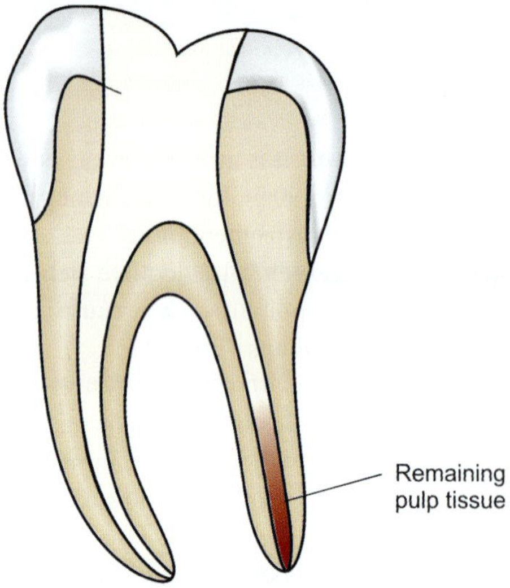


Fig. 20.6: Inadequate debridement of pulp tissue

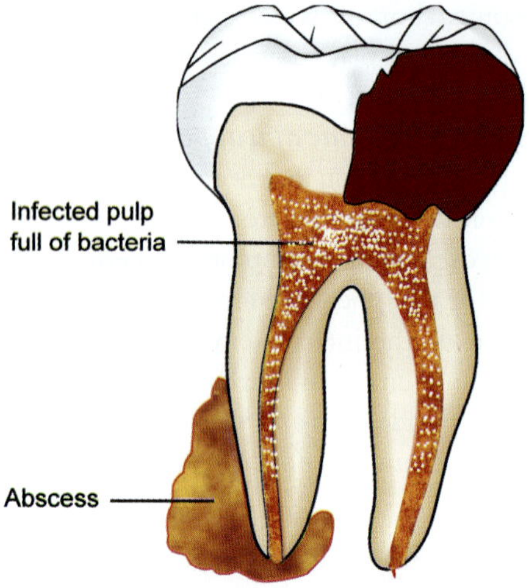


Fig. 20.9: Periapical inocculation of bacteria can cause flare-ups

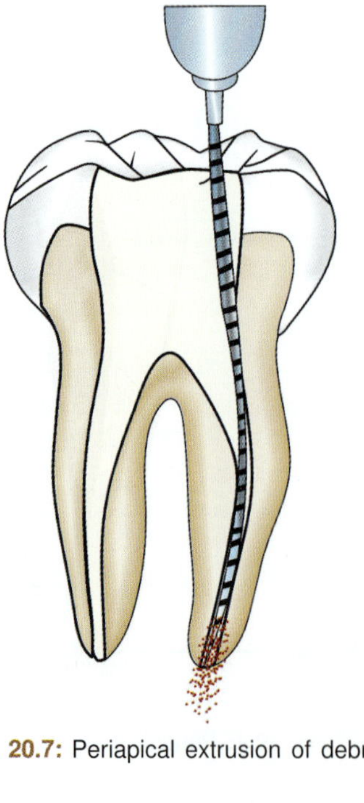

Fig. 20.7: Periapical extrusion of debris

4 ***Overfilling:*** Large overfills of obturating materials like gutta-percha or sealers are responsible for pain (Fig. 20.8). In addition, gross-overfilling can cause nerve damage because of chemical toxicity of obturating materials and also, the mechanical nerve damage can be caused by over extended filling. It has been shown in various studies that extrusion of zinc oxide eugenol sealer causes chronic inflammation.

5 ***Periapical lesion:*** Pulp with larger periapical radiolucency have more bacterial stains and are more infected. These bacteria can cause acute problem if inoculated periapically (Fig. 20.9).

6. ***Retreatment:*** Retreatment cases show more flare-ups (Fig. 20.10). In these cases, host response to extruded filling material and toxic solvents may increase pain.

7. ***Host factors:*** Intensity of preoperative pain and amount of patient apprehension are correlated to degree of post-operative pain. Age, gender, presence of allergies, tooth position, systemic diseases are not shown to have any correlation with flare-ups.

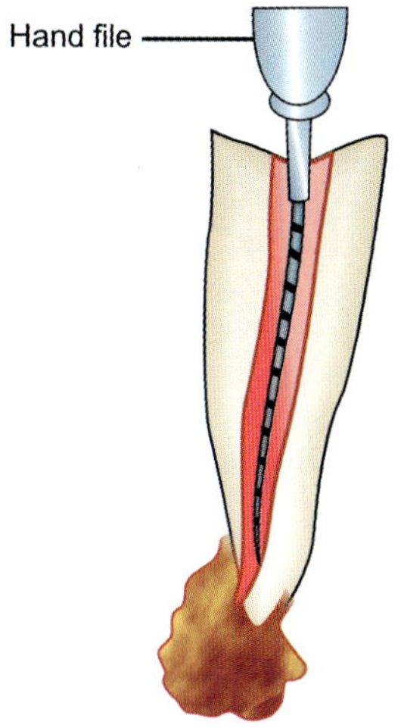


Fig. 20.10: Retreatment cases show more flare-ups

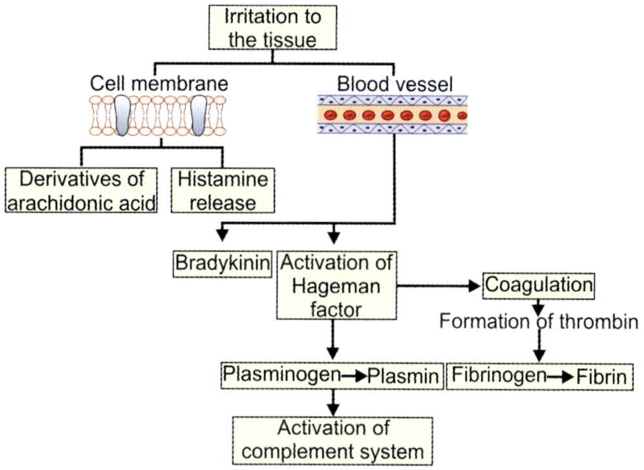


Fig. 20.11: Tissue response to irritation

## MICROBIOLOGY AND IMMUNOLOGY OF FLARE-UPS

### Seven Microbiological and Immunological Factors are Seen to be Responsible for Flare-ups:

- Alteration of local adaptation syndrome
- Changes in periapical tissue pressure
- Microbial factors
- Chemical mediators
- Changes in cyclic nucleotides
- Immunological responses
- Psychological factors

1. ***Alteration of local adaptation syndrome:*** Selye has shown that when a new irritant is introduced in a chronically inflamed tissue, a violent reaction may occur because of disturbance in local tissue adaptation to applied irritants. For example, in case of chronic pulpal diseases, the inflammatory lesion is adapted to irritants but during root canal therapy, a new irritant in form of medicament get introduced in the lesion leading to flare-up.
2. ***Changes in periapical tissue pressure:*** Studies have shown that in teeth with increased periapical pressure, excessive exudate creates pain by causing pressure on nerve endings. Root canals of such teeth when kept open, exudate comes out but in teeth with less periapical pressure, microorganisms and other irritants gets aspirated into periapical area leading to pain.
3. ***Microbial factors:*** It has been shown by many studies that bacteria are main causative factor in the pulpal and periapical disease. After 1970, with the advent of new technique of culture, the role of flora in root canal is clearly shown. Studies have shown that enzymes, endotoxin and other chemicals produced by anaerobes may cause persistence of periapical lesion. Most commonly found anaerobe is Bacteroides melaninogenicus. It produces enzymes which is collagenolytic, fibrinolytic and endotoxin which activates the Hageman factor which further leads to production of bradykinins and pain mediator. Many studies have shown that teichoic acid present in coating of gram-positive bacteria is a potent immunogen producing humoral antibodies like IgM, IgG and IgA which may cause pain.
4. ***Effect of chemical mediators:*** Chemical mediators can be in form of cell mediators, plasma mediators and in form of neutrophils products (Fig. 20.11). Cell mediators include histamine, serotonin, prostaglandins, platelet activating factor and lysosomal components which may lead to pain. The plasma mediators are present in circulation in inactive precursor form and get activated on coming in contact with irritants. For example, Hageman factor when gets activated after in contact with irritants, produce multiple effects like production of bradykinin and activation of clotting cascade which may cause vascular leakage. On instrumentation of root canal, acute inflammatory response is initiated resulting in polymorphonuclear leucocytes infiltration, which on further, release collagenase, peroxidase, amylase, lipase and other lytic enzymes resulting in severe pain and swelling.
5. ***Changes in cyclic nucleotides:*** Bourne et al have shown that character and intensity of inflammatory and immune response is regulated by hormones and the mediators. For example, increased levels of cAMP inhibits mast cell degranulation which helps in reducing pain where as increase in cGMP levels stimulate mast cell degranulation which results in increase in pain (Fig. 20.12). Studies have shown that during flare-up, there is increased level of cGMP over cAMP concentrations.
6. ***Immunological response:*** In chronic pulpitis and periapical disease, presence of macrophages and lymphocytes indicates both cell mediated and humoral response. Despite of their protective effect, the immunologic response also contributes to destructive phase of reaction which can occur, causing perpetuation and aggravation of inflammatory process.
7. ***Psychological factor:*** Anxiety, apprehension, fear and previous history of dental experience appear to play an important role in mid treatment flare-ups.

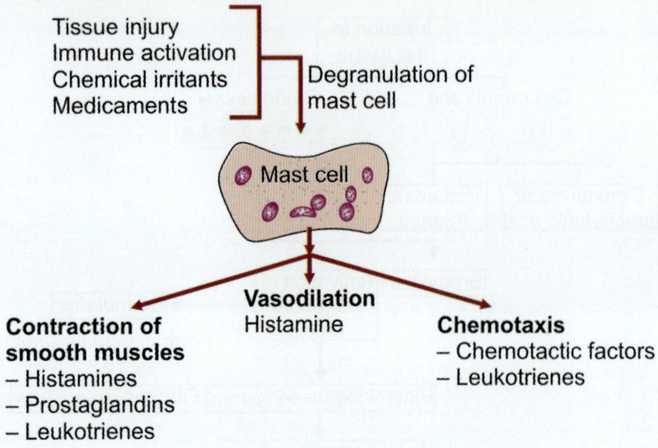


**Fig. 20.12:** Release of inflammatory mediators from mast cell degranulation

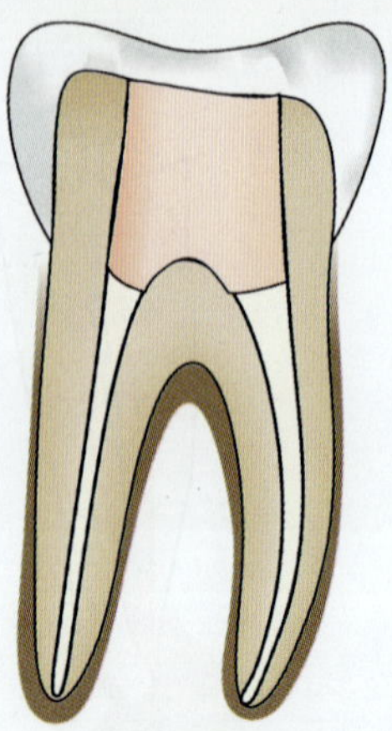

**Fig. 20.13:** Complete debridement of pulp followed by temporary restoration

## DIAGNOSIS AND MANAGEMENT OF FLARE-UPS

Establishing the cause of flare-up is an important step towards management of mid-treatment pain. It is necessary to warn the patient that he or she may experience slight pain after the appointment. So analgesic should be prescribed when patient experience moderate to severe pain after the first appointment. The clinician must review the diagnosis to ensure the tooth under treatment has been identified correctly as the source of pain.

Inter-appointment emergencies are divided into patients with an initial diagnosis of a vital or a necrotic pulp and with or without swelling.

### Previously Vital Pulps with Complete Debridement

In these conditions, chances of flare-ups are less, only patient reassurance and the prescription of mild to moderate analgesic often will suffice.

There is no need of reopening and placing corticosteroids in the canal to reduce the pain and swelling as nothing much is gained by these methods. Studies have shown that flare- ups are not prevented by steroids, whether they are placed intracanally or systemically.

### Previously Vital Pulps with Incomplete Debridement

It is most commonly seen that pulp remnants left during debridement, considered to be a major irritant, causing severe pain.

To manage this condition, the working length should be rechecked and the canals should be carefully cleaned with copious irrigation of sodium hypochlorite. A dry cotton pellet is then placed followed by a temporary filling (Fig. 20.13) and a mild analgesic is prescribed, along the tooth relieving from occlusion.

In some cases, if tooth becomes tender, it indicates that inflammation process has reached periapical tissues. Again the management is same as described above.

#### *Previously Necrotic Pulps without Swelling*

Studies have shown that incidence of flare-ups is higher with necrotic tooth than in vital tooth. Teeth with necrotic pulp often develop as acute apical abscess after the initial appointment. As the lesion is confined to bone, there occurs the severe pain.

The best method of managing the necrotic pulp is to establish accurate working length, complete instrumentation of root canal. In these cases, the tooth is opened and the canal is gently recleaned and irrigated with copious amount of sodium hypochlorite. Drainage must be established if possible. If there is drainage from tooth after opening, then tooth is again cleaned and debrided completely and irrigated with sodium hypochlorite. After drying the canal, calcium hydroxide dressing is placed and access is sealed.

If there is no drainage from the canal, still gently open the tooth, lightly instrument and completely debride the canal. After debridement, copiously irrigate the canal with sodium hypochlorite and place calcium hydroxide paste and close the access. Prescribe analgesics and antibiotics. Leaving the root canal open for drainage is controversial as exposure to oral flora serves no purpose and may lead to flare-ups.

#### *Previously Necrotic Pulp with Swelling*

These cases are best managed by incision and drainage. Also, canals should be opened, debrided and gently irrigated with sodium hypochlorite solution. Then calcium hydroxide paste should be placed and closed.

## GENERAL MANAGEMENT OF FLARE-UPS

Studies have shown that postoperative pain diminishes in 72 hrs. During this patient experiences pain which must be relieved by the clinician.

### General Management of Flare-ups

1. Reassurance to the patient
2. Complete debridement of root canal system
3. Establishment of drainage
4. Relief of occlusion
5. Calcium hydroxide therapy

6. Intracanal medicaments
7. Medications
   a. Analgesic
   b. Antibiotic
   c. Corticosteroid
8. Placebo
1. ***Reassurance to the patient:*** Reassurance is the most important aspect of treatment, so, explain the patient about procedure completely so as to reduce the anxiety and gain confidence of the patient. The explanation should include that the flare-up is not unusual and can be managed effectively. Also, general anesthesia and conscious sedation are also good adjuncts in treating some cases especially uncooperative and fearful patients.
2. ***Complete debridement of root canal system:*** Single most effective method to reduce flare-ups is complete debridement by cleaning and shaping of root canal system (Fig. 20.14). Patency of apex and shaping and cleaning by crown-down technique are two important factors in the management of flare-ups.
3. ***Establishment of drainage:*** In the presence of suppuration, drainage of exudate is the most effective method for reducing pain and swelling (Fig. 20.15). In most cases, accumulated exudate will surge from root canal affording immediate relief. But in some cases, root canal instruments are needed to pass through packed dentinal shavings in the apical third of canal. After exudation, access cavity is closed again to avoid exposure of canal to oral flora and salivary products. These salivary products and oral flora may introduce new microorganisms into the canal which may activate complement system thus leading to exacerbation of pain.
4. ***Relief of occlusion:*** It has been advocated by Cohen for prevention of postoperative pain and/or to reduce intra-appointment pain.
5. ***Calcium hydroxide therapy:*** It is intracanal dressing used for therapeutic purpose for prevention or treatment of flare-ups. It serves following purposes:

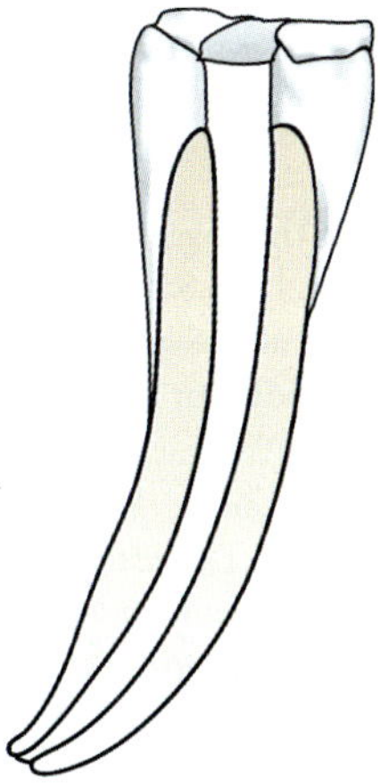

**Fig. 20.14:** Complete cleaning and shaping of root canal system

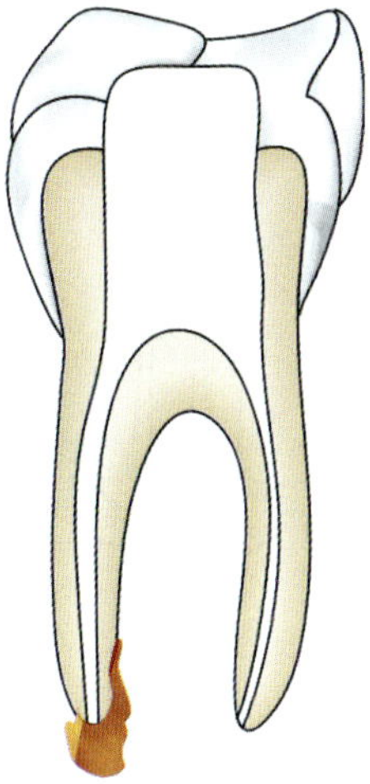

**Fig. 20.15:** Opening of pulp chamber to allow drainage

   - It reduces bacterial colonies and their toxic byproducts. This antimicrobial effect remains in canal for one week.
   - Calcium hydroxide hydroxylates the lipid moiety of bacterial lipopolysaccharide, rendering it incapable of producing biologic effects and complement activation.
   - It absorbs carbon dioxide ($CO_2$), by this action it deprives the capnophilic organism for carbon dioxide in root canal system.
   - It obliterates root canal space which minimizes the ingress of tissue exudate, a potential source of nourishment for remaining bacteria.
   - Extrusion of calcium hydroxide periapically reduces inflammatory reaction by reducing substrate adherence capacity of macrophages.
   - Calcium hydroxide has soft tissue dissolving property because of its high pH. As it can dissolve necrotic tissue, denaturing effect of $Ca(OH)_2$ on protein allows sodium hypochlorite to dissolve remaining tissue more easily.

   Placement of calcium hydroxide in an inflamed canal is shown in Figure 20.16.
6. ***Intracanal medicaments:*** For relief of pain during root canal treatment, commonly used intracanal medicaments are antimicrobial agents, irrigating solutions and corticosteroids. The antimicrobial agents such as formocresol, cresatin, CMCP have been tried to provide relief of pain (Figs 20.17A to C). It has been seen that microorganisms are responsible for exaggeration of inflammation. Among the irrigating solutions, sodium hypochlorite have been proved to provide better effects against the gram-negative anaerobes which are thought to be the main causative factor in flare-up.

   The corticosteroids have been tried because of their anti-inflammatory activity. These inhibit the formation of arachidonic acid from the membrane phospholipids and increases the production of cyclic AMP which further inhibits mast cell degranulation thus reducing the inflammatory response. Corticosteroids also hyperpolarizes the nerve present in inflamed area and thus reduces the nerve impulse transmission. The disadvantage of using

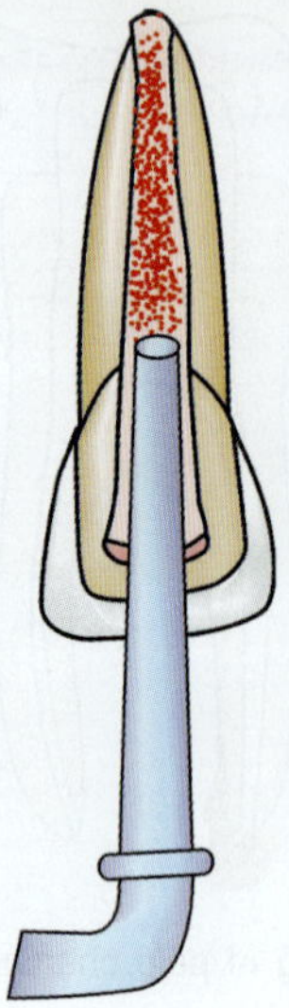

Fig. 20.16: Placement of $Ca(OH)_2$ in canal

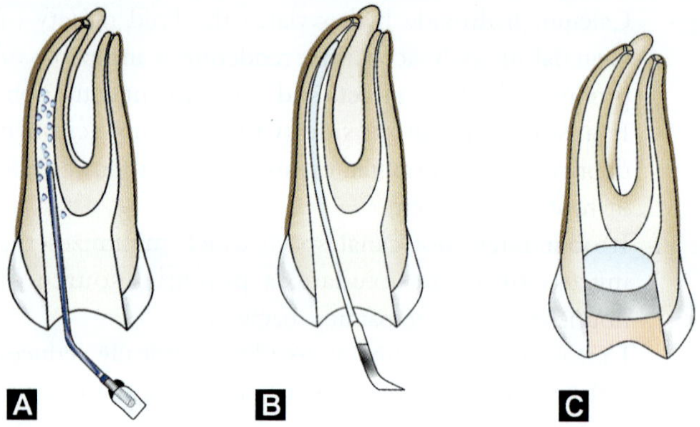


Figs 20.17A to C: A. Irrigation of canal for final cleaning of the canal, B. Drying of the canal using absorbent paper point, C. Placement of intracanal medicament

steroids is that they interfere with phagocytosis and nerve synthesis.

7. *Medications:* Commonly used systemic drugs are:
   a. Analgesic
   b. Antibiotic
   c. Corticosteroid

   Among analgesics, nonsteroidal anti-inflammatory drugs (NSAIDs) are commonly used for relieving the pain. Commonly used drugs are ibuprofen, diclofenac sodium, aspirin and etoricoxib.

   Narcotic analgesics provide relief from pain by acting on neural receptors of brain cells. They raise pain threshold by causing relaxation, apathy and freedom from anxiety. Commonly used drugs are morphine, codeine, meperidine, tramodol and propoxyphene.

   Among antibiotics, pencillins and its derivatives are commonly prescribed. Metronidazole, tinidazole, ornidazole and clindamycin are also used because of their effectivity against anaerobic infections.

8. *Placebo:* Placebos are pharmacologically inert substances which do not have therapeutic effect, they act as analgesics and alleviates anxiety. They mimic the action of active drugs. Studies have shown that patients experience the relief of pain after receiving placebo.

   Placebo effects are based on patients comprehensation and emotional response to drug administration. The observed effects of drug administration are combination of pharma-cological actions and placebo. Clinician himself exerts a potent placebo effect, his conviction that an analgesic is effective, if communicated to anxious patient, increase the expectations of patients relief. Also instruction or suggestions given to patients are powerful aids in controlling pain. Placebos enhance the levels of endorphin productions and thus resulting in pain relief.

## Precautions to be Taken to Prevent Flare-ups

- Proper diagnosis of the case
- Determination of correct working length
- Complete extirpation of the vital pulp
- Avoid filling too close to the radiographic apex
- Reduce tooth from occlusion especially if apex is severely violated by over instrumentation
- Placement of intracanal medicaments
- Prescription of analgesics and antibiotics whenever condition warrants it.

## CONCLUSION

The occurrence of mild pain and discomfort is common even if the treatment rendered is of highest standard. But still psychological preparation of the patient, complete cleaning and shaping of root canal system, use of long acting anesthetic and analgesics decrease the incidence of inter appointment flare-ups in mild to moderate levels.

Prompt and effective treatment of flare-ups is an essential part of overall endodontic treatment.

## QUESTIONS

**Q. Define flare-ups. What are etiological factors for flare-ups?**

**Q. What is microbiology and immunology of flare-ups?**

**Q. How will you manage a case of endodontic flare-up.**

## BIBLIOGRAPHY

1. August DS. Managing the abscessed open tooth: instrument and closed part 2. Endod 1982;8:364.
2. Imura N, Zuolo ML. Factors associated with endodontic flare-ups: A prospective study. Int Endod J 1995;28(5):261-5.
3. Marshall JG, Liesinger AW. Factors associated with endodontic post-treatment pain. J Endod 1993;19:573.
4. Marshall JG, Walton RE. The effect of intramuscular injection of steroid on post-treatment endodontic pain.
5. Seltzer S. Flare-ups in endodontics: Part (etiological factors). J endod 2004;30(7):476-80.
6. Seltzer S, Bender JB, Ehrenreich J. Incidence and duration of pain following endodontic therapy: Relationship to treatment with sulfonamides and to other factors. Oral Surg 1961;14:74.

CHAPTER 21

# Endodontic Emergencies



## INTRODUCTION

It has been seen that more than 80 percent of the patient who report in the dental clinic with emergency symptoms have endodontically related pain (Fig. 21.1). Therefore, the knowledge and skill in various aspects of endodontics are required to achieve successful outcome of endodontic treatment. Incorrect diagnosis and treatment may cause aggravation of the situation. One must have knowledge of pain mechanism, patient management, diagnosis and appropriate treatment measures for both hard and soft tissues. The emergencies are matter of great concern to the both patient and dentists. Emergencies can occur with varying frequencies of pain and swelling in patients before, during and after the root canal treatment. These emergencies are result of combination of various factors which induce severe inflammation in pulp and periapical tissues. The irritation of periradicular tissues result in inflammation and the release of various chemical mediators which initiate inflammation. The pain in endodontic emergencies is mainly related to two factors, chemical mediators and pressure.

*Chemical mediators* cause pain directly by lowering the pain threshold of sensory nerve fibers or by increasing vascular permeability and producing edema.

Increased fluid *pressure* resulting from edema directly stimulates the pain receptors.

In this chapter, we will discuss the diagnosis and treatment of various conditions requiring emergency endodontic treatment.

*Endodontic emergency* is defined as the condition associated with pain and/or swelling which requires immediate diagnosis and treatment. The main *causative factors* responsible for occurrence of endodontic emergencies are:

1. Pathosis in pulp and periradicular tissues
2. Traumatic injuries

**Endodontic emergencies are categorized into three main types**

1. Pretreatment
2. Intra-appointment
3. Postobturation

In pretreatment emergencies, patient initially comes with pain and swelling, while intra-appointment and postobturation emergencies occur during or after the initiation of endodontic therapy. Before managing endodontic emergency, one should differentiate a true emergency and a less critical urgency. A ***true emergency*** is the condition which requires unscheduled visit with diagnosis and treatment at that time. But ***less critical urgency*** indicates a less severe problem in which next visit may be scheduled for mutual convenience of both patient as well as the dentist. These conditions can be differentiated by a system of diagnosis.

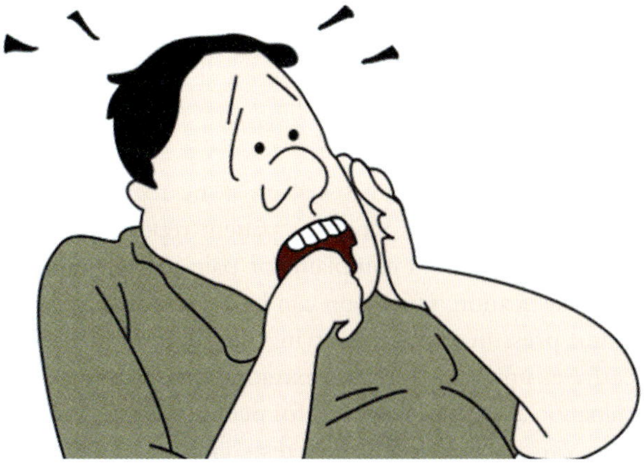

**Fig. 21.1:** Patient in endodontic emergency presents lot of anxiety and apprehension

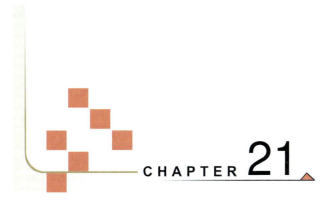

## DIAGNOSIS AND TREATMENT PLANNING

Complete history of the patient along with clinical examination are the two basic steps for successful management of endodontic emergencies. The patient should be asked about the pain, swelling or any other symptom associated with emergency.

The clinician should follow a systematic approach to reach at accurate diagnosis. Certain factors like emotional status of the patient, stress of the clinician and shortage of time, should not affect an orderly approach.

### History of the Patient

Most common component in chief complaint of emergency patient is pain. The initial question should help establish ***two basic components*** of pain; ***time (chronicity)*** and ***severity (intensity).*** The patient should be asked questions such as "How painful the tooth is?", "When does it hurt?" "What makes it worse?", etc. A complete history regarding the pain chronology, i.e. mode, periodicity, frequency and duration, pain quality, i.e. sharp, dull, recurrent stabbing, throbbing should be taken.

Pain is a complex, physiological and psychological phenomenon. The psychological components of pain perception and pain reaction comprise emotional and symbolic factors. The emotional status and anxiety level alter the pain reaction threshold. Thus, for accurate history and to receive cooperation during treatment, the anxiety of patient should be reduced. It can be done by gaining the confidence of the patient, providing attention and sympathy and treating the patient as an important individual. Thus, we can say that psychological management of the patient is the most important factor in emergency treatment. After the patient has provided complete history regarding his or her problem, both subjective questioning and objective examination are performed carefully.

### Subjective Examination

A patient should be asked questions about history, location, duration, severity and aggravating factors of pain. For example, if pain occurs on mastication or when teeth are in occlusion and is localized in nature, it is ***periodontal in origin*** but if thermal stimuli lead to severe explosive pain and the patient is unable to localize, it is ***pulpal in origin***. Basically quality, quantity, intensity, spontaneity and duration of pain should be asked. A tentative diagnosis achieved by means of thorough subjective examination, is confirmed by objective tests and radiographic findings.

### Objective Examination

In objective examination, tests are done to reproduce the response which mimics what the patient reports subjectively. For example, if patient complains of pain to thermal changes and on mastication, same pain can be reproduced by applying cold and pressure, thus identifying the offending tooth. The objective examination includes extraoral examination, intraoral examination and diagnostic tests for periradicular as well as pulp tissues. Various pulp evaluating tests are:

- Thermal tests which include heat and cold test.
- Electric pulp test.
- Direct dentin stimulation.

*The tests done for evaluation of periradicular status include:*

- Periodontal Probing
- Palpation over the apex
- To check the mobility of tooth
- Selective biting on an object

### Radiographic Examination

Radiographs are helpful but have many limitations. Though it is impossible to obtain good information without the use of radiograph but one needs to have excellent quality films for correct interpretation. Also one should not become totally dependent on radiographs. It is mandatory that other tests should be used in conjunction with radiographs. Intraoral periapical and bitewing radiographs may detect caries, restorations, pulp exposures, root resorption-external or internal and periradicular pathologies.

So, we can see that by following the system of diagnosis as mentioned above, the offending tooth and the tissue, i.e. pulpal or periradicular can be identified. If diagnosis is not clear to a general practitioner, the patient should be referred. No treatment is initiated without clear diagnosis.

**Common features of oral pain**

| *Origin* | *Associated sign* | *Useful test* | *Radiograph* |
|---|---|---|---|
| **Pulp** | Deep caries, previous treatment, extensive restoration | Heat or cold test | Caries, extensive restoration |
| **Periradicular tissue** | Swelling, redness, tooth mobility | Percussion palpation probing | Caries, sometimes and periradicular signs |
| **Dentin** | Caries, defective restoration | Hot, cold test, scratching | Caries, poor restorations |
| **Gingiva** | Gingival inflammation | Percussion, visual examination | None |

### Classification of Endodontic Emergencies (According to P Carrotte)

A. Pretreatment
   1. Dentin hypersensitivity
   2. Pain of pulpal origin
      a. Reversible pulpitis
      b. Irreversible pulpitis
   3. Acute apical periodontitis
   4. Acute periapical abscess
   5. Traumatic injury
   6. Cracked tooth syndrome

B. Patients under treatment
   1. Mid treatment flare-ups
   2. Exposure of pulp
   3. Fracture of tooth
   4. Recently placed restoration
   5. Periodontal treatment

C. Post endodontic treatment
   1. Overinstrumentation
   2. Overextended filling

3. Underfilling
4. Fracture of root
5. High restoration

## PRETREATMENT ENDODONTIC EMERGENCIES

***Hot tooth*** refers to a painful tooth and initial therapy for hot tooth refers to what needs to be done to give relief from pain at first appointment for tooth with pulpal or periapical involvement.

Before treatment is given, diagnosis is made, that is whether pain is of odontogenic or nonodontogenic origin. The odontogenic pain can originate from pulp and periradicular tissues while the nonodontogenic pain can result from abnormal neural structures, maxillary sinus, psychogenic or neurovascular structures.

Pulpal pain can be diagnosed by mainly two ways:

a. Clinical findings
b. Histological findings

The aim of clinical diagnosis is to interpret which tooth is responsible for pain and also idea about the histological status of the pulp. Periradicular pain usually results due to extension of pulpal diseases into the surrounding periradicular area. The pain of periradicular origin seems to present little diagnostic challenge as proprioceptors present in the periodontal ligament give exact clue about the location of pressure stimuli. Sometimes periradicular pain may be associated with acute apical periodontitis or acute periradicular abscess.

Before coming to final diagnosis, three clinical determinations are required prior to the initiation of endodontic therapy:

1. Presence or absence of pulp vitality.
2. Presence or absence of pain on percussion.
3. Radiographic evaluation.

The ***patient management*** is the most critical factor which affects the prognosis of treatment. An anxious and frightened patient may lose confidence in clinician and may even assume that extraction is necessary. So, reassurance is the most important aspect of the treatment.

To ***obtain an adequate anesthesia*** of inflamed tissues is the challenge. To provide adequate pulpal anesthesia in the mandible, inferior alveolar, lingual and long buccal injection should be preferred. If anesthesia is required in the lower premolars, canine and incisor, then other alternative such as mental nerve block, periodontal ligament injection (Fig. 21.2), intraosseous anesthesia and intrapulpal injection (Fig. 21.3) are given in painful irreversible pulpitis along with classical nerve block. In contrast to mandible, maxillary anesthesia is easier to obtain by giving infiltration or block injections in the buccal or palatal region. These include posterior superior alveolar (PSA), middle superior alveolar (MSA) and infraorbital nerve block.

## CONDITIONS REQUIRING EMERGENCY ENDODONTIC TREATMENT

1. ***Dentin Hypersensitivity:***
   - Dentin hypersensitivity is defined as "sharp, short pain arising from exposed dentin in response to stimuli typically thermal, chemical, tactile or osmotic and which cannot be ascribed to any other form of dental defect or pathology.
   - The primary underlying cause for dentin hypersensitivity is exposed dentin tubules. Dentin may become exposed by two processes; either by loss of covering periodontal structures (gingival recession), or by loss of enamel.
   - *Two main treatment options* are plug the dentinal tubules preventing the fluid flow and desensitize the nerve, making it less responsive to stimulation.
2. ***Cracked tooth syndrome:***
   - *The crack tooth syndrome means incomplete fracture of a tooth with vital pulp.* The fracture commonly involves enamel and dentin but sometimes pulp and periodontal structure may also get involved (Fig. 21.4).

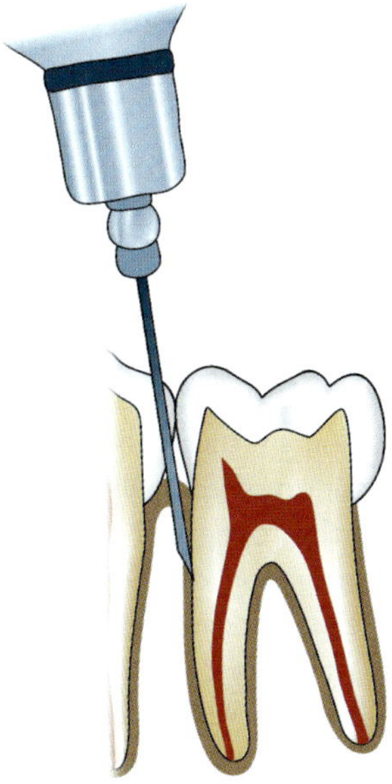

Fig. 21.2: Intraligamentary injection

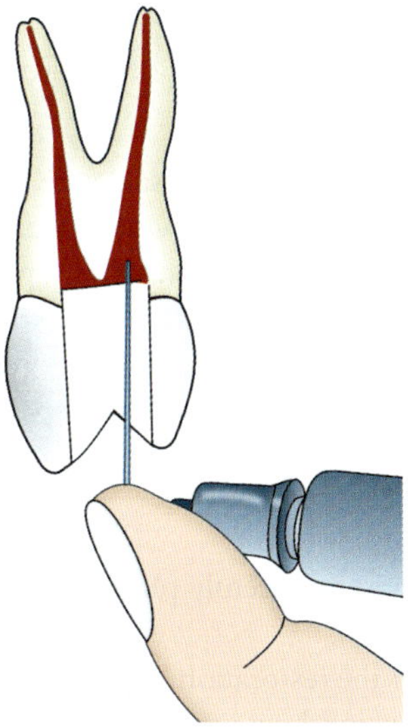

Fig. 21.3: Intrapulpal injection

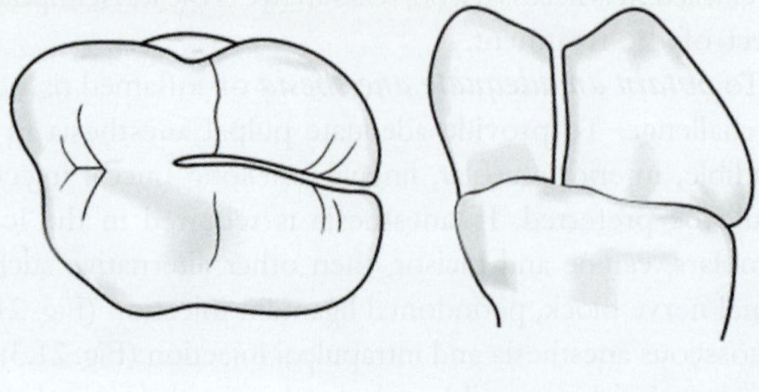

Fig. 21.4: Cracked tooth

- It is commonly seen to be associated in teeth with large and complex restorations.
- Crack tooth can be diagnosed by taking proper history of the patient which includes detailed history regarding dietary and parafunctional habits and any previous trauma.
- During tactile examination, pass the tip of sharp explorer gently along the tooth surface, so as to locate the crack by catch.
- Patient can be asked to bite on Orangewood stick, rubber wheel or the tooth sloth. The pain during biting or chewing especially upon the release of pressure is classic sign of cracked tooth syndrome.

## Treatment

**Urgent care** of the cracked tooth involves the immediate reduction of its occlusal contacts by selective grinding of tooth at the site of the crack or its antagonist.

## Definitive Treatment

Definitive treatment of the cracked tooth aims to preserve the pulpal vitality by providing full occlusal coverage for cusp protection.

- Full coverage crown if fracture involves crown portion only.
- If fracture involves root canal system. Which is superficial to alveolar crest, go endodontic treatment and restoration of tooth.
- If fracture of root extends below alveolar crest extract the tooth.

3. ***Acute reversible pulpitis:*** Acute reversible pulpitis is characterized by the following features:
   1. Localized inflammation of the pulp.
   2. Lowering of threshold stimulation for A-delta nerve fibers.
   3. Exaggerated, non-lingering response to stimuli.

## Management

1. Removal of the cause.
2. Recontouring of recently placed restoration which causes pain.
3. Removal of the restoration and replacing it with the sedative dressing if painful symptoms still persist following the tooth preparation.
4. Relieving the occlusion.

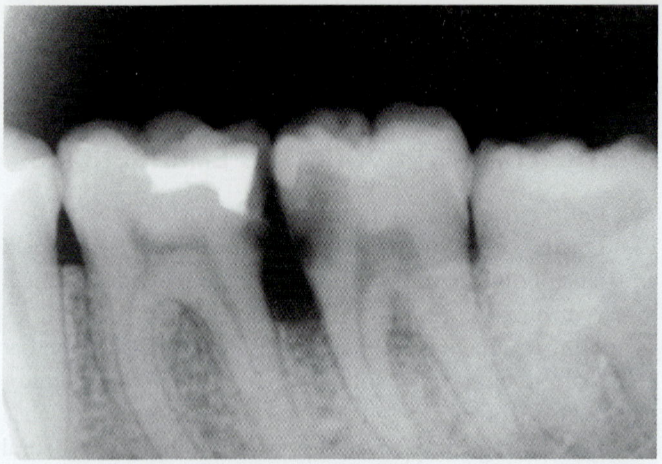

Fig. 21.5: Radiograph showing deep caries resulting in pulpitis and acute pain in patient

4. ***Acute irreversible pulpitis (Fig. 21.5):*** If the inflammatory process progresses, irreversible pulpitis can develop. It is characterized by following:
   1. Presence of inflammatory mediators lowers the threshold of stimulation for all intrapulpal nerves.
   2. History of spontaneous pain and exaggerated response to hot or cold that lingers after the stimulus is removed.
   3. Extensive restoration or caries may be seen in the involved tooth.
   4. Lingering pain occurs after thermal stimulation of A-delta nerve fibers while spontaneous dull, aching pain occurs by stimulation of unmyelinated C-fibers in the pulp.
   5. Mediators of inflammation (bradykinin) directly stimulate the fibers.
   6. Tooth may be responsive to electrical and thermal tests.

In certain cases of irreversible pulpitis, the patient may arrive at the dental clinic sipping a glass of ice water or applying ice to affected area. In these cases, cold actually alleviates the patient's pain removal of the cold causes return of symptoms and can be used as a diagnostic test.

## Management

1. Profound anesthesia of the affected tooth.
2. Application of the rubber dam.
3. Preparation of the access cavity.
4. Extirpation of the pulp from the chamber (Fig. 21.6).
5. Thorough irrigation and debridement of the pulp chamber.
6. Determination of the working length.
7. Total extirpation of the pulp followed by cleaning and shaping of the root canal (Fig. 21.7).
8. Thorough irrigation of the root canal system.
9. Drying of the root canal with sterile absorbent points.
10. Placement of a dry cotton pellet or pellet moistened with CMCP, formocresol or eugenol in the pulp chamber and sealing it with the temporary restoration (Fig. 21.8).
11. Relief of the occlusion.
12. Appropriate analgesics therapy and antibiotics, if needed.

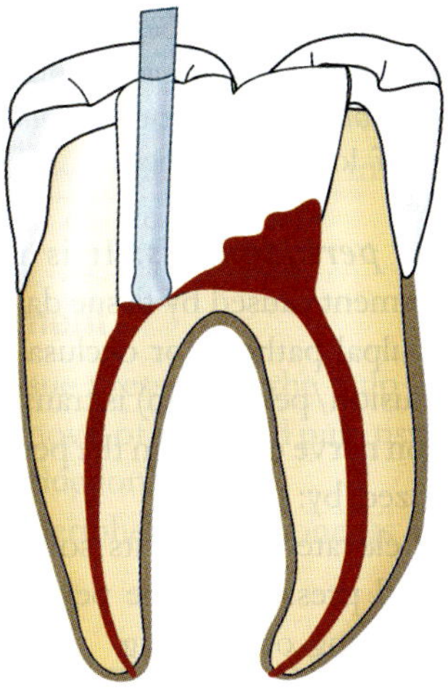

Fig. 21.6: Extirpation of pulp chamber

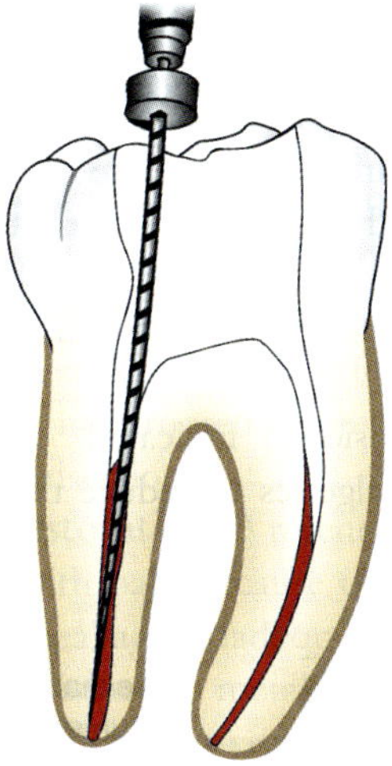

Fig. 21.7: Cleaning and shaping of the root canal

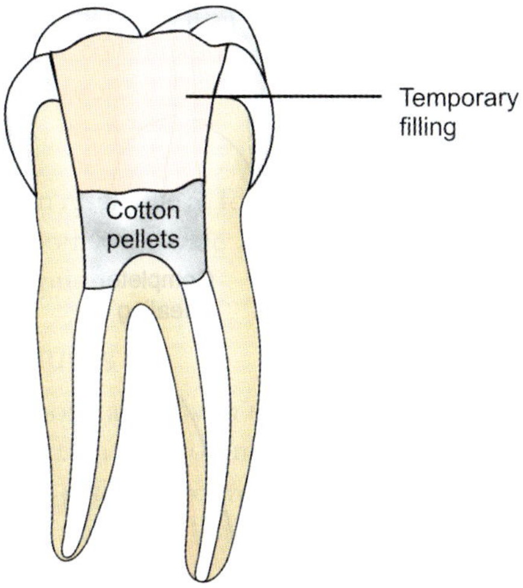


Fig. 21.8: Placement of sedative dressing

5. ***Acute periapical abscess:*** Formation of a periapical abscess implies the breakdown of body's immune system because it should have been able to contain the microbes inside the root canal system. Large numbers of bacteria get past the apex into the periradicular tissues (Fig. 21.9) resulting in local collection of purulent exudates.

   Acute periapical abscess is characterized by following features:

- Clinically, swelling to various degrees is present along with pain and a feeling that tooth is elevated in the socket.
- May not have radiographic evidence of bone destruction because fluids are rapidly spread away from the tooth.
- Systemic features such as fever and malaise may also be present.
- Mobility may or may not be present.

## Management

1. Biphasic treatment:
   a. Pulp debridement (Fig. 21.10)
   b. Incision and drainage (Fig. 21.11)

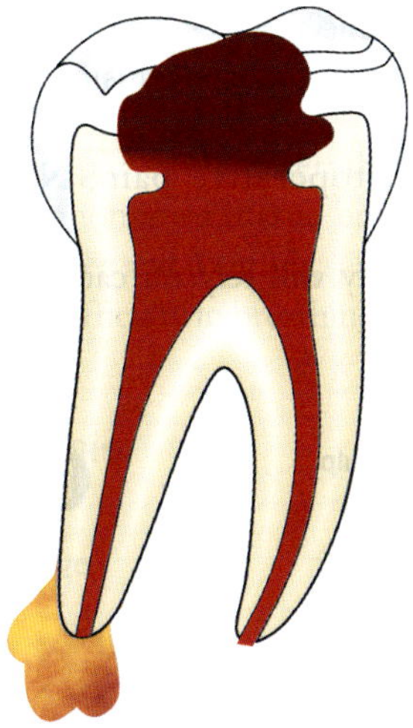

Fig. 21.9: Periapical abscess resulting from tooth decay

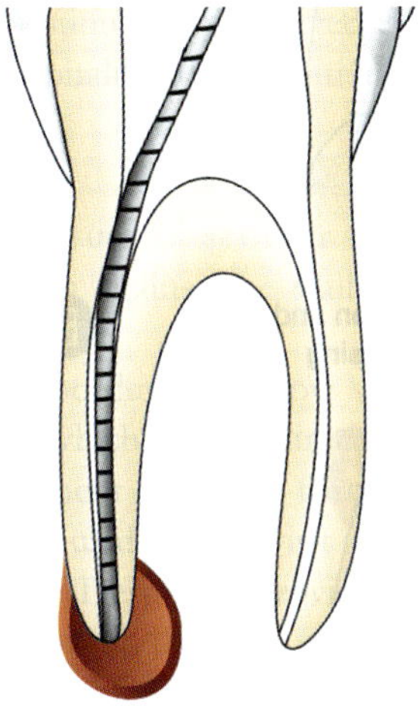

Fig. 21.10: Opening of root canal system for drainage

## To Summarize, Etiology of Mid Treatment Flare-ups

1. Overinstrumentation (Fig. 21.13)
2. Inadequate debridement (Fig. 21.14)
3. Missed canal
4. Hyperocclusion
5. Debris extrusion
6. Procedural complications (Figs 21.15 to 21.17).

## Risk Factors Contributing Inter Appointment Flare-ups

1. Preoperative pain, percussion, sensitivity and swelling.
2. One visit endodontics in cases of acute apical periodontitis.
3. Retreatment
4. Apprehension
5. History of allergies

## Prevention

1. Psychological preparation of the patient.
2. Long acting anesthetics such as Bupivacaine should be preferred.
3. Complete cleaning and shaping of the root canal.
4. Analgesics should be prescribed for relief of pain.

## Treatment

1. Reassure patients.
2. Adjust occlusion if tooth is out of occlusion.
3. Complete debridement along with cleaning and shaping of the root canal system.
4. Analgesics should be given.
5. Antibiotics if required should be given.
6. Never leave the tooth open for drainage.
7. Recall the patient until the painful symptoms subside.

## POSTOBTURATION EMERGENCIES

Following completion of root canal treatment, patients usually complain of pain especially on biting and chewing. Incidence of pain after root canal filling is small and number of visits

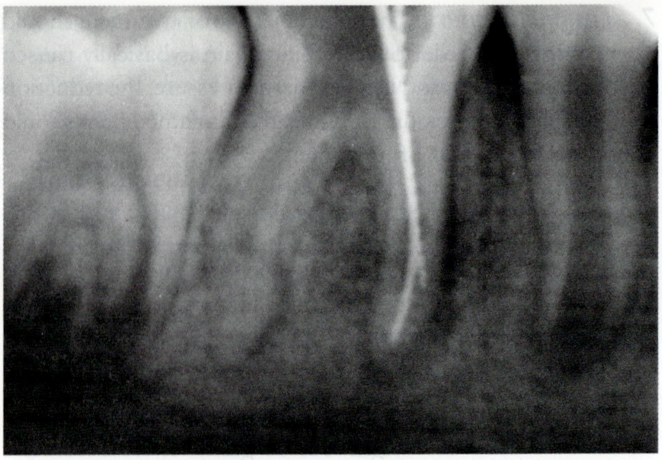

Fig. 21.15: Ledge formed in mesiobuccal canal of 36

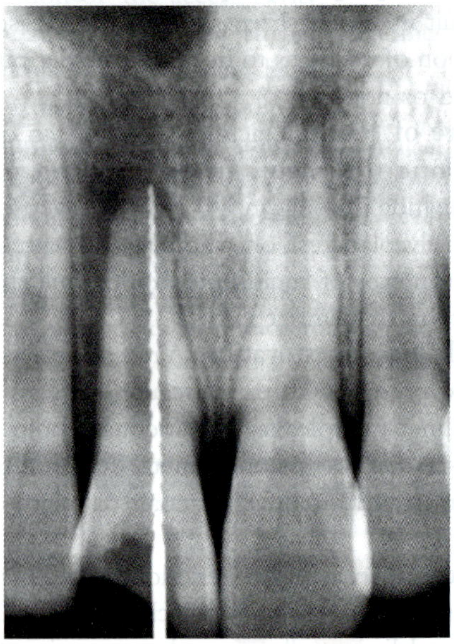

Fig. 21.16: Apical perforation in 11

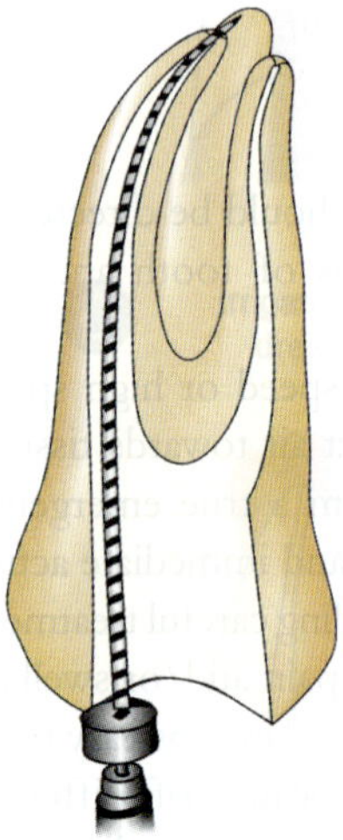

Fig. 21.13: Over-instrumentation

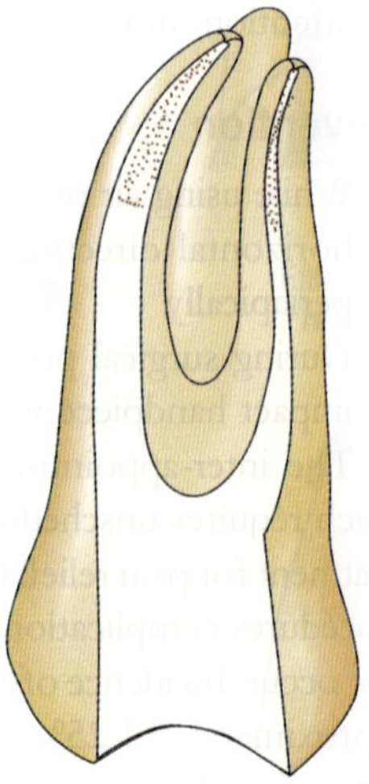

Fig. 21.14: Inadequate debridement

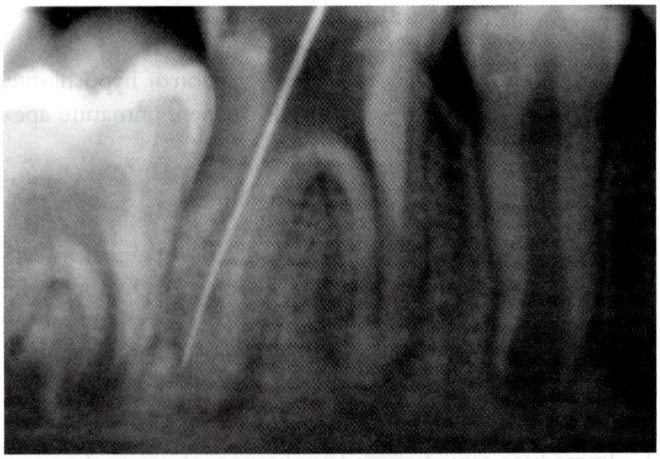

Fig. 21.17: Perforation in distal canal of 36

does not make much difference. There are more chances of experiencing postoperative discomfort when pain is present preoperatively. Also the endodontic treatment of posterior teeth seems to produce more postoperative discomfort. The painful episodes are usually caused by pressure exerted by insertion of root canal filling materials or by chemical irritation from ingredients of root canal cements and pastes.

Various factors resulting in postobturation pain can be enlisted as following:

**Overinstrumentation** is directly proportional to post operative pain. If care of working length is not properly taken overobturation or overfilling may result.

**Overextended obturation** leads to pain. Periapical inflammation results in firing of proprioceptive nerve fibers in the periodontal ligament. These results are short lived and abate in 24-48 hours. No treatment is usually necessary in these cases.

**Persistent pain:** Persistence of pain or sensitivity for longer periods may indicate ***failure of resolution of inflammation***. In rare cases, inflamed but ***viable pulp tissue may be left in root canal*** (Fig. 21.18). Retreatment is then indicated in such cases.

## Vertical Root Fracture (VRF)

Vertical fracture of crown and/or root (Fig. 21.19) can occur:
- During obturation due to wedging forces of spreader or plugger
- During post placement of structurally weakened endodontically treated tooth.
- Due to fracture of coronal restoration because of lack of ferrule effect on remaining root structure.

**Diagnosis:** Periodontal probing may reveal single isolated narrow pocket adjacent to fracture site. Radiograph may show lateral diffuse widening of periodontal ligament.

Surgical exposure of tooth may reveal vertical root fracture.

**Management:** Prognosis of VRF is poor and tooth generally undergoes extraction.

**High restoration:** It is managed by selective occlusal grinding.

**Etiology**
- Overinstrumentation
- Overfilling
- Persistent pain
- Fracture of root
- Hyperocclusion
- Poor coronal seal

## Treatment

Most of the times there is some discomfort following obturation which subsides in two to five days. To manage postobturation endodontic emergencies following can be done:
- Reassurance of the patient
- Prescribe analgesics
- Check occlusion
- Do not retreat randomly. Retreatment is done only in cases of persistent untreatable problems.

Reassurance of the patient is first and foremost step in the treatment of endodontic emergency to control the patient anxiety and overreaction. Retreatment is indicated when prior treatment has been inadequate. Sometimes the patient reports severe pain but there is no evidence of acute apical abscess, and the root canal treatment has been well done. These patients are treated with reassurance and analgesics, again the symptoms subside spontaneously. But if acute apical abscess develops with inadequate root canal treatment, apical surgery may be needed.

## Various Analgesics Used in Endodontic Emergencies

- Mild pain
  - Aspirin 325 mg
  - Ibuprofen 200-400 mg
  - Paracetamol 600-1000 mg

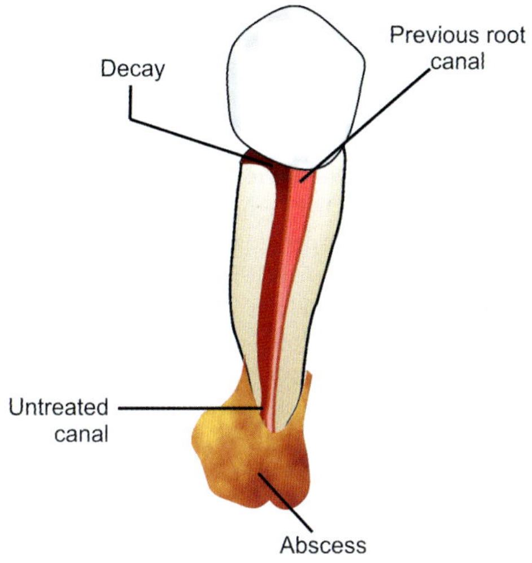


**Fig. 21.18:** Inadequate root canal treatment

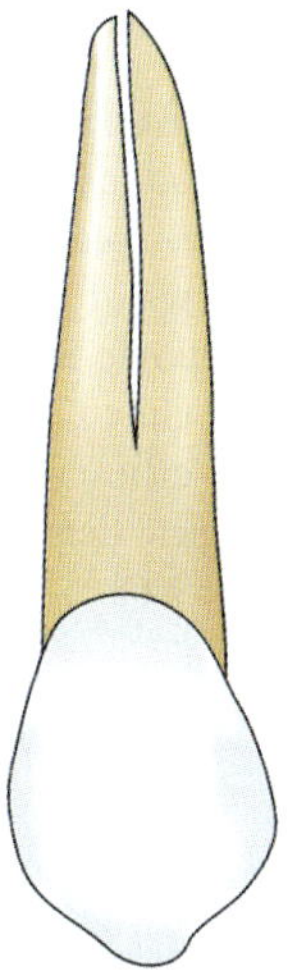

**Fig. 21.19:** Vertical root fracture

- Moderate pain
  - NSAIDs maximum effective dose.
  - Ibuprofen 400-600 mg.
- Severe pain
  - NSAIDs combined with narcotics
  - Ibuprofen 600-800 mg and Codeine 60 mg.

## QUESTIONS

**Q. Define and classify endodontic emergencies.**

**Q. What are pretreatment endodontic emergencies. Discuss their management?**

**Q. Enumerate postobturation emergencies?**

## BIBLIOGRAPHY


1. A Prospective randomized trail on efficacy of antibiotic prophylaxis in asymptomatic teeth with pulpal necrosis and associated periapical pathosis. Oral Surg Oral Med Oral Pathol 1988;66(6):722-33.
2. August D5. Managing the abscessed open tooth instrument and close:Part 2, J Endod 1982;8:364.
3. Auslander WP. The acute apical abscess. NY State Dent J 1970;36: 623.
4. Balaban FS, Skidmore AE, Griffin JA. Acute exacerbations following initial treatment of necrotic pulps. J Endod 1984;10:78.
5. Chestner SB, Selman AJ, Friedman J, Heyman RA. Apical Fenestration: Solution to recalcitrant pain in root canal therapy. J Am Dent Assoc 1968;77:846.
6. Deblanco LP. Treatment of crown fractures with pulp Exposure. Oral Surg Pra Med Oral Pathol Radiol 1996;82:564.
7. DeVore DT. Legal considerations for treatment following trauma to teeth. Dent Clin N Am 1995;39:203.
8. Dummer PH, Hicks R, Huws D. Clinical signs and symptoms in pulp disease. Int Endod J 1980;13:27-35.
9. Ehrmann GH. The effect of triamcinolone with tetracycline on the dental pulp and apical periodontium. J Prosthet Dent 1965;15:149.
10. Elliott JA, Holcomb JB. Evaluation of a minimally traumatic alveolar trephination procedure to avoid pain. J Endod 1988;14(8):405-07.
11. Fazakerley MW, McGowan P, Hardy P, Martin MV. A comparative study of Cephradine, amoxicillin and phenoxymethylpenicillin in the treatment of acute dentoalveolar infection. Br. Dent J 1993;174(10):359-63.
12. Garfunkel A, Sela J, Ulmansky M. Dental pulp pathosis; Clinico-pathological correlations based on 109 cases. Oral Surg 1973;35: 110-17.
13. Genet JM, et al. Preoperative and operative factors associated with pain after the first endodontic visit. Int Endod J 1987;20:53.
14. Gill Y, Scully C. The microbiology and management of acute dentoalveolar abscess: Views of British Oral and maxillofacial surgeons. Br J Oral Maxillofac Surg 1988;26(6):452-57.
15. Habib S, Matthews RW, Scully C, Levers BG, Shepherd JP. A study of the comparative efficacy of four common analgesics in the control of postsurgical dental pain. Oral Surg Oral Med Oral Pathol 1990;70(5):559-63.
16. Hargreaves KM. Case 5, refractory toothache. K Endod 1998;24:699.
17. Harrington GW, Natkin E. Midtreatment flare-ups. Dent Clin North AM 1992;36:409-23.
18. Harrison JW, Bellizzi R, Osetek EM. The clinical toxicity of endodontic medicaments. J Endod 1979;5:42.
19. Jackson DL, Moore PA, Hargreaves KM. Preoperative nonsteroidal anti-inflammatory medication for the prevention of postoperative dental pain. I Am Dent Assoc 1989; 119(5):641-47.
20. Krishnan V, Johnson JV, Helfrick JF. Management of maxillofacial infections: A review of 50 cases. J Oral Maxillofac Surg 1993;51(8):868-73; discussion 873-74.
21. Marshall JG, Liesinger Aw. Factors associated with endodontic posttreatment pain. J Endod 1993; 19(11):573-75.
22. Mehlisch DR, Sollecity WA, Helfrick JF, Leibold DG, Markowitz R, Schow CE Jr, et al. Multicenter clinical trial of ibuprofen and acetaminophen in the treatment of postoperative of dental pain. Jam Dent Assoc 1990;121(2):257-63.
23. Mitchell DF, Tarplee RE. Painful pulpitis: A clinical and microscopic study. Oral Surg 1960;13:1360.
24. Naidorf IJ. Endodontic flare-ups: Bacteriological and immunological mechanisms. J Endod 1985;11:462.
25. Nakamura Y, Hirayama K, Hossain M, Matsumoto K. A case of an odontogenic cutaneous sinus tract. Int Endod J 1999;32(4):328-31.
26. Sac-Lim V, Yuen KW. An evaluation of after-office hour dental trauma in Singapore. Endod Dent Traumatol 1997;13:164.
27. Schuen NJ, Panzer JD, Atkinson WH. A comparison of clindamycin and penicillin V in the treatment of oral infections. J Oral Surg 1974;32(7):503-05.
28. Selden HS. Pain Empowerment—a strategy for pain management in endodontics. J Endod 1993;19:521.
29. Seltzer S, Bender IB, Zionitz M. The dynamics of pulp inflammation: Correlation between diagnostic data and histologic findings in the pulp. Oral Surg 1963;16:846-71, 969-77
30. Seltzer S, Naidorf IJ. Flare-ups in endodontics II. Therapeutic measures. J Endod 1985;11:472.
31. Seltzer S, Naiorf IJ. Flare-ups in endodontics. Etiological factors. J Endod 1985;11:472.
32. Torabinejad M, Cymerman JJ, Frankson M, Lemon RR, Maggio JD, Schilder H. Effectiveness of various medications on postoperative pain following complete instrumentation. J Endod 1994;20(7):345-54.
33. Walton R, Fouad A. Endodontic interappointment flare-ups: A prospective study of incidence and related factors. J Endod 1992.18:172.
34. Walton RE, Chiappinelli J. Prophylactic penicillin: Effect on post-treatment symptoms following root canal treatment of asymptomatic periapical pathosis. J Endod 1993;19(9):466-70.
35. Watts A, Patterson RC. The response of the mechanically exposed pulp to prednisolone and triamcinolone acetonide. Int Endod J 1988;21:16.
36. Woods R. Diagnosis and antibiotic treatment of alveolar infections in dentistry. Int Dent J 1981;31(2):145-51.

# Procedural Accidents

CHAPTER 22



## INTRODUCTION

Like any other field of dentistry, a clinician may face unwanted situations during the root canal treatment which can affect the prognosis of endodontic therapy. These procedural accidents are collectively termed as ***endodontic mishaps.***

Accurate diagnosis, proper case selection, and adherence to basic principles of endodontic therapy may prevent occurrence of procedural accidents. Whenever any endodontic mishap occurs; inform the patient about—

a. The incident and nature of mishap
b. Procedures to correct it
c. Alternative treatment options
d. Prognosis of the affected tooth.

Endodontic mishaps may have dentolegal consequences. Thus, their prevention is the best option both for patient as well as dentist. Knowledge of etiological factors involved in endodontic mishaps is mandatory for their prevention. Recognition of a procedural accident is first step in its management.

Procedural accidents can occur at any stage of the root canal treatments which may lead to endodontic failures.

## VARIOUS PROCEDURAL ACCIDENTS

Grossly we can categorize the procedural errors as following:

1. Inadequately cleaned and shaped root canal system.
   a. Loss of working length
   b. Canal blockage
   c. Ledging of canal
   d. Missed canals
2. Instrument separation
3. Deviation from normal canal anatomy
   a. Zipping
   b. Stripping or lateral wall perforation
   c. Canal transportation
4. Inadequate canal preparation
   a. Overinstrumentation
   b. Overpreparation
   c. Under preparation
5. Perforations
   a. Coronal perforations
   b. Root perforations
      i. Cervical canal perforations
      ii. Mid root perforations
      iii. Apical perforations
   c. Post space perforations

*contd...*

*contd...*

6. Obturation related
   a. Over obturation
   b. Under obturation
7. Vertical root fracture
8. Instrument aspiration

## INADEQUATELY CLEANED AND SHAPED ROOT CANAL SYSTEM

Regardless of the instrumentation technique used for cleaning and shaping of the root canal system, the main objectives of biomechanical preparation are to remove pulp tissue, debris and bacteria, as well as to shape the canal for obturation (Fig. 22.1).

As with access opening preparations, failure to pay close attention to detail during canal cleaning and shaping will result in violation of the principles of biomechanical canal preparation. These procedural errors and their sequelae can adversely affect the prognosis of treatment. The errors that most often occur during canal preparation include:

1. Loss of working length
2. Deviations from normal canal anatomy
3. Inadequate canal preparation
4. Perforations

## LOSS OF WORKING LENGTH

Loss of working length during cleaning and shaping is a common procedural error. The problem may be noted only on the master cone radiograph or when the master apical file is short of established working length (Fig. 22.2).

*Etiology*

- Secondary to other endodontic procedural errors, like blockages, formation of ledges and fractured instruments.
- Rapid increase in the file size.
- Accumulation of dentinal debris in the apical third of the canal (Fig. 22.3). Preventive measures include frequent irrigation with NaOCl, recapitulation and periodic radiographic verification of working length (Fig. 22.4).

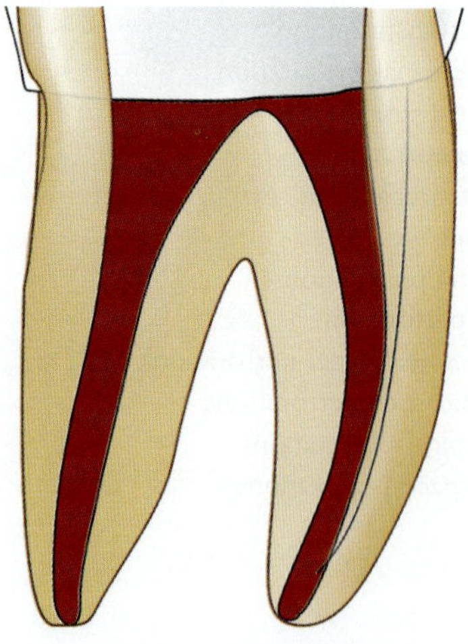

**Fig. 22.1:** Complete cleaning and shaping of root canal system

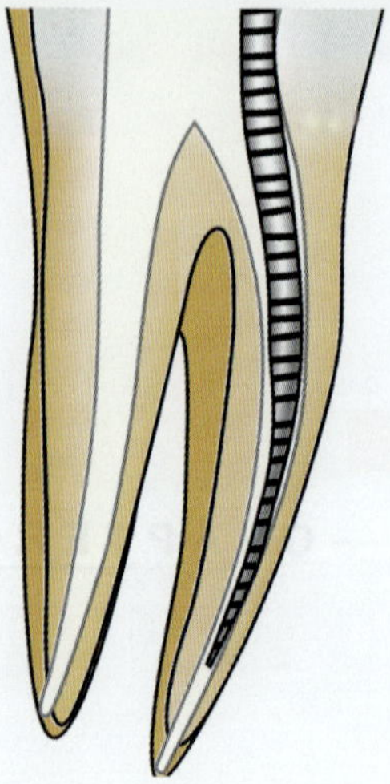

**Fig. 22.2:** Master apical file short of working length

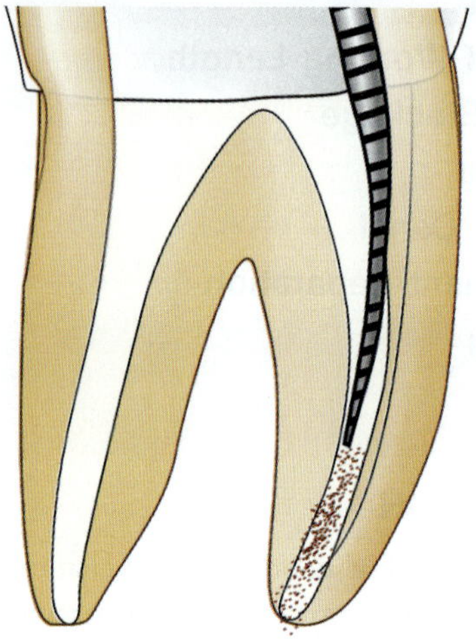

**Fig. 22.3:** Accumulation of dentinal debris in apical third because of loss of working length

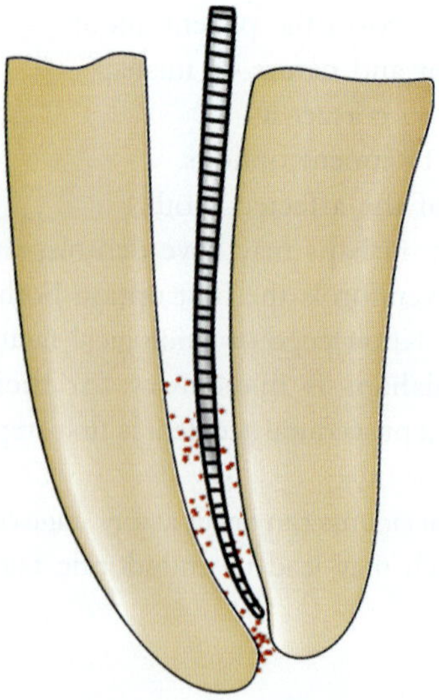

**Fig. 22.4:** Recapitulation

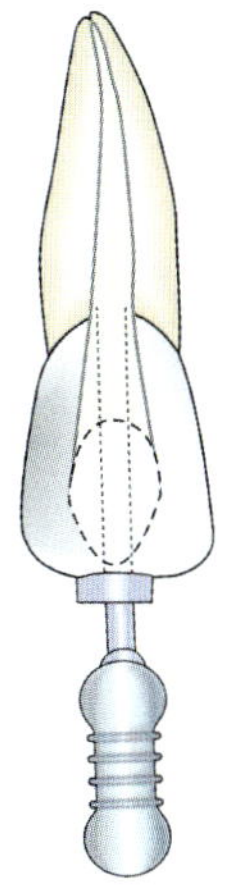

Fig. 22.5: Use of sound reference point

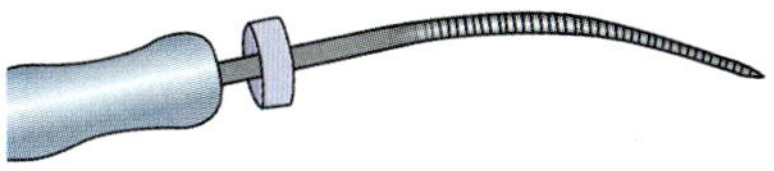

Fig. 22.6: Precuring of a file

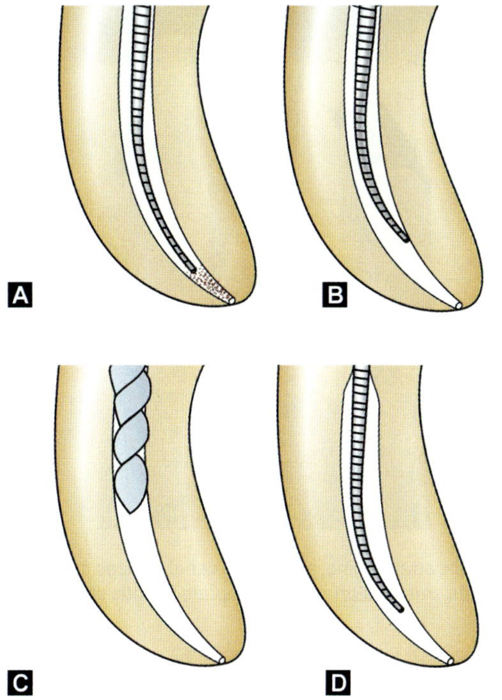


Figs 22.7A to D: Reasons why file does not reach to full working length (A) Dentin chips (B) Wrong angulation of instrument (C) Larger instrument than canal diameter (D) Restriction to instrument making it short of apex

- Lack of attention to details, such as malpositioned instrument stops, variations in reference points, poor radiographic technique and improper use of instruments.

To maintain proper working length during canal cleaning and shaping, adherence to the following specific guidelines is recommended:

1. Use sound and reproducible reference points (Fig. 22.5).
2. Precurve all instruments with sterile 2 × 2 inch gauge (Fig. 22.6).
3. Continually observe the instrument stops as they approach the reference points.
4. Directional instrument stops should be used. The direction of the stop must be constantly observed.
5. When verifying the instrument position radiographically, use consistent radiographic angles.
6. Always maintain the original preoperative shape of the canal and clean and shape within these confines.
7. Use copious irrigation and recapitulation throughout cleaning and shaping procedures.
8. Always use sequential file sizes and do not skip sizes.

## CANAL BLOCKAGE

A blockage is obstruction in a previously patent canal system that prevents access to the apical constriction or apical stop.

*Etiology*

- Common causes of canal blockage can be packed dentinal chips, tissue debris, cotton pellets restorative materials or presence of fractured instruments.
- The instrument does not reach to its full working length if it experiences any kind of restriction during its way to canal apex or if tip of the instrument used is wider than the canal diameter (Figs 22.7A to D).
- Blockage is confirmed by taking radiograph which may show that file is not reaching up to its established working length.

### Treatment

- When a blockage occurs, place a small amount of EDTA lubricant on a fine instrument and introduce into the canal. Use a gentle watch winding motion along with copious irrigation of the canal to remove the dentin chips or tissue debris. One should avoid giving the excessive rotation to the instrument as it may cause instrument separation.
- If this doesn't solve the problem, endosonics may be used to dislodge the dentin chips by the action of acoustic streaming.
- Whatever happens don't force the instrument into the blockage as it may further pack the dentinal debris and worsen the condition. Moreover, forcing instruments may cause the perforation of the canal. In some cases, canal can be obturated to the blockage level such as if patient is asymptomatic with no associated endodontic or periodontal problem.

### Prevention

1. Remove all the caries, unsupported tooth structure, restorations before completion of the access cavity preparation (Fig 22.8).
2. Keep the pulp chamber filled with an irrigant during canal preparation (Fig. 22.9).
3. There should be a straight line access to the canal orifices (Fig. 22.10).
4. All temporary restorations around the outline of the access opening must be removed.
5. Copious irrigation must always be done during pulp space debridement and canal cleaning and shaping. Constant flushing and removal of debris reduces the amount of foreign material present in canal system.
6. Intracanal instruments must always be wiped clean before they are inserted into the canal system.
7. Instruments must be used in sequentially order.
8. Recapitulation must be done during instrumentation.

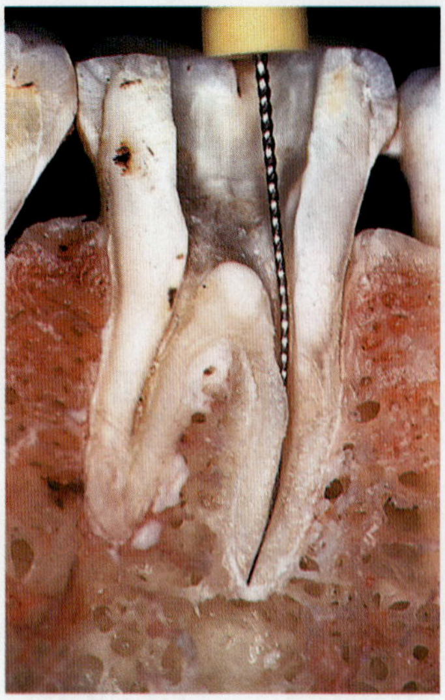

Fig. 22.8: Gain straight line access to canal orifices by removing all caries, restoration and unsupported tooth structure

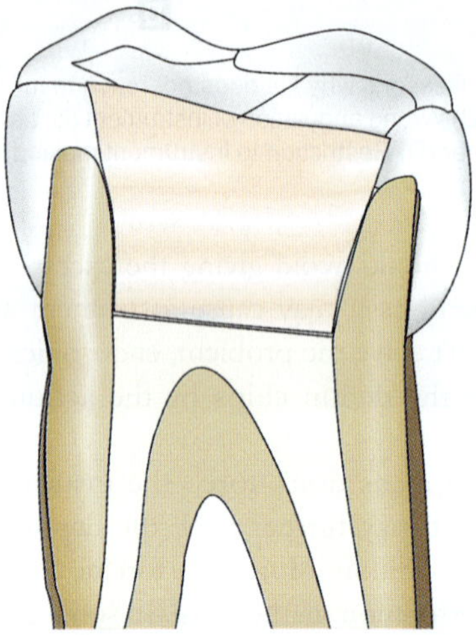

Fig. 22.9: Keep the pulp chamber filled with irrigant during canal preparation

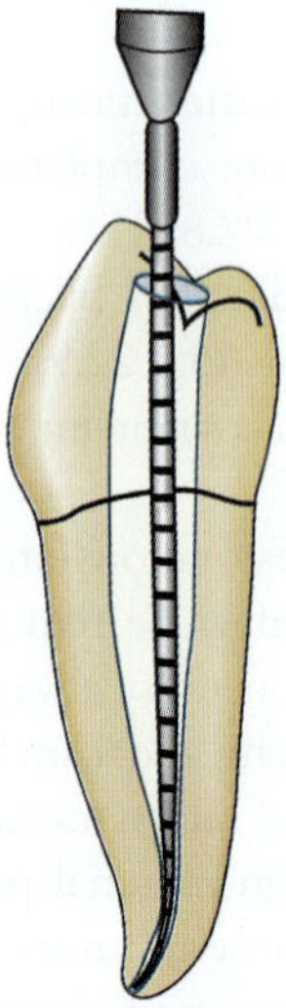

Fig. 22.10: Straight line access to canal orifices

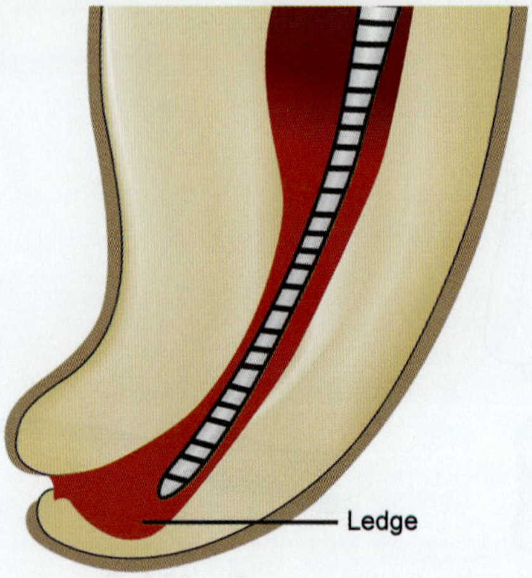


Fig. 22.11: Ledge formation in a curved canal using stiffer files

9. Excessive pressure and rotation of intracanal instruments must be avoided.
10. Never use instruments in a dry canal.
11. Place a sound temporary restoration.

## LEDGING

*Ledge is an internal transportation of the canal which prevents positioning of an instrument to the apex in an otherwise patent canal.*

*Etiology*

- Caused by forcing uncurved instruments apically short of working length in a curved canal (Fig. 22.11).
- Rotating the file at the working length causes deviation from the natural canal pathway, straightening of the canal, and the creation of a ledge in the dentinal wall (Fig 22.12).
- Rapid advancement in file sizes or skipping file sizes.

*Identification of ledge formation*

Ledges occur on the outer wall of the canal curvature. One may get suspicious that ledge has been formed when there is:

- Loss of tactile sensation at the tip of the instrument
- Loose feeling instead of binding at the apex.
- Instrument can no longer reach its estimated working length.
- When in doubt a radiograph of the tooth with the instrument in place is taken to provide additional information.

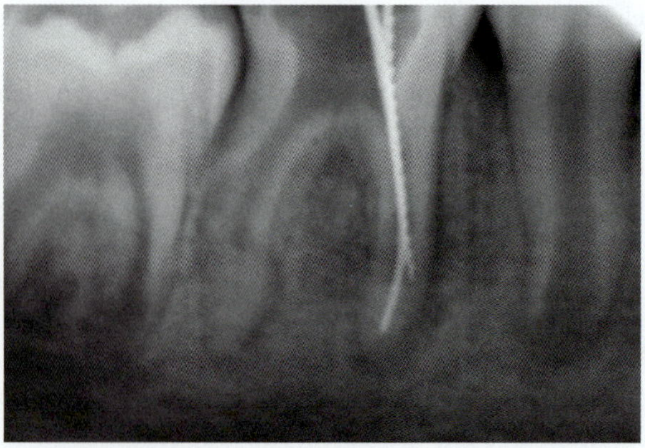

Fig. 22.12: Ledge formation due to use of straight files in curved canal

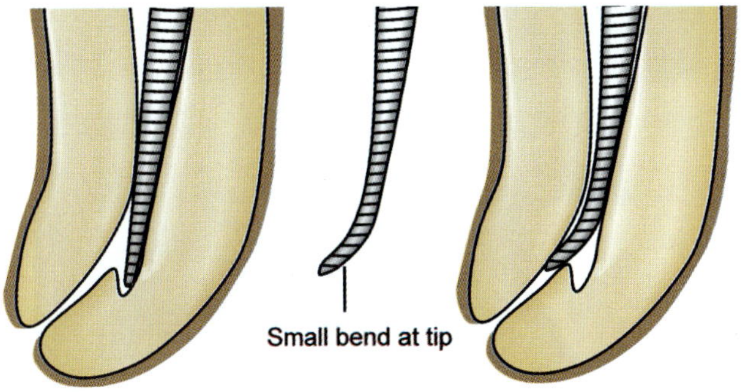


Figs 22.13A and B: A. Formation of ledge by use of stiff instrument in curved canal. B. Correction of ledge; Ledge is bypassed by making a small bend at tip of instrument. Bent instrument is passed along canal wall to locate original canal

### Treatment

To negotiate a ledge, choose a smaller number file, usually No. 10 or 15. Give a small bend at the tip of the instrument (Fig. 22.13) and penetrate the file carefully into the canal. Once the tip of the file is apical to the ledge, it is moved in and out of the canal utilizing ultra short push-pull movements with emphasis on staying apical to the defect. When the file moves freely, it may be turned clockwise upon withdrawal to rasp, reduce, smooth or eliminate the ledge. When the ledge can be predictably bypassed, then efforts are directed towards establishing the apical patency with a No. 10 file. Gently passing 0.02 tapered No. 10 file 1 mm through the foramen ensures its diameter is at least 0.12 mm and makes the way for the No. 15 file. Nowadays, a significant improvement has occurred in ledge management by use of nickel-titanium (NiTi) hand files that exhibit tapers greater than ISO files. Progressively tapered NiTi files can be introduced into the canal when the ledge has been bypassed, the canal negotiated and patency established.

Not all ledges can be removed. Clinicians must weigh risk versus benefit and make every effort to retain maximum amount of remaining dentin.

### Prevention of Ledge Formation

- Use of stainless steel patency files to determine canal curvature.
- Accurate evaluation of radiograph and tooth anatomy.
- Precurving of instruments for curved canals.
- Use of flexible NiTi files.
- Use of safe ended instruments with non cutting tips.
- Use of sequential filing avoid skipping instruments sizes.
- Frequently irrigation and recapitulation during biomechanical preparation.
- Preparation of canals in small increments.

## MISSED CANAL

Sometimes endodontic failure can occur because of untreated missed canals which are store house of tissue, bacteria and other irritants (Figs 22.14A and B). To avoid occurrence of such problem, one should have thorough knowledge of the root canal anatomy.

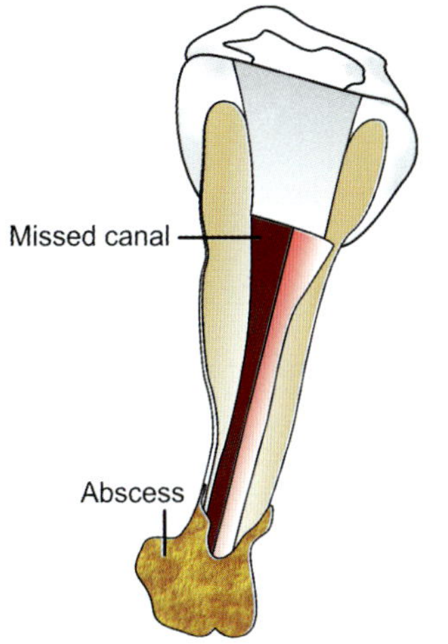


Fig. 22.14A: Missed canal leading to root canal failure

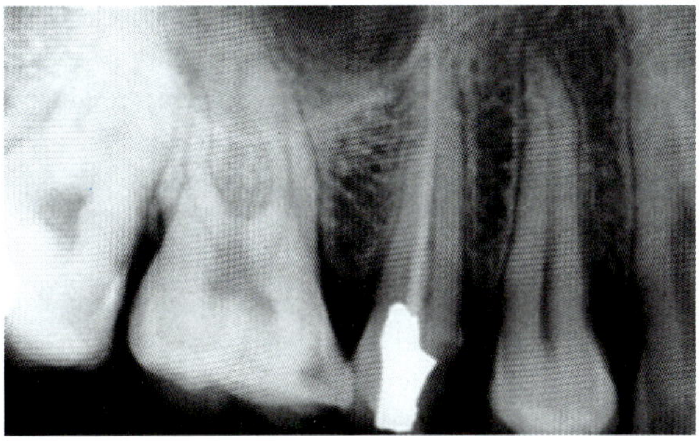

Fig. 22.14B: Radiograph showing missed canal in maxillary second premolar

*Etiology*

1. Lack of thorough knowledge of root canal anatomy along with its variations.
2. Inadequate access cavity preparation.

### Common Sites for Missed Canals

1. During canal exploration, if canal is not centered in the root, one should look for presence of extra canal.
2. There are several teeth which have predisposition for extra canal which might be missed if not explored accurately while treatment. For example:
   - Maxillary premolars may have three canals (mesiobuccal, distobuccal and palatal)
   - Upper first molars usually have four canals
   - Mandibular incisors usually have extra canal
   - Mandibular premolars often have complex root anatomy
   - Mandibular molars may have extra mesial and/or distal canal in some cases.

### Missed Canals can be Located by

1. Taking radiographs.
2. Use of magnifying glasses, endomicroscope.
3. Accurate access cavity preparation.
4. Use of ultrasonics.
5. Use of dyes such as methylene blue.

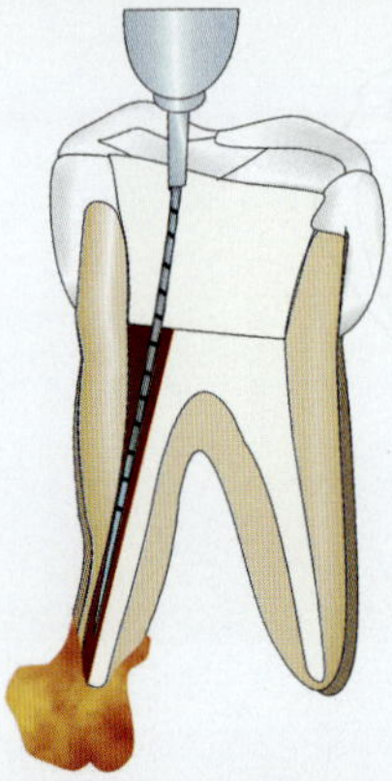

**Fig. 22.15A:** Retreatment of endodontically treated tooth with failure due to poor obturation

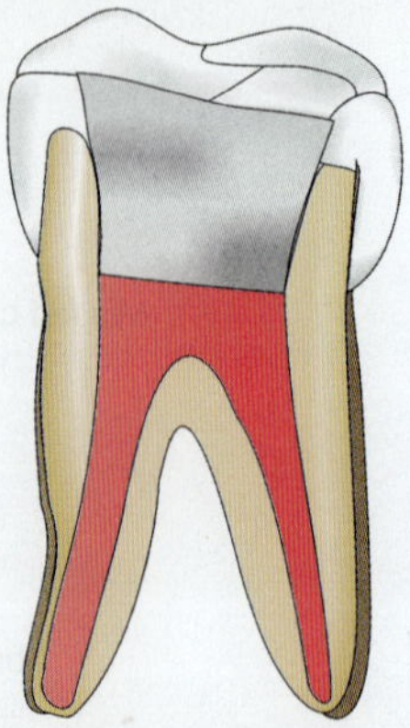

**Fig. 22.15B:** Completion of endodontic retreatment. Three-dimensional obturation of root canal system is main aim of endodontic therapy

6. Use of sodium hypochlorite: After thorough cleaning and shaping, pulp chamber is filled with sodium hypochlorite. If bubbles appear in, it indicates either there is residual tissue present in a missed canal or residual chelator in the prepared canal. This is called as "***Champagne test***".

## Prevention of Missed Canal

1. Good radiographs taken at different horizontal angulations.
2. Good illumination and magnification.
3. Adequate access cavity preparation
4. Clinician should always look for an additional canal in every tooth being treated.

## Significance of Missed Canal

Missed canal can contribute to endodontic failure because it holds the tissue debris, bacteria and other irritants. The tooth should be retreated first conservatively if endodontic failure exists, before going for endodontic surgery procedure (Figs 22.15A and B).

## INSTRUMENT SEPARATION

Instrument breakage is a common and frustrating problem in endodontic treatment which occurs by improper or overuse of instruments. Any time during the cleaning and shaping of root canal file, reamer, broach or Gates Glidden may break especially while working in curved, narrow or tortuous canals (Fig. 22.16).

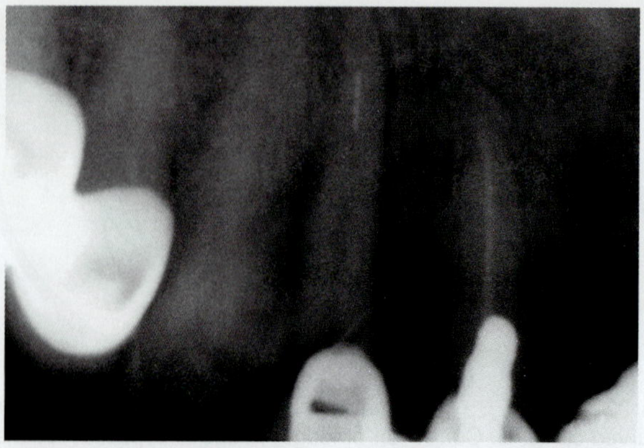

**Fig. 22.17:** Radiography showing fractured instrument in 25

*Etiology*

- Variation from normal root canal anatomy.
- Overuse of damaged instruments.
- Overused of dull instruments.
- Inadequate irrigation.
- Use of excessive pressure while inserting in canal.
- Inadaquate access cavity preparation.

## Management

Always inform the patient immediately. Take a radiograph so as to check the site of fractured instrument (Fig. 22.17).

### *Instrument Retrieval*

Before instrument retrieval one should evaluate the tooth radiographically to check:

1. Curvature and length of canal
2. Accessibility of instrument
3. Location of separated instrument (Fig 22.18)
4. Type of broken instrument that is whether stainless steel or NiTi
5. Amount of dentin present around the instrument.

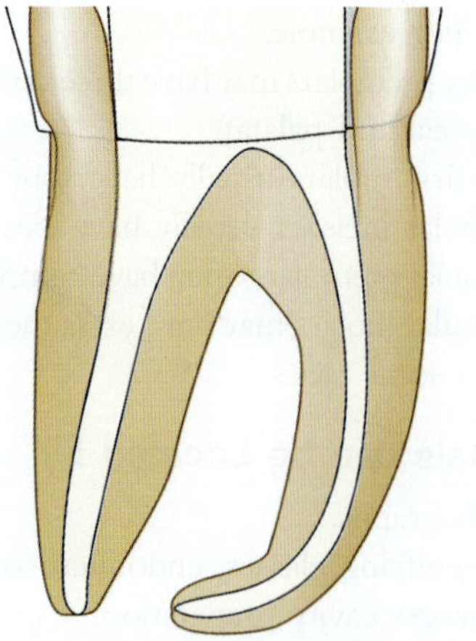

**Fig. 22.16:** Curved, narrow and tortuous canals are more prone for instrument fracture

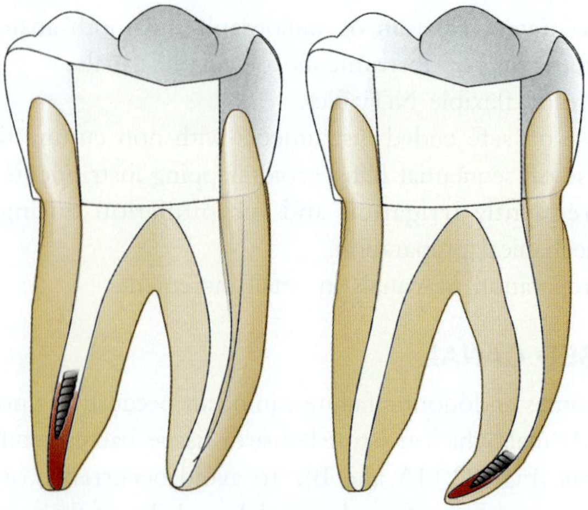

**Fig. 22.18:** Diameter, curvature of canal and location of instrument affects its removal

One should make use the combination of ultrasonics, adequate magnification and illumination for instrument retrieval.

Special instruments used for retrieval of separated instrument are:

1. Wire-loop technique
2. Masserann kit
3. Endoextractor
4. Instrument removal system
5. Separated instrument retrieval

### Masserann Kit

In Masserann kit, an extractor is present into which the instrument to be retrieved as locked. Also it has assorted end cutting trepan burs which are large and rigid meant to be used only in coronal portion of straight canals. These should not be used in curved canals.

Steps for retrieving instruments using Masserann kit:

a. Enlarge the canal orifice using a round bur.
b. Gain a straight line access to fractured instrument using gated glidden drills.
c. Move end cutting trepan burs slowly in anticlockwise direction so as to free 4 mm of the fragment. These burs can be used by hand or with reduction gear contra angle handpiece at the speed of 300-600 rpm.
d. Take extractor and slidely open it over free end of the fragment
e. Firmly hold the extractor in place and rotate the screw head until the fragment is gripped.
f. Once gripped tightly, move extractor in anticlockwise direction for removal of all cutting root canal instruments and in clockwise direction for removing filing instruments.

### Use of Endoextractor

In endoextractor, cyanoacrylate adhesive is placed on it so as to lock the object into the extractor. Technique for removal is same as that for masserann extractor.

### Instrument Removal System (Fig. 22.19)

Instrument removal system consists of different size of microtubes, and inserts wedges which fit into separated instrument. Microtube has 45° bevelled end and a handle.

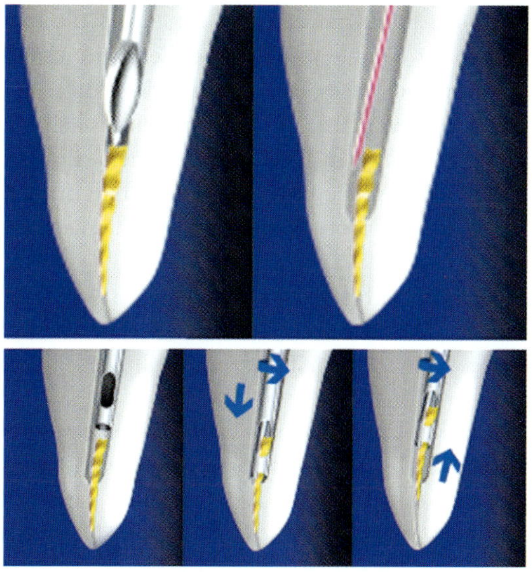

**Fig. 22.20:** Technique of using IRS for removal of fractured instrument

### Technique of Using IRS (Fig. 22.20)

- Gain straight line access to the canal.
- Select a microtube and insert it into the canal.
- After this, guide the head of the broken instruments into the lumen of the microtube.
- Place an insert wedge through the open end of microtube till it comes in contact with separated instrument.
- Turn the insert wedge clockwise to engage the instrument.
- Finally, move the microtube out of canal to retrieve the separated instrument.

## File Bypass Technique

The key to bypass a file is establishing straight line access and patency with small instruments (Fig. 22.21). The initial attempts should be made with number 6 or 8 file. In order to get past the broken instrument fragment, a small sharp bend should be given at the end of the instrument. Insert the file slowly and carefully into the canal. When the negotiation occurs past the fragment, one will find a catch. Do not remove file at this point. Use a small in and out movements along with copious irrigation of the root canal.

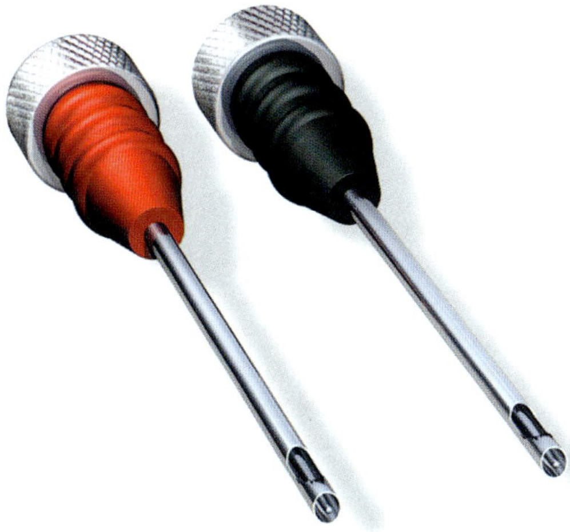

**Fig. 22.19:** Microtubes of instrument removal system

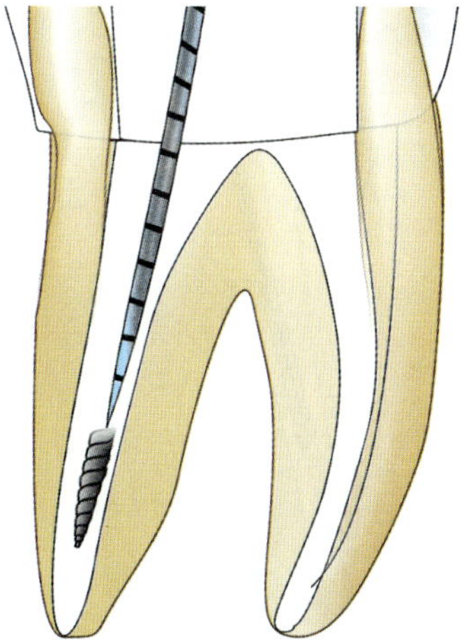

**Fig. 22.21:** Straight line access to instrument is primary requirement

While doing these movements, sometimes file may kink, and one may not be able to place the file in the canal to the same length. In such cases, use new file with similar bend and repeat the above procedure. Once the patency is achieved with No.10 file, stick to it. It may get kinked or bent, discard it and start with new file. While doing this procedure, if patency is lost again repeat the procedure, starting with smaller number files.

Once patency with a No. 15 instrument is achieved, go to K reamers. Use a "place-pull/rotate/withdrawal" movement rather than a filing motion. Two things will occur in response to this:

1. The reamer will be deflected by the fragment and then there is need to find a consistent path of instrument insertion that is probably different than the initial path.
2. Every time one rotates the reamer, there will be a "clicking" sound as the flutes brush up against the file fragment. This is normal. One must avoid placing an instrument directly on top of the broken file. This can push it deeper resulting in loss of patency. If the file is visible at this point, it is possible to use a small tipped ultrasonic instrument or 1/4 turn withdrawal-type handpiece to dislodge and remove it.

In order to attempt file removal, exposure of fragment is mandatory. Instrument can be visualized using microscope. Modified Gates-Gliddens can also be used to expose the instrument.

Gates-Glidden is modified by removing their bottom half and thus creating a flat surface. The crown down technique using Gates-Glidden burs is carried out. Once it is accomplished, use modified Gates-Glidden to enlarge the canal to a point where instrument is located; this way a platform is created which enable to visualize the broken fragment (Fig. 22.22). It creates a flat area of dentin surrounding the file fragment. Thereafter, small tipped ultrasonic instruments can be used around the instrument and eventually vibrate the file out of the canal (Fig. 22.23). The tip is used in a counterclockwise motion to loosen the file. Irrigation combined with ultrasonics can frequently flush it out at this point. If sufficient file is exposed, an instrument removal system can be used.

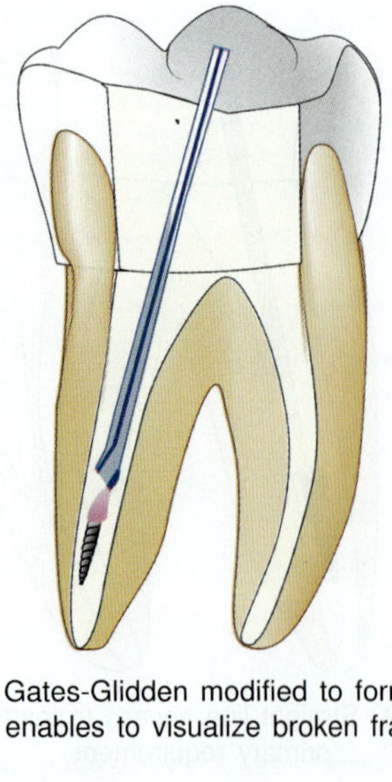

**Fig. 22.22:** Gates-Glidden modified to form a platform which enables to visualize broken fragment

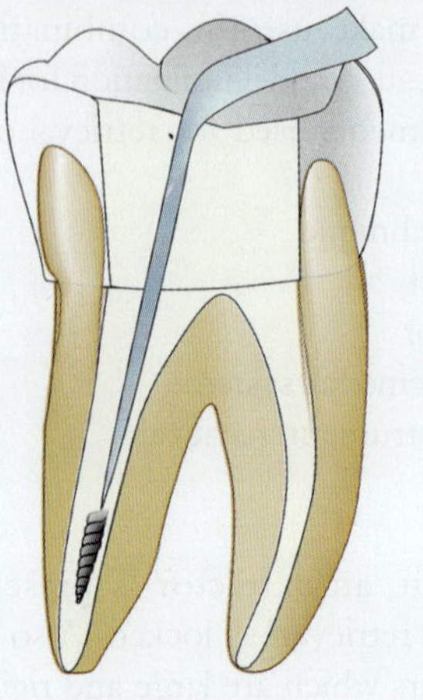

**Fig. 22.23:** Use of ultrasonic instrument to remove fractured instrument

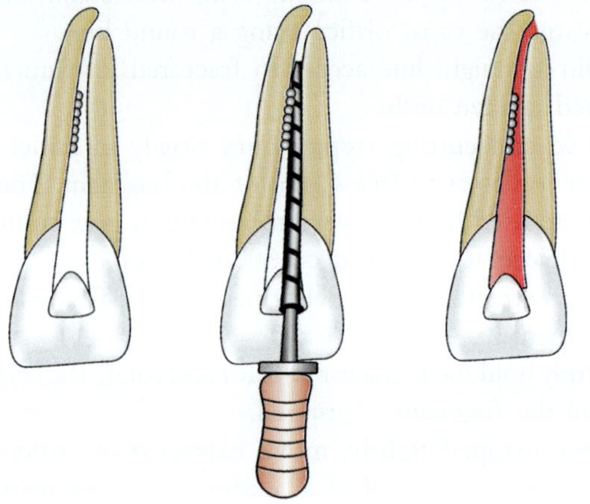

**Fig. 22.24:** If unable to remove the fractured instrument incorporate it in final obturation

If it is very difficult to remove the fractured instrument, incorporate the instrument fragment in the final obturation. (Fig. 22.24).

*Surgical treatment for removal of broken fragment is indicated when:*

1. Broken file is behind the curve.
2. File fragment is not visible because of the curved root.
3. Instrument is in the apical part of the canal and is difficult to retrieve (Fig. 22.25).
4. Much of dentin has to be removed to allow file removal.

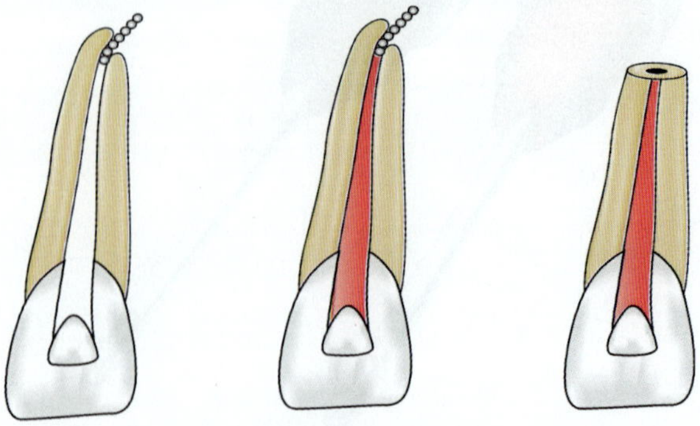

**Fig. 22.25:** Surgical removal of fractured instrument

## Prognosis

Prognosis of separated instrument depends upon following factors:

a. Timing of separation
b. Status of pulp tissue
c. Position of separated instrument
d. Ability to retrieve or bypass the instrument.

## Prevention

1. Examine each instrument before placing it into the canal. One should always discard instrument when there is:
   - Bending of instrument.
   - Corrosion of instrument
   - Unwinding of flutes.
   - Excessively heating of instrument
   - Dulling of NiTi instrument
2. Instead of using carbon steel, use stainless steel files.
3. Use smaller number of instruments only once.
4. Always use the instruments in sequential order.
5. Never force the instrument into the canal.
6. Canals should be copiously irrigated during cleaning and shaping procedure.
7. Never use instruments in dry canals.
8. Always clean the instrument before placing it into the canal. Debris collected between the flutes retard the cutting efficiency and increase the frictional torque between the instrument and canal wall.
9. Do not give excessive rotation to instrument while working with it.

Studies have shown that instrument separation in root filled teeth with necrotic pulps results in a poorer prognosis. But if an instrument can be bypassed and incorporated in the root canal filling, prognosis becomes favorable. Also if instrument separates at later stages of instrumentation and close to apex, prognosis is better than if it separates in undebrided canals, short of the apex or beyond apical foramen. Separated instrument are not the prime cause of endodontic failure but separated instruments impede mechanical instrumentation of the canal, which may cause endodontic failure.

Before going for removal of broken instrument, evaluate the tooth radiographically. Before starting with the instrument retrieval efforts, one should ensure straight line access to the canal orifice.

## ZIPPING

*Zipping is defined as transposition of the apical portion of the canal* (Fig. 22.26).

### *Etiology*

This is commonly seen in curved canals because of following reasons:

1. Failure to precurve the files.
2. Forcing instruments in curved canal
3. Use of large, stiff instruments to bore out a curve canal.

In zipping, apical foramen tends to become a tear drop shape or elliptical, is transported from the curve of the canal.

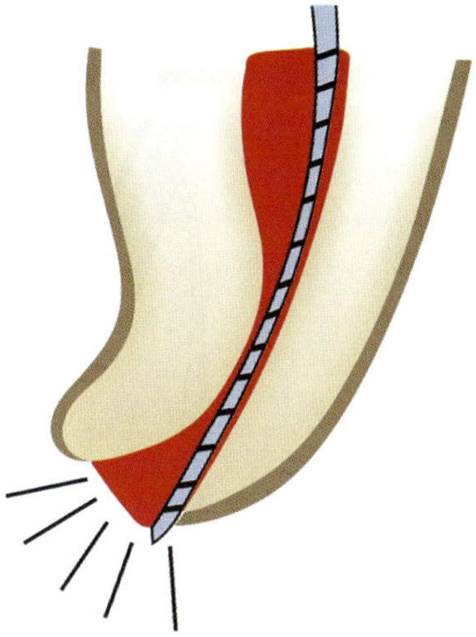

**Fig. 22.26:** Zipping is transposition of apical portion of the canal

File placed in curved canal cuts more on the outer portion of the canal wall at its apical extent, thus causing movement of the canal away from the curve and its natural path. In contrast, the coronal third of the flutes remove more on the inner most aspect of the canal wall causing an uneven reduction of the dentin in the coronal third.

When a file is rotated in a curved canal, a biomechanical defect known as an elbow is formed coronal to the elliptically shaped apical seat. This is the narrowest portion of the canal (Fig. 22.27). In many cases the obturating material terminates at the elbow leaving an unfilled zipped canal apical to elbow. This is the common occurrence with laterally compacted gutta-percha technique. Use of vertical compaction of warm gutta-percha or thermoplasticized gutta-percha is ideal in these cases to compact a solid core material into the apical preparation without using excessive amount of sealer.

Elbow prevents optimal compaction in the apical portion of the canal. Since elbow becomes the apical seat, the obturating material is compacted against the elbow and patient is recalled or regular basis.

*Zipping can be prevented by:*

1. Using precurved files for curved canals.

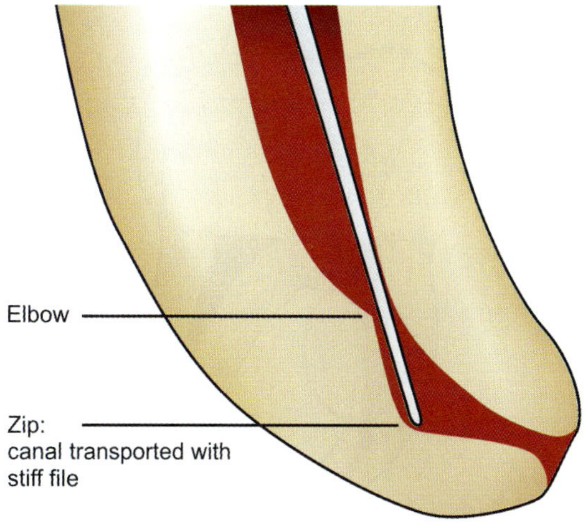


**Fig. 22.27:** Elbow formed in a curved canal

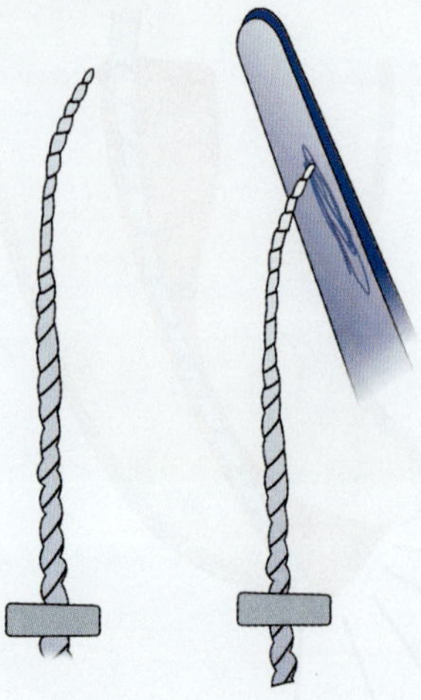

Fig. 22.28: Modification of flutes of file

2. Using incremental filing technique.
3. Using flexible files.
4. Removing flutes of file at certain areas, for example, file portion which makes contact with outer dentinal wall at the apex and portion which makes contact with inner dentinal wall especially in the mid root area (Fig. 22.28).
5. Over curving in apical part of the file specially when working for severely curved canals.

## STRIPPING OR LATERAL WALL PERFORATION

"Stripping" is a lateral perforation caused by over instrumentation through a thin wall in the root and is most likely to happen on the inside or concave wall of a curved canal such as distal wall of mesial roots in mandibular first molars (Fig. 22.29). Stripping is easily detected by sudden appearance of hemorrhage in a previously dry canal or by a sudden complaint by patient.

### Management

Successful repair of a stripping or perforation relies on the adequacy of the seal established by repair material.

Access to mid-root perforation is most often difficult and repair is not predictable. Calcium hydroxide can be used as a biological barrier against which filling material is packed.

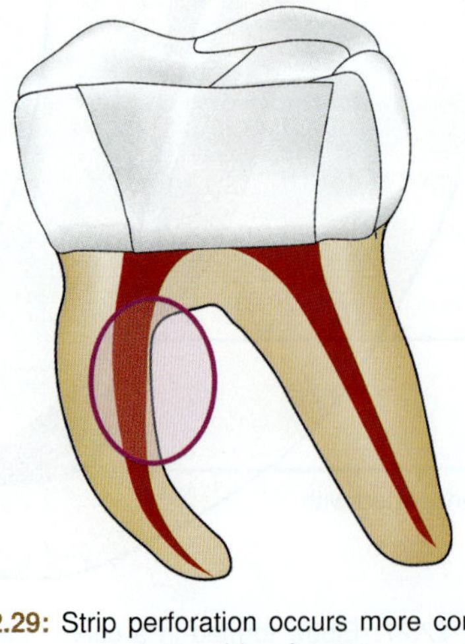

Fig. 22.29: Strip perforation occurs more commonly on inner side of curve

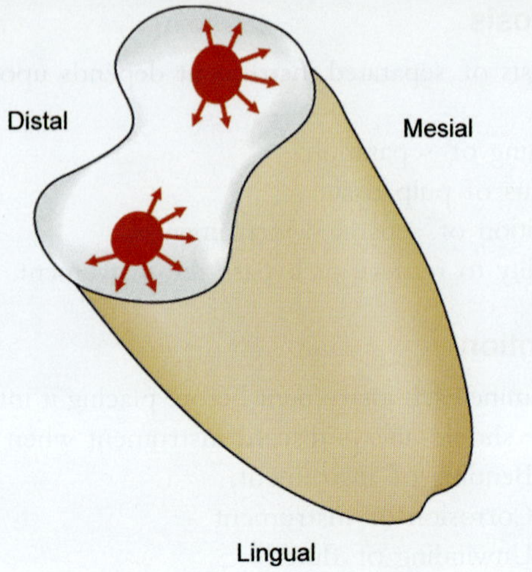


Fig. 22.30: Anticurvature filing

Repair of strip perforation can be done both non-surgically as well as surgically. Majority of techniques however proposed a two step method, where the root canal is first obturated and defect is repaired surgically.

### Prevention

1. Use of pre-curved files for curved canals.
2. Use of modified files for curved canals. A file can be modified by removing flutes of file at certain areas, for example, file portion which makes contact with outer dentinal wall at the apex and portion which makes contact with inner dentinal wall especially in the mid-root area (Fig. 22.29).
3. Using anticurvature filing, i.e. more filling pressure is placed on tooth structure away from the direction of root curvature and away from the invagination, thereby preventing root thinning and perforation of the root structure (Fig. 22.30).

## CANAL TRANSPORTATION

"Apical canal transportation is moving the position of canal's normal anatomic foramen to a new location on external root surface" (Figs 22.31A to C).

In this case, root shows reverse architecture which is difficult to obturate, resulting in poor quality of obturation and thus contributing to endodontic failures.

Canal transportations can be classified into three types, viz. Type I, II and III.

*Type I:* It is minor movement of physiologic foramen. In such cases, if sufficient residual dentin can be maintained, one can try to create positive apical canal architecture so as to improve the prognosis of the tooth (Fig. 22.31A).

*Type II:* Apical transportation of Type II shows moderate movement of the physiologic foramen to a new location (Fig. 22.31B). Such cases compromise the prognosis and are difficult to treat. Biocompatible materials like MTA can be used to provide barrier against which obturation material can be packed.

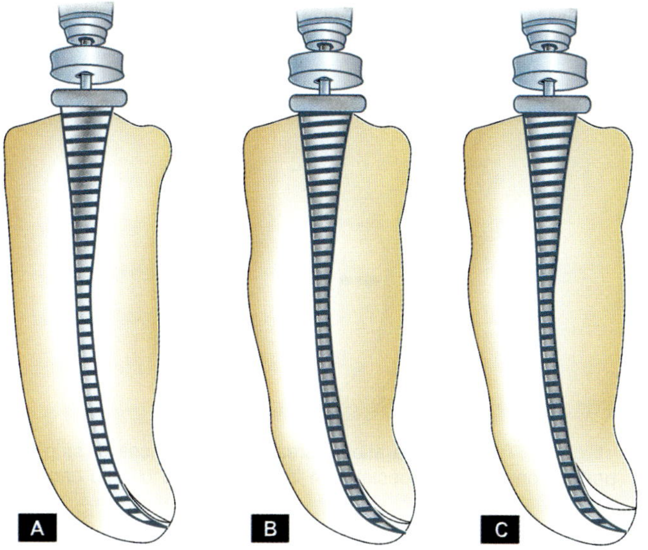


**Figs 22.31A to C:** Type I, II and III canal transportation (A) Minor movement of apical foramen (Type I) (B) Moderate movement of apical foramen (Type II) (C) Severe movement of apical foramen (Type III)

*Type III:* Apical transportation of Type III shows severe movement of physiological foramen (Fig. 22.31C). In such type, prognosis is poorest when compared to Type I and Type II. A three dimensional obturation is difficult in such cases. This requires surgical intervention for correction otherwise tooth is indicated for extraction.

## INADEQUATE CANAL PREPARATION

### Over Instrumentation

Excessive instrumentation beyond the apical constriction violates the periodontal ligament and alveolar bone. Loss of apical constriction creates an open apex with an increased risk of overfilling, lack of an adequate apical seal (Fig 22.32), pain and discomfort for the patient.

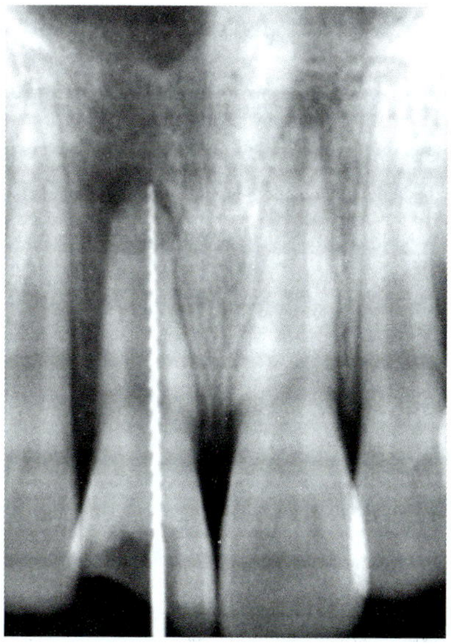

**Fig. 22.32:** Radiograph showing instrument going beyond periapex

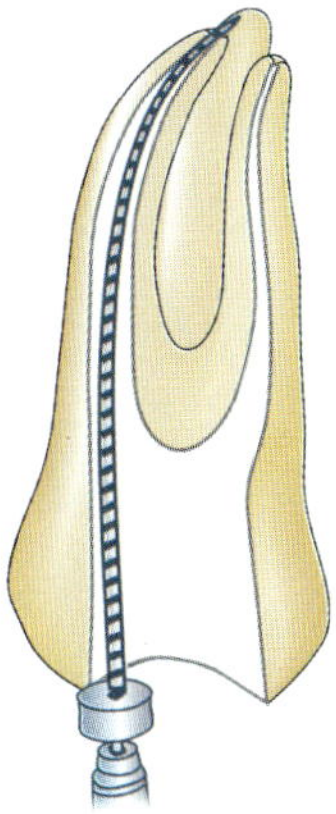

**Fig. 22.33:** Excessive instrumentation

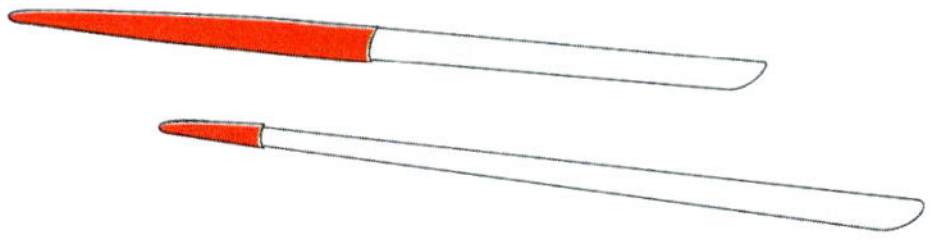

**Fig. 22.34:** Paper point showing hemorrhage at the tip

Over instrumentation is recognized when hemorrhage is evident in the apical portion of canal with or without patient discomfort (Fig. 22.33) and when tactile resistance of the boundaries of canal space is lost. It can be confirmed by taking a radiograph and by inserting paper point in the canal (Fig. 22.34).

### Treatment

Treatment includes re-establishing tooth length short of the original length and then enlarging the canal, with larger instruments, to that length. The canal is then carefully filled to established working length so as to prevent extrusion of the filling beyond apex (Figs 22.35A and B).

Another technique which can be employed to prevent over extrusion of the filling is creating an apical barrier. Materials used for developing such barrier include dentin chips, calcium hydroxide powder, hydroxyapatite and more recently MTA.

### Prevention

Over instrumentation beyond apical constriction can be prevented by:

1. Using good radiographic techniques.

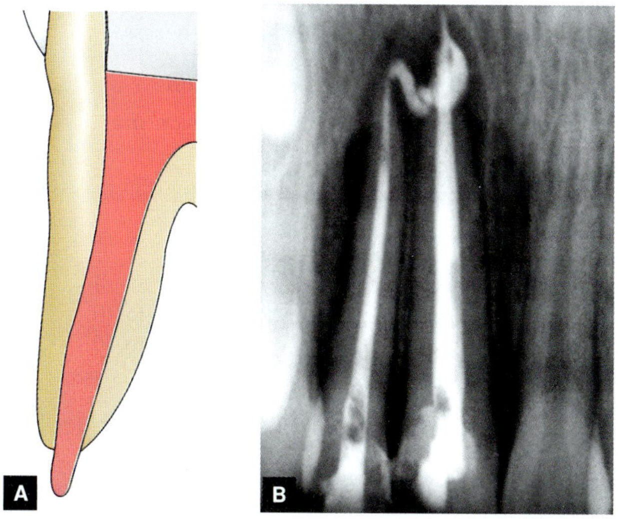


**Figs 22.35A and B:** Overfilling of the canal causing irritation to periapical area

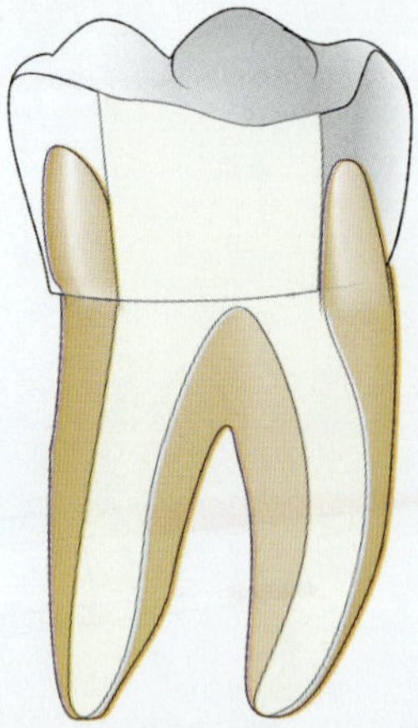

Fig. 22.36: Overpreparation of canal causes excessive removal of root dentin

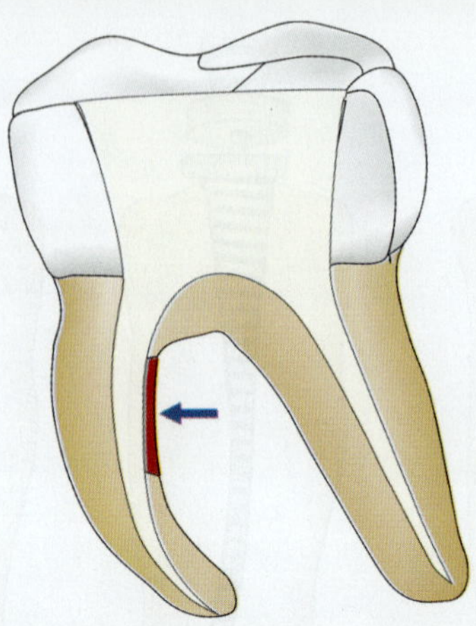

Fig. 22.37: Overpreparation increases the chances of strip perforation (arrow) especially on inner side of a curved canal

2. Accurately determining the apical constriction of the root canal.
3. Using sound reference points.
4. Using stable instrument stops.
5. Maintaining all instruments within the confines of the canal system.
6. Occlusal alterations before determination of the working length.
7. Intermittent radiographic confirmation of the working length.
8. Confirming the integrity of the apical stop with paper points.

### *Overpreparation*

Overpreparation is excessive removal of tooth structure in mesiodistal and buccolingual direction (Fig. 22.36). During biomechanical preparation of the canal, size of apical preparation should correspond to size, shape and curvature of the root. For example, to produce an apical seat equivalent to No. 50 **K-file** in a curved (10°-20°) mesiobuccal canal of a mandibular first molar is likely to cause procedural errors like zipping of root apex, perforation and transportation of the apical foramen. Adherence to the guidelines for the recommended range of size termination for each type of root is mandatory, with modification made as necessary.

**Suggested size for final apical preparation**

| *Tooth group* | *Final apical size* |
|---|---|
| **Maxillary teeth** | |
| Central incisor | 35 to 60 |
| Lateral incisor | 25 to 40 |
| Canine | 30 to 50 |
| Premolar | 25 to 40 |
| Molar | MB/DB 25 to 40 |
| | Palatal 25 to 50 |
| **Mandibular teeth** | |
| Incisors | 25 to 40 |
| Canines | 30 to 50 |
| Premolar | 30 to 50 |
| Molar | |
| MB/ML | 25 to 40 |
| Distal | 25 to 50 |

Over preparation is a commonly seen in the apical portion of the canal system, but it can also occur in middle and coronal portion of the canal. Excessive canal flaring increases the chances of stripping and perforation (Fig. 22.37). One should avoid excessive removal of tooth structure because over prepared canals are potentially weaker and subject to fracture during compaction and restorative procedures.

### *Underpreparation*

Underpreparation is the failure to remove pulp tissue, dentinal debris and microorganisms from the root canal system. Sometimes the canal system is improperly shaped which prevents three dimensional obturation of the root canal space (Fig. 22.38).

*Etiology*

Inadequate preparation of the canal system occurs in the following ways.

1. Insufficient preparation of the apical dentin matrix.
2. Insufficient use of irrigants to dissolve tissues and debris.
3. Inadequate canal shaping, which prevents depth of spreader or plugger penetration during compaction.
4. Establishing the working length short of the apical constriction.

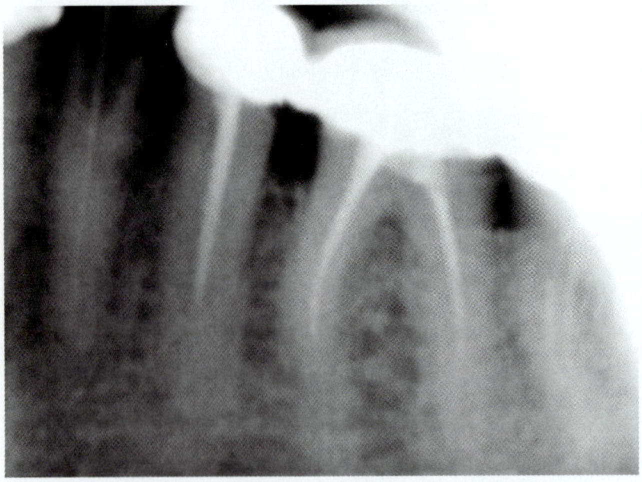

Fig. 22.38: Improperly shaped canal prevents three-dimensional obturation of root canals

5. Creation of ledges and blockages that prevent complete cleaning and shaping.

Underprepared canals are best managed by strictly following the principles of working length determination and biomechanical preparation. Copious irrigation and recapitulation during instrumentation ensure a properly cleaned canal. Before obturation spreaders and pluggers must be pre-fitted to determine their depth of placement and to ensure proper canal shape.

## PERFORATIONS

According to glossary of endodontic terms (by AAE) the *perforation is defined as "the mechanical or pathological communication between the root canal system and the external tooth surface".*

Pathologic conditions such as caries, root resorptions aside, the mechanical or iatrogenic perforation are the procedural mishaps which can significantly affect the long term prognosis of a tooth.

Perforations can occur at any stage while performing endodontic therapy that is during access cavity preparation or during instrumentation procedures leading to canal perforations at cervical, mid-root or apical levels.

*Access cavity perforation* can occur during access cavity preparation (Figs 22.39 to 22.41). If the perforation is above the periodontal attachment, leakage of saliva into cavity or sodium hypochlorite in mouth are the main sign. But if perforation occurs into the periodontal ligament, bleeding is the hallmark feature.

*Root canal perforation* can occur at three levels:

a. *Cervical canal perforation:* It commonly occurs while locating the canal orifice and flaring of the coronal third of the root canal. Sudden appearance of blood from canal is the first sign of perforation.
b. *Mid-root perforation (Fig. 22.42):* It commonly occurs in the curved canal when a ledge is formed during instrumentation along inside the curvature of root canal, as it is straightened out, i.e. strip perforation may result (Fig. 22.43). Usually it is caused by over-instrumentation and over-preparation of the thin wall of root or concave side of the curved canals. Sudden appearance of bleeding is the pathognomic feature.

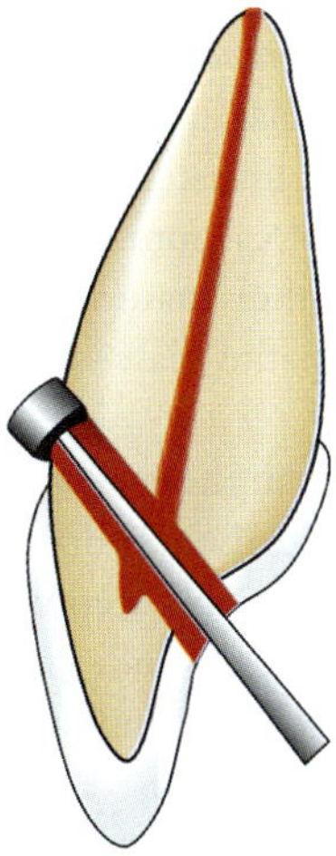

Fig. 22.39: Perforation caused during access cavity preparation

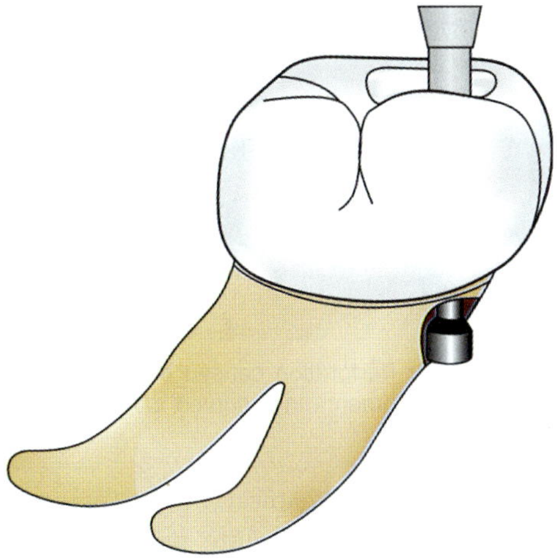

Fig. 22.40: Perforation caused by misdirection of bur during access cavity preparation of a molar with previously placed crown

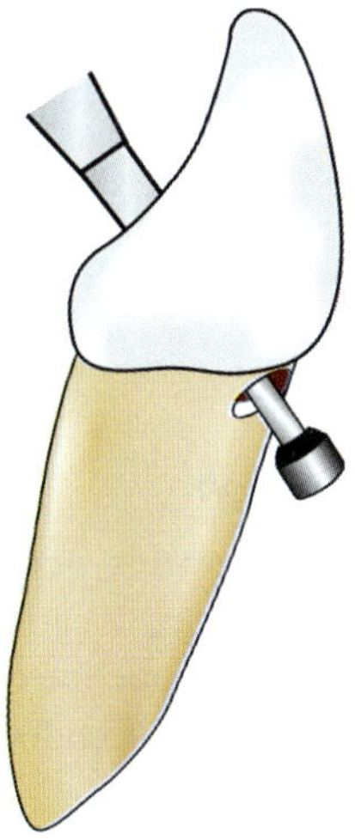

Fig. 22.41: Misorientation of bur causing perforation during access cavity preparation

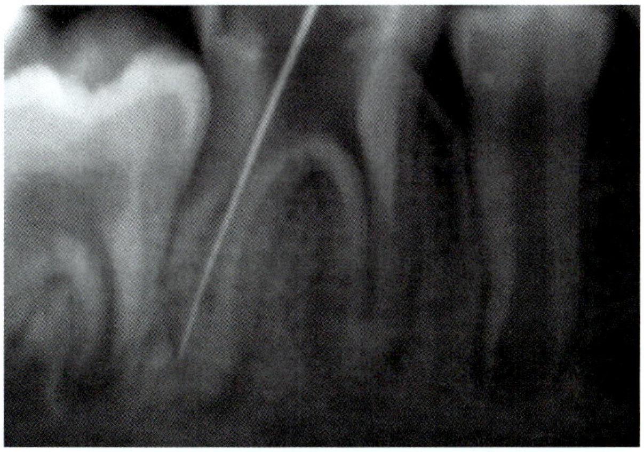

Fig. 22.42: Radiograph showing perforation of distal canal molar of mandibular first molar

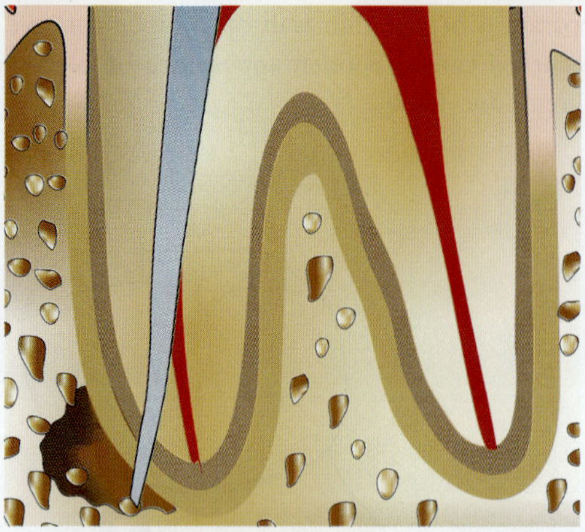

Fig. 22.43: Perforation caused by use of stiff instruments in a curved canal

c. *Apical root perforation:* Apical root perforation can occur.
   I. When instrument goes into periradicular tissue, i.e. beyond the confines of the root canal (Fig. 22.44).
   II. By overuse of chelating agents along with straight and stiffer large sized instruments to negotiate ledging, canal blockage or zipping, etc.

*Occurrence of a perforation can be recognized by:*

1. Placing an instrument into the opening and taking a radiograph.
2. Using paper point.
3. Sudden appearance of bleeding.
4. Complain of pain by patient when instrument touches periodontal tissue.

### Repair of the Perforation

Treatment of the endodontics perforation depends on recognition of the condition, location, size, level of the perforation, timing of therapeutic intervention and clinician's skill and experience. Prognosis of endodontically treated teeth with perforation depends upon prevention of bacterial infection of the perforation site.

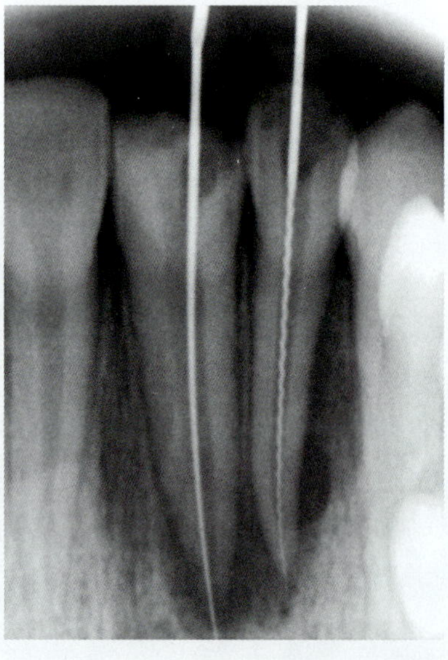

Fig. 22.44: Radiograph showing apical root perforation i.e. instrument is going beyond confines of root canal

***Location*** greatly influences the prognosis. When perforation is located at alveolar crest or coronal to it, prognosis is poor because of epithelial migration and periodontal pocket formation. Perforation in the furcation area has the poor prognosis. Perforation in coronal third of root and surrounded by a healthy periodontium, i.e. which does not communicate with the gingival sulcus has good prognosis. Perforation occurring in mid-root and apical part of root does not have communication with oral cavity and thus has good prognosis.

***Size*** of perforation too affects the prognosis. A small perforation has less tissue destruction and inflammation, thus having better prognosis than larger sized perforation.

***Visibility, accessibility*** also affects the perforation repair.

***Time*** between perforation repair affects the prognosis greatly. The perforation should be repaired as soon as possible to discourage further loss of attachment and prevent sulcular breakdown. Early treatment enhances the success.

***Associated periodontal condition and strategic importance*** of tooth also influence the treatment plan of the perforation. If attachment apparatus is intact without pocket-formation, nonsurgical repair is recommended whereas in case of loss of attachment, surgical treatment should be planned.

In addition **esthetics** influences the perforation repair and material to be used for repair of the perforation.

## MATERIAL USED FOR PERFORATION REPAIR

Various materials have been tried for perforation repair since long with variable degree of the success.

*An Ideal Material for Perforation Repair should*

- Adhere to preparation walls of the cavity and seal the root canal system.
- Be non-toxic
- Be easy to handle
- Be radiopaque
- Be dimensionally stable
- Be well tolerated by periradicular tissue
- Be non-absorbable
- Not corrode
- Not be affected by moisture
- Not stain periradicular tissues.

Some of the most investigated materials for perforation repair include amalgam, calcium hydroxide, IRM, Super EBA, gutta-percha, MTA, other materials tried for repair include dentin chips, hydroxyapatite, glass ionomer cements and plaster of paris.

For perforation repair, hemostatics are needed to control the hemorrhage and make the area dry so that optimal placement of restorative material can be accomplished. Materials which can be used as hemostatics include calcium hydroxide, calcium sulphate, freezed dried bone and/or MTA.

Whichever is the material used, the ultimate goal is to seal the defect with a biocompatible material and maintain an intact periodontal attachment apparatus.

## Management of the Coronal Third Perforations

In these cases esthetics is the main concern. Here the materials used for perforation repair could be calcium sulphate barrier along with composites, glass ionomer cements and white MTA. But in posterior teeth where aesthetics is not the main criteria, super EBA, amalgam, MTA can be tried.

## Management of Perforations in Mid-root Level

In these cases, the success of perforation repair depends on the hemostasis, accessibility and visibility, use of micro-instrumentation techniques and selection of the material for repair.

If the defect is small and hemostasis can be achieved, perforation can be sealed and repaired during three dimensional obturation of the root canal. But in case the perforation defect is large and moisture control is difficult, then one should prepare the canal before going for perforation repair.

Lemon in 1992 gave the internal matrix concept for the repair of inaccessible strip perforations using microsurgical technique. The rationale behind this concept was that a matrix was needed to control the material and thus preventing overfilling of the repair material into the periradicular tissues.

Several materials meet these criteria like cavit, amalgam, zinc oxide, eugenol, gutta-percha and sealer. But none of these can overcome contamination, underfilling and overfilling. According to Lemon, hydroxyapatite could be used for accessible perforations.

*A Material to be Used as Internal Matrix should*

a. Be biocompatible
b. Be sterile
c. Be easy to manipulate
d. Stimulate osteogenesis

## Technique of Placement of Matrix

1. Attain the hemostasis and place files, silver cones or gutta-percha points in the canals to maintain their patency.
2. The hydroxyapatite (HA) particles are wetted with saline and clumped together for their easy transportation.
3. The HA is deposited into perforation and condensed with pluggers. This will stop bleeding (Fig. 22.45).

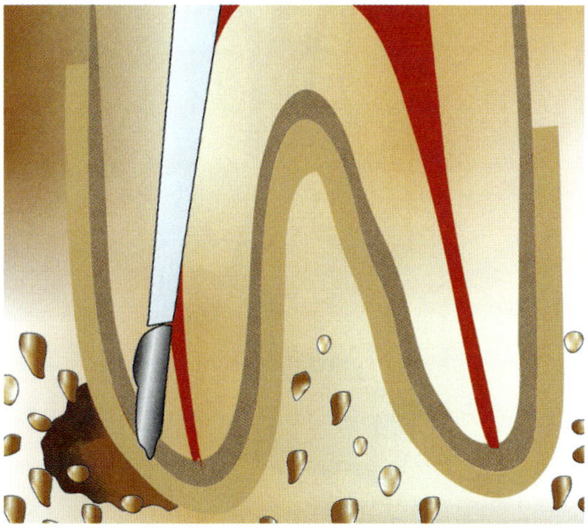

**Fig. 22.45:** Hydroxyapatite crystals are packed and condensed in perforation using pluggers

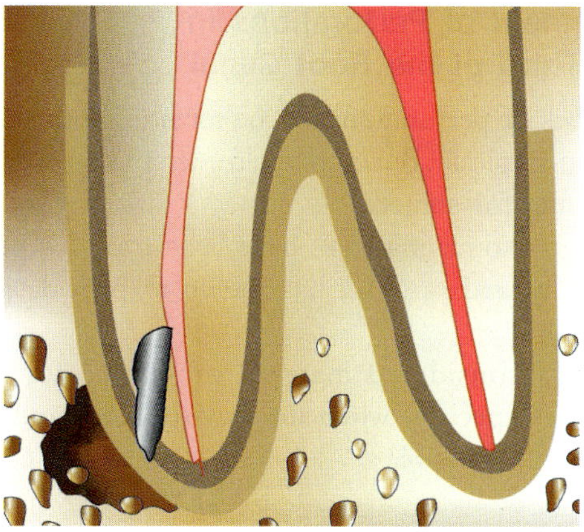

**Fig. 22.46:** Complete packing of HA crystals in canal with perforation

4. Like this, completely fill the defect with HA (Fig. 22.46).
5. Excess material is removed with excavator to the level of periodontal ligament.
6. After that, a bur is used to prepare the perforation site to receive the material. Using a flat instrument, apply restorative material like amalgam or GIC to repair the perforation (Fig. 22.47).

## Indications

1. Accessible perforations (below crestal bone).
2. Larger perforations in middle or apical thirds of the roots with straight canals.

## Contraindications

1. Inaccessible defects.
2. Perforations on external root surface or above the level of crestal bone.

## Disadvantages of Matrix Placement Technique

1. Internal matrix cannot be used in all the cases.
2. Radiographic evaluation of bone fill is difficult especially if radio-densities of materials and bone are same.
3. Special device for placement of matrix, i.e. fiber optic imaging technology is required.

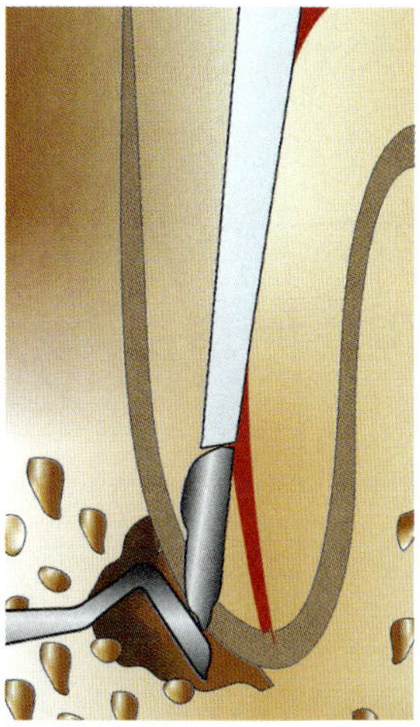

**Fig. 22.47:** A flat instrument is used to pack the restorative material outside the tooth at the site of defect

### Management of Perforations in Apical Third of the Root Canal

These types of perforations can be repaired both surgically as well as non-surgically. But one should attempt non-surgical repair before going for surgery.

Though various materials have been tried for perforation repair but nowadays MTA has shown to provide promising results.

MTA is considered material of choice for repairing perforation especially when dry environment and technical access are not possible.

#### *Technique*

1. Apply rubber dam and debride the root canal system.
2. Dry the canal system with paper points and isolate the perforation site.
3. Prepare the MTA material according to manufacturer's instructions.
4. Using the carrier provided, dispense the material into perforation site. Condense the material using pluggers or paper points.
5. While placing MTA, instrument is placed into the canal to maintain its patency and moved up and down in short strokes till the MTA sets. It is done to avoid file getting frozen in the MTA. Place the temporary restoration to seal chamber.
6. In next appointment, one sees the hard set MTA against which obturation can be done.

MTA is composed of Tricalcium silicate, Dicalcium silicate, Tricalcium aluminate, Tetracalcium aluminaferrite, Calcium sulfate and Bismuth oxide. The main advantage of this material is that being hydrophilic it requires moisture to set. It sets in brick hard consistency and shown to induce cementogenesis, bone deposition with almost absence of inflammatory response. All these make MTA a material of choice in treatment of perforations (Fig. 22.48).

#### *Precautions to Prevent Perforations*

1. Evaluation of the anatomy of the tooth before starting the endodontic therapy.
2. Using the smaller, flexible files for curved canals.
3. Not skipping the file sizes.
4. Recapitulation with smaller files between sizes.
5. Confirming the working length and maintaining the instruments within the confines of working length.
6. Using anticurvature filing techniques in curved canals to selectively remove the dentin.
7. Minimizing the overuse of Gates-Gliddens too deep or too large especially in curved canals.
8. Avoiding overuse of chelating agents, larger stiff files in order to negotiate procedural errors like ledges, canal blockages, etc.
9. Copious irrigation of the canal to prevent the canal blockage by dentin chips or tissue debris.

## POST SPACE PERFORATIONS

Post preparation is an integral part of restoration of endodontically treated tooth. Iatrogenic perforations during post space preparations can severely impair the prognosis of the tooth. They are usually caused by poor clinical judgment and improper orientations of the post preparing drills (Figs 22.49 and 22.50). Perforation can be recognized by sudden appearance of blood in the canal or radiographically. The error of this iatrogenic perforation is compounded when clinician is unaware of the perforation and proceeds with post placement in the perforated site.

Treatment of post space perforation involves the same principles as for repair of other perforations. In other words, sealing of the perforation site is the primary goal. Perforation can be repaired in several ways. The defect can be accessed both surgically as well as non-surgically. Various materials like dental amalgam, calcium hydroxide, glass ionomer, composite

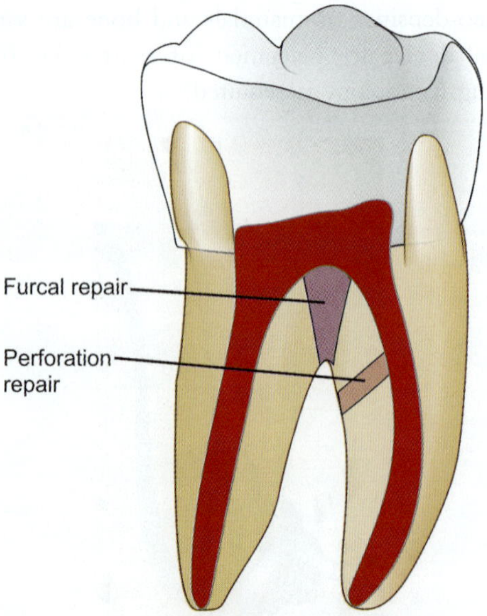


**Fig. 22.48:** Use of MTA for repair of perforation

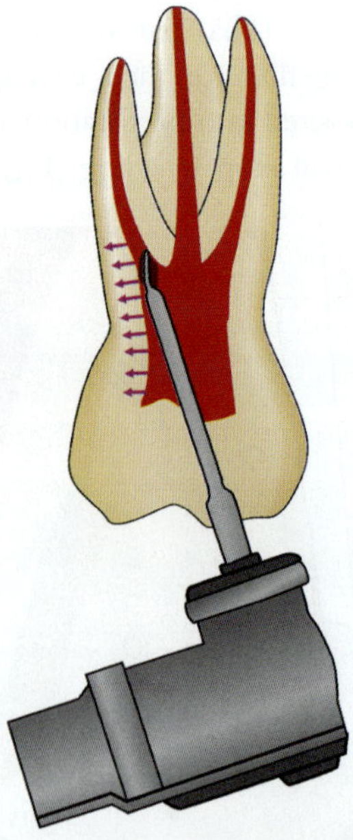

**Fig. 22.49:** Post space perforation caused by misdirection of post preparing drills

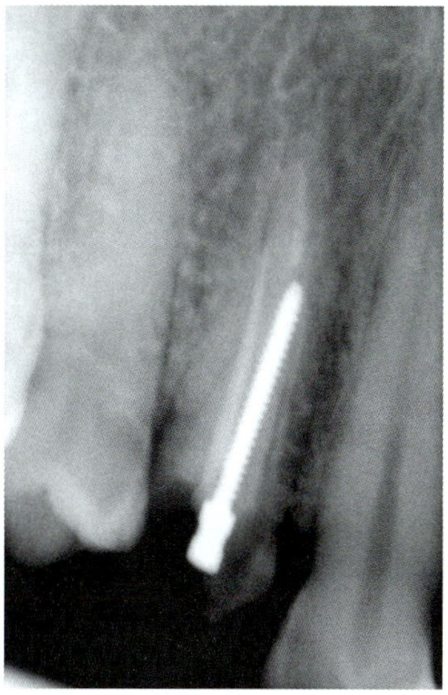

**Fig. 22.50:** Improper post placement due to improper direction of drill

resins, cavity, freezed dried bone and tricalcium phosphate can be used to repair the perforation.

### Prevention of Post-related Perforation

1. One must know anatomic features of root including radicular considerations of root anatomy as well its variations.
2. One should opt preparing post space at the time when obturation of root canal is done.
3. Avoid excessive use of Gates-Gliddens or peeso reamers to cut the dentin.

## UNDERFILLING/INCOMPLETELY FILLED ROOT CANALS

Underfilling, i.e. more than 2 mm short of radiographic apex occurs commonly because of procedural errors like ledge formation, blockage or incomplete instrumentation of the root canal (Fig. 22.51).

Inaccurate working length determination, inadequate irrigation and recapitulation during biomechanical preparation can lead to accumulation of dentin chips and tissue debris which

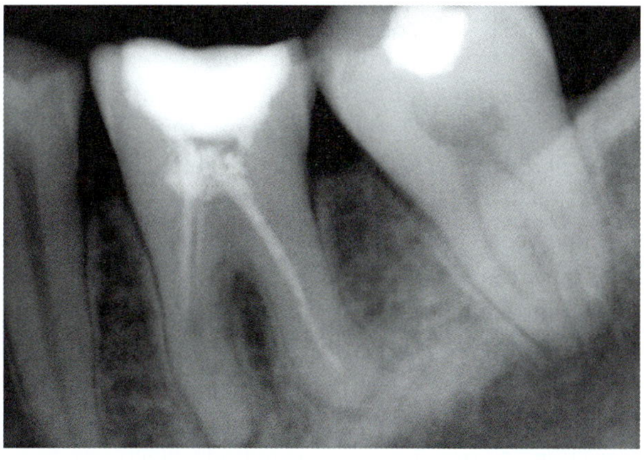

**Fig. 22.51:** Radiograph showing underfilled canals

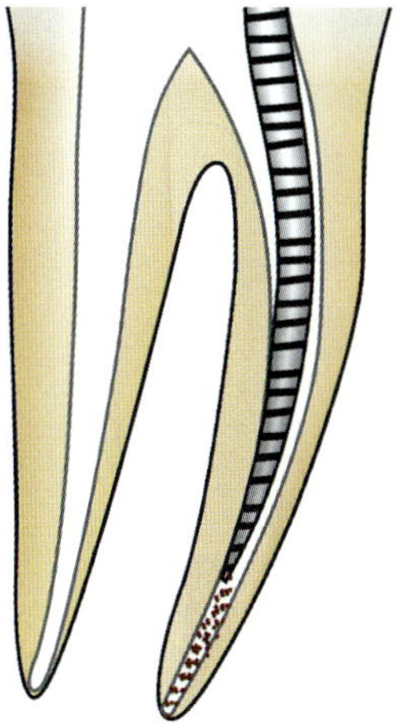

**Fig. 22.52:** Accumulation of dentin chips and tissue debris resulting in incomplete instrumentation

will result in canal blockage and incomplete instrumentation of the canal (Fig. 22.52).

Ledge can be caused by using:
- Large stiff files in curved canals (Fig. 22.53).
- Inadequate straight line access to canals apices.
- Inadequate irrigation.
- Skipping the file sizes during biomechanical preparation.
- Packing dentin chips, tissue debris in apical portion of the canal.

All these lead to inadequate removal of infected necrotic tissue remaining in the apical portion of the root canal. In teeth with periapical pathosis bacteria get colonized at and around the apical foramen. Thus, persistent bacterial infection in the root canal may result in initiation or perpetuation of existing periapical pathosis (Fig. 22.54). Fillings short of apex have shown poorer prognosis, especially in cases with necrotic pulp and periradicular pathosis.

Various research studies have shown that underfillings *per se* don't have direct effect on the success of endodontic treatment but it is the remaining infected necrotic tissue in inadequately instrumented and filled canals which lead to continued irritation to the periradicular tissues (Fig. 22.55).

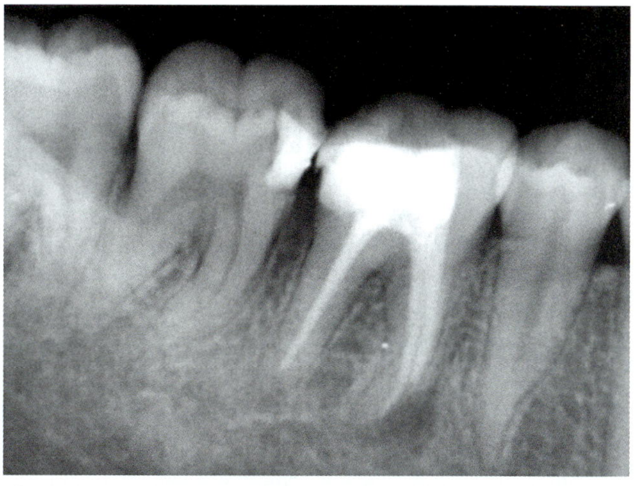

**Fig. 22.53:** Ledge formation in mesiobuccal canal of mandibular first molar results in incomplete obturation of the canal

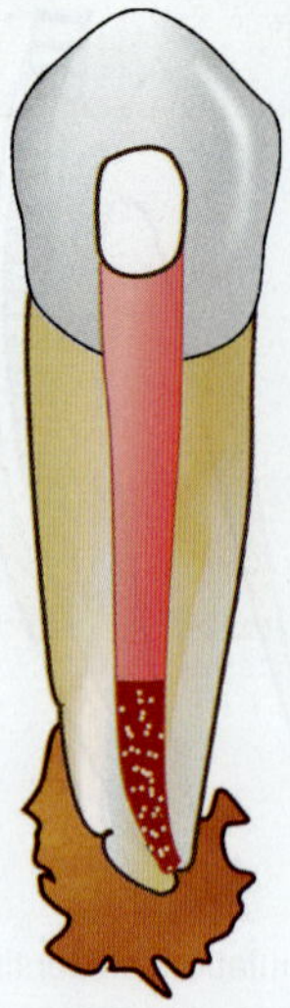

Fig. 22.54: Persistent bacterial infection in root canal with filling short of apex causes treatment failure

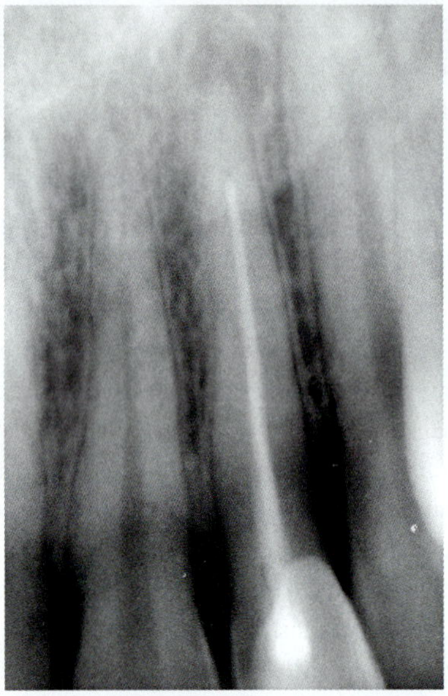

Fig. 22.55: Radiograph showing incomplete obturation (short of the apex)

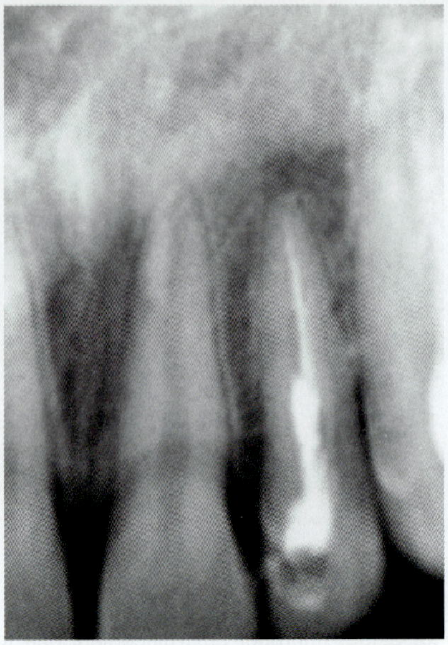

Fig. 22.56: Radiograph showing improper obturation

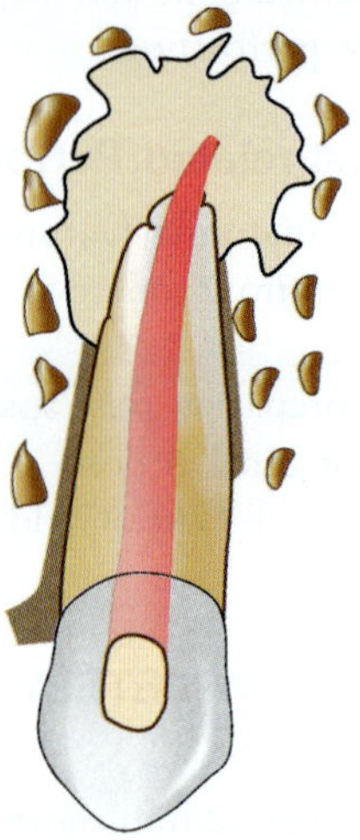

Fig. 22.57: Overfilling of canal causes irritation of periapical tissues

Consequently for the ultimate success of endodontic therapy the practice of underfilling should be avoided (Fig. 22.56).

## Prevention of Underfilling

1. Obtaining straight line access to canal orifices to apex.
2. Precurving the files before using in curved canals.
3. Copious irrigation and recapitulation of the canal.
4. Attaining apical patency.
5. Using EDTA in vital cases especially to emulsify the pulp and remove it completely.
6. Using the files sequentially.
7. Clinician should feel the tensional binding of the file which exists at minor constriction of the apical foramen.

## OVERFILLING OF THE ROOT CANALS

Overfilling of the root canals is filling more than 2 mm beyond the radiographic apex (Fig. 22.57).

*Etiology*

1. Over instrumentation of the root canal.
2. Inadequate determination of the working length (Fig. 22.58).
3. Incompletely formed root apex.
4. Inflammatory apical root resorption.
5. Improper use of reference points for measuring working length.

Not all teeth can lead to endodontic failures. The response of periradicular tissues to root canal filling materials depend on the interaction of the host immune response and properties of the materials.

Over instrumentation often precedes overfilling which inevitably poses risk of forcing infected root canal contents into the periradicular tissues, thereby impairing the healing process.

Studies have shown that overfilling may cause foreign giant call reaction and may act as a foreign body which may support the formation of biofilms. Biofilm is an accumulation of

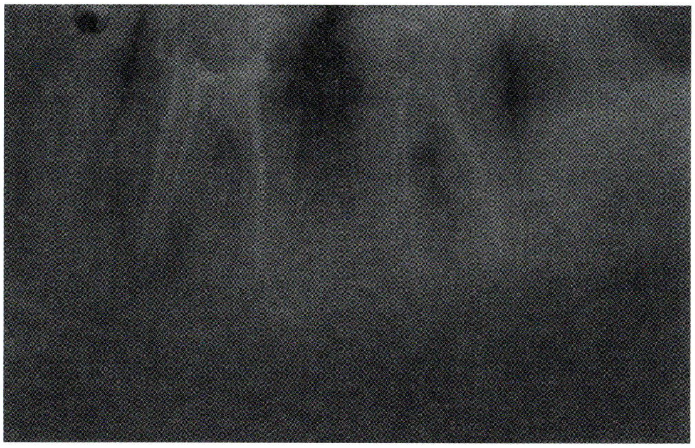

**Fig. 22.58:** Radiograph showing over-extended gutta-percha in 36

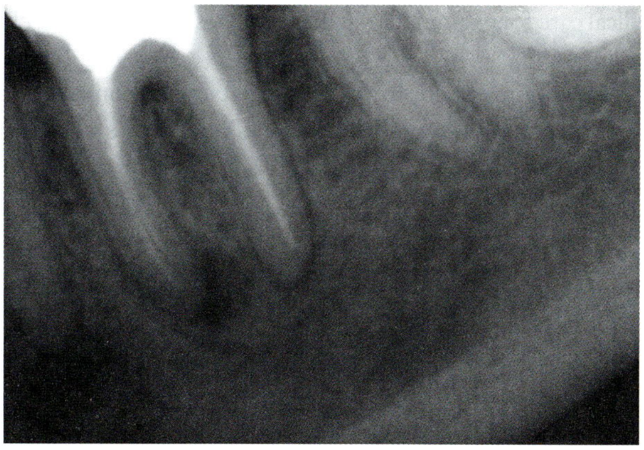

**Fig. 22.60:** Radiograph showing J-shaped radiolucency around mesial root of mandibular molar with vertical root fracture

microorganisms embedded in self produced extracellular polysaccharide matrix adherent to a solid surface. Biofilms constitute the bacterias embedded in them which enable them to survive in a hostile environment.

## VERTICAL ROOT FRACTURE

Vertical root fracture can occur at any phase of root canal treatment that is during biochemical preparation, obturation or during post placement. This fracture results from wedging forces within the canal. These excessive forces exceed the binding strength of existing dentin causing fatigue and fracture (Fig. 22.59).

### Clinical Features

- Vertical root fracture commonly occurs in faciolingual plane.
- Sudden crunching sound accompanied by pain is the pathognomic of the root fracture.
- The fracture begins along the canal wall and grows outwards to the root surface.
- Certain root shapes and sizes are more susceptible to vertical root fracture, for example, roots which are deep facially and lingually but narrow mesially and distally are particularly prone to fracture.

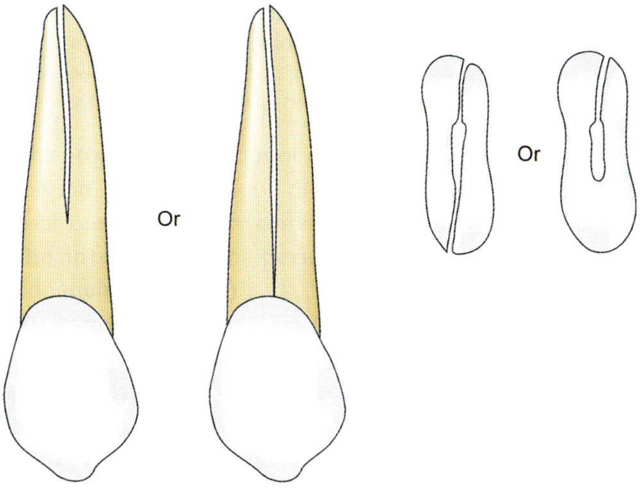


**Fig. 22.59:** Vertical root fracture

- The susceptibility of root fracture increases by excessive dentin removal during canal preparation or post space preparation. Also the excessive condensation forces during compaction of gutta-percha while obturation increases the frequency of root fractures.
- Radiographically vertical root fracture may vary from no significant changes to extensive resorption patterns. In chronic cases, they may show hanging drop radiolucent appearance. According to Cohen, it can be seen radiographically as 'J' shaped radiolucency or may appear as halo shaped defect around the involved root (Fig. 22.60).

***Treatment of vertical root fracture*** involves extraction in most of the cases. In multirooted teeth, root resection or hemisection can be tried.

Other treatment options include retention of the fractured fragment and placement of calcium hydroxide or cementation of the fractured fragments.

Recently, repair of root fracture have been tried by binding them with the help of adhesive resins, glass ionomers and lasers. But to date, no successful technique has been reported to correct this problem.

### Prevention of Root Fracture

Prevention of root fracture basically involves avoidance of the causes of root fracture. The main ***principles*** to prevent root fracture are to:

1. Avoid weakening of the canal wall.
2. Minimize the internal wedging forces.

*To avoid occurrence of vertical root fracture:*

1. Avoid over preparation of the canal.
2. Use less tapered and more flexible compacting instruments to control condensation forces while obturation.
3. Posts should not be used unless they are necessary to retain a tooth.

## INSTRUMENTS ASPIRATION

Aspiration of instruments can occur during endodontic therapy if accidentally dropped in the mouth. It occurs specially in absence of rubber dam. It is a type of emergency which has to be tackled as soon as possible. Patient must be provided

### Radiographic Evaluation

The radiographic criteria for failures are development of radiographic periapical areas of rarefaction after the endodontic treatment, in cases where they were not present before the treatment or persistence or increase in sizes of the radiolucency after the treatment. To predict the success or failure, one should be able to accurately compare the radiographs that are taken at different times.

Prognosis is prediction of whether an endodontic treatment will be successful or a failure and if successful to what degree it will be. Normally, the development of apical periodontitis is indication of endodontic failures. This condition is frequently asymptomatic clinically, and the radiograph is the way to determine the success here.

### Histological Evaluation

Histological criteria for success or failure of endodontic therapy may include absence of inflammation and regeneration of periodontal ligament, bone and cementum following endodontic therapy. Histologically, the success of endodontically treated tooth is reduced because chronic inflammation may persist for long even without any symptoms.

**Histological criteria for success**
- Absence of inflammation
- Regeneration of periodontal ligament fibers
- Presence of osseous repair
- Repair of cementum
- Absence of resorption
- Repair of previously resorbed areas.

## CAUSES OF THE ENDODONTIC FAILURES

Most commonly the causes of root canal failures are directly or indirectly related to bacteria somewhere in the root canal system. The treatment failures can occur despite of the strict adherence to the basic treatment principles. Multitude of factors affect the success or failure of the endodontic treatment but there are certain factors which are common in all the cases for their success or failure and in some cases, success or failure is particularity related to that individual case.

**Factors affecting success or failure of endodontic therapy in every case**
- Diagnosis and the treatment planning
- Radiographic interpretation
- Anatomy of the tooth and root canal system
- Debridement of the root canal space
- Asepsis of treatment regimen
- Quality and extent of apical seal
- Quality of post endodontic restoration
- Systemic health of the patient
- Skill of the operator.

Basically the causes of root canal failures can be broadly divided into local and systemic.

### Local Factors Causing Endodontic Failures

#### *Infection*

Presence of infected and necrotic pulp tissue in root canal acts as the main irritant to the periapical tissues (Fig. 23.2). For success of the endodontic therapy, thorough debridement of the root canal system is required for removal of these irritants. If infected tissue is present, the host parasite relationship, virulence of microorganisms and ability of infected tissues to heal in the presence of microorganisms are the main factors which influence the repair of the periapical tissues following endodontic therapy.

If apical seal or coronal restorations are not optimal (Figs 23.3 and 23.4), reinfection of root canal can occur through them.

#### *Incomplete Debridement of the Root Canal System (Fig. 23.5)*

It is one of the principle factors contributing to the endodontic failures. The main objective of root canal therapy is the complete elimination of the microorganisms and their byproducts from the root canal system. The poor debridement can lead to residual microorganisms, their byproducts and tissue debris which further recolonize and contribute to endodontic failure.

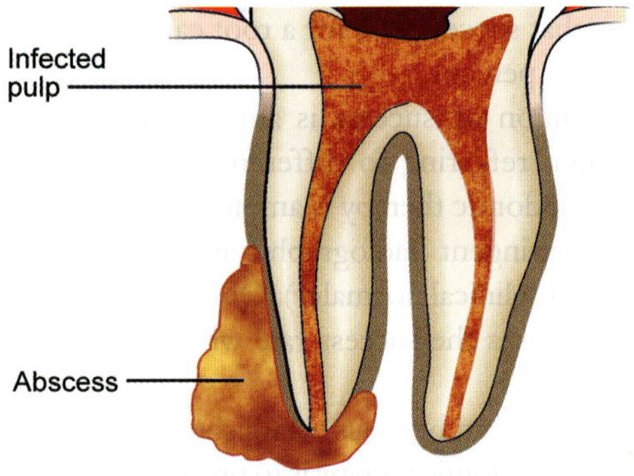


**Fig. 23.2:** Presence of infected pulp acts as main irritant to periapical tissues

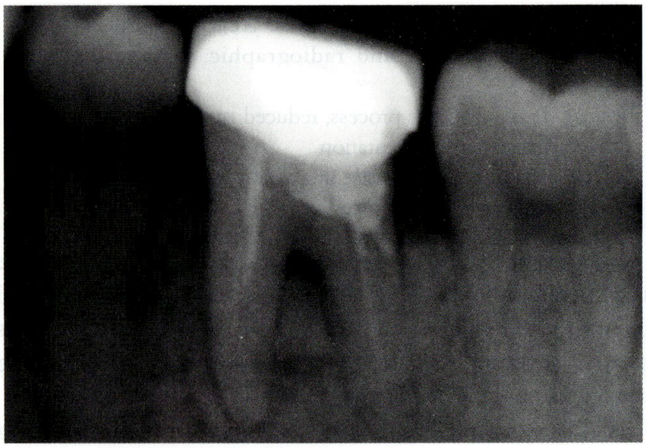

**Fig. 23.3:** Defective root canal obturation results in endodontic failure

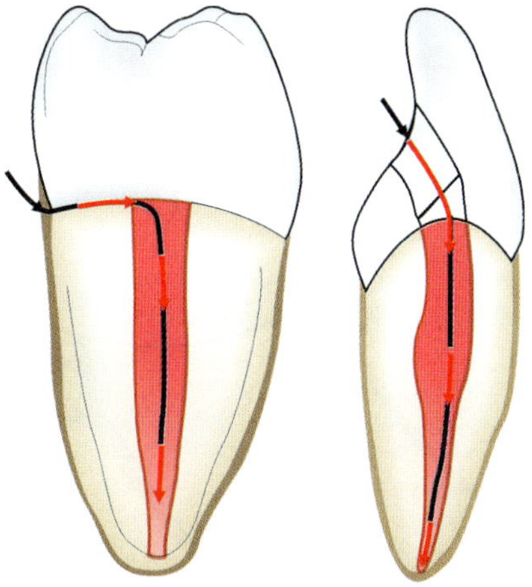

Fig. 23.4: Microleakage because of defective coronal seal can result in endodontic failure

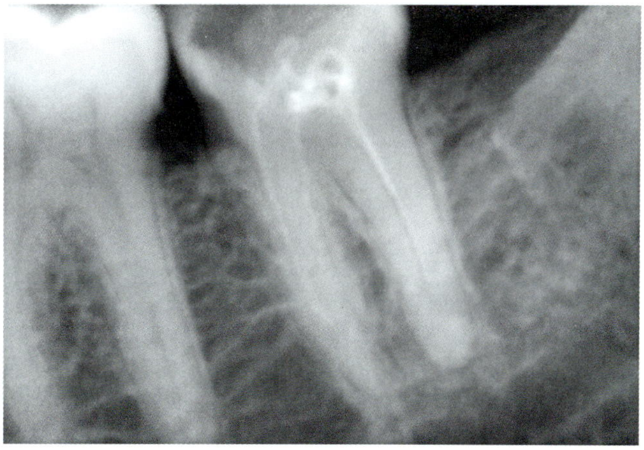

Fig. 23.5: Defective obturation resulting in root canal failure

### Excessive Hemorrhage

Extirpation of pulp and instrumentation beyond periapical tissues lead to excessive hemorrhage. Mild inflammation is produced because of local accumulation of the blood. The extravasated blood cells and fluids must be resorbed because otherwise they act as foreign body. Also the extravasated blood acts as nidus for bacterial growth especially in the presence of infection.

### Overinstrumentation

Instrumentation beyond apical foramen causes decrease in the prognosis of endodontic treatment because of trauma to periodontal ligament and the alveolar bone (Fig. 23.6). Whereas when instrumentation of the root canal system remains within the confines of root canals, the chances of success of endodontic therapy are more (Fig. 23.7).

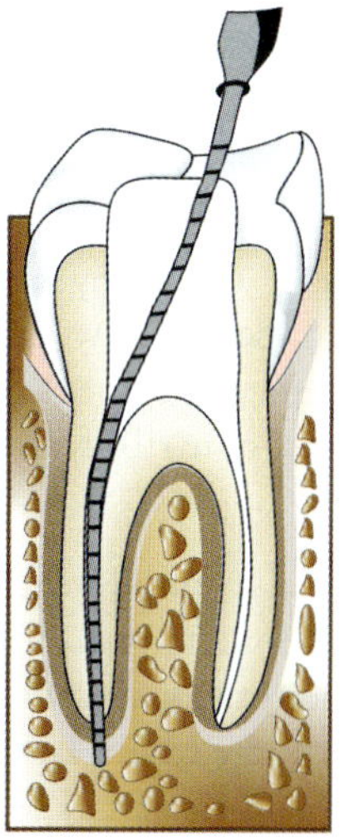

Fig. 23.6: Overinstrumentation results in trauma to periodontal tissue and decreases the prognosis of tooth

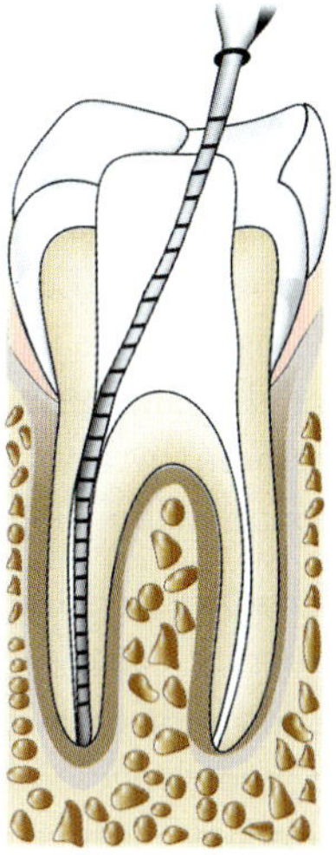

Fig. 23.7: If instrumentation is kept within confines of root canal space, it improves the prognosis

### Chemical Irritants

Chemical irritants in form of intracanal medicaments, irrigating solution decrease the prognosis of endodontic therapy if they get extruded in the periapical tissues. The complete biomechanical preparation of the root canal system does not require the use of these medicaments except in some cases where the chronic inflammation is present. One should take care while using the medicaments to avoid their periapical extrusion.

### Iatrogenic Errors

*Instrument separation:* Instrument separation is caused by improper or overuse of instruments and forcing them in curved and tortuous canals. Seltzer et al reported that prognosis of endodontic therapy was not much affected in teeth in which vital pulps were present before treatment, but if instrument separation occurred in teeth with pulpal necrosis, prognosis was found to be poor after treatment. Basically separated instruments impair the mechanical instrumentation of infected root canals apical to instrument, which contribute to endodontic failure (Fig. 23.8).

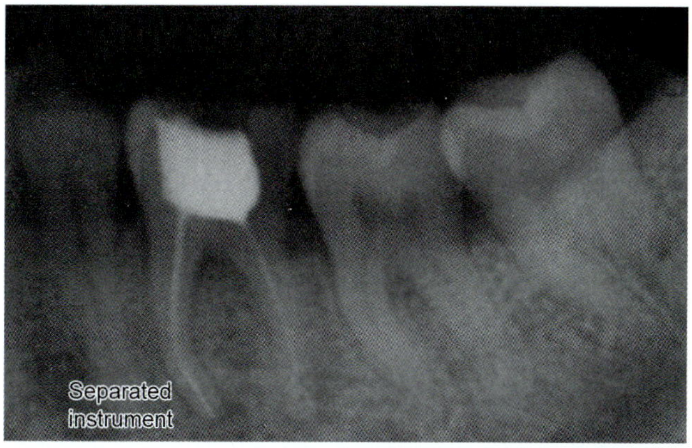


Fig. 23.8: Radiograph showing separated instrument in mesiobuccal canal of 46

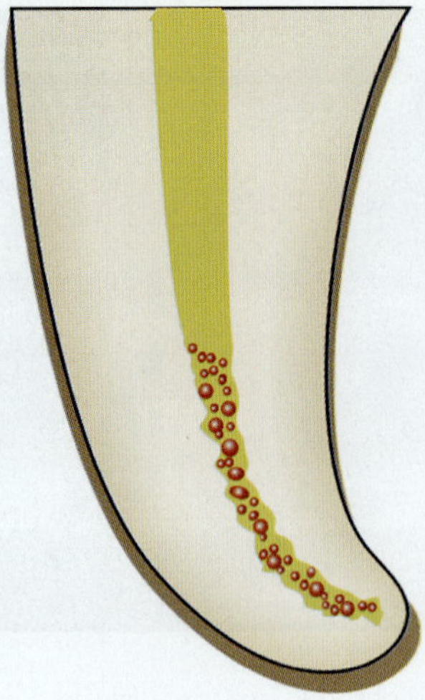

Fig. 23.9: Accumulation of dentin chips and debris causing incomplete instrumentation

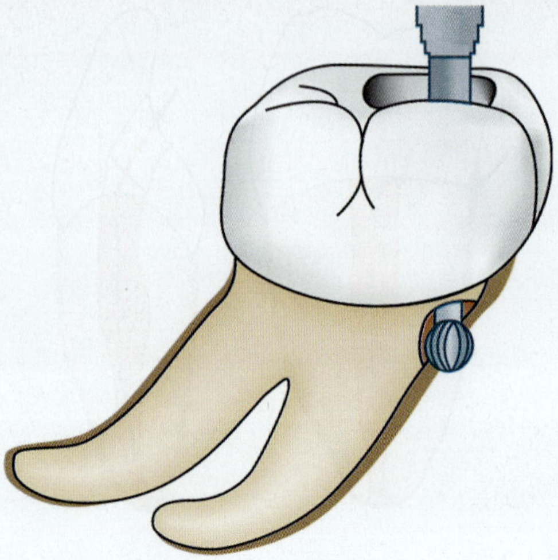

Fig. 23.11: Perforation of molar

*Canal blockage and ledge formation:* In cases with canal blockage and ledge formation, complete cleaning and shaping of the root canal system cannot be accomplished. Canal blockage can occur due to accumulation of dentin chips or tissue debris which prevents the instrument to reach its full working length (Fig. 23.9). Ledge formation usually occurs by using straight instruments in curved canals. All these lead to working short of the canal terminus and thus bacteria and tissue debris may remain in non-instrumented area contributing to endodontic failure (Fig. 23.10).

*Perforations:* Perforation i.e. mechanical communication between root canal system and the periodontium can occur during the root canal therapy. Usually perforations occur by lack of knowledge of internal anatomy of the tooth, lack of attention and misdirection of the instruments (Figs 23.11 and 23.12). Prognosis of endodontically treated tooth with perforations depend on many factors such as location (its closeness to gingival sulcus), time which has elapsed before defect is repaired, adequacy of perforation seal and size of the perforation. Teeth with perforations show poor prognosis because of remaining infected tissue in non-instrumented portion of the canal apical to perforation (Fig. 23.13).

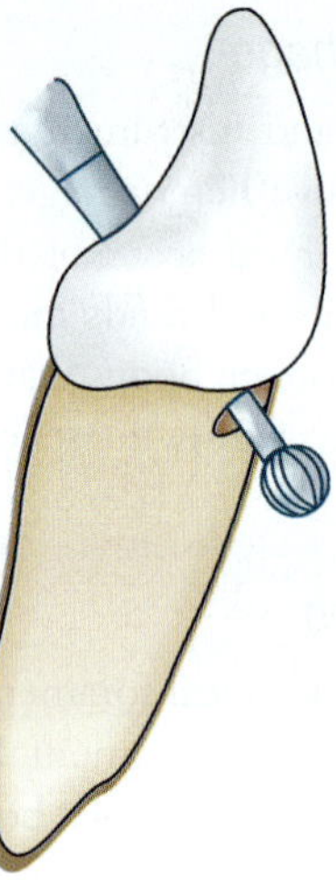

Fig. 23.12: Perforation of anterior tooth due to misdirection of bur

*Incompletely filled teeth:* Incompletely filled teeth are teeth filled more than 2 mm short of apex (Figs 23.14 and 23.15).

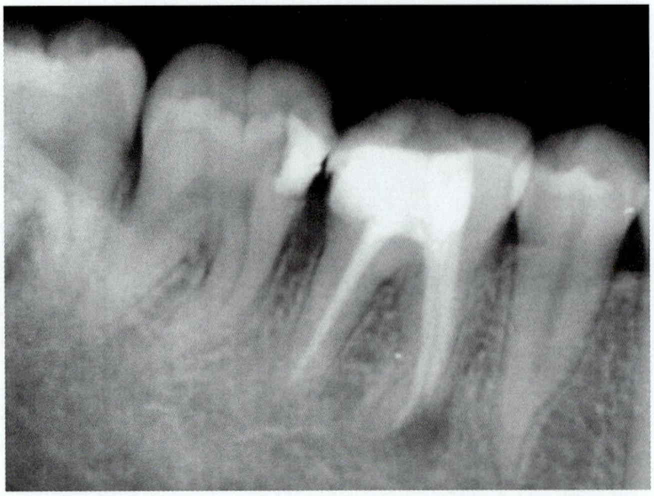

Fig. 23.10: Ledge formation in mesiobuccal canal of 46 resulting in poor prognosis of treatment

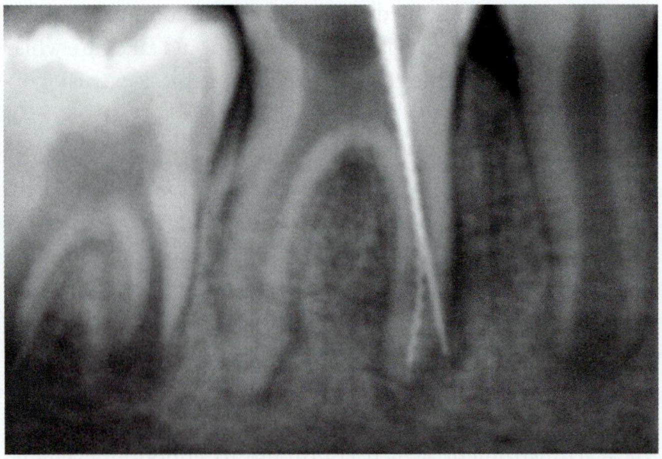

Fig. 23.13: Perforation in mesiobuccal canal of 46 decreasing the prognosis of treatment

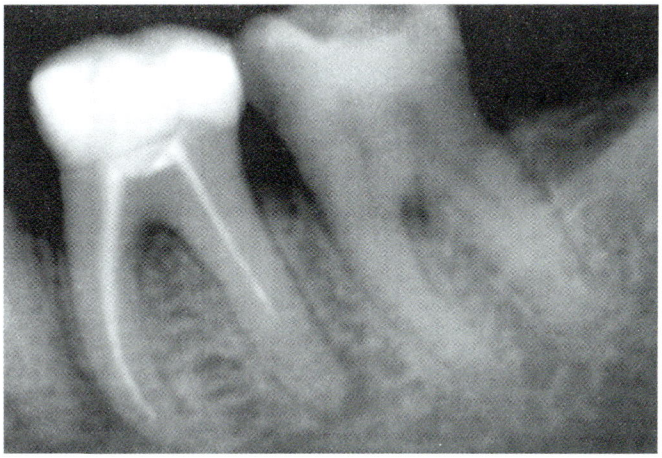

**Fig. 23.14:** Radiograph showing incompletely filled molar

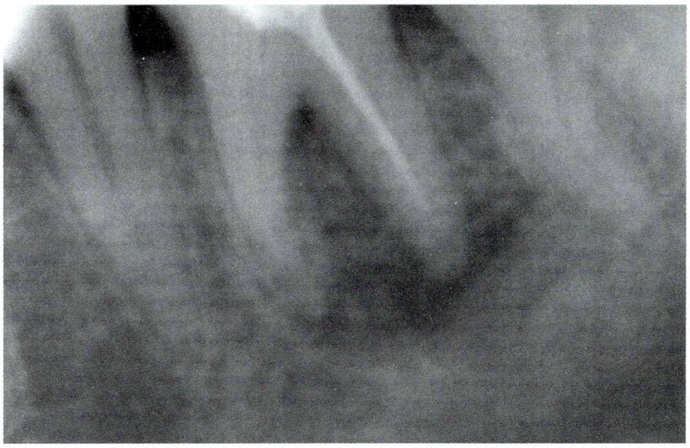

**Fig. 23.15:** Radiograph showing improperly obturated molar

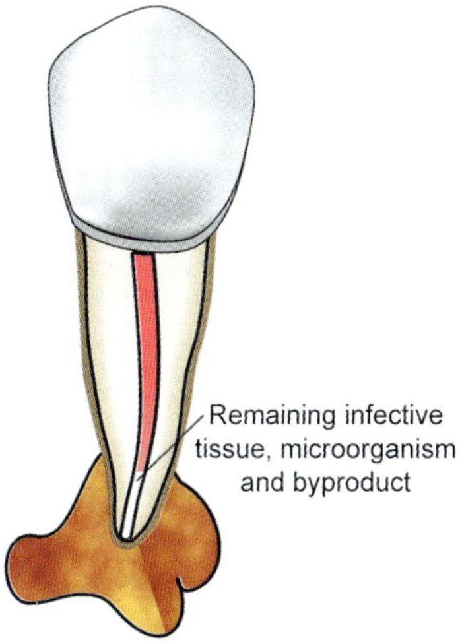


**Fig. 23.16:** Remaining infective tissue, microorganisms and their byproducts of incompletely filled space act as constant irritant

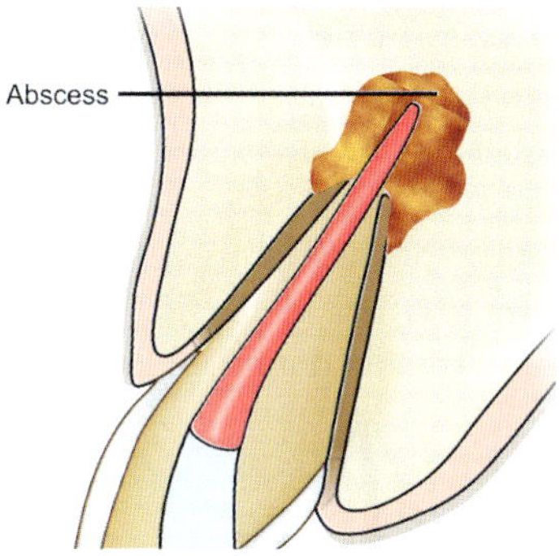


**Fig. 23.17:** Overfilling of canal results in endodontic failure due to constant irritation to periapical tissues

Underfilling can occur due to incomplete instrumentation or ledge formation, blockage of canal by dentin chips, tissue debris and improper measurements of working length. Several studies have shown poorer prognosis of teeth with underfillings especially those with necrotic pulps. Remaining infected necrotic tissue, microorganism and their byproducts in inadequately instrumented and filled teeth cause continuous irritation to the periradicular tissues and thus endodontic failure (Fig. 23.16).

*Overfilling of root canals:* Overfilling of root canals, i.e. obturation of the canal extending more than 2 mm beyond radiographic apex. It can occur because of apical root resorption, incompletely formed roots and overinstrumentation of the root canal system. Overfilling of the root canals may cause endodontic failure because of continuous irritation of the periapical tissues (Fig. 23.17). The filling material acts as a foreign body which may generate immunological response. Biofilms (accumulation of microorganisms embedded in self-produced extracellular polysaccharide matrix, adherent to solid surface) are seen on the extruded material which contains the treatment resistant bacteria.

*Corrosion of root canal fillings:* Corrosion is the tendency of most of the metals to revert to their lower form by oxidation. Silver cones have shown to produce corrosion. The main area of corrosion of silver cones is coronal and the apical portions, the areas which contact tissue fluids either periapical exudation or saliva. The corrosion products are cytotoxic and may act as tissue irritants causing persistent periapical inflammation.

*Anatomic factors:* Presence of overly curved canals, calcifications (Fig. 23.18), numerous lateral and accessory canals, bifurcations, aberrant canal anatomy like C or S-shaped canals may pose problems in adequate cleaning and shaping and

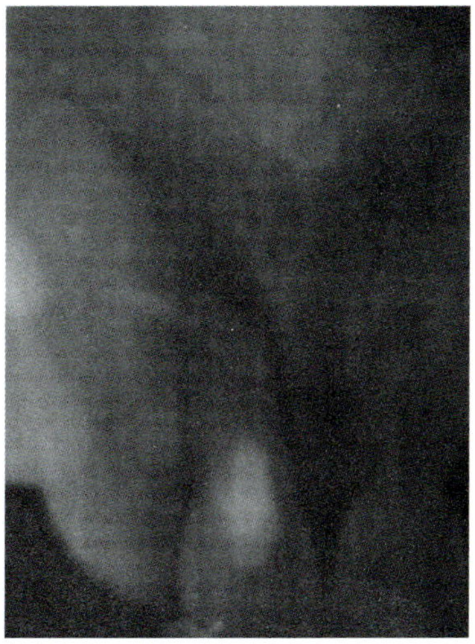

**Fig. 23.18:** Radiograph showing calcified 12

thereby incomplete filling of the root canals. These can lead to endodontic failure.

*Root fractures (Fig. 23.19):* Endodontic failures can occur by partial or complete fractures of the roots. Prognosis of teeth with vertical root fracture is poorer than horizontal fractures.

*Traumatic occlusion:* Traumatic occlusion has also been reported to cause endodontic failures because of its effect on periodontium.

*Periodontal considerations:* An endodontic failure may occur because of communication between the periodontal ligament and the root canal system (Fig. 23.20). Also the recession of attachment apparatus may cause exposure of lateral canals to the oral fluids which can lead to reinfection of the root canal system because of percolation of fluids (Fig. 23.21).

## Systemic Factors

Systemic factors influence the success or failure of the endodontic therapy. The systemic diseases may influence the local tissue resistance and thus interfering with the normal healing process.

When systemic disease is present, the response of the periapical tissues may get intensified if there is increase in concentration of irritants during endodontic therapy. Thus a

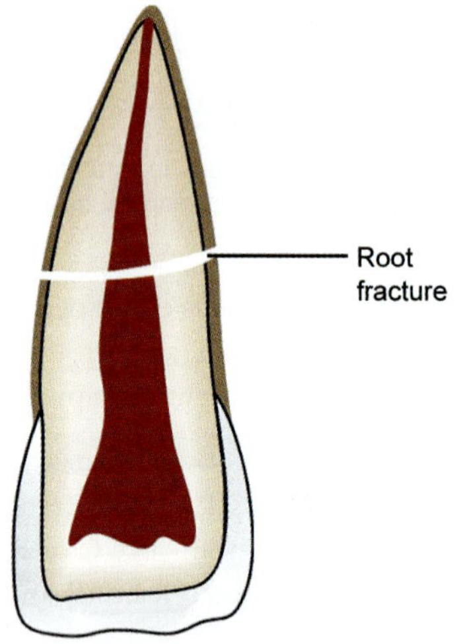


**Fig. 23.19:** Root fracture decreases the prognosis of treatment

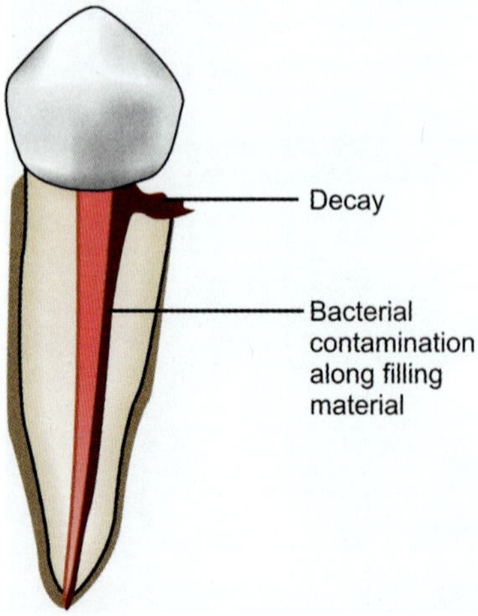


**Fig. 23.20:** Decay at subgingival area below crown can result in contamination of root filling and contribute to endodontic failure

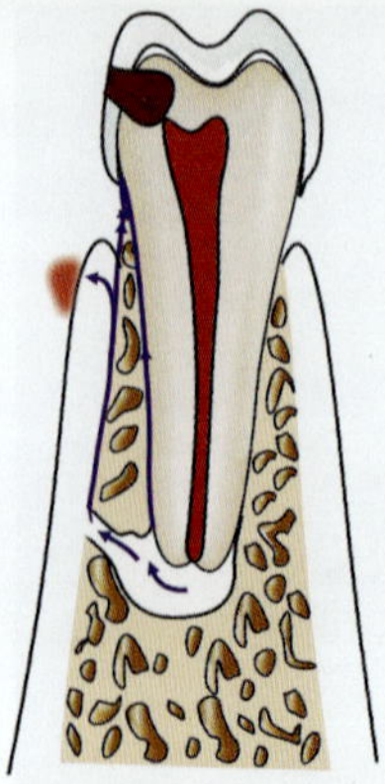

**Fig. 23.21:** Endodontic periodontal communication results in endodontic failure

severe reaction may occur following cleaning and shaping, i.e. mechanical irritation and chemical irritation from medicaments and irrigants, causing dispersion of the microorganisms. Healing is also impaired in patients with systemic disease. Various systemic factors which can interfere in the success of endodontic therapy are nutritional deficiencies, diabetes mellitus, renal failure, blood dyscrasias, hormonal imbalance, autoimmune disorders, opportunistic infections, aging, and patients on long-term steroid therapy.

Thus before starting endodontic therapy, a complete medical history is essential to predict the prognosis of the tooth.

## Factors Responsible for Endodontic Failures

*Local*
- Infection
- Incomplete debridement of the root canal system
- Excessive hemorrhage
- Overinstrumentation
- Chemical irritants
- Iatrogenic errors
  - Separated instruments
  - Canal blockage and ledge formation
  - Perforations
  - Incompletely filled teeth
  - Overfilling of root canals
- Corrosion of root canal fillings
- Anatomic factors
- Root fractures
- Traumatic occlusion
- Periodontal considerations

*Systemic*
- Nutritional deficiencies
- Diabetes mellitus
- Renal failure
- Blood dyscrasias
- Hormonal imbalance
- Autoimmune disorders
- Opportunistic infections
- Aging
- Patients on long-term steroid therapy

The tooth which has experienced the endodontic failure could be treated either by nonsurgical retreatment, surgical or combination of both procedures. In endodontic retreatment, one attempt to eliminate the root canal microorganisms but in case of surgical correction, there is an attempt to confine the microorganisms within the root canal.

### *Before going for endodontic retreatment, following factors should be considered:*

a. When should treatment be considered, i.e. if patient is asymptomatic even if treatment is not proper, the retreatment should be postponed.

b. Patient's needs and expectations.
c. Strategic importance of the tooth.
d. Periodontal evaluation of the tooth.
e. Other interdisciplinary evaluation.
f. Chair time and cost.

Retreatment can be differentiated from the normal endodontic therapy in its unique considerations and techniques.

*Before performing endodontic retreatment following points should be considered:*

a. Retreatment may be performed to prevent the potential disease.
b. To gain access into root canal extensive coronal restoration has to be removed and remade.
c. Technical problems may result from previous treatment or aberrant canal anatomy.
d. Even after retreatment sometimes better results may not be achieved.
e. Root canal filling materials have to be removed during retreatment.
f. Prognosis of retreatment could be poorer than the initial endodontic therapy.
g. Patient might be more apprehensive than with initial treatment.

## CASE SELECTION FOR ENDODONTIC RETREATMENT

Retreatment is usually indicated in symptomatic endodontically treated teeth or in asymptomatic teeth with improperly done, initial endodontic therapy to prevent future emergence of the disease.

1. Careful history of patient should be taken to know the nature of case, pathogenesis and urgency of the treatment, etc.
2. Evaluate the anatomy of root canal in relation to canal curvature, calcifications, unusual configurations, etc.
3. Evaluate the quality of obturation of primary endodontic treatment.
4. Check for iatrogenic complications like separated instruments, ledges, perforations, zipping, canal blockages, etc.
5. Consider the cooperation of the patient which is mandatory for retreatment procedure.

### Factors Affecting Prognosis of Endodontic Treatment

- Presence of any periapical radiolucency (Fig. 23.22)
- Quality of the obturation
- Apical extension of the obturation material (Fig. 23.23)
- Bacterial status of the canal
- Observation period
- Post-endodontic coronal restoration
- Iatrogenic complication.

### Contraindications of Endodontic Retreatment

- Unfavorable root anatomy (shape, taper, remaining dentin thickness)

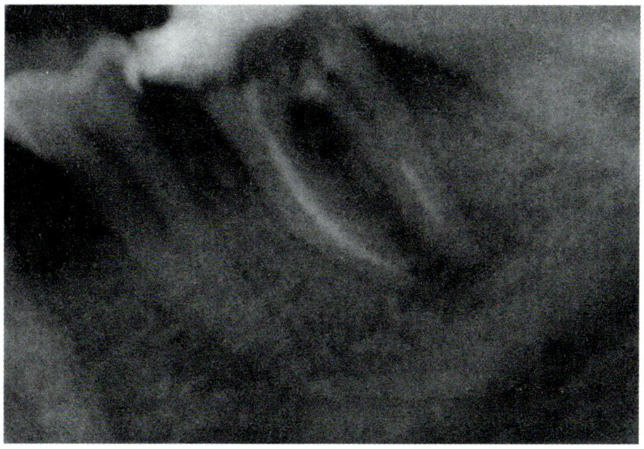

Fig. 23.22: Root canal failure due to separated instrument, poorly obturated canals and poor coronal restoration

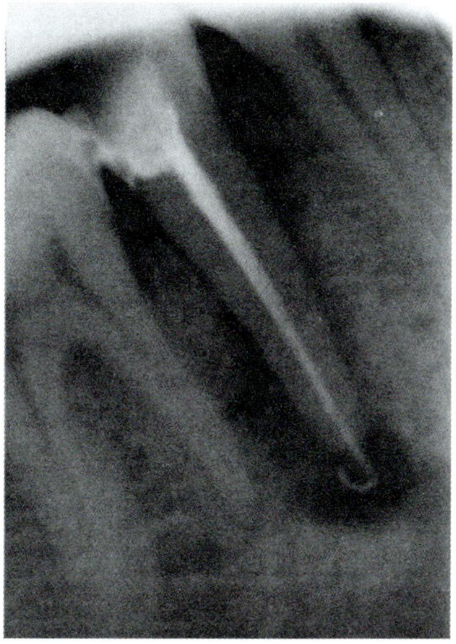

Fig. 23.23: Radiography showing overextended obturation of 35

- Presence of untreatable root resorptions or perforations.
- Presence of root or bifurcation caries.
- Insufficient crown/root ratio.

### Problems Commonly Encountered during Retreatment

- Unpredictable result
- Frustration
- Cost factor
- Time consuming.

## STEPS OF RETREATMENT

- Coronal disassembly
- Establish access to root canal system
- Remove canal obstructions
- Establish patency
- Thorough cleaning, shaping and obturation of the canal.

### Coronal Disassembly

Endodontic retreatment procedures commonly require removal of the existing coronal restoration (Fig. 23.24). But in some

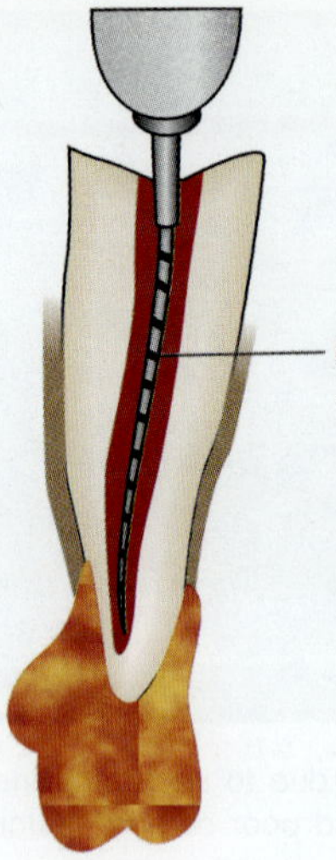


Fig. 23.24: Entry to root canal after coronal dissembly

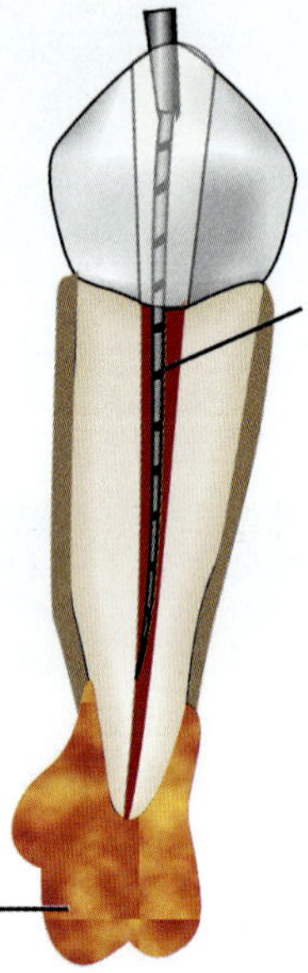


Fig. 23.25: Entry to root canal system through coronal restoration

cases access can be made through the existing restoration (Fig. 23.25).

Gaining access through original restoration helps in:

a. Facilitating rubber dam placement
b. Maintaining form, function and esthetics
c. Reducing the cost of replacement.

But disadvantages of retaining a restoration include:

a. Reduced visibility and accessibility
b. Increased risks of irreparable errors.
c. Increased risks of microbial infection if crown margins are poorly adapted.

It is advisable to remove the existing restoration especially if it has poor marginal adaptation, secondary caries to avoid procedural errors (Fig. 23.26). To maintain form, function and esthetics, temporary crown can be placed.

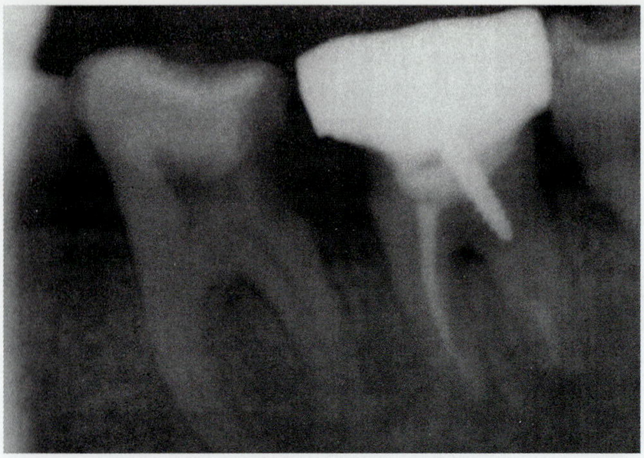

Fig. 23.26: Radiograph showing poor marginal adaptation and secondary caries under coronal restoration. It is advisable to remove such restoration before retreatment

## Establish Access to Root Canal System

In some teeth, post and core needs to be removed for gaining access to the root canal system (Figs 23.27 to 23.29). However, when crown is with good marginal integrity, access can be gained without crown removal (Fig. 23.30).

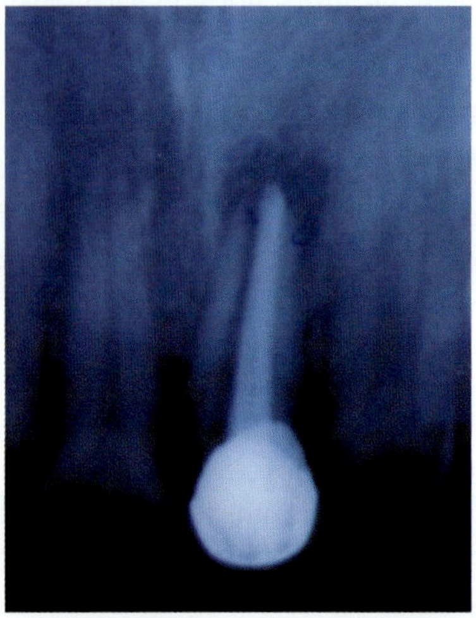

Fig. 23.27: Root canal failure of 11 with crown placed over it

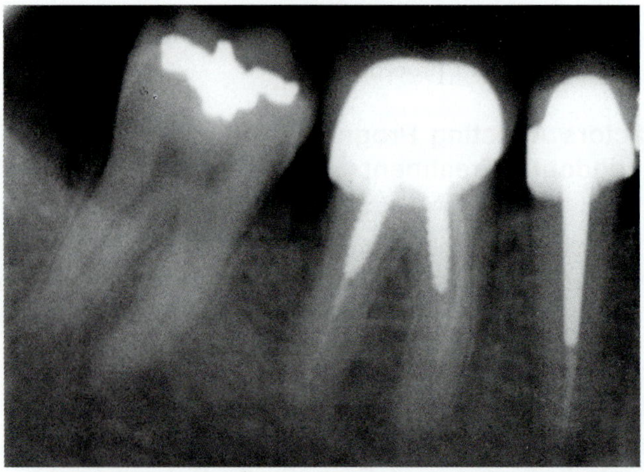

Fig. 23.28: Radiograph showing improperly done root canal treatment in 46 for gaining access to canals coronal dissembly is required here

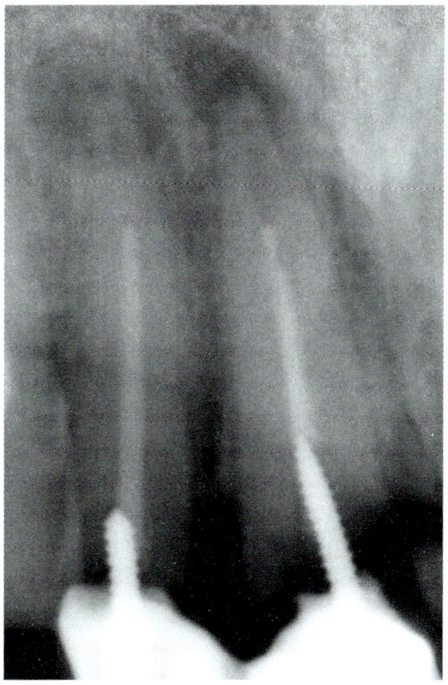

Fig. 23.29: Radiograph showing failure of root canal with improper coronal seel

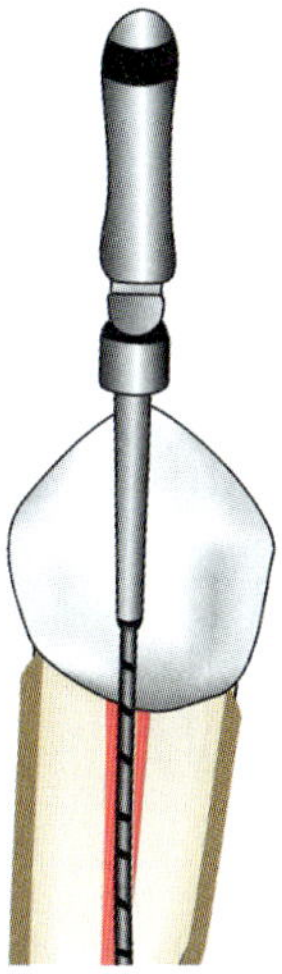

Fig. 23.30: When crown has good marginal seal, entry can be gained through it

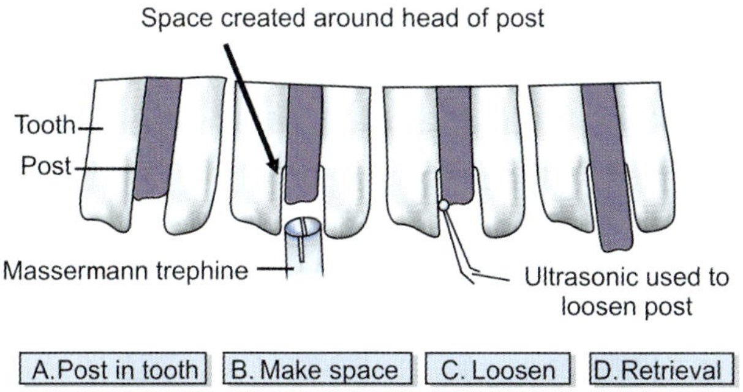


Fig. 23.31: Use of ultrasonics to remove post

Posts can be removed by various methods. These are:

1. Weakening retention of posts by use of ultrasonic vibration (Fig. 23.31).
2. Forceful pulling of posts but it increases the risk of root fracture.

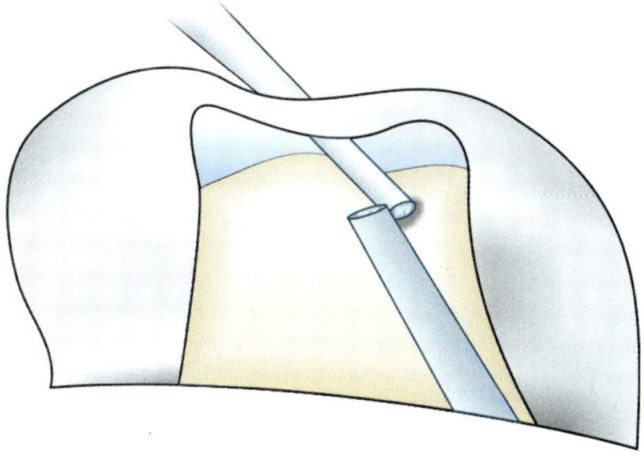

Fig. 23.32: Use of transmeatal bur for dooming head of post head

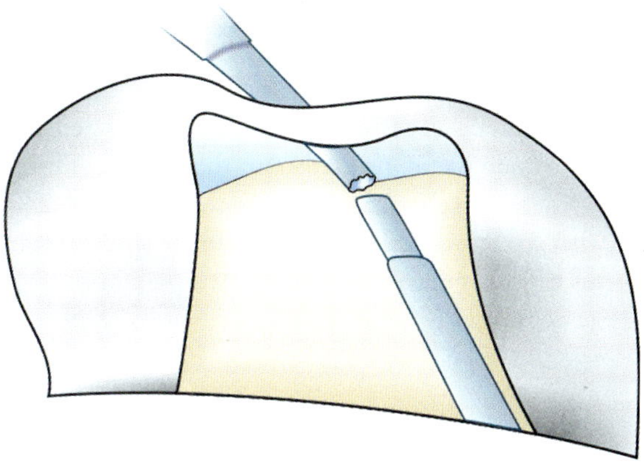

Fig. 23.33: Selection of trephine to engage the 2-3 mm of post head

3. Removing posts with the help of special pliers using post removal systems.
4. Occasionally access can be made through the core for retreatment procedure without disturbing the post.

The recently developed Post Removal System (PRS) simplified the removal of post from the canal. For use of PRS kit, one should have straight line access to the canal and also the post should be easily visualized from the chamber.

PRS kit consists of five variously designed trephines and corresponding taps, a torque bar, a transmeatal bur, rubber bumpers and extracting pliers.

1. Initially a transmeatal bur is used for efficiently dooming of the post head (Fig. 23.32).
2. Then a drop of lubricant such as RC Prep is placed on the post head to further facilitate the machining process.
3. After this select the largest trephine to engage the post and to machine down the coronal 2-3 mm of the post (Fig. 23.33).
4. Followed by a PRS microtubular tap is inserted against the post head and screwed it into post with counter clockwise direction. Before doing this rubber bumper is inserted on the tap to act as cushion against forces (Fig. 23.34).
5. When tubular tap tightly engages the post, rubber bumper is pushed down to the occlusal surface.
6. Mount the post removal plier on tubular tap by holding it firmly with one hand and engaging it with other hand

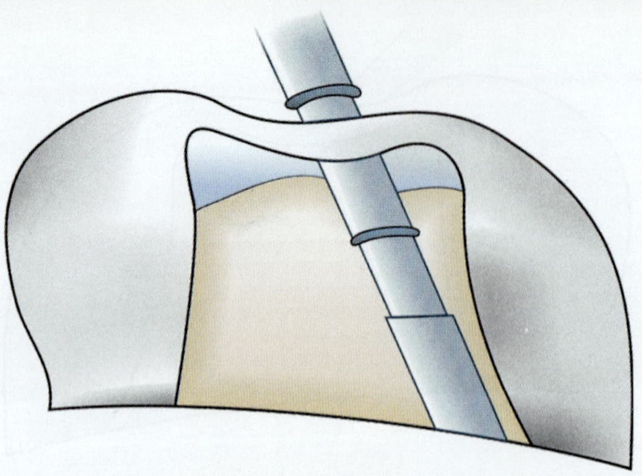

Fig. 23.34: Insert microtubular tap against post head and move it in counter clockwise direction

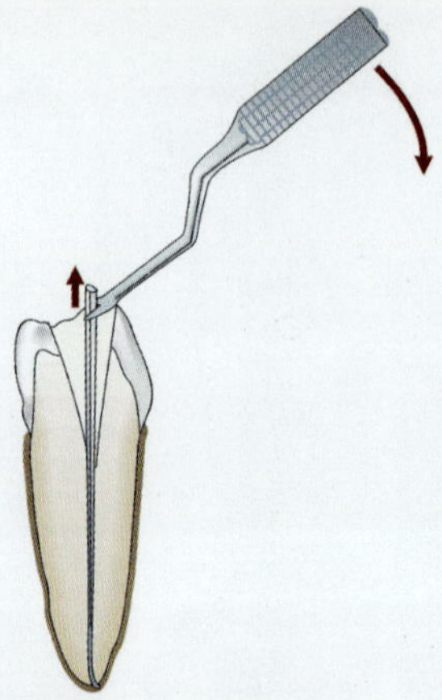

Fig. 23.36: Removal of silver point using microsurgical forcep

by turning screw knob clocking if post is strongly bonded in the canal, then ultrasonic instrument is vibrated on the tap or a torque bar is inserted onto the handle to increase the leverage, thereby facilitating its removal (Fig. 23.35).

7. After that select an ultrasonic tip and vibrate it on the tubular tap, this causes screwed knob to turn further and thus help in post removal.

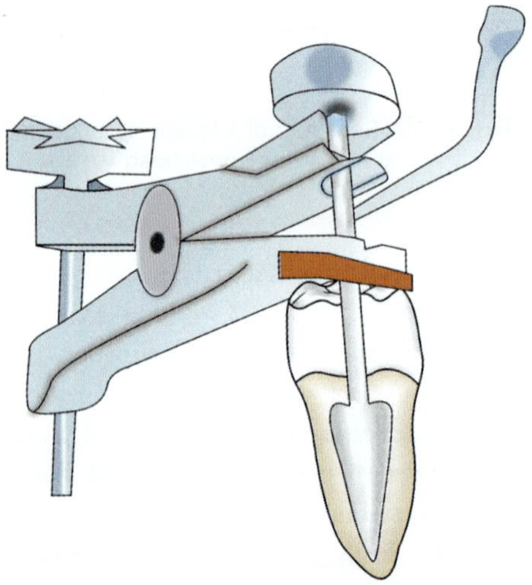

Fig. 23.35: Mount post removal plier on tubular tap and then vibrate ultrasonic instrument on to the tap to increase leverage

## Removing Canal Obstructions and Establishing Patency

Patency of canal can be regained by removing obstructions in the canal which can be in the form of silver points, gutta- percha, pastes, sealers, separated instruments and posts, etc.

### *Silver Point Removal*

They can be bypassed or removed depending upon the accessibility and canal anatomy. Silver points can be retrieved from the canal by:

a. Using microsurgical forceps—Its use is ideal especially when cone heads are sticking up in the chamber (Fig. 23.36).

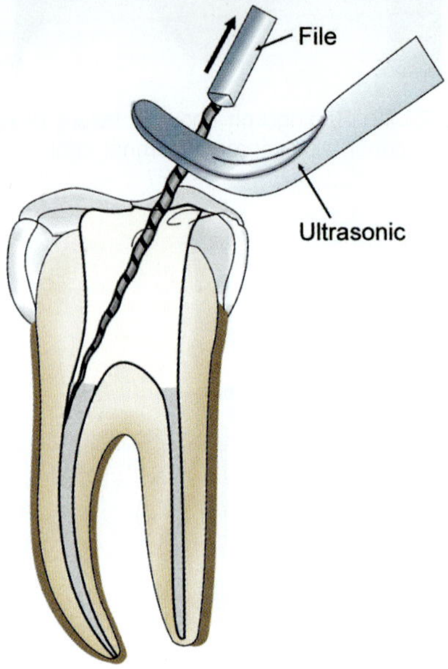


Fig. 23.37: Ultrasonic file is moved around the silver point to loosen it with vibration

b. Using ultrasonic—In this ultrasonic file is worked around the periphery of instrument to loosen it with vibration (Fig. 23.37).
c. Using Hedstroem files—In this Hedstroem files are placed in the canal and are worked down alongside the silver point (Fig. 23.38). These files are twisted around each other by making clockwise rotation. This will make grip around silver point which then can be removed (Fig. 23.39).
d. Using hypodermic needle which is made to fit tightly over the silver point over which cyanoacrylate is placed as an adhesive (Fig. 23.40). When it sets, needle is grabbed with pliers (Fig. 23.41).
e. By tap and thread option using microtubular taps from post removal the post removal system kit.
f. Using instrument removal system.

### *Gutta-percha Removal*

The relative difficulty in removing gutta-percha is influenced by length, diameter, curvature and internal configuration of the

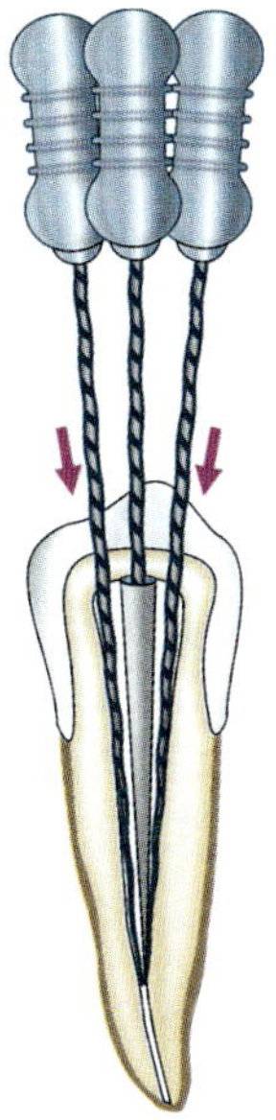

Fig. 23.38: Use of Hedstroem files to remove silver point

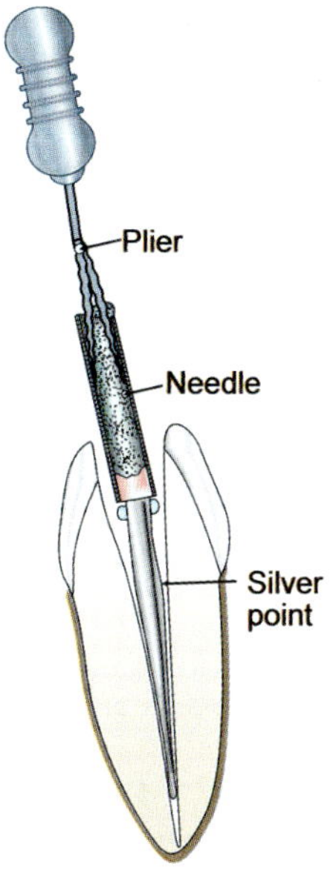


Fig. 23.41: After the cyanoacrylate sets, grab the needle with plier

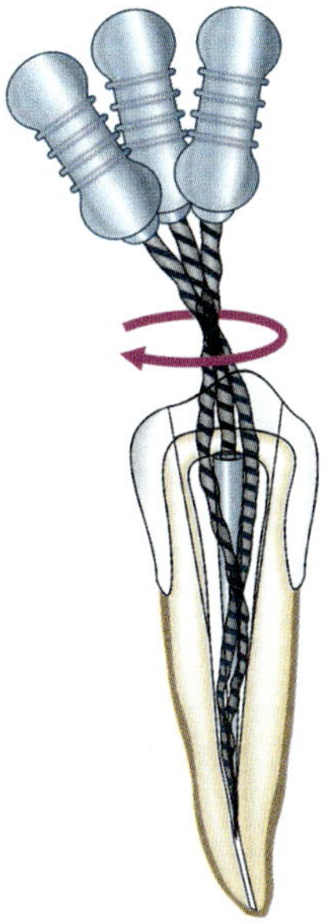

Fig. 23.39: Files are twisted around each other by making clockwise rotation. This will grip the silver point

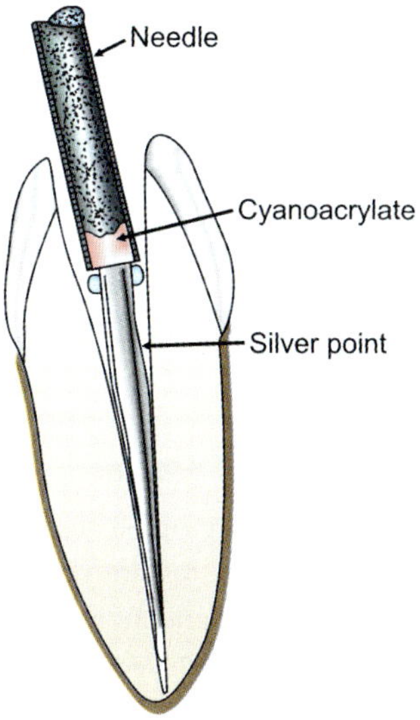


Fig. 23.40: Use of hypodermic needle to fit it tightly over silver point over which cyanoacrylate is placed as adhesive

canal system. Irrespective of the technique gutta-percha is best removed from root canal in progressive manner to prevent its extrusion periapically.

### *Removal of Gutta-percha*

Gutta-percha is best removed is crown down technique. Following factors affect gutta-percha removal:

i. Density of filling
ii. Curvature of canal
iii. Length of canal

Gutta-percha can be removed by:

i. Using solvents
ii. Using hand instruments
iii. Using rotary instruments
iv. Using microdebrider.

*i. Use of solvents to remove gutta-percha:* Since it has been seen that gutta-percha is soluble in chloroform, methyl chloroform, benzene, xylene, eucalyptol oil, halothane and rectified white turpentine, it can removed from the canal by dissolving it among these solvents (Fig. 23.42).

Being highly volatile, chloroform is most effective so commonly used. Since at high concentrations, it has shown to be carcinogenic, its excessive filling in pulp chamber is avoided.

Gutta-percha dissolution has to be supplemented by further negotiation of the canal and removing the dissolved material from it (Fig. 23.43).

*ii. Use of hand instruments:* Hand instruments are mainly used in the apical portion of the canal. Poorly condensed gutta-percha can be easily pulled out by use of files. Hedstroem files are used to engage the cones so that they can be pulled

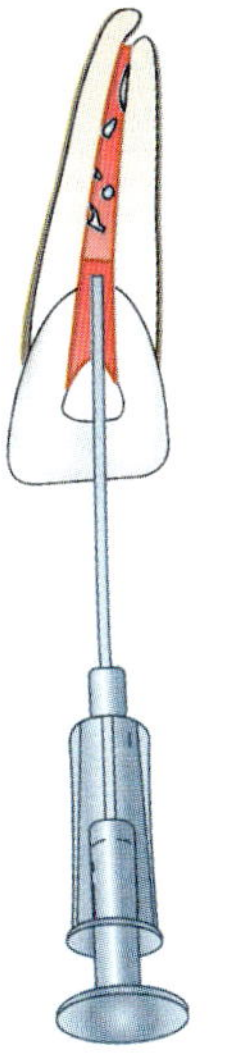

Fig. 23.42: Use of solvents to dissolve gutta-percha

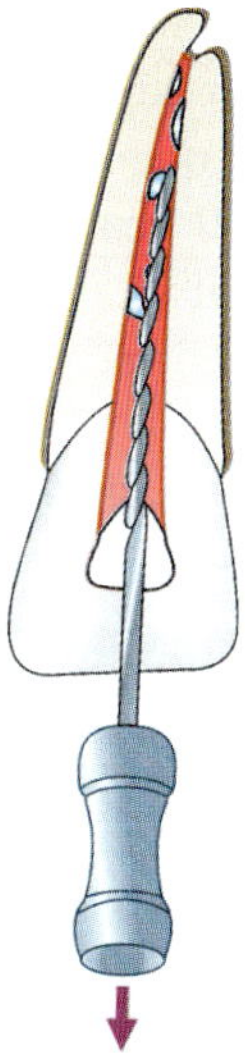

Fig. 23.43: Removal of dissolved gutta-percha using files

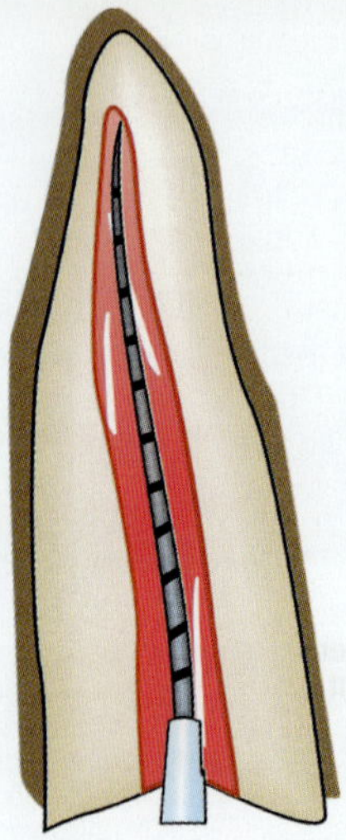

Fig. 23.44: Removal of gutta- percha using H-file

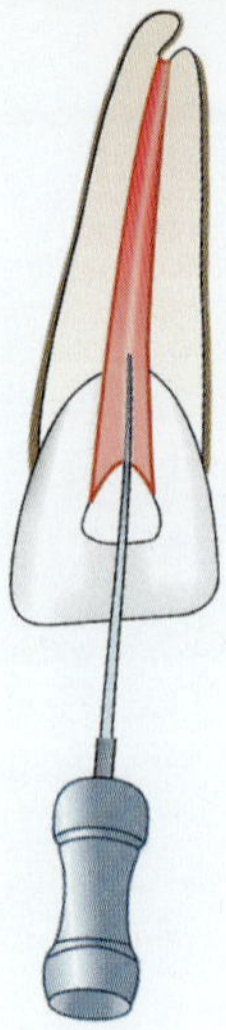

Fig. 23.45: Removal of gutta-percha using hot instrument like reamer or file

out in single piece (Fig. 23.44). Removal of gutta-percha can also be done by using hot endodontic instrument like file or reamer (Fig. 23.45). Reamers or files can be used to bypass the gutta-percha sometimes.

With overextended cones, files sometimes have to be extended periapically to avoid separation of the cone at the apical foramen. Sometimes cones which get separated at apex may not be retrieved.

Coronal portion of gutta-percha should always be explored by Gates-Gliddens so as to:

a. Remove gutta-percha quickly.
b. Provide space for solvents.
c. Improve convenience form.

iii. *Use of rotary instrumentation:* Rotary instruments are safe to be used in straight canals. Recently in May 2006, new ProTaper universal system was introduced consisting of $D_1$, $D_2$, and $D_3$ to be used at 500-700 rpm.

**$D_1$ file:**

- Removes filling from coronal third
- 11 mm handle
- 16 mm cutting surface
- White ring for identification
- ISO 30 active tip for easier penetration of obturation material
- 9 percent taper file.

**$D_2$ file:**

- Removes filling from middle third
- 11 mm handle
- 18 mm cutting blades
- Two white rings for identification
- ISO 25, non-active rounded tip to follow canal path
- 8 percent taper file.

**$D_3$ file:**

- Removes filling from apical third
- 11 mm handle
- 22 mm cutting blades
- Three white rings for identification
- ISO 20 non-active rounded tip to follow canal path
- 7 percent taper file.

iv. *Using microdebriders:* These are small files constructed with 90 degrees bends and are used to remove any remaining gutta-percha on the sides of canal walls or isthmuses after the repreparation.

### *Removal of Resilon*

Resilon can be removed using combination of hand and rotary instruments, similarly as we do for removal of gutta-percha. For effective removal of resilon, combination of chloroform dissolution and rotary instrumentation is recommended. For removal of resilon sealer use of gates glidden drills and H-files is recommended.

## Carrier Based Gutta-percha Removal

Following should be done for removal of carrier based gutta-percha:

1. Grasp the carrier with pliers and try to remove it using fulcrum mechanism rather than straight pulling if from the tooth.
2. Use ultrasonics along the side of the carrier and thermo-soften the gutta-percha. Then move ultrasonics apically and displace the carrier coronally.
3. Use solvents to chemically soften the gutta-percha and then use hand files to loosen the carrier.
4. Use rotary instruments to remove plastic carrier from the canal.
5. Use instrument removal system to remove carrier especially if it is metal carrier.

### *Removal of Paste*

A wide variety of pastes are used to obturate the root canals. In general pastes are divided into soft, hard, penetrable and impenetrable and non-removable type.

*Soft setting pastes* can be removed using the normal endodontic instruments preferably using crown down technique (Fig. 23.46).

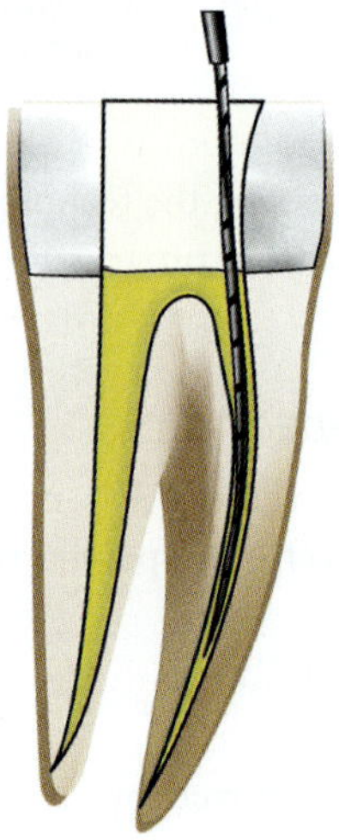

Fig. 23.46: Removal of soft setting paste using normal endodontic instrument in crown down technique

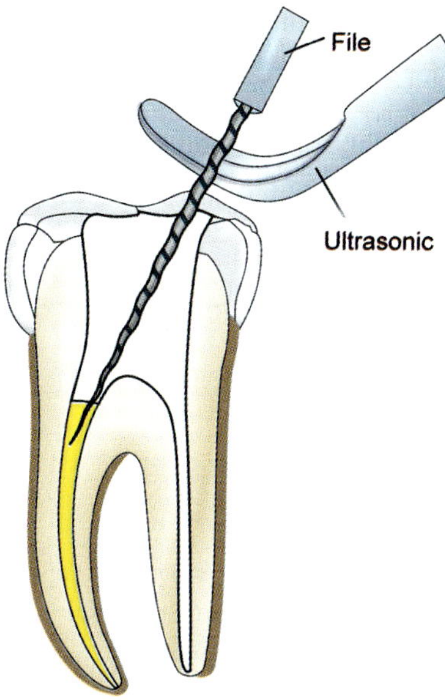


Fig. 23.47: Use of ultrasonic vibration for paste removal

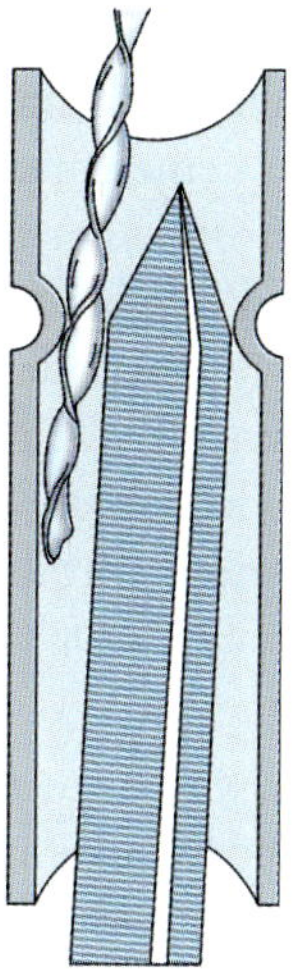

Fig. 23.48: Use of Massermann extractor for removal of separated instrument

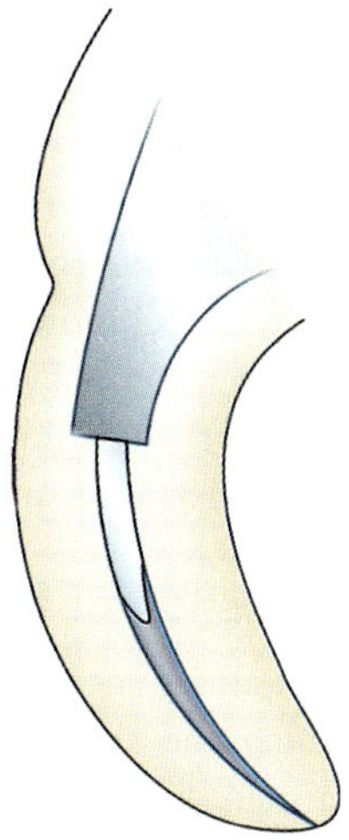

Fig. 23.49: Use of Gates-Gliddens to form a staging platform

*Hard setting cements* like resin cements can be first softened using solvents like xylene, eucalyptol, etc. and then removed using endodontic files. Ultrasonic endodontic devices can also be used to breakdown the pastes by vibrations and thus facilitate their removal (Fig. 23.47).

Following methods can be employed to remove pastes for retreatment cases:

1. Use of heat is employed for some resin pastes for softening them.
2. Use of ultrasonic energy is employed to remove brick hard resin type pastes.
3. Sometime chemicals like Endosolve "R" and Endosolve E are employed for softening hard paste. (R denotes resin based & E denotes eugenol based pastes).
4. Use of microdebriders is done to remove remnants of paste material. These are available in 16 mm length and have Hedstroem type cutting blades with the tip diameter of 0.2 and 0.3 mm and taper of 0.02.
5. Rotary instruments are also used for removal of pastes. Paste filled root canals are first negotiated with 0.02 tapered stainless steel instruments negotiated with 0.02 tapered stainless steel instruments one entry is gained rotary Ni Ti are used to remove the paste coronally. Sometimes end cutting NIT rotary instruments are used to penetrate paste. But time they are more active apically, so to avoid iatrogenic errors, they should be used with caution.

## Separated Instruments and Foreign Objects

Broken instruments or foreign objects can be retrieved from the canals but primary requirement for their removal is their accessibility and visibility. So, we one can say that if root canal is obstructed by foreign object in coronal third then attempt retrieval, in middle third, attempt retrieval or bypass and if it is in apical third leave or surgically treat.

The secret of removing the instruments broken in coronal and middle third is to recognize how much coronal tooth

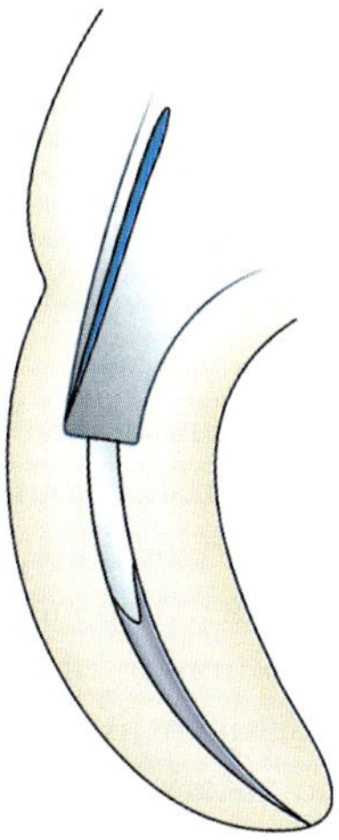

Fig. 23.50: Use of ultrasonic tip to rotate it around instrument and then move it counterclockwise to remove instrument

structure one has to remove to gain access to the instrument. If over preparation of canal compromises the dentin thickness, one should leave the instrument in place rather than compromising the coronal dentin.

If instrument is readily accessible, remove it by holding with instruments like Stieglitz pliers and Massermann extractor. Massermann extractor comprises a tube with a constriction into which a stylet is introduced to grasp the fractured instrument (Fig. 23.48).

Ultrasonics can also be used to remove the instruments by their vibration effect.

Broken instruments can also be attempted for their removal using modified Gates-Glidden bur and then creating a staging platform before using an ultrasonic tip to rotate around the file in a counterclockwise direction to remove it (Figs 23.49 and 23.50).

When it is not possible to remove the foreign objects, attempts should be made to bypass the object and complete biomechanical preparation of the canal system.

Bypassing of instrument can be attempted using hand instruments like reamers and files. These instruments are inserted alongside the broken instrument to soften its cementation and thus facilitating its removal. While making efforts to the bypass the instrument, copious irrigation is needed. Irrigation with sodium hypochlorite, hydrogen peroxide and RC Prep may float the object coronally through the effervescence they create.

Use of ultrasonic K-file No. 15 or 20 with vibration and copious irrigation may also pull the instrument coronally.

### Completion of the Retreatment

After gaining access to the root canal system, with its thorough cleaning and shaping and managing other complications, the treatment is completed using the routine procedures. But sometimes the retreatment may become difficult due to presence of therapy resistant microorganisms like *Enterococcus faecalis*. During retreatment procedures a wide coronal access is needed and canal is slightly over enlarged than the previous one to completely remove the residues of previous treatment.

Clinician may face difficulty in retreating a case especially if:

- Access is to be made through the previously placed restoration
- Post removal is impossible
- There is overextended gutta-percha
- There is presence of foreign objects, or hard setting pastes which are amenable to remove.

The outcome of retreatment can be divided ?into short-term and long-term. The short-term outcome may be associated with postoperative discomfort including pain and swelling. Long-term outcomes of retreatment depend mainly on regaining the canal patency and the obturation of the root canal system. It has been seen that retreatment is most frequently associated with the procedural complications than the primary treatment. Thus, an effective communication is required between clinician and the patient about the potential problems before the treatment is initiated to avoid frustration.

### Radiographic Criteria for Success of Endodontic Treatment

- Normal or slightly thickened periodontal ligament space
- Reduction or elimination of previous rarefaction
- No evidence of resorption
- Normal lamina dura
- A dense three-dimensional obturation of canal space.

### Factors Affecting Success or Failure of a Particular Case

- Pulpal status
- Periodontal status
- Size of periapical radiolucency
- Canal anatomy like degree of canal calcification, presence of accessory or lateral canals, resorption, degree of curvature of canal, etc.
- Crown and root fracture
- Iatrogenic errors
- Occlusal discrepancies if any
- Extent and quality of the obturation
- Quality of the post endodontic restoration
- Time of post-treatment evaluation.

### Occurrence of Endodontic Failures does not Depend on

1. Type of tooth to be treated
2. Location of the tooth
3. Age and sex of the patient
4. Cause of pulpal injury
5. Number of appointment for root canal treatment
6. Type of root canal obturating material
7. Preoperative and postoperative pain.

## QUESTIONS

**Q. What are different criteria's used for evaluation of endodontic treatment?**

**Q. What is etiology of endodontic failures?**

**Q. What is criteria of case selection for endodontic retreatment? Enumerate different steps of retreatment**

**Q. Write short note on:**

a. Gutta-percha removal
b. Silver point removal

## BIBLIOGRAPHY


1. Abbott P. Endodontic management of combined endodontic-periodental lesions. JNZ Soc Periodontol. 1998;(83):15-28.
2. Antrim DD, Bakland LK, Parker MW. Treatment of endodontic urgent care cases. Dent Clin North Am 1986;30(3):549-72. Review.
3. Bondra DLm Hartwell GR, MacPherson MG, portell FR. Leakage in vitro with IRM, high copper amalgam, and EBA cement as retrofilling materials. J Endod 1989;15:157-60.
4. Ford TR, Rhodes JS. Root canal retreatment: I, case assessment and treatment planning. Dent update 2004;31(1):34-39.
5. Goldstein S, Sedaghat-Zandi A, Greenberg M, Fried man S. Apexification and apexogenesis. N Y State Dent J 1999; 65(5):23-25.
6. Gorni FG, Gagliani MM. The outcome of endodontic retreatment A 2 yr follow up. J Endod 2004;30:1-4.
7. Green D. Double canals in single roots. Oral Surg Oral Med Oral Pathol 1973;35:689-96.
8. Montgomery S, Ferguson CD. Endodontics. Diagnostic, treatment planning, and prognostic considerations. Dent Clin North Am 1986;30(3):533-48.
9. Pekruhn RB. The incidence of failure following single-visit endodontic therapy. J Ended 1986;12(2):68-72.
10. Sjogren U, Hagglund B, Sundqvist G, Wing K. Factors affecting the long-term results of endodontic treatment. J Endod 1990;16(10):498-504.

# Endodontic Periodontal Relationship

CHAPTER 24



## INTRODUCTION

The health of periodontium is important for proper function of the tooth. The periodontium consists of gingiva, cementum, periodontal ligament (PDL) and alveolar bone. This is the fact that the periodontium is anatomically interrelated with dental pulp by virtue of apical foramina and lateral canals which create pathways for exchange of noxious agents between these two tissues (Fig. 24.1). When the pulp becomes infected, the disease can progress beyond the apical foramen and affects the PDL. The inflammatory process results in formation of inflammatory tissue, which if not treated can result in resorption of alveolar bone, cementum and dentin.

Besides going through apical foramen, pulpal disease can progress through lateral canals, commonly present in the apical third and the furcation areas.

Not only the interaction between periodontium and pulp, produce or aggravate the existing lesion, they also present challenges in deciding the direct cause of an inflammatory condition. So a correct diagnosis should be made after careful history taking and clinical examination.

### Definition

An endo-perio lesion is one where both pulp and periodium tissues are affected by the disease progress.

### Pathways of Communication between Pulp and Periodontium

#### *Physiologic Pathways*

- Dentinal tubules
- Lateral and accessory canals

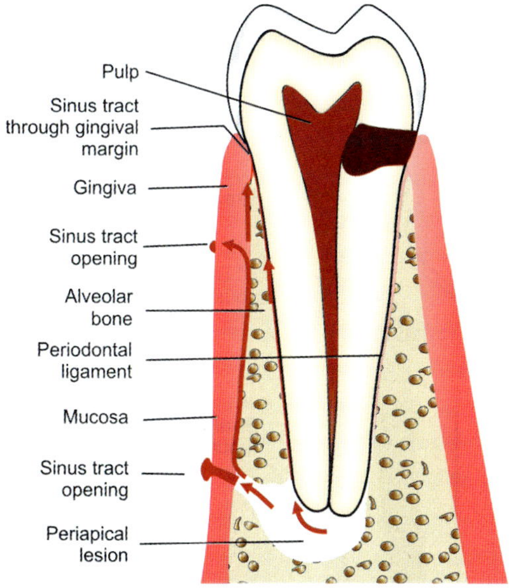


Fig. 24.1: Pathway for exchange of noxious agents between endodontic and periodontal tissue

- Apical foramen
- Palatogingival groove

*Pathological*

- Perforations
- Vertical root fracture
- Loss of cementum

*Iatrogenic*

- Perforation during endodontic therapy.
- Root fracture during root canal therapy
- Exposure of dentinal tubules during root planning

## PHYSIOLOGIC PATHWAYS

### Dentinal Tubules

Dentinal tubules traverse from pulpodentinal junction to cementodentinal or dentinoenamel junction.

Dentin tubules follow a straight course in root dentin whereas in coronal portion they follow S-shaped contours (Fig. 24.2). Usually they are patent but their potency may decrease with age, sclerosis or calcifications. Cementum acts as protective barrier to the dentin but because of periodontal disease, periodontal therapy (root planning) or other irritants, if cementum is destroyed a direct communication between dentinal tubules and the oral cavity may occur.

**Dentinal tubules**

- Traverse from pulpodentinal junction to cementodentinal or dentinoenamel junction.
- In radicular area–straight course.
- In coronal portion–S-shaped course.
- Greater density at pulpodentinal junction than cementodentinal junction (CDJ).
- Congenital absence of cementum, cemental exposure by periodontal disease, caries, root surface instrumentation – exposes dentinal tubules.
- Communication between pulp and periodontium.

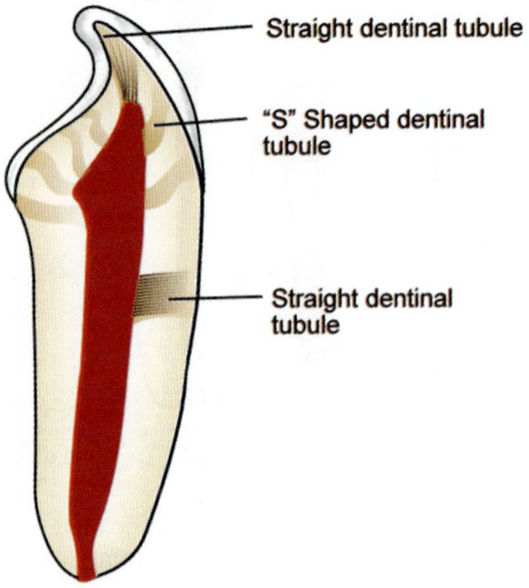


**Fig. 24.2:** Pattern of dentinal tubules

### Lateral or Accessory Canals

Lateral or accessory canals may exist anywhere on the root surface, though majority of them are found in apical third and furcation area of the root. It has been seen that up to 40 percent of teeth have lateral or the accessory canals (Fig. 24.3). As the periodontal disease progresses down the root surface, more of the accessory and lateral canals get exposed to oral cavity. Clinically, positive identification of the presence of lateral canal can be made when an isolated lateral lesion associated with a nonvital tooth is seen radiographically or during obturation, when some of the filling material got extruded into the lateral canal.

### Lateral and Accessory Canals

- Most common in apical third of posterior teeth.
- Difficult to identify on radiographs.
- Identified by isolated defects on the lateral surface of roots or by post-obturation radiographs showing sealer puffs.

Condition when pulp is necrotic and lateral canal is exposed, the periodontal reattachment to root surface can be inhibited if periodontal therapy is done before endodontic treatment. Thus in cases where pulp is nonvital and periodontal prognosis is good, then endodontic treatment should precede the periodontal therapy.

### Apical Foramen

One of the major pathways of communication between the dental pulp and the periodontium is through apical foramen (Fig. 24.4).

**Apical foramen**

- Major pathway of communication
- Inflammatory factors exit through apical foramen and irritate periodontium.

### Palato Gingival Groove

It is developmental anomaly commonly seen in maxillary incisor teeth. The groove begins in the central fossa, crosses the cingulum and extends apically at varying distance.

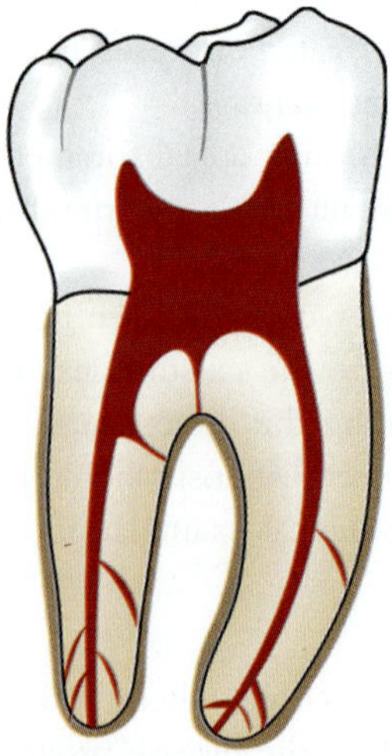

**Fig. 24.3:** Lateral and accessory canals can exist anywhere on the root surface

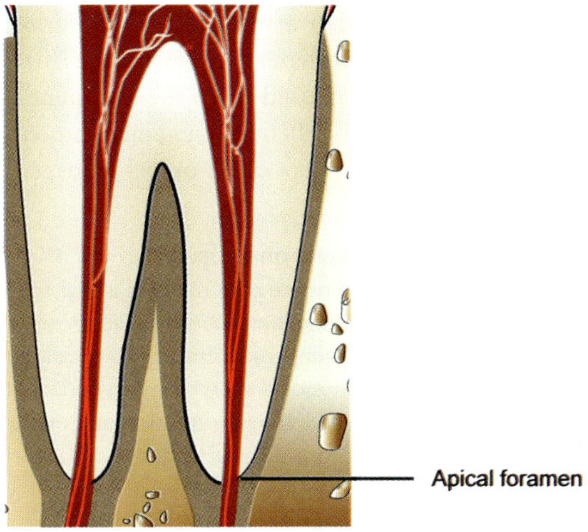


Fig. 24.4: Apical foramen communicating endodontic and periodontal system

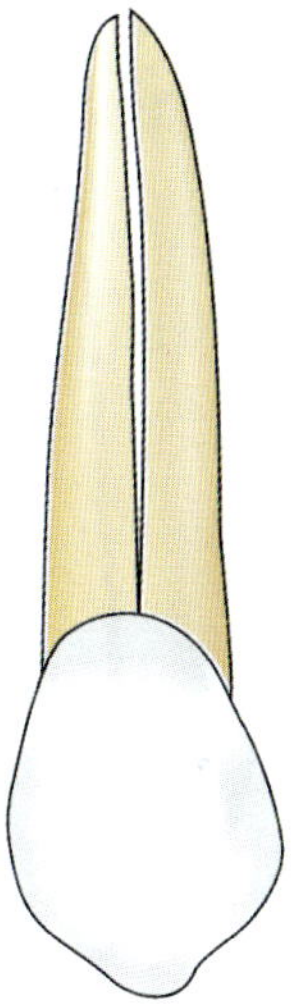

Fig. 24.6: A communication can form between root canal system and periodontium via vertical root fracture

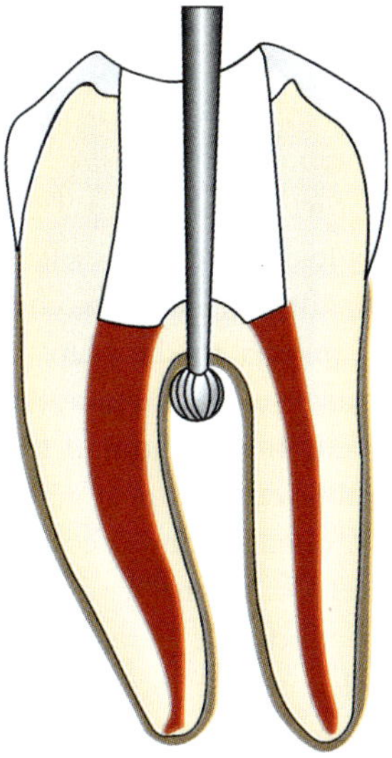

Fig. 24.5: Furcation of root creates communication between root canal system and periodontium

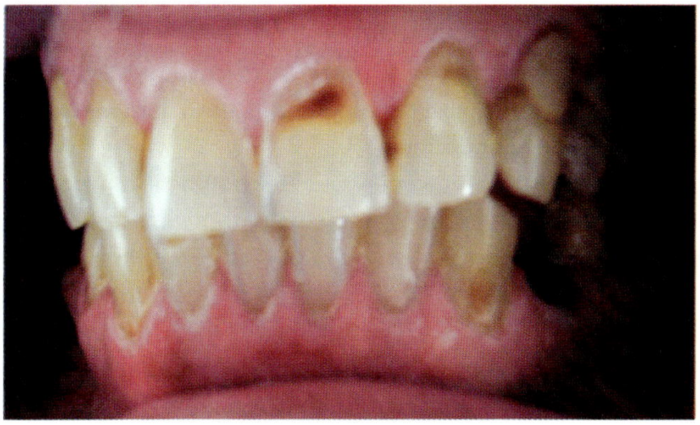

Fig. 24.7: Gingival recession resulting in loss of cementum

## PATHOLOGIC PATHWAYS

### Perforation of the Root (Fig. 24.5)

Perforation creates an artificial communication between the root canal system and the periodontium. Closer the perforation to the gingival sulcus, greater is the chances of apical migration of the gingival epithelium in initiating a periodontal lesion.

### Vertical Root Fracture (Fig. 24.6)

Vertical root fracture can form a communication between root canal system and the periodontium. The fracture site provides entry for bacteria and their toxic products from root canal system to the surrounding periodontium.

### Loss of Cementum

Loss of cementum can occur because of gingival recession, due to presence of inadequate attached gingiva, improper brushing technique, periodontal surgery, overzealous tooth cleansing habits, etc. (Fig. 24.7).

## IATROGENIC

### Perforation During Endodontic Therapy

Perforation is basically a mechanical or pathological communication between the root canal system and the external tooth surface. It can occur at any stage while performing endodontic therapy that is during access cavity preparation or during instrumentation procedures leading to canal perforations at cervical, midroot or apical levels.

### Root Fracture During Root Canal Therapy

Root fracture can occur at any stage of root canal treatment, that is during biochemical preparation, obturation or during post placement. The common reasons for root fracture are excessive dentin removal during biomechanical preparation and weakening of tooth during post space preparation. Whatever is the reason, the fracture site provides entry for bacteria and their toxic products from root canal system to the surrounding periodontium.

### Exposure of Dentinal Tubules During Root Planning

Exposure of dentinal tubules during periodontal surgery or root planning procedures can result in a pathway of communication between pulpal and periodontal space.

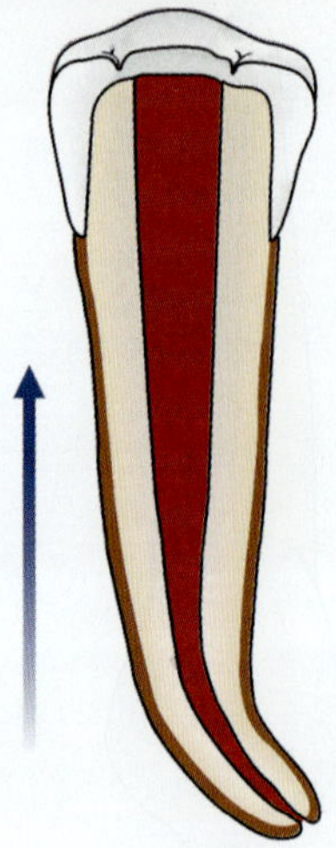

Fig. 24.8: Retrograde periodontitis

## IMPACT OF PULPAL DISEASES ON THE PERIODONTIUM

Pulpal infection may cause a tissue destructive process which may progress from apical region to the gingival margin, termed as "retrograde periodontitis" (Fig. 24.8).

Caries restorative procedures and/or traumatic injuries may cause inflammatory changes in the pulp, though it is still vital. It has been seen that even in presence of significant inflammation, a vital pulp does not affect the periodontium. But necrosis of pulp is frequently seen to be associated with the involvement of the periodontal tissue. Commonly, the areas of bone resorption are seen at apex, furcation areas and on the lateral surface of the root. These lesions can be in form of cyst, granuloma or abscess.

The inflammatory process in periodontium associated with necrotic pulps is similar to periodontal disease, that is an infectious etiology. The only difference lies is the source of infection.

Inflammatory lesions may also form from a root canal infection through lateral and accessory canals present on the lateral surface of root and furcation areas. These lesions are induced and maintained by the bacterial products which reach the periodontium through lateral canals.

## IMPACT OF PERIODONTAL DISEASE ON PULPAL TISSUE

The pathogenic bacteria and inflammatory products of periodontal diseases may enter into the root canal system via accessory canals, lateral canals, apical foramen, dentinal tubules or iatrogenic errors. Though irreversible pulpitis or pulpal necrosis is not the common occurrence, but inflammatory and pathologic changes may occur once the periodontal disease reaches the terminal stage, i.e. when plaque involves the apical foramina. As periodontal disease extends from gingival sulcus towards apex, the auxillary canals get affected which results in pulpal inflammation. It becomes more serious if these canals get exposed to oral cavity because of loss of periodontal tissues by extensive pocket depth.

Periodontal therapy also affects the pulp. Periodontal instruments like ultrasonic scalers, vibrators, curettes may cause harm to the pulp specially if used when the remaining dentin thickness is $< 2$ mm. Also the chemicals and medicaments used during periodontal therapy may cause pulpal damage.

**Effect of periodontal disease on pulp**

- Periodontal disease may involve pulp through apical foramen, lateral and accessory canals, dentinal tubules or iatrogenic errors.
- Periodontal procedures; scaling, root planning, surgically expose dentinal tubules due to removal of cementum and dentin.
- Chemical irritants and medicaments irritate pulpal tissue.
- Effects depend on remaining dentin thickness.

## ETIOLOGY OF ENDODONTIC PERIODONTAL PROBLEMS

It has been proved since ages that primary etiologic agent in periodontitis is bacterial plaque. Besides this primary factor, there are secondary factors which contribute to the disease process either by increasing the chances of plaque accumulation or by altering the response of host to the plaque.

It is also seen that irreversible pulpal disease occurs when trauma inflicted on pulpal tissue exceeds its reparative capacity. Such insult can occur through bacteria, chemical, mechanical, thermal or electrical trauma to the pulp.

Pulpal diseases can result in the periodontal problems and vice versa. It is the length of time that the etiological factor persists in the susceptible environment which is directly related to the probability of occurrence of combined lesions.

1. **Bacterial plaque:** Commonly associated microorganisms associated with endodontic periodontal lesions are A. a. comitans, F. nucleatum, P. intermedia, P. gingivalis and spirochetes sometimes C. albicans, viruses like herpes simplex, cytomegalo virus and E.B.V. have also shown to pay an important role in periapical lesions.
2. **Foreign bodies** like amalgam filling, root canal filling material, dentin or cementum chips and calculus deposits can irritate pulp and periodontium.
3. **Contributing factors:**

**Predisposing factors resulting in combined endodontic periodontal lesions**

- Malpositioned teeth causing trauma.
- Presence of additional canals in teeth.
- Cervical enamel projects into furcation of multirooted teeth.
- Large number of accessory and the lateral canals.
- Trauma combined with gingival inflammation.
- Vertical root fracture.
- Crown fracture.
- Root resorption.
- Perforations
- Systemic factors such as diabetes.

## CLASSIFICATION OF ENDODONTIC PERIODONTAL LESIONS

Various classifications have been proposed for classifying endodontic periodontal lesions.

### Classification

1. **According to weine: Based on etiology and treatment plan:**
   1. Class I: Tooth which clinically and radiographically simulates the periodontal involvement but it is due to pulpal inflammation or necrosis.
   2. Class II: Tooth has both pulpal and periodontal disease occurring concomitantly.
   3. Class III: Tooth has no pulpal problem but requires endodontic therapy for periodontal healing.
   4. Class IV: Tooth that clinically and radiographically simulates pulpal and periapical disease but has periodontal disease.
2. **Classification given by Simon, et al (1972): Based on etiology, diagnosis, prognosis and treatment.**
   - Type 1 : Primary endodontic lesion.
   - Type 2 : Primary endodontic lesion with secondary periodontal involvement.
   - Type 3 : Primary periodontal lesions.
   - Type 4 : Primary periodontal lesion with secondary endodontic involvement.
   - Type 5 : True combined lesion.
3. **Classification given by Grossman (1988)**
   - **Type I:** Lesions requiring endodontic treatment only, e.g.
     - a. Tooth with necrotic pulp reaching periodontium.
     - b. Root perforations
     - c. Root fractures
     - d. Chronic periapical abscess with sinus tract
     - e. Replants
     - f. Transplants
     - g. Teeth requiring hemisection.
   - **Type II:** Lesion that require periodontal treatment only. For example:-
     - a. Occlusal trauma causing reversible pulpitis
     - b. Suprabony or infrabony pockets caused during periodontal treatment resulting in pulpal inflammation.
   - **Type III:** Lesions that require combined endodontic and periodontal treatment. It includes:-
     - a. Any lesion of type I which result in irreversible reaction to periodontium requiring periodontal treatment.
     - b. Any lesion of Type II which results in irreversible damage to pulp tissue requiring endodontic therapy.

## DIAGNOSIS OF ENDODONTIC PERIODONTAL LESIONS

**Diagnosis** of the combined endodontic and periodontal lesions is often multifaceted and exasperating. A growing periapical lesion with secondary involvement of the periodontal tissue may have the similar radiographic appearance as a chronic periodontal lesion which has reached to the apex. Images of bone resorption, including apex furcation and marginal areas may confuse the diagnosis.

Pulp tests may be done sometimes to rule out an endodontic etiology, but they are not always reliable. Partial pulpal necrosis in multirooted teeth can respond positively to the vitality tests indicating pulp vitality despite of a combined lesion.

An endodontically treated tooth or a nonvital tooth associated with periodontal lesion can pose greater diagnostic problem as in such cases pulpal inflammation is frequently associated with inflammation of periodontal tissue.

Thus, a careful history taking, visual examination, diagnostic tests involving both pulpal and periodontal testing and radiographic examination are needed to diagnose such lesions.

**Tooth with combined endodontic periodontal lesions must fulfill the following criteria**
- Tooth involved should be nonvital.
- There must be destruction of the periodontal attachment which can be diagnosed by probing from gingival sulcus to either apex of the tooth or to the level of involved lateral canal.
- Both endodontic therapy and periodontal therapy are required to resolve the lesion completely.

Following clinical tests should be done to diagnose a case of endodontic periodontal problem.

***Chief complaint of patient:*** Patient may tell the pain indicating pulpal or periodontal type. History of patient may reveal previous pulpal exposure or any periodontal treatment.

It is generally seen that pulpal condition is usually acute where as periodontal or secondary pulpal or combined lesions are usually chronic in nature.

***Associated etiology:*** For pulpal disease, caries trauma or pulp exposure is common etiology where as for periodontal disease plaque/calculus is primarily responsible.

***Clinical tests:*** Clinical tests are imperative for reaching at correct diagnosis and differentiation of endodontic and periodontal diseases. Different signs and symptoms can be assessed by visual examination, palpation and percussion (Fig. 24.9). Mobility testing tells the integrity of attachment apparatus or extent of the inflammation in the periodontal ligament (Fig. 24.10).

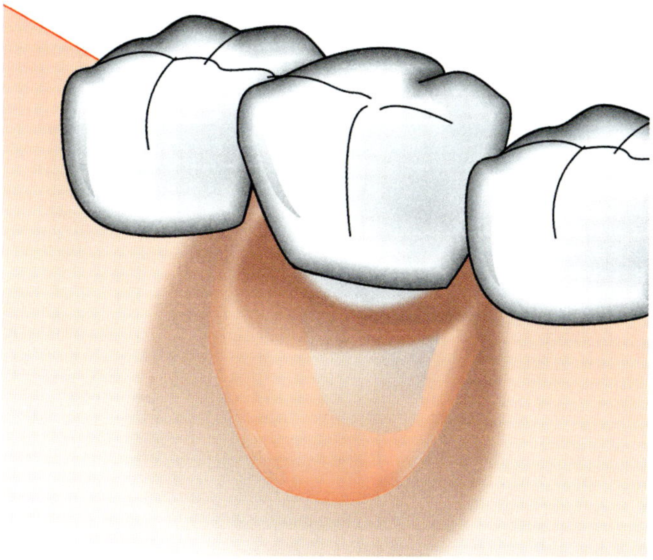

Fig. 24.9: Clinical picture of periodontal abscess

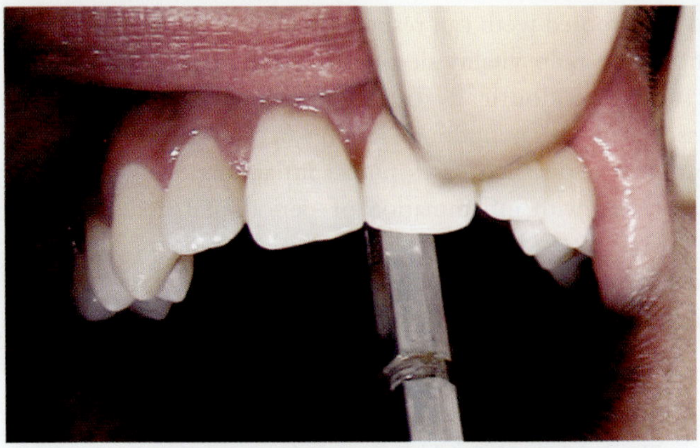

**Fig. 24.10:** Mobility of tooth tells integrity of attachment apparatus

***Radiographs:*** Radiographs are of great help in diagnosing caries, extensive restorations, pulp treatments if done, previous root canal treatments, root form, root resorption, root fracture, stage of root development, root canal obliteration, thickened periodontal ligament space and any changes in the alveolar bone (Figs 24.11 and 24.12). Periodontal disease causing the alveolar bone loss can be effectively detected by radiographs where as integrity of dental pulp can not be determined by looking at radiographs alone.

***Pulp vitality tests:*** Determination of pulp vitality is essential for accurate differential diagnosis of the lesions. Any abnormal response of pulp may indicate degenerative changes occurring in the pulp. Cases associated with nonsvital pulp have pulpal pathology where as teeth associated with vital pulp usually have periodontal disease. Commonly used pulp vitality tests are cold test, electric test, blood flow test and cavity test (Fig. 24.13). Recent advances in the diagnosis include the use of Laser Doppler Flowmetery, pulp oximetery and magnetic resonance imaging.

***Tracking sinus or fistula:*** Tracking the fistula may aid the clinician to differentiate the source (Fig. 24.14).

***Pocket probing:*** Pocket probing helps in knowing location and extent of the pockets, depth of pocket and any furcation involvement if any (Fig. 24.15).

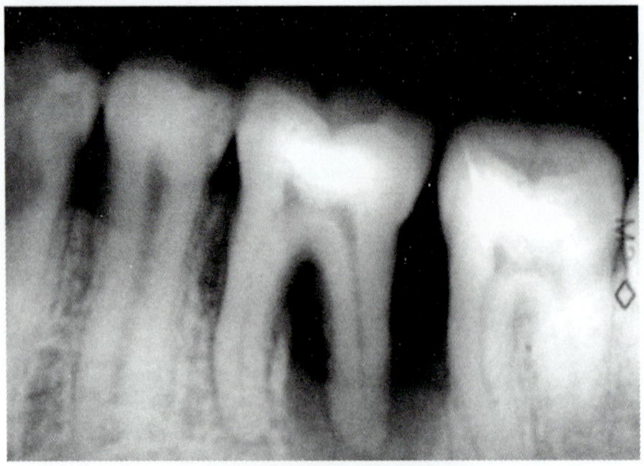

**Fig. 24.11:** Radiographs showing endo-perio lesion with bone resorption in left mandibular molar

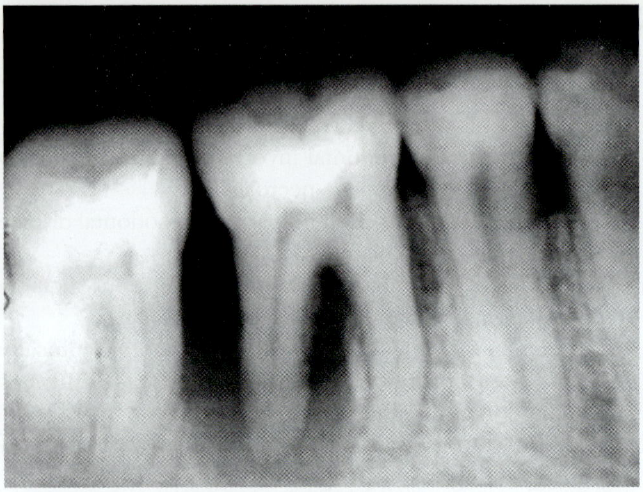

**Fig. 24.12:** Radiograph showing endo-perio lesion with bone resorption in right mandibular molar

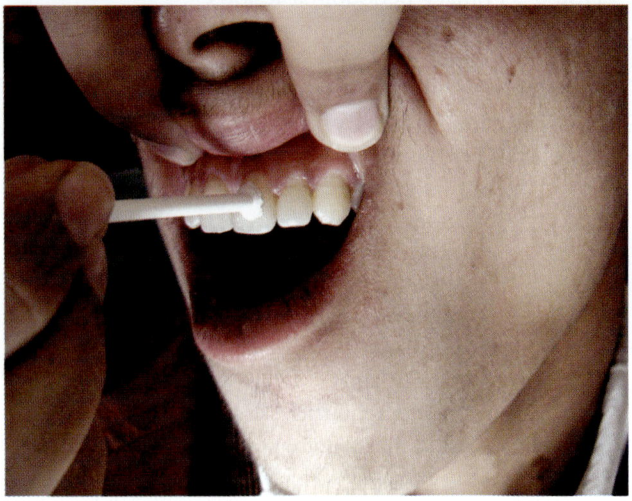

**Fig. 24.13:** Checking vitality of pulp using hot gutta-percha stick

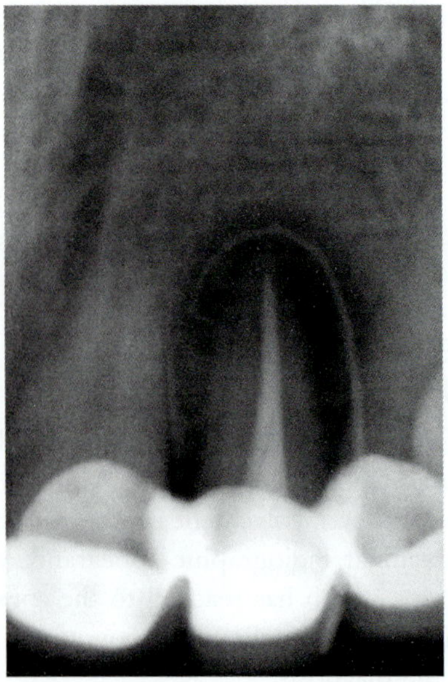

**Fig. 24.14:** Tracking a sinus tract using gutta-percha and then taking radiograph

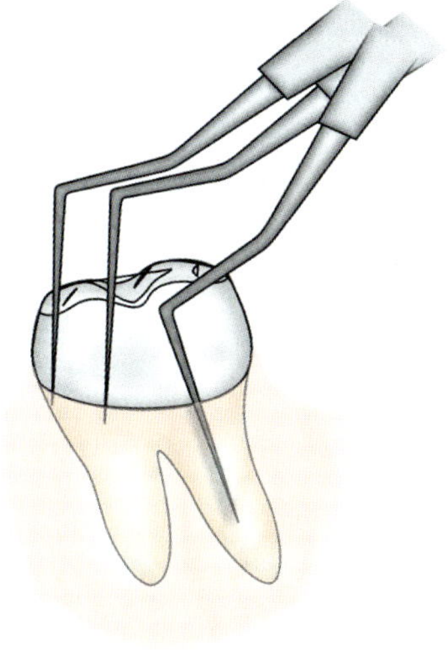

Fig. 24.15: Probing of tooth helps in knowing extent of pockets

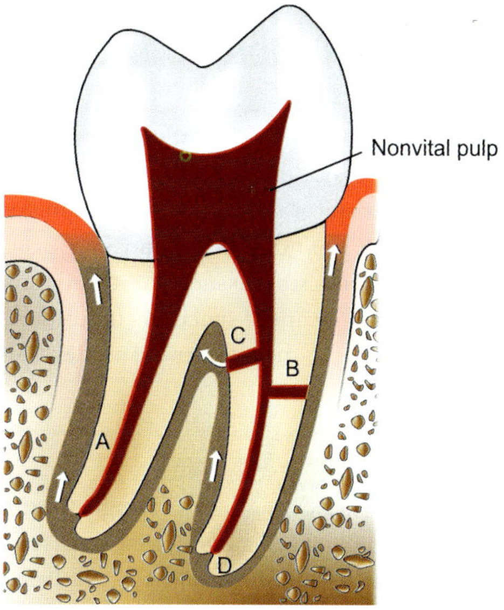


Fig. 24.16: Spread of infection can occur; (A) from apical foramen to gingival sulcus via periodontium; (B) from lateral canal to pocket; (C) from lateral canal to furcation; (D) from apex to furcation

***Microbiological examination:*** Occasionally the microbiological analysis can provide an important information regarding the main source of the problem.

***Distribition:*** Pulpal pathology is usually localized in nature whereas periodontal condition is generally localized.

***Bone loss:*** In pulpal disease, bone loss is generally localized, and wider apically. It is not associated with vertical bone loss. In periodontal disease, bone loss is generalized which is wider coronally. It may be associated with vertical bone loss.

***Pain:*** When pain is associated with pulp pathology, it is usually acute and sharp in nature and patient can not identify the offending tooth. Where as pain associated with periodontal pathology is dull in nature and patient can identify the offending tooth (because of presence of proprioceptive nerve fibers in the periodontal ligament).

***Swelling:*** If swelling is seen on the apical region, it is usually associated with pulpal disease. If it is seen around the margins or lateral surface of teeth, swelling is usually associated with periodontal disease.

### Treatment and Prognosis

Treatment planning and prognosis depend mainly on diagnosis of the specific endodontic and/or periodontal disease. In teeth with combined endodontic-periodontal lesions, the prognosis depends on extent of destruction caused by the periodontal disease. If lesion is of endodontic origin, an adequate endodontic treatment has good prognosis. Thus in combined disease, prognosis depends on efficacy of periodontal therapy.

## PRIMARY ENDODONTIC LESIONS (FIG. 24.16)

Sometimes an acute exacerbation of chronic apical lesion in a nonvital tooth may drain coronally through periodontal ligament into the gingival sulcus, thus resembling clinical picture of periodontal abscess. The lesion presents as an isolated pocket or the swelling on the side of the tooth.

### Etiology

- Dental caries
- Deep restorations close to pulp.
- Traumatic injury
- Poor root canal treatment

### Clinical Features

- Patient is usually asymptomatic, but history of acute exacerbation may be present.
- Since tooth is associated with necrotic pulp, pulp does not show response to vitality tests.
- Sinus tract may be seen from apical foramen, lateral canals or the furcation area.
- Probing shows true pockets. Pocket is associated with minimal plaque or calculus. The significant sign of this lesion is that patient does not have periodontal disease in other areas of oral cavity.

### Diagnosis

- Necrotic pulp draining through periodontal ligament into gingival sulcus.
- Isolated pocket on side of tooth.
- Pocket associated with minimal amount of plaque or calculus.
- Patient asymptomatic with history of acute exacerbations.

### Treatment

- Root canal therapy
- Good prognosis

### Prognosis

The prognosis after endodontic therapy is excellent. In fact, if periodontal therapy is performed without considering pulpal problem, prognosis becomes poor.

## PRIMARY ENDODONTIC LESION WITH SECONDARY PERIODONTAL INVOLVEMENT (Fig. 24.17)

This lesion appears if primary endodontic lesion is not treated. In such case, the endodontic disease continues, resulting in destruction of periapical alveolar bone, progression into the interradicular area, and finally causing breakdown of surrounding hard and soft tissues. As the drainage persists through periodontal ligament space, accumulation of irritants result in periodontal disease and further migration of attachment.

### Clinical Features

- Isolated deep pockets are seen though there may be the presence of generalized periodontal disease.
- In such cases, endodontic treatment will heal part of the lesion but complete repair will require periodontal therapy.

### Diagnosis

- Continuous irritation of periodontium from necrotic pulp or from failed root canal treatment.
- Isolated deep pockets.
- Periodontal breakdown in the pocket.

### Treatment

- Root canal treatment to remove irritants from pulp space.
- Retreatment of failed root canal therapy.
- Concomitant periodontal therapy
- Extraction of teeth with vertical root fracture if prognosis is poor.
- Good prognosis.

### Prognosis

In case, vertical root fracture is causing the endoperio lesions, tooth is extracted, otherwise the prognosis is good.

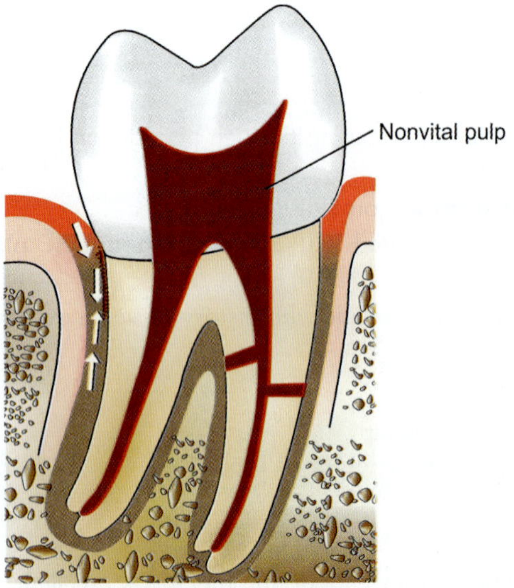


**Fig. 24.17:** Primary endodontic lesion with secondary periodontal involvement

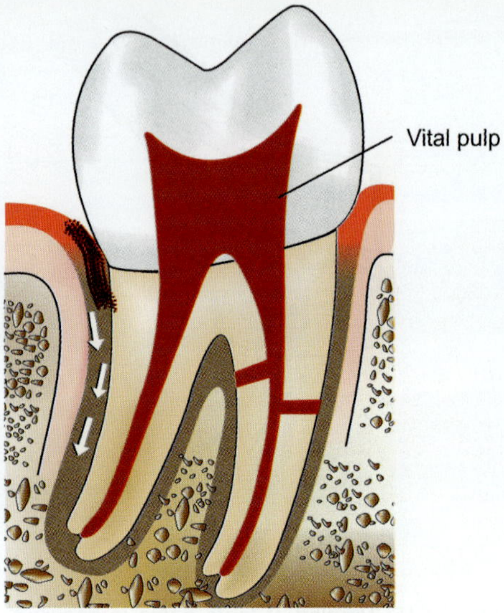


**Fig. 24.18:** Primary periodontal lesion

## PRIMARY PERIODONTAL LESIONS (Fig. 24.18)

Primarily these lesions are produced by the periodontal disease. In these lesions periodontal breakdown slowly advances down to the root surface until the apex is reached. Pulp may be normal in most of the cases but as the disease progress, pulp may become affected.

### Etiology

- Plaque
- Calculus
- Trauma

### Clinical Features

- Periodontal probing may show presence of plaque and calculus within the periodontal pocket.
- Due to attachment loss, tooth may become mobile.
- Usually generalized periodontal involvement is present.

### Diagnosis

- Periodontal destruction associated with plaque or calculus.
- Patient experiencing periodontal pain.
- Pulp may be normal in most of the cases.

### Treatment

- Oral prophylaxis and oral hygiene instructions
- Scaling and root planning.
- Periodontal surgery, root amputation may be required in advanced cases.

### Prognosis

- Prognosis becomes poor as the disease advances.

## PRIMARY PERIODONTAL LESIONS WITH SECONDARY ENDODONTIC INVOLVEMENT (Fig. 24.19)

Periodontal disease may have effect on the pulp through lateral and accessory canals, apical foramen, dentinal tubules or during

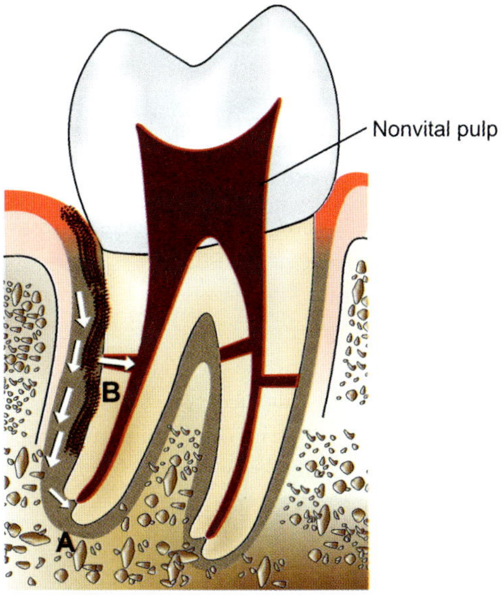


Fig. 24.19: Spread of periodontal lesion into endodontic space via: (A) periodontium into apex (B) lateral canals

iatrogenic errors. Once the pulp gets secondarily affected, it can in turn affect the primary periodontal lesion.

## Etiology

Periodontal procedures such as scaling, root planning, curettage, etc. may open up lateral canals and dentinal tubules to the oral environment, resulting in pulpal inflammation. In such case, patient complains of sensitivity or inflammation after periodontal therapy.

## Clinical Features

- Oral examination of patient reveals presence of generalized periodontal disease.
- Tooth is usually mobile when palpated.
- If severe periodontal destruction exposes the root surface, irreversible pulpal damage can result.
- Radiographically, these lesions become indistinguishable from primary endodontic lesions with secondary periodontal involvement.

## Diagnosis

- Periodontal destruction associated with nonvital tooth.
- Generalized periodontal disease present.
- Patient may complain sensitivity after routine periodontal therapy.
- Usually the tooth is mobile.
- Pocket may show discharge on palpation.

## Treatment

- Root canal treatment
- Periodontal surgery in some cases.

## Prognosis

- Prognosis depends on the periodontal problem.

# INDEPENDENT ENDODONTIC AND PERIODONTAL LESIONS WHICH DO NOT COMMUNICATE

One may commonly see a tooth associated with pulpal and periodontal disease as separate and distinct entities. Both the disease states exist but with different etiological factors and with no evidence that either of disease has impact on the other.

## Clinical Feature

- Periodontal examination may show periodontal pocket associated with plaque or calculus.
- Tooth is usually nonvital.
- Though both periodontal and endodontic lesions are present concomitantly but they cannot be designated as true combined endo-perio lesions because there is no demonstrable communication between these two lesions.

## Treatment

- Root canal treatment is needed for treating pulp space infection.
- Periodontal therapy is required for periodontal problem.

## Prognosis

Prognosis of the tooth depends on the periodontal prognosis.

# TRUE COMBINED ENDO-PERIO LESIONS (FIG. 24.20)

The true combined lesions are produced when one of these lesion (pulpal or periodontal) which are present in and around the same tooth coalesce and become clinically indistinguishable. These are difficult to diagnose and treat.

## Clinical Features

- Periodontal probing reveals conical periodontal type of probing, and at base of the periodontal lesion the probe abruptly drops farther down the root surface and may extend the tooth apex (Fig. 24.21).
- Radiograph may show bone loss form crestal bone extending down the lateral surface of root.

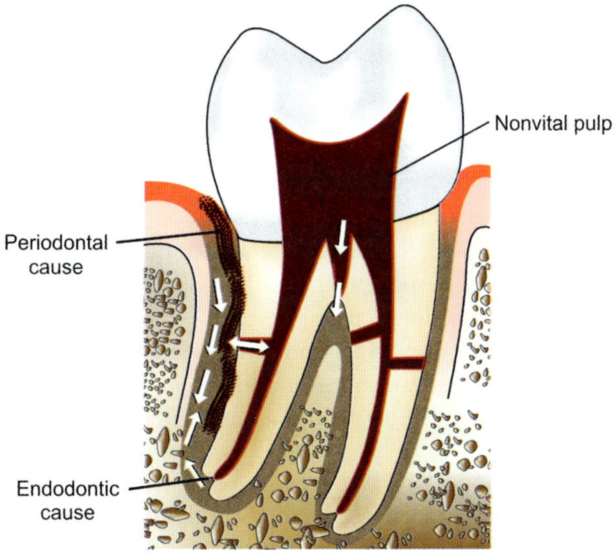


Fig. 24.20: True combined endo-perio lesion

| Differential diagnosis between pulpal and periodontal disease | | |
|---|---|---|
| *Features* | *Periodontal* | *Pulpal* |
| Etiology | Periodontal infection | Pulpal infection |
| Plaque and calculus | Commonly seen | No relation |
| Tooth vitality | Tooth is vital | Non vital |
| Restorations | No Relation | Usually show deep and extensive restoration |
| Periodontal destruction | Usually present, and generalized | If present single, isolated |
| Gingiva and epithelial attachment | Recession of gingival with apical migration of attachment | Normal |
| Pattern of disease | Generalized | Localized |
| Radiolucency | Usually not related | Perapical radiolucency |
| Inflammatory and granulation tissue | Usually present on coronal part of tooth | Commonly seen on apical part of tooth |
| Treatment | Periodontal therapy | Root canal therapy |
| Microbial | Complex | Few |
| Bone loss | Wider coronally | Wider apically |
| Pattern | Generalized | Localized |
| Gingiva | Some recession | Normal |
| pH of saliva | often alkaline | often acidic |

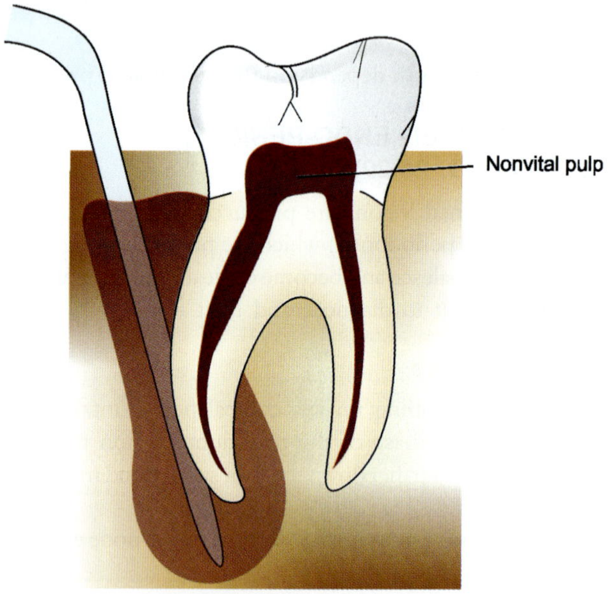


**Fig. 24.21:** In true combined endodontic periodontal lesion, at the base of periodontal lesion the probe abruptly drops farther down the root and extend to tooth apex

## Treatment

- First see whether periodontal condition is treatable, if promising, and then go for endodontic therapy. The endodontic therapy is completed before initiation of the definitive periodontal therapy.
- After completion of endodontic therapy, periodontal therapy is started which may include scaling, root planning, surgery along with oral hygiene instructions.

## Prognosis

It depends upon prognosis of the periodontal disease.

| Different between combined lesion and concomitant lesion | |
|---|---|
| *Combined lesion* | *Concomitant lesion* |
| 1. Chronic and generalized in nature | Acute and localized in nature |
| 2. There is communication between pulpal and periodontal lesion when seen clinically or radiographically | There may not be communication between pulpal and periodontal lesion when seen clinically and radiographically |

## QUESTIONS

**Q. What are etiological factors for endodontic periodontal lesions? How will you diagnose a case of endodontic periodontal lesion?**

**Q. Classify endodontic periodontal lesions?**

**Q. Write in detail about primary endodontic lesion with secondary periodontal involvement.**

**Q. How can you differentiate pulpal and periodontal disease.**

## BIBLIOGRAPHY


1. Adriaens PA. Edwards CA, De Boever JA, Loesche WL Ultrastructural observations on bacterial invasion in cementum and radiation dentin of periodontally diseased human tech, I Periodontal 1988;59:493.
2. Allison RT Electron microscopic study of "Rushton" hyaline bodies in cyst linings.
3. Contreras A, Slots J. Herpesvirus in human periodontal disease. J Periodontal Res 2000;35:3.
4. Contreras A, Umeda M, Chen C, et al. Relationship between herpeviruses and adult periodontitis and periodontopathic bacteria. J Periodontol 1999;70:478.

5. Czarnecki RT, Schilder H. A histologic evaluation of the human pulp in teeth with varying degrees of periodontal disease J. Endod 1979;5:242.
6. Dahle UR, Tronstad L, Olsen I. Observation of an unusually large spirochete in endodontic infection. Oral microbial immunol 1993;8:251.
7. Forabinejad M, Kigar RD. Histologic evaluation of dental pulp tissue of a patient with periodontal disease. Oral Surg oral Med Oral Pathol Oral Radiol Endod 1985;59:198
8. Gold SL, Moskow BS. Periodontal repair of periapical lesions the borderland between pulpal and periodontal disease. J Clin Periodontal 1987;14:251.
9. Grossman LI, Oliet Sm, Del Rio CE. Endodontic-periodontic interrelationship. Endodontic Practice (11th edn). Philadelphia: Lea and Febiger, 1988.
10. Jansson L, Ehnevid H. The influence of endodontic infection on periodontal status in mandibular molars. J periodontol 1998;69:1392.
11. Jansson L, Ehnevid J, lindskog SP, Biomlof LB. Radiographic attachment in periodontitis-prone teeth with endodontic infection. J Periodontol 1993;64:947.
12. Langeland K, Rodrigues H, Dowden W. Periodontal disease bacteria and pulpal histopathology. Oral Surg Oral Med Oral Pathol Oral Radiol Endod 1974:37:257.
13. Mandi FA. Histological study of the pulp changes caused by periodontal disease. J Br. Endod Soc 1972;6:80.
14. Miyashita H, Bergengoltz G, Grondahl K. Impact of endodontic conditions on marginal bone loss. J periodontol 1998;69:158.
15. Nair PNR. New perspectives on radicular cysts: do they heal? Int Endod J 1998; 31: 155.
16. Peterson K, Soderstrom C, Kiani-Anaraki M, Levy G. Evaluation of the ability of thermal and electrical tests to register pulp vitality. Endod dent traumatol 1999;15:127.
17. Ranta K, Haapasalo M, Ranta H. Monoinfection of root canals with Pseudomonas aeruginosa. Endod Dent Traumatol 1988;4:269.
18. Rotstein I, Simon JH. Diagnosis, prognosis and decision making in the treatment of combined periodontal-endodontic lesions. Periodontol 2004;34:265-303.
19. Sen BH, Piskin B, Demirci T. Observations of bacteria and fungi in infected root canal and dentinal tubules by SEM. Endod Dent Traumatol 1995;11:6.
20. Simon JH, Glick DH, Frank AL. The relationship of endodontic-periodontic lesions. J clin periodontol 1972;43:202.
21. Simon JHS, Hemple PL, Rotstein I, Salter PK. The possible role of L-form bacteria in periapical disease. Endodontology 1999;11:40.
22. Siqueira JF Jr, Rocas IN, Souto R, et al. Checkboard DNA-DNA hybridization analysis of endodontic infections.Oral Surg Oral Med Oral Pathol Oral Radiol Endod 2000;89:744.
23. Stock C, Gulabivala K, Walker R. Perio-endo lesions, Endodontics (3rd edn). St. Louis: Mosby, 2004.
24. Sundqvist G, Figdor D, Persson S, Sjogren U. Microbiologic analysis of teeth with failed endodontic treatment and the outcome of conservative re-treatment. Oral Surg Oral Med Oral Pathol Oral Radiol Endod 1998;85:86.
25. Sundqvist G. Ecology of the root canal flora. J Endod 1992;18:427.
26. Tronstad L, Barnett F, Riso K, Slots J. Extraradicular endodontic infections. Endod Dent Traumatol 1987;3:86.
27. Van Winkelhoff AL, Boutaga K. Transmission of periodontal bacteria and model of infection. J Clin periodontol 20051;32 (Suppl 6):16.
28. Waltiimo T, Haapasalo M, Zehnder M, Meyer J. Clinical aspects related to endodontic yeast infections. Endod topics 2005;8:1.
29. Waltimo TM, Siren EK, Torkko HL, et al. Fungi in therapy-resistant apical periodontitis. Int. Endod J 1997;30:96.
30. Wong R, Hirch RS, Clarke NG. Endodontic effects of root planning in humans. Endod Dent Traumatol 1989;5:193.

# Surgical Endodontics

CHAPTER 25



## INTRODUCTION

*Endodontic surgery is defined "as removal of tissues other than the contents of root canal to retain a tooth with pulpal or periapical involvement."* Surgical intervention is required for cases where retreatment has failed or is not an option, and the tooth is to be retained rather than extracted. Endodontic therapy eliminates root canal flora by chemomechanical debridement followed by obturation of the canal to achieve a seal. Clinical radiographic and histological observation are the criteria for evaluating success. The percentage of success reported has been consistently high. Failures may arise due to inadequate control of infection, poor design of the access cavity, inadequate instrumentation and obturation, missed canals and coronal leakage. Factors for persistence of periapical radiolucencies after conventional canal treatment in well-treated cases may be intraradicular infection, extraradicular infection, foreign body reaction and true cysts. Endodontic failures may be retreated, receive endodontic surgery or the problem tooth extracted.

The first cases of endodontic surgery were those performed by *Abulcasis* in the *11th century*. A root-end resection procedure to manage a tooth with a necrotic pulp and an alveolar abscess was documented in 1871 and root end resection with retrograde cavity preparation and filling with amalgam in the 1890s. Endodontic surgery was often considered as an alternative to root canal treatment and indications for surgery were proposed first in the 1930s. The rational for performing surgical treatment has changed over the past 120 years. The current view is that retreatment by conventional methods is the preferred alternative to apicoectomy.

In the 1960s, surgery was indicated in a non-vital tooth if instrument had not reached within 2-3 mm of the root apex. The level of unfilled or poorly filled canal determined the level of resection, and at that time the cut was beveled towards the labial surface to improve visualization and ease of placement of a root and filling. There was little evidence to show any increase in the rate of success by preparing and delaying the root canal filling until two consecutive negative cultures were obtained following antibacterial treatment. At that time appropriate anaerobic culturing techniques were not available, and calcium hydroxide was not in major use as a medicament. Also, in the 1960s it was believed that the main cause of endodontic failure was a poor apical seal.

Radiographic evaluation is important criteria to see the success of endodontic therapy, with increase in size or development of a lesion considered to be a failure. Usually a radiographic follow-up till 4 years is satisfactory for determining success. Biological and technical failures continue to occur as there are parts of root canal where debridement and obturation are not adequate. The reason for persistence of a radiolucency in what seem well-treated cases are not yet fully understood. New developments in root canal treatment in the last 10 years include an increased use of microscopes, preparations using ultrasound, canal preparations.

## OBJECTIVES OF ENDODONTIC SURGERY

1. Removal of diseased periapical tissue like granuloma, cyst, overfilled material, etc.
2. Root inspection for knowing etiology of endodontic failure, fracture, accessory canals, etc.
3. To provide fluid tight seals at apical end by retrograde preparation and obturation.
4. To eliminate apical ramifications by root resections so as to completely remove the cause of failure for endodontic treatment.

## RATIONALE FOR ENDODONTIC SURGERY

It has been seen that an ideal endodontic treatment can offer up to 95 percent of success rate. This success rate is lower in case of retreatment. A root canal may fail because of incomplete removal of bacteria and their byproducts from root canal system, incomplete obturation, presence of resistant granuloma and a true cyst.

The rationale of surgical endodontics is to remove the diseased tissue present in the canal and around the apex, and retrofil the root canal space with biologically inert material so as to achieve a fluid tight seal.

## INDICATIONS

Indications of Endodontic Surgery—As given by *Luebke, Click and Ingle*

1. Need for surgical drainage
2. Failed nonsurgical treatment:
   - Irretrievable root canal filling material.
   - Irretrievable intraradicular post.
   - Continuous postoperative discomfort
   - Recurring exacerbations of nonsurgical endodontic treatment.
3. Calcific metamorphosis of the pulp space.
4. Horizontal fracture at the root tip with associated periapical disease.
5. Procedural errors:
   - Instrument separation
   - Non-negotiable ledging
   - Root perforation
   - Severe apical transportations
   - Symptomatic overfilling
6. Anatomic variations
   - Root dilacerations
   - Apical root fenestrations
   - Non negotiable root curvatures.
7. Biopsy
8. Corrective surgery
   - Root resorptive defects
   - Root caries
   - Root resection
   - Hemisection
   - Bicuspidization.
9. Replacement surgery
   - Intentional replantation
   - Post-traumatic replantation.
10. Implant surgery
    - Endodontic implants
    - Osseointegrated implants.
11. Exploratory surgery.

## CONTRAINDICATIONS

1. Periodontal health of the tooth: Tooth mobility and periodontal pockets are two main factors affecting the treatment plan.
2. Patients health considerations
   - Leukemia or neutropenia in active state leading to more chances of infection after surgery, and impaired healing
   - Uncontrolled Diabetes Mellitus—Defective leukocyte function, defective wound healing commonly occurs in severe diabetic patients
   - Recent serious cardiac or cancer surgery
   - Very old patients—Old age is usually associated with complications like cardiovascular or pulmonary disorders, decreased kidney functions, liver functions.
   - Uncontrolled hypertension
   - Uncontrolled bleeding disorders
   - Immunocompromised patients
   - Recent myocardial infarction or patient taking anticoagulants
   - Patients who have undergone radiation treatment of face because in such cases incidence of osteoradio-necrosis and impaired healing is high
   - Patient in first trimester of pregnancy – It is during this period the fetus is susceptible to insult, injury and environmental influences that may result in postpartum disorders.
3. Patient's mental or psychological status:
   - Patient does not desire surgery
   - Very apprehensive patient
   - Patient unable to handle stress for long complicated procedures.
4. Surgeon's skill and ability—Clinician must be completely honest about their surgical skill and knowledge. Beyond their

abilities, case must be referred to endodontist or oral surgeon.

5. Anatomic considerations such as in mandibular second molar area:
   - Roots are inclined lingually
   - Root apices are much closed to mandibular canal
   - Presence of too thick buccal plate
   - Restricted access to the root tip
6. Short root length in which removal of root apex further compromises the prognosis.
7. Proximity to nasal floor and maxillary sinus—A careful surgical procedure is required to avoid surgical perforation of sinus.
8. Miscellaneous
   - Non restorable teeth
   - Poor periodontal prognosis
   - Vertically fractured teeth
   - Nonstrategic teeth.

## CLASSIFICATION

I. Surgical drainage
   a. Incision and drainage (I and D)
   b. Cortical trephination (Fistula surgery) (Fig. 25.1)

II. Periradicular surgery
   a. Curettage
   b. Biopsy
   c. Root-end resection
   d. Root-end preparation filling
   e. Corrective surgery
      i. Perforation repair
         1. Mechanical (Iatrogenic)
         2. Resorptive (Internal and external)
      ii. Root resection
      iii. Hemisection.

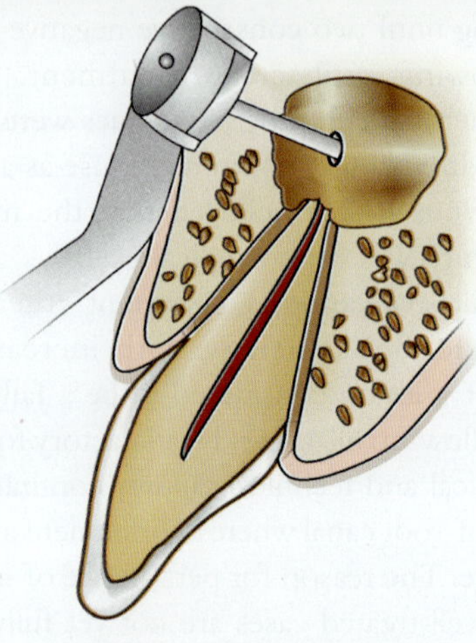

**Fig. 25.1:** Cortical trephination

III. Replacement surgery

IV. Implant surgery
   a. Endodontic implants
   b. Root-form osseointegrated implants.

### Classification of Endodontic Microsurgical Procedures (Fig. 25.2)

It was given by Richard Rubenstein and kim according to assessment of root form osseous integrated implant treatment outcome.

**Class A:** Absence of periradicular lesion but persistent symptoms after nonsurgical treatments.

**Class B:** Presence of small periapical lesion and no periodontal pockets

**Class C:** Presence of large periapical lesion progressing coronally but no periodontal pockets

**Class D:** Any of class B or C lesion with periodontal pocket

**Class E:** Periapical lesion with endodontic and periodontal communication but no root fracture

**Class F:** Tooth with periapical lesion and complete denouement of buccal plate

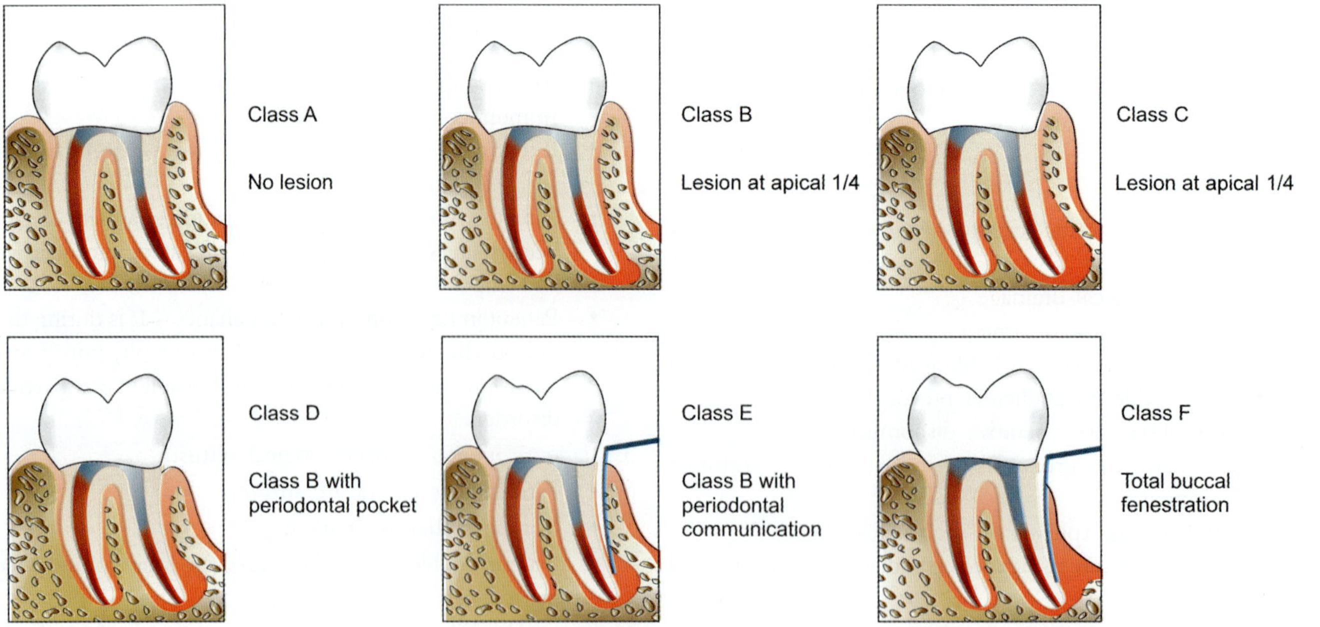


**Fig. 25.2:** Classification of endodontic microsurgical procedures

## PRESURGICAL CONSIDERATIONS

Before initiating the surgical procedure the clinician should evaluate following factors which affect the treatment outcome:

1. Success of surgical treatment versus nonsurgical retreatment.
2. Review of medical history of the patient and consultation with physician if required.
3. Patient motivation.
4. Esthetic considerations like scarring.
5. Evaluation of anatomic factors by taking radiographs at different angles.
6. Periodontal evaluation.
7. Presurgical preparation.
8. Taking informed consent.

## INCISION AND DRAINAGE

### Surgical Drainage

Surgical drainage is indicated when purulent and/or hemorrhagic exudates forms within the soft tissue or the alveolar bone as a result of symptomatic periradicular abscess (Fig. 25.3).

### Protocol of Treatment

1. If swelling is intraoral and localized—Only incision and drainage is required.
2. If swelling is diffuse or has spread into extraoral musculofacial tissues or spaces, then go for surgical drainage and prescribe systemic antibiotics to the patient.
3. If there is hard, indurated and diffuse swelling—Allow it to localize and became soft and fluctuant before incision and drainage.
4. To anesthetize the tooth local anesthesia is given, here nerve block is preferred which is supplemented with infiltration.
5. Use of nitrous oxide analgesia is also advocated sometimes to reduce anxiety and lowering pain.
6. Incision to the most dependent part of swelling is given with scalpel blade, No. 11 or 12. Horizontal incision is placed at dependent base of the fluctuant area for effective drainage to occur (Fig. 25.4).

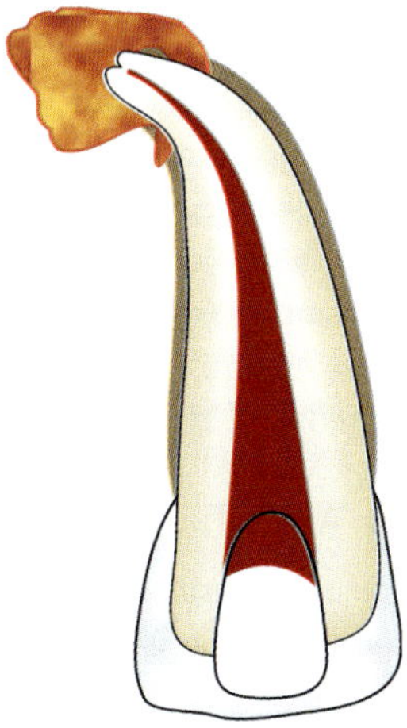

**Fig. 25.3:** A large symptomatic periapical abscess is indicated for incision and drainage

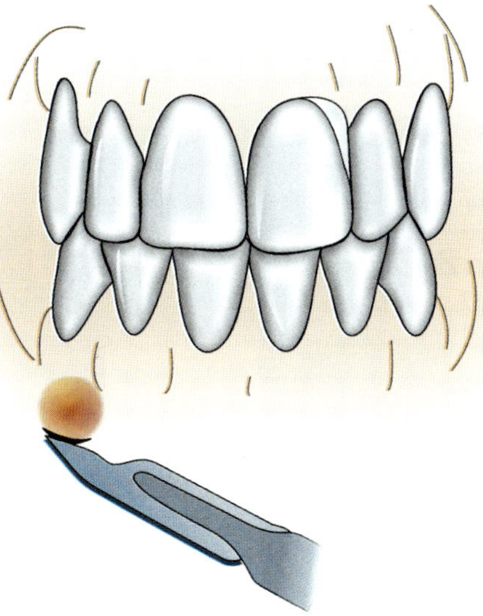

**Fig. 25.4:** Incision is made at most dependent part of swelling

## PERIRADICULAR SURGERY

Before proceeding for periradicular surgery, the clinician must take care of the factors which affect the prognosis of the tooth like taking the complete dental and medical history of the patient, evaluating accessibility to the surgical site, conducting suitable vitality tests and radiographs and assessing the compliance of patient.

### Armamentarium for Periradicular Surgery

It consists of all the sterile instruments needed from start till the completion of the procedure. It includes:

- Anesthesia like lidocaine with adrenaline and disposable syringes
- Sterilized gauze pieces and cotton pellets
- Bard parker handle, No. 15 and 12 blade
- Mirrors
- A periodontal probe
- Endodontic explorer
- Periosteal elevator
- Periodontal and surgical curettes
- Hemostats
- Scissors
- Cotton forceps
- Flap retractor
- Suturing material
- Surgical and regular length burs.

### Local Anesthesia and Hemostasis (Fig. 25.5)

1. Local anesthetics with vasopressors are the main choice in surgical endodontic procedures to obtain profound anesthesia and optimal hemostasis (Fig. 25.6).
2. Lidocaine with vasopressor adrenalin is the local anesthesia of choice for surgical procedures.
3. If amide is contraindicated, then ester agent, i.e. procaine, propoxicaine with levonordeffrin is indicated.
4. For nerve blocks 2 percent lidocaine with 1 : 100000 or 1 : 200000 adrenalin is used. But for obtaining hemostasis adrenalin concentration should be 1 : 50000 (Figs 25.7 to 25.10).

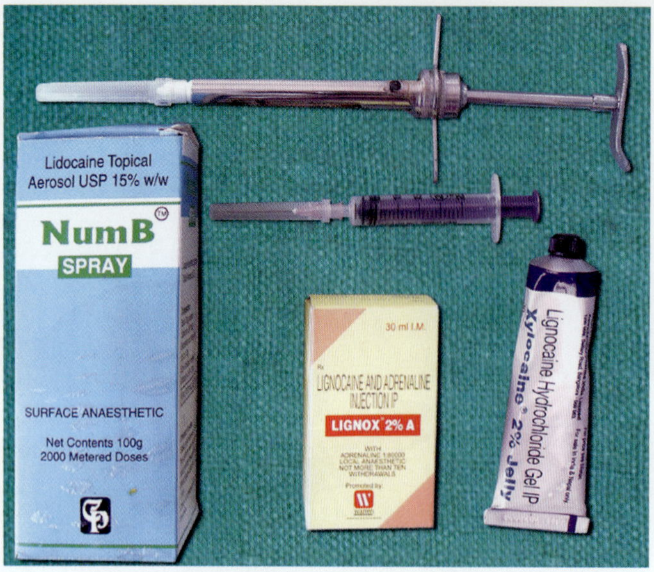


Fig. 25.5: Commonly used materials for local anesthesia

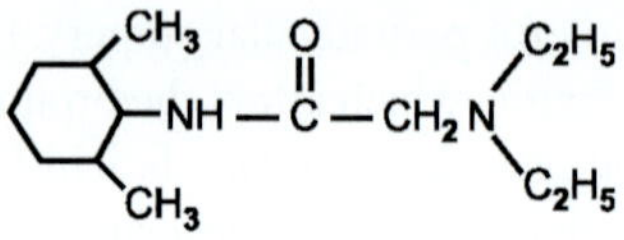

Fig. 25.6: Structure of commonly used local anesthesia

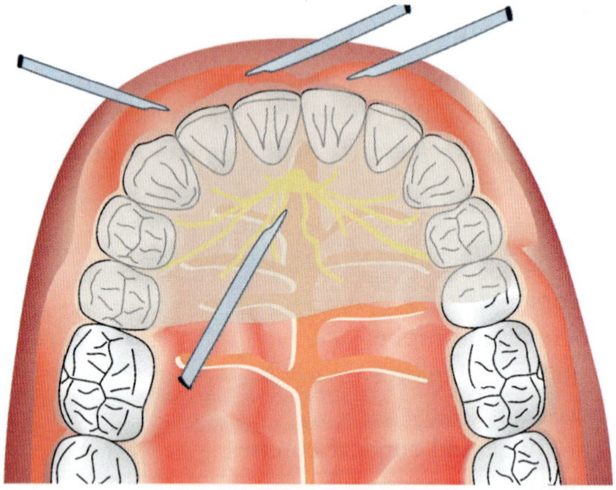

Fig. 25.7: Anesthesia for maxillary anterior teeth

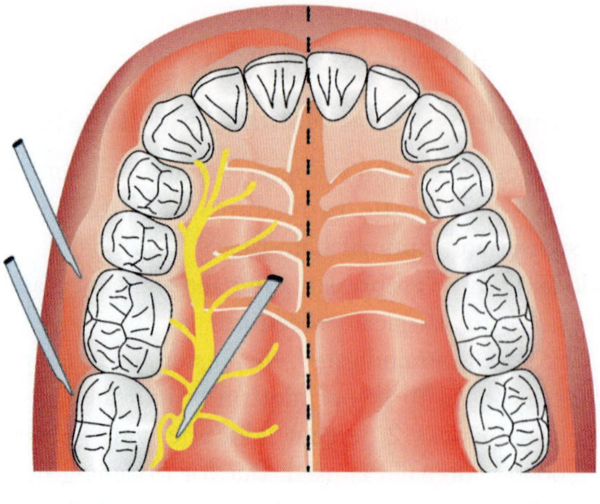

Fig. 25.8: Anesthesia of maxillary posterior area

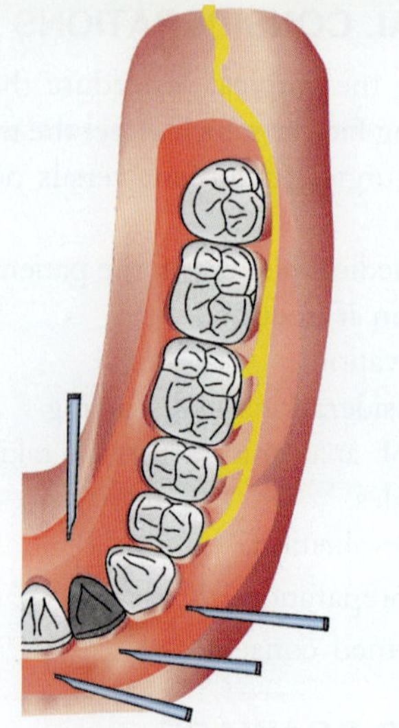

Fig. 25.9: Anesthesizing mandibular anterior region

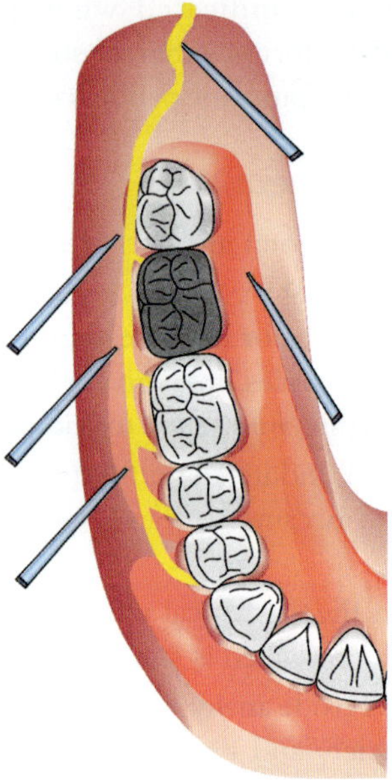

Fig. 25.10: Anesthesizing mandibular posterior area

5. Rate of injection should be 1 ml/minute with maximum safe rate of 2 ml/minute.
6. Submucosal infiltration for hemostasis should be given with 30 gauge needle with the bevel towards bone and penetration just superficial to periosteum at the level of root apices. 0.25-0.5 ml should be injected slowly at a place.
7. Rapid injection produces localized pooling of solution in the injected site resulting in delayed and limited diffusion into the adjacent tissue, thus surface contact with microvasculature reduces, resulting in reduced hemostasis.

## Amount of Local Anesthesia

It depends on the size of surgical site.

- Small site involving only few teeth require 1.8 ml with 1 : 50000 adrenalin.
- For extensive surgery involving multiple teeth, one needs 3.6 ml with 1 : 50000 adrenalin.

- Delay the incision for 4-5 minutes following injection. It is advised so as to have sufficient time for achieving good hemostasis. This is clinically indicated by a blanching of the soft tissues through out the surgical site.

## Receptors and Mechanism of Hemostasis

- There are two types of adrenergic receptors viz. alpha and beta receptors
- *Gage* demonstrated that the action of a vasopressor drug on microvasculature depends on
  a. Predominant receptor type
  b. Receptor selectivity of vasopressor drug.
- Alpha receptor predominate in oral mucosa and gingiva
- Beta receptors predominate in skeletal muscles
- Adrenalin receptor selectivity approximately equal for both alpha and beta
- Stimulation of alpha receptors results in vasoconstriction and thus decrease in the blood flow
- Stimulation of beta receptors causes vasodilatation which results in increased blood flow.

## Reactive Hyperemia: The Rebound Phenomenon

This phenomenon occurs due to rebound from an alpha to a beta response. In this condition concentration of vasoconstrictor decreases so that it does not cause alpha adrenergic response but after some time blood flow increases more than normal leading to reactive hyperemia. Rebound phenomenon is because of localized tissue hypoxia and acidosis caused by prolonged vasoconstriction.

Once this reactive hyperemia occurs, it is impossible to re-establish hemostasis by additional injections. Therefore, in case of long surgical and more complicated procedures which require hemostasis for longer time should be done first and less hemostasis dependent procedures should be kept for last.

## FLAP DESIGNS AND INCISIONS

Good surgical access is fundamentally dependent on appropriate flap design.

## Classification

*I. Full mucoperiosteal flaps*
  a. Triangular (single vertical releasing incision)
  b. Rectangular (double vertical releasing incision)
  c. Trapezoidal (Broad based rectangular)
  d. Horizontal (No vertical releasing incision)

*II. Limited mucoperiosteal flaps*
  a. Submarginal curved (semi-lunar)
  b. Submarginal scalloped rectangular (Luebke-Ochsenbein)

## PRINCIPLES AND GUIDELINES FOR FLAP DESIGNS

1. Avoid horizontal and severely angled vertical incisions, because:
   - Gingival blood supply occurs from supraperiosteal vessels, which follow vertical course parallel to long axis of teeth (Fig. 25.11).

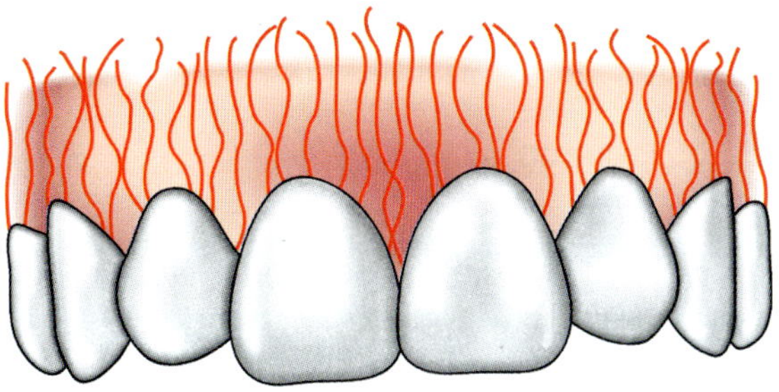

Fig. 25.11: Vertical course of supraperiosteal vessels parallel to long axis of teeth

   - Collagen fibers of gingiva and alveolar mucosa form attachments for crestal bone and supracrestal cementum to the gingiva and periosteum on the buccal and lingual radicular bone
     i. Fibers over crestal radicular bone are parallel to long axis of tooth.
     ii. Tissue in sharp corners become ischemic and delayed healing
2. Avoid incisions over radicular eminences for example in canines and maxillary first premolars.
3. Incisions should be placed and flaps repositioned over solid bone.
   - Incisions should never be placed over areas of periodontal bone loss or periradicular lesions.
   - ***Hooley and Whitacre*** suggested that a minimum of 5 mm of bone should exist between the edge of a bony defect and incision line.
4. Avoid incisions across major muscle attachment.
5. Extent of vertical incisions should be sufficient to allow the tissue retractor to seat on solid bone, thereby leaving the root apex well exposed.
6. Extent of horizontal incision should be adequate to provide visual and operative access with minimal soft tissue trauma.
7. Avoid incisions in the mucogingival junction.
8. The junction of the horizontal sulcular and vertical incisions should either include or exclude the involved interdental papilla.
9. When submarginal incision is used, there must be a minimum of 2 mm of attached gingiva around each tooth to be flapped.
10. The flap should include the complete mucoperiosteum.
11. Avoid improper treatment of periosteum.

## Functions of a Flap

1. Most important function is to raise soft tissue overlying the surgical site to give the best possible view and exposure of the surgical site.
2. To provide healthy tissue that will cover the area of surgery, decrease pain by eliminating bone exposure and aid in obtaining optimal healing.

## FULL MUCOPERIOSTEAL FLAPS

For full mucoperiosteal flaps the entire soft tissue overlying the cortical plate in the surgical site is reflected. Most of the advantages attributed to this type of flap are because of intact supraperiosteal vessels maintained in reflected flap.

## Types of Incision

### Triangular Flap

- It was first described by ***Fischer*** in 1940
- Earlier triangular flap was usually formed by giving two incisions, i.e., horizontal and vertical. Nowadays, intrasulcular incision is also given along with these two incisions. Vertical incision is usually placed towards the midline (Fig. 25.12). Horizontal incision is submarginal curved incision placed along the crowns of the teeth in the attached gingiva so as to preserve the marginal gingiva (Fig. 25.13).

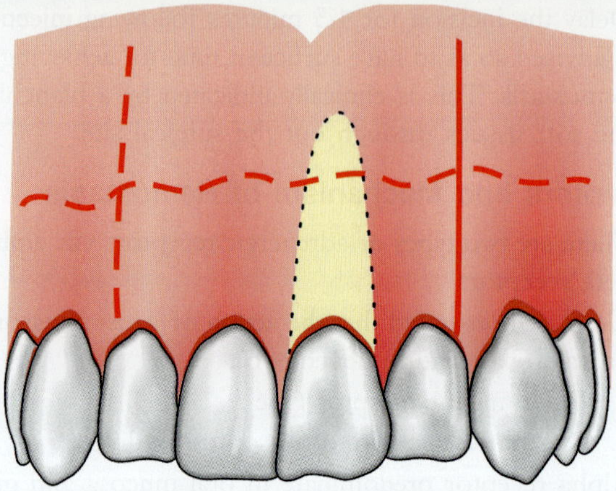

**Fig. 25.12:** Triangular flap

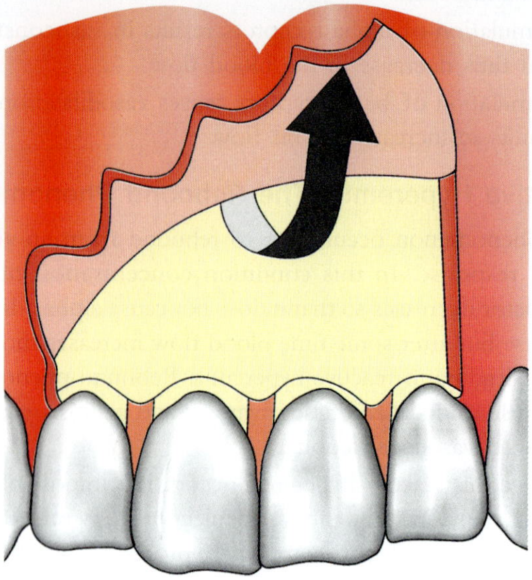

**Fig. 25.13:** Reflection of flap

#### Advantages

1. Enhanced rapid wound healing.
2. Ease of wound closure.

#### Disadvantage

Limited surgical access.

#### Indications

- Maxillary incisor region
- Maxillary and mandibular posterior teeth
- It is the only recommended flap design for posterior mandible region.

***Triangular flap is not recommended for:***

1. Teeth with long roots (maxillary canine).
2. Mandibular anteriors because of lingual inclination of these roots.

### Rectangular Flap (Fig. 25.14)

Earlier a rectangular flap was made by giving only two vertical and a horizontal incision but nowadays, instrasulcular incision has also been added in this design.

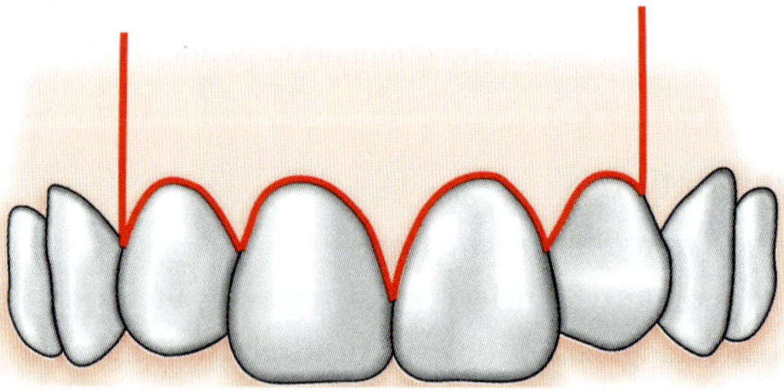

**Fig. 25.14:** Rectangular flap

#### Advantages

1. Enhanced surgical access.
2. Easier apical orientation.

#### Disadvantages

1. Wound closure as flap re-approximation and postsurgical stabilization are more difficult than triangular flap.
2. Potential for flap dislodgement is greater.

#### Indications

1. Mandibular anteriors
2. Maxillary canines
3. Multiple teeth

This flap is not recommended for mandibular posterior teeth.

### Trapezoidal Flap

It was described by ***Neumann and Eikan in 1940***. Trapezoidal flap is formed by two releasing incisions which join a horizontal intrasulcular incision at obtuse angles (Fig. 25.15).

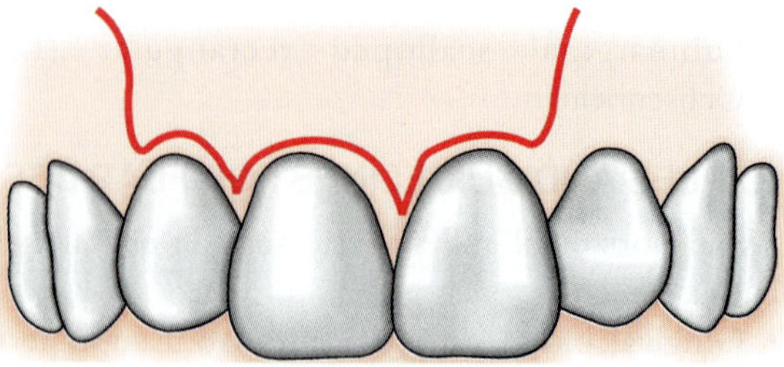

**Fig. 25.15:** Trapezoidal flap

### Disadvantages

- Wound healing by secondary intention
- Pocketing or clefting of soft tissue
- Compromise in blood supply
- Contraindicated in periradicular surgery.

## Envelope Flap

It is formed by a single horizontal intrasulcular incision and is usually recommended for corrective endodontic surgery.

### Indications

1. For repair of perforation defects
2. For root resections
3. In cases of hemisections

### Advantages

1. Improved wound healing
2. Easiness of wound closure and postsurgical stabilization.

### Disadvantages

1. Extremely limited surgical access.
2. Essentially impractical for periradicular surgery. But some use it for palatal surgery.

### Potential Disadvantages of Full Mucoperiosteal Flaps

1. Loss of soft tissue attachment level: A key element in preventing loss is ensuring that root attached tissues are not damaged or removed during surgery.
2. Loss of crestal bone height.
3. Postsurgical flap dislodgement.

# LIMITED MUCOPERIOSTEAL FLAPS

## Semilunar Flap

It was first given by ***Partsch,*** also known as ***Partsch incision.*** It is formed by a single curved incision. This flap is called as semilunar flap because horizontal incision is modified to have a dip towards incisal aspect in center of the flap, giving resemblance to the half moon (Fig. 25.16). This flap has no primary advantage and it is ***not preferred in modern endodontic*** practice because of its numerous disadvantages.

### Disadvantages

1. Limited surgical access
2. Difficult wound closure
3. Poor apical orientation
4. Potential for postsurgical soft tissue defects by incising through tissues unsupported by bone.
5. Maximum disruption of blood supply to un-flapped tissues.

## Ochsenbein-Luebke Flap

This is also known as ***submarginal retaan flap.*** In 1926, Neumann described a surgical technique for management of periodontal diseases which is very much similar to this flap. This flap is modification of the rectangular flap (Fig. 25.17).

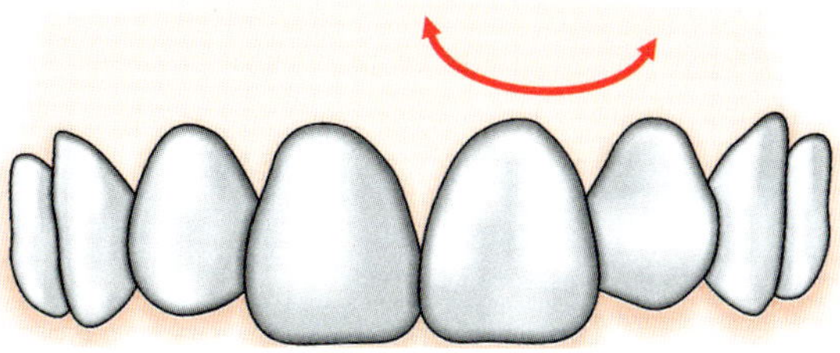

**Fig. 25.16:** Semilunar flap

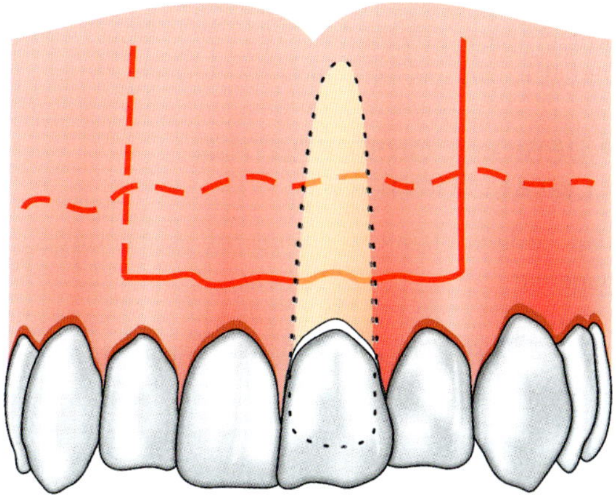

**Fig. 25.17:** Ochsenbein-Luebke flap

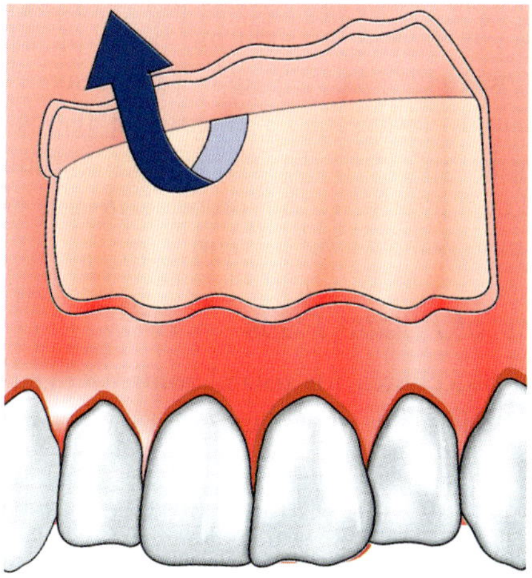

**Fig. 25.18:** Flap design for Ochsenbein-Luebke flap

***Flap design***—in this scalloped horizontal incision is given in the attached gingival which forms two vertical incisions made on each side of surgical site (Fig. 25.18). This flap is developed by an endodontist and periodontist. This flap gives advantage of vertical flap along with semilunar flap.

### Advantages

1. Marginal and inter-dental gingiva are not involved
2. Unaltered soft tissue attachment level
3. Crestal bone is not exposed
4. Adequate surgical access
5. Good wound healing potential—as compared to semi-lunar flap

### *Indications*

1. In presence of gingivitis or periodontitis associated with fixed prosthesis.
2. Where bony dehiscence is suspected

### *Disadvantages*

1. Disruption of blood supply to un-flapped tissues
2. Flap shrinkage
3. Difficult flap re-approximation and wound closure
4. Untoward postsurgical sequelae
5. Healing with scar formation
6. Limited apical orientation
7. Limited or no use in mandibular surgery.

## FLAP DESIGN CONSIDERATION IN PALATAL SURGERY

Two flap designs mainly indicated for palatal surgery are:
1. Triangular
2. Horizontal

In triangular flap, the vertical releasing incision extends from the marginal gingiva mesial to first premolar to a point near the palatal midline and is joined by a horizontal intrasulcular incision which extends distally far as to provide access (Fig. 25.19).

Relaxing incisions are given between first premolar and canine to decrease the chances for severance of blood vessels.

The bony surface of posteriors part of palate is pebblier which makes it difficult area during elevation. In these area, scalpal can be used to partially dissect the tissues for modified thickness flap. In palatal flap, retraction of flap is difficult, so sling suture be given for flap retraction (i.e. suture the edge of flap and tie it tightly to tooth on opposite side of arch when surgery is completed, suture is cut).

### *Indications of Palatal Flaps*

1. Surgical procedures for palatal roots of maxillary molars and premolars for retrofilling, perforation repair or root amputation.
2. Perforation or resorption repair of palatal surfaces of anterior teeth.

## FLAP REFLECTION AND RETRACTION

Without giving proper attention to these simple procedures there can be severe damage to delicate tissues that play an important role in wound closure.

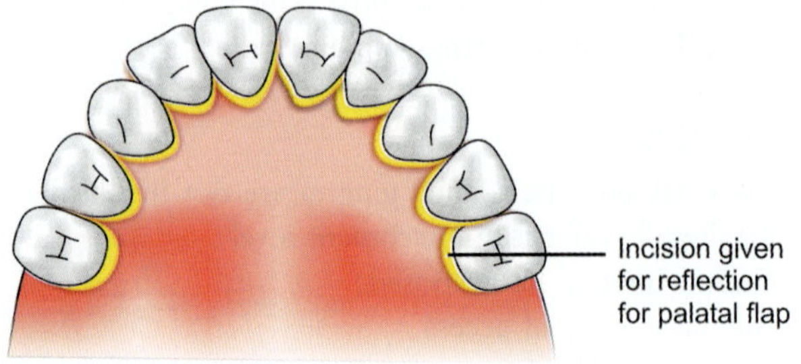


**Fig. 25.19:** Flap for palatal surgery

### For Full Mucoperiosteal Flap

Marginal gingiva is very delicate and easily injured. Therefore, it is not appropriate to begin the reflection process in the horizontal incision. For supracrestal root, attached tissues are of greater clinical significance. These are easily damaged by direct reflective forces. If damaged, they lose their viability causing apical epithelial down growth resulting in increased sulcular depth and loss of soft tissue attachment level.

### For Submarginal Flaps

Here also reflection should not begin in horizontal incision as reflecting forces may damage critical wound edges and delay healing and result in scar formation.

### Flap Reflection

Reflection of a flap is the process of separating the soft tissues (gingiva, mucosa and periosteum) from the surface of alveolar bone.

It should begin in the vertical incision a few millimeters apical to the junction of the horizontal and vertical incisions (Fig. 25.20).

Once these tissues are lifted form cortical plate, then the periosteal elevator can be inserted between them and the bone, the elevator is then directed coronally. This allows the marginal and interdental gingiva to be separated from underlying bone and the opposing incisional wound edge without direct application of dissectional forces. This technique allows for all of the direct reflective forces to be applied to the periosteum and the bone. This elevation is continued until the attached gingival tissues have been lifted from underlying bone to the full extent of horizontal incision (Fig. 25.21).

### Flap Retraction

Retraction of the tissues provides access to the periradicular area. For good quality retraction the retractor should rest on

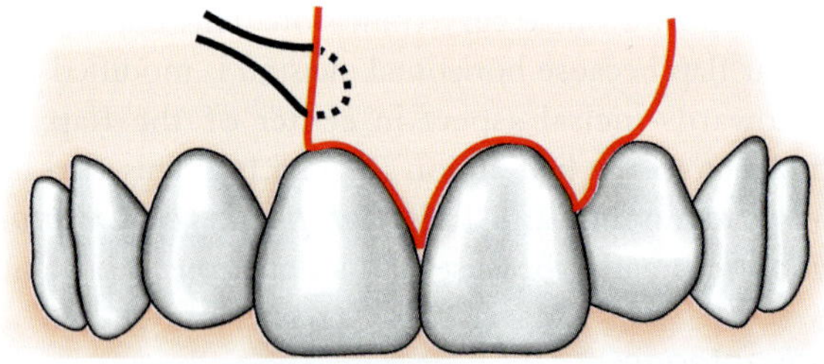

**Fig. 25.20:** Flap reflection begins in the vertical incision, apical to junction of horizontal and vertical incision

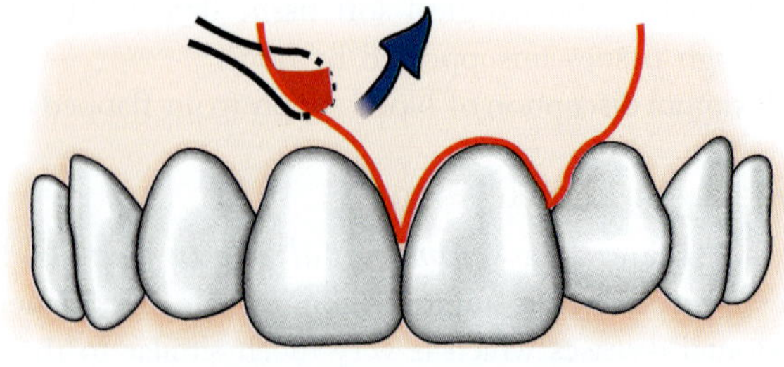

**Fig. 25.21:** Lifting of mucoperiosteum

cortical bone with light but firm pressure directed against the bone. If retractor rests on the base of reflected tissues, it can result in damage to microvasculature of alveolar mucosa and thus delayed healing.

### Time of Retraction

As a general rule longer the flap is retracted, greater are the complications following surgery. This happens because:

- Vascular flow is reduced during retraction
- Tissue hypoxia may result which can further cause the delayed wound healing.

Irrespective of the time of retraction, flap irrigation with normal saline should be frequently done to prevent dehydration of periosteal surface of the flap. Because of severance of the vertically oriented supraperiosteal vessels, limited mucoperiosteal flaps are more susceptible to dehydration and thus require more frequent irrigation than full mucoperiosteal flaps.

## HARD TISSUE MANAGEMENT

After reflection of the flap, root apices are approached by making an access through the cortical plates. In case of presence of radiolucency around the root apex, osseous tissue need not be removed surgically. But when radiolucency is not present periapically, osseous cutting is required to gain access to the root apex.

### Osseous Tissue Response to Heat

Erikson et al in 1982 in their study found the sequence of bone injury and response of osseous tissue to heat. They noted the following response of tissues to heat:

I. Above 40°C, a hyperemia was noted as blood flow increased.
II. 47-50°C for 1 minute—rabbit fat cell resorption and osseous resorption.
III. 50-53°C for 1 minute—blood flow stasis and death of vascular channels within 2 days.
IV. At 56°C, bone alkaline phosphatase undergoes rapid inactivation.
V. At 60°C or more—termination of the blood flow and tissue necrosis.

### Tissue Response to Bone Removal

It depends upon multiple variables. Bone in surgical site has temporary decrease in blood supply because of local anesthetics. This causes bone to become more heat sensitive and less resistant to injury. So, any small changes during bone removal can affect bone physiology and viability.

### Speed of Cutting

1. ***At 8000 rpm:*** Almost similar tissue response are seen when irrigation is done with or without a coolant or with a mixture of blood and saliva or water.
2. ***At high speed (up to 300000 rpm)*** favorable tissue response are noted when other parameters (coolant, pressure, type of bur) are controlled.

### Use of Coolant

- Various studies have supported the use of a liquid coolant (water, saline) to dissipate the heat generated during the cutting osseous tissue, and by keeping the cutting flutes of instrument free of debris there by reducing friction and using cutting efficacy of bur.
- For coolant to be effective, it must be directed on the head of the bur enough to prevent tissue debris from clogging the flutes (Fig. 25.22).
- Use of coolant with high speed rotary instruments can contaminate a sterile field due to back splash effect during cutting.
- There are certain guidelines which helps in controlling the bacterial population:
    1. Thorough rinsing with mouthwash for one minute before surgery.
    2. Waterlines connected to dental unit should be thoroughly clean with sufficient amount of water or hypochlorite solution.
    3. Handpiece should also be flushed with sufficient amount of normal saline.
    4. Handpiece should always be sterilized before every use.

Studies have shown that using high speed handpiece with 45° angled heat increase visibility and efficiency of cutting instead of using slow speed handpiece. ***Impact air 45° high speed handpiece*** has added advantage that air is exhausted to rear of turbine rather towards bur and surgical site. So, it decreases the splatter and chances of tissue emphysema, pyema and pneumomediastinum, etc.

### Bur Types

Shape of bur and flute design plays a very important role.

- Cutting of osseous tissue with a No. 6 or No. 8 round bur produces less inflammation and results in a smoother cut surface and a shorter healing time than when a fissure or diamond bur is used.
- Burs with the ability to cut sharply and cleanly with the largest space between cutting flutes, regardless of the speed of rotation, leave defects that heal in the shortest postsurgical time.
- Cutting bone with a diamond stone is the most inefficient as defects produced by these burs heal at very slow rate.

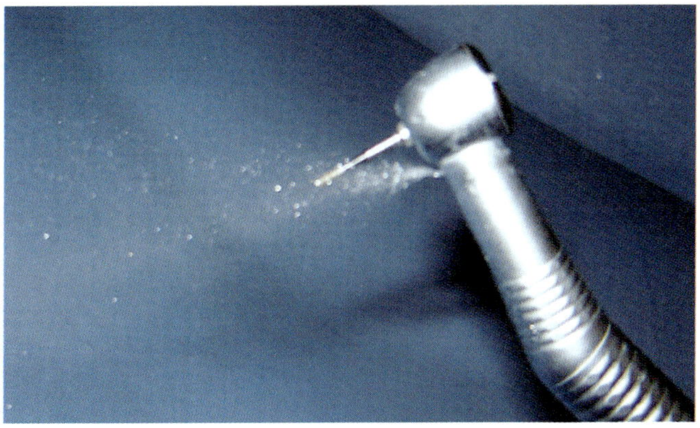

Fig. 25.22: Coolant must be directed on head of bur for efficient action

### *Pressure and Time during Cutting Procedure*

Pressure should be minimum possible and time the bur stays in contact with bone should be as short as possible. This reduced time factor along with light pressure can be achieved by employing the technique of "Brush stroke" cut method.

## PRINCIPLES OF SURGICAL ACCESS TO ROOT STRUCTURE

Normally when radiolucent area is present around apex of tooth, tooth root is visible through cortical plate. It is difficult when bone is to be removed to gain access to tooth especially when no periapical radiolucent area is present. Guidelines which should be strictly followed to accurately determine and locate the root apices are:

1. Angulation of crown of tooth to root should be assessed
2. Measurement of entire tooth to root should be assessed.
3. Locate root from coronal to apex where bone covering root is thinner. Once it is located, then covering bone is removed slowly with light brush strokes working in apical direction.
4. Exposing radiographs from both a mesial and distal angulation in addition to straight view.
5. Probing can be done forcibly using instruments like endodontic explorer or straight curette in the apical region to know whether a small defect is present or not.

When a small defect is present in the bone, then a small piece of lead sheet, gutta-percha point or a plug of alloy can be placed to know the position of apex.

There are some characteristic points (***given by Barnes***) which are helpful in differentiating root surface from surrounding osseous tissue:

1. Root structure is yellowish in color
2. Texture of root is smooth and hard while that of bone is porous and granular
3. Root does not bleed when probed
4. Root is surrounded by periodontal ligament. The methylene blue dye can be used to identify the periodontal ligament.

## PERIRADICULAR CURETTAGE

It is a ***surgical procedure to remove diseased tissue from the alveolar bone in the apical or lateral region surrounding a pulpless tooth.***

### Indications

a. Access to the root structure for additional surgical procedures.
b. For removing the infected tissue from the bone surrounding the root.
c. For removing overextended fillings.
d. For removing necrotic cementum.
e. For removing a long standing persistent lesion especially when a cyst is suspected.
f. To assist in rapid healing and repair of the periradicular tissues.

### Surgical Techniques

1. Inject local anesthetic with vasoconstrictor into soft tissue. This will help in controlling hemorrhage during surgery.
2. Design flap depending upon condition of the patient and preference of the clinician.
3. Expose the surgical site.
4. Use the bone curette to remove the pathologic tissue surrounding the root.
5. Insert the curette between the soft tissue and bone, apply the pressure against the bone.
6. After removing the tissue from the bony area, grasp the soft tissue with the help of tissue forceps.
7. Send the pathological tissue for histopathological examination.

## ROOT-END RESECTION (APICOECTOMY, APICECTOMY)

***It is the ablation of apical portion of the root-end attached soft tissues***

The current indications of root-end resection are:

a. Inability to perform nonsurgical endodontic therapy due to anatomical, pathological and iatrogenic defects in root canal.
b. Persistent infections after conventional endodontic treatment.
c. Need for biopsy.
d. Need to evaluate the resected root surface for any additional canals or fracture.
e. Medical reasons.
f. Lack of time.
g. For removal of iatrogenic errors like ledges, fractured instruments, and perforation which are causing treatment failure.
h. For evaluation of apical seal.
i. Blockage of the root canal due to calcific metamorphosis or radicular restoration.

### Guidelines for Bone Removal

1. Adequate anesthesia and hemostasis is necessary.
2. Always sterilize the handpiece before use.
3. Flush the water lines connected to dental unit thoroughly before use.
4. Use sharp and sterile round burs.
5. Amount of pressure should be light while cutting the bone.
6. Handpiece either high speed or low speed should be used with coolant.
7. Cut bone in a shaving or brush stroke method.
8. Visibility of the operative site should be good in order to increase the success of procedure. Position the handpiece, bur, suction tip and operating light in right direction to increase the visibility.
9. Avoid deep penetration (3-5 mm) during cutting.

***Factors to be considered before root-end resection are:***

1. Instrumentation
2. Extent of resection
3. Angle of resection.

1. ***Instrumentation:*** High speed handpiece with surgical length fissure bur usually results in satisfactory resection. Use of

round bur may result in gouging of root surface where as crosscut fissure burs can lead to uneven and rough surface.

In a study by ***Nedderman et al*** it was found that use of round burs produce ditching of the root surface where as crosscut fissure burs produce the roughest root surface. Use of low speed tissues bur showed to produce the smoothest root surface.

Recently studies have shown the use of Er:YAG laser and Ho:YAG laser for root end resection but among these Er:YAG laser is better as it produces clean and smooth root surface. ***Advantages of use of laser in periradicular surgery over the traditional methods include:***

1. Reduction of postoperative pain.
2. Improved hemostasis.
3. Reduction of permeability of root surface.
4. Potential sterilization of the root surface.
5. Reduction of discomfort.

**2. *Extent of resection***

Historically it was thought that since root-end is surrounded by granulation tissue, failure to remove all foci of infection should result in persistent disease process so it was advised to resect the root surface to the level of healthy bone.

But study by Andreasen and Rud showed no correlation between presence of microorganisms in dentinal tubules and degree of the periapical inflammation.

***Factors to be considered while performing root-end resection are:***

1. Access and visibility of surgical site.
2. Anatomy of the root, i.e. its shape, length, etc.
3. Anatomy of the resected root surface to see number of canals.
4. Presence and location of iatrogenic errors.
5. Presence of any periodontal defect.
6. Presence of any root fracture.
7. Need to place root-end filling into sound tooth structure.

According to Cohen et al the length of root tip for resection depends upon the frequency of lateral canals and apical ramifications at the root-end. They found that when 3 mm of apex is resected, the lateral canals are reduced by 93 percent and apical ramifications decreased by 98 percent (Fig. 25.23). Whereas a root resection of 3 mm at a 0 degree bevel angle eliminates most of the anatomic features that are possible cause of failure (Fig. 25.24).

## Angle of Root-end Resection

Earlier it was thought that root-end resection at 30-45° from long axis of root facing buccally or facially provides:

- Improved visibility of the resected root-end.
- Improved accessibility

Recently, several authors presented evidence that beveling of root-end results in opening of dentinal tubules on the resected root surface that may communicate with the root canal space and result in apical leakage, even when a retrofilling has been placed (Figs 25.25A and B). Nowadays a ***bevel of 0°-10°*** is recommended with ressection at the level of 3 mm.

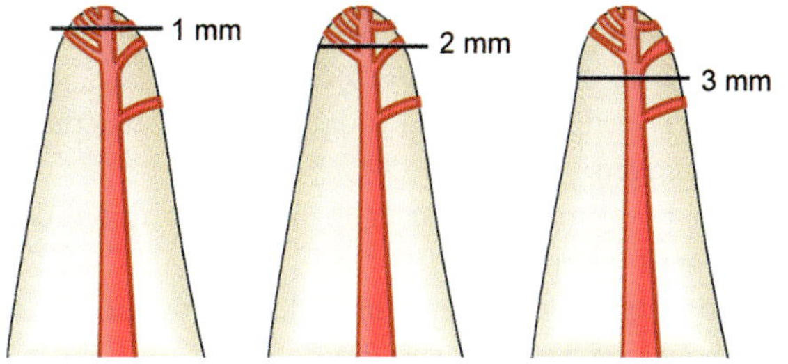


**Fig. 25.23:** Frequency of canals found at different levels of root canals

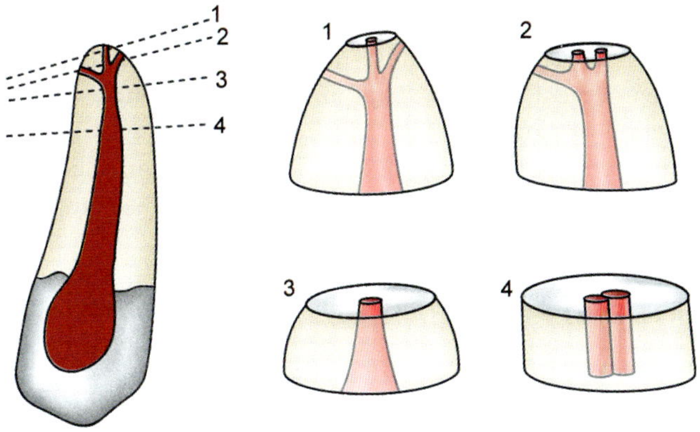


**Fig. 25.24:** Diagram showing root resection at different levels. Fig. shows that root resection of 3 mm at 0° bevel, eliminates most of the anatomic features

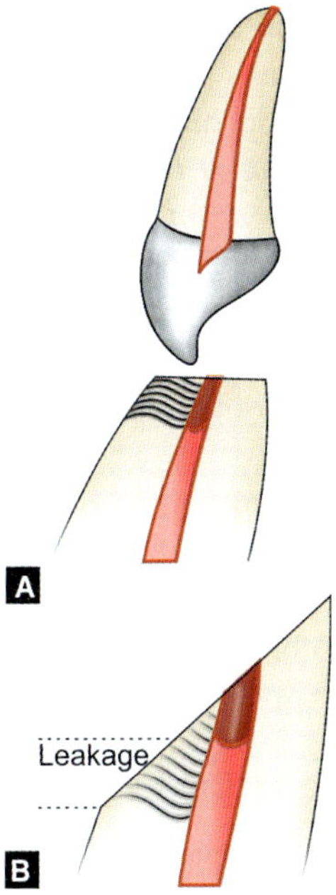


**Figs 25.25A and B:** (A) Zero degree bevel expose less of dentinal tubules to oral environment; (B) Beveling results in opening of dentinal tubules on resected tooth surface, which communicate with root canal space, and result in apical leakage

**Short bevel of 0° is almost perpendicular to long axis of the tooth. It has following advantages:**

1. Short bevel allows inclusion of lingual anatomy with less reduction.

2. If multiple canals are present, increase in bevel causes increase in distance between them.
3. For preparing long bevel more of tooth structure has to be removed.
4. Short bevel makes it easier for the clinician to resect the root end completely.
5. With short bevel more of lingual anatomy can be assessed with less of tooth destruction.
6. With Longer bevel, it is more difficult to keep instruments within long axis of the tooth. It is always preferred to keep instruments with in long axis of the tooth so as to avoid unnecessary removal of radicular dentin. This can be achieved with short bevel.
7. Long bevel exposes more dentinal tubules to the oral environment, this can result in more microleakage over a period of time.

Irrespective of the angle or extent of the resection, the main fundamental of the root resection is that it should be complete and no segment of root is left unresected.

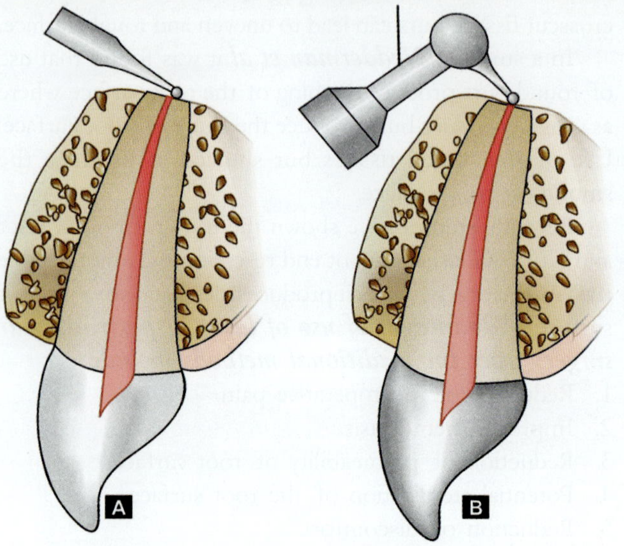


**Figs 25.26A and B:** (A) Root-end preparation using straight handpiece; (B) Root-end preparation using endopiece

## ROOT-END PREPARATION

The main objective of root-end preparation is to create a cavity to receive root-end filling. It is performed with small round or inverted cone burs using a straight or miniature handpiece. The preparation for, and placement of a biocompatible root-end filling is recommended, whenever root-end resection has been performed because root-end resection has shown to disturb the gutta-percha seal. Root-end preparation should accept filling materials so as to seal off the root canal system from periradicular tissues.

***Car and Bentkover*** defined an ***ideal root-end preparation as "a class I preparation at least 3.0 mm into root dentin with walls parallel to a coincident with the anatomic outline of the pulp space".***

***Five requirements*** have been suggested for a root-end preparation to fulfill:

1. The apical 3 mm of root canal must be freshly cleaned and shaped.
2. Preparation must be parallel to anatomic outline of the pulp cavity.
3. Creation of an adequate retention form.
4. Removal of all isthmus tissue if present.
5. Remaining dentin walls should not be weakened.

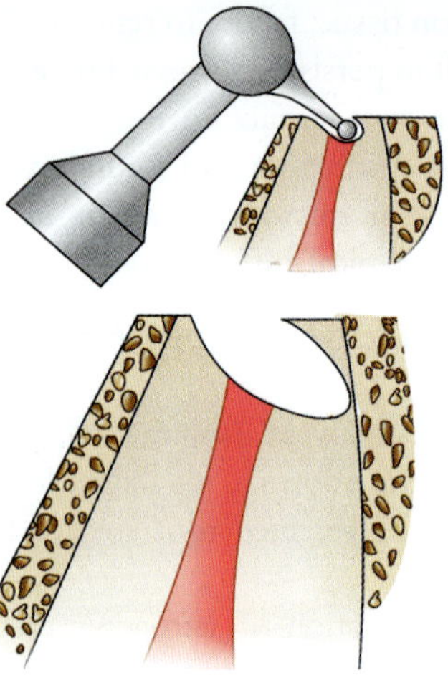

**Fig. 25.27:** Perforation of root caused by misdirection of handpiece

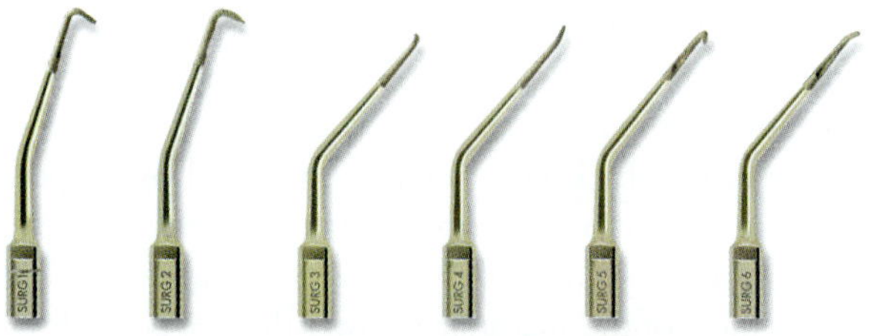


**Fig. 25.28:** Ultrasonic tip for root-end preparation

### Traditional Root-end Cavity Preparation

Miniature contra-angle or straight handpiece, with a small round or inverted cone bur is used to prepare a class I cavity at the root-end within confines of the root canal (Figs 25.26A and B). One of the main problems in root-end preparation is that these preparations seem to be placed in the long axis of the tooth, but they are directed palatally, ultimately causing the perforations (Fig. 25.27).

***Ultrasonic root-end preparation*** was developed to resolve the main shortfalls of bur preparation. For this specially designed ultrasonic root-end preparation instruments have been developed (Figs 25.28 and 25.29).

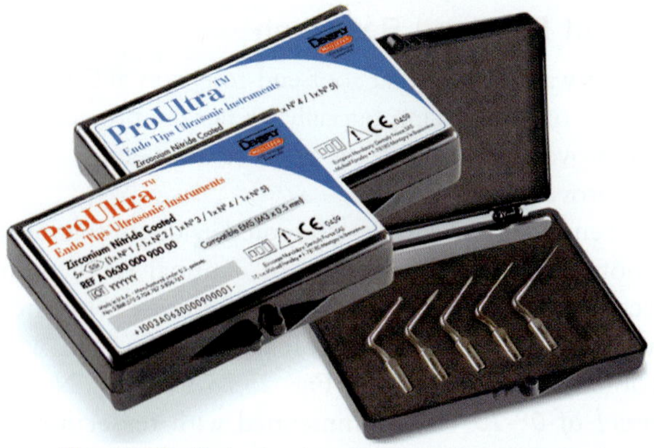


**Fig. 25.29:** Endo tips for ultrasonic instruments

| Difference between traditional and microsurgery | | |
|---|---|---|
| *Procedure* | *Traditional* | *Microsurgery* |
| 1. Apex identification | Difficult | Precise |
| 2. Osteotomy | Large (8-10 mm) | Small (3-4 mm) |
| 3. Angle of bevel | 45-60° | Less then 10° |
| 4. Identification of Isthmus | Almost Impossible | Easy |
| 5. Root surface inspection | None | Always |
| 6. Retropreparation | Approximate | Precise |
| 7. Root-end filling | Imprecise | Precise |
| 8. Root-end preparation | Sometimes inside canal | Always in the canal |
| 9. Suture material (Silk suture) | 3-0 or 4-0 | 5-0 or 6-0 |
| 10. Suture removal (Postoperative) | After 1 week | After 2-3 day |
| 11. Healing | Slow | Fast |

### *Advantages*

1. Smaller preparation size and better access.
2. Less or no need for root-end beveling.
3. A deeper preparation possible, coincident with the anatomic outline of pulp space.
4. More parallel walls for better retention.
5. Less debris and smear layer than those prepared with a bur.

### *Steps of Root-end Preparation by Ultrasonic Instruments*

1. First of all examination is done using magnification and staining.
2. Thereafter cavity design is planned and outlined by sharp point of a CT-S ultrasonic tip, without irrigation (Fig. 25.30).
3. Prepared cavity design is deepened with appropriately sized and angled ultrasonic tip with irrigation (Fig. 25.31).
4. At completion, cavity is thoroughly irrigated with sterile saline, dried and finally examined under magnification.

## RETROGRADE FILLING

The main aim of the endodontic therapy whether nonsurgical or surgical is three-dimensional obturation of the root canal system. Therefore after the apical surgery, placement of a root-end filling material is an equally important step. Root canal filling material is placed in the prepared root-end in a dry field. To place a material in the retropreparation, it is mixed in the desired consistency, carried on the carver (hollenback) and placed carefully into the retropreparation (Fig. 25.32) and compacted with the help of burnisher. After the material is set, excess of it is removed with carver or periodontal curette (Fig. 25.33). Finally the root-end filling is finished with carbide finishing bur and a radiograph is exposed to confirm the correct placement of the filling.

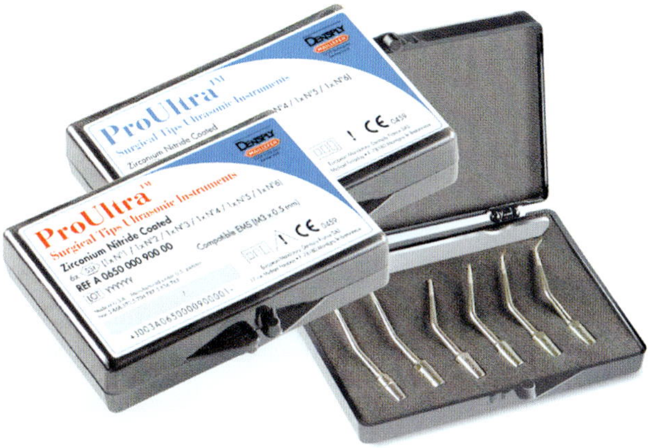


**Fig. 25.30:** Surgical tips for ultrasonic instruments

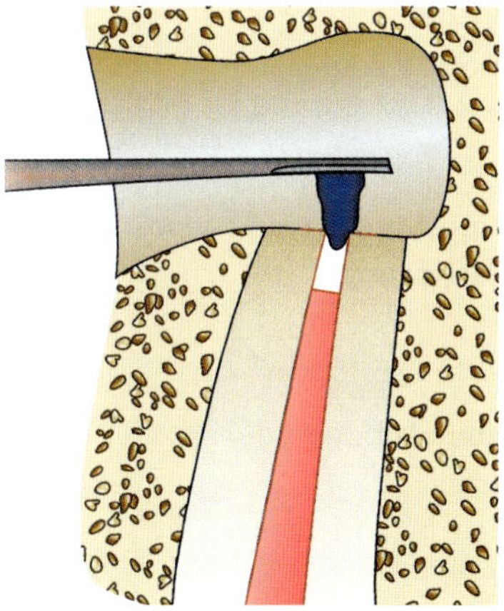

**Fig. 25.32:** Placement of restorative material

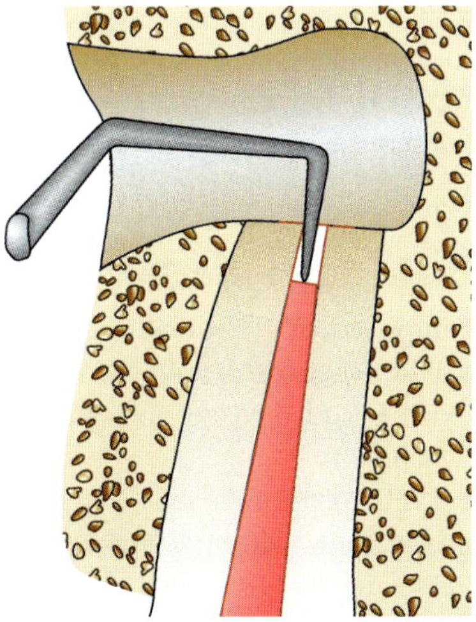

**Fig. 25.31:** Retrograde cavity preparation using ultrasonic handpiece

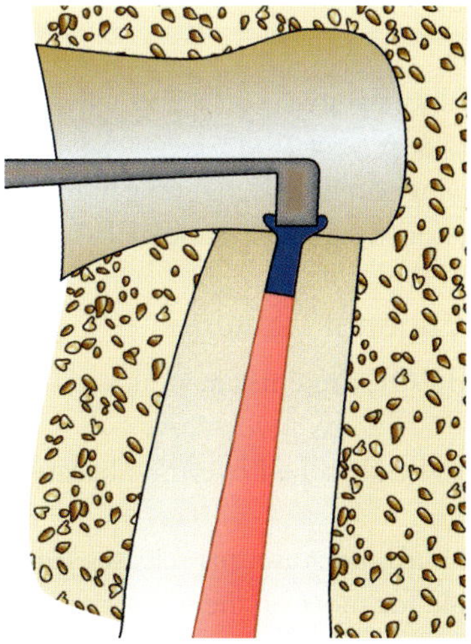

**Fig. 25.33:** Removal of excess material

## ROOT-END FILLING MATERIALS

Ideal properties of a root-end filling material are that it:

1. Should be well tolerated by periapical tissues
2. Should adhere to tooth surface.
3. Should be dimensionally stable
4. Should be resistant to dissolution
5. Should promote cementogenesis
6. Should be bactericidal or bacteriostatic
7. Should be non corrosive
8. Should be electrochemically inactive
9. Should not stain tooth or periradicular tissue
10. Should be readily available and easy to handle
11. Should allow adequate working time, then set quickly
12. Should be radiopaque.

**Commonly used root-end filling materials are:**

1. Amalgam
2. Gutta-percha
3. Gold foil
4. Titanium screws
5. Glass ionomers
6. Zinc oxide eugenol (ZOE)
7. Cavit
8. Composite resins
9. Polycarboxylate cement
10. Poly HEMA
11. Super EBA
12. Mineral trioxide aggregate

### Amalgam

It is one of the most popular and widely used retrograde filling material since last century.

#### *Advantages*

1. Easy to manipulate
2. Readily available
3. Well tolerated by soft tissues
4. Radiopaque
5. Initially provides tight apical seal

#### *Disadvantages*

1. Slow setting
2. Dimensionally unstable
3. It shows leakage
4. Stains overlying soft tissues, resulting in formation of tattoo.
5. More cytotoxic than IRM, super EBA or MTA.

### Zinc Oxide Eugenol Cements

1. Unmodified ZOE cements are weak and have a long setting time.
2. They tend to be absorbed overtime because of high water solubility.
3. On contact with moisture this releases free eugenol which is responsible for most of the effects caused by zinc oxide eugenol cements.

### Effects of Free Eugenol

1. Competitively inhibit prostaglandin synthetase by preventing biosynthesis of cyclooxygenase.
2. Inhibits sensory nerve activity.
3. Inhibits mitochondrial respiration.
4. Kills a range of natural oral microorganisms.
5. Can act as allergen.

### Intermediate Restorative Material (IRM)

1. IRM is a ZOE cement reinforced by addition of 20 percent polymethacrylate by weight to zinc oxide powder.
2. This reinforcement eliminated the problem of absorbability.
3. Milder reaction than unmodified ZOE cements.
4. Mild to zero inflammatory effect after 30 days.
5. Have statistically significant higher success rate compared to amalgam.

### Super EBA

It is a ZOE cement modified with ethoxy benzoic acid (EBA) to alter the setting time and increase the strength of mixture.

***Powder contains:***

- 60 percent zinc oxide
- 34 percent silicone dioxide
- 6l percent natural resin.

***Liquid contains:***

- EBA—62.5 percent
- Eugenol—37.5 percent

#### *Advantages*

1. Neutral pH
2. Low solubility
3. Radiopaque
4. Strongest and least soluble of all ZOE formulations
5. Yield high compressive and tensional strength
6. Significantly less leakage than amalgam
7. Non resorbable
8. Good adaptation to canal walls compared with amalgam

#### *Disadvantages*

1. Difficult to manipulate because setting time is short and greatly affected by humidity.
2. Tends to adhere to all surfaces—Difficult to place and comfort.

### Mineral Trioxide Aggregate (MTA)

1. MTA is composed of Tri-calcium silicate, Tri-calcium aluminate; Tri-calcium oxide and Silicate oxide.
2. Bismuth oxide is added to the mixture for radiopacity.
3. pH-12.5 (when set).
4. Setting time is 2 hr 45 minutes.
5. Compressive strength—40 MPa (immediately after setting) which increases to 70 MPa after 21 days.
6. Insignificant weight loss following settings.

## MTA Placement Technique

1. Preparation of root-end is completed.
2. Bony crypt is packed with sterile cotton pellet.
3. MTA powder and liquid are mixed to put consistency.
4. Mix is carried to the site with amalgam carrier or messing gun and is placed into the preparation (Figs 25.34 and 25.35).
5. MTA is compacted using micropluggers.
6. Cleaning of the surface is done with damp cotton pellet.

## Advantages of MTA

1. Least toxic of all filling materials.
2. Excellent biocompatibility, in contact with periradicular tissues, it forms connective tissue and cementum, causing only very low levels of inflammation.
3. Hydrophilic—Not adversely affected by blood or slight moisture.
4. Radiopaque
5. Sealing ability—Superior to that of amalgam or super EBA.

### *Disadvantages*

- More difficult to manipulate
- Longer setting time
- Expensive

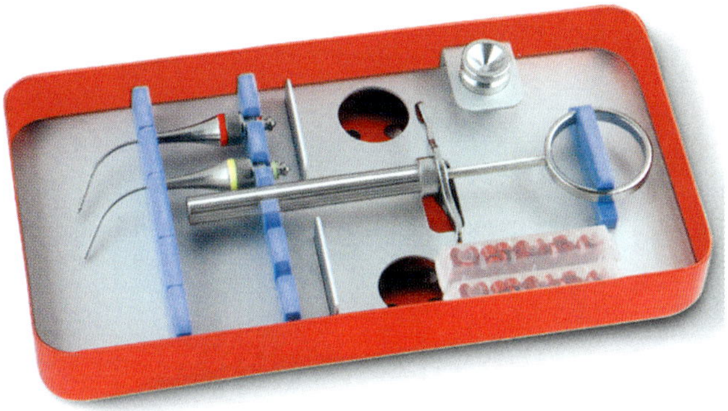

**Fig. 25.34:** Messing gun for MTA placement

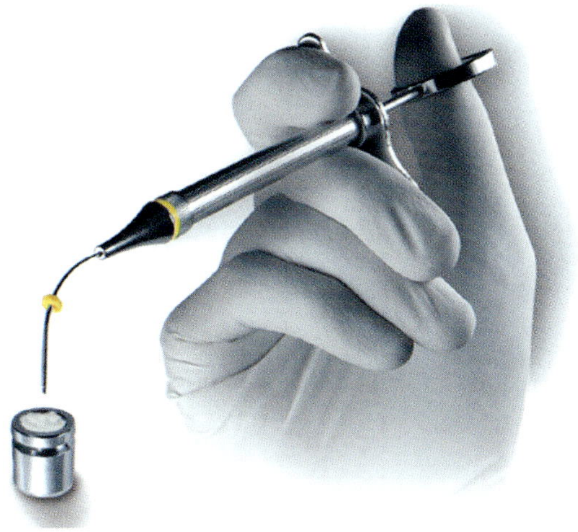

**Fig. 25.35:** Carrying MTA with messing gun or amalgam carrier

## Composite Resins

Though composite resins have shown superior physical properties but they are very technique sensitive. Since, it is very difficult to obtain a total dry field, their use is not encouraged as root-end filling material.

## REAPPROXIMATION OF THE SOFT TISSUE

Following surgery, final inspection of the root-end filling and cleaning of the surgical site is done and a radiograph is taken to assess presence of any root fragments or surplus root-end filling material.

## Repositioning of the Flap

Flap is replaced in the original position with the incision lines approximated as close as possible. Now flap is compacted by applying light yet firm pressure to the flapped tissue for 2-5 minutes with the help of damp surgical gauze. This compression of the flap helps in:

a. Approximation of the wound edges, and their initial adhesion.
b. Augment the formation of thin fibrin clots at the wound site.

## REPLANTATION

Replantation is defined as intentional removal of a tooth and after examination, diagnosis, endodontic therapy and repair, placing it back into the original socket.

## Classification

It can be of two types:

a. Intentional replantation
b. Unintentional replantation

## Indications

1. Nonsurgical endodontic treatment not possible because of limited month opening
2. Calcifications, posts or separated instruments present in canals making nonsurgical endodontics therapy difficult.
3. Persistent infection even after root canal treatment
4. Inaccessibility for surgical approach for periradicular surgery due to anatomic factors
5. Perforations in inaccessible areas where for surgery excessive bone loss is required
6. Accidental avulsion i.e. unintentional replantation.
7. For thorough examination of root defects like crack or perforation.

## Contraindications

1. Curved and flared canals
2. Nonrestorable tooth
3. Moderate to severe periodontal disease
4. Missing interseptal bone

*Factors affecting outline of replantation procedure—*

1. Root surface (with PDL cells) should be kept moist with Hanks balanced salt solution (HBSS) or saline during the time tooth is out of socket

2. Out of socket time should be shortest possible
3. One should take care not to damage PDL cells and cementum. Avoid touching forcep's beaks on cementum.

### Techniques

1. Incise periodontal fibers using No. 15 scalpel blade
2. Gently elevate the tooth using forcep in rocking motion until grade I mobility is achieved. The forcep should be placed away from the cementum so as to avoid damage to periodontal ligament (Figs 25.36 and 25.37).
3. Take out the tooth using forcep whose beaks have been wrapped with a sterile gauze piece which is saturated with HBSS or normal saline.
4. Thoroughly examine the roots for defects or fractures
5. Repair the root defects if indicated. Any repair or procedure should be done as quickly as possible in the bath of normal saline or HBSS solution so as to prevent desiccation (Fig. 25.38).
6. Irrigate the extraction socket using normal saline
7. Gently place the tooth back in the socket
8. After placing tooth back, place a rolled gauze piece on occlusal surface of the tooth and ask patient to bite on it. This will help in seating the tooth into socket. Ask patient to maintain biting pressure for at least 5-10 minutes.
9. Stabilize the tooth using periopak, sutures or splints. Recall the patient after 7-14 days so as to remove the stabilization and to evaluate the mobility.
10. Follow-up after 2, 6, 9 and 12 months is done following surgery.

*Causes of failure of reimplantation:*

1. Extended extraoral time resulting in damage to periodontal cells.
2. Contamination during procedure resulting in infection and resorption.
3. Undetected fracture of tooth.
4. Mishandling of tooth during reimplantation procedure.

## TRANSPLANTATION

It is the procedure of replacement of a tooth in a socket other than the one from which it had been extracted from.

## ROOT RESECTION/AMPUTATION

Root resection is defined as removal of a complete root leaving the crown of tooth intact.

### Indications for Root Resections

1. Extensive bone loss in relation to root where periodontal therapy cannot correct it.
2. Root anatomy like curved canal which cannot be treated
3. Extensive calcifications in root
4. Fracture of one root, which does not involve other root
5. Resorption, caries or perforation involving one root

### Contraindications for Root Resections

1. Fused roots
2. Roots in close proximity to each other

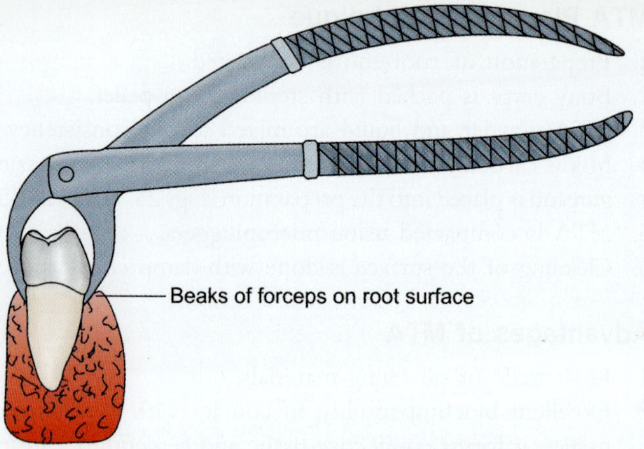


**Fig. 25.36:** Beaks of the forceps should be away from the cementum so as to avoid damage to periodontal ligament

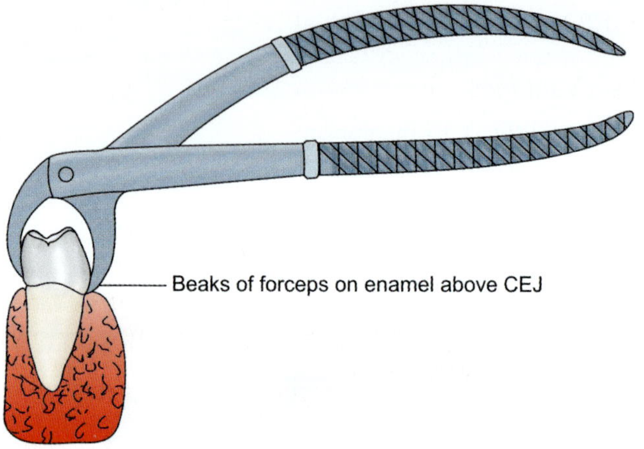


**Fig. 25.37:** Beaks of forcep should rest on cement enamel junction so as to avoid injury to periodontal tissue

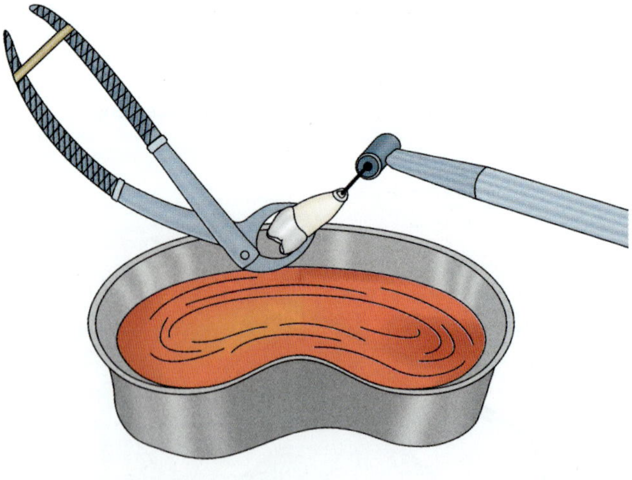

**Fig. 25.38:** Any repair or procedure should be done as quickly as possible in the bath of normal saline or HBSS solution to prevent desiccation

3. Uncooperative patient
4. Lack of optimal bone support for remaining root/roots
5. Endodontically incompatible remaining root/roots

### Technique

Before root resection, endodontic treatment is done on the roots to be retained, once the canals to be retained are obturated, the permanent restoration is done. After this, root resection is carried out. There are basically two approaches for root resections—

a. *Vertical*: Here complete root is ressected along with its associated portion of crown. This procedure also called as hemisection or trisection.

   It is done from mesial to distal in maxillary molars and bucccal to lingual in mandibular molars.

b. *Horizontal/Oblique*: In this, root is ressected at the point where it joins to the crown. It is also called as root resection.

### Presurgical Crown Contouring (Fig. 25.39)

This method involves trimming the portion of crown over the root to be amputated so as to gain access. Before carrying out this technique, roots should be obturated with gutta percha (it acts as an important landmark). It is done with tapered fissure bur. The bur is moved so as to trim the crown portion present above the root to be amputated up to the level of cementoenamel junction.

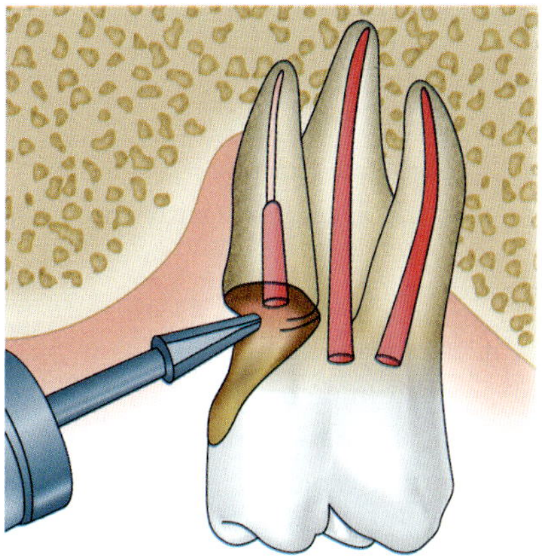

**Fig. 25.39:** In presurgical contouring, crown which is present over root to be amputated is trimmed with bur upto the level of cementoenamel junction

## BICUSPIDIZATION/BISECTION

It is defined as surgical separation of a multirooted tooth into two halves and their respective roots. Each root is then restored with a separate crown. Basically bicuspidization is done to form a more favorable position for the remaining segments which leaves them easier to clean.

### Indications

1. When periodontal disease involves the furcation area and therapy does not improve the condition of tooth.
2. Furcation is transferred to make interproximal space which makes the area more manageable by the patient.

### Contraindications

1. Fused roots
2. Lack of osseous support for separate segments
3. Uncooperative patient

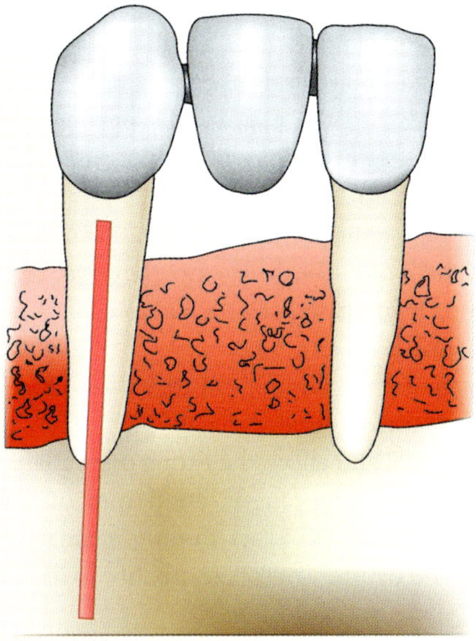

**Fig. 25.40:** Endodontic implant

## ENDODONTIC IMPLANTS

Endodontic implants are used for providing stabilization of teeth in which alveolar support is lost due to endodontic and periodontal disease (Figs 25.40 and 25.41).

It enhances root anchorage by extension of artificial material beyond alveolar socket but within range of alveolar bone.

### Case Selection for Endodontic Implants

1. Teeth with straight canals
2. Presence of sufficient alveolar height
3. Absence of systemic disease
4. Absence of any anatomic complications
5. Absence of any calcifications in canals.

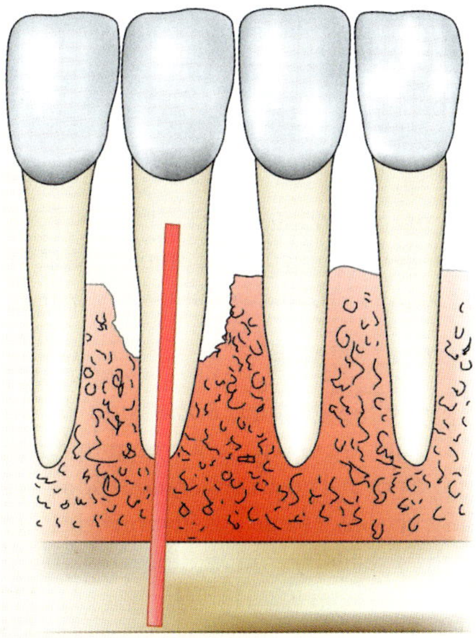

**Fig. 25.41:** Endodontic implant in tooth with severe bone loss

### Indications

1. Horizontal root fracture
2. Unaffordable rootcrown ratio
3. Periodontally involved teeth
4. Endodontically involved teeth with short roots

### Contraindications

1. Presence of calcifications in roots
2. Proximity of anatomic structures
3. Patient suffering from systemic disease
4. Presence of curved canals

### Material Used for Implants

- Titanium
- Chrome cobalt alloys

### Technique

1. After anesthetizing the tooth isolate it using rubber dam.
2. Extirpate the pulp, and take working length radiograph
3. Add 2-3 mm to the estimated working length so that instrument goes periapically with a minimal preparation of ISO size 60
4. Start intraosseous preparation using 40 mm long reamers
5. Ream the bone about 10 mm beyond the apex with sequentially increased sizes so as to achieve round apical preparation.
6. Complete the preparation till atleast ISO No. 70, or until apex is reamed round.
7. Dry the canal and check the fitting of implant. If tugback is there at working length, cut 1 mm of apical end of implant so as to avoid its butting against bone
8. Irrigate and dry the canal, take care not to disturb the apical clot.
9. Fit the canal and cut it at the point below gingival level using carborrundum disk. One should take care that cement is applied only to the part of implant within confines of the canal.
10. Seal the implant using gutta-percha.
11. Do coronal restoration using crown, or composite restoration

### Reasons for Failure of Endodontic Implants

- Extrusion of cementing media
- Inadequate seal at junction of implant and the apex
- Wrong technique of placement.

## POSTSURGICAL CARE

It includes providing genuine expression of concern and reassurance to patient, good patient communication, regarding the expected and normal postsurgical sequelae as well as detailed home care instructions. Home care instructions should be best conveyed both verbally and in writing.

### Instructions

1. No difficult activity or work for the rest of day.
2. No alcohol or any tobacco for next 3 days.
3. Good nutritious diet. Drink lot of liquids for first few days after surgery.
4. Do not lift up lip or pull back check to look where surgery was done – it may pull the stitches loose and cause bleeding.
5. A little bleeding from the surgical site is normal and it should last for a few hours. Little swelling or bruising of face is normal and will last for few days.
6. Application of ice bags on face where surgery was done—20 minutes on and 20 minutes off till 6-8 hours.
7. Next day after surgery— Hot fermentation for 3-5 days.
8. Prescribed medicines should be taken regularly.
9. Rinsing of mouth with chlorhexidine mouthwash twice daily for one week.
10. Suture removal.
11. Follow-up appointment.
12. In case of any problem or any question – Contact the endodontic surgeon.

## SUTURING MATERIALS AND TECHNIQUES

### Definition

***A suture is strand of material used to close the wound.***

The purpose of suturing is to approximate incised tissues and also stabilize the flapped mucoperiosteum until reattachment occurs. Skillful wound closure requires not only knowledge of proper surgical techniques but also knowledge of the physical characteristics and properties of the suture and needle.

### History

- ***Celsus*** recommended ligature in protocol of control of hemorrhage
- ***Gaten*** in 2nd century—used silk for sutures
- ***Dr. Philip Physick*** (1806)—made absorbable suture
- ***Lister*** advocated the chromic acid impregnation of catgut so that its absorption is delayed
- ***Synthetic*** sutures were introduced in 1940s.

#### *Classification of Sutures*

1. It can be classified according to absorbency
   i. Absorbable
   ii. Nonabsorbable
2. It can be classified according to physical property
   i. Monofilament
   ii. Multifilament
   iii. Twisted or braided

### Ideal Suture Characteristics

1. Non-reactive in tissues
2. Easy to handle
3. High tensile strength
4. Sterile
5. Resistant to infection
6. Non-capillary action
7. High knotting quality
8. Economical

**Comparison of monofilament and multifilament sutures**

| *Monofilament* | *Multifilament* |
|---|---|
| 1. Made up of single strand | 1. Made up of several strands |
| 2. Less chances of harboring microorganisms | 2. More chances of harboring microorganisms |
| 3. Less tensile strength | 3. More tensile strength |
| 4. Difficulty in handling and tying | 4. Easy in handling and tying |

## Few Facts About Sutures

- The most important consideration in suturing is not the strength of suture material, but the holding power of tissues to be sutured
- Knotting decreases the strength by 40-50 percent
- The weakest point in the suture is the knot
- Absorbable sutures are digested by enzymatic degration in case of natural materials while synthetic absorbable sutures are digested by hydrolysis
- Capillarity—extent to which absorbed fluid is transferred along the suture
- Knots of skin suture should be placed on one side of the incision to avoid irritation and separation of wound edges
- Medium chromic gut also called type C is not widely used
- Sutures are designated by two Arabic numbers which are separated by hyphen. This is according to United State of Pharmcopia (USP). In this system, numbers are like 3-0, 4-0, and 5-0. The higher the first number, smaller the diameter of suture material
- Monofilament suture is better than multifilament sutures.

## Suture Needle

Most often suture is made available in sterile single pack with or without needle. The needles when present are swaged on to the thread and are of either cutting or non-cutting type.

There are certain characteristics of ideal surgical needle:

- High quality stainless steel should be used
- Should be sharp enough to penetrate tissue with minimal resistance
- Easy to sterile
- Should be corrosion resistant
- It should be stable while holding with needle holder

## Parts of Surgical Needle (Fig. 25.42)

### *The Body*

The body or the shaft section is usually referred as the needle grasping area. This part of needle incorporate the majority of the needle length. The body of the needle is important for interaction with needle holder and also transmits penetrating force to the point.

### *Point*

This portion of the needle extends from the tip to maximum cross-section of the body. The tip can be cutting, round or blunt.

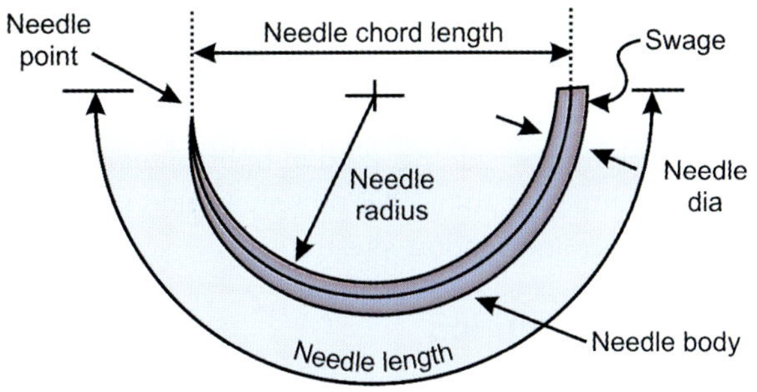


**Fig. 25.42:** Parts of surgical needle

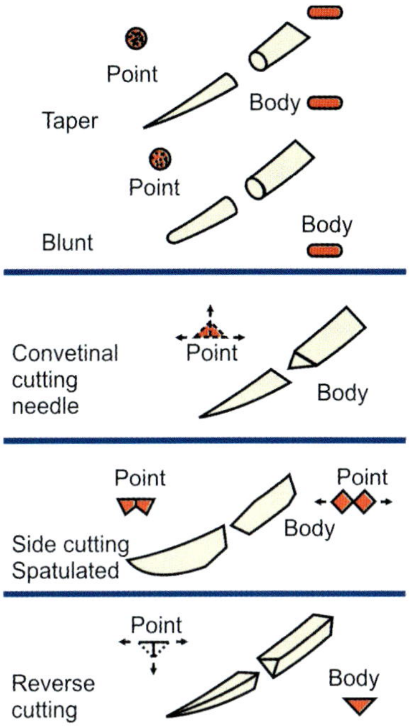


**Fig. 25.43:** Classification of needles according to point geometry

### *The Swage*

There are two types of needles; atraumatic and traumatic. In atraumatic needle, an eyeless needle is attached to a specific length of suture thread forming a continuous unit of suture and needle. The suture manufacturer swages the suture thread to the eyeless atraumatic needle at the factory. In traumatic needle, there is a hole or eye present at its end, to which suture thread is inserted. The suture is threaded on site as is done when sewing at home.

Atraumatic needle some advantages over traumatic needle like the doctor and assistant do not have to spend time threading the suture on needle also it is less traumatic.

Different shapes of surgical needles:

- Straight
- Half curved
- ¼ circle
- 3/8 circle
- ½ circle
- 5/8 circle

*Needles can also be classified according to point geometry (Fig. 25.43)*

- Taper (round)—needle body is sound and tapers smoothly to a point, e.g. used in subcutaneous layers periosteum

- Cutting—needle body is triangular and has sharpened cutting edge present inside.
- Side cutting—flat on top and bottom with a cutting edge present along one side e.g. used in ophthalmic procedures
- Reverse cutting—cutting edge present outside, used for skin, oral mucosa and tendon sheaths.

## Principles of Suturing

1. The needle should enter the mucosal skin perpendicular to the surface of tissue.
2. The needle should always pass from free tissue to fixed tissue.
3. The needle should always be inserted at an equal depth and distance from incision line on both sides.
4. The suture knot should never lie on the incision line.
5. The suture should not be too tight. Sutures are given to approximate the tissues, not to blanch the tissues. If sutures are too tight, there will be local ischemia underneath the suture tracks.
6. The needle should always from thinner to thicker tissues.
7. Tissues should not be closed under tension.
8. The needle should be held in needle holders two thirds of way from needle tip to swage.
9. The needle should take smooth semicircular course to exit at 90 degrees to the wound edge.
10. Sutures should be spaced evenly.
11. After tying, knot should be left to one side.

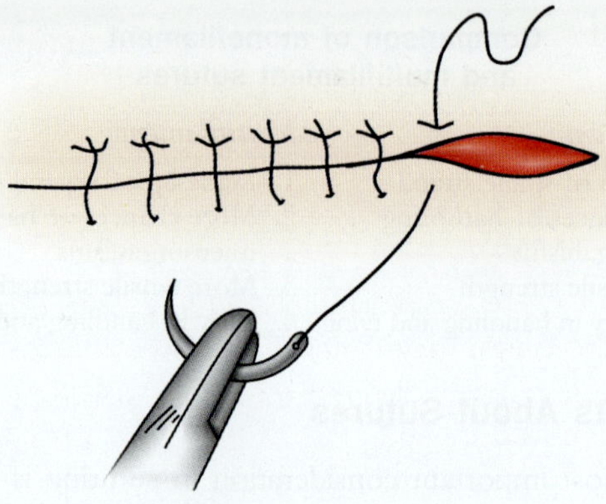

**Fig. 25.44:** Interrupted suture

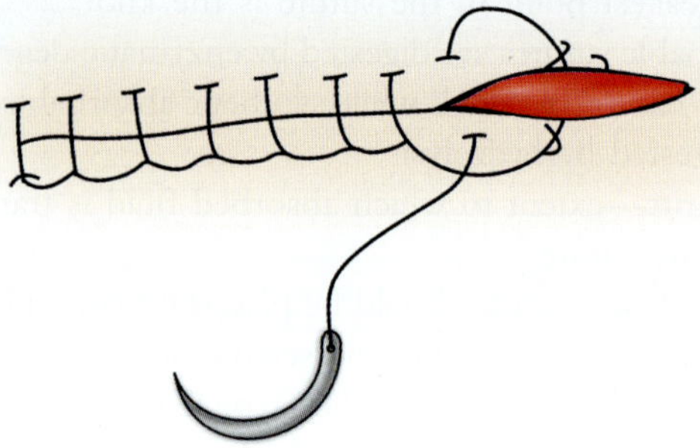

**Fig. 25.45:** Continuous locking suture

## Suturing Techniques

### *Interrupted Suture (Fig. 25.44)*

This is simple technique which is most commonly used. In this suture is passed through both edges of incision line at an equal distance and depth. It is known as an "interrupted suture" because several individual stitches are needed to close wound.

### *Advantages*

1. Usually gives an adequate cosmetic finish if properly done.
2. Simple to learn.
3. Can be used in places of stress.

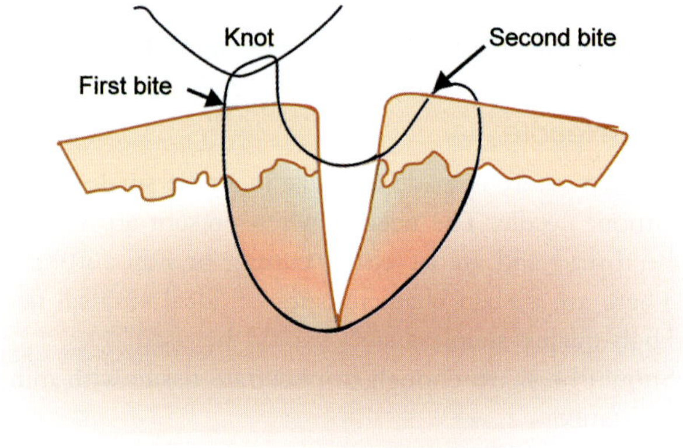


**Fig. 25.46:** Vertical mattress suture

### *Continuous Locking Suture (Fig. 25.45)*

It is similar to simple interrupted suture except there are no individual sutures. It provides watertight closure and is rapid technique for closure. This can be used in scalp and oral cavity.

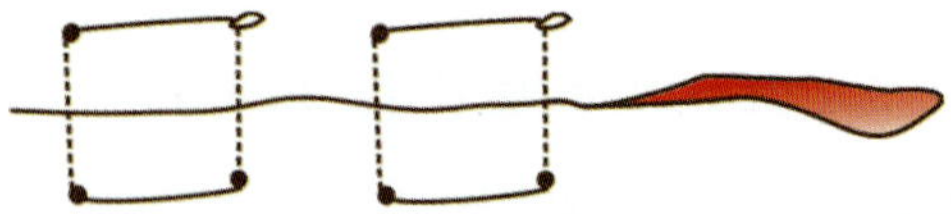

**Fig. 25.47:** Horizontal mattress suture

### *Vertical Mattress Suture (Fig. 25.46)*

This technique is similar to simple suture but a second, superficial bit is taken in the same vertical plane. It produces more eversion of tissues than simple interrupted suture. It can be used in facial skin.

### *Horizontal Mattress Suture (Fig. 25.47)*

This is on similar concept to the vertical suture except that it extends along a horizontal plane, almost like two simple interrupted sutures lying next to each other. It can be used in closing of extraction socket wound.

## COMPLICATIONS OF SUTURING

- Infection
- Tattooing
- Scarring
- Dehiscence

## Suture Removal

- Apply topical anesthesia if necessary
- Clear the incision area with normal saline antiseptic solution before removing the suture
- Instruments required—tissue forcep, suture cutting scissor and surgical blade
- Lift one end of suture lightly to cut under the knot in case of simple interrupted suture
- Suture should be pulled out across the wound rather than away from the wound
- Non-absorbable suture should be removed in time. For example in case of scalp (7-10 days), face (5-7 days)

# POSTSURGICAL COMPLICATIONS

1. *Postoperative swelling:* Postoperative swelling usually reaches maximum after 24 or 48 hours. The patient should be informed earlier about the postoperative swelling. It usually resolves within a week. Proper compression of surgical flap, both before and after suturing reduces postoperative swelling.

## Management

1. Inform the patient earlier as it reduces the anxiety.
2. Application of ice packs should be advocated for next 6-8 hours to decrease the swelling (decreasing the temperature increase the flow of blood in that area and avoids rebound phenomenon).
3. Application of hot moist towel is recommended after 24 hours (decreasing the temperature causes increase in blood flow in that area which enhances inflammatory and healing process).
4. Postoperative bleeding: Slight oozing of blood is usually seen after surgery for several hours. This slight oozing of the blood is normal, but significant bleeding is uncommon and may require attention.

Postoperative bleeding can be reduced by compression of the surgical flap both before and after suturing.

## Management

1. First and foremost step in managing bleeding is apply firm pressure over the area for 10-20 minutes. This can be applied with either moistened cotton gauge or a tea bag or ice pieces placed in cotton gauge.
2. Some prefer pressure to the area along with local anesthetic containing epinephrine (1:50,000 or 1:1,00000).
3. If bleeding still continues, then sutures should be removed and then search for blood vessels causing bleeding. Cauterization should be done either by using thermal (heating an instrument) or electrical method (electrocautery if available). In these cases, local hemostatic agents can also be tried.
   - If bleeding is still unmanageable, then hospitalization of patient is necessary. Review the medical status of the patient.

## Extraoral Ecchymosis (Extraoral discoloration)

Discoloration/ecchymosis usually results when blood has leaked into the surrounding tissues. This condition is self limiting in nature and lasts up to 2 weeks and does not affect the prognosis.

## Management

1. Application of moist hot for 2 weeks is helpful as heat promotes fluid exchange and also speeds up resorption of discoloring agents from tissues.

## Pain

Postoperative pain usually maximum on the day of surgery and it decreases thereafter.

## Management

1. Pain can be managed by prescribing NSAIDs
2. If severe pain is present, opoid analgesics may be combined with NSAIDs
3. Long acting anesthetics like bupivacaine has also been advocated.

**Absorbable suture**

| *Suture* | *Classification* | *Origin* | *Absorption* | *Disadvantages* | *Advantages and properties* | *Uses* |
|---|---|---|---|---|---|---|
| 1. Surgical gut | Natural mono-filament | Formaldehyde treat streps from submucosa of sheep | 70 days<br>90 days | • Inflammatory response<br>• Loss of tensile strength (variable response) | • Elasticity<br>• Knot severity<br>• Can be used in presence of infection | • Suturing in subcutaneous and fatty tissue<br>• Oral surgery |
| 2. Collagen | Natural mono-filament | Bovine flexor tendon<br>• Treated with formaldehyde or chromic salts or both | 50-60 days | • Low tensile strength after 2 weeks | • Limited to use in areas where healing is faster | • Has only ophthalmic use |

*Contd...*

*Contd...*

| *Suture* | *Classification* | *Origin* | *Absorption* | *Disadvantages* | *Advantages and properties* | *Uses* |
|---|---|---|---|---|---|---|
| 3. Vicryl (polyglactin 910) | Synthetic multifilament | • Braided co polymer of glycolic and lactic acid in ratio of 9 : 1 | 56-70 days (minimal absorption in 40 days) | • 50% loss of tensile length after 2 weeks | • Minimal tissue reaction<br>• Coated with calcium stearate for easy passage in tissue and knot placement<br>• Easy to handle | • Can be used in presence of infection<br>• Soft tissue approximation and ligation |
| 4. Polydioxanone (PDS) | Synthetic monofilament | • Polymer of paradioxanone | 180 days (minimal within 90 days) | • 30% loss of strength after 2 weeks | • Slight tissue reaction<br>• Low affinity for microorganisms<br>• Greater flexibility than vicryl<br>• Extremely strong | • Soft tissue approximation in pediatric, ophthalmic and plastic surgery |

| **Non-absorbable suture** | | | | | | |
|---|---|---|---|---|---|---|
| *Suture* | *Classification* | *Origin* | *Absorption* | *Disadvantages* | *Advantages and properties* | *Uses* |
| 1. Silk | Natural multifilament | • Silk fibers from silk worm cocoon | • Absorbed by proteolysis<br>• Undetectable after 2 years | • High inflammatory response<br>• Low knot security | • Easy to handle<br>• Encapsulation within tissues | Used in oral surgery and plastic surgery |
| 2. Surgical cotton | Natural multifilament | • Cotton fibers | Not available | • 50% loss of tensile strength in 6 months | • Encapsulation within tissues<br>• Minimal tissue reaction | Used for ligating and suturing |
| 3. Surgical steel | Natural monofilament, twisted multifilament | • Stainless steel | • Not available | • May break at points of bending during knotting<br>• May cause electrolyte reactions in presence of other metals | • Low tissue reaction<br>• High tensile strength | Used primarily in orthopedic, neurosurgical and thoracic applications |
| 4. Polyamide (Nylon) | Synthetic mono/ multifilament | • Polyamide polymer | • Not available | • Low knot security | • High degree of memory<br>• Good handling characteristics<br>• Minimal acute inflammatory reaction<br>• Stronger than silk suture | • Skin closure, plastic and oral and maxillofacial surgery |
| 5. Polypropylene (prolene) | Synthetic monofilament | • Stereoisomer of linear propylene isomer | Not available | • Difficult in handling | • Biologically inert<br>• Minimal tissue reaction<br>• Resistance to bacterial contamination<br>• Retention of strength (up to 2 years) | • Useful in contaminated and infected wound<br>• Plastic and oral surgery |

## Infection

Postoperative infection usually occurs due to inadequate aseptic technique and improper soft tissue handling, approximation and stabilization. The symptoms usually appear 36-48 hours after surgery. Suppuration, elevated temperature and lymphadenopathy is seen in some cases.

## Management

1. Systemic antibiotics should be prescribed. Antibiotic of choice in these cases is pencillin. If person is allergic to pencillin, then clindamycin should be given (initial dose-600 mg, maintenance 150-300 mg).

## Miscellaneous

i. Maxillary sinusitis
ii. Paresthesia

## QUESTIONS

**Q. Classify various endodontic surgical procedures. What are indications and contraindications of endodontic surgery?**

**Q. What are indications and technique of root end resection. Write in detail about factors to be considered before root end resection.**

**Q. Write short notes on:**

a. Incision and drainage
b. Ochsenbein-Luebke flap.
c. Semilunar flap
d. Hemisection
e. Reimplantation
f. Endodontic implants

**Q. What are different materials used for root-end restoration.**

## BIBLIOGRAPHY


1. Apaydin ES, Shabahang S, Torabinejad M. Hard-tissue healing after application of fresh or set MTA as root-end filling material. J Endod 2003;30:21-24.
2. Aqrabawi JA. Outcome of endodontic treatment of teeth filled using lateral condensation versus certical compaction (Schilder's technique). Contemp Dent Pract 2006;7(1):17-24.
3. Baumgartner KR, Talor J, Walton R. Canal adaptation and coronal leakage: Lateral condensation compared to thermafil. J Am Dent Assoc 1995;126(3):351-56.
4. Belli S, Zhang Y, Pereira P, Pashley D. Adhesive sealing of the pulp chamber. J Endod 2001;27(8):521-26.
5. Bodrumlu E, Tunga U. Apical Leakage of Resilon obturation material. J Contemp Dent Pract 2006;7(4):45-52.
6. Bodrumlu E, Tunga U. The apical sealing ability of a new root canal filling material. Am J Dent 2007;20(5):295-98.
7. Bodrumlu E, Tunga U. Coronal Sealing ability of a new root canal filling material. J Can Dent Assoc 2007;73(7):623.
8. Boyne P. Histologic response of bone to sectioning by high speed rotary instruments. J Dent Res 1966;45:270-76.
9. Brent PD, Morgan La, Marshall JG, Baumgartner IC. Evaluation of diamond-coated ultrasonic instruments for the root end preparation. J Endod 1999;25:672-75.
10. Buckley JA, Ciancio SG, McMullen IA. Efficacy of epinephrine concentration on local anesthesia during periodontal surgery. J Periodontol 1984;55:653-57.
11. Calzonetti KJ, Owanowski T, Komorowski R, Friedman S. Ultrasonic root-end cavity preparation assessed by an in situ impression technique. Oral Surg Oral Med Oral Pathol Radiol Endod 1998;85:210-15.
12. Cambruzzi J, Marshall E. Molar endodontic surgery. J Can Dent Assoc 1983;1:61-66.
13. Carr GB. Microscope in endodontics. J Califf Dent Assoc 1992;20:55.
14. Carr GB. Ultrasonic root-end preparation. Dent Clin North Am 1997;11:55-61.
15. Cheraskin E, Prasertsuntarasai T. Use of epinephrine with local anesthesia in hypertensive patients. IV Effect of tooth extraction on blood pressure and pulse rate. J Am Dent Assoc 1959;58:61-68.
16. Chong BS, Pitt Ford Tr, Hudson MB. A prospective clinical study of mineral trioxide aggregate and IRM when used as root-end filling material in endodontic surgery. Int Endod J 2003;36:520-26.
17. Cohen S, Hargreaves KM. Pathways of the Pulp (9th edn), p.59. St Louis: Mosby, 2006.
18. Cohen S, Burns RC. Pathways of the pulp, 8th edn. St Louis:CV Mosby, 2002.
19. Crane DL, Heuer MA, Kaminski EJ, Moser JB. Biological and physical properties of an experimental root canal sealer with out eugenol. JOE 1980;6:438.
20. Dorn SO, Gartner AH. Retrograde filling materials: A retrospective success-failure study of amalgam, EBA, and IRM. J Endod 1990;16:391-93.
21. Economides E, Pantelidou O, Kokkas A, Tziafas D. Short-term periradicular tissue response to mineral trioxide aggregate (MTA) as root-end filling material. Int Endod J 2003;36: 44-8.
22. Engel TK, Steiman HR. Preliminary investigation of ultrasonic root-end preparation. J Endod 1995;21:443-8.
23. Fisher EJ, Arens Dem Miller CH. Bacterial leakage of mineral trioxide aggregate as compared with zinc-free amalgam, intermediate restorative material, and Super-EBA as a rootened filling material. J Endod 1998;24:176-79.
24. Friedman S, Lustmann J, Shaharabany V. Treatment results of apical surgery in premolar and molar teeth. J Endod 1991; 7:30-33.
25. Gerhards F, Wagner W. Sealing ability of five different retrograde filling materials. J Endod 1996;22:463-6.
26. Gondim E, Zaia AA, Gomes BP, Ferraz CC, Teixeira FB, Souza-Filho FJ. Investigation of the marginal adaptation of root-end filling materials in root-end cavities prepared with ultrasonic tips. Int Endod J 2003;36:491-9.
27. Grossman LI. International replantation of teeth: A clinical evaluation. J Am Dent Assoc 1966;72(5):1111-18.
28. Grossman I, Oliet S, Del Rio C. Endodontic Practice (11th edn), p-253 Varghese Publication, 1991.
29. Grossman LI. A brief history of endodontics. J Endod 1982; 8:536.
30. Gutmann JL, Harrison JW. Posterior endodontic surgery. Anatomical considerations and clinical techniques. Int Endod J 1985;18(1):8-34.
31. Gutmann JL, Pitt Ford TR. Management of the resected root end: A clinical review. Int Endod J 1993;233:273-83.
32. Harrison JW, Johnson SA. Excisional wound healing following the use of IRM as a root-end filling material. J Endod 1997;23:19-27.
33. Harty FJ, Parkins BJ, Wengraf AM. The success rate of apicectomy. Br Dnet J 1970;129:407-13.
34. Hauman CHJ, Love RM. Biocompatibility of dental materials used in contemporary endodontic therapy: a review. Part 2. Root canal-filling material Int. Ended J 2003;36:147-60.
35. Ibarrola JL, Bjorenson JE, Austin BP, Gerstein H. Osseous reaction to three haemostatic agents. J Endod 1985;11:75-83.

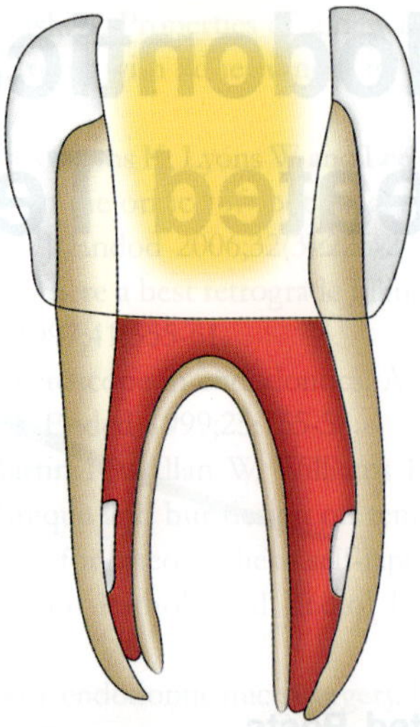

Fig. 26.2: Poor coronal restoration resulting in microleakage and disintegration of obturation

Final restoration of endodontically treated tooth should be done at the earliest so as to long-term success, clinician should evaluate the tooth at regular follow ups because normal leakage can create an impact on success of treatment. One should evaluate signs, symptoms, radiographic changes, defect in coronal restoration like secondary caries, marginal integrity, etc. for better prognosis of treatment.

## EFFECTS OF ENDODONTIC TREATMENT ON THE TOOTH

### Structural Changes

In general the crowns of endodontically treated teeth could be weakened by caries, trauma and/or during access cavity preparation (Fig. 26.3). This weakened crown portion becomes unable to perform its normal function even after successful endodontic therapy. This weakened tooth structure is further prone to fracture. The compromised structural integrity makes the tooth insufficient to perform its function because of loss of occlusion with its antagonist and adjacent teeth. Also the excessive removal of radicular dentin during canal preparation compromises the root (Fig. 26.4).

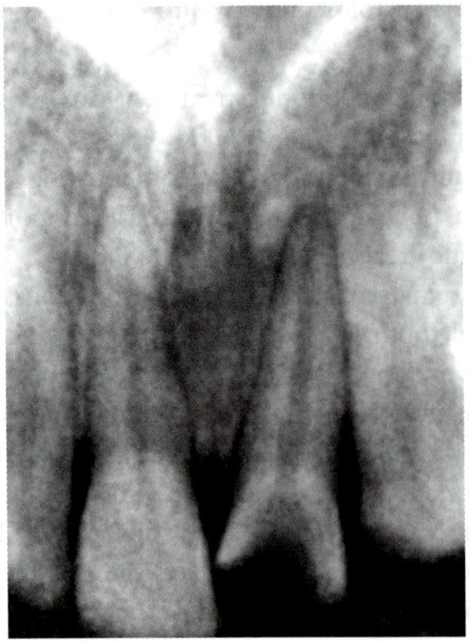

Fig. 26.3: Weakening of tooth structure due to caries

**Effects of endodontic treatment on tooth**

- *Structural changes*
  *Tooth weakening caused by:*
  - Caries
  - Trauma
  - Access cavity preparation
  - Radicular preparation

  Compromised structural integrity.
- *Changes in dentin*
  - A reduced amount of moisture in nonvital teeth.
- *Esthetic considerations*
  - Loss of tooth structure
  - Change in appearance because of alteration in biochemical properties of dentin.
  - *Discoloration because of:*
    - Incomplete debridement
    - Accumulation of sealer or debris.

### *Changes in the Dentin Physical Characteristics*

The endodontic treatment has shown to cause irreversible changes and weakening of the existing tooth structure. Physical chemistry of the dentinal structure also changes following the endodontic therapy. Radicular dentin possesses less of moisture content than the coronal part because of fewer tubules, more inorganic part and anatomically it is intertubular dentin. Moisture content further gets reduced because of aging, decrease in amount of organic content and increased in inorganic components. There are different opinions on whether endodontically treated teeth become more brittle because of moisture loss or caused by loss of pulpal tissue. Helfer et al proved that endodontically treated dog teeth have 9 percent less moisture than normal vital teeth. This should be noted that active retaining posts could induce mechanical stress during cementation and functional loading causing root fracture and failure of postendodontic restorations.

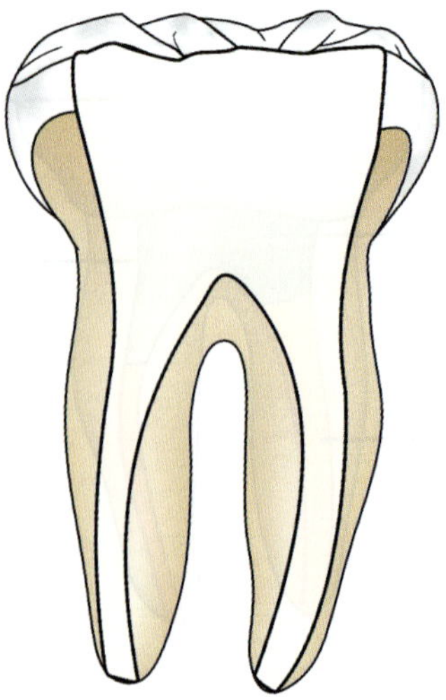

Fig. 26.4: Excessive removal of radicular dentin may result in weakening of roots

## Esthetic Consideration

Devitalization of the normal tooth causes the loss of translucency and discoloration of the crown. These biochemical changes in dentin modify the refraction of light through the tooth and thus changes its appearance. The discoloration of tooth can also result because of incomplete cleaning and shaping of the root canal system, the accumulation of sealer, debris or filling materials left in the chamber.

## PLANNING POSTENDODONTIC RESTORATION PROCEDURE

Various studies of unsuccessful endodontic procedures have shown that failures due to inadequate restoration of the teeth. Restorative treatment of tooth depends upon amount of remaining tooth structure, its functional need and need for the tooth as abutment. After caries is removed and access cavity is prepared, the postendodontic restoration can be planned following the complete visualization of the tooth.

*The restoration plan depends on*:

- Amount of remaining tooth structure
- Functional needs of the patient
- Position/location of tooth in the arch
- Morphology/anatomy of the root canal.

As the remaining tooth structure decreases, and the functional need increases, greater restorative control is needed. Teeth with only little remaining tooth structure have increased risk of fracture, so great care is needed for restorative planning.

### For Anterior Teeth

*Not all endodontically treated teeth require posts*

1. Most teeth with healthy remaining tooth can be restored by direct closure of the access cavity, with usually tooth composite resins or glass ionomer cements (Fig. 26.5).
2. For devitalized, discolored anterior teeth, where more than half of the coronal structure is intact, the preferred treatment should be bleaching and/or composite or porcelain laminate veneers rather than the full coverage crowns or post and core (Fig. 26.6).
3. But if there is doubt regarding the adequacy of resistance form of the coronal portion of the tooth for any restoration, then in such cases post and core is indicated (Fig. 26.7).

### For Posterior Teeth

Since posterior teeth are subjected to greater loading than anterior teeth, these should be treated differently. Also the morphology of posterior teeth is such that the cusps can be wedged apart, which make them more susceptible to fracture.

1. If there are no proximal fillings, caries or unsupported cusps or strong facets, the access cavity of posterior teeth can be easily restored with amalgam or high strength posterior composites (Fig. 26.8).
2. If there is moderate damage of posterior teeth having at least minimum of one sound cusp, the choice of restoration can be:

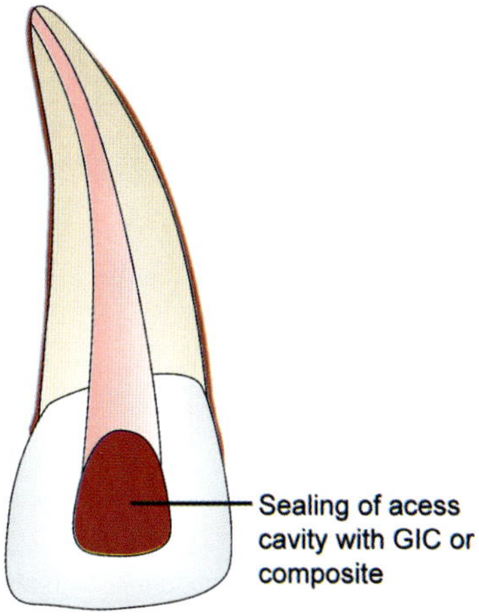


**Fig. 26.5:** In anterior tooth with most of healthy structure remaining access preparation can be sealed with GIC or composite

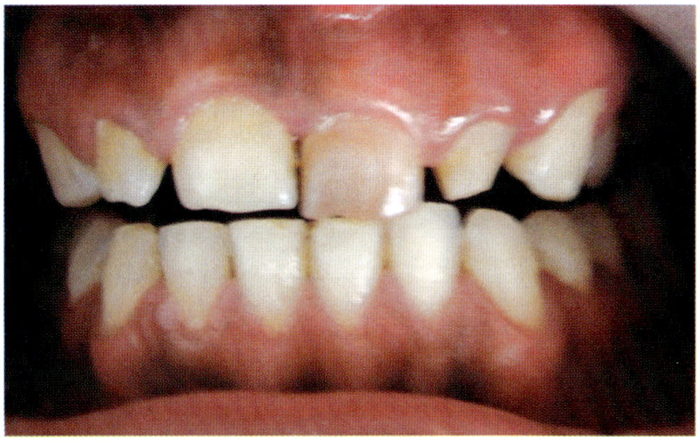

**Fig. 26.6:** In devitalized, discolored anterior tooth, the preferred treatment is bleaching, veneer or porcelain laminate rather than full coverage crown

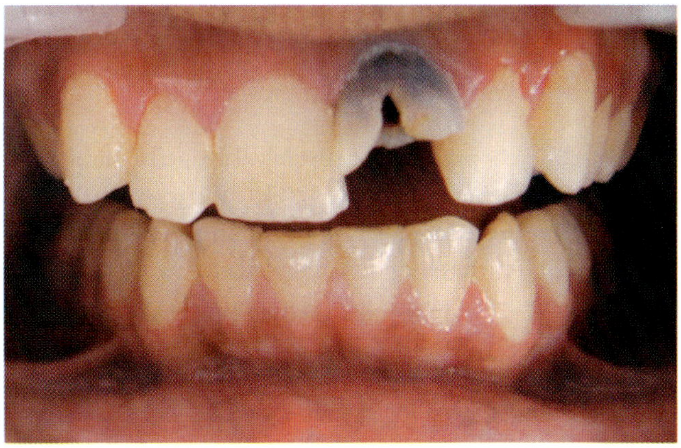

**Fig. 26.7:** When adequate resistance and retention form cannot be achieved from coronal surface, then post and core is indicated

- *Amalgam:* Coronal-radicular core (Nayyers Technique) which is finally restored with cast restoration (Fig. 26.9)
- Pin retained restorations
- Onlay
- Prosthetic crown.

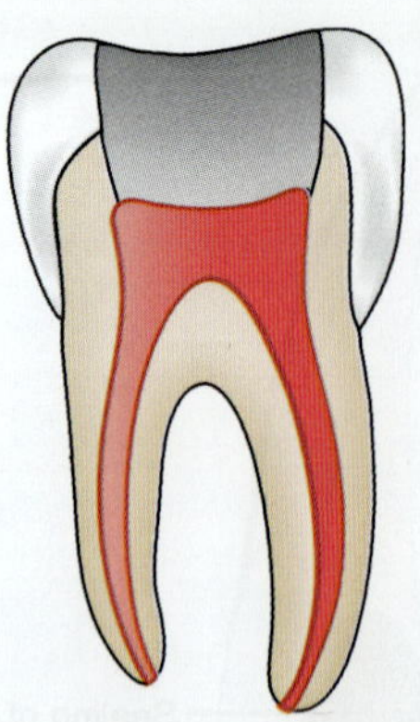

Fig. 26.8: If most of the healthy tooth structure is present, the access preparation should be sealed with amalgam or high strength composite

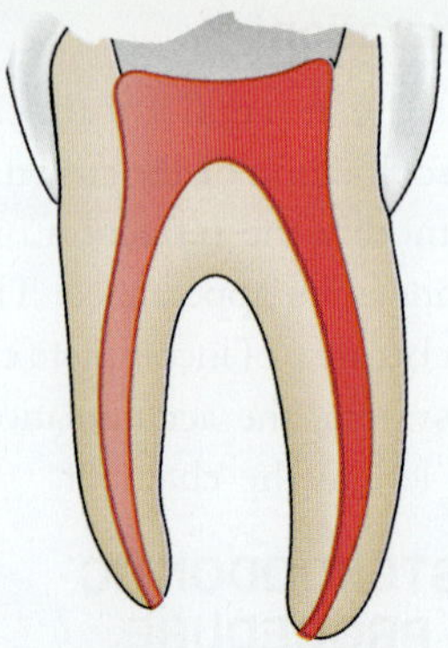

Fig. 26.10: In case of severely damaged crown with no remaining cusps, post is indicated

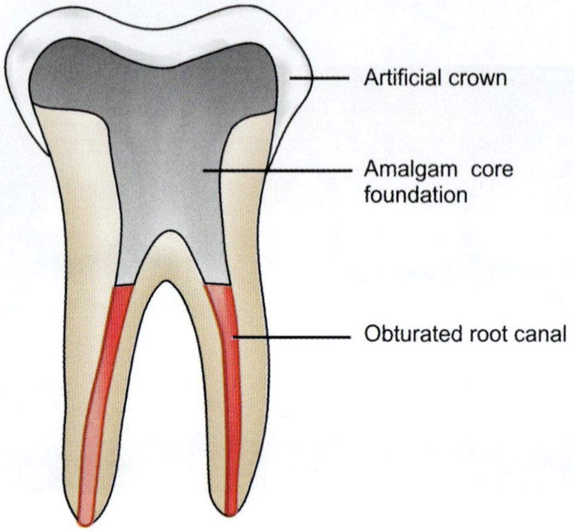


Fig. 26.9: Amalgam core foundation

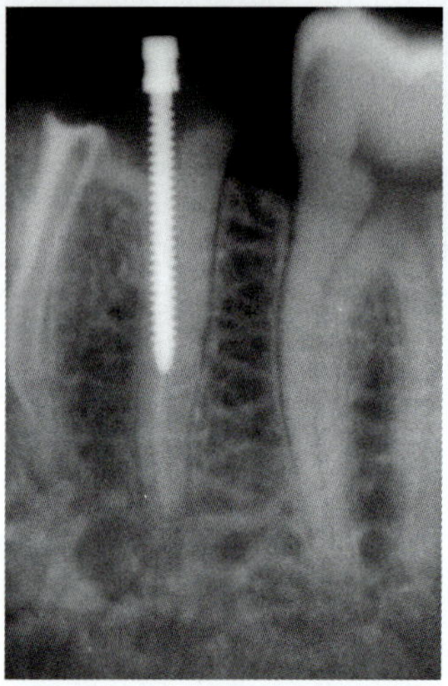

Fig. 26.11: In case of severely damaged crown, root canal space is used for intra-radicular retention. Radiograph showing post placement in distal canal of 36

3. In case there is presence of severely damaged clinical crown with no remaining cusps (Fig. 26.10), the root canal is used as a space for intraradicular retention (Fig. 26.11).

Generally all the endodontically treated teeth should be restored using the crown. A post is indicated in the tooth when it is severely damaged, or it is to serve as an abutment for a removable partial denture. In such cases, the forces which act on teeth are not physiologic, thus a coronal reinforcement is indicated. Post is usually given in palatal canal of maxillary molars and distal canal of mandibular molars.

## Features Evaluated before Going for Post and Core

- Restorability of the tooth
- Role of tooth in the month
- Periodontal considerations
- Functional loading

## Requirements of a Tooth to Accept a Post and Core

- Optimal apical seal
- Absence of fistula or exudate
- Absence of active inflammation
- No sensitivity to percussion
- Absence of associated periodontal disease
- Sufficient bone support around the root
- Sound tooth structure coronal to alveolar crest
- Absence of any fracture of root.

**Component of post and core system (Fig. 26.12)**

1. Residual coronal and radicular tooth structure
2. Post
3. Core
4. Coronal restoration which protect tooth and restores function and esthetics
5. Luting cement

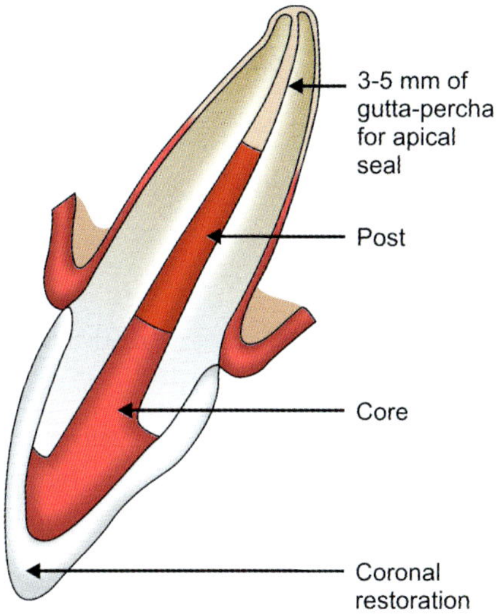

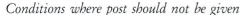

**Fig. 26.12:** Components of post and core

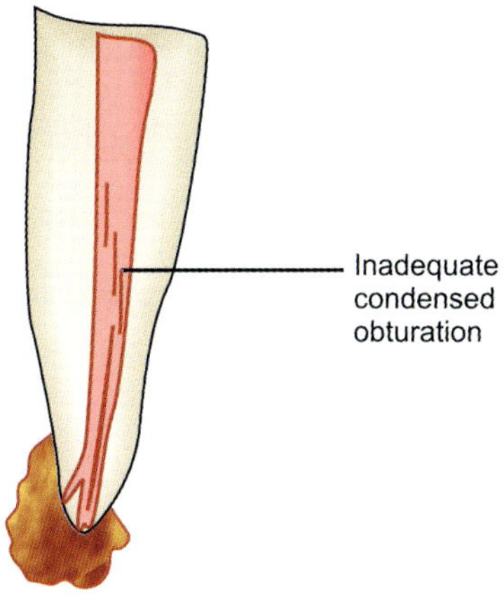


**Fig. 26.13:** A tooth with endodontic failure due to poor quality obturation is not indicated for post and core

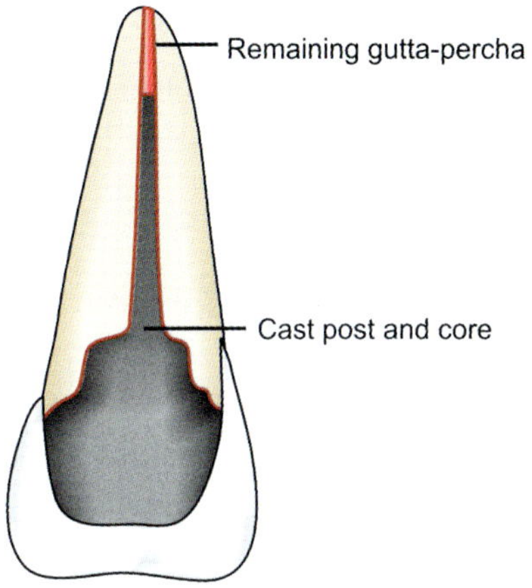


**Fig. 26.14:** Cast post and core system

*Conditions where post should not be given*

1. Any sign of endodontic failures are evident, i.e. tooth exhibits:
   - Poor apical seal and poor quality obturation (Fig. 26.13)
   - Active inflammation
   - Presence of fistula or sinus
   - Tender on percussion.
2. If adequate retention of core can be achieved by natural undercuts of crown.
3. If there are horizontal cracks in the coronal portion of the teeth.
4. When tooth is subjected to excursive occlusal stresses such as when there is presence of lateral stresses of bruxism or heavy incisal guidance.

## Post

It is relatively rigid restorative material placed in the root of a nonvital tooth. It extends coronally to anchor the core material which supports the crown.

## Core

Core is the supragingival portion which replaces the missing coronal tooth structure and forms the center of a new restoration. In other words it acts as a miniature crown (Fig. 26.14).

## Purpose of Use of Post and Core

### *Post Mainly Serves Two Functions*

- Helps in retaining the core
- Helps in favorable distribution of the stresses through the radicular dentin portion of the teeth to apex.

Earlier it was believed that posts strengthen or reinforce the teeth but it has been shown by various studies that posts actually weaken the tooth and increases the risk of root fracture. It has been suggested that endodontically treated teeth are more brittle and may fracture more easily than vital teeth. Subsequently post space preparation or placement of post can further weaken the root and may lead to root fracture. Therefore, a post should be used only when there is insufficient tooth structure remaining to support the final restoration. In other words the main function of post is retention of the core to support the coronal restoration.

## Ideal Requirements of a Post

### *A Post Should:*

- Provide maximum protection of the root to resist root fractures
- Provide maximum retention of the core and crown
- Be easy to place
- Be less technique sensitive
- Have high strength and fatigue resistance
- Be visible radiographically
- Be biocompatible
- Be easily retrievable when required
- Be esthetic
- Be easily available and not expensive.

## CLASSIFICATION OF POSTS

A. *Posts can be classified as:*
   I. Prefabricated (Fig. 26.15)
   II. Custom made (Fig. 26.16).

I. Prefabricated post
   1. Metal prefabricated posts are made up of:
      - Gold alloy
      - High platinum alloys
      - Co-Cr-Mo alloys
      - Stainless steel
      - Titanium and titanium alloys
   2. Carbon fiber post
   3. Quartz fiber post
   4. Zirconia posts
   5. Glass fiber post
   6. Plastic posts.

II. Custom made posts
   They can be cast from a direct pattern fabricated in patient's month or indirect pattern fabricated in the lab.

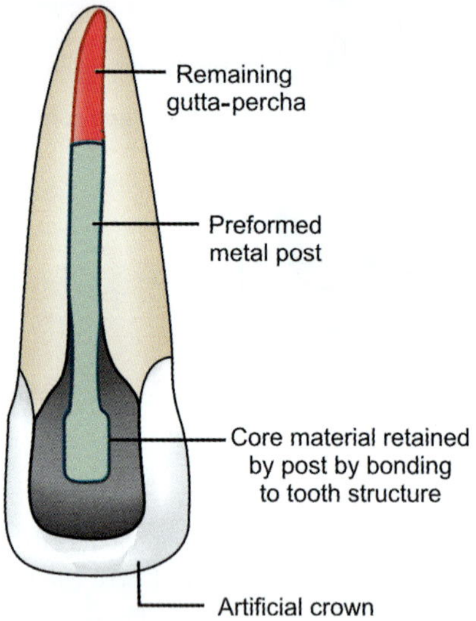


**Fig. 26.15:** Prefabricated post and core

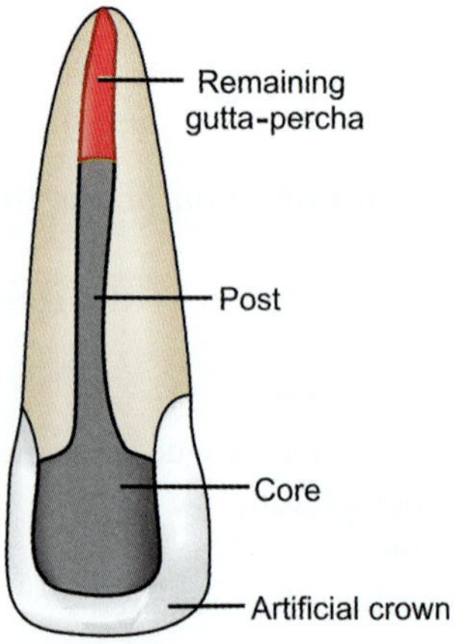


**Fig. 26.16:** Custom made post and core

These can be of two types:

a. *Custom cast metal post and core* are usually made up of:
   - Gold alloys
   - Platinum-palladium alloys
   - Base metal alloys
   - Co-Cr-Mo alloys
   - Ni-Cr alloys.

b. *Ceramic custom made posts* are made up of all ceramic.

B. *Posts can also be classified as:*
   1. *Active post:* Active posts mechanically engage the canal walls. They are retentive in nature but can generate stresses during their placement and functional loading (Fig. 26.17).
   2. *Passive or cemented posts:* Passive posts do not engage the canal walls. They are less retentive but also produce low stresses while placement and functional loading (Fig. 26.18).

C. *According to post design*
   They can be (Fig. 26.19):
   - Smooth
   - Serrated
   - Parallel sided
   - Tapered
   - Combination of above

| *Parallel post* | *Tapered post* |
|---|---|
| • More retentive | • Less retentive |
| • Induce less stresses because of less wedging effects | • Causes more stresses because of wedging effects |
| • Less likely to cause root fracture | • Causes increased chances of root fracture |
| • Require more dentin removal | • Require less dentin removal |

## CUSTOM CAST METAL POST

The custom fabricated cast gold post and core has been used for decades as foundation restoration. Custom cast metal post is post of choice for single rooted teeth especially when remaining coronal tooth structure supporting the artificial crown is minimal. In such case, post must be capable of resisting the rotation which can be better achieved by custom cast posts.

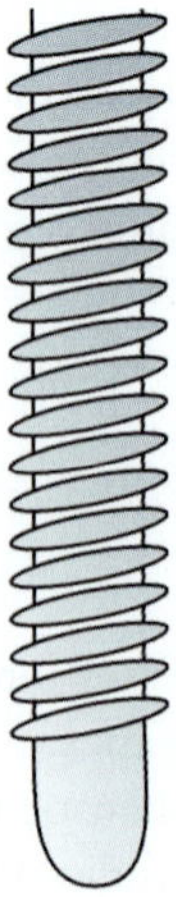

**Fig. 26.17:** Active post mechanically engages the canal walls

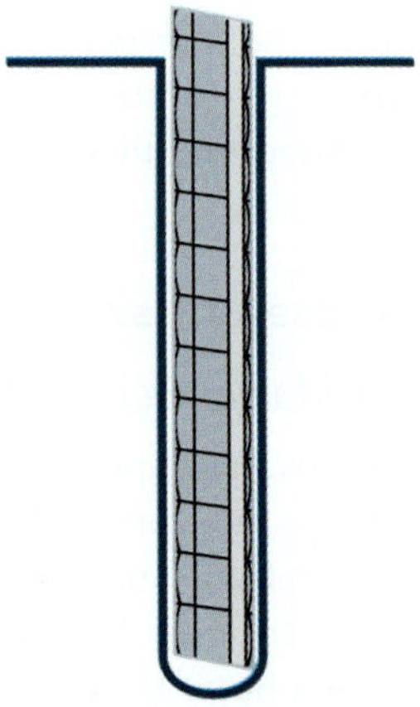

**Fig. 26.18:** Cemented post

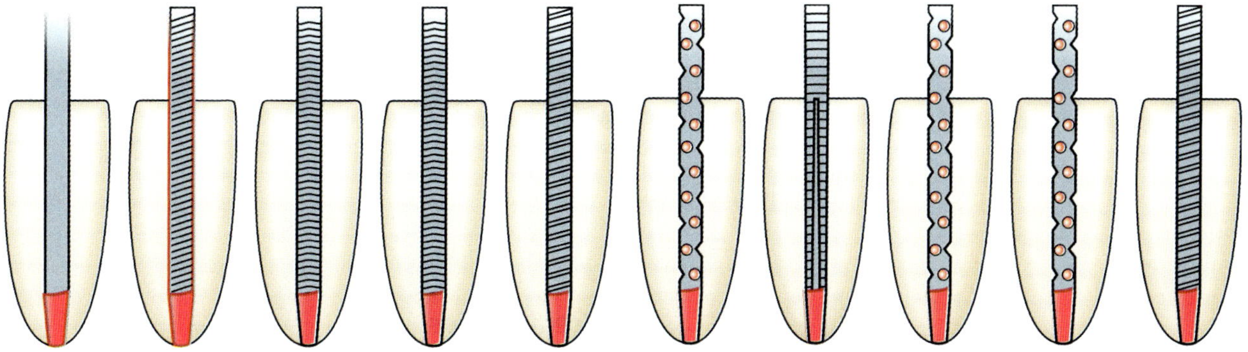

Fig. 26.19: Different types of posts designs like smooth, serrated, parallel, tapered or combination

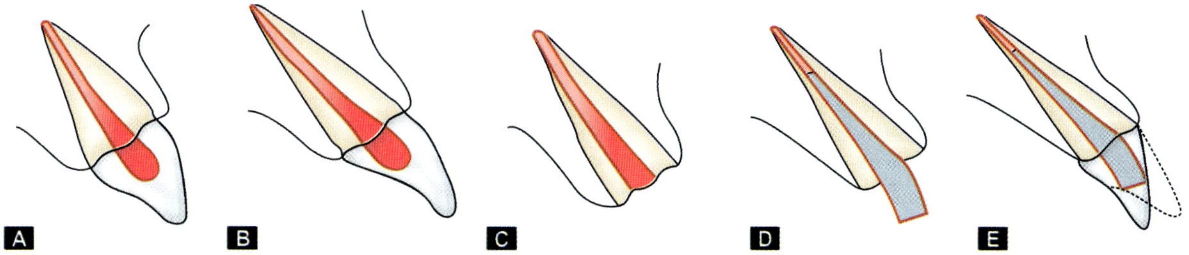


Figs 26.20A to E: Advantage of custom cast metal post when angle of core is to be changed in relation to post

### Advantages

1. Adaptable to large irregularly shaped canals
2. Very strong
3. Better core retention because core is an inherent part of the post
4. In multirooted teeth, they are cost effective
5. Better choice for small teeth
6. Beneficial in cases where angle of the core must be changed in relation to the post (Figs 26.20A to E).

### Disadvantages

1. Requires more chair side time
2. Very rigid so lead to greater stress concentration in root causing root or post fracture
3. Poor aesthetics
4. Require temporization
5. Prone to corrosion
6. Risk of casting inaccuracy
7. Difficult retrieval
8. Hypersensitivity in some cases because of Ni-Cr ions.

## ALL CERAMIC POST AND CORES

### Advantages

1. Excellent aesthetics
2. Biocompatibility
3. Good radiopacity.

### Disadvantages

1. Brittle, so not indicated in high stress conditions like bruxism
2. Very rigid, so more risk of root or post fracture.

## PREFABRICATED POSTS

### *Indications of Prefabricated Posts*

1. Sufficient width and length of root structure is present.
2. Roots are of circular cross-section, for example, roots of maxillary premolars.
3. Gross undercuts in root canals make pattern fabrication for cast posts difficult.

Various forms and shapes of existing prefabricated posts are:

- *Metals posts which are made of:*
  - Stainless steel
  - Titanium alloys or pure titanium
  - Co-Cr-Mo alloys
  - High platinum alloys
  - Zirconia
  - Carbon fiber
  - Glass fiber
  - Fiber reinforced resin based composites

### Prefabricated Metal Posts

These have been widely used for past 20 years. They are available in various metal alloys and can be available in active or passive forms.

### Advantages

1. Simple to use
2. Less time consuming
3. Easy retrieval (of passive posts)
4. Available in various shapes and sizes
5. Retentive within the root specially serrated and parallel sided posts
6. Radiopaque
7. Cost-effective.

### Disadvantages

1. Not conservative because root is designed to accept the post
2. Cannot be placed in tortuous canals
3. Poor aesthetics
4. Very rigid
5. Difficult retrieval of active posts
6. Prone to corrosion
7. Tapered posts can have wedging effect in the canal.

## Carbon Fiber Posts

Carbon fiber posts were introduced by Duret et al in 1996 based on the carbon fiber reinforcement principle. Carbon fiber post consists of bundle of stretched carbon fibers embedded into an epoxy matrix. This was the first nonmetallic post introduced to the dentistry. The original form of carbon post was black and unaesthetic.

### Advantages

1. Clinical procedure is less time consuming
2. Strong but low stiffness and strength than ceramic and metal posts
3. Easily retrievable
4. Less chair side time
5. Modulus of elasticity similar to dentin
6. Biocompatible
7. Good retention.

### Disadvantages

1. Black in color, so unaesthetic
2. Radiolucent, so difficult to detect radiographically
3. Flexture strength decreases by 50 percent by moisture contamination
4. On repeated loading, show reduced modulus of elasticity.

## Glass Fiber Post

It was introduced in 1992. It consists of unidirectional glass fibers embedded in a resin matrix which strengthens the dowel without compromising the modulus of elasticity.

### Advantages

1. Esthetically acceptable
2. Modulus of elasticity similar to dentin
3. Biocompatible
4. Distributes stresses over a broad surface area, thus increasing the load threshold
5. Easy to handle and place
6. Less time consuming
7. Favorable retention in conjunction with adhesive bonding technique
8. High resistance to fracture
9. Easy retrieval.

### Disadvantages

1. Poor radiographic visibility
2. Expensive
3. Technique sensitive.

## Zirconia Post

These were introduced in dentistry in late 1980 by Christel et al. They are made from fine grained tetragonal zirconium polycrystals (TZP).

They possess high flexural strength and fracture toughness.

### Advantages

1. For teeth with severe coronal destruction, zirconia posts provide adequate strength.
2. Smaller zirconia posts can be used for an all ceramic post and core construction for narrower canals.
3. Combination of glass ceramic and zirconia ceramic can be used because of their similarity in coefficient of thermal expansion.

### Disadvantages

1. Adhesion to tooth and composite is compromised which becomes a problem for retreatment.
2. They are brittle with high modulus of elasticity.
3. When used with direct composite resin build up, high stresses and functional forces may lead to microleakage and their deformation because of high polymerization shrinkage and high coefficient of thermal expansion of composites.
4. Expensive.

**Factors to be considered while planning posts**

- Retention and resistance form
- Preservation of tooth structure
- Ferrule effect
- Mode of failure
- Retrievability.

# FACTORS TO BE CONSIDERED WHILE PLANNING POST AND CORE

## Retention and the Resistance Form

Post retention refers to the ability of post to resist vertical dislodging forces. Post resistance refers to the ability of the post and the tooth to withstand the lateral and rotational forces (Fig. 26.21).

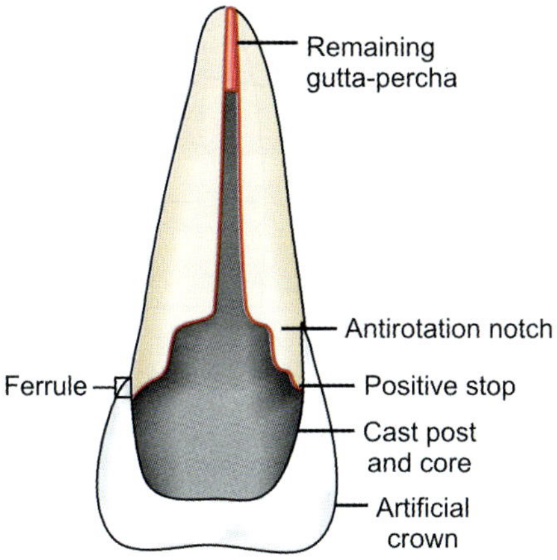


**Fig. 26.21:** Diagram showing post and core placement with ferrule effect, positive stop and antirotation notch

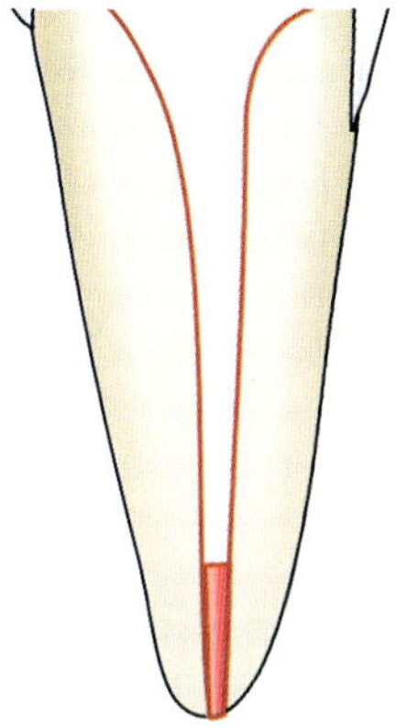

**Fig. 26.22:** 3-6 mm of apical gutta-percha must be preserved to maintain apical seal

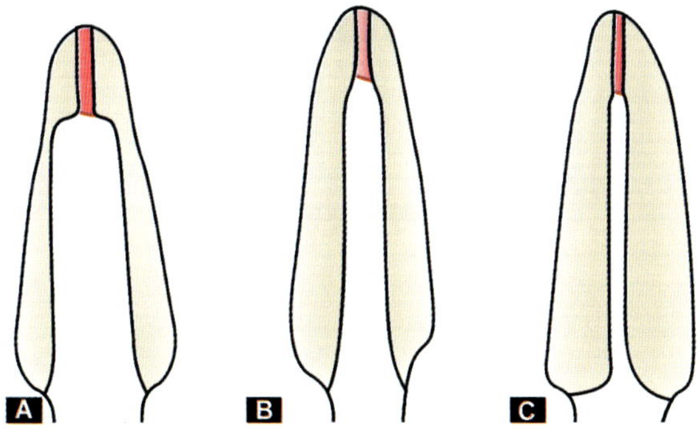


**Figs 26.23A to C:** (A) Too wide diameter of post space; (B) Optimum diameter of post space; (C) Too narrow diameter of post space

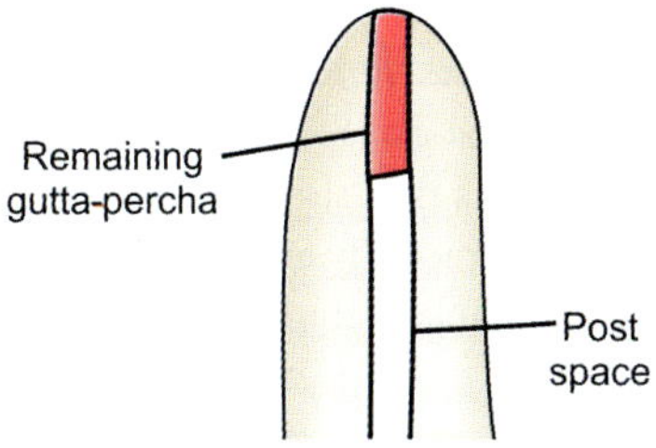


**Fig. 26.24:** Conservationist approach

**Factors affecting post retention**
- Post length
- Post diameter
- Post taper and design
- Luting agent
- Luting method
- Canal shape
- Post position in dental arch.

**Factors affecting post resistance**
- Post length
- Rigidity
- Presence of antirotational features
- Presence of ferrule.

### *Post Length*

There are many guidelines available as suggested by various authors regarding the post length. It is obvious that longer the post in the canal, more retentive it is. But increased length also increases risk of root fracture and perforation.

Generally, it is accepted that apical 3-6 mm of gutta-percha must be preserved to maintain the apical seal (Fig. 26.22).

## Accepted Guidelines for Determining Post Length

These include:
- Post should be equal to clinical crown length.
- Post should be equal to one-half to two-thirds of the length of the remaining root.
- Post should end halfway between the crestal bone and the root apex.
- Post should be as long as possible without disturbing the apical seal.

Since root anatomy varies from tooth to tooth, so post space should be evaluated and planned accordingly.

### *Post Diameter*

It has been seen that post diameter has little difference in the retention of post, but increase in post diameter increases the resistance form but it also increases the risk of root fracture (Figs 26.23 A to C).

Presently there are three different theories/philosophies regarding the post diameter in literature. these are:

*The conservationist:* It suggests the narrowest diameter that allows the fabrication of a post to the desired length. It allows minimal instrumentation of the canal for post space preparation (Fig. 26.24).

According to this, teeth with smaller dowels exhibit greater resistance to fracture.

*The preservationist:* It advocates that at least 1 mm of sound dentin should be maintained circumferentially to resist the fracture (Fig. 26.25).

*The proportionist:* This advocates that post width should not exceed one-third of the root width at its narrowest dimensions to resist fracture (Fig. 26.26). The guideline for determining appropriate diameter of post involves mesiodistal width of the roots.

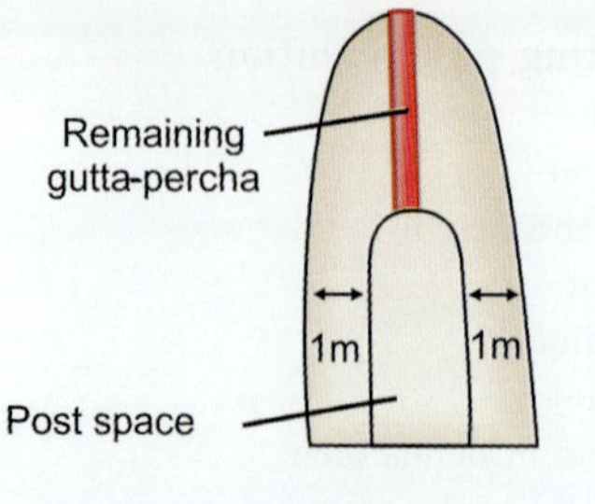


Fig. 26.25: Preservationist approach

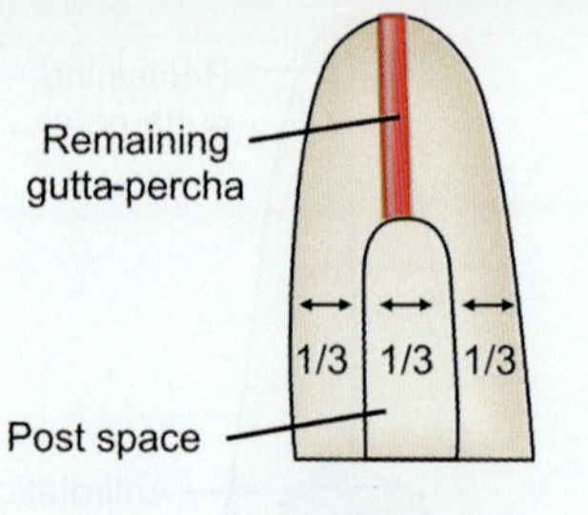


Fig. 26.26: Proportionist approach

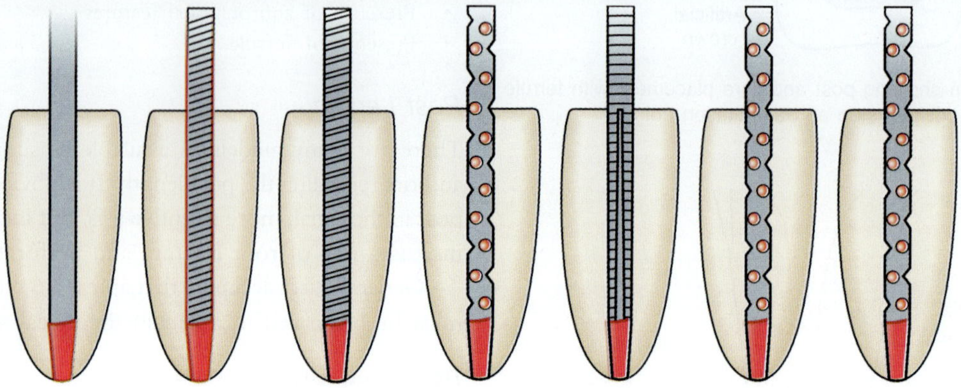

Fig. 26.27: Different types of post designs

### Post Design

Various types of post designs are available in the market (Fig. 26.27). The posts can be:

- Tapered, smooth sided—least retentive
- Tapered, serrated type
- Parallel smooth sided
- Parallel serrated type
- Tapered notched
- Parallel threaded type
- Parallell notched type

**Generally parallel sided are more retentive than tapered ones. Threaded posts are more retentive than cemented ones.*

### Luting Agents

Commonly used dental cements for luting the posts are zinc phosphate, polycarboxylate, glass ionomer cement, resin based composite and hybrid of resin and ionomer.

i. *Zinc phosphate cement* (Fig. 26.28): It has been used for decades to cement and has a long history of success. The primary disadvantages of this cement are solubility in oral fluids, especially in the presence of acids, and lack of true adhesion.

ii. *Polycarboxylate and glass ionomer cements* (Figs 26.29 and 26.30): These are also soluble in oral fluids, but they can chemically bond to dentin. Polycarboxylate cements undergo plastic deformation after cyclic loading which is a major disadvantage. A primary disadvantage of conventional glass ionomer cement is its setting reaction. This cement does not reach its maximal strength for many days. Therefore, any recontouring of the core on the day of cementation of the post can potentially disturb the set of the cement and weaken the immature cement.

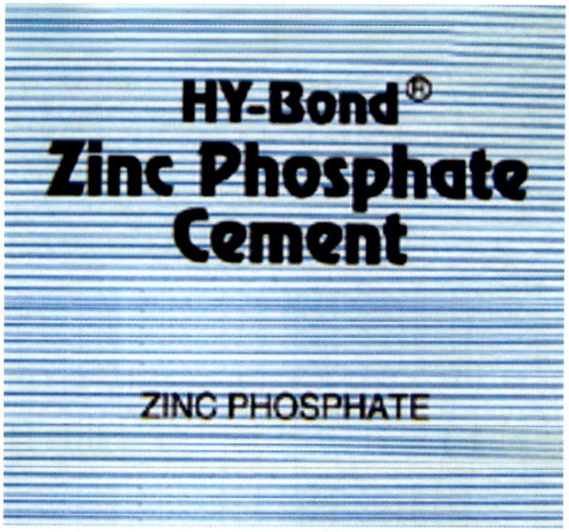


Fig. 26.28: Zinc phosphate cement

iii. *Resin modified glass ionomer cement:* They are stronger than conventional glass ionomer cements, they contain hydrophilic resins that slowly imbibe water, causing the cement film to gradually expand. This expansion would fracture crown relatively soon after cementation.

iv. *Resin cements (Fig. 26.31):* They are essentially insoluble in oral fluids and possess high compressive strengths. Resin cements have some disadvantages. Resin cements

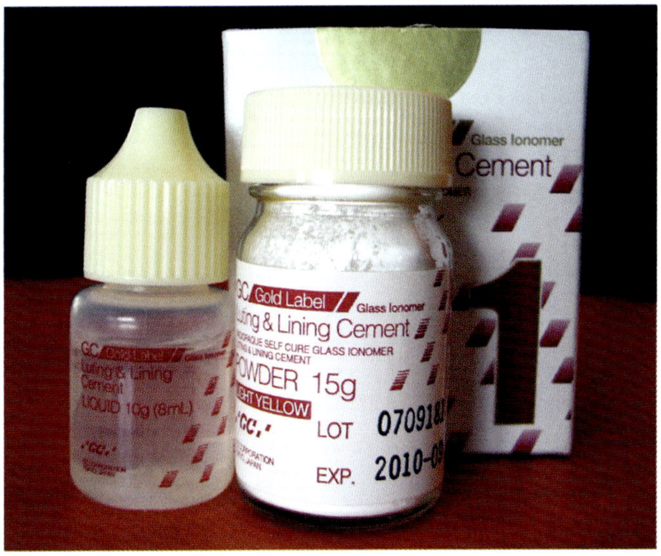


**Fig. 26.29:** Glass ionomer cement

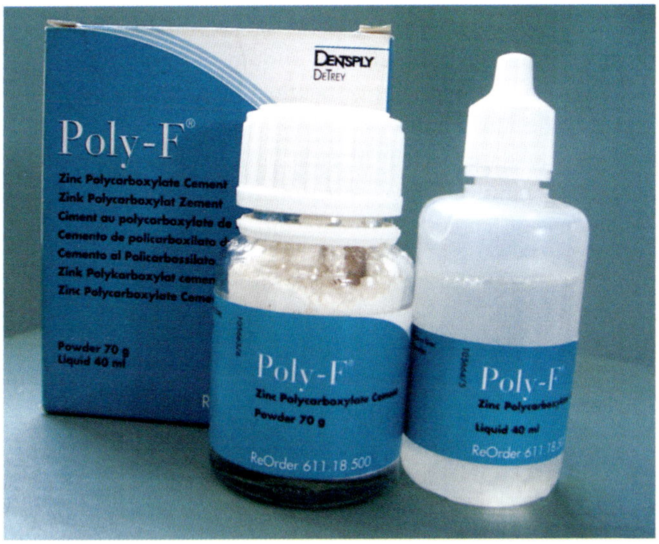


**Fig. 26.30:** Polycarboxylate cement

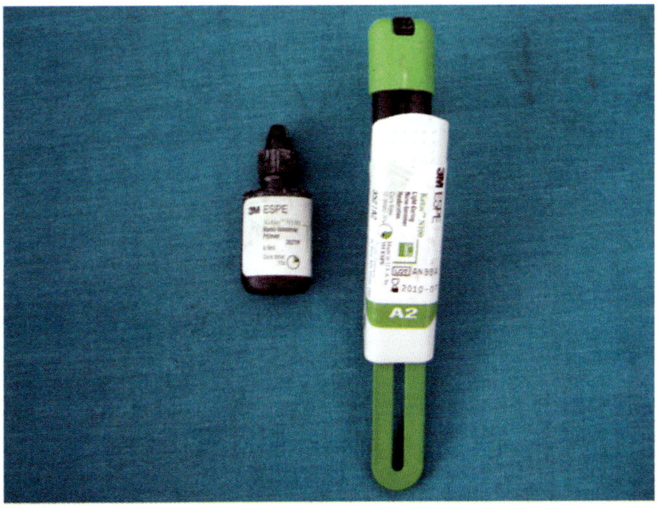


**Fig. 26.31:** Resin cement

are more "technique sensitive" than most of the other luting cements. They require extra steps such as preparing the canal walls with acid or EDTA and placing a dentin-bonding agent.

Contamination of the dentin or post can be a problem. Predictable delivery of etchants and adhesive materials deep into the canal space also be problematic. The post should be cemented with an auto-cure or dual-cure resin cement that is mixed and placed with the post. These steps must be performed quickly and carefully to assure that the post is completely seated. It is generally believed that eugenol-containing root canal sealers inhibit the polymerization of resin cements.

### *Luting Method*

Luting method also affects the retention of post. Since luting agents are susceptible to moisture present in the canal, so canal should be absolute dry.

*Optimal method of cementation of posts is:*
- Dry the canal
- Mix the cement according to instructions
- Uniformly place the cement in the canal
- Place the post into the canal with least possible force to reduce the stress
- Vents should be made to release the hydrostatic pressure when the posts thrust back.

### *Canal Shape*

Since the most common shape of canal is ovoid, and prefabricated posts commonly used are parallel in mature, the majority of prefabricated posts are unlikely to adapt well along their entire interface with canal walls. Knowing the root anatomy of different teeth is important before starting canal preparation for post installation. To determine the appropriate post length and width to avoid root perforation, one must consider conditions such as root taper, proximal root invagination, root curvatures and angle of the crown to the root during preparation of the post space. For this good quality of radiographs provide needed information (Fig. 26.31).

### *Position of Tooth in the Dental Arch*

Location of the tooth in dental arch also affects the post retention, for example, maxillary anterior region is at high risk for failure because of effect of compressive, tensile, shearing and torquing forces specially at the post-dentin interface. If all factors are equal, then post of posterior teeth tends to be more retentive than anterior ones.

## Preservation of the Tooth Structure

One should try to preserve maximum of the coronal and radicular tooth structure whenever possible. Minimal removal of additional radicular dentin for post space preparation should be the criteria. Further enlargement of posts only weakens the tooth. Minimal enlargement of post space means a post must be made of a strong material than can withstand functional and parafunctional forces. Various studies have shown use of bonded posts, but their strengthening effect degrades with time because as the tooth is exposed to functional stress, the resin bond to dentin weakens.

## Ferrule Effect (Fig. 26.32)

*Definition*: Ferrule is defined as band of metal which encircles the external surface of residual tooth. It is formed by walls and margins of the tooth. If artificial crown extends apical to margins of the core, and encircles sound tooth structure for 360°, the crown serves as reinforcing ring. In this way ferrule helps to protect the root from vertical fracture. It has been seen that a ferrule with 1-2 mm of vertical tooth structure doubles the resistance to fracture than in teeth without any ferrule effect. This is called as crown ferrule.

Sometimes when adequate tooth structure is not present crown lengthening or orthodontic eruption is needed of a tooth to provide an adequate ferrule.

For optimal benefits of ferrule, it should fulfill following requirements:

1. Parallel axial walls
2. At least 2-3 mm of axial wall height
3. Margins of preparation on sound tooth structure
4. Restoration completely encircling the tooth
5. Crown and crown preparation should not invade attachment apparatus.

### *Functions of Ferrule*

Lack of ferrule may result in fracture because of forcing core, post and root to high function stresses.

a. Resists lateral forces from post.
b. Resists leverage from crown in function.
c. Increases resistance and retention of the restoration.

### *Secondary Ferrule/core Ferrule*

Sometimes a contra bevel is given on a tooth being prepared for cast post with collar of metal which encircles the tooth. This serves as secondary ferrule independent of ferrule provide by cast crown.

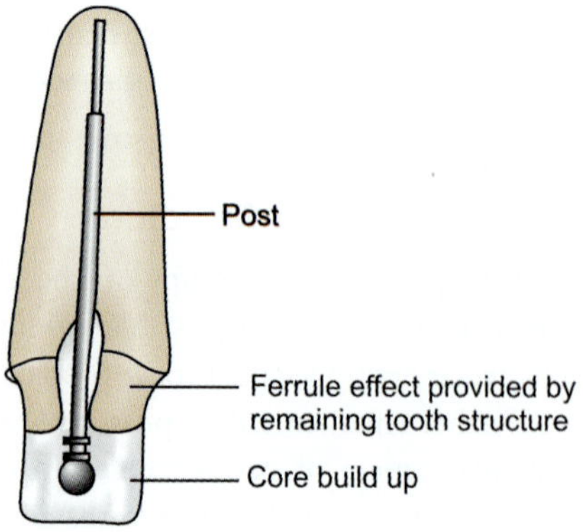


**Fig. 26.32:** Ferrule effect

## Mode of Failure

All post systems show some percentage of failure but with variable range. Post failures are higher in cases of nonrestorable teeth.

## Factors Affecting Clinical Longevity of Post and Core

- Magnitude and direction of force
- Tooth type
- Thickness of remaining dentin
- Post selection
- Quality of cement layer.

*Failures of posts and core can occur in form of*:

- Post fracture
- Root fracture
- Core fracture
- Post dislodgement
- Aesthetic failures.

## Retrievability

Ideally a post system selected should be such that if an endodontic treatment fails, or failure of post and core occurs, it should be retrievable.

Metal posts especially the cast post and core system is difficult to remove. Fiber posts are easy to retrieve whereas zirconium and ceramic posts are difficult to remove.

*Posts can be removed by:*

1. Use of rotary instruments and solvents
2. Use of ultrasonic (Fig. 26.33)
3. Using special kits like Messeran kit, post removal system and endodontic extractors.

## PREPARATION OF THE CANAL SPACE AND THE TOOTH

1. Plan for the length and diameter of the post according to the tooth type (Figs 26.34A to C) and using a proper radiograph.
2. Remove the gutta-percha filling. Whenever possible gutta-percha is removed immediate after obturation, so as not to disturb the apical seal (Fig. 26.35).

   Gutta-percha can be removed using the hot endodontic instrument, rotary instrument, chemical methods or by use of solvents.

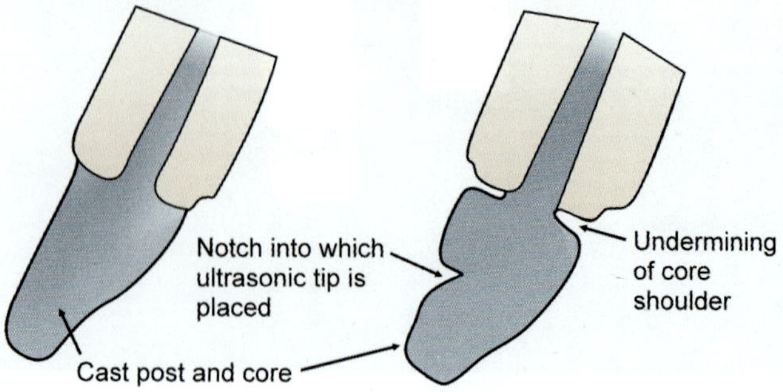


**Fig. 26.33:** Use of ultrasonics to retrieve post

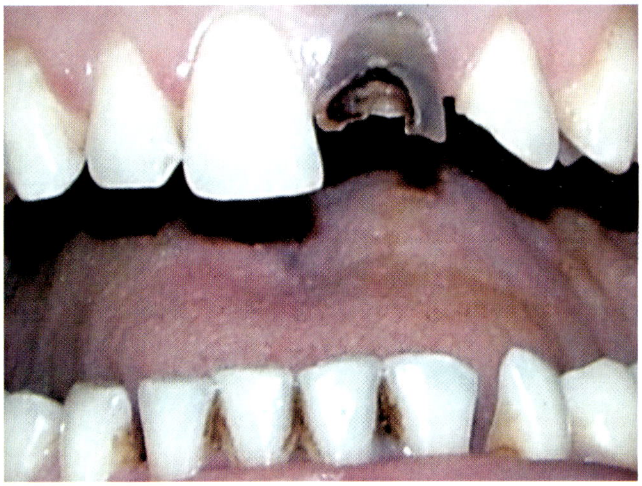

Fig. 26.34A: Grossly carious

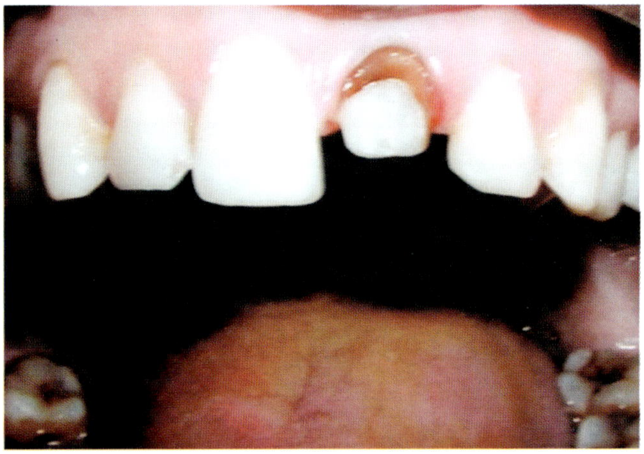

Fig. 26.34B: After endodontic treatment core fabrication in 21

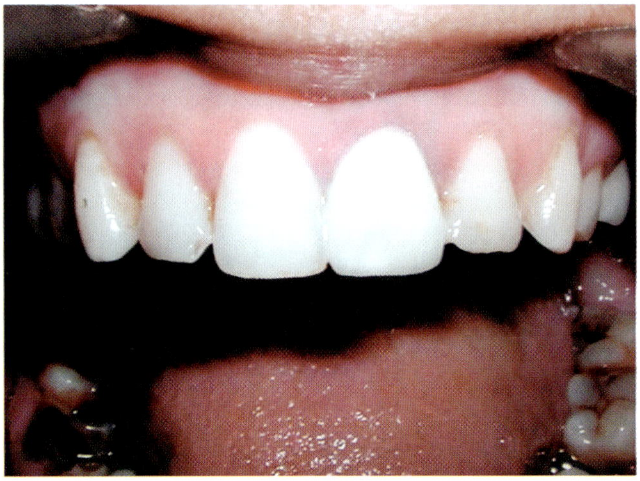

Fig. 26.34C: Tooth restored with final restoration after post and core in 21

3. Prepare the canal space using Gates-Glidden drills or Peeso reamers (Fig. 26.36). The canal space enlargement depends on type of the post. If it is custom made, the main requirement is minimal space preparation without undercuts. For prefabricated post, generally specific penetration drills for each system are supplied for canal preparation.

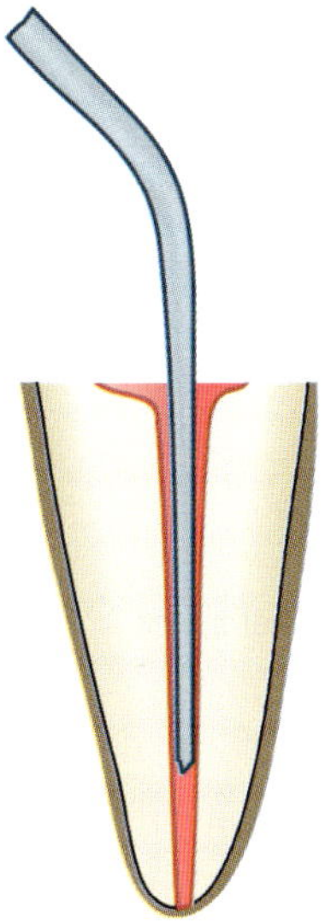

Fig. 26.35: Removal of gutta-percha from root canal

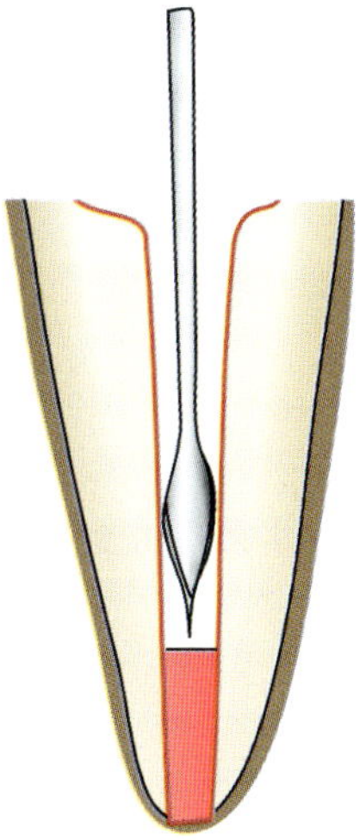

Fig. 26.36: Preparation of root canal space using Gates-Glidden drills

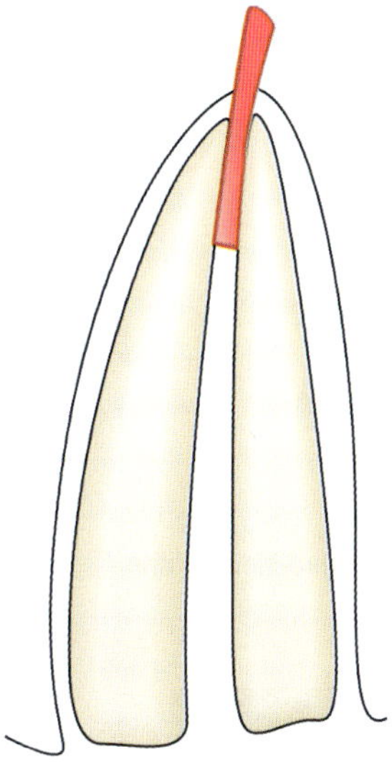

Fig. 26.37: Periapical extrusion of gutta-percha

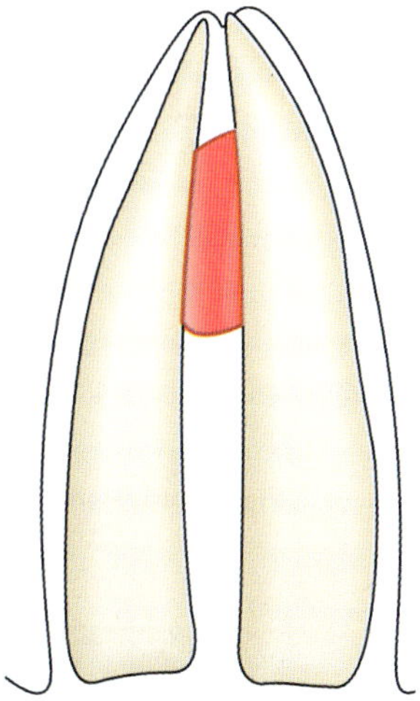

Fig. 26.38: Disturbance of apical seal

Various errors can occur during root canal preparation for post space like periapical extrusion of obturation material (Fig. 26.37), disturbance of apical seal (Fig. 26.38), over enlargement of the canal space (Fig. 26.39) and perforation (Figs 26.40 and 26.41).

4. Following the preparation of canal space, preparation of coronal tooth structure should be prepared in the same manner as if an intact crown irrespective of the remaining tooth structure (Fig. 26.42).
5. Remove all the unsupported tooth structure (Fig. 26.43).
6. Place an antirotational notch with the help of cylindrical diamond or carbide bur. This is done to provide the antirotational stability (Fig. 26.44).
7. Ferrule effect is provided thereafter. The remaining coronal tooth structure is sloped to buccal and lingual surfaces so

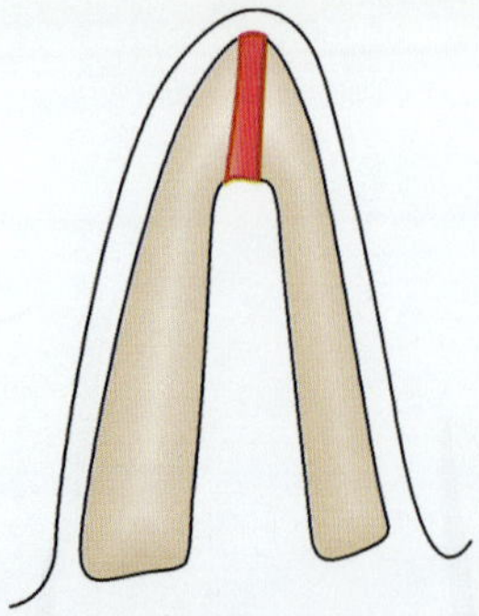

Fig. 26.39: Over enlargement of canal space

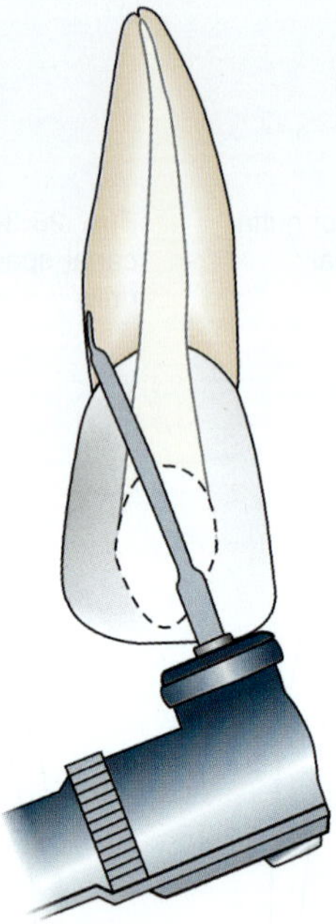

Fig. 26.40: Perforation due to misdirection of drill

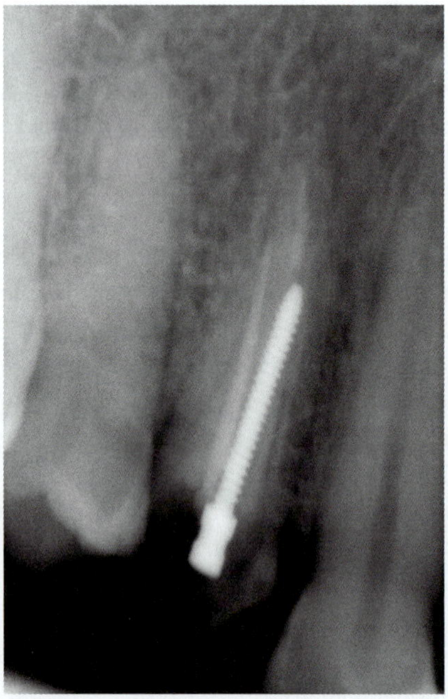

Fig. 26.41: Perforation of root space due to misdirection of drills while preparing post space

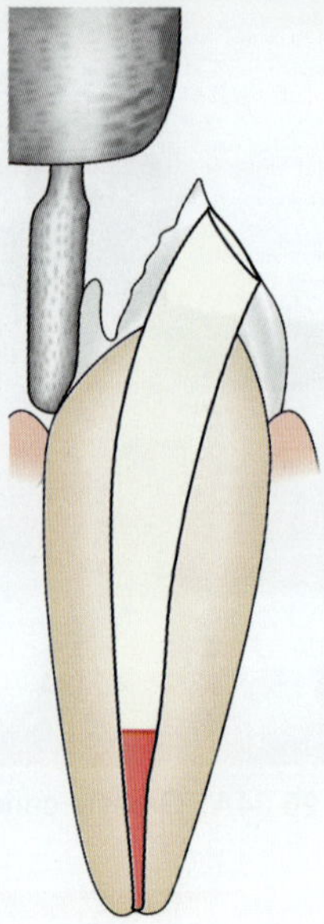

Fig. 26.42: Preparation of tooth structure

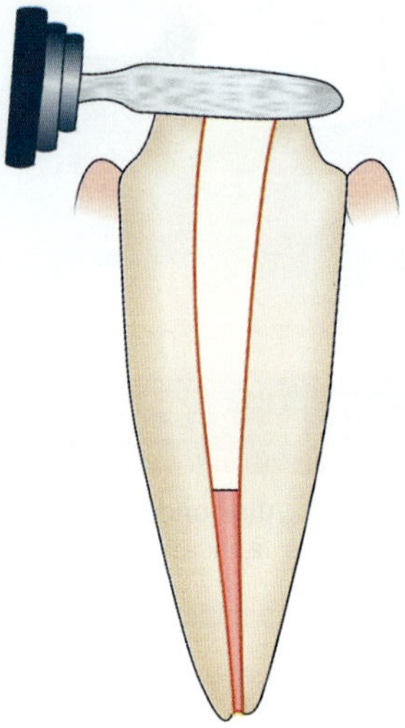

Fig. 26.43: Removal of unsupported tooth structure

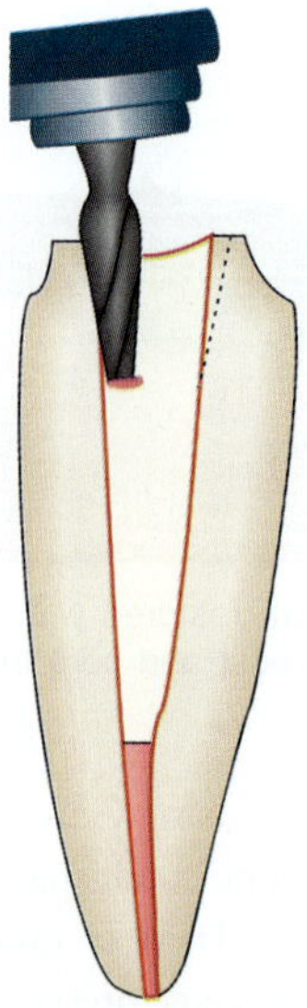

Fig. 26.44: Place antirotational notch with the help of cylindrical diamond bur

as to provide a collar around the occlusal circumference of the preparation (Fig. 26.45). This gives rise to 360° ferrule effect. Ferrule ensures that the final restoration encircles the tooth apical to the core and rests on sound tooth structure. It also presents the vertical root fracture by posts.

8. Finally eliminate all the sharp angles, undercuts and establish a smooth finish line (Figs 26.46 and 26.47).

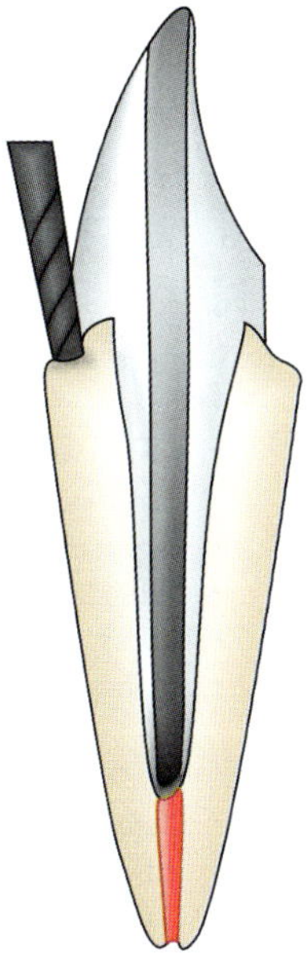

Fig. 26.45: Preparation of ferrule effect

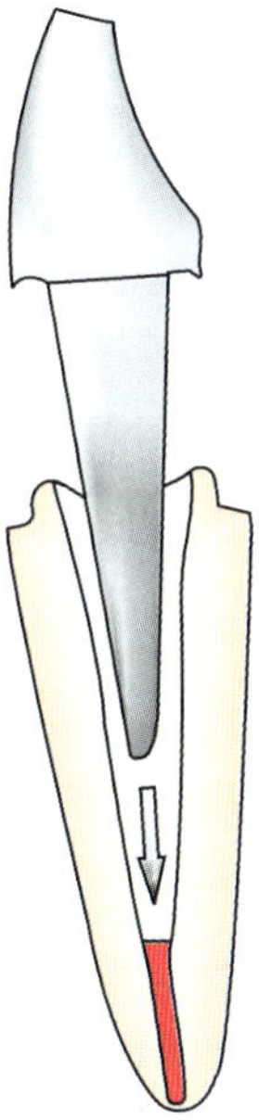

Fig. 26.46: Establish smooth finish line and remove all undercuts

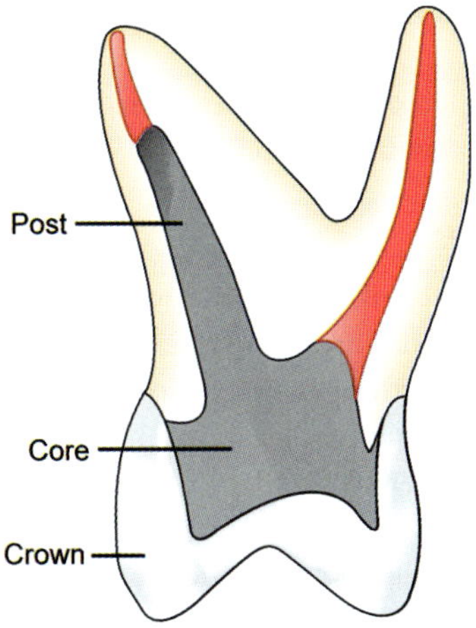


Fig. 26.47: Molar restored with post and core

## CORE

Core is the supragingival portion that replaces the missing coronal tooth structure and forms the center of new restoration. Basically it acts as a miniature crown.

**Various core build up materials**
1. Dental amalgam
2. Resin modified glass ionomers
3. Composite resin
4. Cast core

### Ideal Requirements for a Core Material

- Compressive strength to resist intraoral forces
- Biocompatibility
- Ease of manipulation
- Flexure strength to present core dislodgement
- Ability to bond to tooth structure and post
- Coefficient of thermal expansion similar to dentin
- Minimal water absorption
- Dimensionally stable
- No reaction with chemicals
- Low cost
- Easily available
- Contrasting color to tooth structure except when used for anterior teeth.

Core material include composite resins, cast metal, ceramic, amalgam, glass ionomer resin materials.

### Amalgam Core

- Amalgam has been used as a buildup material, with well recognized strengths and limitations. It has good physical and mechanical properties and works well in high stress area.
- In many cases, it requires the addition of pins or other methods to provide retention and resistance to rotation. Placement can be clumsy when there is minimal coronal tooth structure, and the crown preparation must be delayed to permit the material time to set. Amalgam can cause esthetic problems with ceramic crowns and sometimes makes the gingival look dark. There is a risk of tattooing the cervical gingival with amalgam particles during the crown preparation.
- For these reasons, and potential concern about mercury, it is no longer widely used as a buildup material. Amalgam has no natural adhesive properties and should be used with an adhesive system for buildup.

### Glass Ionomer Cements

The glass ionomer materials, including resin-modified glass ionomer, lack adequate strength and fracture toughness as a

| Available post and core systems | | | | | |
|---|---|---|---|---|---|
| *S.No.* | | *Advantages* | *Disadvantages* | *Indication* | *Precautions* |
| 1. | Amalgam | • Conservation of tooth structure<br>• Easy | • Poor tensile strength<br>• Corrosion | • Posterior teeth with adequate coronal structure | • Not used in anteriors |
| 2. | Glass ionomer | • Conservation of tooth structure<br>• Easy | • Low strength | • Teeth with adequate coronal structure | • Not used in teeth under lateral load |
| 3. | Composite resin | • Conservation of tooth structure | • Low strength<br>• Polymerization shrinkage | • Teeth with adequate coronal structure | • Not used in teeth under lateral load |
| 4. | Custom cast post | • High strength<br>• Better fit | • Time consuming<br>• Complex procedure | • For flared and elliptical canals | |
| 5. | Parallel-sided prefabricated post | • Good retention<br>• High strength | • Less conservation of tooth structure<br>• Corrosion of stainless steel | • Circular canals | |
| 6. | Tapered prefabricated post | • High strength and stiffness<br>• Conservation of tooth structure | • Less retentive | Circular canals | Not used in flared canals |
| 7. | Threaded post | • High retention | • Stress generation is more<br>• Not conservation of tooth structure | Only when more retention is required | |

buildup material and should not be used in teeth with extensive loss of tooth structure. It is also soluble and sensitive to moisture. When there is minimal loss of tooth structure and a post is not needed, GIC works well for block out such as after removal of an MOD restoration.

## Composite Resins

- Composite resin is the most popular core material and has some characteristics of an ideal build up material.

### *Advantages*

Bonded to many of the current posts and to the remaining tooth structure to increase retention.

- High tensile strength and the tooth can be prepared for a crown immediately after polymerization.
- It has fracture resistance comparable to amalgam and cast post and cores, with more favorable fracture pattern when they fail.
- It is tooth colored and can be used under translucent restorations without affecting the esthetic result.

### *Disadvantages*

- Composite shrinks during polymerization, causing gap formation in the areas in which adhesion is weakest. It absorbs water after polymerization, causing it to swell, and undergoes plastic deformation under repeated loads.
- Adhesion to dentin on the pulpal floor is generally not as strong or reliable as to coronal dentin. Strict isolation is an absolute requirement. If the dentin surface is contaminated with blood or saliva during bonding procedures, the adhesion is greatly reduced. Although composite resin is far from ideal, it is currently the most widely used buildup material.

## Cast Core

The core is an integral extension of the post and it does not depend upon the mechanical means of retention on the post. It prevents dislodgement of the core and the crown from the post. But sometimes valuable tooth structure must be removed to create path of withdrawal. Procedure is time consuming and expensive.

## Biomechanical Criteria for Evaluation of Core Materials

### *Bonding (Maximum to Least)*

Resin composites > Glass ionomers > Amalgam

### *Strength*

Amalgam > Resin composite > Glass ionomers

### *Ease of Use*

Resin composites > Amalgam > Glass ionomers

### *Setting Time*

Resin composite > Glass ionomers > Amalgam

### *Dimensional Stability*

Amalgam > Glass ionomers > Composite resins

Following the endodontic treatment, it is necessary to restore the original morphology and function of the tooth which can be achieved by restoration of the endodontically treated teeth.

The restoration should begin at the earliest possible moment because tooth exposed to oral conditions without optimal restoration cannot resist the occlusal forces and oral bacteria for a long period which can result in the treatment failure. Post-endodontic restoration is an important treatment itself because successful treatment cannot be achieved without adequate restoration after endodontic treatment. Proper restoration of endodontically treated tooth begins with understanding of their physical and biomechanical properties and anatomy. Though various new materials have become available for past many years, yet the basic concepts of restoring endodontically treated teeth remains the same.

Most post systems can be used successfully if basic principles are followed. After selection of the post system, finally it is the choice of core material and final restoration which increases the longevity of the treated tooth. The main function of post is retention of the core if insufficient tooth structure is present to support the coronal final restoration. They do not strengthen the tooth, so posts should not be used habitually.

Various types of post systems are available with different strengths and weaknesses. Selection of post should be made by keeping in mind its strength, modulus of elasticity, biocompatibility, retrievability, aesthetics and cost. Though many new materials are available with their indications for use, but long-term evaluations are needed. So care must be taken while selecting these materials.

## QUESTIONS

**Q. Enumerate various changes in a tooth caused by endodontic treatment.**

**Q. Define post and core. What are indications and contraindications of post and core restoration.**

**Q. Classify post. What are advantages and disadvantages of various posts?**

**Q. Enumerate different core materials with their advantages and disadvantages**

**Q. Write short notes on:**

a. Retention and resistance form of a post
b. Preparation of post space
c. Ferrule effect

## BIBLIOGRAPHY


1. Abou-Rass M, Jann JM, Jobe D, Tsutsio F. Preparation of space of posting: Effect on thickness and canal walls and incidence of perforation in molar. J Am Dent Assoc 1982;104:834-37.
2. Asmussen E, Peutzfeldt A, Heitmann T. Stiffness, elastic limit, and strength of newer types of endodontic posts. J Dent 1999;27(4):275-78.
3. Barrieshi- Nusair KM, Hammad HM. Intracoronal sealing comparison of mineral trioxide aggregate and glass ionomer. Quintessence Int 2005;367-8:539-45.
4. Block PL. Restorative margins and periodontal health: A new look at an old perspective. J Prosthet Dent 1987;57:683-89.
5. Bower RC. Furcation development of human mandibular first molar teeth a histologic graphic reconstructional study, J periodontal Res 1983;18:412-19.
6. Calt S, Serper A. Time-dependent effects, of Edta on dentin structures. J Endod 2002;28:17-19.
7. Caputo AA, Standlee JP. Pins and posts-why, when and how. Dent Clin North am 1976;20:299-311.
8. Cohen and burns. Pathways to the pulp. 8th edn; Mosby, St. Louis, 2002.
9. Colley TT, Hampson EL, Lehman MN. Retention of post Crown. Br. Dent J 1968;124:63-69.
10. Cooney IP, Caputo AA, Trabert KC. Retention and stress distribution of Lapered end endodontic posts, J Prosthet Dent 1986;55:540-46.
11. Cruz EV, Shigetani Y, Ishikawa K, Kota K, Iwaku M, Goodis HE. A laboratory study of coronal microleakage using four temporary restorative material. Int endod J 2002;28(2):59-61.
12. DeCleen MJ. The relationship between the root canal filling and post space preparation. Int Endod J 1993;26:53-58.
13. Dickey DJ, Harris GZ, Lemon RR, Luebke RG. Effect of post space preparation on apical seal using solvent techniques and peeso reamers. J endod 1982;8:351-54.
14. Donald E. Vire. Failure of endodontically treated teeth: Classification and evaluation. J Endod 1991;17:338-42.
15. Fernandes A, Rodrigues S, Sar Dessai G, Mehta A, Retention of endodontic post: A review. Endodontology 2001;13:11-18.
16. Freedman GA. Esthetic post and core treatment. Dent Clin N Am, 2001;45:103-16.
17. Gelfand M, Goldman M, Sunderman EJ. Effect of complete veneer crowns on the compressive strength of endodontically treated posterior teeth. J Prosthet Dent 1984;52:635-38.
18. Gutmann JL. The dentin-root complex, anatomic and biologic considerations in restoring endodontically treated teeth. J Prosthet Dent 1992;67:458-67.
19. Ingle and Bakland. Endodontics. 4th edn; Williams and Wilkins, Malvern 1994.
20. Koutayas SO, Kern M. All ceramic posts and cores: The state of the art. Quintessence Int 1999;30:383-92.
21. Pappen AF, Bravo M, Gonzalez-Lopez S, Gonzalez-Rodriguez MP. An in vitro study of coronal leakage after intraradicular preparation of cast-dowel space. J prosthet Dent 2005; 94(3):214-18.
22. Rosenstiel, Land, Fujimoto. Contemporary fixed prosthodontics. 2nd ed. Mosby, St. Louis 1995.
23. Sauaia TS, Gomes BP, Pinheiro ET, Zaia AA, Ferraz CC, Souza-Filho FJ. Microleakage evaluation of intraorifice sealing materials in endodontically treated teeth. Oral Surg Oral Med Oral Pathol Oral Radiol Endod 2006;102(2):242-46. Epub 2006 Apr 21.
24. Verissimo DM, Vale MS. Methodologies for assessment of apical and coronal leakage of endodontic filling materials a critical review. J Oral Sci 2006;48(3):93-98.
25. Weine, Endodontic therapy. 6th edn; Mosby, St. Louis 2004.
26. Wells JD, Pashley DH, Loushine RJ, Weller RN, Kimbrough WF, Pereira ON. Intracoronal sealing ability of two dental cements. J Endod 2002;28(6):443-47.

CHAPTER 27

# Management of Traumatic Injuries

- ❑ Introduction
- ❑ Classification of Dentofacial Injuries
- ❑ Examination of Traumatic Injuries
- ❑ Chief Complaint
- ❑ History of Present Illness
- ❑ Medical History
- ❑ Clinical Examination
- ❑ Clinical Photographs
- ❑ Management of the Traumatic Injuries
- ❑ Crown Fracture
- ❑ Crown Root Fracture
- ❑ Root Fracture
- ❑ Prognosis
- ❑ Luxation Injuries
- ❑ Concussion
- ❑ Subluxation
- ❑ Lateral Luxation
- ❑ Extrusive Luxation
- ❑ Intrusive Luxation
- ❑ Avulsion (Exarticulation)
- ❑ Post Emergency Treatment
- ❑ Assessment of Traumatic Injuries
- ❑ Prevention of Traumatic Injuries
- ❑ Bibliography

## INTRODUCTION

It has been seen that dental traumatic injuries are increasing in their frequency of occurrence, though most of them usually consist of cracked and chipped teeth. A dentist must be prepared to treat not only the minor injuries but also more traumatically destructed crowns, roots, bones, etc.

Though traumatic injuries can occur at any age but most commonly they are seen at the age of 2-5 years during which children are learning to walk. They tend to fall because their judgment and coordination are not fully developed. Another age at which dental injuries are common is 8-12 years when there is increased sports activity, and while learning bicycle, etc. Automobiles accidents, sports mishaps, bad fall may make any body patient of dental trauma.

### Etiology of Traumatic Injuries

- Automobile injury
- Battered child
- Child abuse
- Drug abuse
- Epilepsy
- Fall from height
- Sports related injuries

40-60 percent of dental accidents occur at home. Prior to 1960's, boys to girls ratio in traumatic injuries used to be 3:1 but because of more involvement of females in sports, it has reduced to 2:1.

Type and number of teeth injured in accident vary according to type of accident, impact of force, resiliency of object hitting the tooth, shape of the hitting object and direction of the force. If bone is resilient, tooth will be displaced by trauma but if bone is thick and brittle, tooth will fracture. Maxillary central incisor is most commonly affected tooth followed by maxillary lateral incisor and mandibular incisors (Fig. 27.1).

### Extent of Trauma can be Assessed by Four Factors (Hallet;1954)

- *Energy of impact:* As we know
  Energy = Mass × Velocity
  Thus, the hitting object with more mass or high velocity creates more impact.
- *Direction of impacting force:* Type of fracture depends on the direction of impacting force.
- *Shape of impacting object:* Sharpness or bluntness of object also affect the impact.
- *Resilience of impacting object:* Hardness or softness of the object also affects the extent of the injury.

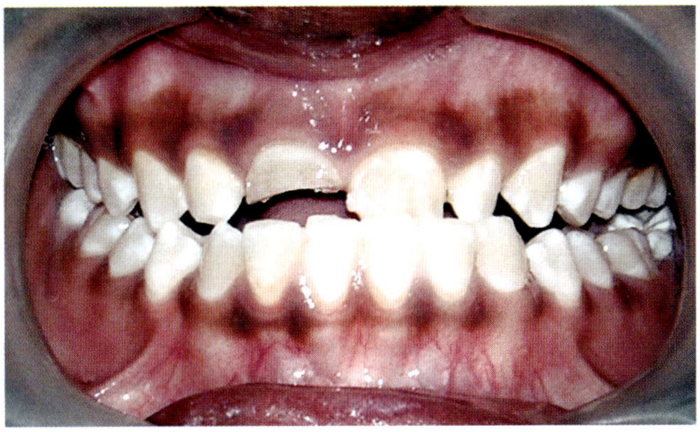

**Fig. 27.1:** Photograph showing traumatized 11

The outcome of dental injury is influenced by patient age, severity, and treatment offered. In most of the cases, immature permanent teeth with injuries have better prognosis than mature teeth with same injuries.

Proper treatment of dental injuries can have a significant effect on outcome and prognosis especially in case of severe injury. For example timely replantation of an avulsed tooth followed by endodontic therapy can improve the prognosis of the tooth.

Follow-up evaluation is also important for example if root resorption is detected early, it can be arrested.

## CLASSIFICATION OF DENTOFACIAL INJURIES

The purpose of classifying dental injuries is to provide description of specific condition allowing the clinician to identify and treat that condition using specific treatment remedies.

**The currently recommended classification is one based on the WHO and modified by Andreasen and Andreasen. This classification is used by International Association of Dental Traumatology.**

*Soft tissues*

| | |
|---|---|
| N873.69 | Lacerations |
| N902.0 | Contusion |
| N910.0 | Abrasions |

*Tooth fractures*

N873.60 Enamel fracture
N873.61 Crown-fractures-uncomplicated (no pulp exposure)
N873.62 Crown-fractures-complicated (with pulp exposure)
N873.64 Crown-root fractures
N873.63 Root fractures

*Luxation injuries*

873.66 - Tooth concussion
873.66 - Subluxation
873.66 - Extrusive luxation
873.66 - Lateral luxation
873.67 - Intrusive luxation
873.68 - Avulsion

*Facial skeletal injuries*

802.20 fracture of alveolar process of mandible
802.40 fracture of alveolar process of maxilla
802.21 fracture of body of mandible
802.41 fracture of body of maxilla

**WHO Classification (1995)**

| | |
|---|---|
| S.O2.5 | Fracture of tooth |
| S.O.2.50 | Fracture of enamel only |
| S.O.2.51 | Fracture of enamel and dentin |
| S.O.2.52 | Fracture of crown with pulp involvement |
| S.O.2.53 | Root fracture |
| S.O.2.54 | Fracture of root and crown with or without pulpal involvement |
| S.O.2.57 | Multiple fracture of tooth |

**Ingle's Classification**

*Soft tissue injury*

Laceration
Abrasion
Contusion

*Laceration injury*

Concussion
Subluxation intrusive luxation
Lateral luxation
Extrusive luxation
Avulsion

*Tooth fractures*

Enamel fractures
Uncomplicated crown fracture
Complicated crown fracture
Crown-root fracture
Root fracture

*Facial skeletal injury*

Alveolar process body of mandible TMJ

**Classification (Rabinowitch ;1956)**

Class I : Enamel fracture
Class II : Enamel and dentin fracture
Class III : Enamel and dentin fracture along with pulpal exposure
Class IV : Root fracture
Class V : Contusion
Class VI : Exarticulation

**Classification Based on Endodontic Treatment (Ulton; 1985)**

Class I : Fracture of enamel
Class II : Fracture of crown with indirect pulp exposure
Class III : Fracture of crown with direct pulp exposure

**Ellis and Davey's Classification (1960)**

- Class I - Simple fracture of the crown involving enamel.
- Class II - Extensive fracture of the crown, with considerable amount of dentin involved but no pulp exposure.
- Class III - Extensive fracture of the crown, with considerable amount of dentin involved, with pulp exposure.
- Class IV - Traumatized tooth becomes nonvital (with or without loss of crown structure.

- Class V - Tooth lost due to trauma.
- Class VI - Fracture of root with or without crown or root structure.
- Class VII - Displacement of the tooth without crown or root fracture.
- Class VIII - Fracture of crown enmass.
- Class IX - Fracture of deciduous teeth.

**Classification by Garcia and Godoy**

I. Enamel crack
II. Enamel fracture
III. Enamel, dentin fracture without pulp exposure
IV. Enamel, dentin fracture with pulp exposure
V. Enamel, dentin cementum fracture without pulp exposure
VI. Enamel, dentin cementum fracture with pulp exposure
VII. Root fracture
VIII. Concussion
IX. Luxation
X. Lateral displacement
XI. Intrusion
XII. Extrusion
XIII. Avulsion

Heitherasy and MARDE recommended a classification of subgingival fracture based on level of tooth fracture in relation to various horizontal planes of periodontium, as follows:

Class I : Fracture line does not extend below level of attached gingivae.
Class II : Fracture line extends below attached gingivae but not below level of alveolar crest.
Class III : Fracture line extends below level of alveolar crest.
Class IV : Fracture line is within coronal third of root but below level of alveolar crest.

**WHO Classification**

WHO gave following classification in 1978 with code no. corresponding to International Classification of Diseases.

- 873.60 - Enamel fracture
- 873.61 - Crown fracture involving enamel, dentin without pulpal involvement
- 873.62 - Crown fracture with pulpal involvement
- 873.63 - Root fracture
- 873.64 - Crown-root fracture
- 873.66 - Luxation
- 873.67 - Intrusion or extrusion
- 873.68 - Avulsion
- 873.69 - Other injuries such as soft tissue lacerations

* ***This classification was modified by Andreasen as following:***

- 873.64 - Uncomplicated crown root fracture without pulp exposure
- 873.64 - Complicated crown root fracture without pulp exposure
- 873.66 - Concussion - injury to tooth supporting structure without loosening or displacement of tooth
- 873.66 - Subluxation - an injury to tooth supporting with abnormal loosening but without displacement of tooth
- 873.66 - Lateral luxation, displacement of tooth in a direction other than maxillary and accompanied by fracture of alveolar socket.

**Classification by Hargreaves and Craig**

Class I : No fracture or fracture of enamel only with or without displacement of tooth
Class II : Fracture of crown involving both enamel and dentin without exposure of pulp, with or without displacement of tooth
Class III : Fracture of crown exposing the pulp with or without displacement of tooth
Class IV : Fracture of root with or without coronal fracture, with or without displacement of tooth
Class V : Total displacement of tooth

Since traumatic injuries are unexpected and inconvenient to reach at accurate diagnosis, a thorough examination is needed. But most of the times examination is not possible so it is essential that one should be prepared to assess such patients rapidly and comprehensively. Patient who has suffered trauma, not only has physical injury but also has emotional distress, so use of comprehensive examination and history should be done at that time.

## EXAMINATION OF TRAUMATIC INJURIES

The examination of trauma patients is similar to the usual examination of all endodontic patients. Medical history is fundamental to all evaluation and treatment of patient.

History includes chief complaint, history of present illness and medical history.

## CHIEF COMPLAINT

Patient should be asked for pain and other symptoms. These should be listed in order of importance to the patient.

## HISTORY OF PRESENT ILLNESS

When, how, where of the trauma are significant. A trauma to lips and anterior teeth can cause crown, root or bone fracture of anterior teeth without injury to posterior region. Another important question to ask is whether treatment of any kind has been given elsewhere for injury before coming to dental office.

## MEDICAL HISTORY

*Patient should be asked for:*

- Allergic reaction to medication
- Disorders like bleeding problems, diabetes, epilepsy, etc.
- Any current medication patient is taking
- ***Condition of Tetanus immunization***—In case of contaminated wound, booster dose should be given if more than 5 years have elapsed since last dose. But for clean wounds, no booster dose needed, if time elapsed between last dose is less than 10 years.

## CLINICAL EXAMINATION

Extraoral examination should rule out any facial bone fracture and should include meticulous evaluation of the soft tissues. Soft tissues such as lips, tongue, cheek, floor of mouth ought to be examined. Lacerations of lips and intraoral soft tissues must be carefully evaluated for presence of any tooth fragments and/or other foreign bodies.

Occlusion and temporomandibular joints should also be examined carefully (Fig. 27.2). Abnormalities in occlusion can indicate fracture of jaws or alveolar process (Fig. 27.3).

Teeth must be checked after proper cleaning of the area. Enamel cracks can be visualized by changing the direction of light beam from side to side. Explore the extent of tooth fracture involvement, i.e. enamel, dentin, cementum and/or pulp. Evaluate the crowns of the teeth for presence of extent of fracture, pulp involvement or change in color. Root fracture can be felt by placing finger on mucosa over the tooth and moving the crown (Fig. 27.4).

Patient's periodontal status can influence the dentist's decision to treat that injury. Teeth and their supporting structures should be examined carefully not only the obviously injured tooth but the adjacent as well as opposite teeth as well.

Reaction to percussion is indicative of the damage to the periodontal ligament. Tooth can show response to percussion in the normal way or it may be tender on percussion when evaluation of periodontal ligament is being done (Fig. 27.5).

Check mobility in all the directions. If adjacent teeth move along with the tooth being tested, suspect the alveolar fracture. In crown fracture, the crown is mobile but tooth will remain in the position.

Condition of pulp should be noted at the time of injury and at various times following traumatic incidence. One should not assume that teeth which give a positive response at initial examination will continue to give positive response and vice versa. Various studies have shown that pulp may take as long as nine months for normal blood flow to return to the coronal pulp of the traumatic tooth.

Vitality tests should be performed at the time of initial examination and recorded to establish a baseline for comparison with subsequent repeated tests in future. Pulp testing procedures require cooperation and a relaxed patient in order to avoid false results. The principle of pulp tests involves transmitting the stimuli to the sensory receptors of the pulp and recording the reaction.

For thermal testing, prefer dry ice over the water ice stick because extremely low temperature of dry ice penetrates deep well in the teeth.

Radiographic examination should be done in the area of suspected injury. An occlusal exposure of anterior region may show lateral luxations, root fractures or alveolar region. Periapical radiographs can assess the crown as well as cervical root fracture (Fig. 27.6). Thus to get maximum information at least one occlusal exposure and three periapical radiographs are needed.

Radiographs help in revealing fractures of teeth, tooth displacements, presence of any foreign objects, root canal

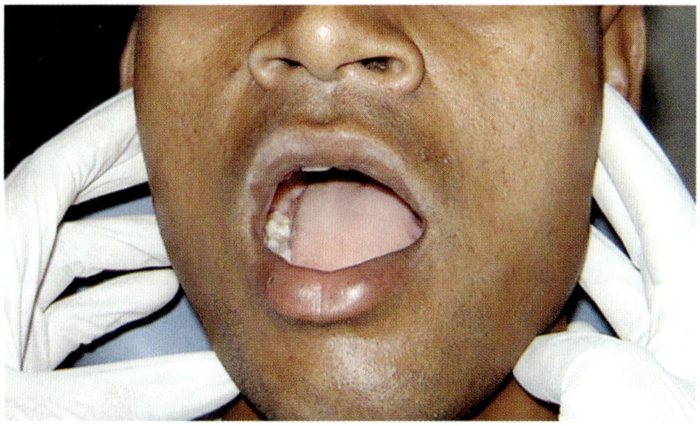

Fig. 27.2: Examination of TMJ

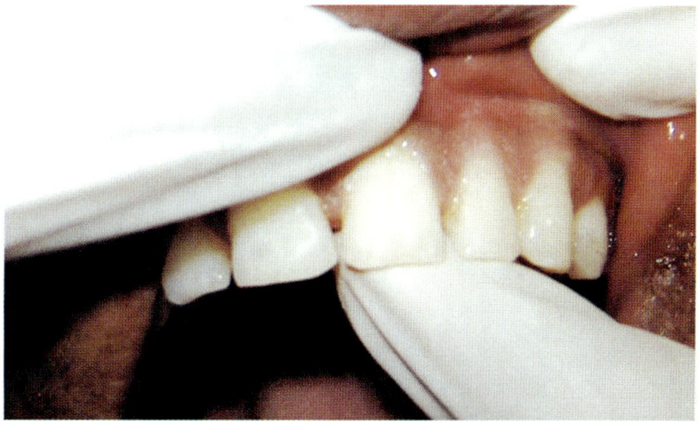

Fig. 27.4: Root fracture can be felt by placing finger on mucosa over tooth and moving the crown

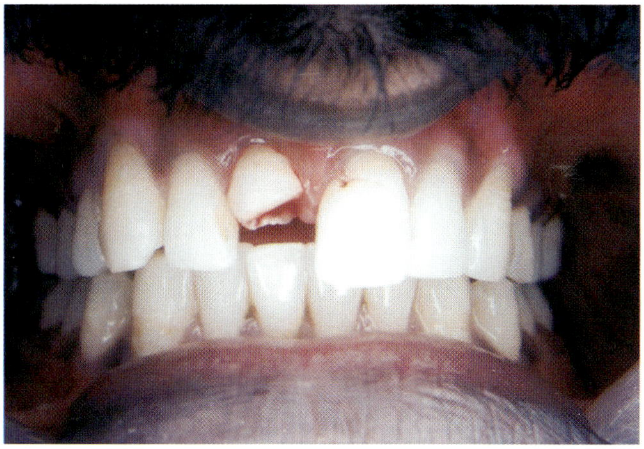

Fig. 27.3: Abnormalities in occlusion may indicate fracture of alveolar process or jaw

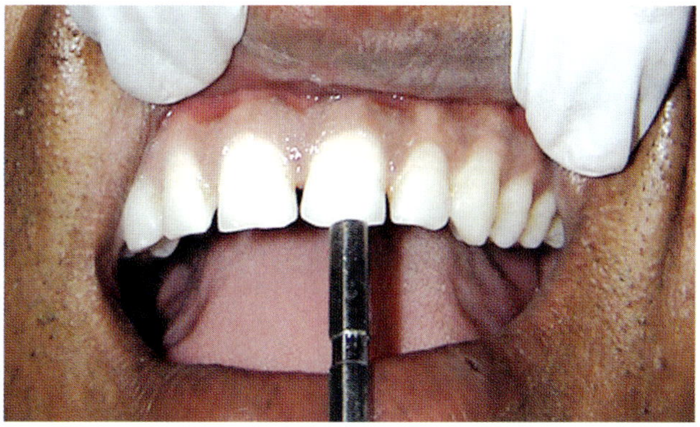

Fig. 27.5: Percussion to check integrity of periodontal ligament

anatomy, apical root development, closeness of fracture to pulp, relationship of root fracture to alveolar crest, etc.

## CLINICAL PHOTOGRAPHS

Clinical photographs are helpful for establishing clinical record for monitoring patient and treatment progress (Fig. 27.7). They also help in being as additional means of documenting injuries for legal purposes and insurance (Fig. 27.8).

Finally record all the findings such as fractures, color changes, pulp injuries or any other associated injuries and treatment planning is made following the final diagnosis.

## MANAGEMENT OF THE TRAUMATIC INJURIES

### Crown Infraction

This type of injury is very common but often unnoticed. A crown infraction is incomplete fracture of enamel without loss of tooth structure. It results from traumatic impact to enamel and appears as craze lines running parallel with direction of enamel rods and ending at dentinoenamel junction.

### Biological Consequence

Fracture lines are the weak points through which bacteria and their products can travel to pulp. Crown infraction can occur alone or can be a sign of a concomitant attachment injury where force taken up by attachment injury leaves enough force to crack the enamel.

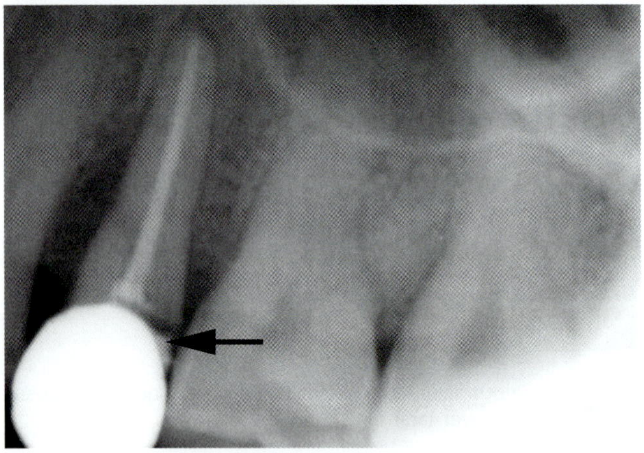

**Fig. 27.6:** Radiograph showing root fracture in premolar

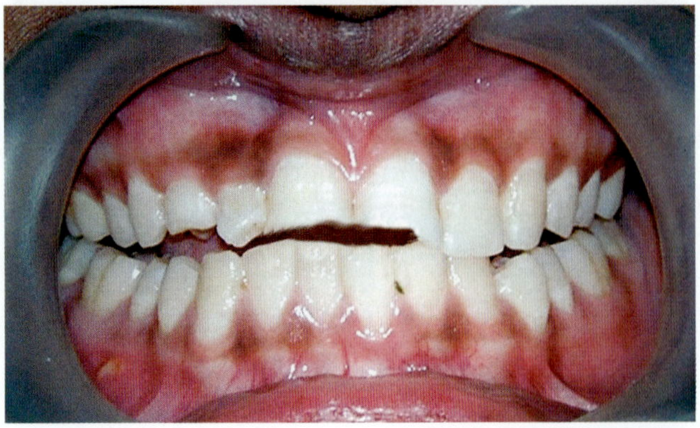

**Fig. 27.7:** Photograph showing traumatized 11 and 21

### Diagnosis

Tooth sustaining fracture is usually vital. Tooth can be:

- Easily recognized by viewing long axis of the tooth from the incisal edge.
- Examined by exposing it to fiber-optic light source, resin curing light, indirect light or by transillumination.

### Treatment

Infracted tooth does not require treatment but vitality tests are necessary to determine extent of pulp damage.

- Smoothening of rough edges by selectively grinding of enamel (Figs 27.9A and B)
- Repairing fractured tooth surface by composite if needed for cosmetic purposes (Fig 27.10).
- Regular pulp testing should be done and recorded for future reference.
- Follow-up of patient at 3, 6 and 12 months interval is done.

### Prognosis

Prognosis is good for infraction cases.

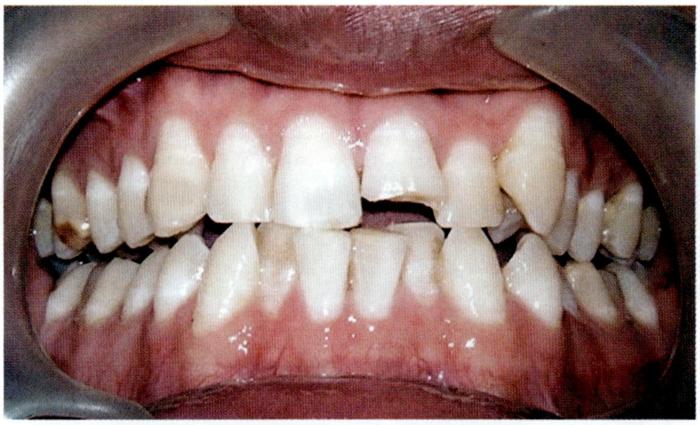

**Fig. 27.8:** Photograph showing fractured 21, can be used as documentation for legal purpose

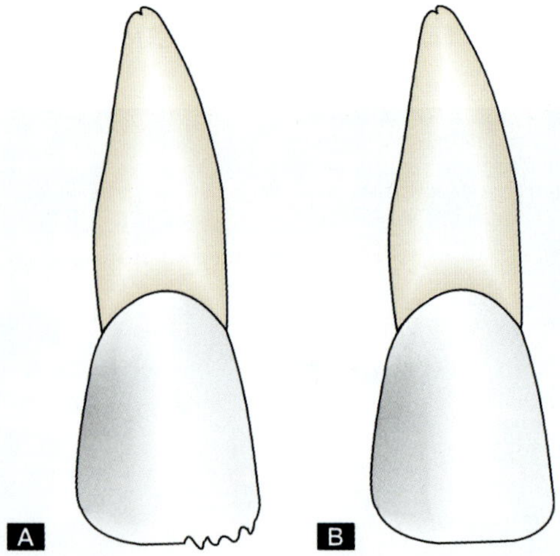


**Figs 27.9A and B:** Smoothening of rough edges by selective grinding of enamel (A) Central incisor with ragged margens (B) Smoothening of rough edges

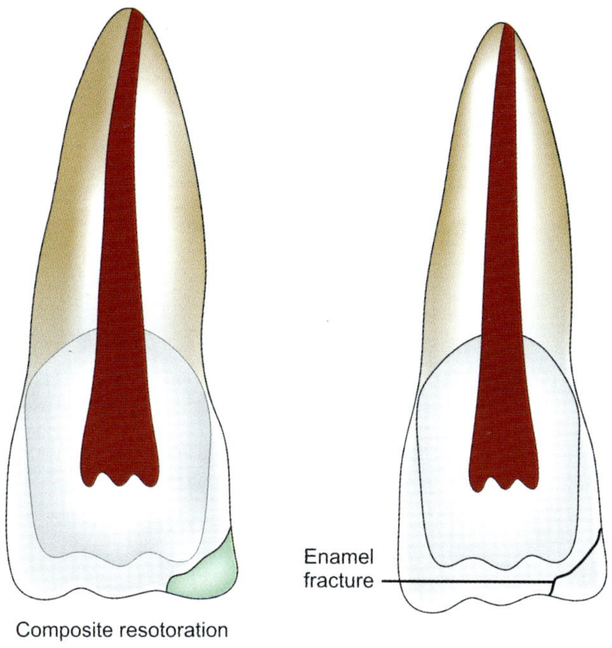


Fig. 27.10: Repairing of fractured tooth surface by composite

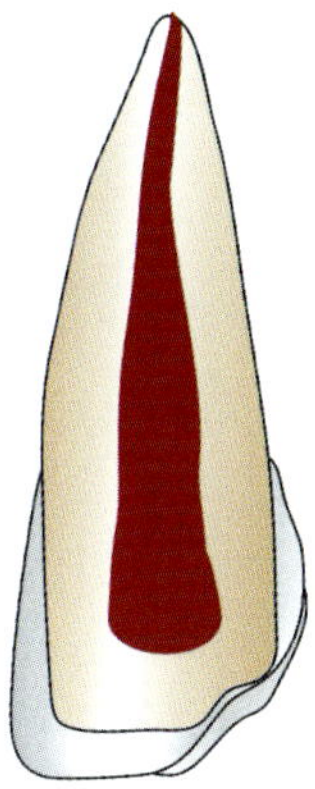

Fig. 27.11: Uncomplicated crown fracture involving enamel and dentin

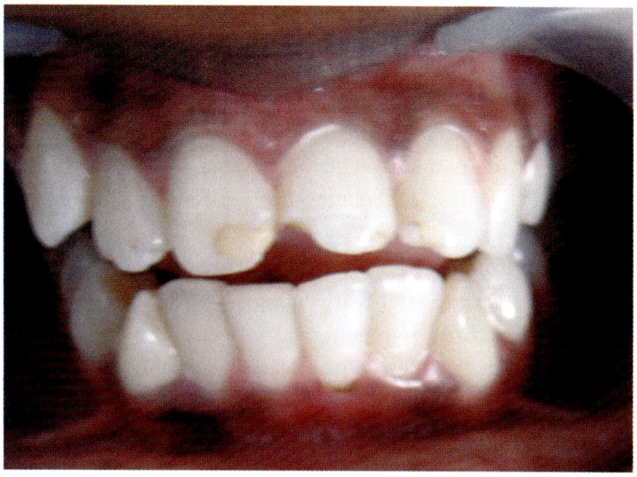

Fig. 27.12: Photograph showing uncomplicated crown fracture in 21 involving enamel and dentin

## CROWN FRACTURE

### Uncomplicated Crown Fracture

Crown facture involving enamel and dentin and not the pulp is called as ***uncomplicated crown fracture*** (Figs 27.11 and 27.12). It occurs more frequently than the complicated crown fracture. This type of fracture is usually not associated with pain and it does not require an urgent care.

### Incidence

Incidence of uncomplicated crown fracture varies from 26-92 percent of all the traumatic injuries of teeth.

### Biological Consequences

Minimal consequences are seen if only enamel is fractured but if dentin is exposed, a direct pathway for various irritants to pass through dentinal tubules to underlying pulp is formed. Pulp may remain normal or may get chronically inflamed depending upon proximity of fracture to the pulp, size of dentinal tubules and time of the treatment provided.

### Diagnosis

It could be easily revealed by clinical examination. If dentin is exposed, sensitivity to heat or cold may be present. Sometimes lip bruise or lacerations are also seen to be associated with injury.

### Treatment

The main objective of the treatment is to protect the pulp by obliterating dentinal tubules.

In case of enamel fractures, selective grinding of incisal edges will be sufficient to remove the sharp edges to prevent injury to lips, tongue, etc.

For esthetic reasons, composite restorations can be placed after acid etching.

***If there is involvement of both enamel and dentin:*** A restoration is needed to seal the dentinal tubules and to restore the esthetics.

Calcium hydroxide placed over exposed dentin helps to disinfect the fractured dentin surface and to stimulate the closure of dentinal tubules.

Dentinal tubules can also be sealed with zinc oxide eugenol cement, glass ionomer cement or dentin bonding agent. Though eugenol cement is very good agent but it should not be used where composite restoration is to be placed as eugenol may interfere with polymerization of composites.

If the fracture fragment of crown is available, reattach it. Reattachment of a fractured crown requires acid etching and application of bonding agent (Fig. 27.13). After removal of any soft tissue remnants, fractured site is disinfected. Following techniques are employed for reattachment of fractured fragment.

1. ***Bevelling of enamel:*** Beveling helps to increase retention of fragment by increasing area for bonding and altering enamel prism orientation.
2. ***Internal dentinal groove:*** In this internal dentinal groove is used as reinforcement for fragment. But this technique

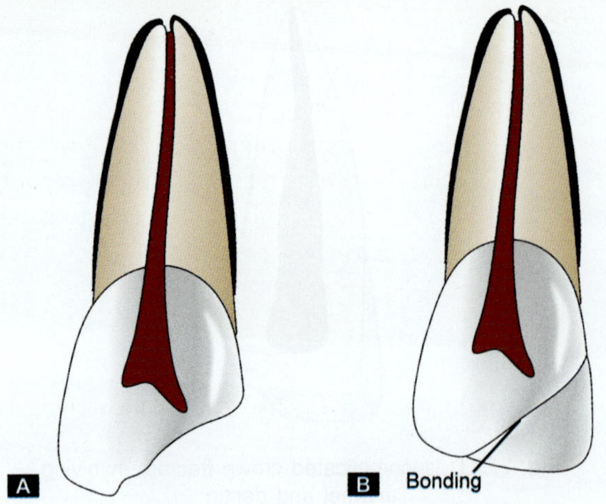


**Fig. 27.13:** Reattachment of fractured crown using etching and bonding technique

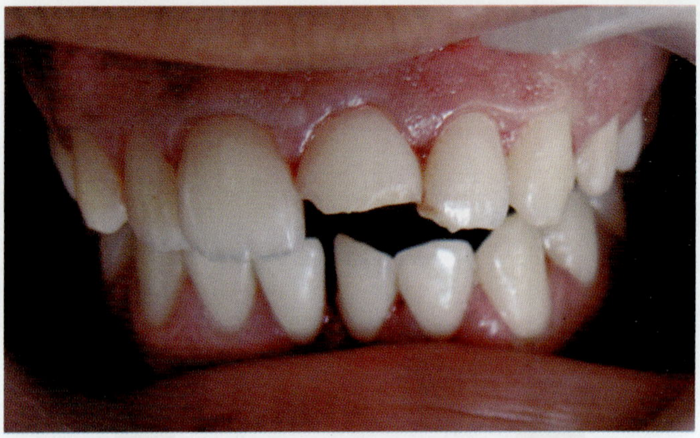

**Fig. 27.14:** Fracture of 21 showing involvement of enamel, dentin and pulp

has shown to compromise esthetics because of internal resin composite.

3. ***Internal enamel groove:*** Here V-shaped retention groove is placed in enamel to which fragment is attached. Due to limited thickness of enamel, this procedure is difficult to perform.
4. ***Overcontouring:*** This technique is used when fracture line is still noticeable after reattachment. In this technique after joining fractured fragment, a composite layer of 0.3 mm is placed superficially on buccal surface. But composite can show abrasion and discoloration with time.
5. ***Simple reattachment:*** In this fragment is reattached using bonding agent without any additional preparation.

### Prognosis

Patient should be recalled and sensitivity testing is done at the regular interval of 3, 6 and 12 months. Prognosis is good.

## Complicated Crown Fracture (Fig. 27.14)

Crown fracture involving enamel, dentin and pulp is called as complicated crown fracture (Fig. 27.15).

### Incidence

This type of fracture occurs in 2-13 percent of all the dental injuries.

### Biological Consequences

Extent of fracture helps to determine the pulpal treatment and restorative needs.

The degree of pulp involvement may vary from pin point exposure to total uncovering of the pulp chamber. If left untreated, it can lead to pulp necrosis. Initially the bacterial contamination of pulp causes both healing and repair, but if further contamination occurs and no treatment is provided, inflammation of pulp results.

### Diagnosis

Diagnosis is made by clinically evaluating the fracture and by pulp testing and taking radiographs (Fig. 27.16).

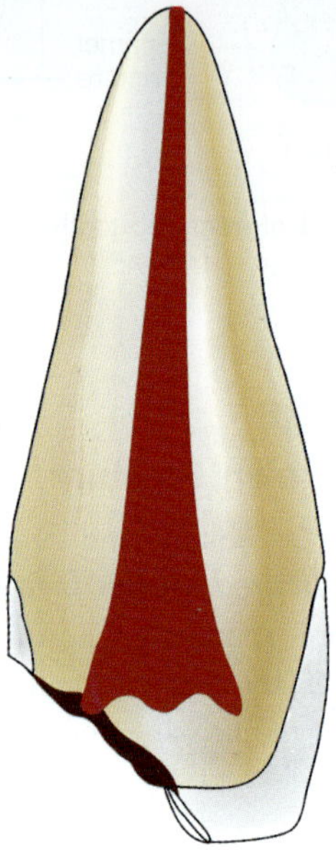

**Fig. 27.15:** Complicated tooth fracture involving enamel, dentin and pulp

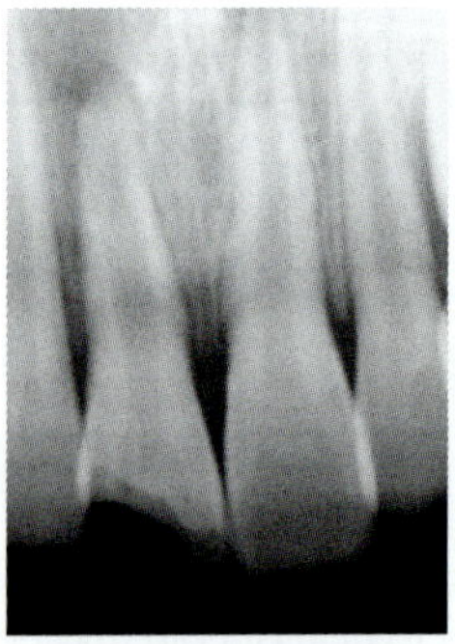

**Fig. 27.16:** Radiograph showing complicated tooth fracture

### Treatment

Factors like extent of fracture, stage of root maturation are imperative in deciding the treatment plane for complicated root fracture.

Maintaining the pulp vitality is main concern in treatment of pulpally involved teeth. In case of immature teeth, apexogenesis, i.e. normal process of root development will not occur unless the pulp remains alive. The pulp produces dentin and if the pulp dies before the apex closes, root wall development will be permanently arrested. The roots of immature teeth become increasingly thin and fragile near the apex. The goal of treatment is to allow the apex to mature and the dentin walls to thicken sufficiently to permit successful root canal therapy.

## Factors Affecting Pulpal Survival

Optimal blood circulation is necessary to nourish the pulp and keep it healthy. The type of injury, the stage of root development and the degree of infection are factors that affect circulation to the injured area and pulp vitality. Bacteria may invade the pulp through crack, causing inflammation and pulp necrosis.

Vitality testing will not be useful in determining the status of immature apex. Until apical closure occurs, teeth do not respond normally to pulp testing. Also, a traumatic injury sometimes temporarily alters the conduction potential of the nerve endings in the pulp leading to false readings. One must relate experience, radiographs, clinical signs or symptoms and knowledge of the healing process to assess pulp vitality.

## Pulp Capping and Pulpotomy

Pulp capping and pulpotomy are the measures that permit apexogenesis to take place and may avoid the need for root canal therapy. The choice of treatment depends on the size of the exposure, the presence of hemorrhage and the length of time since the injury.

## Pulp Capping

Pulp capping implies placing the dressing directly on to the pulp exposure (Figs 27.17A and B).

### *Indications*

On a very recent exposure (< 24 hours) and probably on a mature, permanent tooth with a simple restorative plan.

### *Technique*

After adequate anesthesia, a rubber dam is placed. Crown and exposed dentinal surface is thoroughly rinsed with saline followed by disinfection with 0.12 percent chlorhexidine or betadine. Pure calcium hydroxide mixed with anesthetic solution or saline is carefully placed over the exposed pulp and dentinal surface. The surrounding enamel is acid etched and bonded with composite resin.

### *Follow-up*

Vitality tests, palpation tests, percussion tests and radiographs should be carried out for 3 weeks; 3, 6 and 12 months; and every twelve months subsequently. Continued root development of the immature root is evaluated during this periodic radiographic examination.

### *Prognosis*

It depends on ability of $Ca(OH)_2$ to disinfect the superficial pulp and dentin and to necrose the zone of superficially inflamed pulp. Along with it, quality of bacteria tight seal provided by restoration is an important factor. Prognosis is up to 80 percent.

## Pulpotomy

Pulpotomy refers only to coronal extirpation of vital pulp tissue.

### *Two Types*

- Partial pulpotomy
- Full (cervical) pulpotomy

## Partial Pulpotomy

Partial pulpotomy also termed as "Cvek Pulpotomy", it implies removal of the coronal pulp tissue to the level of healthy pulp (Figs 27.18A to C).

### *Indications*

It is indicated in young permanent teeth with incomplete root formation.

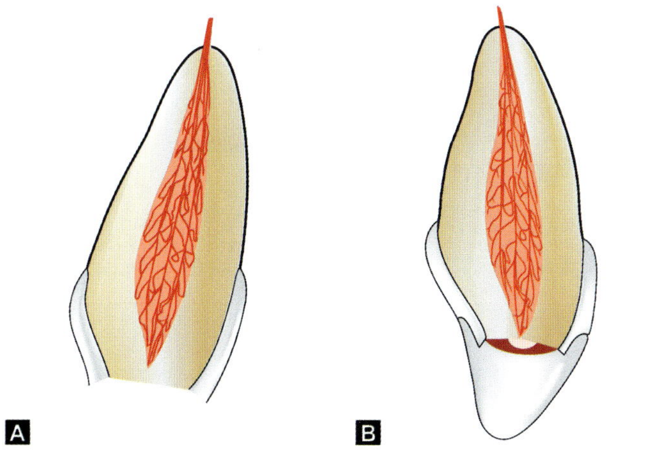


**Figs 27.17A and B:** Pulp capping of done by placing directly on to the pulp

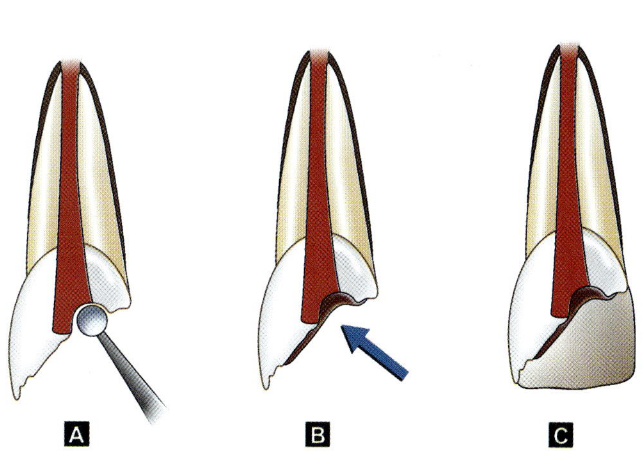


**Figs 27.18A to C:** (A) Removal of coronal pulp with round bur. (B) Placement of $Ca(OH)_2$ dressing over it. (C) Restoration of tooth using hard setting cement

### Technique

After anesthetizing the area rubber dam is applied.

A 1-2 mm deep cavity is prepared into the pulp using a diamond bur. Wet cotton pellet is used to impede hemorrhage and thereafter a thin coating of calcium hydroxide mixed with saline solution or anesthetic solution is placed over it. The access cavity is sealed with hard setting cement like IRM.

### Follow-up

Satisfactory results and evaluation following pulpotomy should show:

1. Absence of signs or symptoms
2. Absence of resorption either internal or external
3. Evidence of continued root formation in developing teeth.

### Prognosis

Prognosis is good (94-96%).

## Cervical Pulpotomy/Deep Pulpotomy

Cervical pulpotomy involves removal of entire coronal pulp to the level of root orifices (Fig. 27.19).

### Indications

- When the gap between traumatic exposure and the treatment provided is more than 24 hrs.
- When pulp is inflamed to deeper levels of coronal pulp.

### Technique

Coronal pulp is removed same as in partial pulpotomy except that it is up to level of root orifice.

### Follow-up

It is same as pulp capping and partial pulpotomy. Main disadvantage of this treatment is that sensitivity tests cannot be done because of loss of coronal pulp. Thus radiographic examination is important for follow-up.

### Prognosis

80-95 percent success rate.

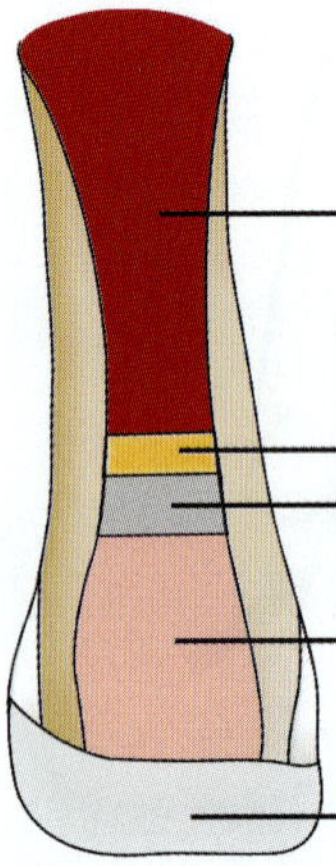


**Fig. 27.19:** Deep pulpotomy involves removal of entire coronal pulp, placement of $Ca(OH)_2$ dressing and restoration of the tooth

## Prerequisites for Success

Vital pulp therapy has an extremely high success rate if the clinician strictly adheres to the following requirements:

1. ***Treatment of a non-inflamed pulp:*** Treatment of a non inflamed pulp is found to be better than the inflamed pulp. Therefore the optimal time for treatment is in the first 24 hours when pulp inflammation is superficial. As time increases between the injury and therapy, the prognosis of vital pulp therapy decreases.
2. ***Pulp dressing:*** Currently, calcium hydroxide is the most common dressing used for vital pulp therapy because of its ability to form hard tissue and antibacterial property. Calcium hydroxide causes the necrosis of superficial layers of pulp, which results in mild irritation to the adjacent vital pulp tissue. This mild irritation initiates an inflammatory response and leads to formation of hard tissue barrier.

   Many materials such as zinc oxide eugenol, tricalcium phosphate and composite resin have been proposed as medicaments for vital pulp therapy. Mineral trioxide aggregate (MTA), a recent material has also been shown to produce the optimal results. Because of its hydrophilic nature it requires moisture for setting. It is a biocompatible material which produces normal healing response without inflammation. Other properties of MTA are its radiopacity and bacteriostatic nature.
3. ***Bacteria tight seal:*** A bacteria tight seal is the most significant factor for successful treatment, because introduction of bacteria during the healing phase causes failure.

## Apexification

It is always desirable to allow root to develop in an immature tooth. However, apexogenesis does not occur unless some vital pulp tissue remains in the root canal. If the pulp tissue is necrotic, apexification is the process which stimulates the formation of a calcified barrier across the apex (Fig. 27.20). Apexification is done to stimulate the hard tissue barrier. For this, initially all canals are disinfected with sodium hypochlorite solution to remove any debris and bacteria from the canal. Following this

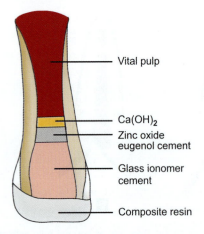

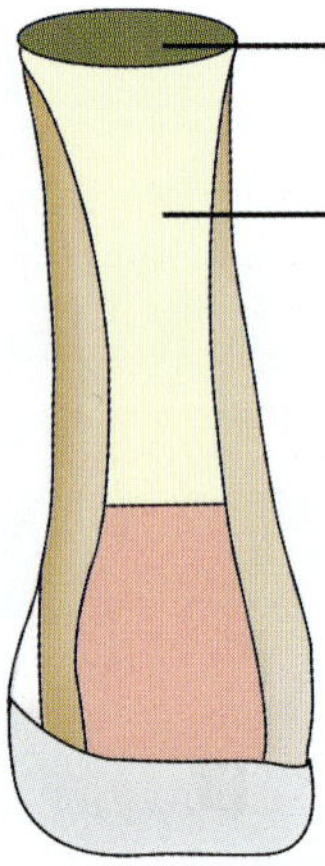


**Fig. 27.20:** Apexification stimulates hard tissue barrier across the apex

calcium hydroxide is packed against the apical soft tissue and later backfilling with calcium hydroxide is done to completely obturate the canal.

When completion of hard tissue is suspected (after 3-6 months), remove calcium hydroxide and take radiograph. If formation of hard tissue is found satisfactory, canal is obturated using softened gutta-percha technique. One should avoid excessive lateral forces during obturation because of thin walls of the root.

Nowadays, MTA, i.e. mineral trioxide aggregate is also used in place of calcium hydroxide. Pulp response to this material is favorable. Since this material does not appear to disintegrate with time, it might not be necessary to replace the restoration after dentin bridge formation as it is done in case of calcium hydroxide (Fig. 27.21).

## CROWN ROOT FRACTURE

Crown root fracture involves enamel, dentin and cementum with or without the involvement of pulp (Fig. 27.22). It is usually oblique in nature involving both crown and root (Fig. 27.23). This type of injury is considered as more complex type of injury because of its more severity and involvement of the pulp (Figs 27.24A to C).

### Incidence

It contributes 5 percent of total dental injuries. In anterior teeth, it usually occurs by direct trauma causing chisel type fracture

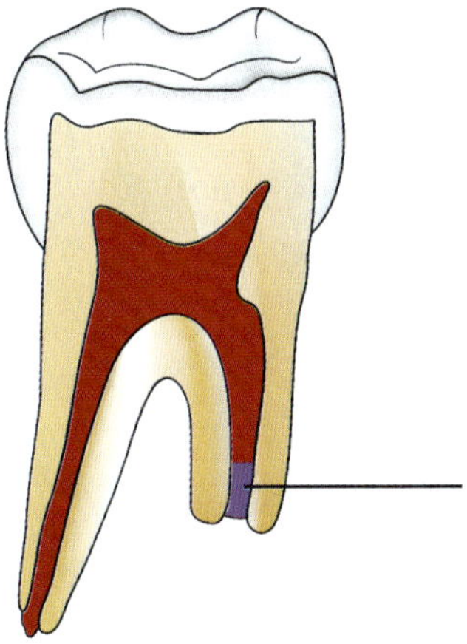


**Fig. 27.21:** Apexification using MTA

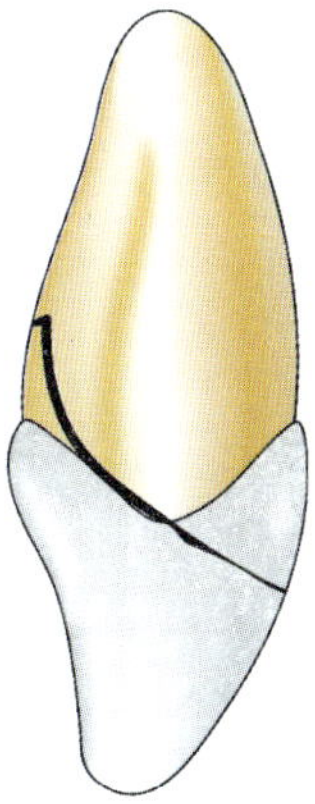

**Fig. 27.22:** Crown root fracture

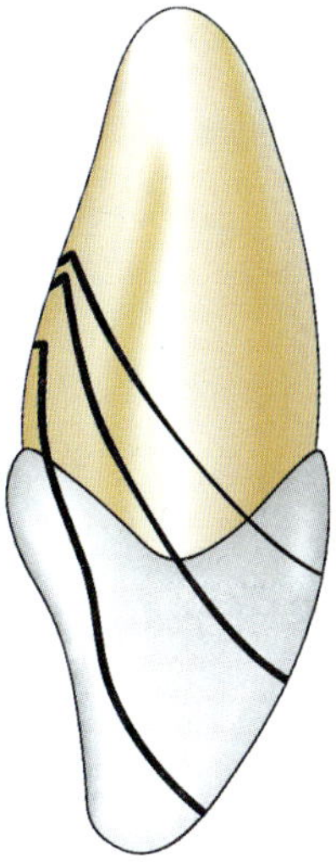

**Fig. 27.23:** Crown root fracture is usually oblique in nature

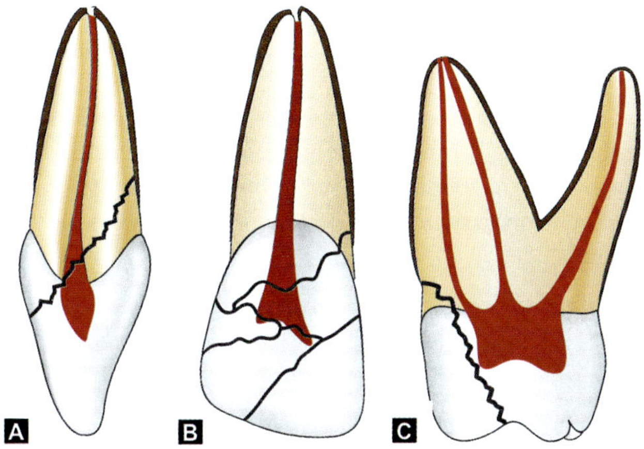


**Figs 27.24A to C:** Oblique type of fracture is considered as more complex because of its severity and pulp involvement

which splits crown and root Figure 27.25. In posterior teeth, fracture is rarely seen but it can occur because of indirect trauma like large sized restorations and high speed instrumentation, etc.

### Biological Consequences

Biological consequences are similar to as that of complicated or uncomplicated fracture depending upon the pulp involvement. In addition to these, periodontal complications are also present because of encroachment of the attachment apparatus.

### Diagnosis

Crown root fractures are complex injuries which are difficult both to diagnose as well as treat. The fracture line in such cases is usually single but multiple fractures can also occur, often originating from the primary fracture.

A tooth with crown root/fracture exhibits following features:

- Coronal fragment is usually mobile. Patient may complain of pain from mastication due to movement of the coronal portion.

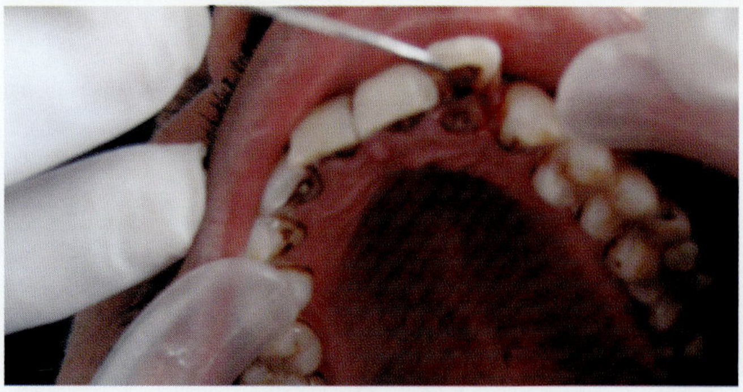

Fig. 27.25: Chisel shaped fracture of 22 splitting crown and root

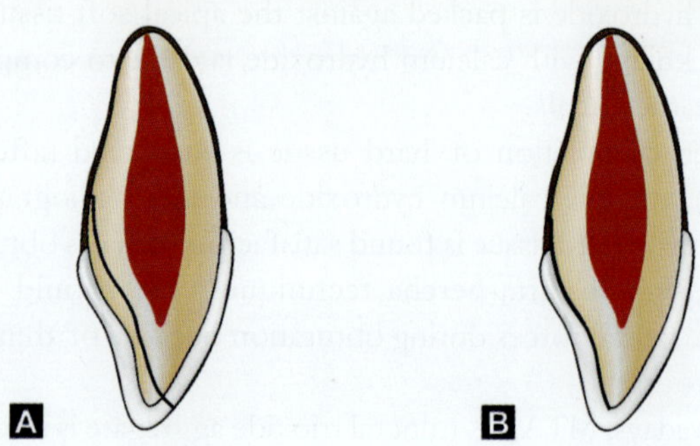

Figs 27.27A and B: Root fracture without pulp involvement

- Inflammatory changes in pulp and periodontal ligament are seen due to plaque accumulation in the line of fracture.
- Patient may complain of sensitivity to hot and cold.

Radiographs are taken at different angles to assess the extent of fracture (Fig. 27.26). Indirect light and transillumination can also be used to diagnose this type of fracture.

## Treatment

The primary goal of the treatment is the elimination of pain which is mainly because of mobile crown fragment. It can be done by applying bonding agents to bond the loose fragments together, temporary crown placement or by using glass ionomer cement.

***The main objective of the treatment is to:***

a. Allow subgingival portion of the fracture to heal.
b. Restoration of the coronal portion.

***Following should be considered while management of crown root fracture:***

- If there is no pulp exposure, fragment can be treated by bonding alone or by removing the coronal structure and then restoring it with composites (Figs 27.27A and B).
- If pulp exposure has occurred, pulpotomy or root canal treatment is indicated depending upon condition of the tooth.
- When remaining tooth structure is adequate for retention, endodontic therapy and crown restoration are possible with the help of crown lengthening procedures.
- When root portion is long enough to accommodate a post retained crown, then surgically removal of the coronal fragment and surgical extrusion of the root segment is done (Figs 27.28A and B).
- To accommodate a post retained crown, after removal of the crown portion, orthodontic extrusion of root can also be done (Figs 27.29A and B).
- When the fracture extends below the alveolar crest level, the surgical repositioning of tissues by gingivectomy, osteotomy, etc. should be done to expose the level of fracture and subsequently restore it.

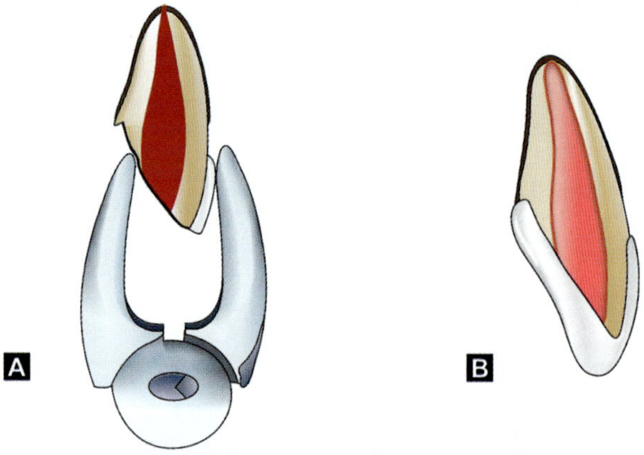

Figs 27.28A and B: When root portion is long enough to accommodate post supported crown, remove the coronal segment, extrude root fragment and perform endodontic therapy

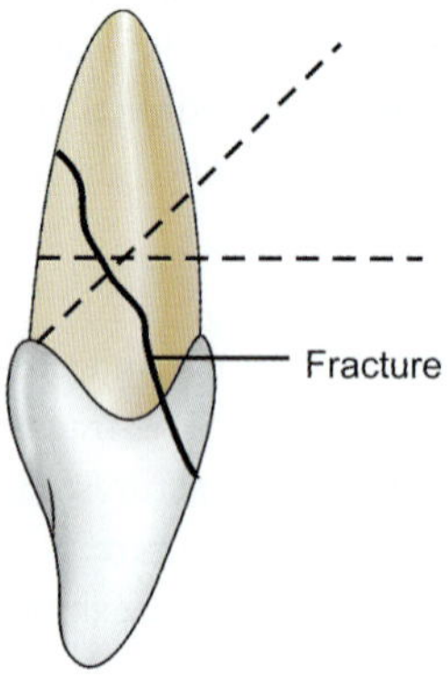


Fig. 27.26: Radiographs taken at more than one angle can show the extent of fracture

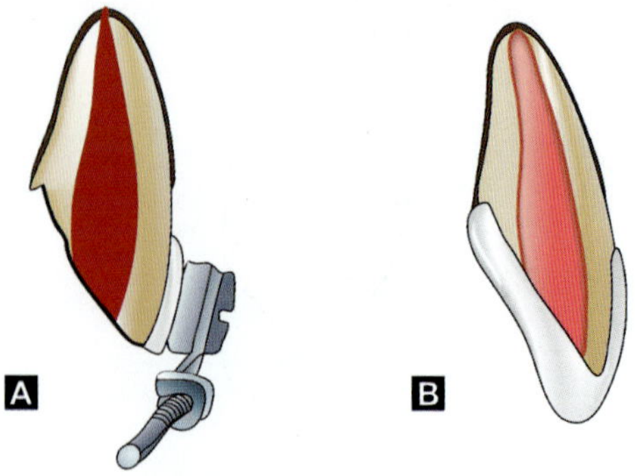

Figs 27.29A and B: Orthodontic extrusion of root (B) Restoration of tooth after endodontic therapy

## Prognosis

Long term prognosis depends on quality of coronal restoration. Otherwise the prognosis is similar to complicated or uncomplicated fracture.

# ROOT FRACTURE

These are uncommon injuries but represent a complex healing pattern due to involvement of dentin, cementum, pulp and periodontal ligament (Figs 27.30 and 27.31).

## Incidence

They form the 3 percent of the total dental injuries. These fractures commonly result from a horizontal impact. Root fractures are usually transverse to oblique in nature (Fig. 27.32). These fractures require radiographs at different angles for their accurate identification.

## Biological Consequences

When root fractures occur horizontally, coronal segment is displaced to varying degrees. If vasculature of apical segment is not affected, it rarely becomes necrotic.

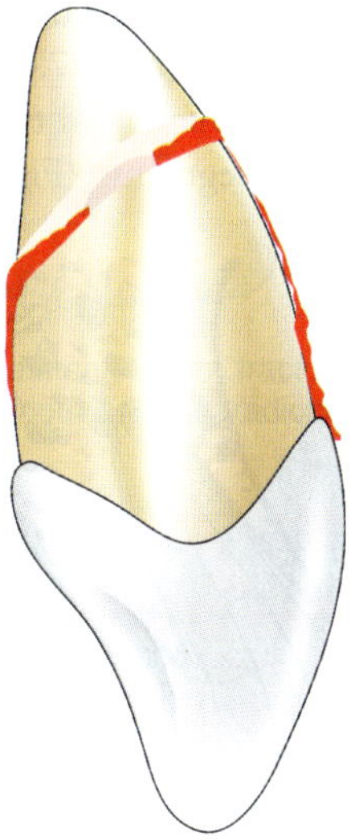

Fig. 27.30: Root fracture

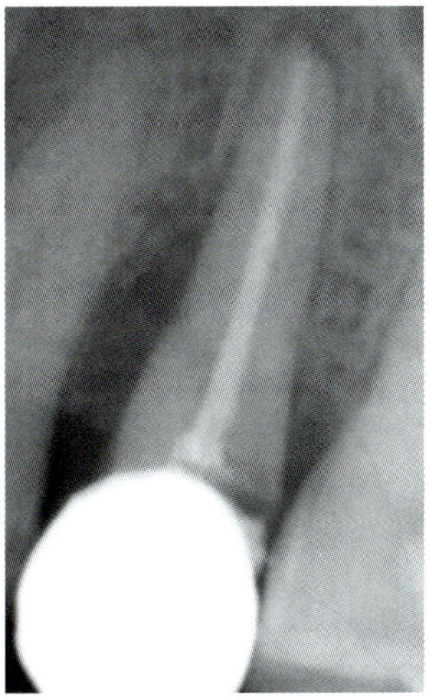

Fig. 27.31: Root fracture at cervical third

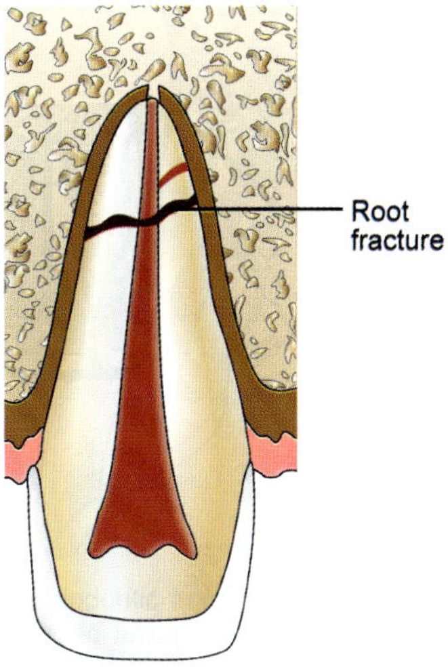


Fig. 27.32: Root fracture is usually oblique in nature

## Diagnosis

Displacement of coronal segment usually reflects the location of fracture (Fig. 27.33A to D).

Radiographs at varying angles (usually at 45°, 90° and 110°) are mandatory for diagnosing root fractures (Fig. 27.34).

## Treatment of Root Fractures

If there is no mobility of tooth and tooth is asymptomatic, only apical third fracture is suspected. In this case to facilitate pulpal and periodontal ligament healing, displaced coronal portion should be repositioned accurately (Fig. 27.35). It is stabilized by splinting for 2-3 weeks (Fig. 27.36).

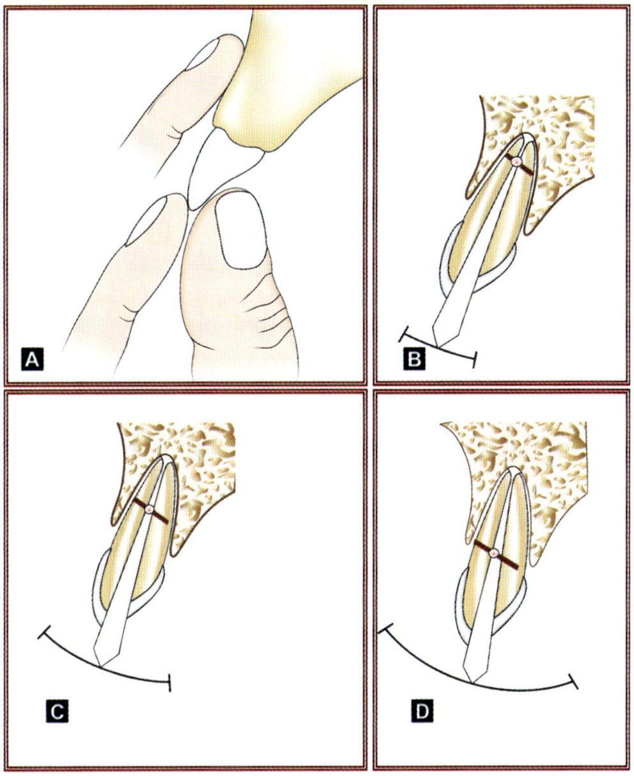


Figs 27.33A to D: Diagnosis of location of root fracture A. Palpating the facial mucosa with one finger and moving crown with other finger B. to D. Arc of mobility of incisal segment of tooth with root. As fracture moves incisally, arc of mobility increases

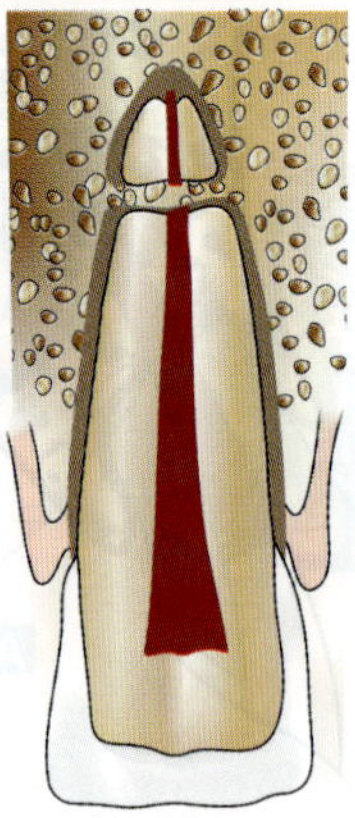

Fig. 27.46: Healing of root fracture by interproximal bone

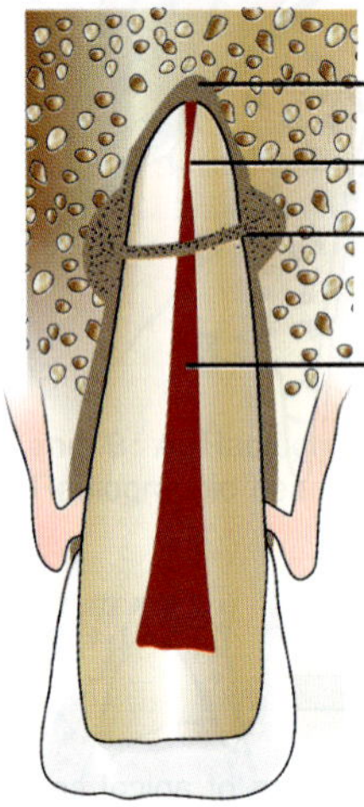


Fig. 27.47: Healing of root fracture by formation of connective tissue between the segments

- Radiographs are taken to predict healing of root fracture. Resorption within the root canal originating at fracture line indicates healing following pulpal damage after trauma. But resorption within the bone at the level of fracture line indicates pulp necrosis which requires endodontic therapy.

## LUXATION INJURIES

Luxation injuries cause trauma to supporting structures of teeth ranging from minor crushing of periodontal ligament and neurovascular supply of pulp to total displacement of the teeth.

They are usually caused by sudden impact such as blow, fall or striking a hard object.

### Incidence

They form 30-40 percent of all the dental injuries.

## CONCUSSION

**In concussion (Fig. 27.48):**

- Tooth is not displaced.
- Mobility is not present.
- Tooth is tender to percussion because of edema and hemorrhage in the periodontal ligament.
- Pulp may respond normal to testing.

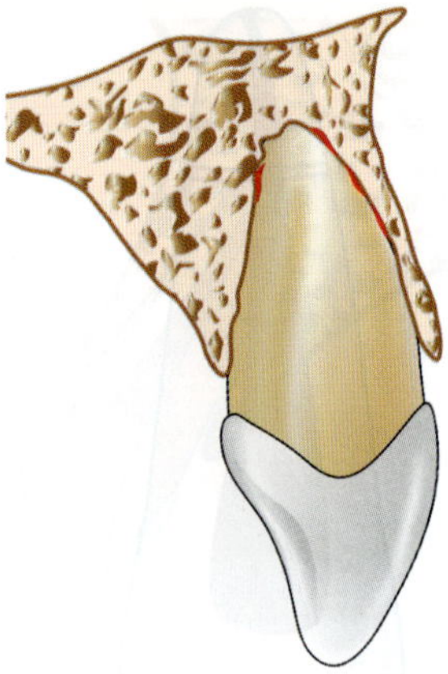

Fig. 27.48: Concussion

## SUBLUXATION

In subluxation (Fig. 27.49)

- Teeth are sensitive to percussion and have some mobility.
- Sulcular bleeding is seen showing damage and rupture of the periodontal ligament fibers.
- Pulp responds normal to testing.
- Tooth is not displaced (Fig. 27.50).

### Treatment of Concussion and Subluxation

- Rule out the root fracture by taking radiographs.
- Relief the occlusion by selective grinding of opposing teeth (Fig. 27.51).
- Immobilize the injured teeth.
- Endodontic therapy should not be carried out at first visit because both negative testing results and crown discoloration can be reversible.

  ***Follow-up*** is done at 3 weeks, 3, 6 and 12 months.

  ***Prognosis*** there is only a minimal risk of pulp necrosis and root resorption.

## LATERAL LUXATION

In lateral luxation:

- Trauma displaces the tooth lingually, buccally, mesially or distally, in other words out of its normal position away from its long axis (Fig. 27.52).

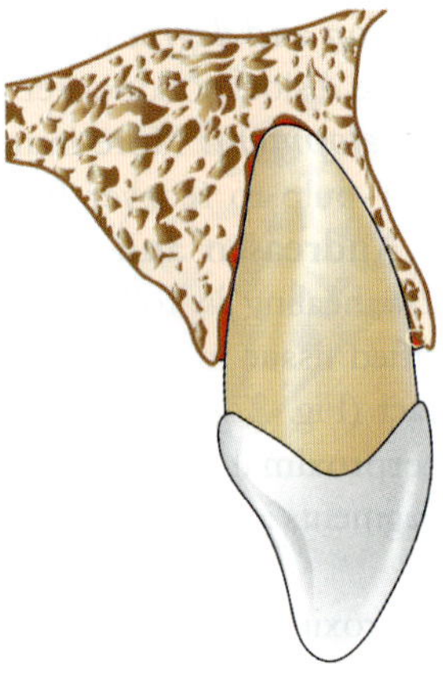

Fig. 27.49: Subluxation

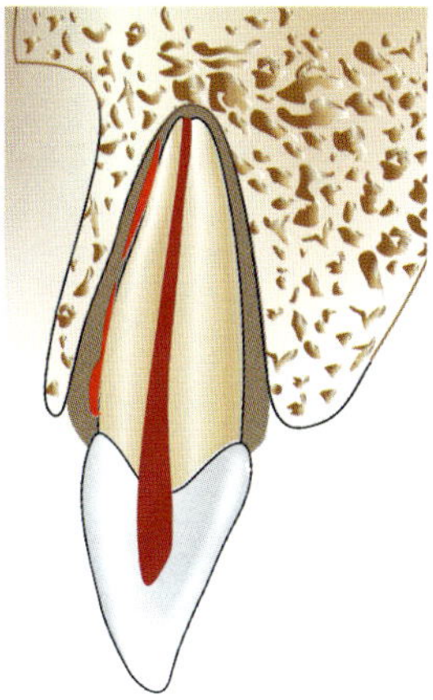

Fig. 27.50: Subluxation showing injury to periodontium

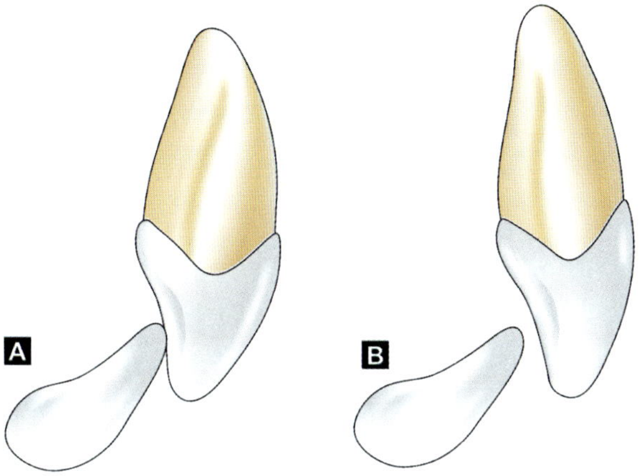

Fig. 27.51: Treatment of injury by selective grinding of tooth

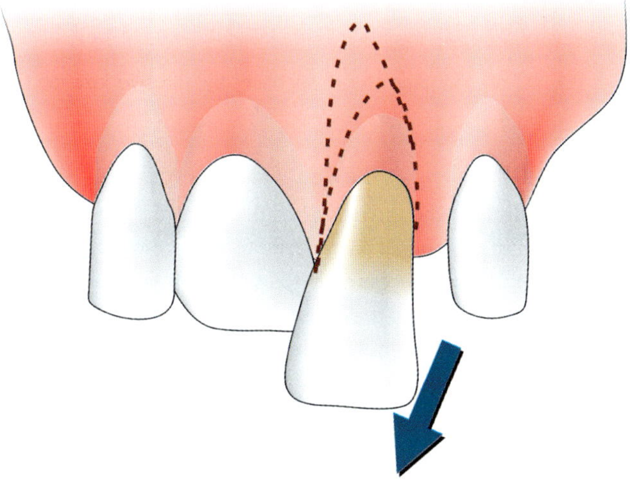

Fig. 27.52: Lateral luxation

- Sulcular bleeding is present indicating rupture of PDL fibers (Fig. 27.53).
- Tooth is sensitive to percussion.
- Clinically, crown of laterally luxated tooth is usually displaced horizontally with tooth locked firmly in the new position. Here percussion may elicit metallic tone indicating that root has forced into the alveolar bone.

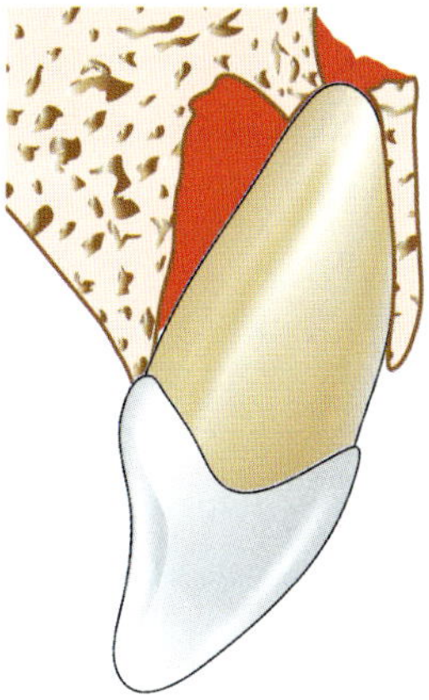

Fig. 27.53: Lateral luxation resulting in injury to periodontium

## EXTRUSIVE LUXATION

In extrusive luxation

- Tooth is displaced from the socket along its long axis (Fig. 27.54)
- Tooth is very mobile
- Radiograph shows the displacement of tooth.

### Treatment of Lateral and Extrusive Luxation

Treatments of these injuries consist of a traumatic repositioning and fixation of teeth which prevents excessive movement during healing.

*Repositioning of laterally luxated teeth* require minimal force for repositioning. Before repositioning laterally luxated teeth, anesthesia should be administrated. Tooth must be dislodged from the labial cortical plate by moving it coronally and then apically. Thus tooth is first moved coronally out of the buccal plate of bone and then fitted into its original position (Fig. 27.55).

*For repositioning of extruded tooth*, a slow and steady pressure is required to displace the coagulum formed between root apex and floor of the socket (Fig. 27.56). After this tooth is immobilized, stabilized and splinted for approximately 2 weeks. Local anesthesia is not needed while doing this.

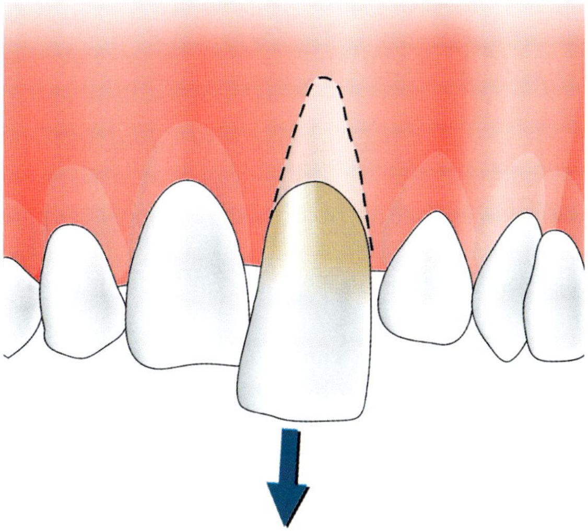

Fig. 27.54: Extrusive luxation

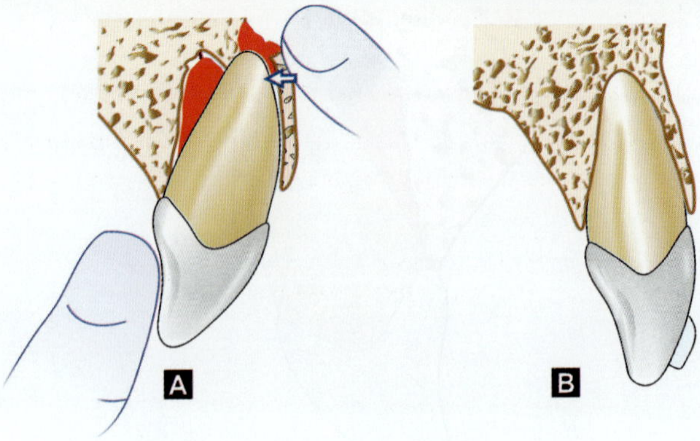


**Fig. 27.55:** Treatment of lateral luxation

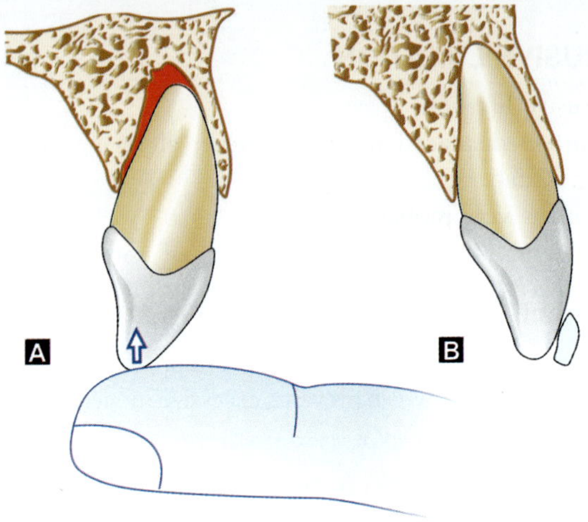


**Fig. 27.56:** Treatment of extrusive luxation

***Follow-up:*** Splint is removed 2 weeks after extrusion. If tooth has become nonvital, inflammatory root resorption can occur, requiring immediate endodontic therapy.

Pulp testing should be performed on regular intervals.

## Prognosis

It depends on stage of root development at the time of injury. Commonly seen sequel of luxation injuries are pulp necrosis, root canal obliteration and root resorption.

## INTRUSIVE LUXATION

In intrusive luxation

- Tooth is forced into its socket in an apical direction (Fig. 27.57).
- Maximum damage has occurred to pulp and the supporting structures (Fig. 27.58).
- When examined clinically, the tooth is in infraocclusion (Fig. 27.57).
- Tooth presents with clinical presentation of ankylosis because of being firm in socket.
- On percussion metallic sound is heard.
- In mixed dentition, diagnosis is more difficult as intrusion can mimic a tooth undergoing eruption.
- Radiographic evaluation is needed to know the position of tooth.

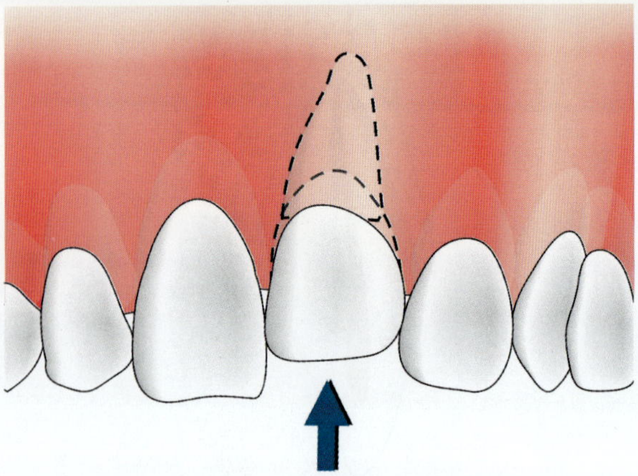

**Fig. 27.57:** Intrusive luxation

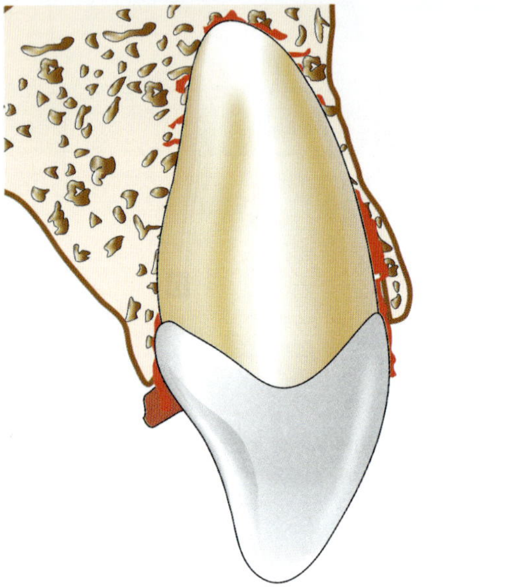

**Fig. 27.58:** Damage to periodontium by intrusive luxation

## Treatment

Healing following the intrusive luxation is complicated because intensive injury to the PDL can lead to replacement resorption and further dentoalveolar ankylosis. Pulp is also affected by this type of injury. So the main objective of treatment is to reduce the extent of these complications. Treatment mainly depends upon stage of root development.

In immature teeth, spontaneous re-eruption is seen. If re-eruption stops before normal occlusion is attained, orthodontic movement is initiated before tooth gets ankylosed (Fig. 27.59).

If tooth is severely intruded, surgical access is made to the tooth to attach orthodontic appliances and extrude the tooth.

Tooth can also be repositioned by loosening the tooth surgically and aligning it with the adjacent teeth.

## Follow-up

Regular clinical and radiographic evaluation is needed in this case because of frequent occurrence of pulpal and periodontal healing complications.

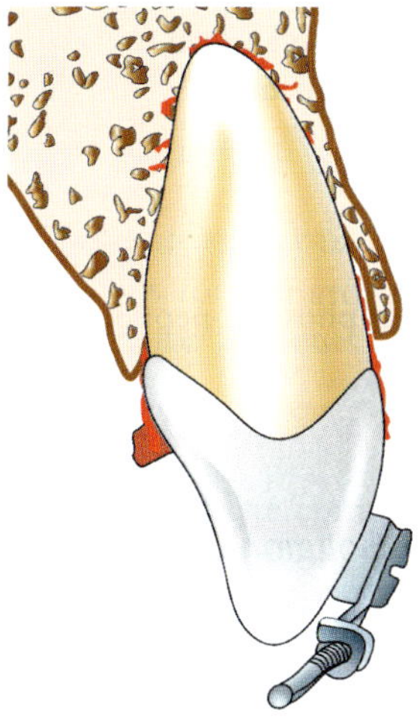

Fig. 27.59: Orthodontic extrusion of intruded tooth

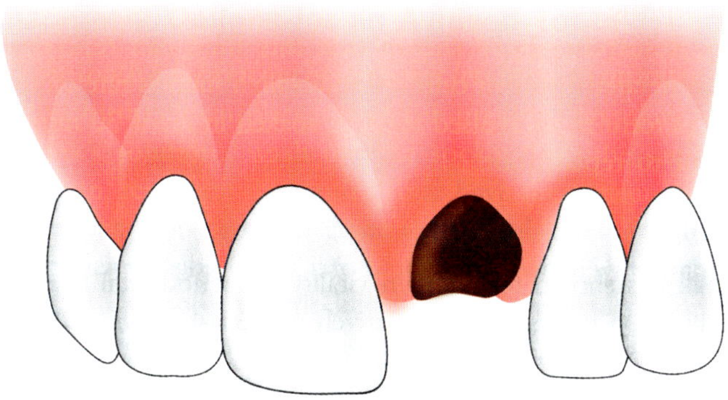

Fig. 27.60: Avulsion of tooth

## AVULSION (EXARTICULATION)

### Definition

It is defined as complete displacement of the tooth out of socket (Fig. 27.60). The common cause is a directed force sufficient to overcome the bond between the affected tooth and the periodontal ligament within the alveolar socket (Fig. 27.61).

Losing a tooth can be physically and emotionally demanding, as a result vacant place is not esthetically agreeable and is difficult to fill and replace. Long-term consequences include shifting of adjacent teeth resulting in misalignment and periodontal disease.

As early as 400 BCE, Hippocrates suggested that dislodged teeth should be replaced and fixed firmly to adjacent teeth with wire. Modern emergency techniques focus on reimplanting the tooth as soon as possible, minimizing periodontal damage, and preventing infection of the pulp tissue.

### Incidence

- It usually occurs in age group of 7-10 years.
- 1-16 percent of all traumatic injuries occur to permanent dentition.

Sports, fall from height and automobile accidents are most frequent cause.

Trauma to the teeth is not life threatening; but when coupled with maxillofacial injuries and fractures, can compromise the airway. Morbidity to the teeth may be individualized to primary or permanent teeth.

**Consequences of trauma to primary teeth**

- Infection
- Abscess
- Loss of space in the dental arch
- Ankylosis
- Failure to continue eruption
- Color changes
- Injury to the permanent teeth

**Consequences of injury to permanent teeth**

- Infection
- Abscess
- Loss of space in the dental arch
- Ankylosis
- Resorption of root structure
- Abnormal root development
- Color changes

### Biologic Consequences

There are several sequelae to avulsion injury of tooth. The predominant and most consistent sequelae seen in such cases are as follows:

1. ***Pulpal necrosis:*** This usually occurs due to disruption of blood supply to the tooth. Pulp testing and frequent monitoring of pulp vitality should be done at regular interval.
2. ***Surface resorption:*** It is non-invasive process which occurs after avulsion injury. Small superficial resorption cavities occur within cementum and the outer dentin (Fig. 27.62). It is repair process of physical damage to calcified tissue by recruitment of cells following removal of damaged tissues by macrophages.
3. ***Inflammatory resorption:*** This resorption occurs as a result of the necrotic pulp becoming infected in the presence of severely damaged cementum. This infected pulp allows bacterial toxins to migrate out through the dentinal tubules into the periodontal ligament causing resorption of both root and adjacent root (Fig. 27.63).
4. ***Replacement resorption:*** Replacement resorption occurs when there is extensive damage to periodontal ligament and cementum. Healing occurs from the alveolar side creating a union between tooth and bone. It is incorporation of the root into the normal remodeling process of alveolus with gradual replacement by bone. As a result, the root is ultimately replaced by bone (Fig. 27.64). Radiographically, there is an absence of the lamina dura and the root assumes a moth-eaten appearance as dentin is replaced by bone. Clinically the tooth will not show any sign of mobility and on percussion, a metallic sound is heard. Replacement resorption in younger patients may interfere with the growth and development of alveolar process which subsequently results in infraocclusion of that tooth.

- Hemorrhage/bleeding from nose/ears/oral cavity
- Nausea
- Vomiting
- Headache
- Amnesia
- Spontaneous dental pain
- Pain on medication

## Extraoral Examination

- Abrasions/contusions/lacerations/Ecchymosis
- Asymmetry
- Bones
  - i. Mobility
  - ii. Crepitus
  - iii. Tenderness
- Swelling
- Hemorrhage
- Presence of foreign bodies
- Check whether any injury to lips, cheeks, nose, ear and eyes.

## TMJ Assessment

- Deviation
- Tender on palpation
- Intraoral opening whether restricted or not
- Deflection pain on opening

## Intraoral Examination (Check any injury present)

- Buccal mucosa
- Gingiva
- Tongue
- Floor of the mouth
- Palate
- Periodontal status

## Occlusion

- Classification
- Molar
- Canine
  - i. Overjet
  - ii. Overbite
- Crossbite; deviation

## Teeth

- Color
- Mobility (mm)
- Pain
  - i. On percussion
  - ii. Response to cold
  - iii. On biting
- Pulp testing
  - i. Electrical
  - ii. Thermal
- Pulp exposure
- Size
- Appearance
- Infarction
- Crown fracture/root fracture
- Luxation
  - i. Direction
  - ii. Extent
- Avulsion
  - i. Extraoral time
  - ii. Storage medium
- Carries/previous restorations

## Radiograph

- Pulp size
- Periodontal ligament space
- Crown/root fracture
- Periapical pathology
- Alveolar fracture
- Foreign body

## Photographs

### *Treatment*

- Repositioning and stabilization
- Soft tissue management
- Pulp therapy
- Medications
- Instructions
  - i. Follow-up
  - ii. Diet
  - iii. Medicines
  - iv. Complications

## PREVENTION OF TRAUMATIC INJURIES

Children with untreated trauma to permanent teeth often exhibit greater impacts on their daily living than those without any traumatic injury. The incidence of dental and orofacial trauma is more in sports affecting the upper lip, maxilla and maxillary incisors. Use of mouthguard may protect the upper incisors. However studies have shown that even with mouthguard in place, 25 percent of dentoalveolar injuries still occur.

A dental expert may be able to alter certain risk factors such as patient's dental anatomy and occlusion. The frequency for dental trauma is significantly higher for children with increased overjet and insufficient lip coverage. Instigating preventive orthodontic treatment in early to mixed dentition of patients with an overjet > 3 mm has shown to prevent traumatic injuries to permanent incisors. Although some sports related traumatic injuries are unavoidable, most can be prevented by means of helmets, face masks and mouthguards. These appliances reduce both the frequency and severity of dental and orofacial trauma. The mouthguard has been used as a protective device in sports like boxing, soccer, wrestling and basketball.

The mouthguard, also referred to as gumshield or mouth protector is "a resilient device or appliance placed inside the mouth to reduce oral injuries, particularly to teeth and surrounding structures".

Mouthguard can be classified into 3 categories (given by the American Society for Testing and Materials).

1. **Type I**
   - Stock mouthguards are purchased over the counter.
   - Designed to use without any modification.
2. **Type II**
   - Mouth-formed, made from thermoplastic material adapted to the mouth by finger tongue and biting pressure after immersing the appliance in hot water.
   - Commonly used by athletes.
3. **Type III**
   - Custom-fabricated mouthguards.
   - Produced on a dental model by either vacuum forming or heat pressure lamination technique.
   - Should be fabricated for maxillary class I and II occlusions and mandibular class III occlusions.
   - Best in performance.

## Functions of Mouthguard

1. Protect the lips and intraoral structures from bruising and laceration.
2. Act as cushion and distribute forces so that crown fractures, root fractures, luxation and avulsions are avoided.
3. Protect jaw from fracture and dislocation of the mandible.
4. Protect against neck injuries.
5. Provide support for edentulous space.
6. Prevent the teeth in opposing arches from violet contract.

## Treatment Options for Teeth with Root Fractures with Necrotic Pulp

1. Root canal treatment for both apical and coronal segment.
2. Root canal treatment for coronal part and no treatment for apical segment.
3. Surgical removal of apical segment, while root canal treatment of coronal part.
4. Root canal treatment for coronal part with apexification procedure in apical part of this segment, but no treatment for apical portion of the teeth.
5. Use of splints.
6. Endodontic implant after extraction.
7. Root extrusion in teeth with fracture at the level of alveolar crest.

## Mainly Five Types of Luxation Injuries are seen:

- Concussion
- Subluxation
- Lateral luxation
- Extrusive luxation
- Intrusive luxation

## Biologic Consequences

- Pulpal necrosis
- Surface resorption
- Inflammatory resorption
- Replacement resorption.

## Contraindications of Replantation

- Compromised medical status of the patient
- Extensive damage to supporting tissues of the tooth
- Child's stage of dental development in which there are chances of ankylosis are more.

Name of the Patient : ...................................................
Age of the patient : ...................................................
Sex of the patient : ...................................................
Date : ...................................................
Time : ...................................................

## Legal Consequences

- Delaying reimplantation
- Improper handling and transportation of the tooth
- Reimplanting a primary tooth
- Not providing the tetanus prophylaxis
- Incomplete examination of the surrounding traumatized tissue for tooth fragments
- Failure to warn patients that any trauma to teeth may disrupt the neurovascular supply and lead to long-term pulp necrosis or root resorption.

## QUESTIONS

**Q. Classify traumatic injuries. How will you diagnose a case with traumatic injury.**

**Q. How will you manage a case of root fracture? How does healing takes place for a root fracture?**

**Q. Define exarticulation/avulsion. How will you manage if patient comes with avulsed tooth in your clinic?**

a. Crown fracture
b. Crown root fracture
c. Luxation injuries

## BIBLIOGRAPHY


1. Anderson FM, Anderson JO, Bayer T. Prognosis of root fractured permanent incisors-prediction of healing modalities. Endod dent Traumatol 1989;15:11-22.
2. Anderson JO, Anderson FM, Anderson L, Textbook and color Atlas of Traumatic Injuries to the teeth (4th ed). Copenhagen: Blackwell Publishing 2007.
3. Anderson JO, Borum MK, Jaconsen HL, Andreasen FM. Replantation of 400 avulsed permanent incisors. Factors related to PDL healing. Endod Dent traumatol 1995;11:76-89.
4. Anderson JO. Effect of extra-alveolar period and storage media upon periodontal and pulpal healing after replantation of mature permanent incisors in monkeys. Int J Oral Surg 1981;10:43-53.
5. Andreasen FM, Zhijie Y, Thomsen BL, Andreasen PK. Occurrence of pulp canal obliteration after luxation injuries in the permanent dnetition. Endodon Dent. Traumatol 1987;3:103.
6. Andreasen FM. Pulpal healing after luxation injuries and root fracture in the permanent dentition. Endodon dent traumatol 1989;5:111.
7. Andreason JO, Andreasen FM. Textbook and colour Atlas of traumatic injuries to the teeth (3rd ed). Copenhagen: Munkshaard, 1994.
8. Bancks F, Trope M. Revascularization of immature permanent teeth with apical periodontitis. New treatment protocol? J Endodon 2004;30:196.
9. Barret EJ, Kenny DJ. Avulsed permanent teeth review of literature and treatment guidelines. Endod Dent traumatol 1997;13:153-63.

10. Baume LJ, Holz J. Long term clinical assessment of direct pulp capping. Int Dent 1981;31:251-60.
11. Caliskan MK Turkun M. Clinical investigation of traumatic injuries of permanent incisors in Izmir, Turkiye. Endod Dent. Traumatol 1995;11:210-13.
12. Cavalleri G, Zerman N. Traumatic Crown fractures in permanent incisors with immature roots: a follow-up Study. Endod. Dent. Traumatol 1995;11:294-96.
13. Cohenca N, Stabholz A. Decoronation-A conservative method to treat ankylosed teeth for preservation of alveolar ridge prior to permanent prosthetic reconstruction literature: review and case presentation. Dent Traumatol 2007;23:87-94.
14. Crona-Larson G, Bjarnason S, Noren JG. Effect of luxation injuries on permanent teeth. Endod. Dent. Traumatol 1991;7:199-206.
15. Cvek M, Cleaton-Jones, Austin J, Lownie J, Kling M, Fatti P. Effect of topical application of doxycycline on pulp revascularization and periodontal healing in reimplanted money incisors. Endod Dent traumatol 1990;6:170-77.
16. Cvek M. Cleaton Jones P, Austin P, Andreasen JO. Pulp reactions to exposure after experimental crown fractures or grinding in adult monkeys. J Endod 1982;8:391.
17. Cvek M, Andreasen JO, Bonum MK. Healing of 208 intraalveolar root fractures in patients aged 7-17 years. Dental Traumatology 2001;17:53-62.
18. DCNA Traumatic injuries to the teeth. 1993;39.
19. Donaldson M, Kinirons MJ. Factors affecting the time of onset of resorption in avulsed and replanted incisor teeth in children. Dental Traumatology 2001;17:205-09.
20. Doyle DL, Dumsha TC, Syndiskis RJ. Effect of Soaking in Hank's balanced salt solution (or) milk on PDL cell viability of dry stored human teeth. Endod Dent. Traumatol 1998;14:221-24.
21. Duggal MS, Toumba KJ, Russell JL, Paterson SA. Replantation of avulsed permanent teeth with avital periodontal ligaments. Endod. Dent. Traumatol 1994;10:282-85.
22. Feiglin B. Dental Pulp response to traumatic injuries a retrospective analysis with case reports. Endod Dent Traumatol 1996;12:1-8.
23. Finn. Clinical Pedodontics 4th edition, 1988.
24. Flores MT, Anderson JO. Guidelines for the management of traumatic dental injuries. Part II. Avulsion of permanent teeth. Dent Traumatol 2007;23:130-36.
25. Flores MT, Andreasen JO, Bakland JK. Guidelines for the evaluation and management of traumatic dental injuries. Dent Traumatol 2001;17:145-48.
26. Forman PC, Barnes IE. Review of calcium hydroxide. Int Endod J 1990;23:283-97.
27. Gopikrishna V, Thomas T, Kandaswamy D. Quantitative analysis of coconut water: a new storage media for avulsed tooth. OOOE 2008;15:61-65.
28. Heide S, Kerekes K. Delayed direct pulp capping in permanent incisor of monkey's. Int Endod J 1987;20:65-74.
29. Hiltz J, Trope M. Vitality of human lip fibroblasts in milk, Hank's balanced salt solution and viaspan storage media. Endod Dent Traumatol 1991;7:69-72.
30. Kernohan. Conservative treatment of severely displaced permanent Endod Dent traumatol 1995;11:51-58.
31. Lee JY, Yanpiset K, Sigurdsson A, Van Jr WF. Laser Doppler Flowmetry for Monitoring traumatized teeth. Dental Traumatology 2001;17:231-35.
32. Leroy RLRG, Aps KM, Rates FM, Martens LC, De Boever JA. A Multidisciplinary treatment approach to a complicated maxillary dental trauma. A case report. Endod Dent Traumatol 2000;16:138-42.
33. McDonald. Dentistry of child and adolescent. 5th edition, Mosby, Harwurt Asia, 1987.
34. Muskgaard EC. Enamel-Dentin Crown fractures Bonded with various bonding agents. Endod dent traumatol 1991;7:73-77.
35. Otuyemi OD. Traumatic anterior dental injuries related to incisor overjet and lip competence in 12 year old Nigerian children. International Journal of Paediatric Dentistry 1994;4:81-85.
36. Oulis C, Vadiakas G, Siskos G. Management of intrusive luxation injuries. Endod Dent Traumtol 1996;12:113-19.
37. Oulis CJ, Berdouses ED. Dental injuries of permanent teeth treated in private practice in Athens. Ended. Dent. Traumatol. 1996;12:60-65.
38. PC Lekic, DJ Kenney, EJ Barrett. The influence of storage conditions on the clonogenic capacity of periodontal ligament cells: implications for tooth replantation. International Endodontic Journal 1998;31:137-40.
39. Roberston A, Andreasen FM, Bergenholtz G, Andreasen JO. Long-term prognosis of crown fractures. Effect of stage of root development and association luxation. Int pedo Dent 2000;10:191-99.
40. Rosenstiel SF, et al. Dental luting agents: A review of the current literature. Int J Pedo Dent 2007;17:134-38.
41. Schatz JP, Joho JP. A retrospective study of dento-alveolar injuries. Endod. Dent. Traumatol 1994;10:11-14.
42. Sjorgen U, Hagglund B, Sundqvist G, Wing K. Factors affecting the long term results of endodontic treatment. J Endod 1990;16:498.
43. Spasser HF. Repair and restoration of a fractured, pulpally involved anterior tooth: A case report. J Am Dent Assoc 1977;94:519-20.
44. Torabinejad M, Hong CU, McDonald F, Pitt Ford TR. Physical and chemical properties of a new root end filling material. J Endod 1995;21:349.
45. Torabinejad M, Pitt Ford TR. Bacterial leakage of MTA as a root and filling material. J Endod 1995;21:109.
46. Trope M. Clinical management of avulsed tooth: present strategies and future direction. Dent Traumatol 2002;18:1-11.
47. Yucel Vilmaz, Cigdem Zehir, Ozge Eyuboglu, Nihal Belduzet. Evaluation of success in the reattachment of coronal fractures traumatology. Dent traumatol 2008;24:151-58.

# Pulpal Response to Caries and Dental Procedure

CHAPTER 28



## INTRODUCTION

By definition, pulp is a soft tissue of mesenchymal origin residing within the pulp chamber and root canals of teeth (Fig. 28.1). Some important features of pulp are as follows:

- Pulp is located deep within the tooth, so defies visualization.
- It gives radiographic appearance as radiolucent line (Fig. 28.2).
- Pulp is a connective tissue with several factors making it unique and altering its ability to respond to irritation.
- Normal pulp is a coherent soft tissue, dependent on its normal hard dentin shell for protection and hence, once exposed, extremely sensitive to contact and temperature but this pain does not last for more than 1-2 seconds after the stimulus removed.
- Pulp is totally surrounded by a hard tissue, dentin which limits the area for expansion and restricts the pulp's ability to tolerate edema.

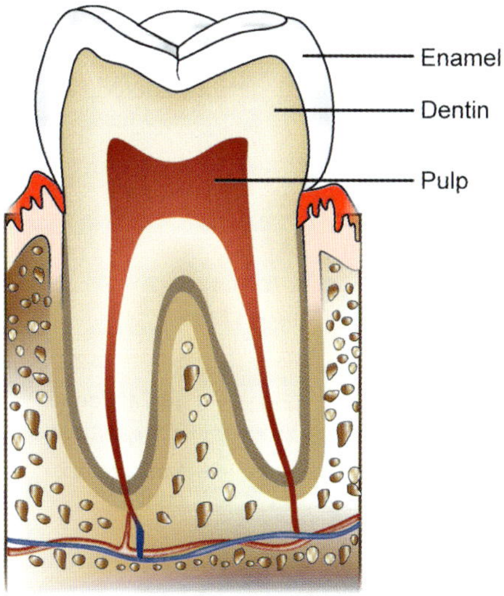


Fig. 28.1: Diagram showing pulp and its relation to surrounding tissues

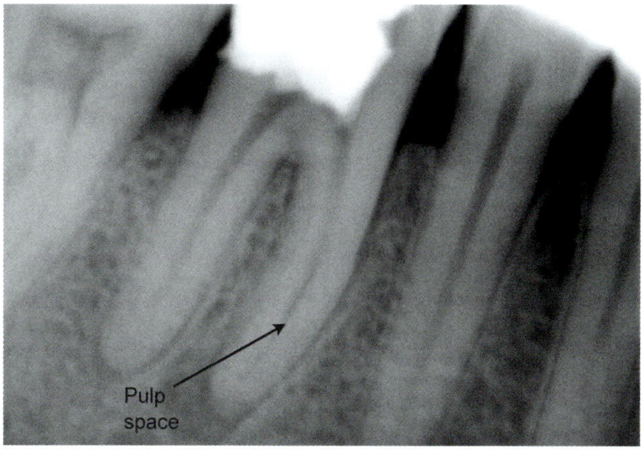


Fig. 28.2: Radiographic appearance of pulp space

- The pulp has almost a total lack of collateral circulation, which severely limits its ability to cope with bacteria, necrotic tissue and inflammation.
- The pulp possesses unique cells the odontoblasts, as well as cells that can differentiate into hard-tissue secreting cells that form more dentin and/or irritation dentin in an attempt to protect itself from injury.

**Why pulp is unique?**
- Enclosed by rigid mineralized dentin so a low compliance environment
- Lacks true collateral blood supply
- Ability to form dentin throughout life
- Potential for regeneration and repair diminishes with age

## PULPAL IRRITANTS

Various pulpal irritants can be:
- **Bacterial irritants:** Most common cause for pulpal irritation are bacteria or their products which may enter pulp through a break in dentin either from:
  - Caries
  - Accidental exposure
  - Fracture
  - Percolation around a restoration
  - Extension of infection from gingival sulcus
  - Periodontal pocket and abscess
  - Anachoresis (Process by which microorganisms get carried by the bloodstream from another source localize on inflamed tissue).
- **Traumatic**
  - Acute trauma like fracture, luxation or avulsion of tooth
  - Chronic trauma including parafunctional habits like bruxism.
- **Iatrogenic:** Various iatrogenic causes of pulpal damage can be:
  - Thermal changes generated by cutting procedures, during restorative procedures, bleaching of enamel, microleakage occurring along the restorations, electrosurgical procedures, laser beam, etc. can cause severe damage to the pulp, if not controlled.
  - Orthodontic movement
  - Periodontal curettage
  - Periapical curettage
  - Use of chemicals like temporary and permanent fillings, liners and bases and use of desiccants such as alcohol.
- **Idiopathic**
  - Aging
  - Resorption—internal or external.

## EFFECT OF DENTAL CARIES ON PULP

Dental caries is the most common route for causing irritation to the pulp. Dental caries is localized, progressive, decay of the teeth characterized by demineralization of the tooth surface by organic acids, produced by microorganisms (Fig. 28.3). From the carious lesion, acids and other toxic substances penetrate through the dentinal tubules to reach the pulp. The following defense reactions take place in a carious tooth to protect the pulp (Fig. 28.4):

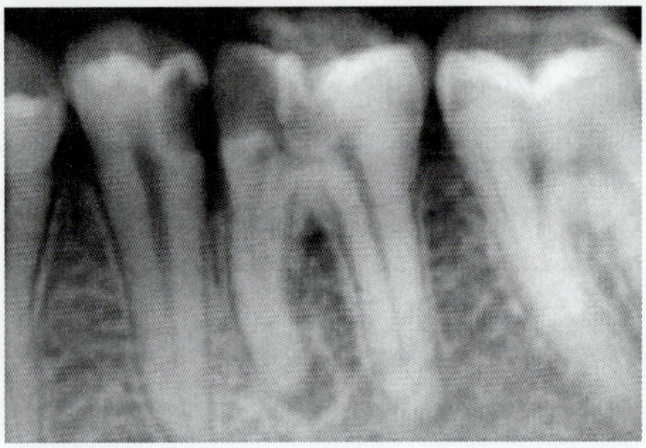

**Fig. 28.3:** Carious exposure of pulp in premolar and molar

1. Formation of reparative dentin.
2. Dentinal sclerosis, i.e. reduction in permeability of dentin by narrowing of dentinal tubules.
3. Inflammatory and immunological reactions.

The rate of reparative dentin formation is related to rate of carious attack. More reparative dentin is formed in response to slow chronic caries than acute caries. For dentin sclerosis to take place, vital odontoblasts must be present within the tubules. In dentin sclerosis, the dentinal tubules are partially or fully filled with mineral deposits, they reduce the permeability of dentin. Therefore, dentinal sclerosis acts as a barrier for the ingress of bacteria and their products.

## INFLAMMATION UNDER CARIES

The bacterial toxins, enzymes, organic acids and the products of tissue destruction show inflammatory response in the pulp. The degree of pulpal inflammation beneath a carious lesion depends on closeness of carious lesions with pulp and permeability of underlying dentin.

The pulp underlying reparative dentin remains relatively normal until the carious process comes close to it. The bacteria are seldom seen in unexposed pulp. When the pulp is exposed, bacteria penetrate the infected dentinal tubule and cause beginning of inflammation of the pulp. The pulp does not become inflamed until the reparative dentin is invaded and wide areas of dentinal tubules are demineralized.

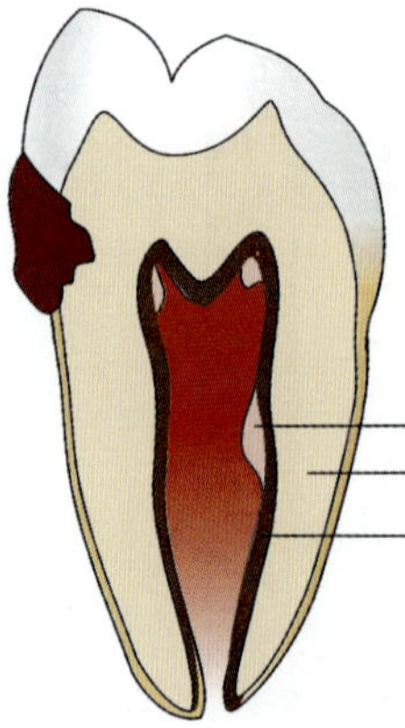


**Fig. 28.4:** Various defense reactions which take place in a carious tooth to protect pulp

The diagnosis of extent of pulpal inflammation under the carious lesion is difficult. Many factors play an important role in determining the nature of carious process in hard dental tissues. The rate of carious process is influenced by following factors:

a. Cariogenicity of the diet
b. Composition of the tooth
c. Salivary flow
d. Type of bacterial flora
e. Oral hygiene
f. Age of the person
g. Buffering capacity of the saliva
h. Antibacterial substances present in saliva.

The early evidence of pulpal reaction to caries is seen in underlying odontoblastic layer. There is reduction in number and size of odontoblast cell bodies, change in the shape of odontoblasts, i.e. from tall and columnar to flat and cuboidal before any inflammatory changes seen in pulp. Concomitant with the changes in odontoblastic layer, hyperchromatic line may develop along the pulpal margin of the dentin, which indicates disturbance in normal equilibrium of the odontoblasts. In addition to dentinal changes, antibodies are also produced by the pulp. These antibodies act against the antigenic component of dental caries. Immunoglobulins IgG, IgM, IgA, complement components, etc. found in the odontoblasts and adjacent pulp cells are capable of reacting against the invading microorganisms. The presence of bacterial antigens and immunoglobulins emphasize the involvement of specific immunologic reactions during carious process. The persistence of dental caries provides a continuous stimulus for an inflammatory response in dental pulp. The pulp protects itself in many ways like by formation of sclerotic dentin and elaboration of reparative dentin, etc.

In acute caries, the caries progress more rapidly than the formation of reparative dentin and chronic inflammatory cells become apparent in the pulp tissue. Initially they are small in number but as the carious lesion comes closer to pulp, more and more plasma cells, macrophages and lymphocytes are seen in pulp. Finally, the pulp gets exposed (Figs 28.5A to C).

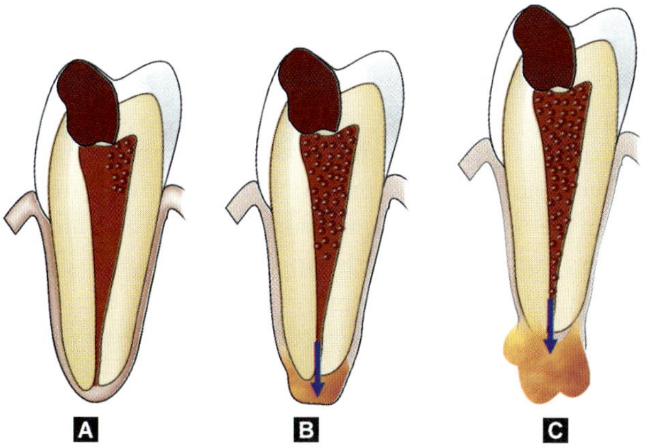


**Figs 28.5A to C:** Sequele of caries: (A) Small number of bacteria close to pulp, (B) As caries progress close to pulp, inflammation starts with more of plasma cells, macrophages and lymphocytes, (C) Exposure of pulp by caries. Site of exposure shows small abscess consisting of dead inflammatory cells and other cells

The pulp reacts at site of exposure with infiltration of inflammatory cells. In the region of exposure, small abscess develops consisting of dead inflammatory cells and other cells. The remainder of the pulp may be uninflamed or if the exposure is present for a long-time, the pulp gets converted into granulation tissue. The chronic inflammation can be partial or complete, depending upon the extent and amount of pulp tissue involved.

As the exposure progresses, partial necrosis of pulp may be followed by total pulp necrosis (Fig. 28.6). The drainage is one of the important factors which determines whether partial or total necrosis of the pulp occurs. If pulp is open to oral fluids, the drainage occurs and apical pulp tissue remains uninflamed. But if the drainage is not possible, entire pulp may become necrotic.

## RESPONSE OF PULP TO TOOTH PREPARATION

The principle aim of operative dentistry is to preserve as much of healthy tissue as possible to enable pulp to respond to future episodes of disease or iatrogenic trauma. Pulpal inflammation resulting from the operative procedures is often termed as ***dentistogenic pulpitis***.

**Factors affecting response of pulp to tooth preparation**

- Pressure
- Heat
- Vibration
- Remaining dentin thickness
- Thermal and mechanical injury
- Speed
- Nature of cutting instruments.

### Irritating Agents of Tooth Preparation

A tooth preparation introduces a number of irritating factors to the pulp (Fig. 28.7). The actual cutting of dentin, in as much as every square mm contains 30,000 to 45,000 dentinal tubules can irritate many millions of odontoblasts.

The ***pressure*** of instrumentation on exposed dentin characteristically causes the aspiration of the nuclei of the odontoblasts or the entire odontoblasts themselves or nerve endings from pulp tissues into the dentinal tubules. This will

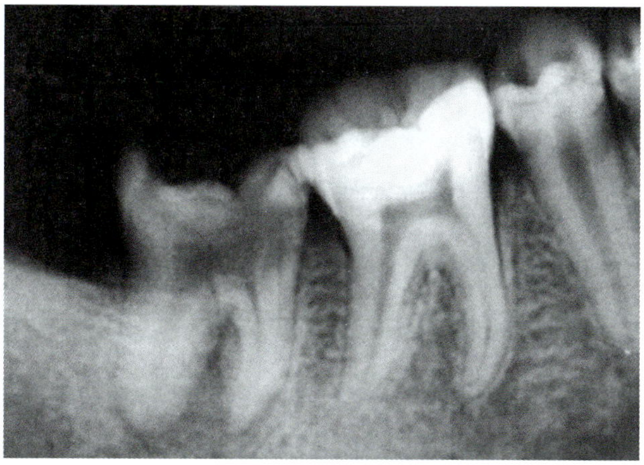

**Fig. 28.6:** Radiograph showing necrotic 37

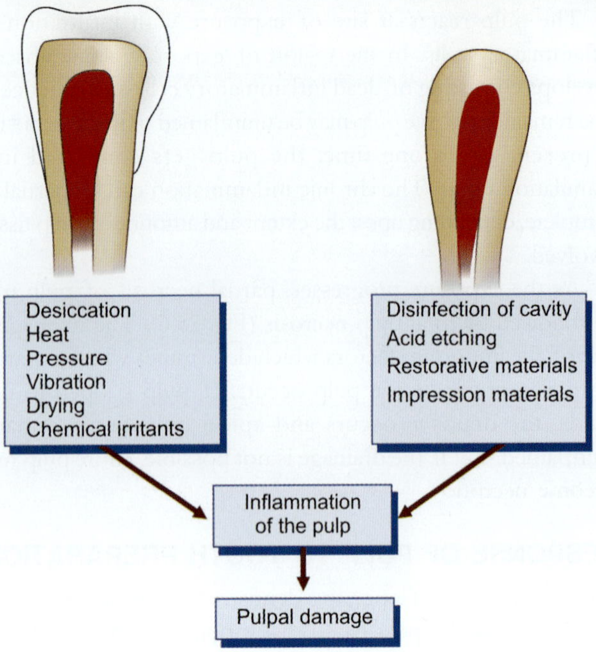


**Fig. 28.7:** Effect of irritants on pulp

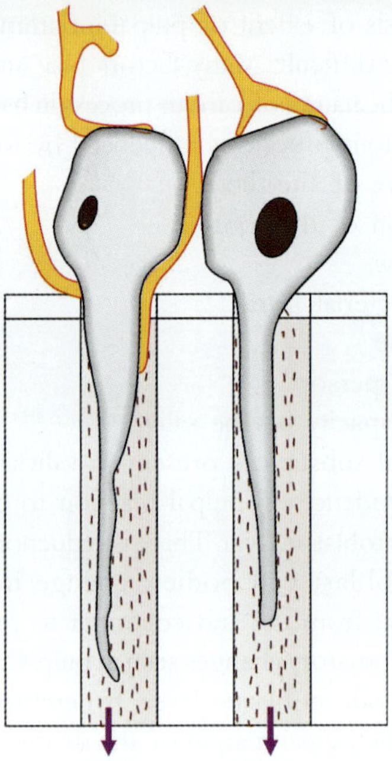

**Fig. 28.8:** Aspiration of odontoblasts into tubules due to desiccation

obviously stimulate odontoblasts, disturb their metabolism and may lead to their complete degeneration and disintegration. This can occur by excessive pressure of hand or rotary instruments, especially in decreased effective depths. Sometimes this pressure may move some microorganisms from infected cavity floor or wall into the pulp, leading to its irritation.

The type of cutting instruments used has variable irritating factors. Sharp hand-cutting instruments in which the energy used with them is completely dissipated in the actual cutting are the most biologically acceptable cutting instruments.

Rotary cutting instruments are also biologically acceptable, if used over effective depths of 2 mm and more, and with proper coolants. This is true with carbide than with steel burs, as the former are more cool-cutting than the latter. Rotary abrasive instruments are not recommended for cutting in vital dentin, as their abrasive action elevates the temperature of surrounding dentin. This is because the energy used to abrade is more than that used to cut. Rotary abrasive instruments may also crush vital dentin much more than any other cutting instruments. Therefore, abrasive actions should be confined to the enamel and the superficial 1 mm of the dentin, as much as possible.

The depth of the cavity is the most disadvantageous exasperating factor to the pulp. Most important is the thickness of the dentin bridge between the floor of the cavity and the roof of the pulp chamber, also termed as the effective depth. Lesser is the effective depth, more destructive the pulpal response will be.

***Heat production*** is the second most damaging factor. If the pulp temperature is elevated by 11°F, destructive reaction will occur even in a normal, vital periodontal organ. Lesser temperatures can precipitate similar responses in already irritated organs. That ***"heat"*** is a function of:

a. *RPM,* i.e. more the RPM more is the heat production. The most deleterious speed is from 3,000 to 30,000 rpm. In deep penetrations of dentin without using coolants, e.g. pin holes, the cutting speed must not exceed 3,000 rpm.
b. ***Pressure*** is directly proportional to heat generation. Whenever, the RPM's are increased, pressure must be correspondingly reduced. Instrumentation pressure should not be more than four ounce when using high speed and twelve ounce when using low speed.
c. ***Surface area of contact***, which is related to the size and shape of the revolving tool. The more the contact between the tooth structures and revolving tool, the more is the heat generation. Heat creates destruction in the pulp tissues, coagulate protoplasm, and burn dentin if the temperature is amply elevated.
d. ***Desiccation***, if occurring in vital dentin such that water in the protoplasm of Tome's fibers is eliminated, can cause aspiration of the odontoblasts into the tubules (Fig. 28.8). The subsequent disturbances in their metabolism may lead to the complete degeneration of odontoblasts. Desiccation increases the permeability of the vital dentin to irritants like microorganisms or restorative materials. So care must be taken to keep a prepared tooth moist during preparation. If air alone is applied, remove only debris and extra moisture from the operative field, and not the dentin's own moisture. A spray of air and water is satisfactory coolant to dislodge attached debris. Coolant sprays should be used even in non-vital or devitalized tooth structures, since the heat will burn the tooth structures, and these burnt areas will be sequestrated later leaving a space around the restoration where failures can occur.

***Vibrations*** which are measured by their amplitude or their capacity and frequency (the number/unit time) are an indication of eccentricity in rotary instruments. The higher the amplitude, the more destructive may be the response of the pulp. The reaction is termed as the ***rebound response*** which is due to the effect of the ultrasonic energy induced. It is characterized by:

1. Disruption of the odontoblasts in the opposite side of the pulp chamber from where the cavity is prepared.
2. Edema
3. Fibrosis of pulp tissues proper.
4. Changes in ground substance.

In addition to affecting the pulp tissues, vibration can create microcracks in enamel and dentin. These cracks may transmit and coalesce, directly joining the oral environment with pulp and periodontal tissues. Vibrations also increase the permeability of the dentin and enamel. The extensiveness of preparation or preparation time is directly related to the extensiveness of the reaction of the periodontal organ, for example a crown preparation will cause more response in the pulp than a Class I preparation. Not all persons will have the same reaction towards the same irritant. Also the individual variations in pulpal response can occur that is teeth in the same person can react in a different way towards the identical irritant. This is because of multiple factors like cellularity and vascularity of the pulp, age, heredity, and other unknown factors. The ultimate effect on periodontal organ is due to a cumulative effect of decay, cavity preparation, instrumentation, placement of the restorative materials and finishing procedures. So during a tooth preparation it should always be remembered that the periodontal organ has been already irritated before the instrumentation and it is going to be more irritated by the restoration procedures.

### Factors Affecting the Response of Pulp to Irritants

- Cellularity of the pulp
- Vascularity of the pulp
- Age
- Heredity
- Unknown factors.

## REMAINING DENTIN THICKNESS

Remaining dentin thickness (RDT) between the floor of the cavity preparation and the pulp chamber is one of the most important factors in determining the pulpal response. This measurement differs from the depth of cavity preparation since the pulpal floor in deeper cavities on larger teeth may be far from the pulp than that in shallow cavities on smaller teeth.

- In human teeth dentin is approximately 3 mm thick.
- Dentin permeability increases with decreasing RDT.
- RDT of 2 mm or more effectively precludes restorative damage to the pulp.
- At RDT of 0.75 mm, effects of bacterial invasion are seen.
- When RDT is 0.25 mm odontoblastic cell death is seen.

The amount of remaining dentin underneath the cavity preparation plays the most important role in the incidence of a pulp response. Generally, 2 mm of dentin thickness between the floor of the cavity preparation and the pulp will provide an adequate insulting barrier against irritants (Fig. 28.9). As the dentin thickness decreases the pulp response increases. It is seen that response of cutting occurs only in areas beneath freshly cut dentinal tubules not lined with reparative or irregular dentin. In presence of reparative dentin only minimal response will occur.

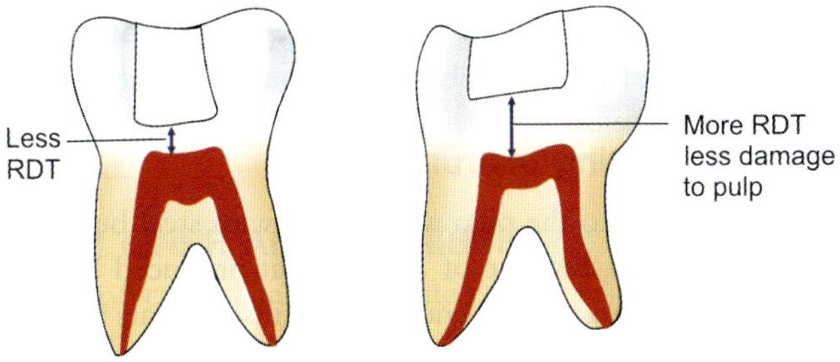

Fig. 28.9: As the remaining dentin thickness decreases, the pulp response increases

**Pulp protection according to remaining dentin thickness (RDT)**

| Value of RDT | Pulp protection |
|---|---|
| ≥ 2 mm | Use of varnish only |
| 1.5 – 2 mm | Varnish + Base |
| < 1.5 mm | Varnish + Base |
| 0.5 mm | Sub base + Base + Varnish |

## THERMAL AND MECHANICAL INJURY

Cutting of dentin with bur or stone always produces some amount of heat which is determined by several factors such as:

i. Size and shape of the cutting instrument.
ii. Speed of rotation.
iii. Length of time, the instrument is in contact with dentin.
iv. Amount of pressure exerted.

To reduce the effect of heat on the pulp, proper cooling should be done along with cutting. As the thermal conductivity of dentin is relatively low, there are less chances of injury to the pulp in deep tooth preparation than shallow tooth preparation. Production of heat is most severe stress for pulp. If higher temperature is reached during cutting procedures, there are chances of severe damage of pulp. If damage is extensive, cell rich zone would be destroyed and chances of reparative dentin formation become less.

Blushing of teeth during or after cavity or crown preparation has been seen in teeth after cutting. After dentin is cut, the coronal dentin develops pinkish hue and this hue is due to vascular stasis in the sub-odontoblastic layer.

### Speed of Rotation

Ultra high speed should be used for removal of enamel and superficial dentin. A speed of 3,000 to 30,000 rpm without coolant can cause pulpal damage. It should be kept in mind that without the use of coolant there is no safe speed. High speed cutting is disadvantageous when burs are countersunk into the dentin, since water is excluded in a confined region.

oxide eugenol has been used as an anodyne for pulpal pain. The sedative effects are apparently because of ability of eugenol to block or reduce nerve impulse activity. This effect is obtained only when a reasonably thin mix of ZOE is used. Another advantage of ZOE is that there is no heat rise during setting.

Its disadvantages as a temporary filling material are:

a. Its softness
b. Long setting time
c. The ease with which it may be displaced by biting stress before setting.

## Zinc Phosphate

Zinc phosphate cement can cause severe pulpal damage because of its irritating properties. Toxicity is more pronounced when the cement is placed in deep cavity preparations. In deep cavities, zinc phosphate cement should not be used without an intervening liner of zinc oxide eugenol or calcium hydroxide. Thick mixes should be used to minimize pulp irritation and marginal leakage. The pulp may be affected by the components of the material, the heat that is liberated in setting, and the marginal leakage that permits the ingress of irritants from saliva. The pulpal injury from the cement is mainly due to marginal leakage rather than to its toxic chemical properties.

Effect of zinc phosphate on pulp are due to:

- Components of zinc phosphate
- Acidic nature
- Heat produced during setting
- Marginal leakage.

## Routes of Microleakage

- Within or via the smear layer
- Between the smear layer and the cavity varnish/cement
- Between the cavity varnish/cement and restorative material

## Zinc Polycarboxylate Cements (Fig. 28.14)

Zinc polycarboxylate cement contains modified zinc oxide powder and an aqueous solution of polyacrylic acid. It chemically bonds to enamel and dentin and has antibacterial properties. Polycarboxylate cement is well tolerated by the pulp, being roughly equivalent to zinc oxide eugenol cements in this respect.

## Glass Ionomer Cement

It possess anticariogenic properties and is well tolerated by the pulp. Toxicity diminishes with setting time. Its pH at mixing is 2.33 and after 24 hours it is 5.67.

## Amalgam

Amalgam has been used in dentistry since ages. It is considered one of the safest filling materials with least irritating properties. Even if varnish is not employed, within a period of a few weeks, marginal seal develops between the tooth and the restoration due to its corrosion products. It has been shown to produce discomfort due to its high thermal conductivity. So liners or bases are necessary to provide thermal insulation.

## Effects of Amalgam on Pulp

- Mild to moderate inflammation in deep caries
- Harmful effects due to corrosion products
- Inhibition of reparative dentin formation due to damage to odontoblasts
- Copper in high copper alloy is toxic
- High mercury content exerts cytotoxic effects on pulp
- Postoperative thermal sensitivity due to high thermal conductivity.

## Precautions to be taken while using Amalgam as a Restorative Material

1. Use of cavity liner or base under the silver-amalgam restoration (Fig. 28.15).
2. Use of varnish at the margins of preparation (Fig. 28.16).

Postoperative sensitivity of amalgam occurs because of expansion and contraction of fluid present in the gap between amalgam and the cavity wall. This fluid communicates with fluid in subjacent dentinal tubule. Any variation in temperature will cause axial movement of fluid in the tubules which further stimulates the nerve fibres, thus causing pain.

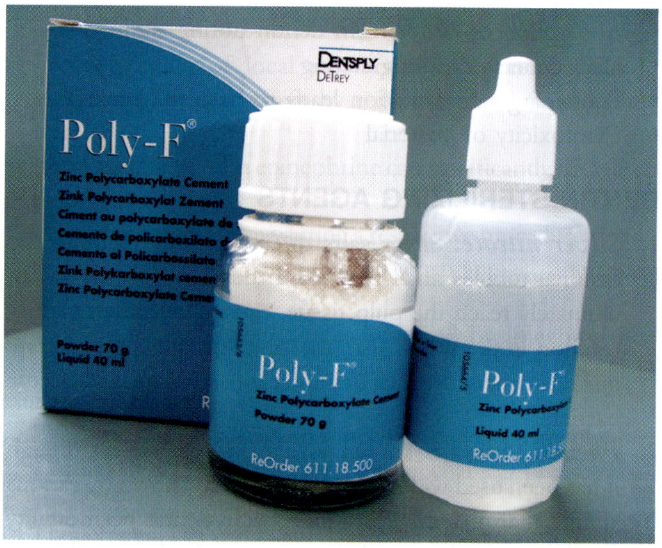


**Fig. 28.14:** Zinc polycarboxylate cement

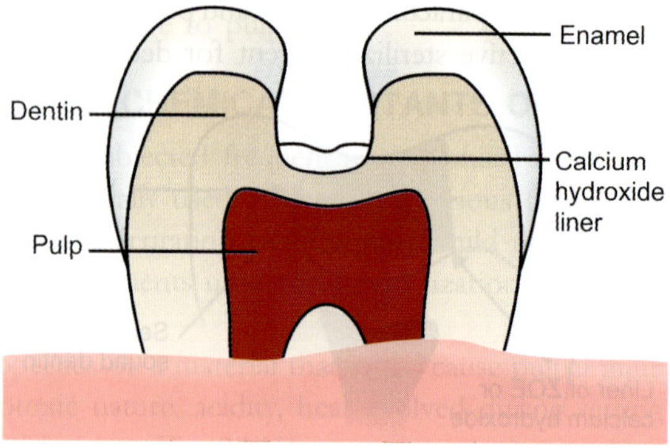


**Fig. 28.15:** Use of liner under amalgam restoration

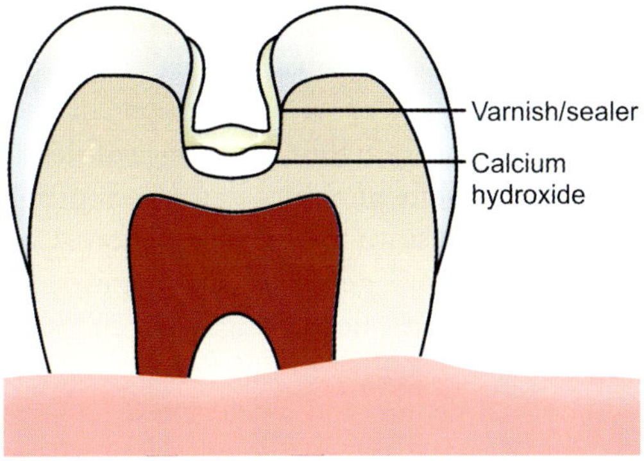


Fig. 28.16: Use of varnish at the walls of preparation

## RESTORATIVE RESINS

Restorative resins have been used in dentistry for past many years. Despite having several advantages, they are not considered best materials because of their high coefficient of thermal expansion and polymerization shrinkage, which results in marginal leakage, subsequently the recurrent caries and ultimately the pulp damage. Monomer present in composite resins also acts as an irritant to the pulp. Though marginal seal can be improved by acid etching of beveled enamel and the use of bonding agent or primer, studies have shown that initial marginal leakage tends to deteriorate as the etched composite restoration ages.

Newer composite materials, filler systems, catalysts and methods of curing, have shown improvement in polymerization characteristics and lower coefficient of thermal expansion but still many researches have shown that all composite resins irritate pulp though to different degrees. Some have been found more irritating than the others. It has been seen that unlined composite resins are harmful to the pulp because of bacterial contamination beneath the restoration so the use of cavity liner is advocated under composite restoration (Fig. 28.17).

**Prevention of pulpal injury**

| *Irritant/Procedure* | *Method to prevent pulpal injury* |
|---|---|
| Tooth preparation | • Effective cooling<br>• High speed ration<br>• Intermittent cutting |
| Restorative material | Use material after considering physical and biological properties according to tooth preparation. |
| Marginal leakage | • Pulp protection using liners and bases<br>• Use of bonding agents |
| While insertion | Avoid application of excessive forces of restoration |
| While polishing | Effective cooling to avoid heat generation during polishing |
| Irritants to dentin | Avoid application of any irritant, desiccant on freshly cut dentin |

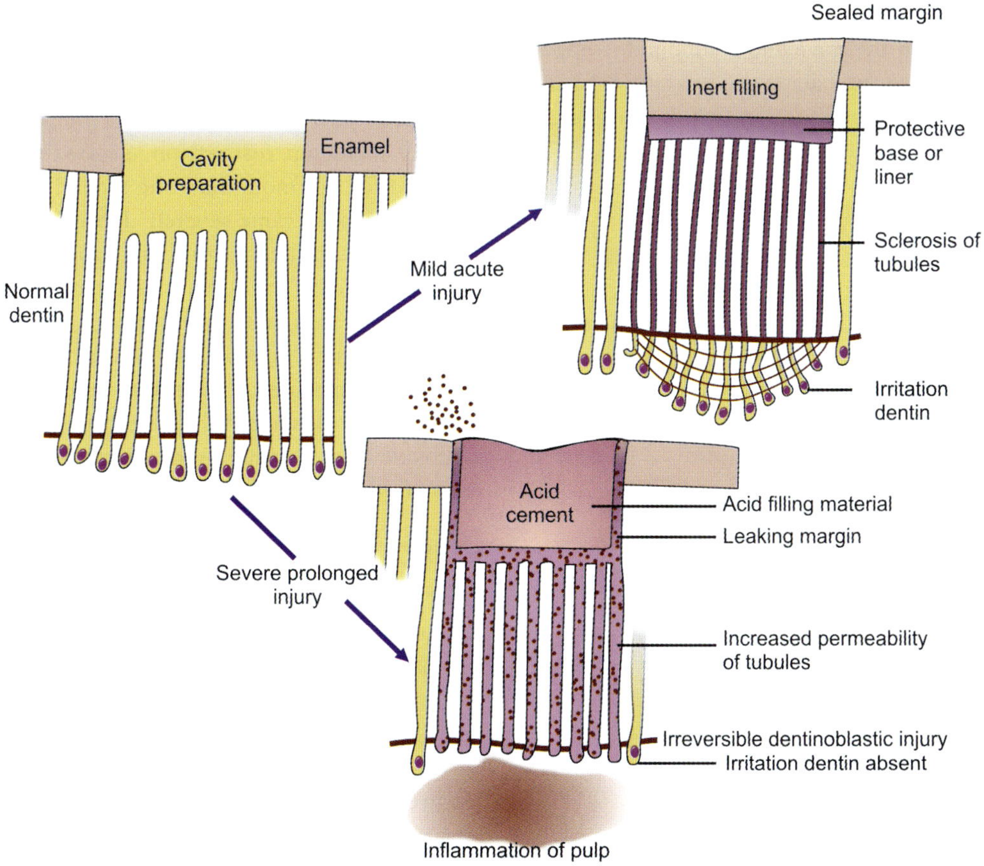


Fig. 28.17: Response of pulpodentinal complex to mild and severe injury

Liners containing calcium hydroxide have shown to provide good protection against bacteria. Zinc oxide eugenol liners should not be used with composite resins since they interfere with polymerization of composites.

### Acid Etchants

Acid etching is an important step in the placement of composite restorations. Commonly used acid etchant is 37 percent phosphoric acid. It has been shown that acid etching does not cause pulpal injury. Etching results in opening of the dentinal tubules and increases dentin permeability. On the contrary acid etching also enhances bacterial penetration of dentinal tubules.

## EFFECTS OF PIN INSERTION

Pins are used in amalgam restoration for building up badly broken tooth or to support amalgam restoration (Fig. 28.18). The insertion of pin results in:

i. Dentinal fractures and unnoticed pulp exposure.
ii. Increases the pulp irritation of already stressed pulp (inflammation of pulp directly proportioned to depth, extensiveness of decay).
iii. Cements used for pins add more irritation to the pulp.

To reduce continued irritation from the pins, use of calcium hydroxide is recommended.

## IMPRESSION MATERIAL

The taking of impressions for inlay and crown fabrication also exposes the pulp to serious hazards. Seltzer et al showed that pulpal trauma can occur when more pressure is applied while taking impression. When the modeling compound is applied to the cavity or full crown preparation, a pressure is exerted on pulp. Also the negative pressure created in removing an impression may cause odontoblastic aspiration.

## EFFECTS OF RADIATIONS ON PULP

The basic cellular effect of ionizing radiation is interference with cell division. Radiation damage to teeth depends on dose, source, and type of radiation, exposure factors, and stage of tooth development at the time of irradiation. In developing human teeth, the extent of damage depends on the amount of radiation and the stage of tooth development at the time of irradiation. Heavy doses at the earliest stage of development can cause complete failure of the tooth to develop; mild doses can result in root end distortions and dilacerations. Circulatory disturbances in the tooth germ are also manifested by the presence of dilated vessels, hemorrhages and endothelial cells swelling. The odontoblasts fail to function normally and may elaborate abnormal dentin, and amelogenesis is retarded or ceases. In the later stages, fibrosis or atrophy of the pulp may occur. The pulps of fully formed human teeth may be affected in patients who are exposed to radiation therapy. Relative dosage, mature odontoblasts appear to be extremely radioresistant. However, in time, the pulp cells exposed to the ionizing radiation may become necrotic. The effects appear to be related to vascular damage and interference with mitosis of cells. The salivary glands are also affected.

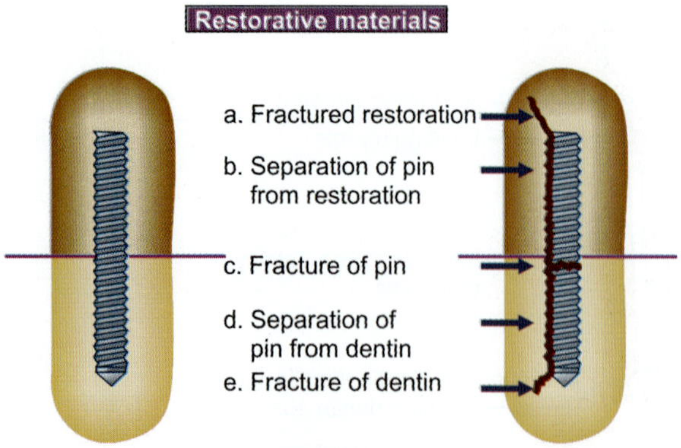


**Fig. 28.18:** Five different locations where pin-restoration failures can occur

### Effects of Radiations

- Interference with cell division
- Mild dose can cause root end distortions and dilacerations
- Heavy doses at the earliest stage of development can cause complete failure of tooth to develop
- Abnormal dentin formation is seen in some cases
- Retardation or cessation of enamel formation
- Fibrosis or atrophy of the pulp
- Salivary glands are also affected.

## EFFECT OF HEAT FROM ELECTROSURGERY

Heat may be delivered to the pulp by electrosurgical gingivoplasty. In a study it was seen that when the electrode tip contacted Class V amalgam restoration electrosurgical current was delivered for not more than one second with a fully rectified unit, the pulps became severely damaged. But no damage to the pulp was noticed from the application of current to unrestored teeth. The contact of the activated electrode with the gingival restorations to no more than 0.2 to 0.4 seconds would be more compatible with clinical usage. However, longer periods of exposure to the electrosurgical currents produced severe pulpal damage. Even the placement of the calcium hydroxide base, covered by copal varnish, under the metallic restorations did not prevent pulpal damage.

## EFFECT OF LASERS ON PULP

Laser damage to pulps varies with the intensity of the energy. Larger doses consistently produced pulp necrosis. Pulp damage was manifested by coagulation necrosis of the odontoblast, edema and occasional inflammatory cell infiltration. Commonly used lasers in operative dentistry are Nd: YAG and $CO_2$ laser. They are used to remove caries, modify dentin to treat hypersensitivity and to eliminate pit and fissures. Mode of action in hypersensitivity teeth is by altering dentin surface, blocking dentinal tubules and by melting and glazing dentin. It may be also due to the transient anesthesia due to permanent damage to sensory nerves.

## DEFENSE MECHANISM OF PULP

### Tubular Sclerosis

The peritubular dentin becomes wider gradually filling the tubules with calcified material progressing with the dentinoenamel junction pulpally. These areas are harder, denser, less sensitive and more protective to the pulp against subsequent irritation. Sclerosis resulting from aging is physiological dentin sclerosis and resulting from mild irritation is reactive dentin sclerosis.

### Smear Layer

Smear layer is an amorphous debris layer consisting of both organic and inorganic constituents which are formed during operative procedures. Smear layer decreases both sensitivity and permeability of dentinal tubules. Smear layer is an iatrogenically produced layer that reduces permeability better than any of the varnishes.

**Defense mechanism of the pulp**

- Tubular sclerosis
- Smear layer
- Reparative dentin formation
  - i. Healthy reparative reaction
  - ii. Unhealthy reparative reaction
  - iii. Destructive reaction.

### Reparative Dentin Formation (Fig. 28.19)

1. ***Healthy reparative reaction:*** This is the most favorable response and it consists of stimulating the periodontal organ to form sclerotic dentin. These are followed by normal secondary dentin containing dentinal tubules. Secondary dentin is different from primary dentin, in that the tubules of secondary dentin are slightly deviated from the tubules of the primary dentin. The healthy reparative reactions occur without any disturbances in the pulp tissues.
2. ***Unhealthy reparative reaction:*** This response begins with degeneration of the odontoblasts. This is followed by the formation of the dead tract in the dentin and complete cessation in the formation of secondary dentin. The unhealthy reparative response is accompanied by mild pathological and clinical changes of a reversible nature in the pulp tissues, resulting in the formation of an irregular type of tertiary dentin. The tertiary dentin formation is considered to be the function of the pulp tissue proper. However, tertiary dentin has certain limitations. It is not completely impervious like the calcific barrier. Also, the rapid formation of tertiary dentin will lead to the occupation of part of the pulp chamber with tissues other than those normally responsible for repair, metabolism and innervations. Thus tertiary dentin is said to "age the pulp", reducing its capacity for further defensive action against irritation. This is very important clinically, because if this reaction occurs as a result of a carious process, the restoration of this tooth may not be favorable, received by the periodontal organ.
3. ***Destructive reaction:*** This is the most unfavorable pulpal response to irritation. It begins with the loss of odontoblasts and the outer protective layer of the pulp which ultimately involves the pulp tissue proper, exceeding its reparative capacity. The resulting tissue reaction will be inflammation, which may progress to abscess formation, chronic inflammation and finally, complete necrosis of the pulp. In any event, the pulp tissues cannot recover from these pathologic changes and removal of these tissues or the whole tooth becomes necessary.

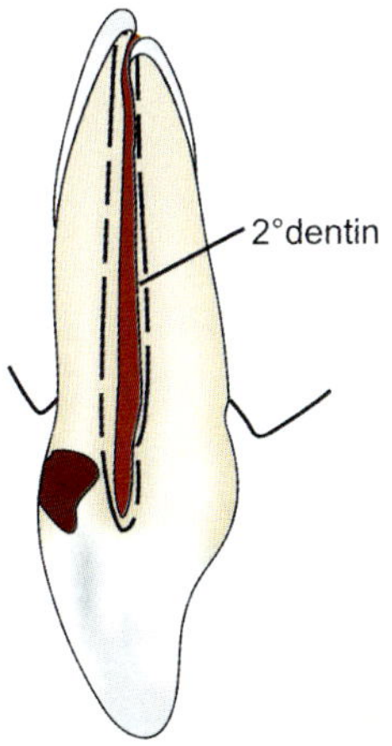


**Fig. 28.19:** Formation of secondary dentin in response to irritation

#### *Prevention of Pulpal Damage due to Operative Procedure*

- To preserve the integrity of the pulp, the dentist should observe certain precautions while rendering treatment.
- Excessive force should not be applied during insertion of restoration.
- Restorative materials should be selected carefully, considering the physical and biological properties of the material.
- Excessive heat production should be avoided while polishing procedures.
- Avoid applying irritating chemicals to freshly cut dentin.
- Use varnish or base before insertion of restoration.
- Patient should be called on recall basis for periodic evaluation of status of the pulp.

## HOW DOES PULP RECOVER?

- As tissue pressure increases from increased blood flow, arteriovenous anastomoses (AVAs) open and shunt blood before it reaches an inflamed region, thus preventing a further increase in blood flow and tissue pressure.
- Increase in tissue pressure pushes macromolecules back into bloodstream via venules in the adjacent healthy pulp.
- Once macromolecules and excess fluid leave the extracellular tissue space via venule, tissue pressure decreases and normal blood flow is restored.

## QUESTIONS

**Q. What is defence mechanism of pulp to various irritants?**

**Q. Write short notes on:**

a. Pulpal response to caries
b. Effect of tooth preparation on pulp.

## BIBLIOGRAPHY


1. Bergenholtz G, Cox CF, Loesche WJ, Syed SA. Bacterial leakage around dental restorations: Its effect on the dental pulp. J Oral Pathol 1982;11:439-50.
2. C Ehreli ZC, Onur MA, Tas, Man E, Gümrükeüoglu A, Artuner H. Effects of current and potential dental etchants on nerve compound action potentials. J Endod 2002;28:149-51.
3. Costa CAS, Hebling J, Hanks CT. Current status of pulp capping with dentin adhesive systems: a review. Dent mater 2000;16:188-97.
4. Costa CAS, Teixeira HM, Nascimento ABL, Hebling J. Biocompatibility of two current adhesive resins. J Endod 2000;26:512-16.
5. Cox CF; Sü Bay RK, Ostro E, Suzuki SH. Tunnel defects in dentin bridges; their formation following direct pulp capping. Oper Dent 1996;21:4-11.
6. Demarco FF, Tarquino SBC, Jaeger MMM, Araujo VC, Matson E. Pulp response and cytotoxicity evaluation of 2 dentin bonding agents. Quintessence. Int 2001;32:211-20.
7. Goldberg M, Six N, Decup F, Lasfargues JJ, Salih E, Tompkins K, Veis A. Bioactive molecules and the future of pulp therapy. Am J Dent 2003;16:66-76.
8. Hafez AA, Cox CF, Tarim B, Otsuki M, Akimoto N. An in vivo evaluation of hemorrhage control using sodium hypochlorite and direct capping with a one- or two-component adhesive systems in exposed non-human primate pulps. Quintessence Int 2002;33:261-72.
9. Hebling J, Aparecida EM, de Souza Costa CA. Biocompatibility of an adhesive system applied to exposed human dental pulp. J Endod 1999;25:676-82.
10. Heys DR, Fitzgerald M, Heys RJ, Chiego DJ. Healing of primate dental pulps capped with Teflon. Oral Surg Oral Med Oral Pathol Oral Radiol Endod 1990;69:227-37.
11. Kitamura C, Ogawa Y, Morotomi T, Terashita M. Differential induction of apoptosis by capping agent during pulp wound healing. J Endod 2003;29:41-43.
12. Kitasako Y, Inokoshi S, Tagami J. Effects of direct resin capping techniques on short-term mechanically exposed pulps. J Dent 1999;27:257-63.
13. Pereira JC, Segala AD, Costa CAS. Human pulpal response to direct pulp capping with an adhesive system. Am J Dent 2000;13:139-47.
14. Pitt Ford TR. Pulpal response to a calcium hydroxide material for capping exposures. Oral Surg Oral Med Oral Pathol Oral Radiol Endod 1985;59:194-97.
15. Schöder U. Effects of calcium hydroxide-containing pulp capping agents on pulp cell migration proliferation and differentiation. J Dent Res 1985;64:541-48.
16. Schuurs AHB, Gruythuysen RJM, Wesselink PR. Pulp capping with adhesive resin-based composite vs. calcium hydroxide: a review. Endod Dent Tramatol 2000;16:240-50.
17. Stanley HR. Pulp capping. Conserving the dental pulp. Can it be done? Is it worth it? Oral Surg Oral Med Oral Pathol Oral Radiol Endod 1989;68:628-39.
18. Yoshiba K, Yoshiba N, Nakamura H, Iwaku M, Ozawa H. Immunolocalization of finronectin during reparative dentinogenesis in human teeth after pulp capping with calcium hydroxide. J Dent Res 1996;75:1590-97.

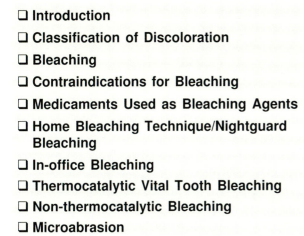

# Management of Discolored Teeth

CHAPTER 29



## INTRODUCTION

In the pursuit of looking good, man has always tried to beautify his face. Since, the alignment and appearance of teeth influence the personality, they have received considerable attention.

Tooth discoloration varies in etiology, appearance, localization, severity and adherence to tooth structure. It may be classified as intrinsic, extrinsic and combination of both. Intrinsic discoloration is caused by incorporation of chromatogenic material into dentin and enamel during odontogenesis or after tooth eruption. Exposure to high levels of fluoride, tetracycline administration, inherited developmental disorders and trauma to the developing tooth may result in pre-eruptive discoloration. After eruption of the tooth, aging and pulp necrosis are the main causes of intrinsic discoloration.

Coffee, tea, red wine, carrots and tobacco give rise to extrinsic stains. Wear of the tooth structure, deposition of secondary dentin due to aging or as a consequence of pulp inflammation and dentin sclerosis affect the light-transmitting properties of teeth, resulting in a gradual darkening of the teeth.

Scaling and polishing of the teeth removes many extrinsic stains. For more stubborn extrinsic discoloration and intrinsic stain, a variety of tooth whitening options are available today, these include over-the-counter whitening systems, whitening tooth pastes and the latest option laser tooth whitening.

Currently available tooth whitening options are:

1. Office bleaching procedures.
2. At home bleaching kits.
3. Composite veneers.
4. Porcelain veneers.
5. Whitening toothpastes.

Among these procedures, bleaching procedures are more conservative than restorative methods, simple to perform and less expensive.

This chapter reviews discoloration and its correction. Following aspects of discoloration and bleaching procedures are discussed in this chapter:

1. Etiology and types of discoloration.
2. Commonly used medicaments for bleaching.
3. External bleaching technique, i.e. bleaching in teeth with vital pulp.
4. Internal bleaching technique, i.e. usually performed in nonvital teeth.
5. Efficacy and performance of each procedure.
6. Possible complications and safety of various procedures.

Before discussing, bleaching of the discolored teeth, we should be familiar with the color of natural healthy teeth. Teeth are polychromatic so color varies among the gingival, incisal and cervical areas according to the thickness, reflections of different colors and translucency of enamel and dentin

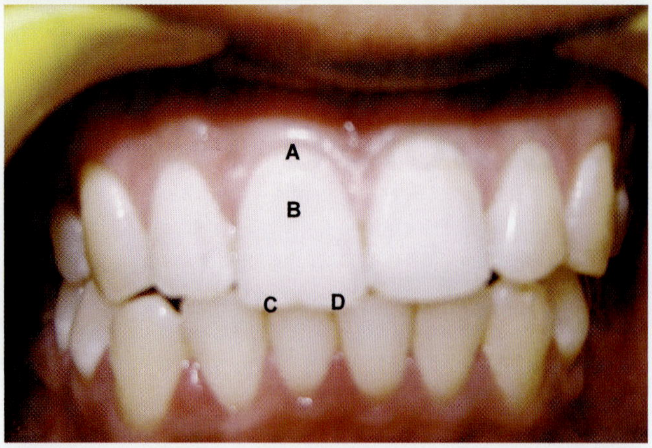

Fig. 29.1: Normal anatomical landmarks of tooth; (A) Cervical margin; (B) Body of tooth; (C) Incisal edge; (D) Translucency of enamel

(Fig. 29.1). Color of healthy teeth is primarily determined by the translucency and color of dentin and is modified by:
- Color of enamel covering the crown.
- Translucency of enamel which varies with different degrees of calcification.
- Thickness of enamel which is greater at the occlusal/incisal edge of the tooth and thinner at the cervical third. That is why teeth are more darker on cervical one-third than at middle or incisal one-third.

Normal color of primary teeth is bluish white whereas color of permanent teeth is grayish yellow, grayish white or yellowish white.

## CLASSIFICATION OF DISCOLORATION

Tooth discoloration varies with etiology, appearance, localization, severity and adherence to the tooth structure. It may be classified as extrinsic or intrinsic discoloration or combination. Feinman et al 1987, describes extrinsic discoloration as that occurring when an agent or stain damages the enamel surface of the teeth. Extrinsic staining can be easily removed by a normal prophylactic cleaning. Intrinsic staining is defined as endogenous staining that has been incorporated into the tooth matrix and thus cannot be removed by prophylaxis. Combination of both is multifactorial in nature, e.g. nicotine staining.

**Classification of discoloration**
- Intrinsic discoloration.
- Extrinsic discoloration.
- Combination of both.

**Etiology of tooth discoloration**

*Intrinsic Stains*

1. ***Pre-eruptive causes***
   a. *Disease*
      i. Alkaptonuria
      ii. Hematological disorders
      iii. Disease of enamel and dentin
      iv. Liver diseases.

   b. *Medications*
      i. Tetracycline stains and other antibiotic use
      ii. Fluorosis stain.
2. ***Posteruptive causes of discoloration***
   a. Pulpal changes
   b. Trauma
   c. Dentin hypercalcification
   d. Dental caries
   e. Restorative materials and operative procedures
   f. Aging
   g. Functional and parafunctional changes.

*Extrinsic Stains*

1. ***Daily acquired stains***
   a. Plaque
   b. Food and beverages
   c. Tobacco use
   d. Poor oral hygiene
   e. Swimmer's calculus
   f. Gingival hemorrhage.
2. ***Chemicals***
   a. Chlorhexidine
   b. Metallic stains.

### Intrinsic Stains

#### *Pre-eruptive Causes*

These are incorporated into the deeper layers of enamel and dentin during odontogenesis and alter the development and appearance of the enamel and dentin.

*Alkaptonuria:* Dark brown pigmentation of primary teeth is commonly seen in alkaptonuria. It is an autosomal recessive disorder resulting into complete oxidation of tyrosine and phenylalanine causing increased level of homogentisic acid.

*Hematological Disorders*

1. *Erythroblastosis fetalis:* It is a blood disorder of neonates due to Rh incompatibility. In this, stain does not involve teeth or portions of teeth developing after cessation of hemolysis shortly after birth. Stain is usually green, brown or bluish in color.
2. *Congenital porphyria:* It is an inborn error of porphyrin metabolism, characterized by overproduction of uroporphyrin. Deciduous and permanent teeth may show a red or brownish discoloration. Under ultraviolet light, teeth show red fluorescence.
3. *Sickle cell anemia:* It is inherited blood dyscrasia characterized by increased hemolysis of red blood cells. In sickle cell anemia infrequently the stains of the teeth are similar to those of erythroblastosis fetalis, but discoloration is more severe, involves both dentitions and does not resolve with time.

*Disease of Enamel and Dentin*

**Developmental defects in enamel formation**
- Amelogenesis imperfecta
- Fluorosis
- Vitamin and mineral deficiency

- Chromosomal anomalies
- Inherited diseases
- Tetracycline
- Childhood illness
- Malnutrition
- Metabolic disorders.

*Amelogenesis imperfecta (AI):* It comprises of a group of conditions, that demonstrate developmental alteration in the structure of the enamel in the absence of a systemic disorders. Amelogenesis imperfecta (AI) has been classified mainly into hypoplastic, hypocalcified and hypomaturation type (Fig. 29.2).

*Fluorosis:* In fluorosis, staining is due to excessive fluoride uptake during development of enamel. Excess fluoride induces a metabolic change in ameloblast and the resultant enamel has a defective matrix and an irregular, hypomineralized structure (Fig. 29.3).

*Staining manifests as:*

1. Gray or white opaque areas on teeth.
2. Yellow to brown discoloration on a smooth enamel surface (Fig. 29.4).
3. Moderate and severe changes showing pitting and brownish discoloration of surface (Fig. 29.5).
4. Severely corroded appearance with dark brown discoloration and loss of enamel.

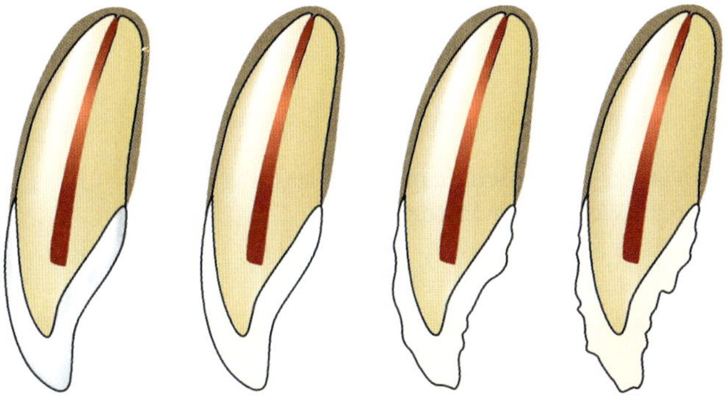


**Fig. 29.2:** Amelogenesis imperfecta

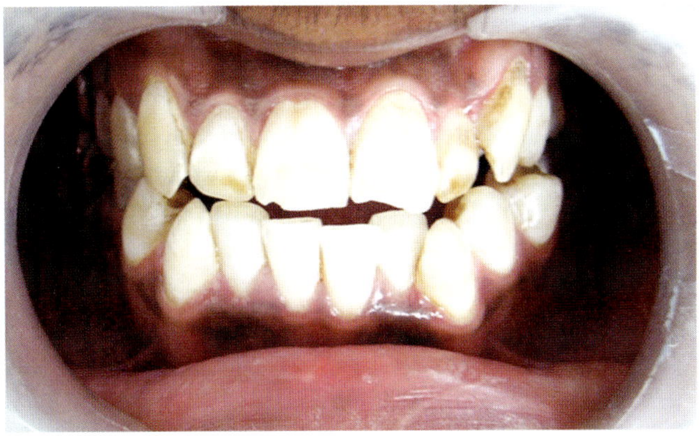

**Fig. 29.3:** Fluorosis of teeth

*Enamel Hypoplasia and Hypocalcification due to Other Causes (Figs 29.6A to C):*

1. Vitamin D deficiency results in characteristic white patch hypoplasia in teeth.
2. Vitamin C deficiency together with vitamin A deficiency during formative periods of dentition resulting in pitting type appearance of teeth.
3. Childhood illnesses during odontogenesis, such as exanthematous fever, malnutrition, metabolic disorder, etc. also affect teeth.

**Defects in dentin formation**

- Dentinogenesis imperfecta.
- Erythropoietic porphyria.
- Tetracycline and minocycline (excessive intake).
- Hyperbilirubinemia.

*Dentinogenesis imperfecta (DI) (Figs 29.7A to C):* It is an autosomal dominant development disturbance of the dentin which occurs along or in conjunction with amelogenesis imperfecta. Color of teeth in DI varies from gray to brownish violet to yellowish brown with a characteristic usual translucent or opalescent hue.

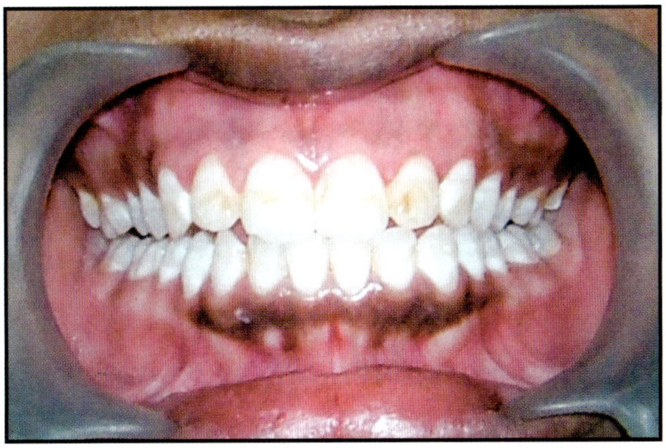

**Fig. 29.4:** Fluorosis of teeth showing yellow to brown discoloration of teeth

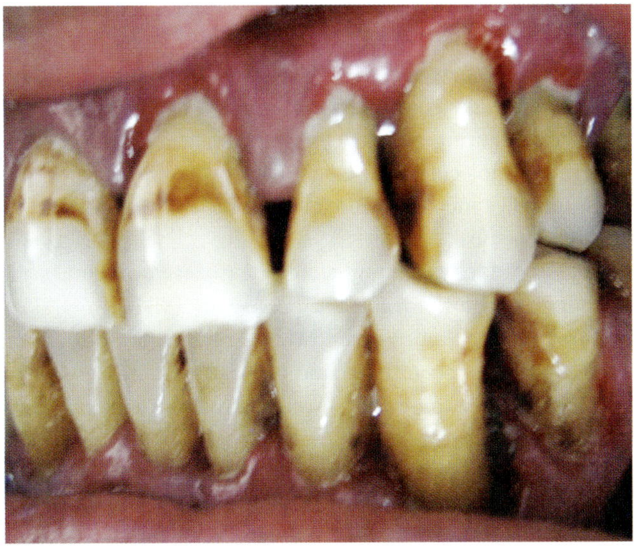

**Fig. 29.5:** Dark brown discoloration caused by fluorosis

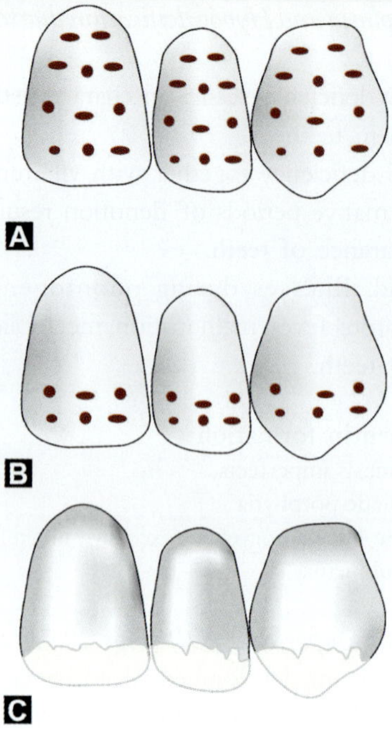


**Figs 29.6A to C:** (A) Amelogenesis imperfecta (hypoplastic, pitted); (B) Acquired enamel hypoplasia; (C) Amelogenesis imperfecta (snow-capped)

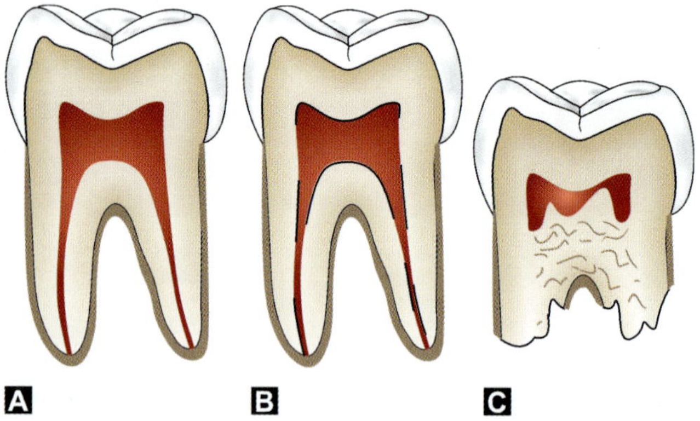


**Figs 29.7A to C:** (A) Normal tooth; (B) Dentinogenesis imperfecta; (C) Dentin dysplasia

*Tetracycline and minocycline:* Unsightly discoloration of both dentition results from excessive intake of tetracycline and minocycline during the development of teeth. Chelation of tetracycline molecule with calcium in hydroxyapatite crystals forms tetracycline orthophosphate which is responsible for discolored teeth.

Classification of staining according to developmental stage, banding and color (Jordun and Boksman 1984).

1. First degree (mild)—yellow to gray, uniformly spread through the tooth. No banding.
2. Second degree (moderate)—yellow brown to dark gray, slight banding, if present.
3. Third degree (severe staining)—blue gray or black and is accompanied by significant banding across tooth.
4. Fourth degree—stains that are so dark that bleaching is ineffective, totally.

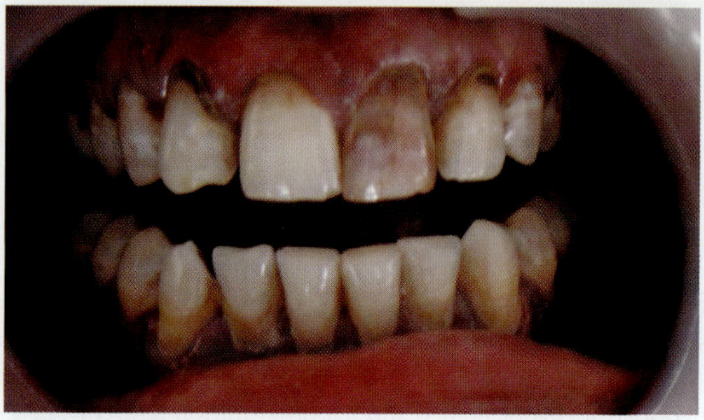

**Fig. 29.8:** Discoloration of 21 due to pulp necrosis

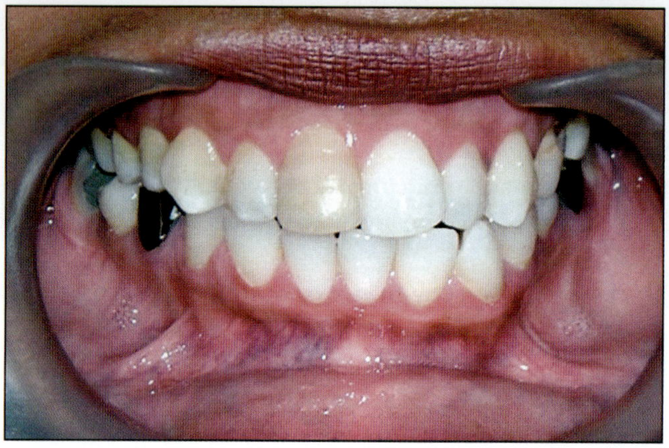

**Fig. 29.9:** Loss of translucency of 11 due to pulp necrosis

**Severity of pigmentation with tetracycline depends on three factors**

- Time and duration of administration.
- Type of tetracycline administered.
- Dosage.

### *Posteruptive Causes*

a. ***Pulpal changes:*** Pulp necrosis usually results from bacterial, mechanical or chemical irritation to pulp. In this disintegration products enter dentinal tubules and cause discoloration (Figs 29.8 and 29.9).

b. ***Trauma:*** Accidental injury to tooth can cause pulpal and enamel degenerative changes that may alter color of teeth (Fig. 29.10). Pulpal hemorrhage leads to grayish discoloration and nonvital appearance. Injury causes hemorrhage which results in lysis of RBCs and liberation of iron sulphide which enter dentinal tubules and discolor surrounding tooth.

c. ***Dentin hypercalcification:*** Dentin hypercalcification results when there are excessive irregular elements in the pulp chamber and canal walls. It causes decrease in translucency and yellowish or yellow brown discoloration of the teeth.

d. ***Dental caries:*** In general, teeth present a discolored appearance around areas of bacterial stagnation and leaking restorations (Fig. 29.11).

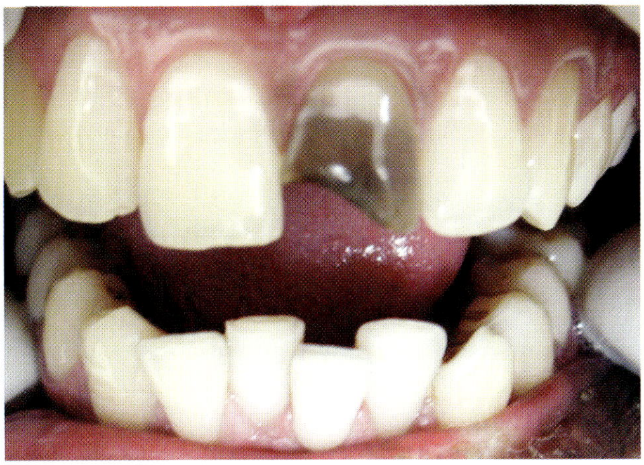

Fig. 29.10: Discolored 21 due to traumatic injury followed by pulp necrosis

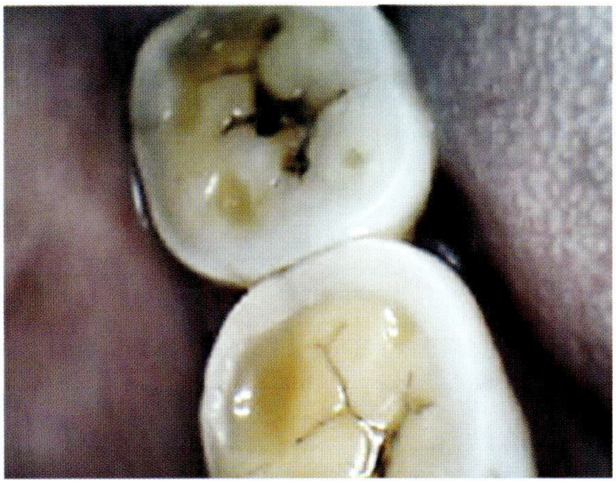

Fig. 29.12: Yellowish discoloration of teeth due to secondary and tertiary dentin deposition

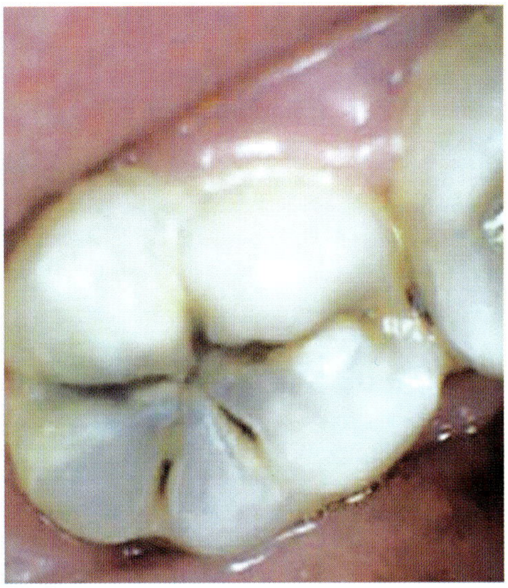

Fig. 29.11: Discolored appearance of teeth due to caries

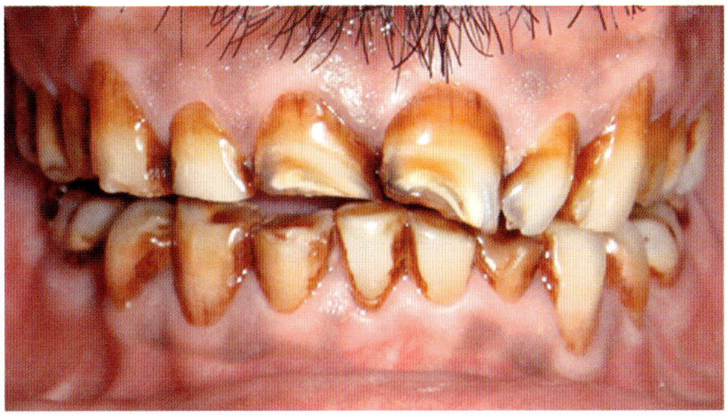

Fig. 29.13: Discoloration of teeth resulting from tooth wear and aging

e. ***Restorative materials and dental procedures:*** Discoloration can also result from the use of endodontic sealers and restorative materials.
f. ***Aging:*** Color changes in teeth with age result from surface and subsurface changes. Age related discoloration are because of:
   – *Enamel changes:* Both thinning and texture changes occur in enamel.
   – *Dentin deposition:* Secondary and tertiary dentin deposits, pulp stones cause changes in the color of teeth (Fig. 29.12).
g. ***Functional and parafunctional changes:*** Tooth wear may give a darker appearance to the teeth because of loss of tooth surface and exposure of dentin which is yellower and is susceptible to color changes by absorption of oral fluids and deposition of reparative dentin (Fig. 29.13).

## Extrinsic Stains

### *Daily Acquired Stains*

1. ***Plaque:*** Pellicle and plaque on tooth surface gives rise to yellowish appearance of teeth.
2. ***Food and beverages:*** Tea, coffee, red wine, curry and colas if taken in excess cause discoloration.
3. Tobacco use results in brown to black appearance of teeth.
4. ***Poor oral hygiene manifests as:***
   - Green stain
   - Brown stain
   - Orange stain
5. ***Swimmer's calculus:***
   - It is yellow to dark brown stain present on facial and lingual surfaces of anterior teeth. It occurs due to prolonged exposure to pool water.
6. Gingival hemorrhage.

## Chemicals

1. ***Chlorhexidine stain:*** The stains produced by use of chlorhexidine are yellowish brown to brownish in nature.
2. ***Metallic stains:*** These are caused by metals and metallic salts introduced into oral cavity in metal containing dust inhaled by industry workers or through orally administered drugs.

**Stains caused by different metals**

- Copper dust—Green stain.
- Iron dust—Brown stain.
- Mercury—Greenish black stain.
- Nickel—Green stain.
- Silver—Black stain.

**Classification of extrinsic stains (Nathoo in 1997)**

- N1 type dental stain (Direct dental stain)—Here colored materials bind to the tooth surface to cause discoloration. Tooth has same color, as that of chromogen.
- N2 type dental stain (direct dental stain)—Here chromogen changes color after binding to the tooth.
- N3 type dental stain (Indirect dental stain)—In this type prechromogen (colorless) binds to the tooth and undergoes a chemical reaction to cause a stain.

## BLEACHING

Bleaching is a procedure which involves lightening of the color of a tooth through the application of a chemical agent to oxidize the organic pigmentation in the tooth.

### History of Tooth Bleaching

Bleaching of discolored, pulpless teeth was first described in 1864 and a variety of medicaments such as chloride, sodium hypochlorite, sodium perborate and hydrogen peroxide has been used, alone or in combination, with or without heat activation.

The Walking Bleach technique was introduced in 1961, involving placement of a mixture of sodium perborate and water into the pulp chamber. This technique was later modified and water replaced by 30-50 percent hydrogen peroxide. Now, the popular technique night guard vital bleaching technique describes the use of 10 percent carbamide peroxide in mouthguard to be worn overnight for lightening tooth color. Later in 1996, Reyto done the tooth whitening by lasers.

## CONTRAINDICATIONS FOR BLEACHING

### *Poor Case Selection*

1. Patient having emotional or psychological problems is not right choice for bleaching.
2. In case selection, if clinician has opinion that bleaching is not in patient's best interest, he should decline doing that.

### *Dentin Hypersensitivity*

Hypersensitive teeth need to provide extraprotection before going for bleaching.

### *Extensively Restored Teeth*

These teeth are not good candidate for bleaching because:

1. They do not have enough enamel to respond properly to bleaching.
2. Teeth heavily restored with visible, tooth colored restorations are poor candidate as composite restorations do not lighten, infact they become more evident after bleaching.

### *Teeth with Hypoplastic Marks and Cracks*

Application of bleaching agents increase the contrast between white opaque spots and normal tooth structure:

In these cases, bleaching can be done in conjunction with:

1. Microabrasion
2. Selected ameloplasty
3. Composite resin bonding.

### *Defective and Leaky Restoration*

Defective and leaky restorations are not good candidate for bleaching.

1. ***Discoloration from metallic salts particularly silver amalgam:*** The dentinal tubules of the tooth become virtually saturated with alloys and no amount of bleaching with available products will significantly improve the shade.
2. ***Defective obturation:*** If root canal is not well obturated, then refilling must be done before attempting bleaching.

**Contraindications of bleaching**

1. Poor patient and case selection
   a. Psychologically or emotionally compromised patient.
2. Dentin hypersensitivity.
3. Extensively restored tooth.
4. Teeth with hypoplastic marks and cracks.
5. Defective and leaky restorations.
   a. Discoloration from metallic salts particularly mercury.
   b. Defective obturation.

## MEDICAMENTS USED AS BLEACHING AGENTS

**An ideal bleaching agent should**

- Be easy to apply on the teeth.
- Have a neutral pH.
- Lighten the teeth efficiently.
- Remain in contact with oral soft tissues for short periods.
- Be required in minimum quantity to achieve desired results.
- Not irritate or dehydrate the oral tissues.
- Not cause damage to the teeth.
- Be well controlled by the dentist to customize the treatment to the patient's need.

Tooth bleaching today is based upon hydrogen peroxide as an active agent. Hydrogen peroxide may be applied directly or produced in a chemical reaction from sodium perborate or carbamide peroxide. Hydrogen peroxide acts as a strong oxidizing agent through the formation of free radicals, reactive oxygen molecules and hydrogen peroxide anions. These reactive molecules attack the long chained, dark colored chromophore molecules and split them into smaller, less colored and more diffusible molecules.

Carbamide peroxide also yields urea which is further decomposed to $CO_2$ and ammonia. It is the high pH of ammonia which facilitates the bleaching procedure.

This can be explained by the fact that in basic solution, lower activation energy is required for formation of free radicals from hydrogen peroxide and the reaction rate is higher, resulting in improved yield rate compared with an acidic environment.

The outcome of bleaching procedure depends mainly on the concentration of bleaching agents, the ability of the agents to reach the chromophore molecules and the duration and number of times the agent is in contact with chromophore molecules.

**Constituents of bleaching gels**

- Carbamide peroxide.
- Hydrogen peroxide and sodium hydroxide (Li, 1998).
- Sodium perborate.
- Thickening agent-carbopol or carboxy polymethylene.
- Urea.
- Surfactant and pigment dispersants.
- Preservatives.
- Vehicle-glycerine and dentifrice.
- Flavors.
- Fluoride and 3 percent potassium nitrate.

### Carbamide Peroxide ($CH_6N_2O_3$)

It is a bifunctional derivative of carbonic acid. It is available as:

1. ***Home bleaching***
   a. 5 percent carbamide peroxide.
   b. 10 percent carbamide peroxide.
   c. 15 percent carbamide peroxide.
   d. 20 percent carbamide peroxide.
2. ***In-office bleaching***
   a. 35 percent solution or gel of carbamide peroxide.

### Hydrogen Peroxide ($H_2O_2$)

$H_2O_2$ breaks down to water and nascent oxygen. It also forms free radical perhydroxyl ($HO_2$) which is responsible for bleaching action.

### Sodium Perborate

It comes as monohydrate, trihydrate or tetrahydrate. It contains 95 percent perborate, providing 10 percent available oxygen.

### Thickening Agents

*Carbopol (Carboxy polymethylene):* Addition of carbopol in bleaching gels results in:

1. Slow release of oxygen.
2. Increased viscosity of bleaching material, which further helps in longer retention of material in tray and need of less material.
3. Delayed effervescence–thicker products stay on the teeth for longer time to provide necessary time for the carbamide peroxide to diffuse into the tooth.
4. The slow diffusion into enamel may also allow tooth to be bleached more effectively.

### Urea

It is added in bleaching solutions to:

- Stabilize the $H_2O_2$
- Elevate the pH of solution.
- Anticariogenic effects.

### Surfactants

Surfactant acts as surface wetting agent which allows the hydrogen peroxide to pass across gel tooth boundary.

### Preservatives

Commonly used preservatives are phosphoric acids, citric acid or sodium stannate. They sequestrate metals such as Fe, Cu and Mg which accelerate breakdown of $H_2O_2$ and give gels better durability and stability.

### Vehicle

1. ***Glycerine:*** It is used to increase viscosity of preparation and ease of manipulation.
2. Dentifrice.

### Flavors

They are added to improve patient acceptability.

### Fluoride and 3 percent Potassium Nitrate

They are added to prevent sensitivity of teeth after bleaching.

**Mechanism of bleaching**

Mechanism of bleaching is mainly linked to degradation of high molecular weight complex organic molecules that reflect a specific wavelength of light that is responsible for color of stain. The resulting degradation products are of lower molecular weight and composed of less complex molecules that reflect less light, resulting in a reduction or elimination of discoloration (Fig. 29.14).

**Rate of color change is affected by**

- Frequency with which solutions are to be changed.
- Amount of time, the bleach is in contact with tooth.
- Viscosity of material.
- Rate of oxygen release.
- Original shade and condition of the tooth.
- Location and depth of discoloration.
- Degradation rate of material.

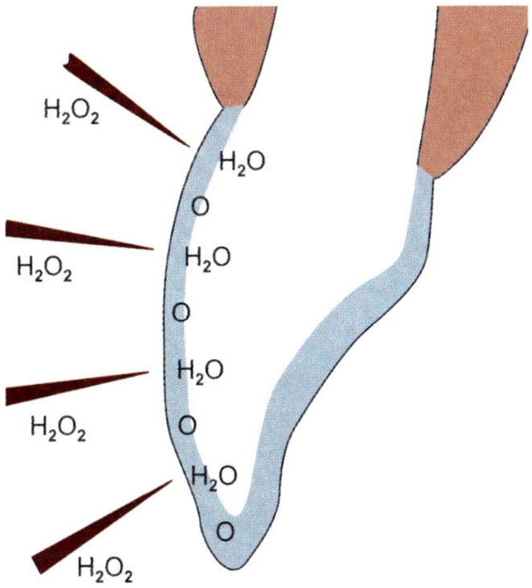


**Fig. 29.14:** Mechanism of bleaching

**Bleaching technique**

1. For vital teeth
   a. Home bleaching technique/Nightguard vital bleaching.
   b. In-office bleaching
   i. Thermocatalytic
   ii. Non-thermocatalytic
   iii. Microabrasion.
2. For nonvital teeth
   a. Thermocatalytic in-office bleaching.
   b. Walking bleach/Intracoronal bleaching
   c. Inside/outside bleaching
   d. Closed chamber bleaching/Extracoronal bleaching.
3. Laser assisted bleaching.

## HOME BLEACHING TECHNIQUE/ NIGHTGUARD BLEACHING

### Indications for Use

- Mild generalized staining.
- Age related discolorations.
- Mild tetracycline staining.
- Mild fluorosis.
- Acquired superficial staining.
- Stains from smoking tobacco.
- Color changes related to pulpal trauma or necrosis.

### Contraindications

- Teeth with insufficient enamel for bleaching.
- Teeth with deep and surface cracks and fracture lines.
- Teeth with inadequate or defective restorations.
- Discolorations in the adolescent patients with large pulp chamber.
- Severe fluorosis and pitting hypoplasia.
- Noncompliant patients.
- Pregnant or lactating patients.
- Teeth with large anterior restorations.
- Severe tetracycline staining.
- Fractured or malaligned teeth.
- Teeth exhibiting extreme sensitivity to heat, cold or sweets.
- Teeth with opaque white spots.
- Suspected or confirmed bulimia nervosa.

### Advantages of Home Bleaching Technique

- Simple method for patients to use.
- Simple for dentists to monitor.
- Less chair time and cost-effective.
- Patient can bleach their teeth at their convenience.

### Disadvantages of Home Bleaching Technique

- Patient compliance is mandatory.
- Color change is dependent on amount of time the trays are worn.
- Chances of abuse by using excessive amount of bleach for too many hours per day.

### Factors that Guard the Prognosis for Home Bleaching

- History or presence of sensitive teeth.
- Extremely dark gingival third of tooth visible during smiling.
- Extensive white spots.
- Translucent teeth.
- Excessive gingival recession and exposed root surfaces.

***Commonly used solution for nightguard bleaching:***

- 10 percent carbamide peroxide with or without carbopol.
- 15 percent carbamide peroxide
- Hydrogen peroxide (1-10%).

### Steps of Tray Fabrication

- Take the impression and make a stone model.
- Trim the model.
- Place the stock out resin and cure it.
- Apply separating media.
- Choose the tray sheet material.
- Nature of material used for fabrication of bleaching tray is flexible plastic. Most common tray material used is ethyl vinyl acetate.
- Cast the plastic in vacuum tray forming machines.
- Trim and polish the tray.
- Checking the tray for correct fit, retention and over-extension.
- Demonstrate the amount of bleaching material to be placed.

### Thickness of Tray

- Standard thickness of tray is 0.035 inch.
- Thicker tray, i.e. 0.05 inch is indicated in patients with breaking habit.
- Thinner tray, i.e. 0.02 inch thick is indicated in patients who gag.

### Treatment Regimen

When and how long to keep the trays in the mouth, depends on patients lifestyle preference and schedule. Wearing the tray during day time allows replenishment of the gel after 1-2 hours for maximum concentration. Overnight use causes decrease in loss of material due to decreased salivary flow at night and decreased occlusal pressure. Patient is recalled 1-2 weeks after wearing the tray.

### Maintenance After Tooth Bleaching

Additional rebleaching can be done every 3-4 years if necessary with rebleaching duration of 1 week.

### Side Effects of Home Bleaching

- Gingival irritation—Painful gums after a few days of wearing trays.
- Soft tissue irritation—From excessive wearing of the trays or applying too much bleach to the trays.
- Altered taste sensation—Metallic taste immediately after removing trays.
- Tooth sensitivity—Most common side effect.

## IN-OFFICE BLEACHING

## THERMOCATALYTIC VITAL TOOTH BLEACHING

Equipment needed for in-office bleaching are:

- Power bleach material.
- Tissue protector.
- Energizing/activating source.
- Protective clothing and eye wear.
- Mechanical timer.

### Light Sources Used for In-office Bleach

Various available light sources are:

1. Conventional bleaching light.
2. Tungsten halogen curing light.
3. Xenon plasma arc light.
4. Argon and $CO_2$ lasers.
5. Diode laser light.

#### *Conventional Bleaching Light*

- Uses heat and light to activate bleaching material.
- More heat is generated during bleaching.
- Causes tooth dehydration.
- Uncomfortable for patient.
- Slower in action.

#### *Tungsten-Halogen Curing Light*

- Uses light and heat to activate bleaching solution
- Application of light 40-60 seconds per application per tooth
- Time consuming.

#### *Xenon Plasma Arc Light*

- High intensity light, so more heat is liberated during bleaching.
- Application requires 3 seconds per tooth.
- Faster bleaching.
- Action is thermal and stimulates the catalyst in chemicals.
- Greater potential for thermal trauma to pulp and surrounding soft tissues.

#### *Argon and $CO_2$ Laser*

- True laser light stimulate the catalyst in chemical so there is no thermal effect
- Requires 10 seconds per application per tooth.

#### *Diode Laser Light*

- True laser light produced from a solid state source
- Ultra fast
- Requires 3-5 seconds to activate bleaching agent
- No heat is generated during bleaching.

#### *Indications of In-office Bleaching*

- Superficial stains.
- Moderate to mild stains.

#### *Contraindications of In-office Bleaching*

- Tetracycline stains.
- Extensive restorations
- Severe discolorations.
- Extensive caries.
- Patient sensitive to bleaching agents.

#### *Advantages of In-office Bleaching*

- Patient preference.
- Less time than overall time needed for home bleaching.
- Patient motivation.
- Protection of soft tissues.

#### *Disadvantages of In-office Bleaching*

- More chair time.
- More expensive.
- Unpredictable and deterioration of color is quicker.
- More frequent and longer appointment.
- Dehydration of teeth.
- Serious safety considerations.
- Not much research to support its use.
- Discomfort of rubber dam.

#### *Procedures (Fig. 29.15)*

1. Pumice the teeth to clean off any debris present on the tooth surface.
2. Isolate the teeth with rubber dam.
3. Saturate the cotton or gauze piece with bleaching solution (30-35% $H_2O_2$) and place it on the teeth.
4. Depending upon light, expose the tooth/teeth.
5. Change solution in between after every 4 to 5 minutes.
6. Remove solution with the help of wet gauge.
7. Repeat the procedure until desired shade is produced.
8. Remove solution and irrigate teeth thoroughly with warm water.
9. Polish teeth and apply neutral sodium fluoride gel.
10. Instruct the patient to avoid coffee, tea, etc. for 2 weeks.
11. Second and third appointment is given after 3-6 weeks. This will allow pulp to settle.

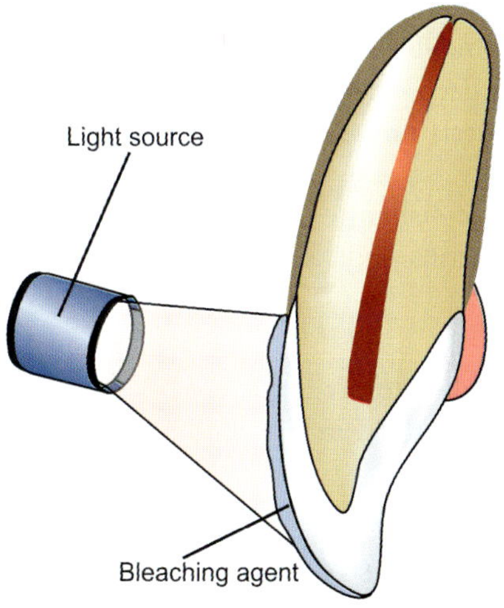


**Fig. 29.15:** Thermocatalytic technique of bleaching for vital teeth

## NON-THERMOCATALYTIC BLEACHING

In this technique, heat source is not used.

**Commonly used solutions for bleaching**

| *Name* | *Composition* |
|---|---|
| 1. Superoxol | 5 parts $H_2O_2$:1 part ether |
| 2. McInnes solution | a. 5 part $H_2O_2$ (30%) |
| | b. 5 part HCl (36%) |
| | c. 1 part ether (0.2%) |
| 3. Modified McInnes solution | a. $H_2O_2$ (30%) |
| | b. NaOH (20%) |

Mix in equal parts, i.e. (1:1) along with either (0.2%)

### Steps

- Isolate the teeth using rubber dam.
- Apply bleaching agent on the teeth for five minutes.
- Wash the teeth with warm water and reapply the bleaching agent until the desired color is achieved.
- Wash the teeth and polish them.

## MICROABRASION

It is a procedure in which a microscopic layer of enamel is simultaneously eroded and abraded with a special compound (usually contains 18% of hydrochloric acid) leaving a perfectly intact enamel surface behind.

### Indications

- Developmental intrinsic stains and discolorations limited to superficial enamel only.
- Enamel discolorations as a result of hypomineralization or hypermineralization.
- Decalcification lesions from stasis of plaque and from orthodontic bands.
- Areas of enamel fluorosis.
- Multicolored superficial stains and some irregular surface texture.

### Contraindications

- Age related staining.
- Deep enamel hypoplastic lesions.
- Areas of deep enamel and dentin stains.
- Amelogenesis imperfecta and dentinogenesis imperfecta cases.
- Tetracycline staining.
- Carious lesions underlying regions of decalcification.

### Advantages

- Minimum discomfort to patient.
- Can be easily done in less time by operator.
- Useful in removing superficial stains.
- The surface of treated tooth is shiny and smooth in nature.

### Disadvantages

- Not effective for deeper stains.
- Removes enamel layer.
- Yellow discoloration of teeth has been reported in some cases after treatment.

### Protocol

1. Clinically evaluate the teeth.
2. Clean teeth with rubber cup and prophylaxis paste.
3. Apply petroleum jelly to the tissues and isolate the area with rubber dam.
4. Apply microabrasion compound to areas in 60 seconds intervals with appropriate rinsing.
5. Repeat the procedure if necessary. Check the teeth when wet.
6. Rinse teeth for 30 seconds and dry.
7. Apply topical fluoride to the teeth for four minutes.
8. Re-evaluate the color of the teeth. More than one visit may be necessary sometimes.

## BLEACHING OF NONVITAL TEETH

## THERMOCATALYTIC TECHNIQUE OF BLEACHING FOR NONVITAL TEETH

1. Isolate the tooth to be bleached using rubber dam
2. Place bleaching agent (superoxol and sodium perborate separately or in combination) in the tooth chamber.
3. Heat the bleaching solution using bleaching stick/light curing unit.
4. Repeat the procedure till the desired tooth color is achieved.
5. Wash the tooth with water and seal the chamber using dry cotton and temporary restorations.
6. Recall the patient after 1-3 weeks.
7. Do the permanent restoration of tooth using suitable composite resins afterwards.

## INTRACORONAL BLEACHING/WALKING BLEACH OF NONVITAL TEETH

It involves use of chemical agents within the coronal portion of an endodontically treated tooth to remove tooth discoloration.

### Indications of Intracoronal Bleaching

- Discoloration of pulp chamber origin (Figs 29.16A and B).
- Moderate to severe tetracycline staining.
- Dentin discoloration.
- Discoloration not agreeable to extracoronal bleaching.

### Contraindications of Intracoronal Bleaching

- Superficial enamel discoloration.
- Defective enamel formation.
- Presence of caries.
- Unpredictable prognosis of tooth.

### Steps

1. Take the radiographs to assess the quality of obturation. If found unsatisfactory, retreatment should be done.

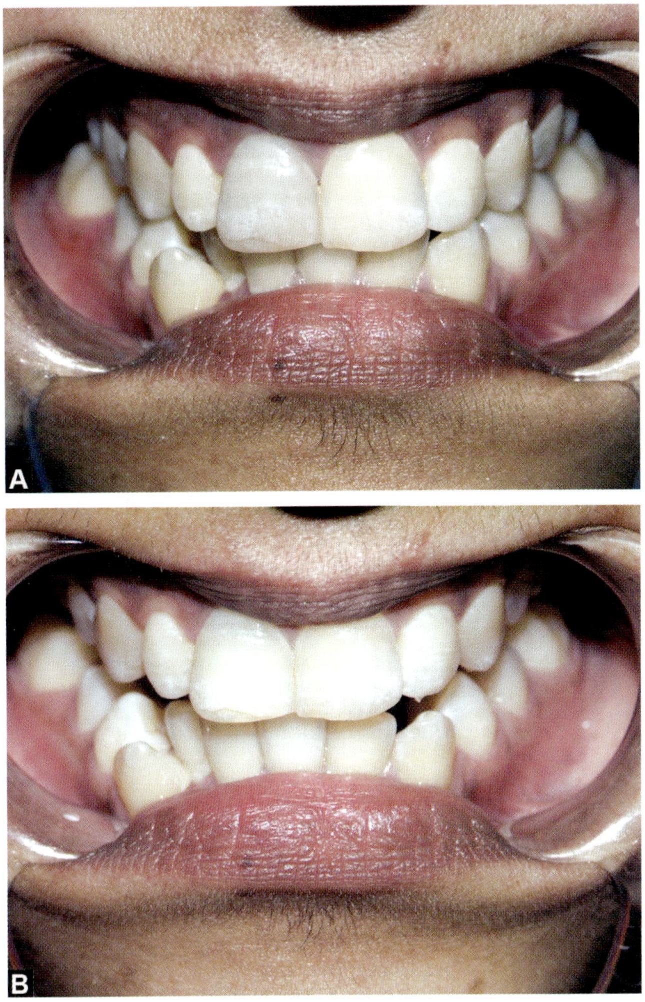

Figs 29.16A and B: (A) Preoperative and (B) Postoperative photograph of nonvital bleaching of maxillary right central incisor (11)

2. Evaluate the quality and shade of restoration if present. If restoration is defective, replace it.
3. Evaluate tooth color with shade guide.
4. Isolate the tooth with rubber dam.
5. Prepare the access cavity, remove the coronal gutta-percha, expose the dentin and refine the cavity (Fig. 29.17).
6. Place mechanical barriers of 2 mm thick, preferably of glass ionomer cement, zinc phosphate, IRM, polycarboxylate cement on root canal filling material (Fig. 29.18). The coronal height of barrier should protect the dentinal tubules and conform to the external epithelial attachment.
7. Now mix sodium perborate with an inert liquid (local anesthetic, saline or water) and place this paste into pulp chamber (Fig. 29.19).
8. After removing the excess bleaching paste, place a temporary restoration over it.
9. Recall the patient after 1-2 weeks, repeat the treatment until desired shade is achieved.
10. Restore access cavity with composite after 2 weeks.

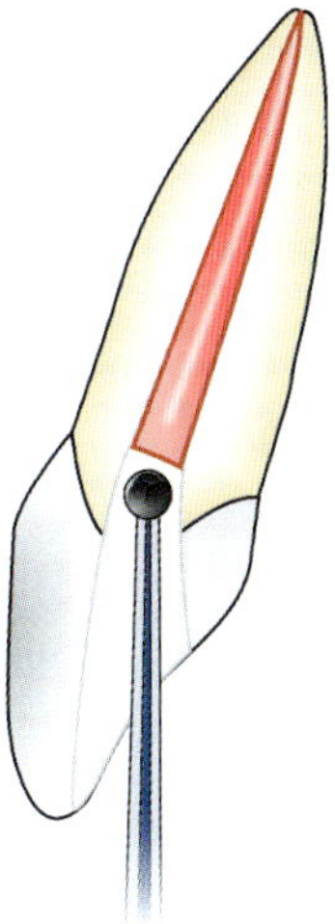

Fig. 29.17: Removal of coronal gutta-percha using rotary instrument

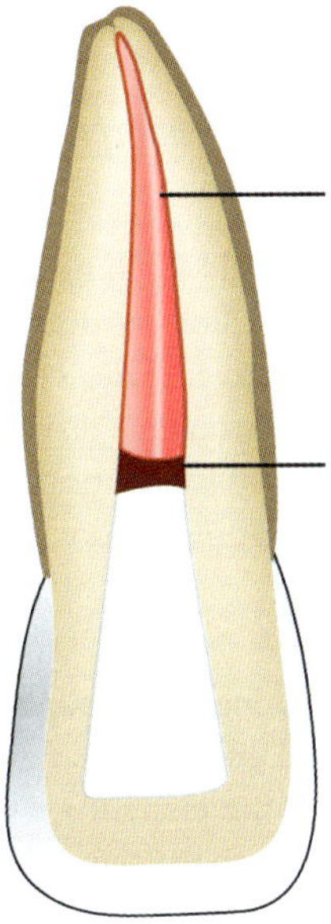


Fig. 29.18: Placement of protective barrier over gutta-percha

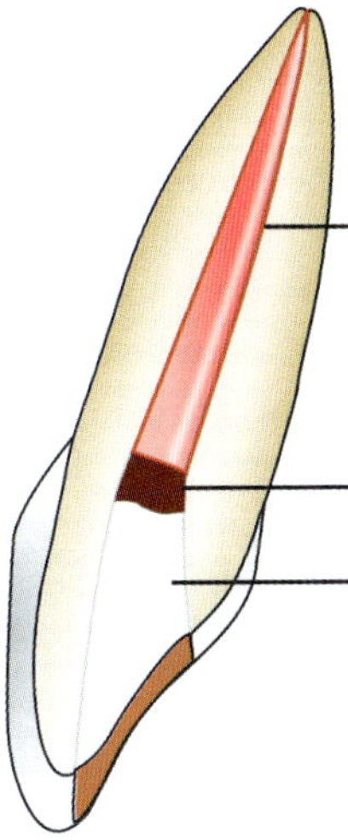

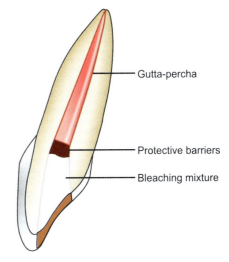

Fig. 29.19: Placement of bleaching mixture into pulp chamber and sealing of cavity using temporary restoration

### Complications of Intracoronal Bleaching

- External root resorption.
- Chemical burns if using 30-35 percent $H_2O_2$.
- Decrease bond strength of composite.

### Precautions to be Taken for Safer Nonvital Bleaching

1. Isolate tooth effectively.
2. Protect oral mucosa.
3. Verify adequate endodontic obturation.
4. Use protective barriers.
5. Avoid acid etching.
6. Avoid strong oxidizers.
7. Avoid heat.
8. Recall periodically.

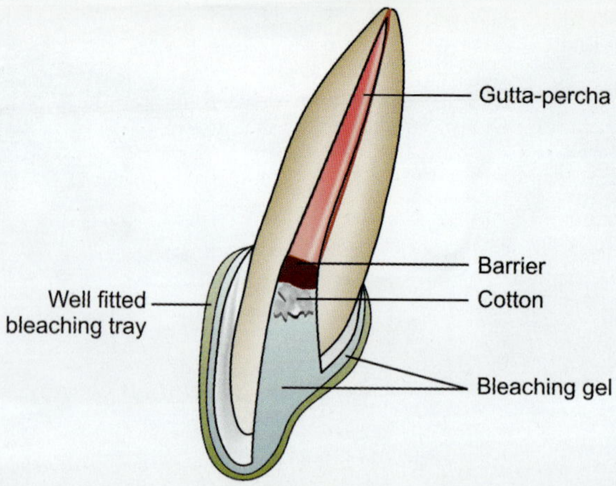


Fig. 29.20: Inside/outside techniques in this tray is sealed over an open internal access opening, with a cotton pellet placed in open access cavity

## INSIDE/OUTSIDE BLEACHING TECHNIQUE

### Synonyms

### Internal/External Bleaching, Modified Walking Bleach Technique

This technique involves intracoronal bleaching technique along with home bleaching technique. This is done to make the bleaching program more effective. This combination of bleaching treatment is helpful in treating difficult stains, for specific problems like single dark vital or nonvital tooth and to treat stains of different origin present on the same tooth.

### Procedures

1. Assess the obturation by taking radiographs.
2. Isolate the tooth and prepare the access cavity by removing gutta-percha 2-3 mm below the cementoenamel junction.
3. Place the mechanical barrier, clean the access cavity and place a cotton pellet in the chamber to avoid food packing into it.
4. Evaluate the shade of tooth.
5. Check the fitting of bleaching tray and advise the patient to remove the cotton pellet before bleaching.
6. Instructions for home bleaching. Bleaching syringe can be directly placed into chamber before seating the tray or extrableaching material can be placed into the tray space corresponding to tooth with open chamber (Fig. 29.20).
7. After bleaching, tooth is irrigated with water, cleaned and again a cotton pellet is placed in the empty space.
8. Re-assessment of shade is done after 4-7 days.
9. When the desired shade is achieved, seal the access cavity initially with temporary restoration and finally with composite restoration after atleast two weeks.

### Advantages

- More surface area for bleach to penetrate.
- Treatment time in days rather than weeks.
- Decreases the incidence of cervical resorption.
- Uses lower concentration of carbamide peroxide.

### Disadvantages

- Noncompliant patients.
- Over-bleaching by overzealous application.
- Chances for cervical resorption is reduced but still exists.

## CLOSED CHAMBER BLEACHING/ EXTRACORONAL BLEACHING

In this technique, instead of removing the existing restoration, the bleaching paste is applied to the tooth via bleaching tray.

**Indications of closed chamber technique**

- In case of totally calcified canals in a traumatized tooth.
- As a maintenance bleaching treatment several years after initial intracoronal bleaching.
- Treatment for adolescents with incomplete gingival maturation.
- A single dark nonvital tooth where the surrounding teeth are sufficiently light or where other vital teeth are also to be bleached.

## LASER ASSISTED BLEACHING TECHNIQUE

This technique achieves power bleaching process with the help of efficient energy source with minimum side effects. Laser whitening gel contains thermally absorbed crystals, fumed silica and 35 percent $H_2O_2$. In this, gel is applied and is activated by light source which in further activates the crystals present in gel, allowing dissociation of oxygen and therefore better penetration into enamel matrix. Following LASER have been approved by FDA for tooth bleaching:

1. Argon laser.
2. $CO_2$ laser.
3. GaAlAs diode laser.

### Argon Laser

- Emits wavelength of 480 nm in visible part of spectrum.
- Activates the bleaching gel and makes the darker tooth surface lighter.
- Less thermal effects on pulp as compared to other heat lamps.

### $CO_2$ Laser

- Emits a wavelength of 10,600 nm.
- Used to enhance the effect of whitening produced by argon laser.
- Deeper penetration than argon laser thus more efficient tooth whitening.
- More deleterious effects on pulp than argon laser.

### GaAlAs Diode Laser (Gallium Aluminium–Arsenic)

Emits a wavelength of 980 nm.

## EFFECTS OF BLEACHING AGENTS ON TOOTH AND ITS SUPPORTING STRUCTURES

### Tooth Hypersensitivity

Tooth sensitivity is common side effect of external tooth bleaching. Higher incidence of tooth sensitivity (67-78%) are seen after in-office bleaching with hydrogen peroxide in combination with heat. The mechanism responsible for external tooth bleaching though is not fully established, but it has been shown that peroxide penetrates enamel, dentin and pulp. This penetration was more in restored teeth than that of intact teeth.

### Effects on Enamel

Studies have shown that 10 percent carbamide peroxide significantly decreased enamel hardness. But application of fluoride showed improved remineralization after bleaching.

### Effects on Dentin

Bleaching has shown to cause uniform change in color through dentin.

### Effects on Pulp

Penetration of bleaching agent into pulp through enamel and dentin occur resulting in tooth sensitivity. Studies have shown that 3 percent solution of $H_2O_2$ can cause:

- Transient reduction in pulpal blood flow.
- Occlusion of pulpal blood vessels.

### Effects on Cementum

Recent studies have shown that cementum is not affected by materials used for home bleaching. But cervical resorption and external root resorption in teeth has been seen in teeth treated by intracoronal bleaching using 30-35 percent $H_2O_2$.

### Cervical Resorption

More serious side effects such as external root resorption may occur when a higher than 30 percent concentration of hydrogen peroxide is used in combination with heat. Hydroxyl groups may be generated during thermocatalytic bleaching, especially where ethylenediaminetetraacetic acid has been used previously to clean the tooth. Hydroxyl ions may stimulate cells in the cervical periodontal ligament to differentiate into odontoclasts, which begin root resorption in the area of the tooth below the epithelial attachment. Cervical resorption is usually painless until the resorption exposes the pulp, necessitating endodontic therapy. Intracanal dressings of calcium hydroxide are often successful in halting further tooth resorption, but severe external root resorption often necessitates extraction of the tooth. Moderate root resorption can be treated by orthodontically extruding the tooth and restoring it with a post-retained crown, but the prognosis of this treatment can be doubtful. Mild cervical resorption can be treated by surgical access, curettage, and placement of a restoration.

### Effects on Restorative Materials

*Application of Bleaching on Composites has Shown Following Changes*

- Increased surface hardness.
- Surface roughening and etching.
- Decrease in tensile strength.
- Increased microleakage.
- No significant color change of composite material itself other than the removal of extrinsic stains around existing restoration.

*Effect of Bleaching Agents on Other Materials*

- No effect on gold restorations.
- Microstructural changes in amalgam.
- Alteration in the matrix of glass ionomers.
- IRM on exposure to $H_2O_2$ becomes cracked and swollen.
- Provisional crowns made from methyl methacrylate discolor and turn orange.

### Mucosal Irritation

A high concentration of hydrogen peroxide (30-35%) is caustic to mucous membrane and may causes burns and bleaching of the gingiva. So the bleaching tray must be designed to prevent gingival exposure by use of firmly fitted tray that may has contact only with teeth.

### Genotoxicity and Carcinogenicity

Hydrogen peroxide shows genotoxic effect as free radicals released from hydrogen peroxide (hydroxy radicals, perhydroxyl ions and superoxide anions) are capable of attacking DNA.

### Toxicity

The acute effects of hydrogen peroxide ingestion are dependent on the amount and the concentration of hydrogen peroxide solution ingested. The effects are more severe, when higher concentrations are used.

Signs and symptoms usually seen are ulceration of the buccal mucosa, esophagus and stomach, nausea, vomiting, abdominal distention and sore throat. It is therefore important to keep syringes with bleaching agents out of reach of children to prevent any possible accident.

**Effects of bleaching agents on tooth and its supporting structures**

- Tooth sensitivity.
- Alteration of enamel surface.
- Effects on dentin.
- Effects of bleaching on pulp.
- Effects on cementum.
- Effects on restorative materials.
- Mucosal irritation.
- Genotoxicity and carcinogenicity.
- Toxicity.

Bleaching is safe, economical, conservative and effective method of decoloring the stained teeth due to various reasons.

It should always be given a thought before going for more invasive procedure like veneering or full ceramic coverage, depending upon specific case.

## QUESTIONS

**Q. What are different etiological factors responsible for discoloration of teeth.**

**Q. Define bleaching. Explain the mechanism of bleaching and classify different bleaching procedures.**

**Q. How will you bleach a nonvital central incisor tooth?**

**Q. Write short notes on:**

a. Contraindication of bleaching
b. Nightguard vital bleaching technique
c. Walking bleach
d. In-office bleach
e. Effects of bleaching on teeth

## BIBLIOGRAPHY


1. Abou-Rass M. The elimination of tetracycline discoloration by intentional endodontics and internal bleaching. J Endod 1982;8:101.
2. AT Hara, LAF Pimenta. Nonvital tooth bleaching: A 2 years case report. Quintessence Int, 1999;30:748-54.
3. C Hegedus, et al. An atomic force microscopy study on the effect of bleaching agent on the enamel surface. J Dent 1999;27:509-15.
4. Croll TB. Enamel microabrasion: the technique. Quint Int 1989;20:395-400.
5. Croll TP, Cavanaugh RR. Enamel color modification by controlled hydrochloric acid-pumice abrasion-Part I: Technique and examples. Quintessence Int 1986;17:81.
6. Curtis WJ, Dickinson GL, Downey MC, Russel CM, Haywood VB, Myers Ml, Johnson MIL. Assessing the effects of 10 percent carbamide peroxide on oral soft tissues. J Am Dent Assoc 1996;12:1218-223.
7. Dean HT. Chronic endemic dental fluorosis. J Am Med Assoc 1932;107:1269.
8. Dederich DN, Bushick RD. Lasers in dentistry. J Am Dent Assoc 2004;135:204-12.
9. Haywood Van B. History safety and effectiveness of current bleaching techniques and applications of the nightguard vital bleaching technique. Quintessence Int 1992;23:471-88.
10. Haywood VB, Heymann HO. Nigthguard vital bleaching: How safe is it? Quintessence Int 1991;22:515-23.
11. Jorgensen MG, Carroll WB. Incidence of tooth sensitivity after home whitening treatment. J Am Dent Assoc 2002;133:1076-82.
12. Laser assisted bleaching: An update. JADA 1998;129:1484-87.
13. Leonard Settembrim, et al. A technique for bleaching nonvital teeth. JADA 1997;1283-85.
14. Mokhils GR, Matis BA, Cochran MA, Eckert GJ. A clinical evaluation of carbamide peroxide and hydrogen peroxide whitening agents during daytime use. J Am Dent Assoc 2000; 31:1269-77.
15. Nageswar Rao R, Nangrani V. Estimation of dissolution of calcium by Old McInnes and New Mcinnes solution. Endodontology 1998;50-53.
16. Nathanson D. Vital tooth bleaching: Sensitivity and pulpal considerations. J Am Dent Assoc 1997;1281:41-44.
17. New man SM, Bottone PW. Tray-forming technique for dentist-supervised home bleaching. Quintessence Int 1995;26:447-53.
18. Reinhardt JW, Eivins SE, Swift EJ, Denchy GE. A clinical study of nigthguard vital bleaching. Quintessence Int 1993;25:379-84.
19. Ronald E Goldstein. Bleaching teeth: New materials-new role. JADA 1987;43-52.
20. Tredwin CJ, Scully C, Bagan-Sebastian JV. Drug induced disorders of teeth. J Dent Res 2005;84(7):596-602.
21. Van B Harywood. Historical development of Whiteners: Clinical safety and efficacy. Dental update, 1997 April.
22. Watts A, Addy M. Tooth discolouration and staining: A literature review. Br Dent J 2001;190:309-16.

# Tooth Resorption

CHAPTER 30



## INTRODUCTION

Pulp and periodontal tissues are unique in many aspects. A number of researches have been conducted to study the reparative, formative and protective reactions of the pulp and the periodontal tissues. Tooth resorption is one such reactive mechanism of these tissues to various forms of injuries. Roots of teeth undergo resorption under many circumstances. But unlike bone, which undergoes resorption and apposition as a part of continual remodeling process, the roots of permanent teeth are not normally resorbed.

If resorption occurs, it is because of some pathologic reasons but deciduous teeth show physiologic resorption before they are shed off.

## DEFINITION

According to the American Association of Endodontics in 1944, (Glossary – Contemporary Terminology for Endodontics) *resorption is defined as* "A condition associated with either a physiologic or a pathologic process resulting in the loss of dentin, cementum or bone."

*Root-resorption* is the resorption affecting the cementum or dentin of the root of tooth.

Resorption is a perplexing problem for all dental practitioners. The etiologic factors are vague, diagnosis is like educated guesses and often the treatment does not prevent the rapid resorption of dental tissues.

The occurrence of resorption cannot be predicted, it can be identified radiographically. But even this diagnostic tool has limitation because resorption on buccal or lingual surface of tooth usually cannot be seen until 20-40% of the tooth structure has been demineralized. Since, the etiological factors, diagnosis, treatment and prognosis differ for the various types of resorption defects, the practitioners must be able to diagnose resorption radiographically or clinically, distinguish internal from external resorption and instigate appropriate treatment to stop the progress of the resorption process.

## CLASSIFICATION OF RESORPTION

The area of root resorption is poorly understood and confusing. Many authors have used their own terminology to classify resorptive area.

### Classification

- *Physiologic tooth resorption* is seen in deciduous teeth during eruption of permanent teeth
- *Pathologic tooth resorption* is seen in both deciduous as well as permanent teeth due to underlying pathology.
  a. *Internal Resorption*
     – Root canal replacement resorption
     – Internal inflammatory resorption
  b. *External Resorption*
     – Surface resorption
     – Inflammatory resorption
     – Replacement resorption
     – Dentoalveolar ankylosis

### Classification of Resorption

- *Inflammatory*
  a. Internal
  b. External

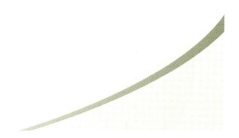

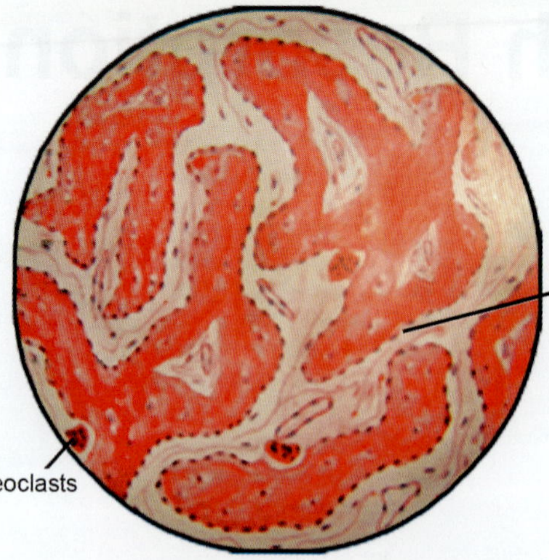


**Fig. 30.1:** Structure of bone showing osteoclasts and osteoblasts

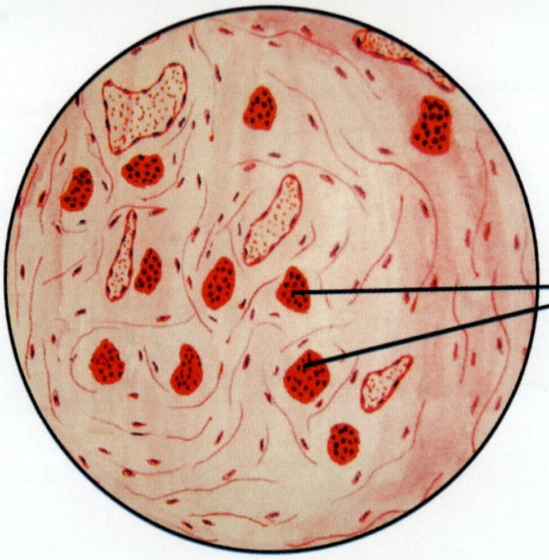


**Fig. 30.2:** Diagram showing giant cells

- *Non-inflammatory*
  a. Transient
  b. Pressure
  c. Replacement

## CELLS INVOLED IN TOOTH RESORPTION

### Clast Cells

*Odonoclasts, dentinoclasts, osteoclasts and cementoclasts*, all these cells belong to the group of clast cells and they have a common origin. They are derived from the circulating monocytes which form macrophages. When the inflammation gets out of control of the monocytes macrophages, they join together to form *giant cells* (Fig. 30.1). Osteoclasts have a lifespan of approximately 2 week. They are highly vacuolated and contain numerous mitochondria. Majority of odontoclasts have 10 or fewer nuclei, i.e. 96 percent are multinucleated and rest 4 percent are mono-nucleated.

Oligonuclear odontoclasts are cells with fewer than 5 nuclei. They resorb more dentin per nucleus when compared with cells with higher number of nuclei. Osteoclasts usually have 20 to 30 nuclei. Clear zone gives indication of the resorption activity.

*Monocytes and macrophages*: Monocytes and macrophages along with osteoclasts, play an important role in bone and tooth resorption. They are found in tissue surfaces adjacent to bone, for example, in resorpting surfaces of rheumatoid arthritis, periodontal diseases, periradicular granulomas, cysts, and in metastatic bone tumors. Although macrophages have a structure (Fig. 30.2) similar to that of osteoclasts, and like osteoclasts, can also become multinucleated giant cells, but macrophages lack a ruffled border that is attached to hard tissue substrates during resorption and do not create lacunae on the dentinal surface.

When there is an irritation of some kind, the tissue responds by the process of inflammation in which, the blood supply to the area is increased. There will be migration of monocytes to the site of inflammation, where they differentiate into macrophages. These processes are regulated by chemotactic factors like c-AMP and calcium.

## MECHANISM OF TOOTH RESORPTION

Resorption of hard tissue takes place in *two events*.

1. There is the degradation of inorganic crystal structures – hydroxyapatite
2. Degradation of the organic matrix.

### Degradation of the Inorganic Crystal Structures

The degradation of the inorganic structures is initiated by the creation of an acidic pH of 3 to 4.5 at the site of resorption. This is created by the polarized proton pump which is produced within the ruffled border of the clast cells. Below the pH of 5, the dissolution of hydroxyapatite occurs.

Enzymes carbonic anhydrase II which catalyses the conversion of $CO_2$ and $H_2CO_3$ intracellularly also maintains an acidic environment at the site of resorption which is a readily available source of $H^+$ ions. The enzyme acid phosphatase also favors the resorption process.

$$CO_2 + H_2O \rightleftharpoons H_2CO_3$$
$$H_2CO_3 \rightleftharpoons H^+ + HCO_3^-$$

### Degradation of the Organic Matrix

Three main enzymes involved in this process are collagenase, matrix metalloproteinases (MMP) and cysteine proteinases

### Enzymes Involved in Degradation of Organic Matrix

1. Collagenase
2. Matrix metalloproteinases (MMP)
3. Cysteine proteinases

Collagenase and MMP act at a neutral or just below neutral pH–7.4. They are found more towards the resorbing bone surface where the pH is near neutral, because of the presence of the buffering capacity of the resorbing bone salts. MMP is more involved in odontoblastic action. Cysteine proteinases are secreted directly into the osteoclasts into the clear zone via the ruffled border. Cysteine proteinases work more in an acidic pH and near the ruffled border, the pH is more acidic.

## Inhibitory Mechanisms of Resorption

### *Cementum*

The innermost layer of cementum is lined by the cementoid tissue and the cementoblasts. The cementoid is less mineralized and so it is more resistant to resorption. Clastic cell are attracted or can attach themselves only to mineralized tissues. The innermost layer of cementum is a highly calcified layer, acts as a barrier between the dentinal tubules and the Sharpey's fibers. They do not allow the passage of toxic products or micro-organisms under normal circumstances. Cementoblasts favor cementum formation. Continuity of root cementum is an important factor to be taken into consideration in various pathologies of resorption.

### *Dentin*

Predentin layer is uncalcified layer of dentin, the just formed dentin, lined by odontoblasts favor dentin deposition. Wedenberg et al has demonstrated it as an anti-invasive factor in dentin.

According to Silva et al, dentin contains numerous polypeptide signaling molecules which may affect the healing and resorption of dental and periodontal tissues.

# FACTORS REGULATING TOOTH RESORPTION

## Systemic Factors

*Parathyroid hormones (PTH)* favor resorption. They stimulate osteoclasts; favor the formation of multinucleated giant cells.

*1, 2, 5 dihydroxy Vit $D_3$* increases the resorption activity of the osteoblasts.

*Calcitonin* inhibits the resorption by suppressing the osteoclastic cytoplasmic mobility of the ruffled border.

## Local Factors

These are secreted from inflammatory cells and osteoblasts as a result of stimulation by bacteria, tissue breakdown products and cytokines themselves.

## Factors Regulating Tooth Resorption

| *Local factors* | *Systemic factors* |
|---|---|
| Macrophage colony stimulating factor (M-CSF) | Parathyroid hormone |
| Interleukin 6 | 1, 2, 5 dihydroxy Vit $D_3$ |
| Interleukin 1 | Calcitonin |
| TNF - alpha | |
| Prostaglandin – $PGE_2$ | |
| Bacteria and toxins | |

# INTERNAL RESORPTION

**Synonym of internal resorption**

- Chronic perforating hyperplasia of the pulp
- Internal granuloma
- Odontoblastoma
- Pink tooth of mummery

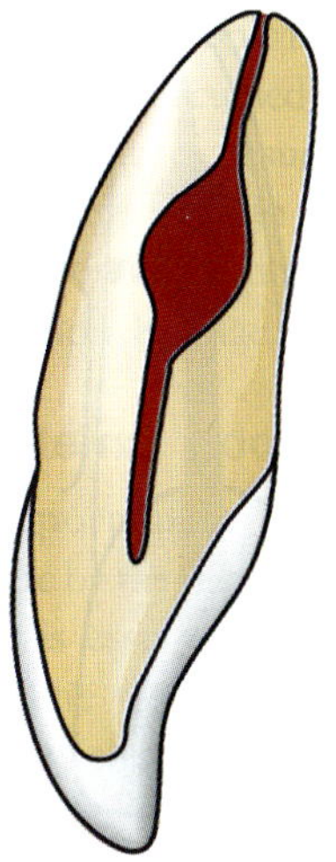

Fig. 30.3: Internal resorption

According to *Shafer*, "Internal resorption is an unusual form of tooth resorption that begins centrally within the tooth, apparently initiated in most cases by a peculiar inflammation of the pulp." It is characterized by oval shaped enlargement of root canal space (Fig. 30.3). It is usually asymptomatic and discovered on routine radiographs. Internal resorption may progress slowly, rapidly or intermittently with period of activity and inactivity.

## Etiology

Internal resorption is pulpally related problem that triggers resorption of the dentin from the pulp outward (Fig. 30.4). The tooth often has a history of trauma or pulp cap. Discoloration may or may not be present. Pulp tests may indicate vitality or necrosis. The abnormal pulpal response results in *dentinoclastic* activity that generates an increase in the size of the chamber and canal space.

Internal resorption may also be caused while doing restorative procedure like preparation of tooth for crown, deep restorative procedures, application of heat over the pulp or pulpotomy using calcium hydroxide, i.e. iatrogenic in origin. Internal resorption can also be idiopathic in origin.

**Etiology of internal resorption**

- Long standing chronic inflammation of the pulp
- Caries related pulpits
- Traumatic injuries
  a. Luxation injuries
- Iatrogenic injuries
  a. Preparation of tooth for crown
  b. Deep restorative procedures
  c. Application of heat over the pulp
  d. Pulpotomy using $Ca(OH)_2$
- Idiopathic

## Clinical Features

The pulp usually remains vital and asymptomatic until root has been perforated and become necrotic. Patient may present pain

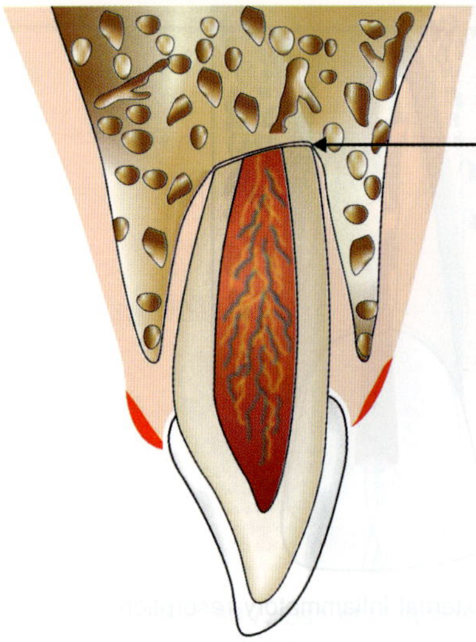


**Fig. 30.13:** Orthodontic tooth movement resulting in inflammatory resorption

- Trauma leads to pulpal necrosis which may further cause periodontal inflammation due to the passage of the toxins and microorganisms from the infected pulp, lateral canals, apical foramen, accessory canals, dentinal tubules where there is a discontinuity of cementum
- Orthodontic tooth movement using excessive forces (Fig. 30.13)
- Trauma from occlusion – leading to periodontal inflammation
- Avulsion and Luxation injuries
- Pressure resorption occurring from pressure exerted by tumors, cysts and impacted teeth
- In the initial stages bowl shaped lacunae are seen in cementum and dentin, if not controlled it may resorb the entire root in latter stages (Figs 30.14A to C).

### *Clinical Features*

- Patient gives history of trauma – recent or past
- Necrotic pulp/irreversible pulpitis are frequently seen.
- Tooth is usually mobile in most of the cases.
- Inflammation of the periodontal tissues is commonly seen.
- Percussion sensitivity is present.

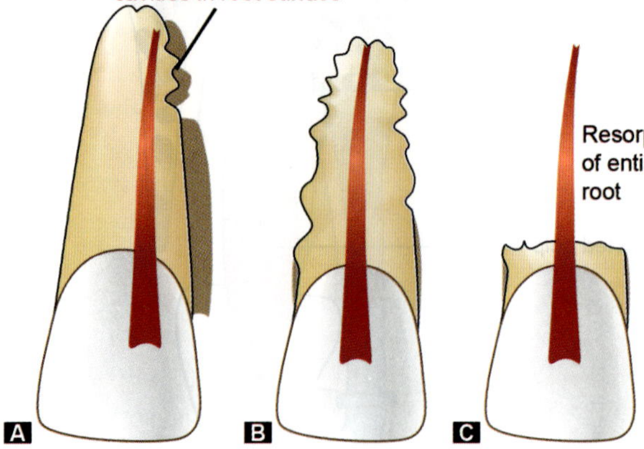


**Figs 30.14A to C:** External inflammatory root resorption (A) In initial stages, bowl shaped resorption cavities are seen in root surface; (B) More of resorption; (C) Complete resorption of root in latter stages

- Pocket formation may or may not be there. If the resorption area communicates with the gingival sulcus, it can lead to pocket formation.

### *Radiographic Feature*

Bowl like radiolucency with ragged irregular areas on the root surface is commonly seen in conjunction with loss of tooth structure and alveolar bone. Small lesions of external root resorption usually go undetected.

### *Treatment*

Treatment for inflammatory resorption is based on removal or reduction of source of infection.

In case of infected gingival tissues, appropriate periodontal care consisting of removal of plaque and calculus followed by periodontal maintenance is indicated.

If the sustaining infection is pulpal, root canal therapy has been shown to be a very successful means of treating inflammatory resorption. It has been recommended to include a Calcium hydroxide paste in the root canal therapy to enhance the success of treatment outcome.

Calcitonin has also been suggested as an interim root canal medicament to assist in the inhibition of osteoclastic bone and dentin resorption. Presumably, Calcitonin penetrates the dentinal tubules in the outward direction, thus exerting a direct effect. Prevention of inflammatory resorption depends primarily on its early detection. A careful program of radiographic control, pulpal evaluation and clinical observation should be followed.

A suggested protocol for monitoring of injured teeth would be as follows:

1. Schedule initial examination as soon as possible after the traumatic event.
2. Re-evaluate the tooth by conducting pulp tests and radiographs every 4 to 6 weeks for the first six months.
3. Afterwards re-evaluate yearly for several years.
4. Begin treatment at any point when there is evidence of resorption. It would also be prudent to recommend root canal therapy if pulp necrosis can be ascertained even in the absence of resorption.

## Replacement Resorption/Dentoalveolar Ankylosis

This is similar to ankylosis, but there is presence of an intervening inflamed connective tissue, always progressive and highly destructive. This is a serious condition for the teeth involved because the teeth become part of the alveolar bone remodeling process and they are therefore, progressively resorbed. It occurs most frequently as a result of complications following avulsions in which the periodontal ligament dries and loses its vitality.

It has also been observed in primary mandibular molars. Ankylosis may be transient or progressive. In the transient type, less than 20 percent of the root surface becomes ankylosed. In such cases, reversal may occur, resulting in reestablishment of a periodontal ligament connection between tooth and bone.

In the progressive type, tooth structure is gradually resorbed and replaced with the bone.

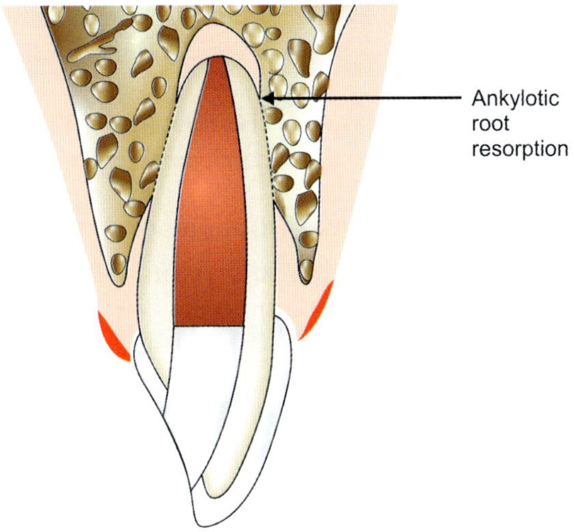


**Fig. 30.15:** Replacement resportion resulting in ankylosis

### Etiopathogenesis

- Traumatic injuries to teeth—In cases of intrusive luxation and reimplantation of avulsed tooth, especially with long extraoral dry time
- The rate of progression of ankylosis is directly related to—the amount of damage to the root surface
- Progression of the ankylosis is very rapid in young individuals as compared to adults.

According to *Tronstad L* the chances of progressive ankylosis increase if more than 20 percent of the root surface is damaged. In dentoalveolar ankylosis, the injury results in damage to periodontal ligament cells and cementum, causing discontinuity in the cementum. Cells present in vicinity of the denuded root try to repopulate it. Bone precursor cells are more active than the slower moving periodontal ligament cells. They move across the socket wall and populate the damaged root without an intermediate attachment apparatus.

Because of this, the bone comes in direct contact with root without an intermediate attachment apparatus. This results in **dentoalveolar ankylosis** (Fig 30.15).

### Histological Examination

It shows a direct fusion between dentin and bone without separating cemental or periodontal ligament layer. Active resorption lacunae with osteoclasts are seen in conjunction with apposition of normal bone laid by osteoblasts.

### Clinical Features

A tooth with dentoalveolar ankylosis shows:

- Lack of mobility
- Dull metallic sound on percussion (may be evident even before the appearance of the radiograph)
- Infraocclusion because of lack of the normal growth of the alveolar process
- Lack of mesial drift.

### Radiographic Appearance

Radiographically one can observe the moth eaten appearance with irregular border, absence of periodontal ligament and lamina dura.

### Diagnosis

Diagnosis can be made from clinical evaluation and radiographic observation. Lack of mobility and high pitched metallic sound on percussion of tooth are often the characteristic features of ankylosis.

Radiographically, the loss of periodontal ligament space with replacement by bone in association with an uneven contour of root is indicative of ankylosis.

### Treatment

Currently there is no treatment offered for replacement resorption. It may be possible to slow the resorptive process by treating the root surface with fluoride solution prior to replantation if it is known that extraoral time for tooth was more than two hours and it was not kept moist to protect the periodontal ligament. One should not view replacement resorption as total failure. A replanted tooth undergoing replacement resorption can see many years before root is fully resorbed.

### Prevention

To prevent ankylosis following points should be considered in cases of avulsion:

- Immediate replantation without much extraoral dry time
- Proper extraoral storage to prevent dehydration
- Incase of extended period of extraoral time, soak the tooth in fluoride gel.

## Recently Introduced Enamel Product "Emdogain"

Emdogain was developed in 1992 with the purpose of regenerating lost periodontium. When it is applied, amelogenin rich protein matrix precipitate out of the solution and forms an insoluble layer on the root surface promoting the attachment of mesenchymal cells. These cells then produce new matrix component and growth factors, which play major role in formation of new periodontal attachment. Emdogain also inhibits epithelial cell growth which could interfere the regenerative process. It promotes both proliferation and differentiation of osteoblastic cells and inhibits the formation of osteoclasts by stimulating the effect of osteoprotegerive (OPG).

Emdogain may also act as growth factor which prolongs the osteoblast growth and maintain their morphology.

There are *two schools* of thoughts of its use as an adjunct in treatment of replacement resorption.

*One school* says the main cause of replacement resorption is damage to periodontal tissue during replantation. Emdogain accumulates in the cell at the root surface and promotes regeneration of PDL tissues.

However, *other school* of thought does not support is use. In a clinical study, avulsed and previously ankylosed teeth replanted with Emdogain developed the subsequent ankylosis after six months leading to conclusion that Emdogain could not prevent or cure ankylosis.

Further studies are needed to prove the efficacy of Emdogain in prevention of replacement resorption.

## CERVICAL ROOT RESORPTION (EXTRACANAL INVASIVE RESORPTION)

According to Cohen, it is the type of inflammatory root resorption occurring immediately below the epithelial attachment of tooth. Epithelial attachment need not be always exactly at the cervical margin but can also be apical to the cervical margin (Fig. 30.16). So the term "Cervical" is a misnomer.

### Etiology

According to *Heithersay*, cervical root resorption is caused by various factors. These can be as following:

- Orthodontic treatment – 24.1 percent
- Trauma – 15.1 percent
- Bleaching of non vital teeth – 3.9 percent
- Periodontal treatment
- Bruxism
- Idiopathic.

### Etiopathogenesis

It is a relatively common occurrence, but not well recognized and often classified as idiopathic resorption because of difficulty in establishing a cause and effect relation. It appears to originate in the cervical area of the tooth below the epithelial attachment and often proceeds from a small surface opening to involve a large part of dentin between the cementum and the pulp.

The resorption can proceed in several direction and often has an invasive quality, hence the term *invasive resorption.* It can extend coronally under the enamel, giving the tooth a pink spot appearance. Because cervical resorption is not always associates with infected or necrotic pulp, the treatment options vary accordingly.

### Clinical Features of Cervical Root Resorption

- Initially asymptomatic
- Pulp vital in most cases
- Normal to sensitivity tests

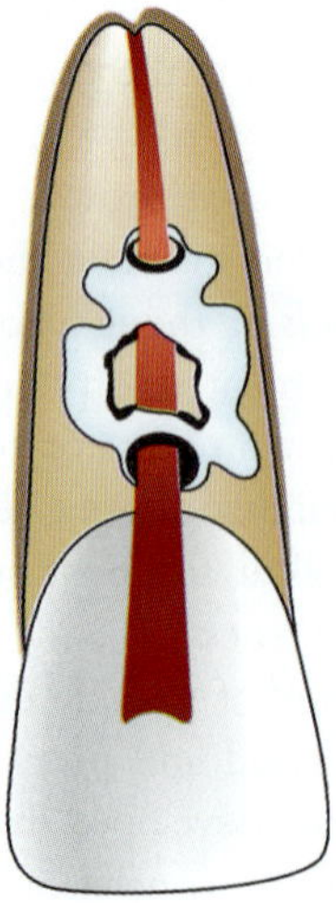

**Fig. 30.16:** Extracanal invasive resorption

- Long standing cases give pink spot appearance Clinically, misdiagnosed as internal resorption but confirmed radiographically
- In due course, it spreads laterally along the root, i.e. apical and coronal direction "enveloping" the root canal.

### Theories of Cervical Root Resorption

i. Some procedures and events (bleaching, trauma, orthodontic treatment) cause alteration in the organic and inorganic cementum, finally making it more inorganic. This makes the cementum less resistant to resorption.

ii. Immunological system senses the altered root surface, as a different tissue, attacks as a foreign body.

### Clinical Features

- Initially the cervical root resorption is asymptomatic in nature
- Pulp if present will be vital in most cases of cervical root resorption. The pulp responds normal to sensitivity tests
- Long standing cervical root resorption cases show extensive loss of tooth structure replaced by granulation tissues which undermines the enamel in due course giving rise to pink spot appearance clinically. It is misdiagnosed as internal resorption, but confirmed with a radiograph. It initially starts as a small lesion, progress and reaches the predentin. Predentin is more resistant to resorption, spreads laterally in apical and coronal direction "enveloping" the root canal.

Rarely, it perforates into the tooth causing secondary involvement of pulp. In most of the cases, it occurs at the immediate subgingival level.

### Heithersay's Classification

*Class I:* A small invasive resorptive lesion near cervical area with shallow penetration into dentin.

*Class II:* Well defined resorptive defect close to coronal pulp chamber, but little or no involvement of radicular dentin.

*Class III:* Deep resorptive lesion involving coronal pulp and also coronal third of the root.

*Class IV:* Resorptive defective extending beyond coronal third of root canal.

### Franks's Classification of Cervical Root Resorption

- *Supraosseous* — Coronal to the level of alveolar bone (Fig. 30.17).
- *Intraosseous* — Not accompanied by periodontal breakdown (Fig. 30.18).
- *Crestal* — At the level of alveolar bone (Fig. 30.19).

### Radiographic Feature

Radiographically one can see the moth-eaten appearance with the intact outline of the canal. Because bone is often

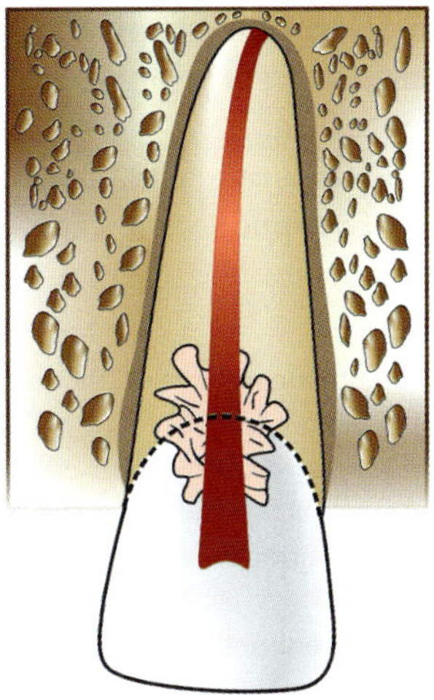

Fig. 30.17: Supraosseous extracanal invasive resorption

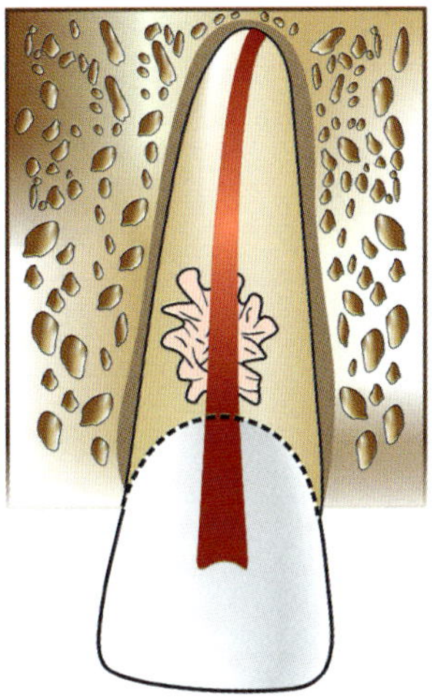

Fig. 30.18: Intraosseous extracanal invasive resorption

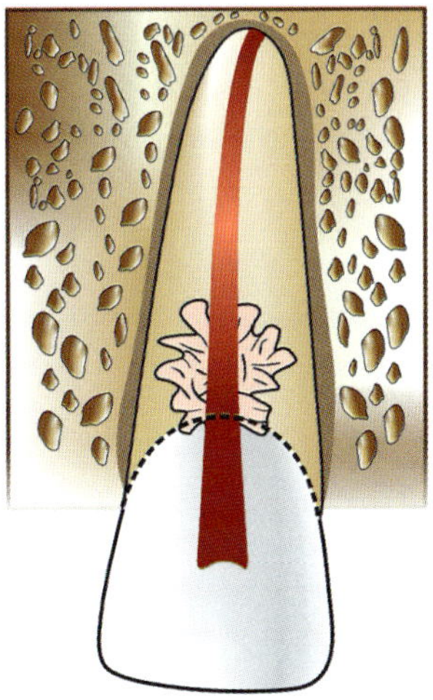

Fig. 30.19: Crestal extracanal invasive resorption

involved, resorption may give the appearance of an infrabony pocket.

### Treatment

The *main aim* of the treatment is to restore the lost tooth structure and to disrupt the resorptive process. A traditional approach is to treat the tooth endodontically first, followed by repair of the resorbed area either from an internal approach or an external one.

A combination of internal restoration followed by a surgical approach to smoothen and finish the surface of filling material where it exits through the original resorptive entry, may provide acceptable results.

*Another treatment* approach has been recommended because the pulp is often vital in a tooth with invasive resorption, the repair of resorbed area may be accomplished without removing the pulp. The clinical procedure consists of surgically exploring the resorbed lacuna and curetting the soft tissue from the defect, which can then be the prepared for restoration. The advantage of such a non endodontic approach is that, it is more conservative than the more common approach of including root canal therapy in the treatment. If pulpal symptoms develop later, root canal therapy can be done when needed. Other treatment options are intentional replantation or root amputation of affected tooth.

There is not known method for prevention of invasive resorption, early detection will allow more conservative treatment. The prognosis after treatment is uncertain because clinical experience has shown that, even after restoration of resorptive defects, new foci of resorption just apical to the previous lacunae may recur.

## TRANSIENT APICAL BREAKDOWN

It is a temporary phenomenon in which the apex of the tooth displays radiographic appearance of resorption—followed by surface resorption and/or obliteration of the pulp canal (Figs 30.20A and B).

- Repair takes place within a year. It is commonly seen in mature teeth with completely closed apex
- Usually it occurs after moderate injuries to the tooth for example—subluxation, extrusion, lateral luxation
- Infections, orthodontic treatment, trauma from occlusion, etc.
- No treatment is recommended.

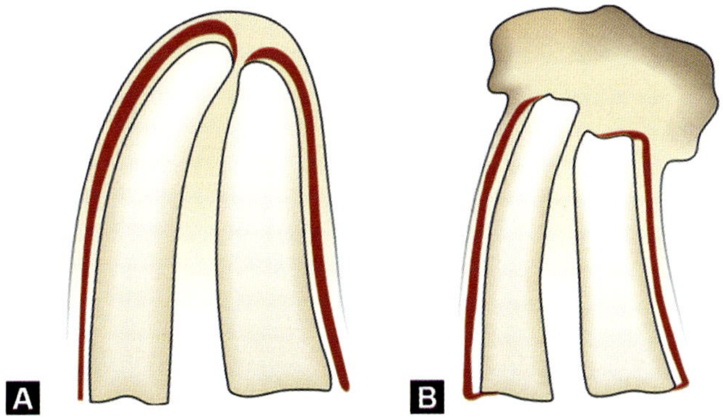


Figs 30.20A and B: A. Normal root apex B. Apical root resorption

## CONCLUSION

Tooth resorption is a perplexing problem where the etiologic factors are vague and less clearly defined. For the best treatment outcome, the clinician should have a very good knowledge of the etiopathology of resorptive lesions. Early diagnosis and prompt treatment in such cases are the key factors which determine the success of the treatment. More clinical studies and research with animal models are required to explain more about this phenomenon scientifically.

## QUESTIONS

**Q. Define and classify root resorption write in detail about internal resorption.**

**Q. Classify external root resorption. Write in detail about replacement resorption.**

**Q. Write short notes on:**

a. Differential diagnosis of internal and external resorption.
b. Cervical root resorption

## BIBLIOGRAPHY


1. Andreasen JO. Traumatic injuries of the teeth, second edition. Philadelphia, WB Saunders 1981.
2. Grossman. Endodontic practice, 11th edition.
3. Heithersay GS, Morile AJ. Australian Dental Journal 1982;27:368.
4. Martin Trope. Root resorption due to dental trauma: Endodontic Topics 2002;79.
5. Oliet S. Journal of Endodontics 1984;10:391.

# Tooth Infractions

CHAPTER 31

- Tooth Infractions
- Vertical Root Fracture (VRF)
- Bibliography

Tooth fracture can be divided into following five categories according to American Association of Endodontists (AAE):

a. *Craze line* — It is confined to enamel only.
b. *Cuspal fracture* — Diagonal fracture not involving pulp.
c. *Cracked tooth* — Incomplete vertical fracture involving pulp.
d. *Split tooth* — It is complete vertical fracture.
e. *Vertical root fracture* — It includes complete longitudinal fracture, usually seen in endodontically treated tooth.

**Synonyms of tooth infraction**

1. Incomplete tooth fracture
2. Cracked tooth syndrome
3. Split tooth syndrome
4. Green stick fracture
5. Hairline fracture
6. Cuspal fracture odontalgia

So we can say that there are mainly two main categories of cracked teeth:

a. Tooth infractions which include craze line, cracked teeth and cuspal fracture
b. Vertical root fracture which usually occur in endodontically treated teeth.

## TOOTH INFRACTIONS

Tooth infraction is defined as "incomplete tooth fracture extending partially through a tooth." The fracture commonly involves enamel and dentin but sometimes pulp and periodontal structure may also get involved (Fig. 31.1).

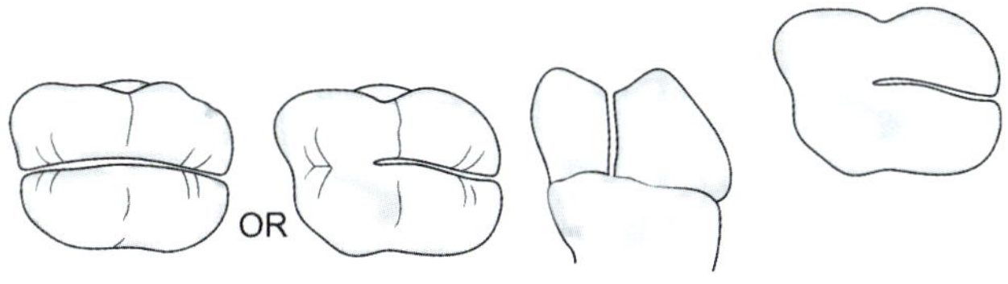


**Fig. 31.1:** Diagrammatic representation of cracked teeth

### Etiology

The etiology of cracked tooth syndrome is not specific but is commonly seen to be associated in teeth with large and complex restorations, leaving the teeth more susceptible to cracks. Moreover, stressful lifestyle, parafunctional habits and high masticatory forces are important contributing factors. So we can enlist etiological factors for cracked teeth as following:

- Extensively large restoration.
- Improperly designed restoration
- Excessive use of pins for restoration
- Age changes in enamel and dentin making teeth more brittle and prone to infraction.
- Deep abrasion, erosion and caries
- Accidental biting on hard object
- High masticatory forces
- Oral habits like bruxism
- Acute trauma to tooth.

### Classification of Cracked Teeth

Cracked teeth can be classified on the basis of pulpal or periodontal involvement and the extent of crack.

*Class A:* Crack involving enamel and dentin but not pulp.
*Class B:* Crack involving pulp but not periodontal apparatus.
*Class C:* Crack extending to pulp and involving periodontal apparatus.
*Class D:* Complete division of tooth with pulpal and periodontal apparatus involvement.
*Class E:* Apically induced fracture.

### Diagnosis

The patient with cracked tooth syndrome gives history of variable signs and symptoms which are difficult to diagnose. Even the radiographs are inconclusive. The careful history of the patient, examination, diagnostic tests, radiographs and sometimes surgical exposure are needed for accurate diagnosis of cracked tooth syndrome.

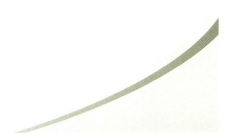

## Clinical Examinations

To reach at definite diagnosis, one should obtain adequate information from patient history and clinical examination.

## Chief Complaint

Patient usually complains of pain on chewing and sensitivity to cold and sweets. If these symptoms are associated with noncarious teeth, one should consider the possibility of infraction.

## History of Patient

Patient with an infracted tooth should be asked about:

a. Previous trauma if any.
b. Details regarding dietary habits.
c. Presence of abnormal habits like bruxism, etc.

## Visual Examination

One should look for presence of:

a. Large restoration
b. Wear facets and steep cusps
c. Cracked restoration
d. Gap between tooth structure and restoration
e. Sometimes removal of restoration is required for examination of fracture line in a cavity.

## Tactile Examination

While carrying out tactile examination, one should gently pass the tip of sharp explorer along the tooth surface, it may catch the crack.

## Periodontal Probing

Thorough periodontal probing along the involved, tooth may reveal a narrow periodontal pocket.

## Bite Test

Orange wood stick, rubber wheel or the tooth slooth are commonly used for detection of cracked tooth. Tooth slooth is small pyramid shaped, plastic bite block with small concavity at the apex which is placed over the cusp and patient is asked to bite upon it with moderate pressure and release. The pain during biting or chewing especially upon the release of pressure is classic sign of cracked tooth syndrome.

## Transillumination

The use of fiberoptic light to transilluminate a fracture line is also a method of diagnosing cracked tooth syndrome.

## Use of Dyes

Staining of fractured teeth with a dye such as methylene blue can aid in diagnosis. Dye can be directly applied to the tooth to identify fracture (Fig. 31.2), or it can be incorporated into a temporary restoration like ZOE and placed in the prepared cavity (Fig. 31.3) or patient can be asked to chew a disclosing tablet (Fig. 31.4). The dark stain present on the fracture line helps in detecting the fracture.

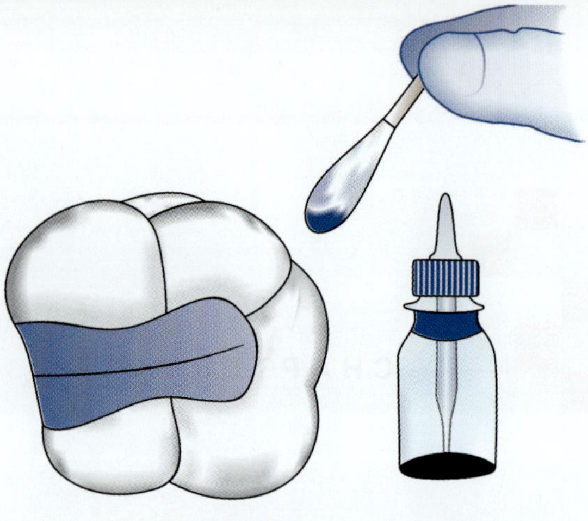

**Fig. 31.2:** To identify a cracked tooth, dye can be directly applied to the tooth

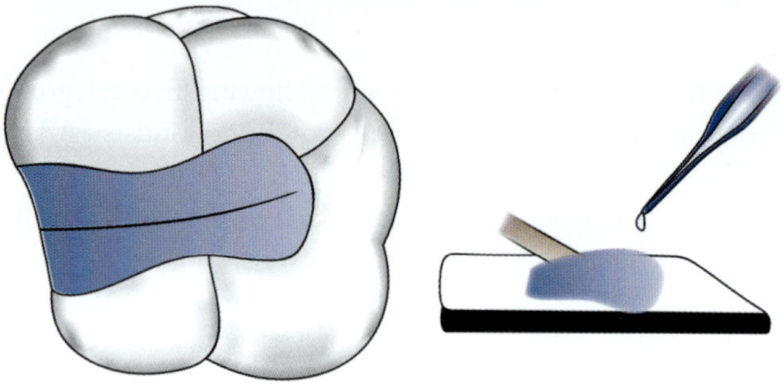

**Fig. 31.3:** Dye can be incorporated in a temporary restoration like ZOE and placed in prepared cavity

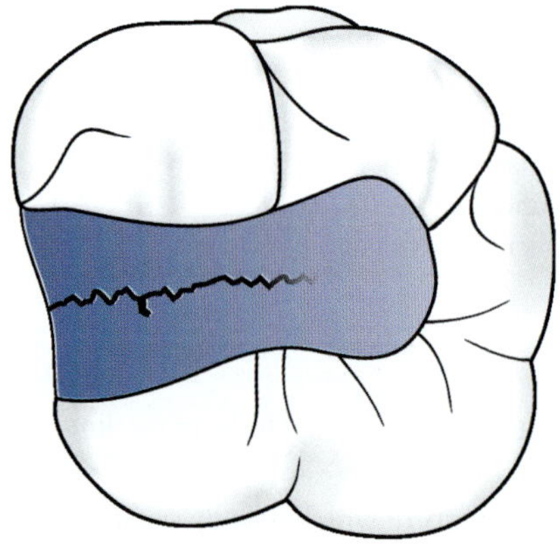

**Fig. 31.4:** Patient can be asked to chew a disclosing tablet, dark line on fracture area indicates crack

## Radiographs

1. Radiographs are not of much help especially, if, crack is mesiodistal in direction. Even the buccolingual cracks will only appear if there is actual separation of the segments or the crack happens to coincide with the X-ray beam.
2. Taking radiographs from more than one angle can help in locating the crack (Fig. 31.5).
3. A thickened periodontal ligament space, a diffused radiolucency especially with elliptical shape in apical area may indicate crack.

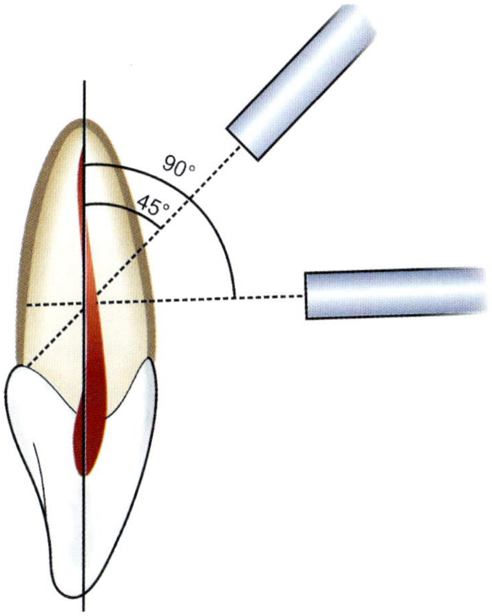


Fig. 31.5: Taking radiographs at more than one angle can help in locating the crack

## Surgical Exposure

If a fracture is suspected, a full thickness mucoperiosteal flap should be reflected for visual examination of root surface.

## Differential Diagnosis of Cracked Tooth Syndrome

The crack is commonly invisible to naked eye and symptoms may vary; these may include pain on chewing, varied patterns of referred pain and sensitivity to thermal changes. Furthermore, inconclusive radiographs make the diagnosis of cracked tooth difficult. There must be differentiation of a cracked tooth from a fractured cusp. The tooth crack occurs more towards the center of the occlusal surface as compared to the cusp fracture which is more peripheral in position.

- If the crack has progressed to involve the pulp or periodontium, patient may have thermal sensitivity which lingers after removal of the stimulus or slight to very severe spontaneous pain consistent with irreversible pulpitis, pulp necrosis or apical periodontitis.
- When crack is mesiodistal across both the marginal ridges, splitting the tooth in two segments, patient may complain of pain on chewing and soreness of gums of the affected area. It should be differentiated from periodontal abscess.

## Treatment of Cracked Teeth

The treatment plan for cracked teeth varies with location and extent of the crack. Even when crack can be located, the extent is still difficult to determine.

- Urgent care of the cracked tooth involves the immediate reduction of its occlusal contacts by selective grinding of tooth at the site of the crack or its antagonist.
- Definitive treatment of the cracked tooth aims to preserve the pulpal vitality by providing full occlusal coverage for cusp protection.
- When crack involves the pulpal floor, endodontic access is needed but one should not make attempts to chase down the extent of crack with a bur, because the crack may become invisible long before it terminates. Endodontic treatment can alleviate irreversible pulpal symptoms.
- If the crack is partially visible across the floor of the chamber, the tooth may be bonded with a temporary crown or orthodontic band. This will aid in determining the prognosis of the tooth and protect it from further deterioration till the endodontic therapy is completed (Figs 31.6A to C).
- Apical extension and future migration of the crack apically onto the root determines the prognosis. If the fracture is not detected, pulpal degeneration and periradicular pathosis may be the initial indication, that complete vertical fracture is present. Depending upon the extensions of the crack and symptoms, the treatment may involve extractions, root resection, or hemisection.

To conclude, it can be stated that the diagnosis of a cracked tooth can be difficult, but it should be done without the sense of urgency, so as to alleviate the painful symptoms, initiate an appropriate treatment plan and to improve the prognosis of the cracked tooth.

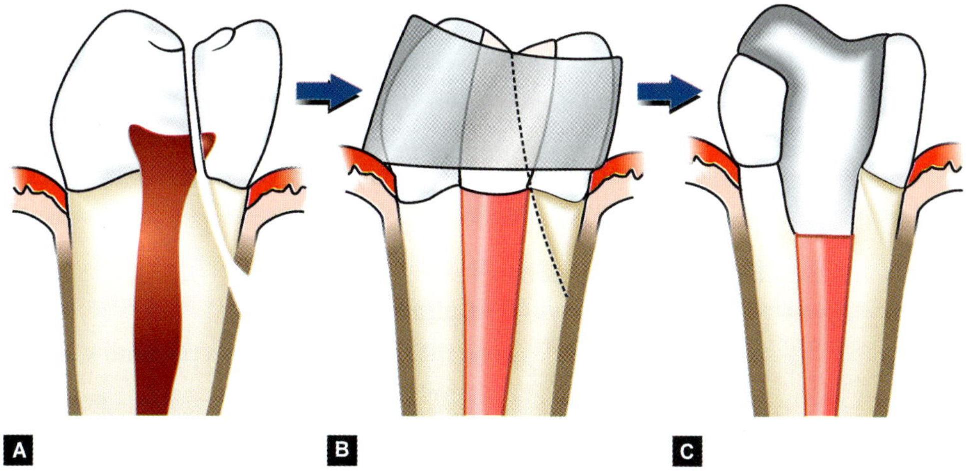


Figs 31.6A to C: (A) If crack is visible across the floor of pulp chamber; (B) tooth may be bonded with orthodontic band; (C) till endodontic therapy is completed

## VERTICAL ROOT FRACTURE (VRF)

According to American Association of Endodontists (AAE), VRF is a longitudinally oriented fracture of root that originates from the apex of tooth and progresses to the coronal part of tooth.

Vertical root fracture can occur at any phase of root canal treatment that is during biochemical preparation, obturation or during post placement. This fracture results from wedging forces within the canal. These excessive forces exceed the binding strength of existing dentin causing fatigue and fracture (Fig. 31.7).

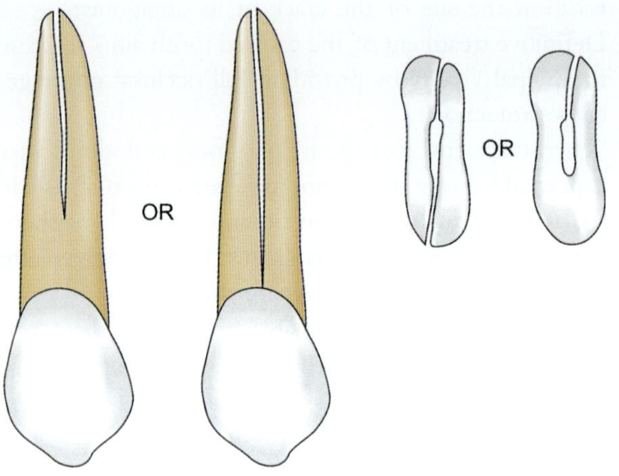


Fig. 31.7: Diagrammatic representation of vertical root fracture

### Etiology

Since they are commonly seen in endodontically treated teeth, the common reasons for vertical root fracture are:

a. Excessive dentin removal during biomechanical preparation.
b. Weakening of tooth during post space preparation.

Other factors which predispose the vertical root fracture are:

a. Anatomy of root: Roots with narrow mesiodistal diameter than buccolingual dimensions, are more prone to fracture. For example, roots of premolars and mesial roots of mandibular molar presence of root curvatures and depression can also predispose the fracture.
b. Amount of remaining tooth structure: Lesser is the amount of remaining tooth structure, more are the chances of VRF.
c. Presence of pre-existing cracks: Cracks present in dentin before treatment may latter propagate to result in VRF.
d. Loss of moisture in dentin: Though loss of moisture is not a main etiological factors, but it can be a predisposing factor for VRF.

Chances of VRF also increase with the use of spreaders during obturation. Use of spreaders result in generation of stresses during lateral compaction of gutta percha due to wedging effect of spreader on canal walls or through gutta-percha.

### Signs and Symptoms

Usually a tooth with vertical root fracture presents with following signs and symptoms:

1. Vertical root fracture commonly occurs in faciolingual plane. The fracture begins along the canal wall and grows outwards to the root surface.
2. Sudden crunching sound accompanied by pain is the pathognomic of the root fracture.
3. Presence of sinus tract near cervical area.
4. If fracture line propagates coronally and laterally to periodontal ligament (PDL), local inflammation in PDL. Causes periodontitis, resulting in deep osseous defect and periodontal type abscess formation.
5. Certain root shapes and sizes are more susceptible to vertical root fracture; for example, roots which are deep facially and lingually but narrow mesially and distally are particularly prone to fracture.
6. The susceptibility of root fracture increases by excessive dentin removal during canal preparation or post space preparation. Also the excessive condensation forces during compaction of gutta-percha while obturation increases the frequency of root fractures.

### Radiographic Examination

VRF is detected radiographically only when:

a. There is evidence of separation of root segments as a radiolucent area surrounding the bone between the roots.
b. Hair line radioleucency in radiographs. To confirm a case of VRF, one should take two or three radiographs at different angles. Most common feature of radiograph of VRF is "halo" appearance, a combined periapical and periradicular radioleucency on one or both sides of the involved root (Fig. 31.8).

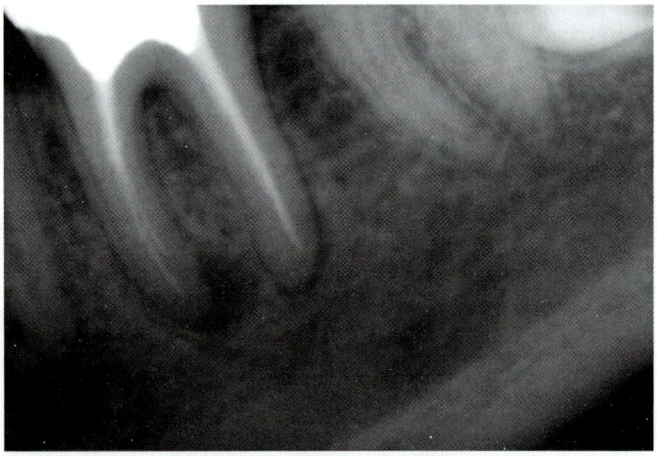

Fig. 31.8: Halo appearance of mesial root of 36 with VRF

### Diagnosis

It is difficult to diagnose a case with VRF because of following reasons:

a. Signs and symptoms commonly present in VRF like pain on mastication, mobility, presence of sinus tract, bony radiolucency and spontaneous dull pain can also be seen in failed root canal treatment or in periodontal disease.

b. Usually VRF is not detected during or immediately after root canal treatment. It may take years to diagnose VRF.
c. It is difficult to detect the crack radiographically.

## Treatment of Vertical Root Fracture

It involves extraction in most of the cases. In multirooted teeth root resection or hemisection can be tried.

Other treatment options include retention of the fractured fragment and placement of calcium hydroxide and then cementation of the fractured fragments.

Recently, repair of root fracture have been tried by binding them with the help of adhesive resins, glass ionomers and lasers. But to date, no successful technique has been reported to correct this problem.

## Prevention of Root Fracture

As we know the prognosis for VRF is poor, as far as possible, it should be tried to prevent the occurrence of VRF. Prevention of root fracture basically involves avoidance of the causes of root fracture. The main *principles* to prevent root fracture are to:

1. Avoid weakening of the canal wall.
2. Minimize the internal wedging forces.

Following points should be kept in mind before, during, and after endodontic therapy:

a. Evaluate the tooth anatomy before taking treatment
b. Preserve as much tooth structure as possible during biomechanical preparation.
c. Use only optimal force during obturation for compaction of gutta-percha.
d. Use posts and pins if indicated.
e. Use posts with passive fits and round edges so as to reduce stress generation.

## QUESTIONS

**Q. What is cracked tooth syndrome? How can you diagnose a case with cracked tooth?**

**Q. What is vertical root fracture? What are signs and symptoms, radiographic features of VRF?**

## BIBLIOGRAPHY


1. Ailor JE. Managing incomplete tooth fractures. J Am Dent Assoc 2000;131:1168-74.
2. Cameron CE. Cracked-tooth syndrome. J Am Dent Assoc 1964;68:405-11.
3. Caufield JB. Hairline tooth fracture: A clinical case report. J Am Dent Assoc 1981;102:501-2.
4. Cohen S, Blanco L, Berman L. Vertical root fractures clinical and radiographic diagnosis. J Am Dent Assoc 2003;134:434-41.
5. Coppens CRM, DeMoor RJG. Prevalence of vertical root fractures in extracted endodontically treated teeth. Int Endod J 2003;36:926.
6. Culjat MO, Singh RS, Brown ER, et al. Ultrasound crack detection in a simulated human tooth. Dentomax Radiol 2005;34:80-5.
7. Fuss Z, Lastig J, Tamse A. Prevalence of vertical root fractures in extracted endodontically treated teeth. Int Endod J 1999;32:283-6.
8. Geursten W, Schwarze T, Günay H. Diagnosis, therapy and prevention of cracked tooth syndrome. Quintessence Int 2003;34:409-17.
9. Gluskin AH, Radke RA, Frost SL, Watanbe LG. The mandibular incisor: Rethinking guidelines for post and core design. J Endod 1995;21:33.
10. Gutamann JL. The dentin-root complex anatomic and biologic considerations in restoring endodontically treated teeth. J Prosthet Dent 1992;67:458-67.
11. Hanning C, Dullin C, Hülsmann M, Heidrich G. Three-dimensional, non destructive visualization of vertical root fracture using flat panel volume detector computer tomography: An ex vivo in vitro case report. Int Endod J 2005;38:904-13.
12. Letchirakarn V, Palamara J, Messer HH. Patterns of vertical fractures: Factors affecting stress distribution in the root canal. J Endod 2003;29:523-8.
13. Lin LM, Langeland K. Vertical root fracture. J Endod 1982;8:558-62.
14. Lommel TJ, Meister F, Gerstein H, et al. Alveolar bone loss associated with vertical root fractures-report or six cases. Oral Surg Oral Med Oral Pathol Oral Radiol Endod 1978;45:909-19.
15. Lustig JP, Tamse A, Fuss Z. Pattern of bone resorption in vertically fractured endodontically treated teeth. Oral surg Oral Med Oral Pathol Oral Radiol Endod 2000;90:224-7.
16. Pilo R, Tamse A. Residual dentin thickness in mandibular premolars prepared with Gates-Glidden and Parapost drills. J Prosthet Dent 2000;83:617-23.
17. Pitts DL, Natkin E. Diagnosis and treatment of vertical root fractures. J Endod 1983;9:338-46.
18. Polson AM. Periodontal destruction associated with vertical root fracture. J Periodontol 1977;48:27-32.
19. Sornkule E, Stannard JG. Strength of roots before and after endodontic treatment and restorations. J Endod 1992;18:440-3.
20. Swepston JH, Miller AW. The incompletely fractured tooth. J Prosthet Dent 1985;55:413-16.
21. Testori T, Badino M, Castagnola M. Vertical root fractures in endodontically treated teeth: A clinical survey of 36 cases. J Endod 1993;19:87-90.
22. Trabert KC, Caputo AA, Abou-Rass M. Tooth fracture. A comparison of endodontic and restorative treatments. J Endod 1978;4:341-5.
23. Yeh C-J. Fatigue root fracture: A spontaneous teeth. Br Dent J 1997;1882:261-6.

# CHAPTER 32

# Tooth Hypersensitivity



## INTRODUCTION

The term tooth hypersensitivity, dentinal sensitivity or hypersensitivity often used intermittently to describe clinically condition of an exaggerated response to an exogenous stimulus.

The exogenous stimuli may include thermal, tactile or osmotic changes. While extreme stimuli can make all the teeth hurt, the term hypersensitivity means painful response to stimuli not normally associated with pain. The response to a stimulus varies from person to person due to difference in pain tolerance, environment factors and psychology of patient. Tooth hypersensitivity can fit the criteria of several pain terms described by Merskey (1979), for the International Association for the study of pain (IASP). Pain is described "as an unpleasant sensory and emotional experience associated with actual or potential tissue damage".

## DEFINITION

Dentin hypersensitivity is defined as "sharp, short pain arising from exposed dentin in response to stimuli typically thermal, chemical, tactile or osmotic and which cannot be ascribed to any other form of dental defect or pathology (Holland et al, 1997)."

**Historic review**

- Leeuwenhoek (1678) described "tooth canals in dentin".
- JD White (1855) proposed that dentinal pain was caused by movement of fluid in dentinal tubules.
- Lukomsky (1941) advocated sodium fluoride as a desensitizing obtundent.
- Brannstrom (1962) described hydrodynamic theory of dentinal pain.
- Kleinberg (1986) summarized different approaches that are used to treat hypersensitivity.

Tooth hypersensitivity is not associated with actual tissue damage in the acute sense but can involve potential tissue damage with constant erosion of the enamel or cementum along with the concomitant pulpal response.

## NEUROPHYSIOLOGY OF TEETH

The dental pulp is richly innervated. According to conduction velocities, the nerve units can be classified into A group—having the conduction velocity more than 2 m/s and C group—with conduction velocity less than 2 m/s.

The sharp, better localized pain is mediated by A delta fibers, whereas C fibers activation seems to be connected with the dull radiating pain sensation. Myelinated A fiber seems to be responsible for dentin sensitivity.

## MECHANISM OF DENTIN SENSITIVITY

**Theories of dentin sensitivity**

- Neural theory.
- Odontoblastic transduction theory.
- Hydrodynamic theory.

### Theories of Dentin Sensitivity

#### *Neural Theory*

The neural theory attributes to activation of nerves ending lying within the dentinal tubules. These nerve signals are then conducted along the parent primary afferent nerve fibers in the pulp, into the dental nerve branches and then into the brain (Fig. 32.1). Neural theory considered that entire length of tubule contains free nerve endings.

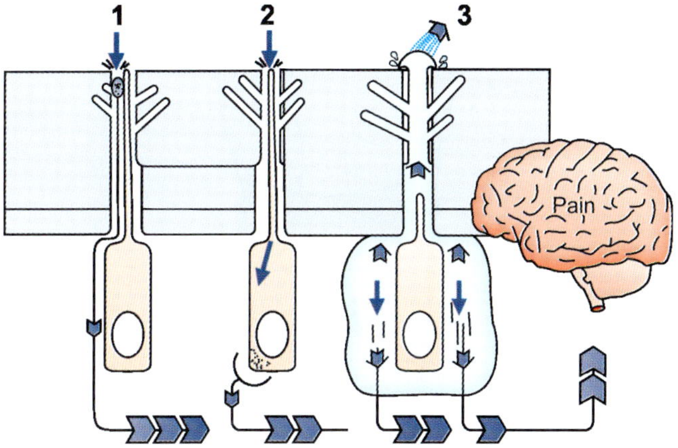


Fig. 32.1: Theories of dentin hypersensitivity; (1) Neural theory: Stimulus applied to dentin causes direct excitation of the nerve fibers; (2) Odontoblastic transduction theory: Stimulus is transmitted along the odontoblast and passes to the sensory nerve endings through synapse; (3) Hydrodynamic theory: Stimulus causes displacement of fluid present in dentinal tubules which further excite nerve fibers

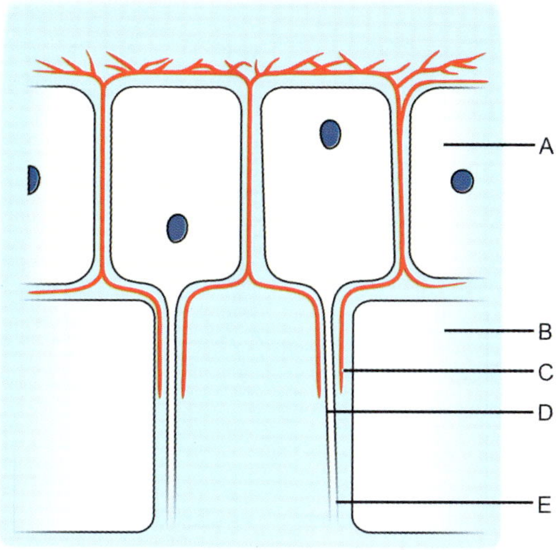


Fig. 32.2: Hydrodynamic theory; (A) Odontoblast; (B) Dentin; (C) A-δ nerve fiber; (D) Odontoblastic process; (E) Stimulation of A-δ nerve fiber from fluid movement

### *Odontoblastic Transduction Theory*

The theory assumed that odontoblasts extend to the periphery. The stimuli initially excite the process or body of the odontoblast. The membrane of odontoblasts may come into close apposition with that of nerve endings in the pulp or in the dentinal tubule and the odontoblast transmits the excitation of these associated nerve endings. However, in the most recent study; Thomas (1984) indicated that the odontoblastic process is restricted to the inner third of the dentinal tubules. Accordingly it seems that the outer part of the dentinal tubules does not contain any cellular elements but is only filled with dentinal fluid.

### *Hydrodynamic Theory*

This theory proposes that a stimulus causes displacement of the fluid that exists in the dentinal tubules. The displacement occurs in either an outward or inward direction and this mechanical disturbance activates the nerve endings present in the dentin or pulp.

***Brannstrom* (1962)** suggested that the displacement of the tubule contents is rapid enough to deform nerve fiber in pulp or predentin or damage odontoblast cell. Both of these effects appear capable of producing pain.

Currently most investigators accept that dentin sensitivity is due to the hydrodynamic fluid shift, which occurs across exposed dentin with open tubules. This rapid fluid movement in turn activates the mechanoreceptor nerves of A group in the pulp (Fig. 32.2).

***Mathews et al* (1994)** noted that stimuli such as cold causes fluid flow away from the pulp, produces more rapid and greater pulp nerve responses than those such as heat, which causes an inward flow. This certainly would explain the rapid and severe response to cold stimuli compared to the slow dull response to heat.

The dehydration of dentin by air blasts or absorbent paper causes outward fluid movement and stimulates the mechanoreceptor of the odontoblast, causing pain. Prolonged air blast causes formation of protein plug into the dentinal tubules, reducing the fluid movement and thus decreasing pain (Fig. 32..3A).

The pain produced when sugar or salt solutions are placed in contact with exposed dentin can also be explained by dentinal fluid movement. Dentinal fluid is of relatively low osmolarity, which have tendency to flow towards solution of higher osmolarity, i.e. salt or sugar solution (Fig. 32.3B).

## INCIDENCE AND DISTRIBUTION OF DENTIN HYPERSENSITIVITY

The prevalence studies for dentin hypersensitivity are limited in number. The available prevalence data vary considerably and dentin hypersensitivity has been stated to range from 8 to 30 percent of adult population.

- Most sufferers range from 20-40 years of age and a peak occurrence is found at the end of the third decade.
- In general, a slightly higher incidence of dentin hypersensitivity is reported in females than in males.
- The reduced incidence of dentin hypersensitivity in older individuals reflects age changes in dentin and the dental pulp. Sclerosis of dentin, the laying down of secondary dentin and fibrosis of the pulp would all interfere with the hydrodynamic transmission of stimuli through exposed dentin.

### Intraoral Distribution

- Hypersensitivity is most commonly noted on buccal cervical zones of permanent teeth. Although all tooth type may be affected, canines and premolars in either jaw are the most frequently involved.

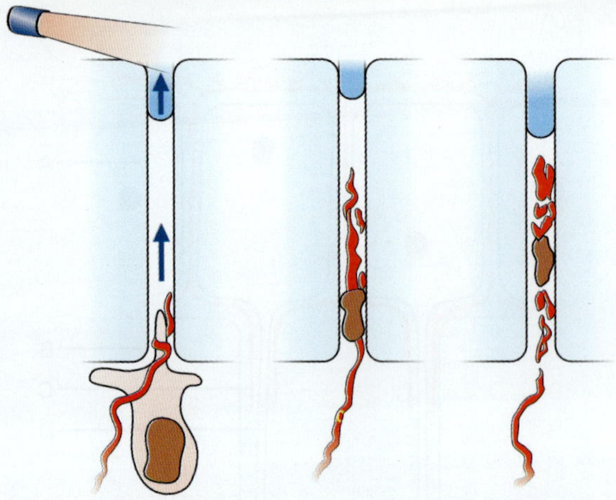

Fig. 32.3A: Effect of air blast on dentin

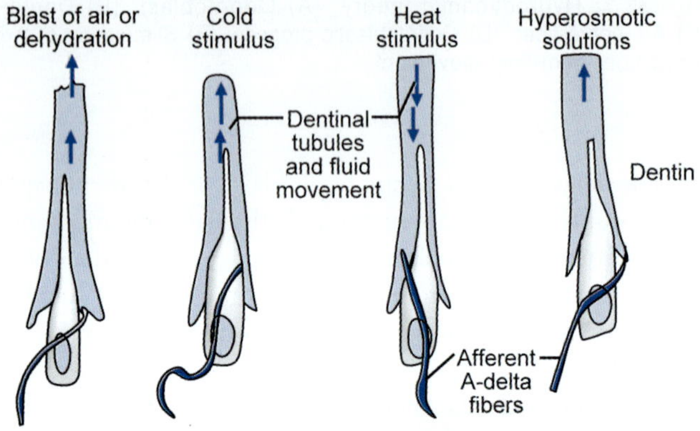


Fig. 32.3B: Pain produced by different stimuli

- Regarding the side of mouth, in right handed tooth brushers, the dentin hypersensitivity is greater on the left sided teeth compared with the equivalent contralateral teeth.

## ETIOLOGY AND PREDISPOSING FACTORS

The primary underlying cause for dentin hypersensitivity is exposed dentin tubules. Dentin may become exposed by two processes; either by loss of covering periodontal structures (gingival recession), or by loss of enamel.

The most common clinical cause for exposed dentinal tubules is gingival recession (Fig. 32.4). Various factors which can cause recession are inadequate attached gingiva, improper brushing technique, periodontal surgery, overzealous tooth cleansing habits, oral habits, etc.

**Common reasons for gingival recession**

- Inadequate attached gingiva.
- Prominent roots.
- Toothbrush abrasion.
- Oral habits resulting in gingival laceration, i.e. traumatic tooth picking, eating hard foods.
- Excessive tooth cleaning.
- Excessive flossing.
- Gingival recession secondary to specific diseases, i.e. NUG, periodontitis, herpetic gingivostomatitis.
- Crown preparation.

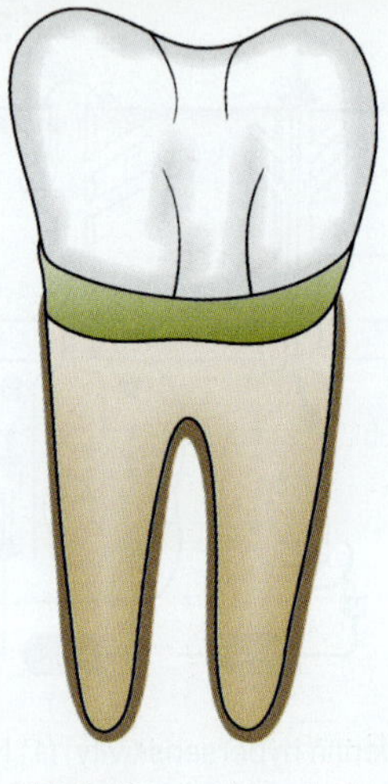

Fig. 32.4: Recession of gingiva

The recession may or may not be associated with bone loss. If bone loss occurs, more dentinal tubules get exposed. When gingival recession occurs, the outer protective layer of root dentin, i.e. cementum gets abraded or eroded away (Fig. 32.5).

This leaves the exposed underlying dentin, which consists of protoplasmic projections of odontoblasts within the pulp chamber (Fig. 32.6). These cells contain nerve endings and when

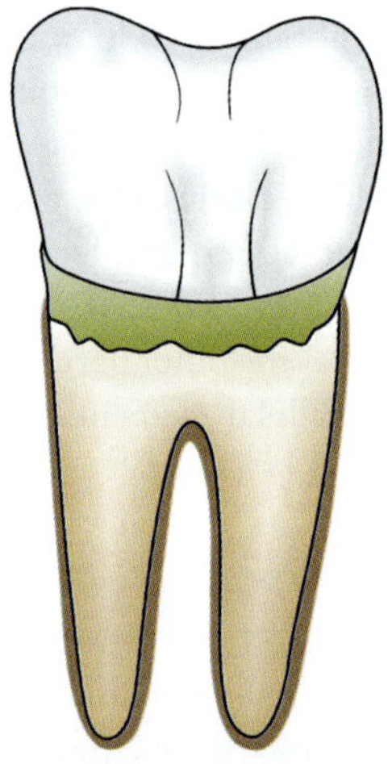

Fig. 32.5: Erosion of cementum

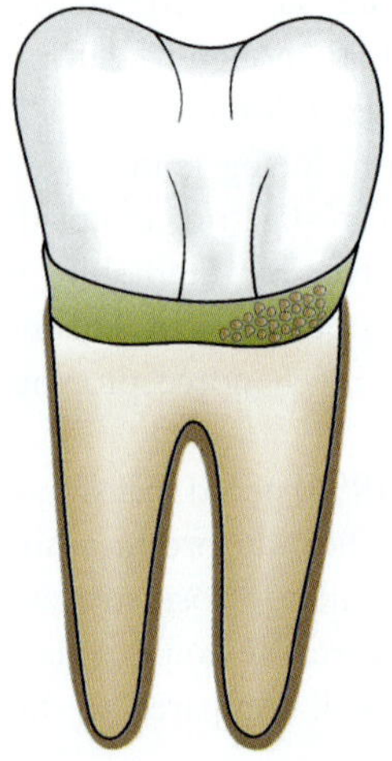

Fig. 32.6: Exposure of dentinal tubules

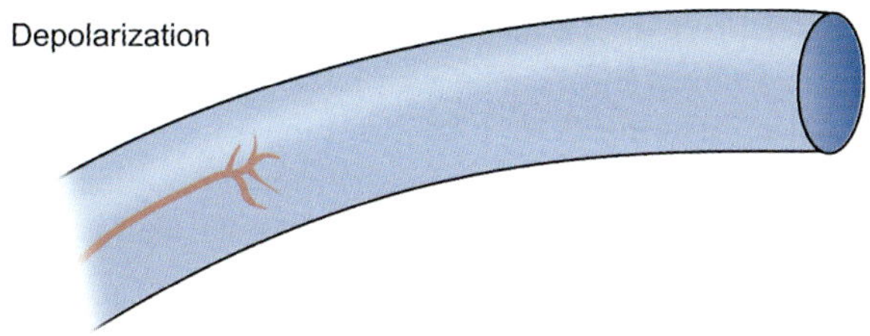


**Fig. 32.7:** Depolarization of nerve ending causing pain

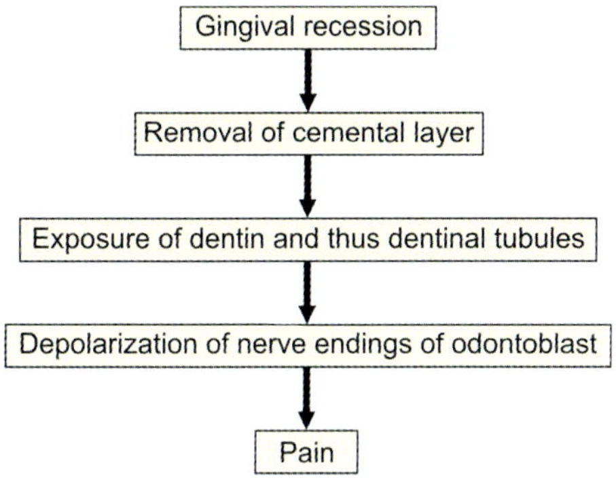


disturbed, nerves depolarize and this is interpreted as pain (Fig. 32.7).

Once the dentinal tubules are exposed, there are oral processes which keep them exposed. These include poor plaque control, enamel wear, improper oral hygiene technique, cervical erosions, enamel wear and exposure to acids.

**Reasons for continued dentinal tubular exposure**

- Poor plaque control, i.e. acidic bacterial byproducts.
- Excess oral acids, i.e. soda, fruit juice, swimming pool chlorine, bulimia.
- Cervical decay.
- Toothbrush abrasion.
- Tartar control toothpaste.

The other reason for ***exposure of dentinal tubules is due to loss of enamel***.

**Causes of loss of enamel**

- Attrition by exaggerated occlusal functions like bruxism.
- Abrasion from dietary components or improper brushing technique.
- Erosion associated with environmental or dietary components particularly acids.

Since dentinal tubules get sclerosed of their own and plug themselves up in the oral environment, treatment should focus on eliminating factors associated with continued dentinal exposure.

## DIFFERENTIAL DIAGNOSIS

Dentin hypersensitivity is perhaps a symptom complex rather than a true disease and results from stimulus transmission across exposed dentin. A number of dental conditions are associated with dentin exposure and therefore, may produce the same symptoms.

Such conditions include:

- Chipped teeth.
- Fractured restoration.
- Restorative treatments.
- Dental caries.
- Cracked tooth syndrome.
- Other enamel invaginations.

## DIAGNOSIS

- A careful history together with a thorough clinical and radiographic examination is necessary before arriving at a definitive diagnosis of dentin hypersensitivity. However, the problem may be made difficult when two or more conditions coexist.
- Tooth hypersensitivity differs from dentinal or pulpal pain. In case of dentin hypersensitivity, patient's ability to locate the source of pain is very good, whereas in case of pulpal pain, it is very poor.
- The character of the pain does not outlast the stimulus; the pain is intensified by thermal changes, sweet and sour.
- Intensity of pain is usually mild to moderate.
- The pain can be duplicated by hot or cold application or by scratching the dentin. The pulpal pain is explosive, intermittent and throbbing and can be affected by hot or cold.

## TREATMENT STRATEGIES

Hypersensitivity can resolve without the treatment or may require several weeks of desensitizing agents before improvement is seen. Treatment of dentin hypersensitivity is challenging for both patient and the clinician mainly for two main reasons:

1. It is difficult to measure or compare pain among different patients.
2. It is difficult for patient to change the habits that initially caused the problem.

### Management of Tooth Hypersensitivity

It is well known that hypersensitivity often resolves without treatment. This is probably related to the fact that dentin permeability decrease spontaneously because of occurrence of natural processes in the oral cavity.

### Natural Process Contributing to Desensitization

1. Formation of reparative dentin by the pulp.
2. Obturation of tubules by the formation of mineral deposits (dental sclerosis).
3. Calculus formation on the surface of the dentin.

**Two principal treatment options are:**

1. Plug the dentinal tubules preventing the fluid flow.
2. Desensitize the nerve, making it less responsive to stimulation.

All the current modalities address these two options.

**Treatment of dentin hypersensitivity can be divided into:**
1. Home care with dentifrices.
2. In-office treatment procedure.
3. Patient education.

**Management of dentin hypersensitivity**
1. *Home care with dentifrices:*
   a. Strontium chloride dentifrices.
   b. Potassium nitrate dentifrices.
   c. Fluoride dentifrices.
2. *In-office treatment procedure:*
   a. Varnishes.
   b. Corticosteroids.
   c. Treatments that partially obturate dentinal tubules.
      - Burnishing of dentin
      - Silver nitrate
      - Zinc chloride—potassium ferrocyanide
      - Formalin
      - Calcium compounds
        – Calcium hydroxide
        – Dibasic calcium phosphate
      - Fluoride compounds
        – Sodium fluoride
        – Sodium silicofluoride
        – Stannous fluoride
      - Iontophoresis
      - Strontium chloride
      - Potassium oxalate.
   d. Tubule sealant
      - Restorative resins
      - Dentin bonding agents.
   e. Miscellaneous
      - Laser.
3. Patient education:
   a. Dietary counseling
   b. Toothbrushing technique
   c. Plaque control.

## Home Care with Dentifrices (Fig. 32.8)

Dentifrice has been defined as a substance used with a toothbrush to aid in cleaning the accessible surfaces of the teeth. Dentifrice components include abrasive, surfactant, humectant, thickener, flavor, sweetener, coloring agent and water.

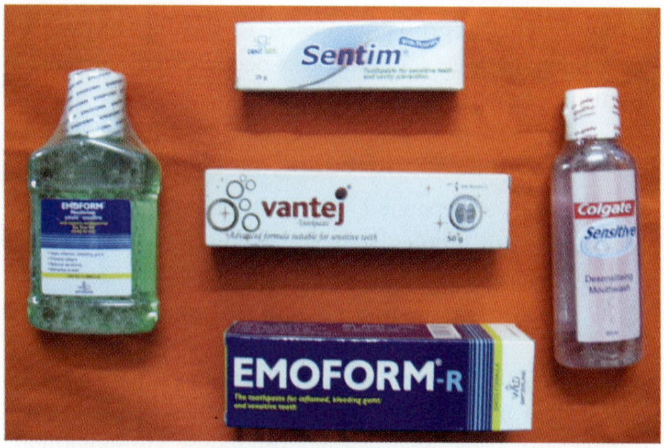


**Fig. 32.8:** Commonly used home care products for dentin hypersensitivity

After professional diagnosis, dentinal hypersensitivity can be treated simply and inexpensively by home use of desensitizing dentifrices. The habit of toothbrushing with a dentifrice for cosmetic reasons is well established in the population, thus compliance with this regimen can be easily made.

### *Strontium Chloride Dentifrices*

Ten percent strontium chloride desensitizing dentifrices have been found to be effective in relieving the pain of tooth hypersensitivity.

### *Potassium Nitrate Dentifrices*

Five percent potassium nitrate dentifrices have been found to alleviate pain related to tooth hypersensitivity.

### *Fluoride Dentifrices*

Sodium monofluorophosphates dentifrices are the effective mode of treating tooth hypersensitivity.

## In-office Treatment Procedure

### *Rationale of Therapy*

According to hydrodynamic theory of hypersensitivity, a rapid movement of fluid in the dentinal tubules is capable of activating intradental sensory nerves. Therefore, treatment of hypersensitive teeth should be directed towards reducing the anatomical diameter of the tubules, obliteration of the tubules or to surgically cover the exposed dentinal tubules so as to limit fluid movement (Figs 32.9A to C).

**Criteria for selecting desensitizing agent**
- Provides immediate and lasting relief from pain.
- Easy to apply.
- Well tolerated by patients.
- Not injurious to the pulp.
- Does not stain the tooth.
- Relatively inexpensive.

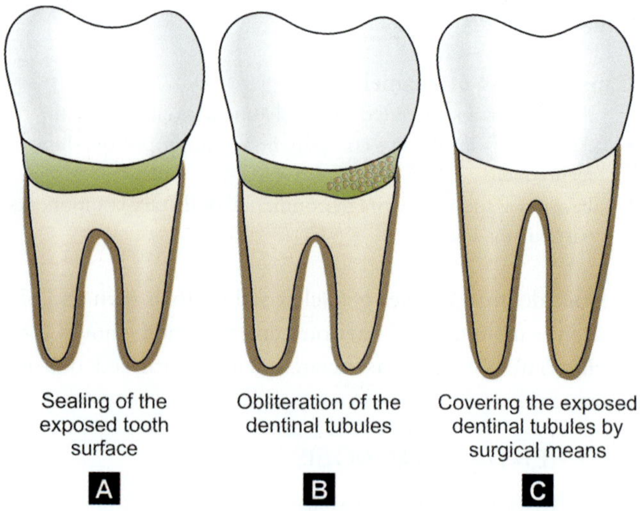


**Figs 32.9A to C:** In-office treatment procedures for dentin hypersensitivity

**Treatment options to reduce the diameter of dentinal tubules can be:**

1. Formation of a smear layer by burnishing the exposed root surface (smear layer consists of small amorphous particles of dentin, minerals and organic matrix—denatured collagen).
2. Application of agents that form insoluble precipitates within the tubules.
3. Impregnation of tubules with plastic resins.
4. Application of dental bonding agents to seal off the tubules.
5. Covering the exposed dentinal tubules by surgical means.

It must be recognized that single procedure may not be consistently effective in the treatment of hypersensitivity; therefore, the dentist must be familiar with alternative methods of treatment. Prior to treating sensitive root surfaces, hard/soft deposits should be removed from the teeth. Root planning on sensitive dentin may cause considerable discomfort, in this case, teeth should be anesthetized prior to treatment and teeth should be isolated and dried with warm air.

### *Varnishes*

Open tubules can be covered with a thin film of varnish, providing a temporary relief; varnish such as copalite can be used for this purpose. For more sustained relief a fluoride containing varnish Duraflor can be applied.

### *Corticosteroids*

Corticosteroids containing 1 percent prednisolone in combination with 25 percent parachorophenol, 25 percent methacresylacetate and 50 percent gum camphor was found to be effective in preventing postoperative thermal sensitivity.

The use of corticosteroids is based, on the assumption that hypersensitivity is linked to pulpal inflammation; hence, more information is needed regarding the relationship between these two conditions.

## Partial Obliteration of Dentinal Tubules

***Burnishing of dentin:*** Burnishing of dentin with a toothpick or orange wood stick results in the formation of a smear layer which, partially occludes the dentinal tubules and thus resulting in decreased hypersensitivity.

***Formation of insoluble precipitates to block tubules:*** Certain soluble salts react with ions in tooth structure to form crystals on the surface of the dentin. To be effective, crystallization should occur in 1-2 minutes and the crystals should be small enough to enter the tubules and must also be large enough to partially obturate the tubules.

- ***Calcium oxalate dihydrate crystals*** are formed when potassium oxalate is applied to dentin; these crystals are very effective in reducing permeability.
- ***Silver nitrate ($AgNO_3$)*** has ability to precipitate protein constituents of odontoblast processes, thereby partially blocking the tubules.
- ***Zinc chloride–potassium ferrocyanide:*** When applied forms precipitate, which is highly crystalline and covers the dentin surface.
- ***Formalin 40 percent*** is topically applied by means of cotton pellets or orangewood sticks on teeth. It had been proposed by Grossman in 1935 as the desensitizing agent of choice in treating anterior tooth because, unlike $AgNO_3$, it does not produce stain.
- ***Calcium compounds*** have been popular agent for many years for the treatment of hypersensitivity. The exact mechanism of action is unknown but evidence suggests that:
  a. It may block dentinal tubules.
  b. May promote peritubular dentin formation.
  c. On increasing the concentration of calcium ions around nerve fibers, may results in decreased nerve excitability. So, calcium hydroxide might be capable of suppressing nerve activity.
     – A paste of $Ca(OH)_2$ and sterile distilled water applied on exposed root surface and allowed to remain for 3-5 minutes, can give immediate relief in 75 percent of cases.
     – Dibasic calcium phosphate when burnished with round toothpick forms mineral deposits near the surface of the tubules and found to be effective in 93 percent of patients.
- ***Fluoride compounds:*** Lukomsky (1941) was the first to propose sodium fluoride as desensitizing agent, because dentinal fluid is saturated with respect to calcium and phosphate ions. Application of NaF leads to precipitation of calcium fluoride crystals, thus, reducing the functional radius of the dentinal tubules.
  – *Acidulated sodium fluoride:* Concentration of fluoride in dentin treated with acidulated sodium fluoride is found to be significantly higher than dentin treated with sodium fluoride.
  – *Sodium silicofluoride:* Silicic acid forms a gel with the calcium of the tooth and produces an insulating barrier. Thus application of 0.6 percent sodium silicofluoride is much more potent than 2 percent solution of sodium fluoride as desensitizing agent.
  – *Stannous fluoride*: Ten percent solution of stannous fluoride forms dense layer of tin and fluoride containing globular particles blocking the dentinal tubules. 0.4 percent stannous fluoride is also an effective agent, however, requires prolonged use (up to 4 weeks) to achieve satisfactory results.
- ***Fluoride Iontophoresis:*** Iontophoresis is a term applied to the use of an electrical potential to transfer ions into the body for therapeutic purposes. The objective of fluoride iontophoresis is to drive fluoride ions more deeply into the dentinal tubules that cannot be achieved with topical application of fluoride alone.
- ***Strontium chloride:*** Studies have shown that topical application of concentrated strontium chloride on an abraded dentin surface produces a deposit of strontium that penetrates dentin to a depth of approximately 10-20 μm and extend into the dentinal tubules.

- ***Oxalates:*** Oxalates are relatively inexpensive, easy to apply and well tolerated by patients. Potassium oxalate and ferric oxalate solution make available oxalate ions that can react with calcium ions in the dentin fluid to form insoluble calcium oxalate crystals that are deposited in the apertures of the dentinal tubules.

### Dental Resins and Adhesives

The objective in employing resins and adhesives is to seal the dentinal tubules to prevent pain producing stimuli from reaching the pulp. Several investigators have demonstrated immediate and enduring relief of pain for periods of up to 18 months following treatment. Although not intended for treatment of generalized areas of root sensitivity, this can be an effective method of treatment when other forms of therapy have failed.

GLUMA is a dentin bonding system that includes glutaraldehyde primer and 35 percent HEMA (hydroxyethyl methacrylate). It provides an attachment to dentin that is immediate and strong. GLUMA has been found to be highly effective when other methods of treatment failed to provide relief (Fig. 32.10).

### Lasers

*Treatment of Dentin Hypersensitivity by Lasers*

***Kimura Y et al (2000)*** reviewed treatment of dentin hypersensitivity by lasers. The lasers used for the treatment of dentin hypersensitivity are divided into two groups:

1. *Low output power (low level) lasers:* Helium-neon [He-Ne] and gallium/aluminum/arsenide (GaAlAs) [diode] lasers.
2. *Middle output power lasers:* Nd:YAG and $CO_2$ lasers.

Laser effects are considered to be due to the effects of sealing of dentinal tubules, nerve analgesia or placebo effect. The sealing effect is considered to be durable, whereas nerve analgesia or a placebo effects are not.

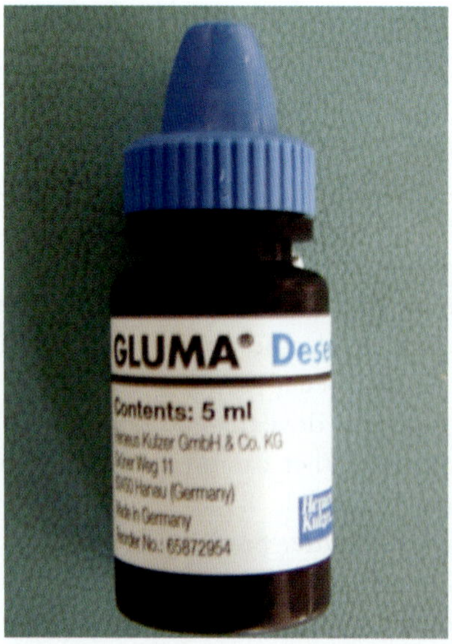


**Fig. 32.10:** GLUMA desensitizing solution

## Patient Education

### Dietary Counseling

Dietary acids are capable of causing erosive loss of tooth structure, thereby removing cementum and resulting in opening of the dentinal tubules. Consequently, dietary counseling should focus on the quantity and frequency of acid intake and intake occurring in relation to toothbrushing. Any treatment may fail if these factors are not controlled. A written diet history should be obtained on patients with dentinal hypersensitivity in order to advise those concerning eating habits.

Because of the presence of a smear layer on dentin, teeth are not usually sensitive immediately following scaling and root planning. However, removal of the smear layer may result from exposure to certain components of the diet. Studies have shown that citrus fruit juices, apple juice and yoghurt are capable of dissolving the smear layer.

Because loss of dentin is greatly increased when brushing is performed immediately after exposure of the tooth surface to dietary acids. Patients should be cautioned against brushing their teeth soon after ingestion of citrus food.

### Toothbrushing Technique

Because incorrect toothbrushing appears to be an etiologic factor in dentin hypersensitivity, instruction about proper brushing techniques can prevent further loss of dentin and the hypersensitivity.

### Plaque Control

Saliva contains calcium and phosphate ions and is therefore able to contribute to the formation of mineral deposits within exposed dentinal tubules. The presence of plaque may interfere with this process, as plaque bacteria, by producing acid, are capable of dissolving any mineral precipitates that form, thus opening tubules.

Professional interest in the causes and treatment of dentinal hypersensitivity has been evident in the dental literature for approximately 150 years or more. Dentinal hypersensitivity satisfies all the criteria to be classified as a true pain syndrome. Myelinated A fibers mostly A-delta type seems to be responsible for the sensitivity of dentin. Of the various theories proposed, the hydrodynamic theory is the most accepted explanation for the mechanism of dentin hypersensitivity. Management of the condition requires determination of etiologic factors and predisposing influences. Desensitizing toothpastes containing potassium nitrate, strontium chloride and sodium monofluorophosphate have proven to be effective in the management of hypersensitivity. Partial obturation of open tubules is the most widely practiced in office treatment of dentinal hypersensitivity.

## QUESTIONS

**Q. Define dentin hypersensitivity?**

**Q. How will you manage a case of dentin hypersensitivity?**

CHAPTER 33

# Pediatric Endodontics



## INTRODUCTION

Preservation of dental arch and its functions is main motive behind pediatric dentistry. The retention of the primary teeth is needed until they are naturally exfoliated. There are several advantages of preserving the natural primary teeth (Fig. 33.1). Primary teeth help in preserving the arch length, play an important role in mastication, esthetics, appearance, speech and act as space maintainers for permanent teeth.

### Importance of Pulp Therapy

- Maintains arch length
- Prevents abnormal habits
- Maintains esthetics
- Helps in mastication
- Prevents infection
- Prevents speech problems
- Helps in timely eruption of permanent tooth.

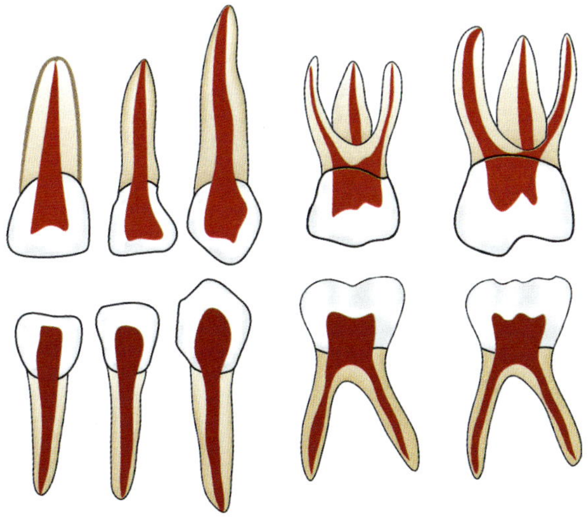

Fig. 33.1: Pulp anatomy of primary teeth

### Why Endodontic Treatment of Primary Teeth is Challenging?

Endodontic therapy of primary teeth is considered more challenging and difficult than adults teeth due to various reasons

1. Lesser patient cooperation
2. Reduced mouth opening
3. More chances of injury to permanent tooth bud
4. Behavioral management
5. Anatomic differences between primary and permanent teeth.

## ANATOMY OF PRIMARY TEETH

In primary teeth, enamel and dentin are thinner with pulp horns closer to the cusps when compared with permanent teeth (Figs 33.2 and 33.3). Floor of the pulp chamber is thin and there is more number of accessory canals in primary teeth than in permanent teeth. Roots of the primary teeth are long, slender and flared apically (Fig. 33.4). Roots are in close relation with permanent successor and undergo physiologic resorption during the exfoliation phase (Fig. 33.5).

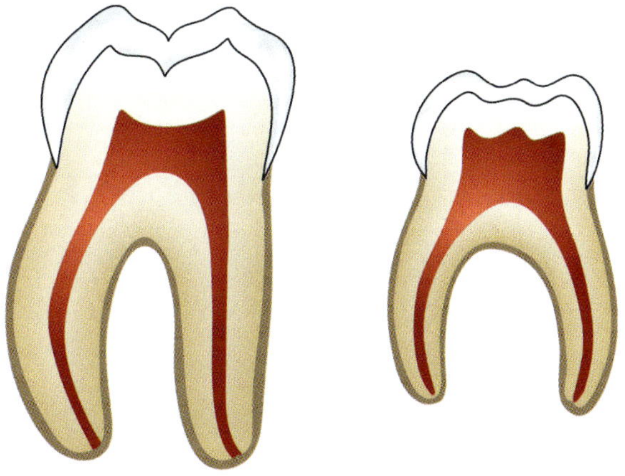

Fig. 33.2: Difference between anatomy of permanent and primary teeth

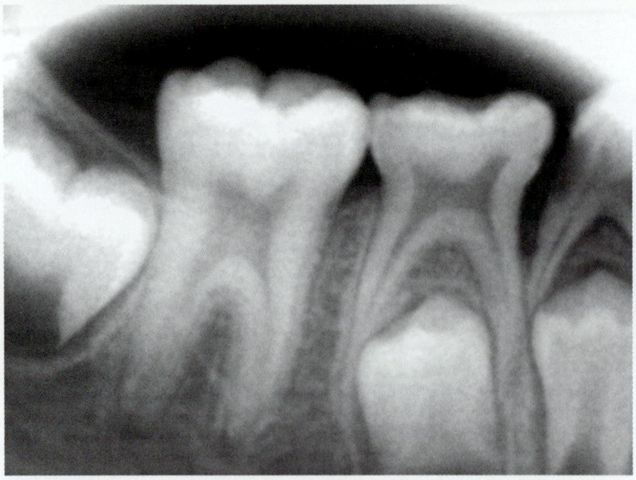

**Fig. 33.3:** Thin enamel and dentin and high pulp horns of primary teeth

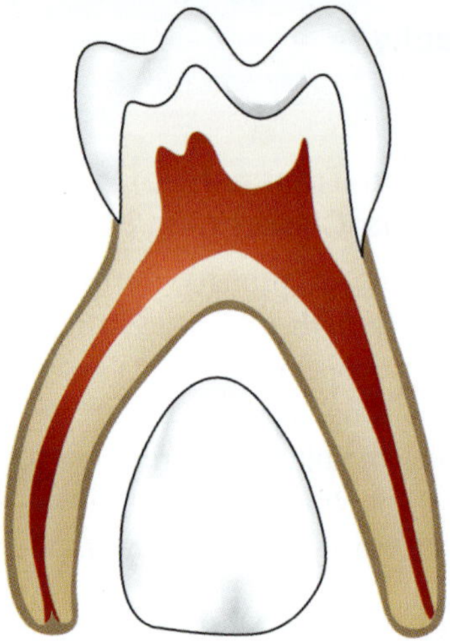

**Fig. 33.4:** Roots of primary teeth are long, slender and are flared apically

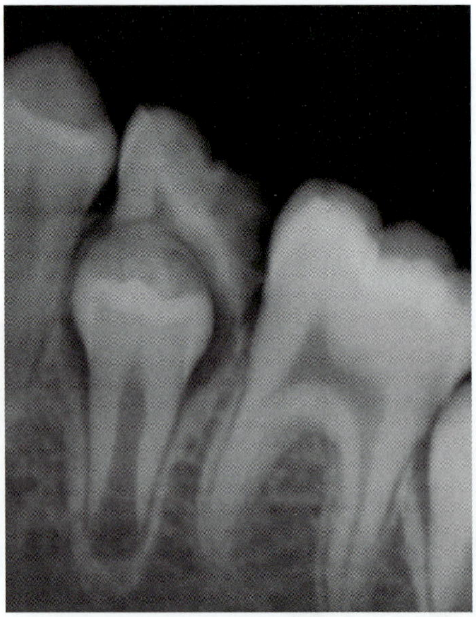

**Fig. 33.5:** Physiologic resorption of primary teeth during exfoliation stage

## Anatomic Differences between Primary and Permanent Teeth

1. Pulp horns are closer to cusps in primary teeth than in the permanent tooth particularly mesial pulp horn
2. Enamel and dentin thickness is less in deciduous teeth, thus increases the risk of exposure.
3. Pulp chamber anatomy in primary teeth resembles outer surface of crown and pulp volume is relatively larger than permanent teeth.
4. Roots of primary tooth are longer and slender.
5. Number of accessory canals are more in primary teeth.
6. Roots of primary teeth are more flared apically than permanent teeth.

## PULP TREATMENT PROCEDURES

### Indirect Pulp Capping

Indirect pulp capping is a procedure performed in a tooth with deep carious lesion adjacent to the pulp (Fig. 33.6). In this procedure, caries near the pulp is left in place to avoid pulp exposure and is covered with a biocompatible material.

#### *Indications*

1. Deep carious lesion near the pulp tissue but not involving it.
2. No mobility of tooth.
3. No history of spontaneous toothache.
4. No tenderness to percussion.
5. No radiographic evidence of pulp pathology.
6. No root resorption or radicular disease should be present radiographically.

#### *Contraindications*

1. Presence of pulp exposure.
2. Radiographic evidence of pulp pathology.
3. History of spontaneous toothache.
4. Tooth sensitive to percussion.
5. Mobility present.
6. Root resorption or radicular disease is present radiographically.

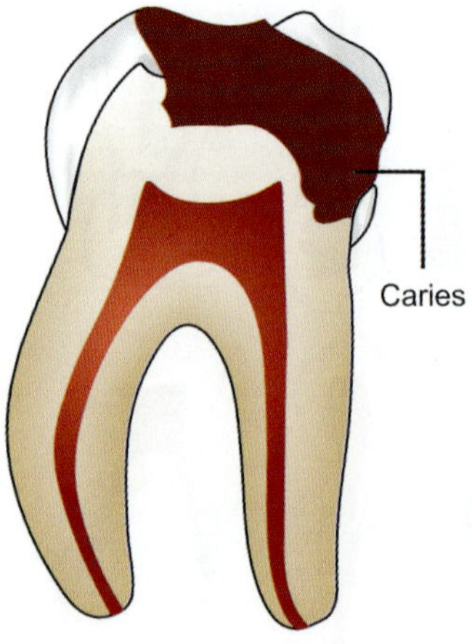


**Fig. 33.6:** Indirect pulp capping is done in cases when carious lesion is quite close to the pulp

### Clinical Techniques

1. Band the tooth if tooth is grossly decayed.
2. Anesthetize the tooth.
3. Apply rubber dam to isolate the tooth.
4. Remove soft caries either with spoon excavator or round bur.
5. Use fissure bur and extend it to sound tooth structure.
6. A thin layer of dentin and some amount of caries is left to avoid exposure.
7. Place calcium hydroxide paste on the exposed dentin.
8. Cover the calcium hydroxide with zinc oxide eugenol base (Fig. 33.7).
9. If restoration is to be given for a longer time, then amalgam restoration should be given (Fig. 33.8).
10. Tooth should be evaluated after 6-8 weeks.

## Direct Pulp Capping

Direct pulp capping procedure involves the placement of biocompatible material over the site of pulp exposure to maintain vitality and promote healing.

When a small mechanical exposure of pulp occurs during cavity preparation or following a trauma, an appropriate protective base should be placed in contact with the exposed pulp tissue so as to maintain the vitality of the remaining pulp tissue.

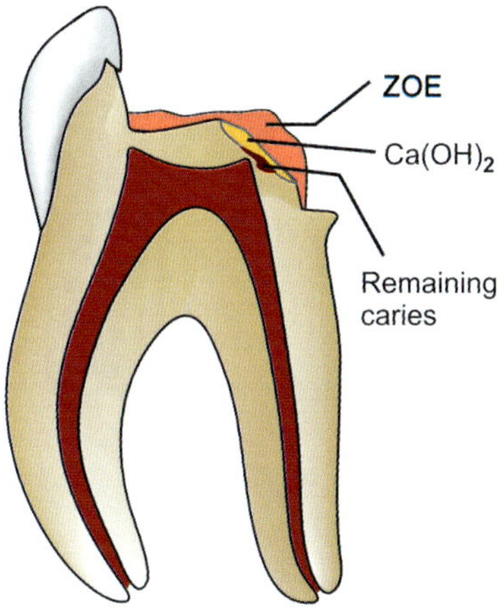


**Fig. 33.7:** Placement of calcium hydroxide and zinc oxide eugenol dressing after excavation of soft caries

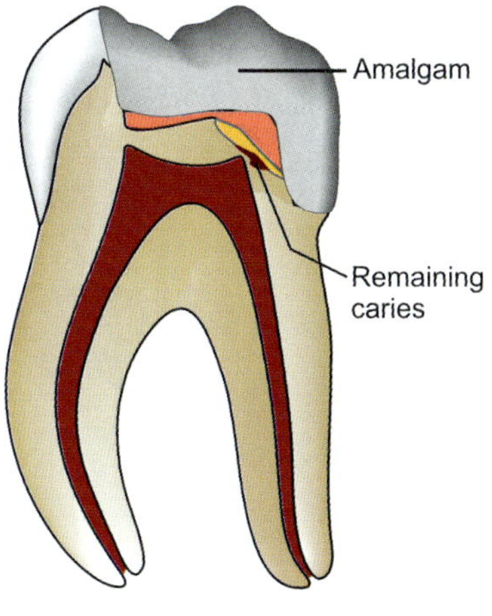


**Fig. 33.8:** Permanent restoration of tooth

### Indications

1. Small mechanical exposure of pulp during
   i. Cavity preparation
   ii. Traumatic injury.
2. No or minimal bleeding at the exposure site.

### Contraindications

1. Wide pulp exposure.
2. Radiographic evidence of pulp pathology.
3. History of spontaneous pain.
4. Presence of bleeding at exposure site.

### Clinical Procedure

1. Administer local anesthesia.
2. Isolate the tooth with rubber dam.
3. Clean and dry the exposure site.
4. Apply calcium hydroxide (preferably Dycal) over the exposed area.
5. Give interim restoration such as zinc oxide eugenol for 6-8 weeks.
6. After evaluation, replace the interim restoration with permanent restoration.

# PULPOTOMY

Pulpotomy refers only to coronal extirpation of vital pulp tissue.

## Objectives of Pulpotomy

1. To preserve the vitality of pulp.
2. To promote apexogenesis by retaining pulp in the canal of an immature young permanent tooth.
3. To provide pain relief in case of acute pulpitis.

## Rationale of Pulpotomy

As we know bacterial contamination causes inflammatory response in the pulpal tissue. This inflammation transmits from coronal to apical part with time. The rational of pulpotomy is to save the remaining pulp when only superficial part of it is infected. By this we preserve the vitality of the tooth.

This partial excision of pulp, i.e. pulpotomy offers following advantages over complete removal of pulp, i.e. pulpectomy:

a. Preserves structural integrity of tooth as endodontically treated tooth becomes brittle and more prone to fracture.
b. Pulpectomy in young permanent tooth can interrupt growth of root, resulting in short root without apical constriction.

## Criteria for Successful Pulpotomy

- No indication of root resorption should be present
- No radiographic signs of periradicular periodontitis
- Tooth should respond to pulp testing
- Tooth should be asymptomatic

- Continued root development should be evident radiographically.

## Calcium Hydroxide Pulpotomy

Mechanism of action of calcium hydroxide:

Calcium hydroxide has high alkaline pH of 11 which is responsible for its antibacterial activity and its ability to form hard tissue (Figs 33.9 and 33.10). Though calcium ions from calcium hydroxide do not directly contribute to formation of hard tissue but the stimulate the repair process.

Mechanism of hard tissue formation is though not known yet it can be because of one of following:

a. By increasing blood derived concentration of calcium ions in healing area.
b. By neutralizing lactic acid produced by osteoclasts. This stops further demineralization.
c. By increasing the action of enzyme alkaline phosphatase.
d. The short roots of young permanent teeth show unfavorable crown-root ratio resulting in periodontal problems and mobility of teeth.
e. Wide root canals of these teeth are usually more prone to fracture because of less radicular dentin.

So we can say when only superficial pulp is involved, one should always try for a conservative procedure like pulpotomy rather than pulpectomy.

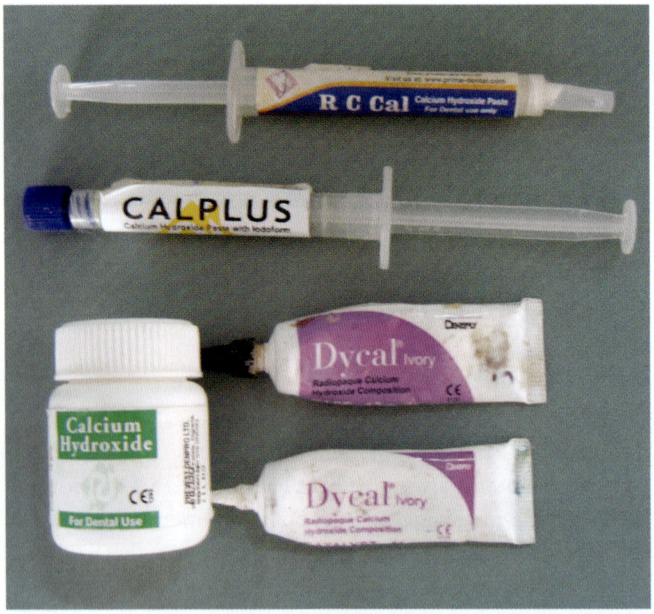


**Fig. 33.9:** Different forms of calcium hydroxide available commercially

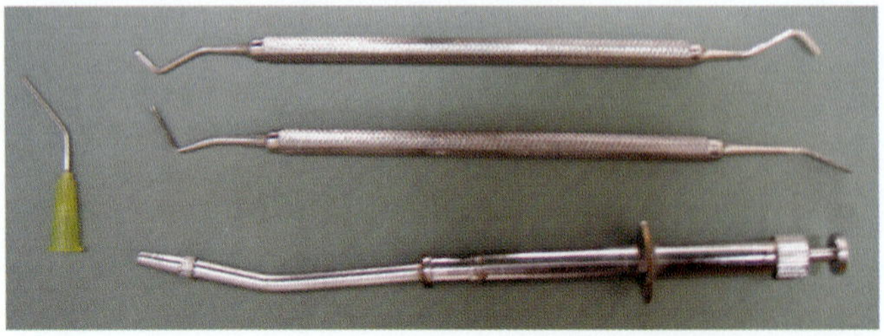

**Fig. 33.10:** Instruments for carrying $Ca(OH)_2$

### *Indication*

It is indicated in young permanent teeth with incomplete root formation to promote apexogenesis (Fig. 33.11).

## Partial Pulpotomy

It implies removal of the coronal pulp tissue to the level of healthy pulp. Calcium hydroxide is material of choice for pulpotomy in young permanent teeth to stimulate the formation of dentin bridge in cariously exposed pulp.

### *Techniques*

- After anesthetizing the tooth, rubber dam is applied.
- After this, 1-2 mm deep cavity into the pulp is prepared using a diamond bur (Fig. 33.12).
- A thin coating of calcium hydroxide mixed with saline solution or anesthetic solution is placed over it (Fig. 33.13) and the access cavity is sealed with a temporary restoration like IRM (Fig. 33.14).

## Cervical or Complete Pulpotomy

Cervical or complete pulpotomy involves removal of entire coronal pulp to the level of root orifices. It is performed when pulp is inflamed to deeper levels of coronal pulp.

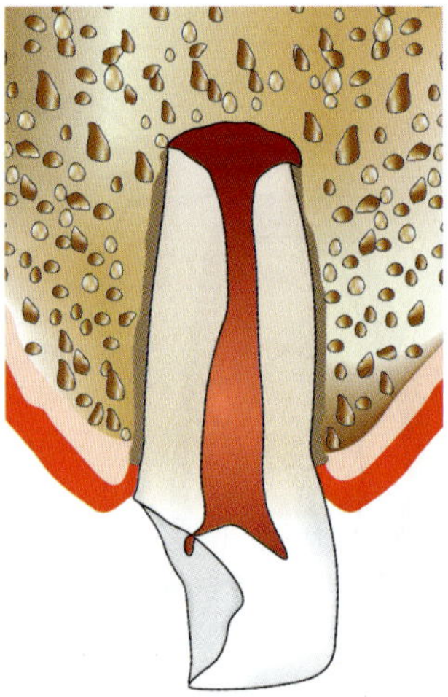

**Fig. 33.11:** Partial pulpotomy is indicated in patients with incomplete root formation

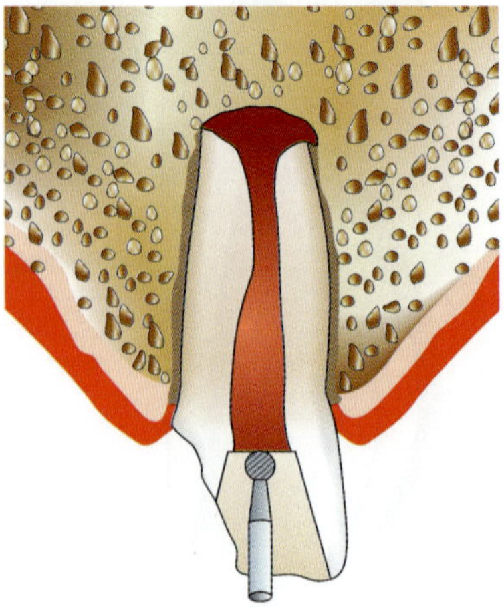

**Fig. 33.12:** Preparation of cavity 1-2 mm deep into pulp

### Technique

Coronal pulp is removed same as in partial pulpotomy except that it is up to level of root orifice (Figs 33.15 and 33.16).

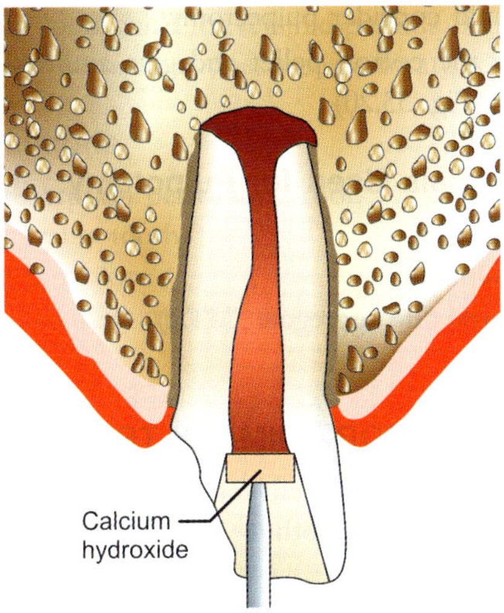


Fig. 33.13: Placement of calcium hydroxide over pulp

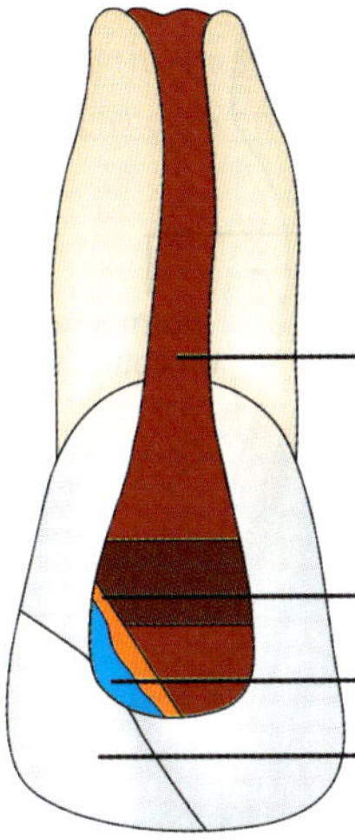

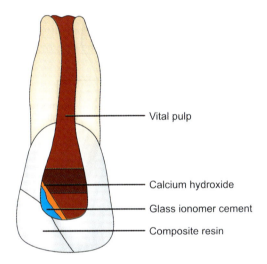

Fig. 33.14: Completed partial pulpotomy

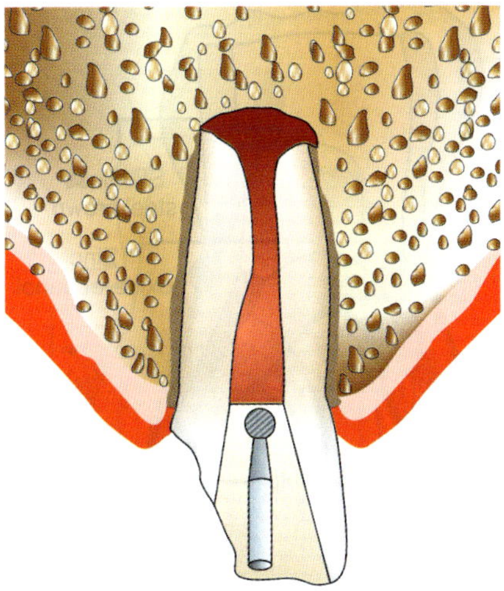

Fig. 33.15: Removal of coronal pulp up to the level of roof orifices

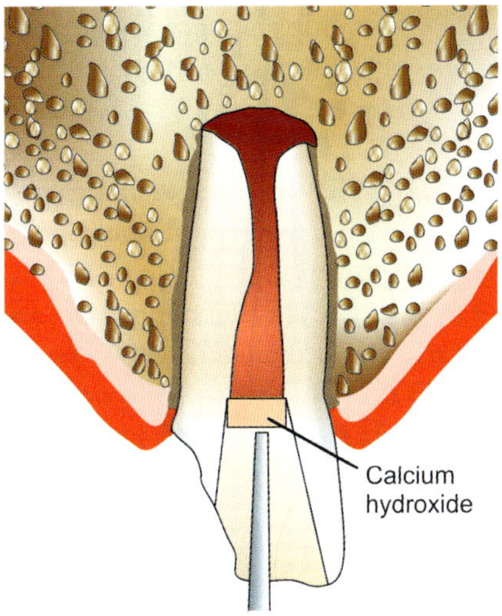


Fig. 33.16: Placement of $Ca(OH)_2$ over exposed pulp

| | *Partial pulpotomy (Fig. 33.17)* | *Cervical pulpotomy (Fig. 33.18)* |
|---|---|---|
| Indication | • Carious/traumatic exposure<br>• When 1-2 mm of coronal pulp is involved in vital tooth | • Carious/traumatic exposure<br>• When entire coronal pulp is involved in a vital tooth |
| Pulp tissue removal | • It is done only in superficial 1-2 mm | • Entire pulp tissue is removed from the chamber |
| Healing potential | • Better because it preserves cell rich zone of coronal pulp | • Depends on radicular pulp because of excision of cell rich zone of coronal pulp |
| Technique | • Relatively simple | • More difficult than partial pulpotomy |
| RCT | • Not done if there is formation of calcific bridge | • More often it is done |
| Pulp vitality tests | • Better results | • Because of loss of coronal pulp, tests are not reliable. |

## Formocresol Pulpotomy

Sweet popularized this technique in 1930. Clinical and radiographic success rate of 98 percent has been reported in teeth with formocresol pulpotomy which is considered much higher than calcium hydroxide pulpotomy. Formocresol is preferred in primary teeth because of high success rate.

### Indications

- Vital primary tooth with carious or accidental exposure
- No evidence of pulpal pain
- Clinical signs of normal pulp.

### Contraindications

- Presence of spontaneous pain
- Tooth tender on percussion
- Presence of bleeding at exposure site
- Any abnormal mobility

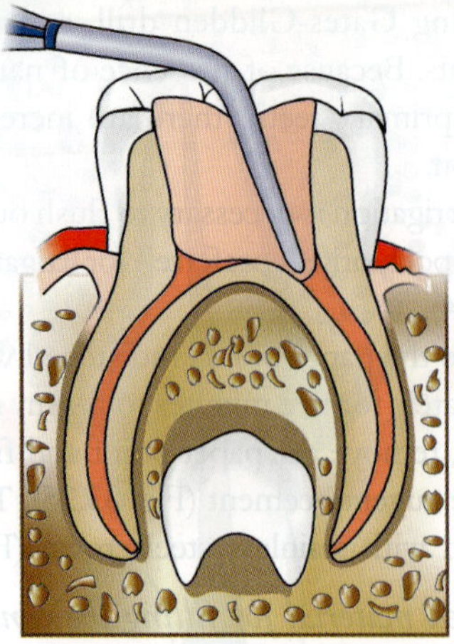

**Fig. 33.25:** Placement of ZOE cement in the canal

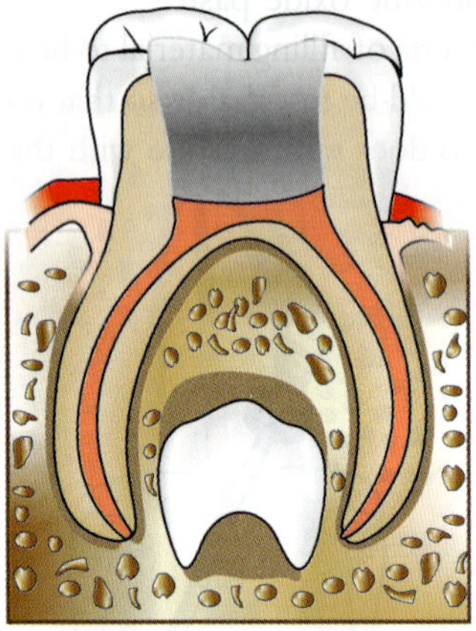

**Fig. 33.26:** Complete restoration of the tooth

The root canal filling material is carried into the pulp chamber and then into the canal with the help of pluggers or lentulospirals. Care should be taken to avoid overfilling of the root canals.

## Follow-up after Pulpectomy

Deciduous teeth with pulpectomy should be checked for the success of the treatment. The treatment would be considered successful if:

a. Tooth is asymptomatic.
b. There is absence of pain, sinus, mobility or swelling associated with tooth.
c. Preoperative radiographs show success.
d. There is simultaneous resorption of filling material and the deciduous roots.
e. There is normal radiographic appearance.

# APEXIFICATION

Apexification is the process of inducing the development of the root and the apical closure in an immature pulpless tooth with an open apex. It is different from apexogenesis in that in latter, root development occurs by physiological process.

In young permanent teeth with nonvital pulp, apexification is advantageous over the conventional root canal treatment because—

a. Apex is funnel shaped with apical part wider than canal.
b. Canal walls are thin and fragile.
c. Absolute dryness of canal is difficult to achieve.

## Objectives of Apexification

The main objective of apexification is to achieve an apical stop for obturating material. This apical stop can be obtained by:

a. Inducing natural calcific barrier at apex or short of apex.
b. Forming an artificial barrier by placing a material at or near the apex.
c. Inducing the natural root lengthening by stimulating Hertwig's epithelial root sheath.

## Rationale of Apexification

The main aim of apexification is to preserve the Hertwig's root sheath and apical pulp tissue. It is based on the fact that after completion of root formation, Hertwig's epithelial root sheath disintegrated and its remnants remain at apical end of root. HERS is considered to be highly resistant to infection so even if tooth is nonvital, viable HERS may be present at the apex which can help in further root development.

In apexification, it is always suggested to complete biomechanical preparation 2 mm short of the radiographic apex so as to avoid any trauma to apical pulp or HERS tissue present in that area.

In cases when damage has already occurred to HERS, root formation cannot take place of its own. In such cases, an artificial barrier is created by placing a material in the apical portion.

Hard barrier or calcific barrier which is formed in apexification has shown to possess "Swiss cheese configuration". It may mimic dentin, cementum or bone.

## Indications

In young permanent teeth with blunderbuss canal (Fig. 33.27) having following symptoms:

a. Symptoms of irreversible pulpitis
b. Teeth with necrotic pulp
c. Teeth with pulpoperiapical pathology showing swelling, tenderness or sinus.

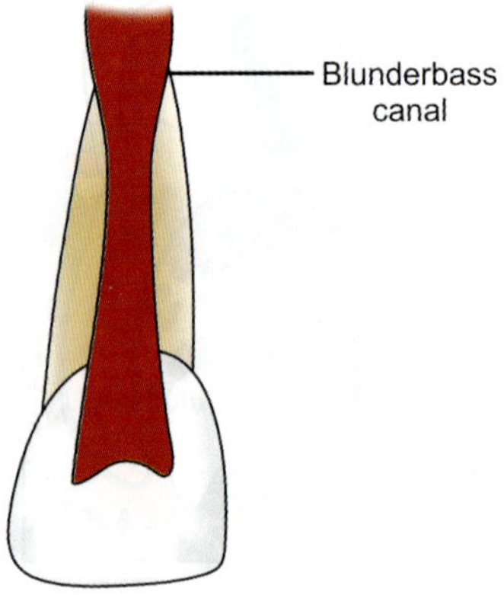


**Fig. 33.27:** Blunderbass canal

### Materials Used for Apexification

1. Calcium hydroxide
2. Calcium hydroxide in combination with other drugs like:
   a. Camphorated paramonochlorophenol
   b. Cresanol
   c. Anesthetic solution
   d. Normal saline
   e. Ringer's solution.
3. Zinc oxide paste
4. Antibiotic paste
5. Tricalcium phosphate
6. Collagen calciumphosphate gel
7. Mineral trioxide aggregate
8. Osteogenic protein I and II.

### Techniques

1. Anesthetize the tooth and isolate it with rubber dam.
2. Gain the straight line access to canal orifice.
3. Extirpate the pulp tissue remnants from the canal and irrigate it with sodium hypochlorite.
4. Establish the working length of canal. The final working length should be adjusted 2 mm short of the radiographic apex (Fig. 33.28).
5. Complete cleaning and debridement of canal, irrigate and then dry the canal. The main reason for biomechanical preparation is debridement and not the shaping of the canal. Because the canal is already very wide, thus care should be taken further not to thin down the fragile dentinal walls.
6. Place calcium hydroxide in the canal for apexification procedure. Thick paste of calcium hydroxide can be carried out in the canal using amalgam carrier (Fig. 33.29). Place a dry cotton pellet over the material and seal it with temporary restorative material.
7. Second visit is done at the interval of three months for monitoring the tooth. If tooth is symptomatic, canal is cleaned and filled again with calcium hydroxide paste.
8. Patient is again recalled until there is radiographic evidence of root formation.
9. Clinically check the progress of apexification by passing a small instrument through the apex after removal of calcium hydroxide.
10. If apexification is incomplete, repeat the above said procedure again. If apexification is complete, radiograph is taken to confirm it (Figs 33.30A to C). If seal is found satisfactory, final obturation of canal is done with gutta-percha points.

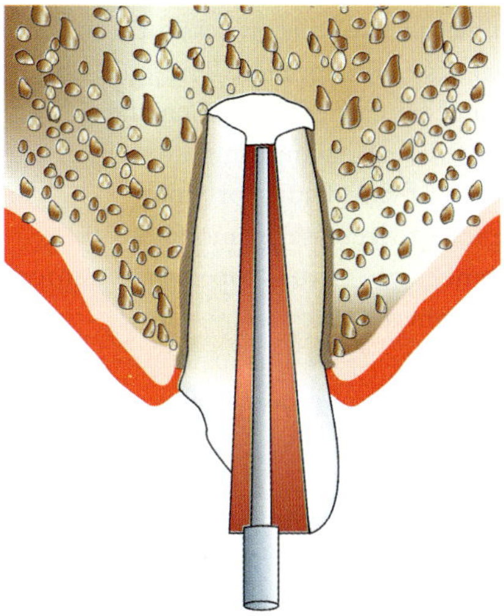

**Fig. 33.28:** Adjust the final working length 2 mm short of radiographic apex

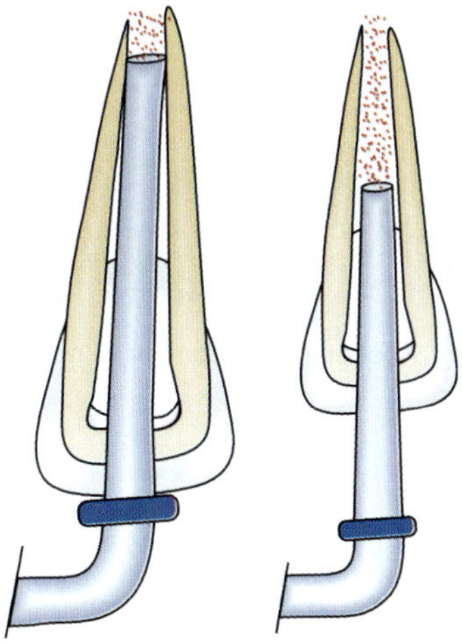

**Fig. 33.29:** Packing of calcium hydroxide paste in canal

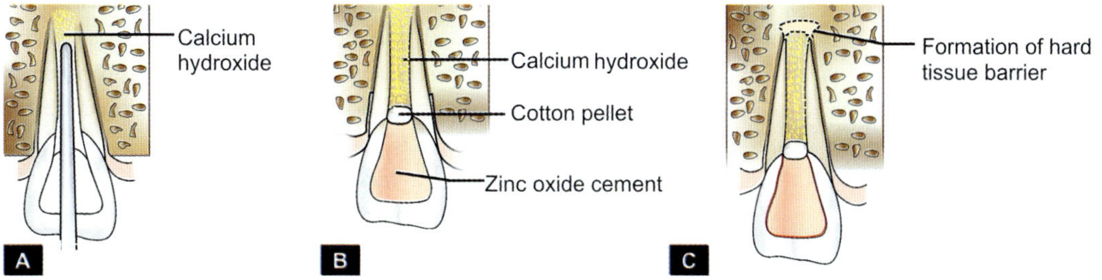


**Figs 33.30A to C:** (A) Placement of calcium hydroxide in the canal; (B) Restoration of the tooth with zinc oxide cement; (C) Formation of hard tissue barrier at apex

### *Types of Closure which can Occur during Apexification*

1. Root-end development in normal pattern (Fig. 33.31).
2. Apex closes but is wider at the apical end (Fig. 33.32).
3. Development of calcific bridge just coronal to apex (Fig. 33.33).
4. Formation of thin barrier at or close to the apex (Fig. 33.34).

The time taken for this process for completion may range from 6 weeks to 18 months. The final obturation of the canal should be carried out when there is:

a. Absence of any symptoms
b. Absence of any fistula or sinus.
c. Absence or decrease in mobility.
d. Evidence of firm stop both clinically as well radiographically.

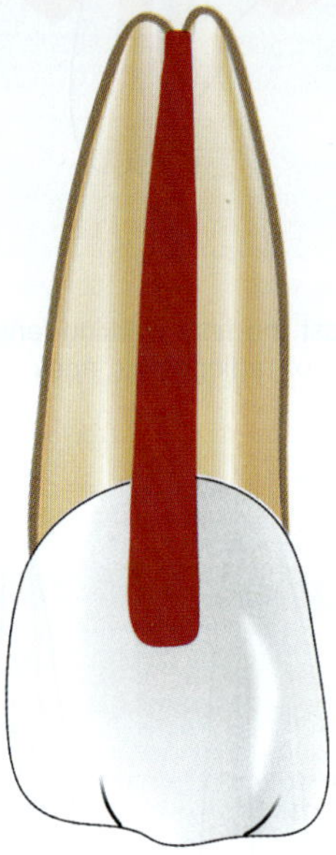

**Fig. 33.31:** Root-end development in normal pattern

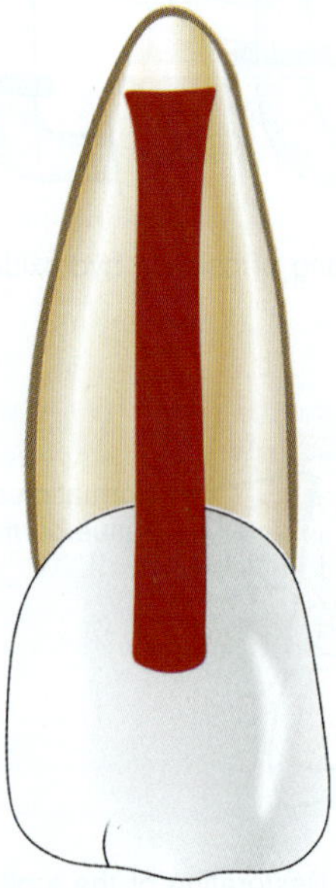

**Fig. 33.32:** Apex closes but wider at apical end

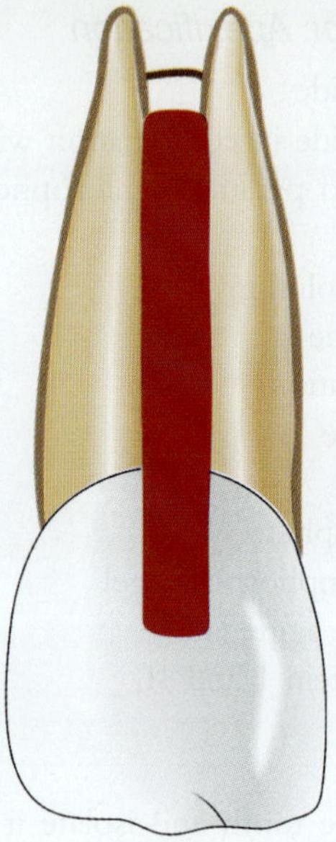

**Fig. 33.33:** Development of calcific bridge coronal to apex

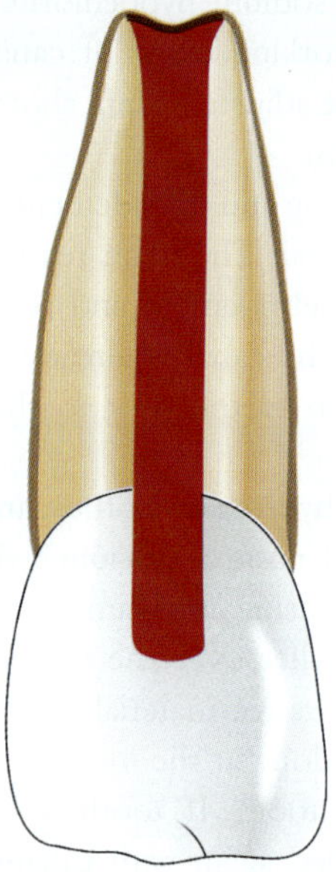

**Fig. 33.34:** Formation of thin barrier close to apex

Obturation in such teeth using lateral condensation is not advocated because the lateral pressure during compaction of gutta-percha may fracture the teeth. In such teeth, vertical compaction method of obturation is preferred.

Since, the dentinal walls are weak in such cases, restoration should be designed to strengthen the tooth. To strengthen the root, gutta-percha should be removed below the alveolar crest, the dentin is acid etched and then composite resin is placed. Placement of posts in such cases should be avoided as far as possible.

MTA a recently introduced material is also used in the apexification procedure. MTA is considered choice of material for apexification because it creates a permanent apical plug at the outset of treatment. To place MTA in the canal isolate the tooth, mix MTA and compact it to the apex of the tooth, creating a 2 mm thickness of plug (Fig. 33.35). Take a radiograph

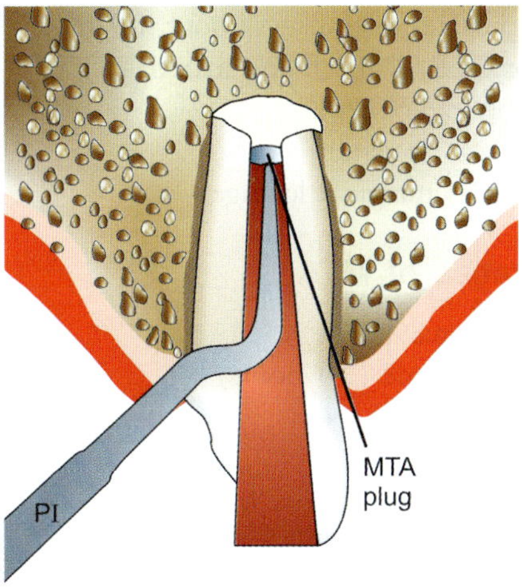


**Fig. 33.35:** Placing MTA at apex of tooth, creating a 2 mm thickness of the plug

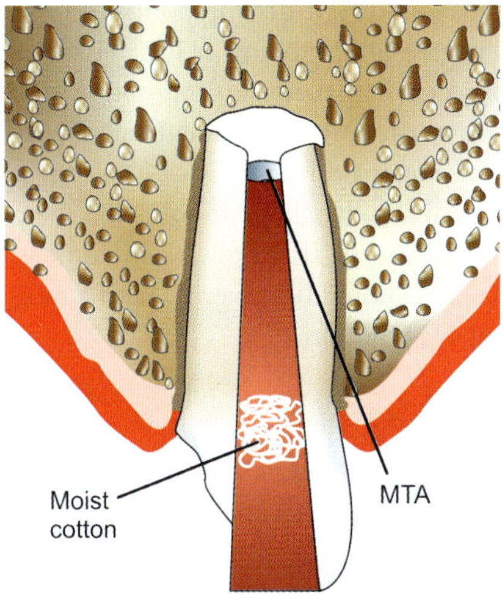


**Fig. 33.36:** Cavity is sealed with moist cotton since MTA needs moisture for setting

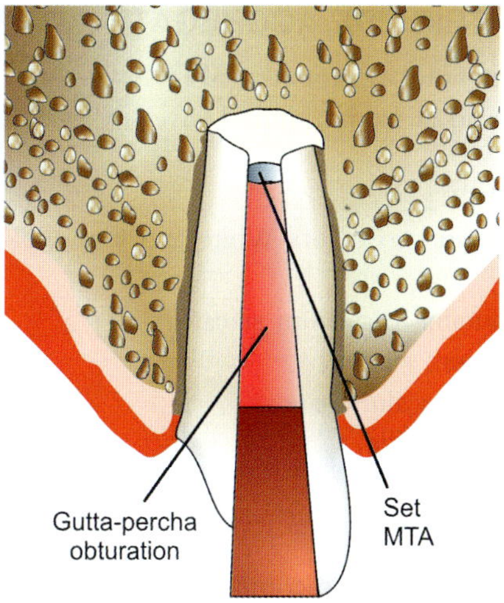


**Fig. 33.37:** After confirming final set of MTA, canal is obturated using gutta-percha

to confirm its placement. Since MTA needs moisture for setting, the cavity is sealed with moist cotton pellet (Fig. 33.36). After 48 hours, confirm the final set of MTA, and obturate the remaining canal using gutta-percha (Fig. 33.37).

Basically the rationale behind the pediatric endodontic therapy is to maintain the integrity of dental arch. A successful pediatric outcome should fulfill the following aims:

a. Re-establishment of healthy periodontium tissue.
b. Maintaining the primary teeth free of infection and acting as space maintainers for their permanent successors.
c. Maintaining the vitality of pulp in young permanent teeth and thus enhancing the root dentin formation.
d. Freedom from pathologic root resorption.

So we can say that pediatric endodontics may prove helpful in providing the health benefits to the child.

| | *Calcium hydroxide* | *Mineral trioxide aggregate* |
|---|---|---|
| Discovery | In 1920 by Herman. It is time tested material | In 1993 by torabinajed. It is still being evaluated. |
| Availability | As powder, settable and nonsettable paste system | As powder which is mixed with water or saline. |
| pH | 11-12 | 10.5 initially, reaches 12.5 in 3 hours. |
| Solubility | High so disintegrates with time | Low, so does not change over time. |
| Compressive strength | Low | High |
| Marginal leakage | More | Less |
| Manipulation | Easy | Difficult because mix is grainy and difficult to handle |
| Adherence of dentin | Does not adhere | Adheres to dentin |
| Calcific bridge | Forms hard tissue barrier slowly which is not very thick and uniform | Forms hard tissue barrier faster. It is thick, uniform and resembles normal structure. |
| While using on pulp | Bleeding should be stopped | Bleeding need not be stopped, infact moisture is required for setting. |
| Inflammation | Causes inflammation to pulp and periapical tissues | Does not cause inflammation as it is highly biocompatible. |
| Replenishment | Needs to be replenished at 3-6 months interval | Can be used in single visit apical barrier technique. Need not be replenished. |
| Antibacterial efficacy | Good | Poor |
| Cost factor | Not expensive | Expensive |

## MINERAL TRIOXIDE AGGREGATE (MTA)

Mineral trioxide aggregate (MTA) was developed by Dr Torabinejad at Loma Linda University in 1993.

### Composition

It is available in two colors White and Gray color

*Gray color*

- It contains tricalcium silicate,
- Dicalcium silicate,
- Tricalcium aluminate
- Bismuth oxide
- Calcium sulfate
- Tetracalcium aluminoferrite

*White color:* It has same composition as that of gray color MTA except the lack of tetracalcium aluminoferrite. Thus, it is white in color.

### Properties

1. pH of MTA is 12.5 (When set) so, it has biological and histological properties similar to calcium hydroxide.
2. Setting time is 2 hours and 45 minutes.
3. Compressive strength is 40 MPa immediately after setting and 70 MPa after 21 days.
4. Contrast to $Ca(OH)_2$, it produces hard setting non-resorbable surface.
5. It sets in a moist environment (hydrophilic in nature).
6. It has low solubility.
7. It shows resistance to marginal leakage.
8. It also reduces bacterial migration.
9. It exhibits excellent biocompatibility in relation with vital tissues.
10. The compressive strength of MTA is equal to IRM and SuperEBA but less than that of amalgam.
11. MTA is also known as ***Portland's cement*** except for addition of bismuth oxide which is added for modifying its setting properties. Its consistency is similar to very hard cement, which can be compared to concrete.

Commercially it is available under the name ProRoot MTA (Dentsply).

### Manipulation of MTA

To prepare MTA, a small amount of *liquid and powder are mixed to putty consistency*. Since, MTA mixture is a *loose granular aggregate* (like concrete cement) it *doesn't stick* very well *to any instrument*. It cannot be carried out in cavity with normal cement carrier and thus has to be *carried with Messing gun, amalgam carrier* or *specially designed carrier*. Once MTA is placed, it is *compacted with burnishers and micropluggers*. Unless compacted very lightly, the loosely bound aggregate will be pushed out of the cavity. Next, a *small damp cotton pellet is used to gently clean the resected surface* and *to remove any excess MTA from cavity*.

### Advantages of MTA

1. Water based chemistry, so requires moisture for setting
2. Excellent biocompatibility
3. Normal healing response without inflammation
4. Least toxic of all the filling materials
5. Reasonably radiopaque
6. Bacteriostatic in nature
7. Resistance to marginal leakage.

### Disadvantages of MTA

1. Difficult to manipulate
2. Long setting time (3-4 hours)
3. Costly.

### Precautions to be taken for MTA

1. MTA material should be kept in closed container to avoid moisture.
2. MTA must be stored in dry area.
3. MTA material should be immediately placed after mixing with liquid, to prevent dehydration during setting.
4. Do not irrigate after placing MTA, remove excess water with moist cotton pallet.
5. Adding too much or too little liquid will reduce the ultimate strength of the material.
6. MTA material usually takes 3-4 hours but the working time is about five minutes. If more working time is needed, the mixed material should be coverted with a moist gauge pad to prevent evaporation.

### Indications of use of MTA

1. As a pulp capping material.
2. For the repair of root canals as an apical plug during apexification.
3. For the repair of root perforations during root canal therapy.
4. For the repair of root resorptions.
5. As a root-end filling material.

### Clinical Applications of MTA

1. ***Pulp capping:*** Vital pulp therapy is indicated in some cases. By placing MTA over the exposed area often allows healing and preservation of vital pulp without further treatment. Rinse the cavity with sodium hypochlorite to disinfect the area. Mix the MTA with enough sterile water to give it a putty consistency. Apply it over the exposed pulp and remove the excess. Blot the area dry with a cotton pellet and restore the cavity with an amalgam or composite filling material.
2. ***Apexification:*** MTA is excellent material for apexification because it creates a permanent apical plug at the outset of treatment.

   *Vital pulp:* Isolate the tooth with a rubber dam and perform a pulpotomy procedure. Place the MTA over the pulp stump and close the tooth with temporary cement until the apex of the tooth closes up.

   *Nonvital pulp:* Isolate the tooth with a rubber dam and perform root canal treatment. Mix the MTA and compact it to the apex of the tooth, creating a 2 mm thickness of plug. Wait for it to set; then fill in the canal with cement and gutta-percha.

3. ***Internal and external root resorption:*** The root resorption is an idiopathic condition resulting in the breakdown or destruction of the root structure. In the case of *internal root resorption*, isolate the tooth and perform RCT in the usual manner. Once the canal has been cleaned and shaped, prepare a putty mixture of MTA and fill the canal with it, using a plugger or gutta-percha cone and obturate the canal. In the case of *external resorption*, complete the root canal therapy for that tooth. Raise a flap and remove the defect on the root surface with a round bur. Mix the MTA in the same manner as above and apply it to the root surface. Remove the excess cement and condition the surface with tetracycline. Graft the defect with decalcified freeze dried bone allograft and a calcium sulfate barrier.
4. ***Perforation:*** Perforations are the result of procedural error in which communication between the pulp canal and periodontal tissues occur. First finish cleaning and shaping of the perforated canal. Irrigate the canal really well with sodium hypochlorite and dry it with a paper point. If the perforation is down at the mid to apical third, then follow the directions for treating an internal resorption. If the perforation is closer to the coronal third, then obturate the canal with gutta-percha as usual. Next, remove the gutta percha below the perforation using the Pesso reamer. Mix the MTA and fill the rest of the canal up with a plugger.
5. ***Root-end filling:*** Root-end filling is required when an endodontic case can best be treated or retreated with a surgical (extraradicular) rather than intraradicular approach. MTA has shown excellent sealing ability and allows periradicular healing when used as a root-end filling material during periradicualr surgery. First, gain access to the root-end and resect the root-end with a surgical bur. Prepare a class I cavity preparation. Isolate the area and achieve hemostasis. Mix the MTA according to manufacture's instructions. Condense the MTA material into the cavity using a small plugger. Excess cement is removed with the help of moist gauge. Confirm with the help of radiograph.

## QUESTIONS

**Q. What are indications and contraindications of pulpotomy?**

**Q. What is apexification? Explain in detail about the technique of apexification.**

**Q. Write short notes on:**

a. Indirect pulp capping
b. Direct pulp capping
c. MTA

## BIBLIOGRAPHY


1. Accorinte ML, Holland R, Reis A, Bortoluzzi MC, Murata SS, Dezan (Ir) E, Souza V, Alessandro LD. Evaluation of mineral trioxide aggregate and calcium hydroxide cement as pulp-capping agents in human teeth. J Endod 2008;34(1):1-6.
2. Andelin WE, Shabahang S, Wright K, Torabinejad M. Identification of hard tissue after experimental pulp capping using dentin sialoprotein (DSP) as a marker. J Endod 2003;29 (10):646-50.
3. Bakland LF. Endodontic considerations in dental trauma, in JF Ingle and IF Bakland (eds), Endodontics London: BC Decker (5th edn) 2002;829-31.
4. Bakland LK. Management of traumatically injured pulps in immature teeth using MTA. J Calif Dent Assoc 2000;28(11): 855-58.
5. Barrieshi-Nusair KM, Qudeimat MA. A prospective clinical study of mineral trioxide aggregate for partial pulpotomy in cariously exposed permanent teeth. J Endod 2006;32(8):731-35.
6. Blanco L, Cohen S. Treatment of crown fractures with exposed pulps. J Calif Dent Assoc 2002;30(6):419-25.
7. Carrotte P. Endodontic Part 9. Calcium hydroxide root resorption, endo-perio lesions. Br Dent J 2004;197(12):735-43.
8. Chosak A, Sefa J, Cleaton-Jones P. A histological and quantitative histomorphometric study of apexification of nonvital permanent incisors of velvet monkeys after repeated root filling with a calcium hydroxide paste. Endod Dent Traumatol 1997;13:211-17.
9. Chueh LH, Huang GT. Immature teeth with periradicular periodontitis or abscess undergoing apexogenesis: A Paradigm Shift. J Endod 2006;32(12):1205-13.
10. Cvek M. A clinical report on partial pulpotomy and capping with calcium hydroxide in permanent incisors with complicated crown fracture. J Endod 1978;4(8):232-37.
11. De Leimburg ML, Angeretti A, Ceruti P, Lendini M, Pasqualini D, Berutti E. MTA obturation of pulpless teeth with open apices: Bacterial leakage as detected by polymerase chain reaction assay. J Endod 2004;30(12):883-86.
12. De-Deus G, Coutinho-Filho T. The use of white Portland cement as an apical plug in a tooth with a necrotic pulp and wide-open apex; A case report. Int Endod J 2007;40:653-60.
13. Erdogan G. The treatment of nonvital immature teeth with calcium hydroxide-sterile water Paste: Two case reports. Quintessence Int 1997;28(10):681-86.
14. Farhad A, Mohammadi Z. Calcium hydroxide: A review. Int Dent J 2005;55(5):293-301.
15. Felippe MCS, Felippe WT, Marques MM, Antoniazzi JH. The effect of the renewal of calcium hydroxide paste on the apexification and periapical healing of teeth with incomplete root formation. Int Endod J 2005;38:436-42.
16. Fong CD, Davis MJ. Partial pulpotomy for immature permanent teeth, its present and future. Pediatr Dent 2002; 24(1):29-32.
17. Giuliani V, Baccetti T, Pace R, Pagavino G. The use of MTA in teeth with necrotic pulps and open apices. Dent Traumatol 2002;18:217-21.
18. Grossman LI. Endodontic Practice (11th edn). Philadelphia: Lea and febiger, 1998.
19. Gupta S, Sharma A, Dang N. Apical bridging in association with regular root formation following single-visit apexification. A case report. Quintessence Int 1999;30:560-62.
20. Hayashi M, Shimizu A, Ebisu S. MTA for obturation of mandibular central incisors with open apices. Case report. J Endod 2004;30(2):120-22.
21. Kontham UR, Tiku AM, Damle SG, Kalaskar RR. Apexogenesis of a symptomatic mandibular first permanent molar with calcium hydroxide pulpotomy. Quintessence Int 2005;36(8):653-57.
22. Mackie IC, Hill FJ. A clinical guide to the endodontic treatment of nonvital immature permanent teeth. Br Den J 1999; 186(2):54-58.
23. Metzger Z, Solomonov M, Mass E. Calcium hydroxide retention in wide root canals with flaring apices. Dent Traumatol 2001;17:86-92.

24. Mjör IA. Pulp-dentin biology in restorative dentistry. Part 7: The exposed pulp. Quintessence Int 2002;33(2):113-35.
25. Nosrat IV, Nosrat CA. Reparative hard tissue formation following calcium hydroxide application after partial pulpotomy in cariously exposed pulps of permanent teeth. Int Endod J 1998;31(3): 221-26.
26. Pitt Ford TR. Apexification and apexogenesis, in RE Walton and M Torabinejad (eds), Principles and practice of Endodontcis (3rd edn), Philadelphia: WB Saunders Co., 2002.
27. Rafter M. Apexification: A review. Dent Tramatol 2005;21:1-8.
28. Roberts HW, Toth JM, Berzins DW, Charlton DG. Mineral trioxide aggregate material use in endodontic treatment: A review of the literature. Dent Mater 2008;24:149-64.
29. Seldon Hs. Apexification: An interesting case. J Endod 2002; 28(1):44-45.
30. Siqueira JF Jr, Lopes HP. Mechanisms of antimicrobial activity of calcium hydroxide: A critical review. Int Endod J 1999;32: 361-69.
31. Svizero Nadia R, Bresciani E, Francischone CE, Franco EB, Pereira JC. Partial pulpotomy and tooth reconstruction of a crown-fractured permanent incisor: A case report. Quintessence Int 2003;34(10):740-47.
32. Teixeira LS, Demarco FF, Coppola MC, Bonow ML. Clinical and radiographic evaluation of pulpotomies performed under intrapulpal injection of anesthetic solution. Int Endod J 2001;34(6):440-46.
33. Torabinejad M, Chivian N. Clinical applications of mineral trioxide aggregate. J Endod 1999;25(3):197-205.
34. Torabinejad M, Hong CU, McDonald F, Pitt Ford TR. Physical and chemical properties of a new root-end filling material. J Endod 1995;21(7):349-53.
35. Torabinejad M, Watson TF, Pitt Ford TR. Sealing ability of a mineral trioxide aggregate when used as a root-end filling material. J Endod 1993;19(12):591-95.
36. Whittle M. Apexification of an infected untreated immature tooth. J Endod 2000;26(4):245-47.
37. Witherspoon DE, Small JC, Harris GZ. Mineral trioxide aggregate pulpotomies: A case series outcomes assessment. J Am Dent Assoc 2006;137(9):610-18.

# CHAPTER 34

# Geriatric Endodontics



Human beings are a part of nature and thus are amenable to all natural laws. Aging is a normal, genetically dictated physiological process. It is a state of interplay between the physiological and pathological process. It leads to gradual impairment in performance of various systems, hence of the individual as a whole.

Today people tend to live longer than before because of increasing medical progress and steady rise in living standards; consequently there are enough older people to command for attention, in the science of medicine and dentistry.

DCNA 1989 defined Geriatric dentistry as the provision of dental care for adult persons with one or more chronic debilitating, physical or mental illness with associated medication and psychosocial problems.

## ORAL ASPECTS OF AGING

**Dental problems in the aged include**

- Delayed wound healing
- Tissue friability
- Abnormal taste sensation
- Stomatodynia
- Postmenopausal osteoporosis
- Excessive bone resorption
- Fungal infection
- Causalgia
- Vague fears
- Pains

### Age Changes in Bone Tissue

- *Cortical thinning:* The cortex thins and porosity increases from about an age of 40–80.
- *Loss of trabeculae*
- *Cellular atrophy*
- *Sclerosis* of bone

## AGE CHANGES IN THE TEETH

### Macroscopic Changes

- Changes in form and color.
- Wear and attrition of teeth (Figs 34.1 and 34.2).
- Causes for change in color of teeth:
  - Decrease in thickness of dentin.
  - General loss of translucency.

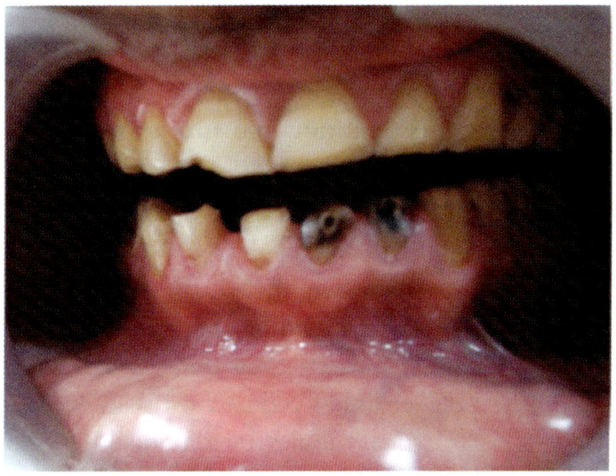

Fig. 34.1: Physiological wear of teeth

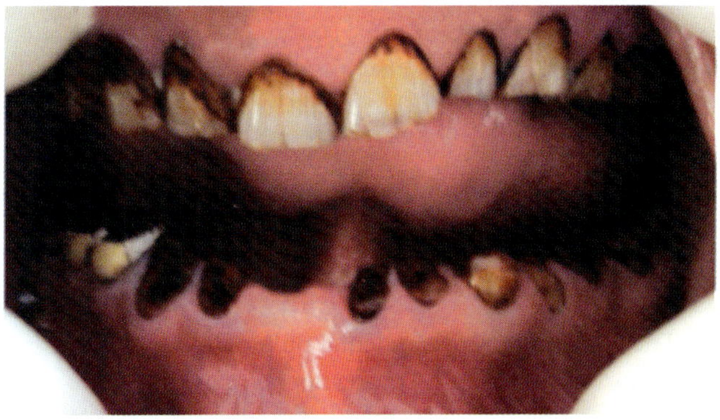

Fig. 34.2: Attrition of teeth resulting in multiple pulp exposure

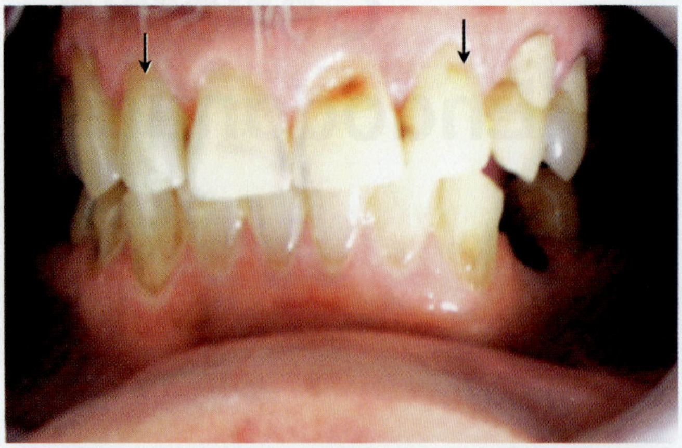

**Fig. 34.3:** Abrasion of teeth

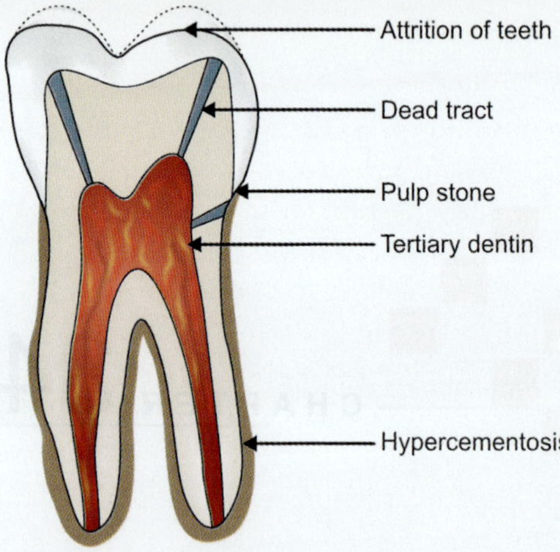


**Fig. 34.4:** Age changes in enamel, pulp, dentin and cementum

- Pigmentation of anatomical defects.
- Corrosion products.
- Inadequate oral hygiene.

## Age Changes in Enamel

All changes in enamel are based on ionic exchange mechanism.

- Decrease in permeability of enamel
- Enamel becomes more brittle with age.
- The nitrogen content in enamel increases with age.
- Enamel exhibits attrition, abrasion and erosion (Fig. 34.3).

## Age Changes in Cementum

- Cementum gradually increases in thickness with age.
- Cementum becomes more susceptible to resorption.
- There is increased fluoride and magnesium content of cementum with age.

## Age Changes in Dentin

- Physiologic secondary dentin formation.
- Gradual obliteration of dentinal tubules
- Dentin sclerosis.
- Size of the pulp chamber reduces with age
- Occlusion of dentinal tubules by a gradual deposition of the peritubular dentin

## Clinical Implications of Age Changes in Dentin

- Obliteration of the tubules leads to reduction in sensitivity of the tissue.
- Reduction in dentin permeability prevents the ingress of toxic agents.
- Addition of more bulk to the dentin prevents pulpal reactions and decreases the chances of pulp exposures.

## Age Changes in Pulp (Fig. 34.4)

- The difference between dental pulp of old individuals and young teeth is due to more fibers, and less cells.
- Blood supply to the tooth decreases with age.
- The prevalence of pulp stones increases with age.

## Age Changes in Oral Mucosa

The oral cavity is lined by stratified squamous epithelium which forms a barrier between internal and external environment, thus providing protection against:

- Entry of noxious substances and organisms
- Mechanical damage
- Fluid exchange.

### *Clinical Changes in Epithelium*

With age, oral mucosa has been reported to become increasingly thin, smooth, and dry to have edematous appearance with loss of elasticity and stippling and thus becomes more susceptible to injury.

Tongue exhibits loss of filliform papillae, and deteriorating taste sensation with occasional burning sensation.

### *Histological Changes in Oral Mucosa*

1. Epithelial changes
2. Connective tissue changes.

### *Epithelial Changes*

These are

- Decreased thickness of epithelial cell layer.
- Reduced keratinization
- Alteration in the morphology of epithelial-connective tissue interface.
- Decrease in the length of retepegs of oral epithelium have been reported with age.
- Rate of cell renewal in human oral epithelia decreases with aging.

### *Connective Tissue Change*

There is increase in number and density of elastin fibers. Cellular changes are also reported, which include:

- Cells becoming shrunken
- Cells becoming inactive
- Reduction in number of cells.

## Age Changes in Periodontal Connective Tissue

### Structural Changes

- Gingival connective tissue becomes denser and coarsely textured upon aging.
- Decrease in the number of fibroblasts.
- Decrease in the fiber content.
- Increase in the size of interstitial compartments containing blood vessels.
- Evidence of calcification on and between the collagen fibers.

## Age Changes in Salivary Glands

A common generalized association with aging oral cavity is the diminished function of salivary glands.

Saliva exists principally to protect oral cavity and performs important functions such as:

- Lubricating proteins in saliva help to keep the oral mucosa pliable and hydrated.
- Antibacterial factors regulate the oral microorganisms.
- Inorganic and organic buffers neutralize proton produced by cariogenic bacteria.
- Helps in proper sensation to taste buds.
- Contributes to food bolus formation, thus aiding initial stages of deglutition.

The most recognizable age change is reduced salivation or xerostomia. The main consequences of xerostomia include dry mouth, generalized mouth soreness, burning or painful tongue, taste changes, chewing difficulty, problems with swallowing, talking, and reduced denture retention.

# ENDODONTICS IN GERIATRIC PATIENTS

The primary function of teeth is mastication, thus the loss of teeth leads to detrimental food changes and reduction in health. The needs, expectations, desire, demands of older patients thus exceeds for those of any age group (Fig. 34.5).

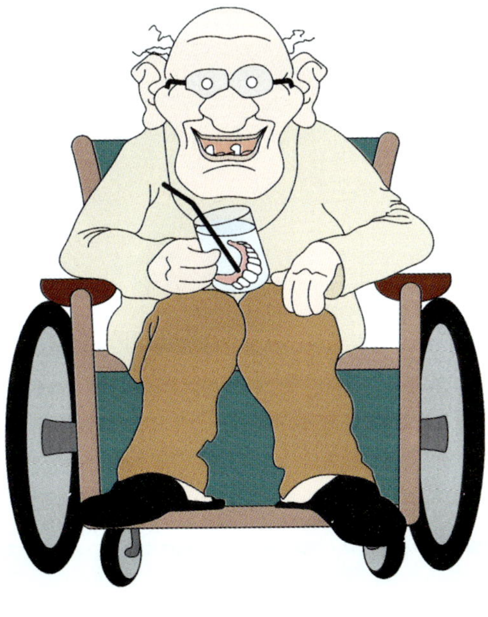

Fig. 34.5: Geriatric patient

The quality of life for older patients can be improved by preventing the loss of teeth through endodontic treatment and can add a large and impressive value to their overall dental, physical, mental health. Endodontic treatment is the treatment of a damaged or necrotic pulp in a tooth, to allow the tooth to remain functional in the dental arch.

Most of the endodontic procedures can be carried out with high rate of success. The objective of the endodontic treatment is to clean the root canal system of infected and toxic debris and to shape the canal to receive an obturation material, which will seal the entire canal system from periodontal tissues and from oral cavity. This creates an environment, which is aimed at preserving normal periradicular tissues or restoring, these tissues to health.

The desire for root canal treatment is increasing considerably amongst aging patients. Root canal treatment can be offered as a favorable alternative to the terms of extraction and cost of replacement.

## Medical History

Dentists should recognize that the biologic or functional age of an individual is far more important than chronological age. As most of the old aged people suffer from one or the other medical problems, a medical history should be taken prior to starting any treatment for geriatric patients.

A standardized form should be used to identify any disease or therapy that would alter treatment plan or it's outcome. Aging usually causes changes in cardiovascular, respiratory, central nervous system that result in most drug therapy needs. The renal and liver function of the patients should be considered while prescribing drugs as they have some action on these organs. Consultation can be taken from the patient's family, guardian, and physician to complete the history including information on compliance with any prescribed treatment and sensitivity to medications.

Root canal treatment is certainly far less traumatic in the extremes of age or health than is extraction, but still a thorough medical history is mandatory.

## Chief Complaint of Geriatric Patients

Most common reason for pain in old age patients is pulpal or periapical problem that requires either root canal treatment or extraction. The dentist should listen to the patient and allow the patient to explain the problem in his own words. This will help to analyze the patient's level of dental knowledge and ability to communicate.

In the chief complaint patient usually informs his reason of visit, teeth he feels are problematic, and severity of the problem. By listening to patient's chief complaint, the dentist can diagnose or he can be directed to diagnose pulpal or periapical disease if present and which tooth is the source.

Older patients are more likely to have already had root canal treatment and have a more realistic perception about treatment comfort. These patients rarely complain about signs and symptoms of pulpal/periapical disease as they may consider them to be minor with other health concerns what they might be facing. In the older patients just the presence of teeth indicates proper maintenance and resistance to disease.

Usually the pain associated with vital pulps seems to be reduced with aging, and severity seems to diminish over time suggesting a reduced pulp volume. Since pulp healing capacity reduces with age, the necrosis may occur quickly after microbial invasion thus reducing the symptoms of pulpitis.

## Past Dental History

The dentist should ask the patients past dental history so as to access the patient's dental status and plan future treatment accordingly. Patient can give history as recent pulp exposure and restoration, or it may be as subtle as a routine crown preparation 15-20 years ago. From dental history, the clinician can assess the patient's knowledge about dental treatment and his psychological attitude, expectations from dental treatment.

## Subjective Symptoms

Subjective symptoms are described by patient. Patient explains regarding their complaint, stimulus or irritant that causes pain, nature of pain, its relationship to the stimulus or irritant. This information is useful in determining whether the source is pulpal or periapical and if these problems are reversible or not.

From this information the dentist can determine the type of diagnostic tests to be done to confirm findings. In older patients the pulpal symptoms are usually chronic. For these patients other sources of orofacial pain should be ruled out when pain is not quickly localized.

## Objective Symptoms

Objective symptoms are the one diagnosed by the dentist by clinical examination. Extraoral and intraoral clinical examination provides dentist useful information regarding the disease and previous treatment done. Dentist should examine the overall oral condition and all abnormal conditions should be recorded and investigated.

Common observations in geriatric patients are:

- In older patients, usually some of teeth get extracted. Missing teeth indicate the decrease in functional ability, resulting in loss of chewing ability. This reduced chewing ability leads to a higher intake of more refined soft carbohydrate diet, and sugar intake to compensate for loss of taste and xerostomia. All these lead to increased susceptibility to dental decay.
- Gingival recession: It results in exposure of cementum and dentin thus making them more prone to decay and sensitivity (Fig. 34.6).
- Root caries (Figs 34.7A and B): It is very common in older patients and is difficult to treat; the caries excavation is irritating to the pulp and often results in pulp exposures or reparative dentin formation that might affect the negotiation of canal, if root canal treatment is needed.
- Attrition, abrasion, erosion expose the dentin and allows the pulp to respond with dentinal sclerosis and reparative dentin which may completely obliterate the pulp (Fig. 34.8).

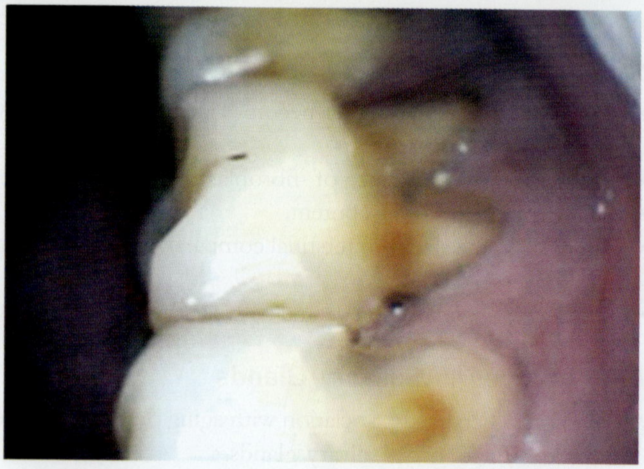

**Fig. 34.6:** Gingival recession is commonly seen in geriatric patients

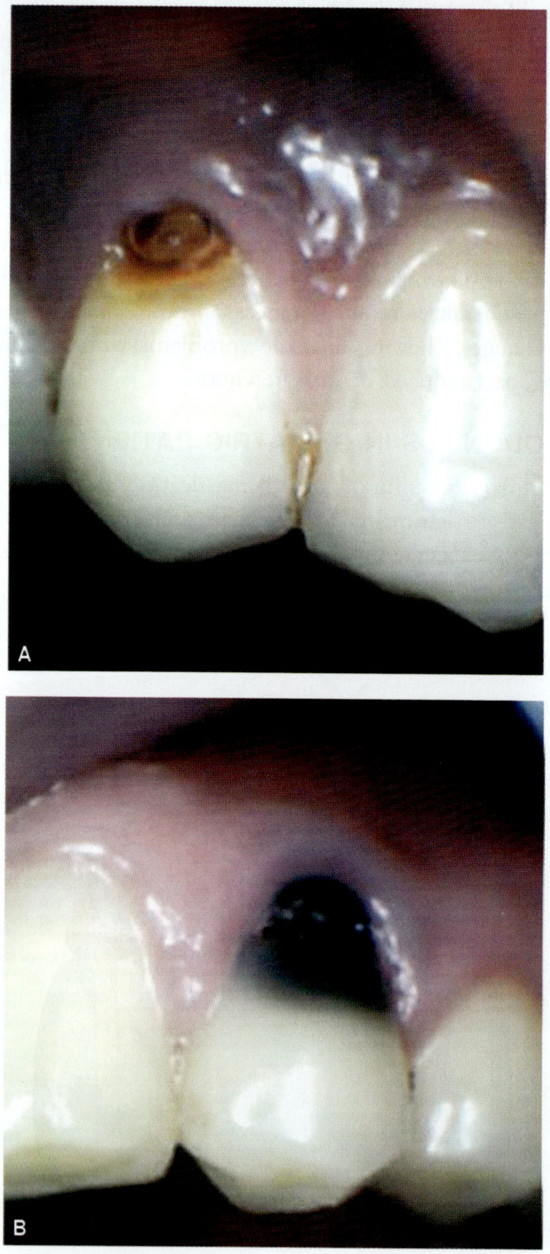

**Figs 34.7A and B:** Root caries

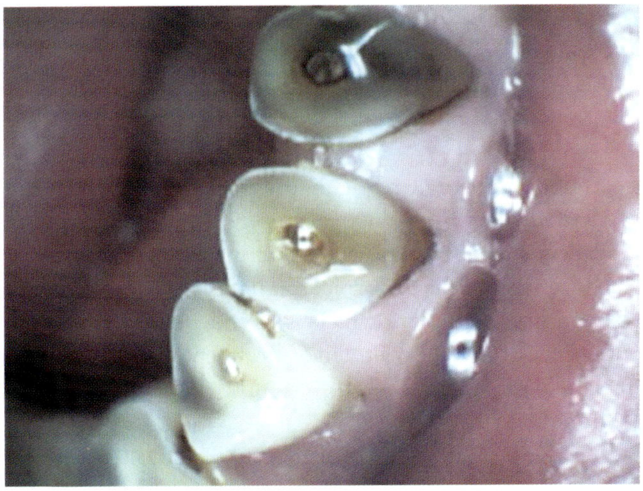

**Fig. 34.8:** Attrition of teeth

- With the increasing age, the pulp cavity size decreases.this decrease in volume can be due to formation of reparative dentin resulting from recurrent caries, restorative procedures and trauma.
- Continued cementum deposition is seen with increasing age thus moving cementodentinal junction (CDJ) farther from the radiographic apex (Figs 34.9A to C).
- Calcification is observed in the pulp cavity which can be due to caries, pulpotomy or trauma and is more of linear type. The lateral and accessory canals can be calcified, thus decreasing their clinical significance.
- Reduced tubular permeability is seen as the dentinal tubules become occluded with advancing age.
- The missing and titled teeth in older patients result in change in the molar relationship, biting pattern in older patients due to can cause TMJ disorders or loss of vertical dimension.
- Reduced mouth opening in older patients increases working time and decreases the space needed for instrumentation.
- The presence of multiple restorations indicates a history of repeated dental treatment.
- Pulpal injury in older age patients is the mainly because of marginal leakage and microbial contamination of cavity walls.

In older patients, improper tooth preparation causes an increased susceptibility to cracks and cuspal fractures. These cracks or craze lines become more evident as a result of staining, but they do not always indicate pulp exposure.

In older patients, pulp exposures caused by tooth infractions usually do not present acute symptoms. Infact, the crack penetrates the sulcus to create a periodontal defect, along with periapical defect. If incomplete cracks are not detected early in older patients, the prognosis for cracked teeth becomes questionable.

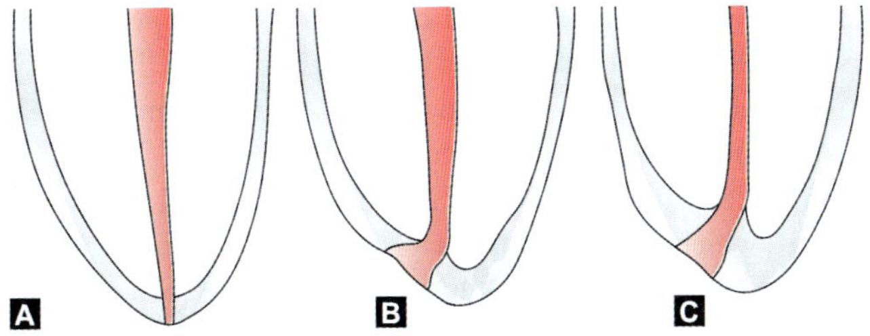


**Figs 34.9A to C:** As the age advances, due to continued deposition of cementum, CDJ moves away from radiographic apex

- With age in older patients, the size and number of apical and accessory foramen reduced, even the permeability of dentinal tubules.
- Periodontal disease is also a major concern for the tooth of old age patients. The periodontal disease must be considered as a pathway for sinus tracts. In teeth with nonvital pulp, the narrow pockets usually represent sinus tracts. These teeth can be resistant to root canal therapy alone when with time they become chronic periodontal pockets. In such cases periodontal treatment plays an important role along with endodontic therapy.
- Root canal treatment is commonly indicated before root amputations are performed.

Sinus tracts should be examined with gutta-percha cones to establish tractsorigin. Sinus tracts usually indicate presence of chronic periapical inflammation, and sinus tracts disappearance, indicates healing. Sinus tract reduces the risk of inter appointment or postoperative pain, although drainage may follow canal debridement or filling.

## Pulp Vitality Tests in Geriatric Patients

The dentist should determine which tooth or teeth are the objects of the complaint by testing the pulp vitality. Vitality responses must correlate with clinical and radiographic findings and should be used in developing the diagnosis. Pulpal and periapical status should be examined.

Pulp vitality can be examined by

a. Thermal pulp tests
b. Cold test
c. Heat test
d. Electric pulp tests

However, these pulp vitality tests are not very accurate because of extensive calcification and reduced size of pulp cavity.

Test cavity is not of much use in determining pulp vitality because the cutting of dentin does not produce the same level of response in an older patient.

## Radiographs

Geriatric endodontics deals with periapical and pulpal tissue which cannot be examined clinically thus, radiographs play a vital role in the diagnosis of the pulpal and periradicular lesions. They help the dentist in identifying the tooth condition/status and the treatment to be advised.

### *Problems Encountered*

- *Tori*: In the elder patients, film placement is affected by tori but this can be solved by the apical position of muscle attachments that increase the depth of the vestibule.
- The presence of tori, exostoses, denser bone requires increased exposure times for proper diagnostic contrast.
- Older patients may be less capable of assisting in film placement; the holders that secure the position should be used.

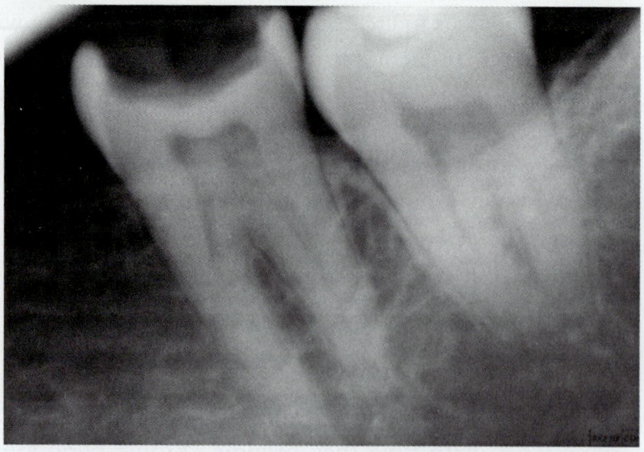

**Fig. 34.10:** Radiograph showing reduced size of pulp cavity of geriatric patients

### Common Radiographic Observations in Geriatric Patients

- Receded pulp cavity which is accelerated by reparative dentin formation (Fig. 34.10)
- Presence of pulp stones and dystrophic calcification
- Receding pulp horns can be noted in the radiograph
- Deep proximal or root decay and restorations that may cause calcification between the observable chamber and root canal.

The periapical area must be included in the diagnostic radiograph as it the most important area of consideration. Radiovisiography (RVG) out powers conventional radiography in detecting early bone changes.

In older patients the examination should be started by examining the canals for their number, size, shape, and curvature. Radiographs of teeth of older patients usually show narrow and sclerotic canals. Canals may show calcification evenly throughout their length. A mid-root disappearance of a detectable canal may indicate bifurcation rather than calcification.

In cases where the vitality tests do not correlate with the radiographic findings, one should consider the presence of odontogenic and nonodontogenic cysts and tumors.

In teeth with root resorption along with apical periodontitis, shape of apex and anatomy of foramen may change due to inflammatory osteoclastic activity.

In teeth with hypercementosis, the apical anatomy may become unclear.

## DIAGNOSIS AND TREATMENT PLAN

The proper diagnosis can be determined based on patient's complaint, history, signs, symptoms, clinical examination, radiographs, vitality of the pulp and presence of periapical pathologic conditions.

Considerations for endodontic treatment in geriatric patients:

- Single appointment procedures are better, as these patients may have physical problems. These patients also need transportation or physical assistance to get into the office or operatory.
- Root canal treatment must be considered when cusps have fractured or when supraerupted or malaligned teeth, intracoronal attachments, guide planes for partial significant tooth reduction.
- Because of reduced blood supply, pulp capping is not as successful in older teeth as in younger ones therefore not recommended.
- Endodontic surgery in geriatric patients is not as viable alternative as for a younger patient.

Patient should be explained about the treatment procedure which is going to be performed on him. It is better to obtain a signed consent form, which is useful in further records. Irrespective of age, the main aim of treatment should be removal of pain and infection so as to restore teeth to normal health and function.

A patient's limited life expectancy should not alter treatment plans and is no excuse for extractions or poor root canal treatment. All the older patients should be explained about the risks and alternatives in prior. For medically compromised or cognitively impaired patients, cardiac patients, neuropsychiatric patients, it is safe and better to start treatment only after a valid consent is obtained from the particular doctors.

The time of appointment should be according to the physical and mental evaluation of the patient. Patient's daily personal, eating, resting habits should be considered along with medication schedule. Depending on the length of the appointment, morning appointments are preferable though some patients prefer late morning or early afternoon visits to allow "morning stiffness" to dissipate. Chair positioning and comfort may be more important for older adults than younger patients. Patients should be offered assistance into operatory and into or out of chair and chair adjustments should be made slowly.

The patient's eyes should be shielded for the intensity of dental chair light. If patient feels tiring of jaws while treatment, procedure should be terminated as soon as possible. Bite blocks are useful in comfortably maintaining free way space and reducing jaw fatigue.

For geriatric patients, the dentist should never immediately start the treatment, first some social exchange of words and personal interest should be shown to develop a good rapport and it also makes the patient more confident towards the dentist and treatment procedure.

It is a fact that the root canal therapy is far less traumatic than extraction for older patients. *Anesthesia* should be given taking into consideration of the pulp vitality status and cervical positioning of the rubber dam clamp. The anatomic landmarks in older patients are more easily noticed. The anesthetics should be slowly deposited without much pain.

Older patients are often less anxious about dental treatment because of low threshold and conduction velocity of nerves, and limited extension of nerves into the dentin, also the dentinal tubules are more calcified so painful response may not be encountered until there is actual pulp exposure.

In older patients, the width of the periodontal ligament is reduced which makes the needle placement for intraligamentary injection more difficult. Only smaller amounts of anesthetic should be deposited and the depth of anesthesia should be checked before repeating the procedure.

Intrapulpal anesthesia is difficult in older patients as the volume of pulp chamber is reduced.

## Isolation

Isolation is very important. Rubber dam is the best method of isolation. If the tooth to be treated is badly mutilated making the placement of rubber dam clamp difficult, then an alternative mode of isolation should be considered which can be multiple tooth isolation with saliva ejector. Other method is one in which canals are identified and their access maintained if restorative procedures are indicated for isolation.

The dentist should not attempt isolation and access in a tooth with questionable marginal integrity of its restorations.

For teeth in which it is difficult to isolate defects produced by root decay, initial preparation should be done using endosonic which use flow through water as an irrigant.

## Access to Canal Orifice

One of the most difficult parts in the treatment of older patients is the identification of the canal orifices.

Obtaining access to the root canal and making the patients to keep their mouth open for a longer period of time is a real problem in older patients. Usually in geriatric patients due to the effect of aging and multiple restorations, the volume and coronal extent of chamber or canal orifices may be reduced but its buccolingual and mesiodistal positions is maintained.

Radiographs/RVG should be used to determine canal position, root curvature, axial inclinations of roots and crowns and involvement of caries, periapical extent of lesion. If there is a restoration on the tooth in the path of access, the patient should be explained about it and the need for removal of restoration.

In case of compromised access for preparation, coronal tooth structure or restorations need to be sacrificed. Endodontic microscopes can be of greater help in identifying and treating narrow geriatric canals (Figs 34.11A & B and 34.12).

### *Biomechanical Preparation*

The calcified canals in geriatric patients are more difficult to locate and penetrate and are also time consuming. The instrument used for initial penetration is DG 16 explorer, this won't get struck in solid dentin but it will resist dislodgment in the canal. Use of broaches for pulp tissue extirpation is usually not done in older patients, since very few canals of older teeth have adequate diameter to allow safe and effective uses of broaches. Older pulps may give clinical appearance that reflects they are calcified, atrophic state with the stiffened, fibrous consistency of a wet toothpick.

In older patients, calcifications are usually more linear in nature (Fig. 34.12). Flaring of root canals is done using instruments with no rake angle in crown down technique. It helps in reduced binding of instrument and provides space for irrigating solutions in narrow, sclerotic canals. It is difficult to locate apical constriction in these patients because of reduced periapical sensitivity in older patients, reduced tactile sense of the clinician and limited use of apex locator in heavily restored teeth.

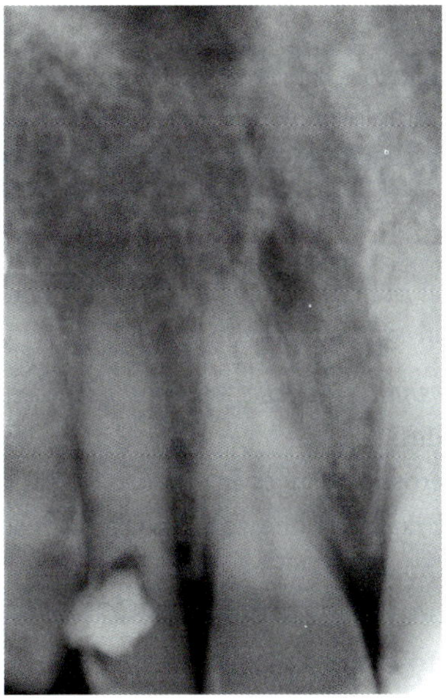

**Fig. 34.11A:** Carious 22 with narrow canal

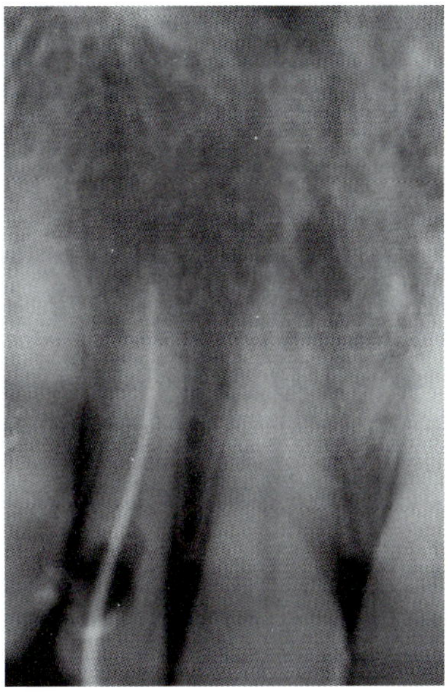

**Fig. 34.11B:** Gaining access in narrow canal of 22

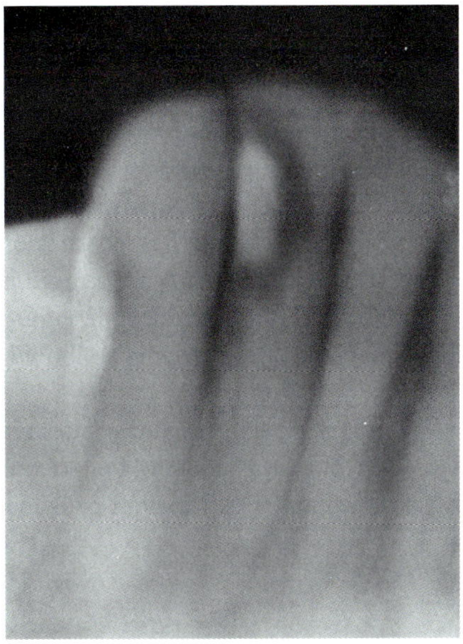

**Fig. 34.12:** Radiograph showing calcified canals of mandibular teeth

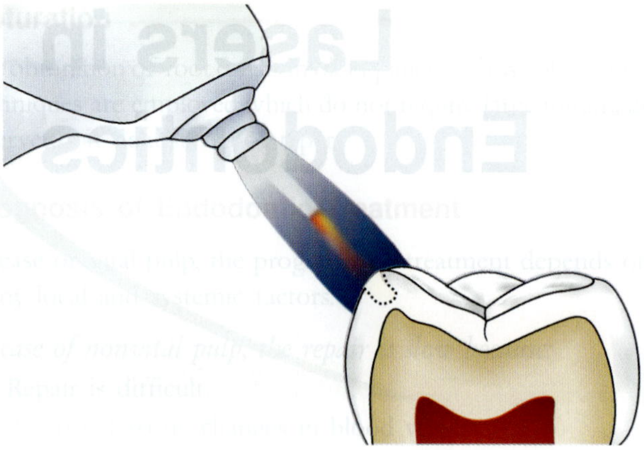

Fig. 35.1: Laser beam produces precised and clean cavity cutting with minimal tooth loss

## CLASSIFICATION OF LASER

1. *According to ANSI and OHSA standards lasers are classified as:*
   **Class I**
   These are low powered lasers that are safe to use, e.g. Laser beam pointer
   **Class II**
   Low powered visible lasers that are hazardous only when viewed directly for longer than 1000 seconds, e.g. He–Ne lasers.
   **Class IIb**
   Low powered visible lasers that are hazardous when viewed for more than 0.25 seconds.
   **Class IIIa**
   Medium powered lasers that are normally hazardous if viewed for less than 0.25 seconds without magnifying optics.
   **Class IIIb**
   Medium powered lasers that can be hazardous if viewed directly.
   **Class IV**
   These are high powered lasers (>0.5W) that produce ocular skin and fire hazards.
2. *Based on the wavelength of the beam:*
   i. **Ultraviolet rays** –140 to 400 nm
   ii. **Visible light** – 400 to 700 nm
   iii. **Infrared** – 700 to microwave spectrum
3. *Based on penetration power of beam:*
   i. **Hard:** Increased penetration power
   For example, Nd:YAG, Argon.
   ii. **Soft lasers:** Decreased penetration power.
   For example, diode, Gallium-Sa, He-Ne lasers.
4. *Based on pulsing:*
   i. **Pulsed:** The beam is not continuous, i.e. of short durations.
   ii. **Nonpulsed:** The beam is continuous and of fixed duration.
5. *According to type of laser material used:*
   i. **Gas lasers:** $CO_2$ lasers, Argon lasers, He-Ne lasers
   ii. **Liquid lasers:** Ions of rare earth or organic fluorescent dyes are dissolved in a liquid, e.g. Dye lasers.
   iii. **Solid state lasers:**
   – Ruby lasers
   – Nd: YAG lasers.
   iv. **Semiconductor lasers:**
   – Gallium
   – Arsenide.

## LASER PHYSICS

The basic units or quanta of light are called photons. Photons behave like a tiny wavelets similar to sound wave pulses. A quantum of light can be depicted as an electromagnetic wave with an electric field oscillating up and down. There is also a magnetic field associated with the photon that moves in and out.

The common principles on which all lasers work is the generation of monochromatic, coherent and collimated radiation by a suitable laser medium in an optical resonator (Fig. 35.2).

**Common principles of laser**
- Monochromatic
- Coherence
- Collimation.

*Monochromatic* means that the light produced by a particular laser will be of a characteristic wavelength. If the light produced is in the visible spectrum (400 nm to 750 nm), it will be seen as a beam of intense color. It is important to have this property to attain high spectral power density of the laser (Fig. 35.3).

*Coherence* means that the light is all perfectly in phase as they leave the laser. That means that unlike a normal light source, their individual contributions are summated and reinforce each other. In an ordinary light source, much of the energy is lost as out of phase, waves cancel each other.

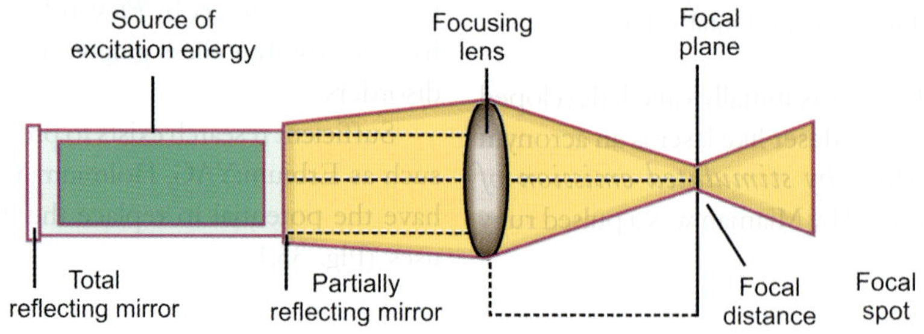


Fig. 35.2: Laser physics

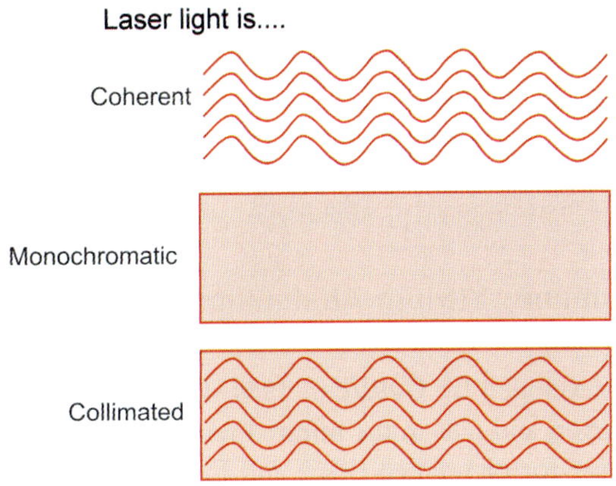


**Fig. 35.3:** Common principles on which all lasers work is generation of monochromatic, coherent and collimated beam

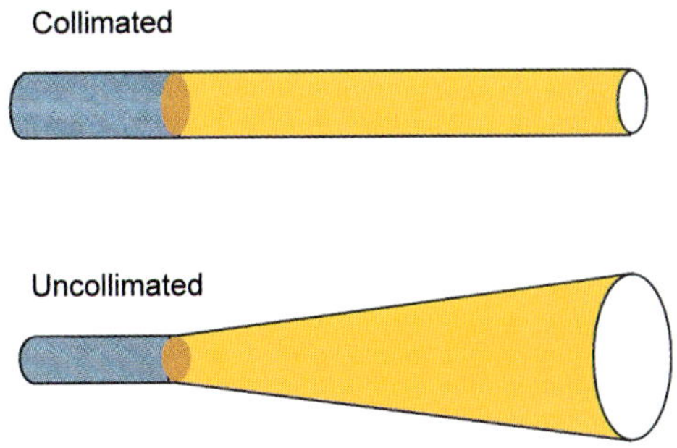


**Fig. 35.4:** Collimated and uncollimated beam

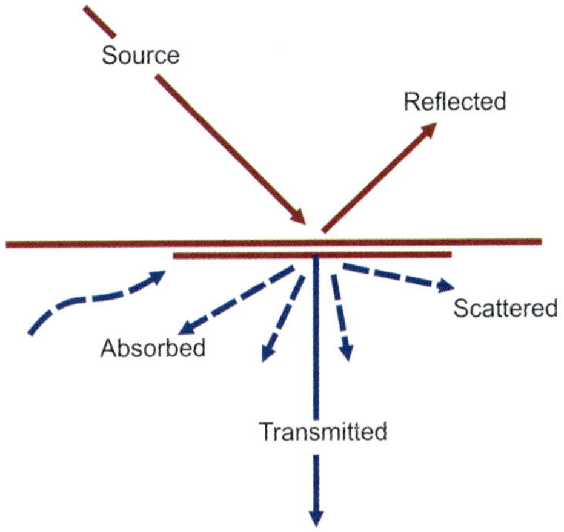


**Fig. 35.5:** When light encounters matter, it can be reflected, scattered, absorbed or transmitted

***Collimation*** means that the laser light beam is perfectly parallel when leaving the laser aperture (Fig. 35.4). This property is important for good transmission through delivery systems.

The main differentiating characteristic of lasers is wave length which depends on the laser medium and excitation diode, i.e. continuous wave or pulsed mode. The different wavelengths can be classified into three groups.

Ultraviolet (UV range) approx 140-400 nm

Visible light (VIS range) approx 400-700 nm

Infrared (IR range) approx 700-microwave spectrum

The shorter the wavelength, more energetic is the light.

## Light Absorption and Emission

When light encounters matter, it can be deflected (reflected or scattered) or absorbed (Fig. 35.5). If a photon is absorbed, its energy is not destroyed, but rather used to increase the energy level of the absorbing atom. The photon then ceases to exist and an electron within the atom, jumps to a higher energy level. This atom is thus pumped up to an excited state from the resting ground state. In the excited state, the atom is unstable and will soon spontaneously go back to the ground state, releasing stored energy in the form of an emitted photon. This process is called spontaneous emission. The spontaneously emitted photon has a longer wavelength and less energy than the absorbed photon. The difference in the energy is usually turned into heat.

## Light Amplification by Stimulated Emission of Radiation

The process of lasing occurs when an excited atom can be stimulated to emit a photon before the process occurs spontaneously. When a photon of exactly the right energy enters the electromagnetic field of an excited atom, the incident photon triggers the decay of the excited electron to a lower energy state. This is accompanied by release of the stored energy in the form of a second photon. The first photon is not absorbed but continues to encounter another excited atom. Stimulated emission can only take place when the incident photon of the identical wavelength travelling in the same direction.

If a collection of atoms is more that are pumped up into the excited state than remain in the resting state, the spontaneous emission of a photon of one atom will stimulate the release of a second photon in a second atom and these two photons will trigger the release of two more photons. These four then yield eight, eight yields sixteen and the cascading reaction follows to produce a brief intense flash of a monochromatic and coherent light.

## Beam Profile and Spot Geometry

The projection of the beam on the target is called the spot. A cross-section of the beam is called the beam profile. The diameter of the spot is called the spot size.

## Power Density

Power density is simply the concentration of photons in a unit area. Photons concentration is measured in watts and area in square cm

Therefore PD $= w/cm^2$

$= w/pr^2$ (r beam diameter/2)

From the beam profile, we know that the power density in the center of the spot is higher and that at the edge of the spot, it approaches zero.

Power density can be increased significantly by placing a lens in the beam path because the light is monochromatic and collimated.

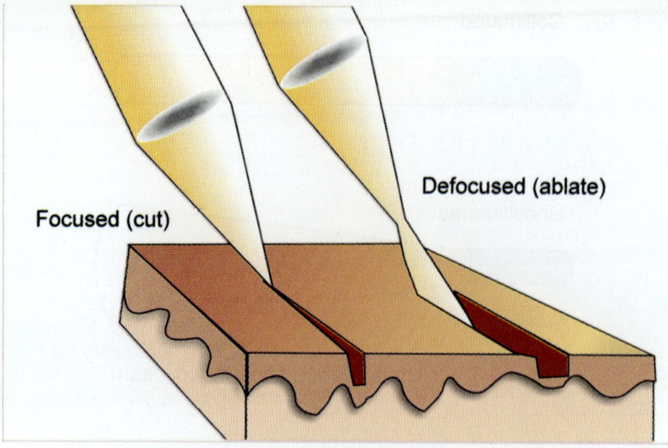


Fig. 35.6: Focused and defocused laser beam

Power density can be increased by the wattage but increasing the power by 10 changes the power density by 10. But decreasing area by 10 increases the power density by 100.

The size and shape of the lens determine the focal length and the spot size at the focal length.

The term focused and defocused refers to the position of the focal point in relation to the tissue plane. The laser beam can be focused through a lens to achieve a converging beam, which increases in intensity to form a focal spot or hot spot, the most intense part of the beam. Past the focal spot, the beam diverges and the power decreases (Fig. 35.6).

When working on tissue, the laser should always be used either with the focal point positioned at the tissue surface or above the tissue surface. The laser should never be positioned with the focal spot deep or within tissue as this can lead to deep thermal damage and tissue effects.

## TYPES OF LASERS

### Carbon Dioxide Lasers

It was developed by Patel et al in 1964. It has a wavelength of 10.6 microns and falls into infrared range on the spectrum. In the United States, the $CO_2$ laser was the first laser approved by the food and drug administration for dental soft-tissue surgical procedures. $CO_2$ laser energy is readily absorbed by tissues high in water content.

When $CO_2$ laser is focused to a fine point, most of its energy in dense state can be used to perform fine dissection. As the beam is defocused and widened its effect on the tissue changes. Instead of a definitive cutting action, the laser ablates the tissue by superficial vaporization of cells and coagulates blood vessels smaller than the diameter of the beam.

#### Uses

It has been used successfully in soft tissue surgeries such as

1. Gingivectomies
2. Soft tissue surgeries
3. Frenectomies
4. Removal of benign and malignant lesions
5. Excisional biopsies
6. Incisional biopsies.

**$CO_2$ LASER**
- Developed by Patel et al in 1964
- Wavelength-10.6 microns
- Limited penetration depth (0.2-0.3 mm)
- Focused beam-fine dissection
- Defocused beam-ablates the tissue.

### Neodymium: Yttrium Aluminium-garnet Lasers (Nd: YAG)

It was developed by ***Geusic*** in 1984. It has a wavelength of 1.06 micron and falls in the infrared range. Nd:YAG laser has an affinity for pigmented tissue and for this reason, prior to using the laser on teeth, the tooth surface is marked with a black dye. The Nd:YAG laser light transmits through water and thus penetrates wet tissues more deeply than $CO_2$ laser. Depending on the mode of delivery, Nd:YAG laser energy can penetrate from 0.5 to 4 mm in oral tissues.

#### Uses

Nd:YAG lasers have been used to

- Vaporize carious tissue
- Sterilize tooth surfaces
- Cutting and coagulation of dental soft tissue
- Sulcular debridement.
- Treat dentinal hypersensitivity
- Remove extrinsic stains
- Prepare pits and fissures for sealants.

**Neodymium: Yttrium Aluminium-Garnet Laser**
- Developed by Geusic in 1964
- Wavelength-1.06 micron
- Penetration depth-0.5-4 mm
- Affinity for pigmented tissues
- Penetrates wet tissues more rapidly.

### Argon Lasers

Argon lasers operate at 488 to 510 nm. The blue wavelength of 488 nm is used mainly for composite curing, while the green wavelength is used for soft tissue procedures and coagulation. The argon laser when used to polymerize photo-activated dental resin materials, can reduce polymerization shrinkage and cure to depths as great as three centimeters in one fourth the time of conventional curing lights.

Argon laser light is not readily absorbed by water but it is absorbed by hemoglobin tissue, melanin cells and similarly dark pigmented tissues. The argon laser may be well suited for selective destruction of blood clots and hemangiomas with minimal damage to adjacent tissue.

#### Uses

1. Light activated whitening gels, impression materials and composite curing (blue wavelength).
2. Green wavelength has excellent hemostatic capabilities, so it is used in acute inflammatory periodontal disease and hemangioma.

3. Caries detection – both wavelength – when argon laser illuminates the tooth, the diseased carious area appears as a dark orange-red color.

**Argon lasers**
- Two emission wavelength used in dentistry
- Blue wavelength-488 nm—composite curing
- Green wavelength-510 nm—soft tissue procedure and coagulation
- Absorbed by hemoglobin tissue and melanin cells

**Uses**
- Composite curing
- Acute inflammatory periodontal lesion
- Hemangioma
- Caries detection

## LASER INTRACTION WITH BIOLOGICAL TISSUES

The essential elements of laser light are that determine its interaction with matter are:

i. Wavelength of the radiant energy emitted by the laser
ii. Power density of the beam
iii. Difference in delivery systems.

The optical properties of tissue element that determine the nature and extent of tissue response:

i. Chemical composition
ii. Spatial structure
iii. Isotopic composition.

***Radiant energy interacts with tissues in four ways:***

i. A portion of the incident beam may be reflected off the surface without penetration or interaction of the light energy with the tissue.
ii. A portion of the light may be transmitted through the tissue.
iii. Some of the light may be absorbed into a component of the tissue.
iv. The remaining light may penetrate the tissue and be scattered without producing a noticeable effect on the tissues.

In multifaceted biologic systems consisting of great diversity of cellular elements and tissues fluids having different optical absorption characteristics, predicting the effect of lasers is quite challenging. But oral soft tissue is largely composed of water which predominantly controls the tissue effects of laser emissions within the infrared spectrum. Tissue elements that exhibit a high co-efficient of absorption for particular wavelength are called chromophores. Other chromophores within tissues such as hemoglobin and melanin pigments also exert a significant influence. Hemoglobin readily interacts with 488-514 nm wavelengths thus accounting for the greater ability of the argon laser for coagulation and hemostasis. In soft tissue, the effects of laser are quite predictable as compared to lasers interaction with hard tissues.

### Tissue Effects of Laser Irradiation

When the radiant energy is absorbed by tissue, four basic types of interaction or responses can occur which may be further subdivided according to how they manifest in clinical application:

*1. Photochemical interaction: this includes*
- *Biostimulation*
- *Photodynamic therapy.*

*2. Photothermal interactions: this includes*
- Photoablation
- Photopyrolysis.

*3. Photomechanical interaction, this includes*
- Photodisruption/photodissociation
- Photoacoustic interactions.

*4. Photoelectrical interaction, this includes*
- Photoplasmolysis.

The biological interaction of laser photon with tissue occurring along the path of radiation is termed a linear effect and can be categorized broadly into photochemical, photothermal and photomechanical. The ability of the laser photon to produce a biological response after being reflected, deflected, scattered or absorbed is termed non-linear effects.

#### *Photochemical Effects*

The basis of the photochemical effect is the absorption of the laser light without any thermal effect leading to change in the chemical and physical properties of atoms and molecules.

A specific wavelength or photon can be absorbed by a molecular chromophore and convert that molecule to an excited state, thus converting laser energy into stored form of chemical energy. The excited state can subsequently participate in a chemical reaction.

The molecular chromophore may be endogenous such as amino acid side chain group, heme pigments, etc. or exogenous molecules introduced into the body.

*Biostimulation:* It is the stimulatory effect of lasers on biochemical and molecular processes that normally occur in the tissues such as healing and repair.

#### *Photothermal Interaction*

This class of interaction is the basis for the most types of surgical laser applications.

In this interaction, radiant light energy absorbed by tissue substances and molecules become transformed into heat energy which produces the tissue effect.The amount of laser light absorbed into the tissue depends on:

1. The wavelength of radiant energy from the laser
2. Power density
3. Pulse duration
4. Spot size
5. Composition of target tissue.

High water content of most oral tissue is responsible for absorption of radiant energy in the target region. The $CO_2$ laser is highly attenuated by intracellular water within the oral soft tissue. This high absorption leads to rapid vaporization of the water component and pyrolysis of the organic matter within the tissue target.

Another important factor, influencing the extent of the thermal damage zone is the relative degree of absorption and scattering of the beam once it enters the tissue. Scattering can directly increase the extent of collateral tissue damage by spatial redistribution of the beam into a larger volume of the surrounding tissue. Much of the scattered beam is transformed into heat energy since it has insufficient power density to cause vaporization.

Laser induced changes in the composition and other optical properties of tissue such as charring, coagulation of blood elements and protein denaturation can alter the nature of subsequent interactions.

The thermal damage can be controlled by
1. Controlling the laser operating parameters
2. By cooling the target area
3. By combining the laser: Nd:YAG with the air water spray.

Thermal effects of laser irradiation range in intensity depending on the level of temperature rise within the target tissue.

**Thermal effects of laser irradiation**
- Temperature < 60°C
  a. Tissue hyperthermia
  b. Enzymatic changes
  c. Edema
- Temperature > 60°C
  a. Protein denaturation
- Temperature < 100°C
  a. Tissue dehydration
  b. Blanching of tissue
- Temperature > 100°C
  a. Superheating
  b. Tissue ablation and shrinkage.

When a single pulse of laser is applied to the oral mucosa vaporization of water at tissue surface occurs. Rapid expansion at the exposure site causes elevation of the superficial epithelium which subsequently ruptures releasing both vapor and tissue particles. The net effect is ablation of tissue resulting in the form of crater defect.

### *Photomechanical and Photoelectrical Interaction*

The high energy levels and rapid absorption that occurs during photoablation results in rapid generation of shockwaves that is capable of rupturing intermolecular and atomic bonds. Mechanical disruption or breaking a part of matter is accomplished by conversion of high energy light energy to vibrational energy. Photodisruption occurs whenever the photon energy of the incident beam exceeds target tissues.

The process involved for the photodisruption can be divided into three interrelated mechanisms or phases:
1. Ionization
2. Plasma formation
3. Shockwave generation.

***Ionization*** can occur in tissue at very high energy densities, when the electric field strength of the beam becomes high enough to ionize atoms. Once ionization occurs, a hot electrically charged gas of free electrons and positive ions or plasma is formed.

As the temperature fluctuates within the electric field from the laser electrons within the plasma begin to vibrate creating a rapid expansion and contraction that leads to the generation of the shockwaves. The pressures exerted by the shockwaves on the target are responsible for the mechanical breaking or shattering of the target material observed during photoplasmolysis.

## Laser Effects on Dental Hard Tissues

In the field of mineralized tissues, the most thoroughly investigated interactions are photothermal and thermo-mechanical interactions and the ablative photodecomposition.

The absorption and transmission of laser light in human teeth is mainly dependent on the wavelength of the laser light. The theory that dentinal tubules work as optical fibers transmitting high energy densities to a pulpal tissues could explain the unpredictable side effects when lasing dental tissues. The absorption of the laser energy in the superficial tissue layer can alter the optical properties of the affected tissue causing a variation in the intensity of the penetration energy. Therefore laser effects are changing in dependence from the depth of penetration.

### *Thermal Effects*

The laser energy is converted into thermal energy or heat that destroys the tissue. The laser beam couples to the tissue surface and this absorption leads to heating with denaturation at about 45 to 60°C. Above 60°C coagulation and necrosis can be observed accompanied by desiccation of the tissue. At 100°C the water inside the tissue vaporizes.

### *Mechanical Effects*

High energetic and short pulsed laser light can lead to a fast heating of the dental tissue. The energy dissipates explosively in a volume of expansion that may be accompanied by fast shockwaves. These mechanical shockwaves can lead to high pressures so that adjacent tissue will be destroyed or damaged.

### *Chemical Effects*

The basis of the photochemical effect is the absorption of laser light without any thermal effect which leads to an alteration in the chemical and physical properties of the irradiated tissue.

## Laser Effects on the Dental Pulp

Characteristically pulp tissue cannot survive on environment of elevated temperature for protracted periods when tooth structure is irradiated with lasers.

The use of combination of air and water spray before during or immediately after laser irradiation to enamel and dentin may be a more effective method for temperature control and reduction of heat transfer to the pulp and other vital structure surrounding the teeth.

Precooling by air and water spray prior to lasing may be used with laser systems such as $CO_2$, Holmium, Erbium-which are more readily absorbed by water. Lasers with limited transmission through enamel and dentin may also be effectively cooled with the application of an air water spray immediately after lasing.

## LASER SAFETY IN DENTAL PRACTICE

The surgical lasers currently used in dentistry generally fall in class IV category which is considered the most hazardous group of lasers. The types of hazards that may be encountered within the clinical practice of dentistry may be grouped:

1. Ocular injury
2. Tissue damage
3. Respiratory hazards
4. Fire and explosion
5. Electrical shock.

1. ***Ocular hazards:*** Injury to the eye can occur either by direct emission from the laser or by reflection from a mirror like surface. Dental instruments have been capable of producing reflections that may result in tissue damage in both operator and patients.

   Irreversible retinal burns can occur by conversion of incident radiation to heat energy within a fraction of a second resulting in permanent radiation.
2. ***Tissue hazards:*** Laser induced damage to skin and other non-target tissue can result from the thermal interaction of the energy with the tissue proteins. Temperature elevations of 21°C above normal body temperature can produce destruction by denaturation of cellular enzymes and structural proteins which interrupt basic metabolic processes.
3. ***Environmental hazards:*** These secondary hazards belong to a group of potential laser hazards referred to as non-beam hazards. Most surgical lasers used in dentistry are capable of producing smoke, toxic gases and chemicals.

   The generation of smoke during surgery can be a danger to both operator and patient. Inhalation of toxic or infectious matter in the form of aerosols and particles has been found to be potentially damaging to the respiratory system. The greatest producers of smoke are $CO_2$ and Erbium lasers followed by Nd:YAG lasers.
4. ***Combustion hazards:*** Flammable solids, liquids, gases used within the surgical setting can be easily ignited if exposed to the laser beam.
5. ***Electrical hazards:*** Because class IV surgical lasers often use very high currents and high voltage power supplies. There are several associated hazards that may be potentially lethal. Electrical hazards can be in form of electric shock, fire or explosion.

### Fire and Electrical Control Measures

To avoid an electrical hazard, the operatory must be kept dry. The control panel and its electrical power unit should be protected from any kind of splashing.

### Personal Protective Equipment

#### *Eye Protection*

Light produced by all class IV lasers by definition presents a potential hazards for ocular damage by either direct viewing or reflection of the beam. Therefore all people must wear adequate eye protection, including the patient.

***When selecting appropriate eye wear several factors should be considered:***

1. Wavelength permissible emission
2. Restriction of peripheral vision
3. Maximum permissible exposure limits
4. Degradation of the absorbing media
5. Optical density of the eye wears
6. Need for corrective lenses
7. Comfort and fit.

### Control of Airborne Contamination

Airborne contamination must be controlled by ventilation, evacuation or other method of respiratory protection. Adequate suction should be maintained at all times especially when treating a pathologic condition as it can spread through laser plume.

### Procedural Controls

1. Highly reflective instruments and those with mirror surfaces should be avoided.
2. Tooth protection is needed, whenever, the beam is directed at angles other than parallel to the tooth surface.
3. A No. 7 wax spatula can be inserted into the gingival sulcus to serve as an effective shield for the teeth.
4. If anesthesia is required, in place of standard PVC tubes, rubber or silastic tubes should be used. For further protection the tube should be wrapped with an aluminum tape.

## SOFT AND HARD TISSUE APPLICATIONS OF LASERS IN DENTISTRY

### Soft Tissue Applications

1. Incise, excise, remove or biopsy of tumors and lesions such as fibromas, papillomas and epulides.
2. Vaporize excess tissue as in gingivoplasty, gingivectomy and labial/lingual frenectomy.
3. Remove or reduce hyperplastic tissues.
4. Remove and control hemorrhaging of vascular lesions such as hemangiomas.

### Hard Tissue Applications

1. Vaporize carious lesions;
2. Desensitize exposed root surfaces;
3. Roughen tooth surfaces, in lieu of acid etching in preparation for bonding procedures;
4. To arrest demineralization and promote remineralization of enamel.
5. Debond ceramic orthodontic brackets.

**Advantages of lasers**
1. Less bleeding
2. Less pain
3. No need for anesthesia
4. No noise
5. Faster healing
6. Less chances of infection

## APPLICATION OF LASERS IN ENDODONTICS

1. ***Diagnosis—Laser Doppler Flowmetry (LDF):***
   a. LDF was developed to assess blood flow in microvascular systems, e.g. in the retina. Electrical vitality testing works on stimulating nerve ending but LDF detects blood circulation in pulp potentially a much more reliable and less uncomfortable for the patient.
   b. Diagnodent
   c. *Thermal testing:* In this pulsed Nd: YAG laser is applied instead of hot burnisher or hot gutta-percha. Pain produced by laser is mild and tolerable when compared to conventional pulp tester.

      Differential diagnosis of normal pulp and acute pulpitis:

      On stimulation by Nd: YAG laser at 2 W and 20 pulses per second, at distance of 1 cm from the tooth, pain occurs within 20-30 seconds but also disappears soon after laser is removed. But in case of acute pulpitis pain lingers on even after removal of laser.
2. ***Pulp capping and pulpotomy:***
   Melcer et al in 1987 first described laser treatment of exposed pulp tissues using the $CO_2$ laser in dogs to achieve hemostasis.

   The first laser pulpotomy was performed using $CO_2$ lasers in dogs in 1985. Following this, studies have been done using Nd:YAG, Ga-As semiconductor and Ar lasers.
3. ***Root canal treatment:***
   a. *Modification of root canal walls*:
      Endodontic instrumentation produces organic and mineral debris on the walls of the root canal. Although this smear layer can be beneficial in that it provides obstruction of the tubules and decreased dentinal permeability. It may also harbor bacteria and bacterial byproducts. For these reasons, use of laser for the removal of the smear layer and its replacement with the uncontaminated chemical sealant or sealing by melting the dentinal surface has become a goal.

      The removal of smear layer and debris by lasers is possible however, it is hard to clean all root canal walls because the laser is emitted straight ahead, making it impossible to irradiate lateral wall.
   b. *Sterilization of root canals*:
      All lasers have a bactericidal effect at high power. There appears to exit a potential for spreading bacterial contamination from the root canal to the patient and the dental team via the smoke produced by the laser. Thus protections such as strong vacuum pumps should be used.

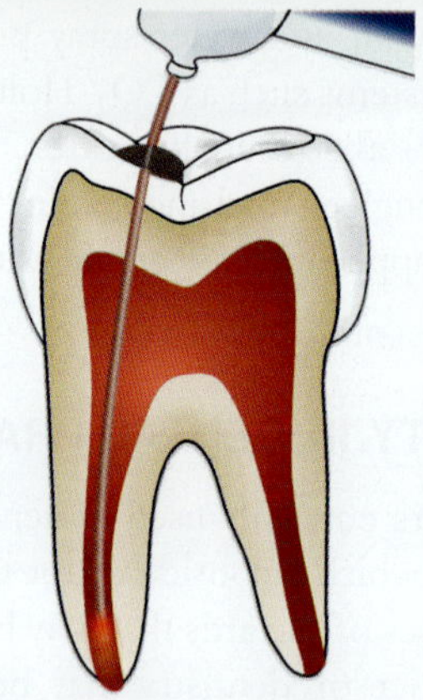

**Fig. 35.7:** Laser beam is directed towards root canal for endodontic therapy

      *Sterilization:* Commonly used laser are Nd: YAG, argon $CO_2$, Er: YAG and semiconductor diode.

      *PAD (Photoactivated Disinfection of root canals):* Initially He-Ne lasers was used in PAD, but it has been replaced with high efficiency diode lasers. Commonly used lasers lie with a range of visible red and infrared lasers.
   c. *Root canal shaping and obturation*:
      Root canal shaping represents an important step in the endodontic procedure as it aids in removal of organic tissues and facilitates irrigation and canal obturation (Fig. 35.7). Ar, $CO_2$ and Nd:YAG laser have been used to soften gutta-percha.

      The 308 nm excirmer laser is the only system that offers precise ablation of tissue, fiber delivery and bactericidal effects. Good transmission through water and enamel surface conditioning in one system.

      It is useful to use lasers as adjuncts to conventional treatment, but it is not possible to use lasers alone for treatment.
4. ***Treatment of incomplete fracture:***
   Lasers are using in repairing incomplete vertical fractures by causing fusion of the fracture.
5. ***Apicoectomy:***
   If laser is used for surgery, a bloodless surgical field should be easier to achieve. If the cut surface is irradiated, it gets sterilized and sealed.

   Clinically the use of Er: YAG laser resulted in improved healing and diminished postoperative discomfort.
6. ***Treatment of dental hypersensitivity:***
   The lasers used for the treatment of dental hypersensitivity are divided into two groups:
   i. Low output power lasers (He-Ne and Ga Al As lasers)
   ii. Middle output power lasers-Nd:YAG and $CO_2$ lasers.

   The mechanism causing a reduction in hypersensitivity is most unknown but is thought that the mechanism for each laser is different.

   In case of low output power lasers, a small fraction of the laser energy is transmitted through enamel or dentin to reach the pulp tissue. He-Ne laser affects the peripheral A-delta or C-fiber nociceptor.

Laser energy of Nd:YAG are indicating thermally mediated effects and pulpal analgesia. $CO_2$ lasers mainly seal the dentinal tubules as well as reduce the permeability.

7. ***Sterilization of instruments:***
   Argon, $CO_2$ and Nd:YAG lasers have been used successfully to sterilize dental instruments.
8. ***Bleaching:***
   The whitening effect of the laser is achieved by a chemical oxidation process. Once the laser energy is applied, $H_2O_2$ breaks down to $H_2O$ and free $O_2$ radical which combines with and thus remove stain molecules.

   The energy of $CO_2$ laser is emitted in the form of heat. This energy can enhance the effect of the whitening after initial argon laser process.

## CONCLUSION

Laser advantages such as a bloodless operative and postoperative course, usually requiring no suturing, minimal to absent postoperative pain, and high patient acceptance make lasers a highly advantageous alternative to conventional treatment modalities such as the scalpel or electrosurgery. As more and more clinicians and researchers discover the advantages, lasers have to offer, the presence of lasers in the dental office will become increasingly common.

Some clinicians are still doubtful of entering this exciting field because of the size and cost of equipment. Lasers will continue to get smaller in size and less costly, but this is true of all technology—consider the history of computers and pocket calculators. The original lasers were not only large but had six-figure price tags. Today's dental lasers are smaller, lightweight, highly portable and more reasonably priced. The future of dental lasers is bright. When used ethically and efficaciously, it results in increase on income which comes from greater patient acceptance of certain treatments. Patients experience minimal discomfort post-procedure, leading to increased referrals.

## QUESTIONS

**Q. Define and classify lasers**

**Q. Write short notes on:**

a. Common principles on which laser work.
b. Tissue effects of laser
c. Role of lasers in endodontics

## BIBLIOGRAPHY


1. Ando N, Hoshino E. Predominant obligate anaerobes invading the deeper layers of the root canal dentin. Int Endod J 1990;23(1):20-27.
2. Anic I, Matsumoto K. Dentinal heat transmission induced by a laser-softened gutta-percha obturation technique. Journal of Endodontics 1995;21:470-74.
3. Arakawa S, Cobb CM, Repley JWm Killoy WJ, Spencer P. Treatment of root fracture by $CO_2$ and Nd: YAG lasers: An in vitro study. Journal of Endodontics 1996;22:662-67.
4. Bader G, Lejeune S. Prospective study of two retrograde endodontic apical preparations with and without the use of $CO_2$ laser. Endodontics and Dental Traumatology 1998;14:75-78.
5. Bender IB, Rossman LE. International replantation of endodontically treated teeth. Oral Surg Oral Med Oral Pathol 1993;76(5):623-30.
6. Berutti E, Marini R, Angeretti A. Penetrationability of different irrigants into dentinal tubules. J Endod 1997;23(12): 725-27.
7. Hardee MW, Miserendino LJ, Kos W, Walia H. Evaluation of the antibacterial effects of intracanal Nd: YAG laser Irradiation. Journal of Endodontics 1994;20:377-80.
8. Kaba K, Kimura Y, Matsumoto K, Takeuchi T, Ikarugi T, Shimizu T. A histopathological study of the morphological changes at the apical seat and in the periapical region after irradiation with a pulsed Nd: YAG laser. International Endodontic Journal 1998;31:415-20.
9. Komori T, Yokoyama K, Taka T, Matsumoto K. Clinical application of the erbium: YAG laser for apicoectomy. J Endod 1997;23(12):748-50.
10. Kouchi Y, Ninomiya J, Yasuda H, Fukui J, Moriyama T, Okamoto H. Location of streptococcus mutans in the dentinal tubules of open infected root canals. J Dent Res 1980;59(12): 2038-46.
11. Levy G. Cleaning and shaping the root canal with a Nd: YAG laser beam: A comparative study. Journal of Endodontics 1992;18:123-27.
12. McKinley IB, Ludlow MO. Hazards of laser smoke during endodontic therapy. Journal of Endodontics 1994;20:558-59.
13. Midda M, Renton-Harper P. Lasers in dentistry. British Dental Journal 1991;168:343-46.
14. Moritz A, Schoop U, Goharkhay K, Sperr W. The $CO_2$ laser as an aid in direct pulp capping. Journal of Endodontics 1998;24:248-51.
15. Moshonov J, Orstavik D, Yamaunchi S, Pettiette M, Trope M. Nd: YAG laser irradiation in root canal disinfection. Endodontics and Dental Traumatology 1995;11:220-24.
16. Paghdiwala AF. Root resection of endodontically treated teeth by erbium: YAG laser radiation. Journal of Endodontics 1993;19:91-94.
17. Potts TV, Petrou A. Laser photopolymerization of dental of materials with potential endodontic applications. Journal of endodontics 1990;16:265-68.
18. Schoop U, Moritz, Kluger W, Starzengruber P, Goharkhay K, Wernisch, Sperr W. Laser-assisted apex scaling: Results of a pilot study. J Oral Lasere Appl 2004;4(3):175-82.
19. Stabholz A, Khayat A, Ravanshad SH, McCarthy DW Neev J, Torabinejad M. Effects of Nd: YAG laser on apical seal of teeth after apicoectomy and retrofill. Journal of Endodontics 1992;18:371-75.
20. Takeda FH, Harashima T, Kimura Y, Matsumoto K. A comparative study of the removal of smear layer by three endodontic. Journal 1999;32:32-39.
21. Takeda FH, Harashima T, Kimura Y, Matsumoto K. Efficacy of Er: YAG laser irradiation in removing debris and smear laser on root canal walls. Journal of Endodontics 1998;24:548-51.
22. Wigdor H, Abt E, Ashrafi S, Walsh JT. The effect of lasers on dental hard tissues. Journal of American Dental Association 1993;124:65-70.
23. Zhang C, Kimura Y, Matsumoto K, Harashima T, Zhou H. Effects of pulsed Nd: YAG laser irradiation on root canal wall dentin with different laser initiators. Journal of Endodontics 1998;24:352-55.

# CHAPTER 36

# Magnification

- ❑ Introduction
- ❑ Loupes
- ❑ Surgical Operating Microscope (SOM)
- ❑ Endoscope
- ❑ Orascope
- ❑ Bibliography

## INTRODUCTION

To visualize operating site, earlier we were dependent only on two dimensional radiographic picture of a three-dimensional tooth system. But nowadays, many advancements have been done to improve the visualization and magnification. Introduction of loupes, microscopes, endoscopes, etc. enables the clinician to magnify an object beyond that perceived by a human eye.

**Magnification:** It is defined as making an object bigger in size
**Differentiation:** It is defined as making something distinct.

## LOUPES

These are most commonly used for improving magnification. Loupes can be of single-lens loupes and multi-lens loupes. All loupes employ convergent lenses so as to form a magnified image (Figs 36.1 and 36.2).

***In single-lens loupes***, there is fixed focal length and working distance.

### *Advantages*

- Light weight
- Economical

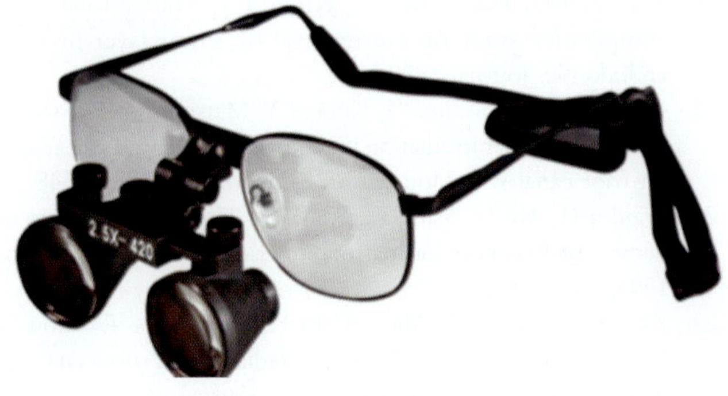


Fig. 36.1: Loupes for endodontics

### *Disadvantages*

- Poor resolution
- Because of fixed working distance, dentist has to adjust according to them.

### Multi-lens Loupes

They provide better magnification and have improved working distance. This type of glass with multi-lens system is known as **Galilean optical system**. It offers magnification up to 2.5 times.

### *Advantages*

- Good magnification
- Adjustable working distance

### *Disadvantage*

Bulky

## SURGICAL OPERATING MICROSCOPE (SOM)

Use of microscope in endodontics was first introduced in 1990s and since its introduction in endodontics, there has been made

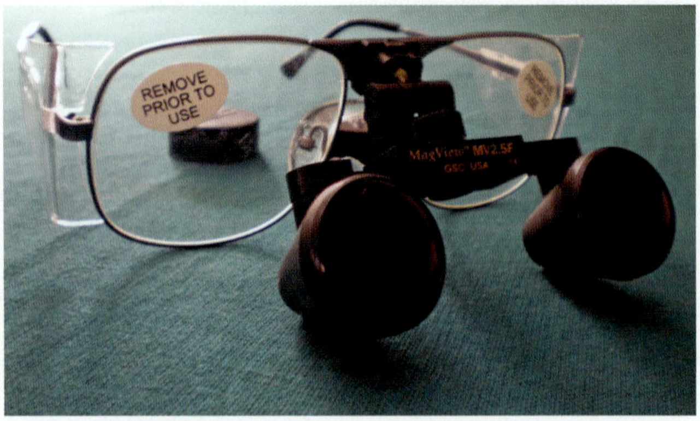


Fig. 36.2: Loupes used in endodontics

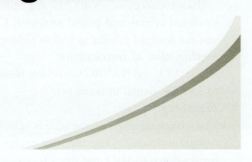

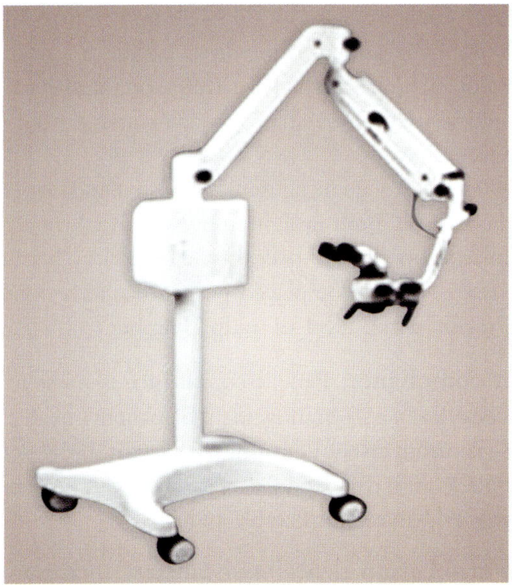

Fig. 36.3: Endomicroscope (floor type)

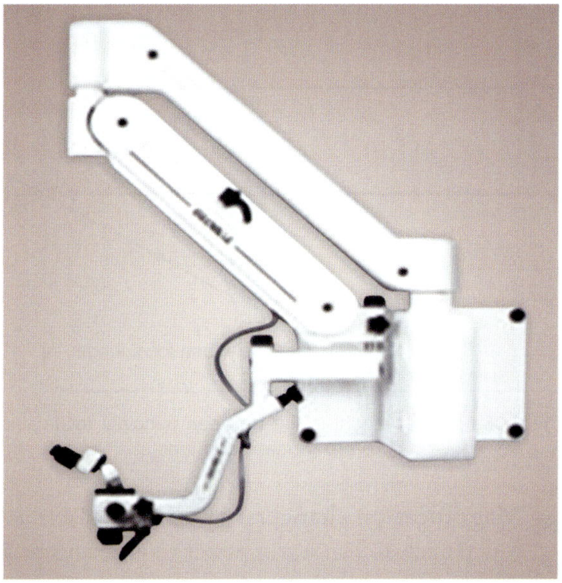

Fig. 36.5: Wall mounted endomicroscope

great change in the way endodontics is done and has also affected the success rate of endodontic therapy (Figs 36.3 to 36.5).

Most of surgical microscope come with **three to five steps** of magnification ranging from 3x to 27x. The light source is usually 100 to 150 watt halogen bulb connected to the microscope via a high efficiency fiberoptic cable.

To use SOM in endodontics, one should have specially designed microinstruments for example files specially designed for this are called microopeners, similarly other instruments like micromirrors are used with SOM.

Before using SOM, rubber dam placement is necessary because direct viewing through the canal with microscope is difficult, so a mirror is needed to reflect the canal. But without the use of rubber dam, mirror will fog soon.

To maximize the access and quality of view there should be 45° angle between the microscope and the mirror.

Following are the areas where surgical operating microscope can have great impact:

a. For visualization of surgical field
b. For evaluation of surgical technique

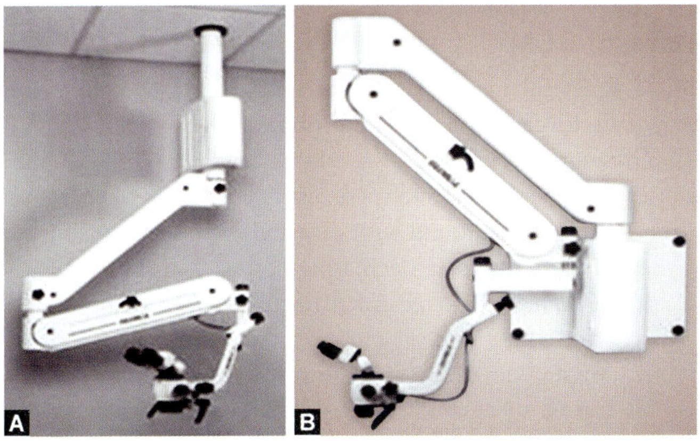

Figs 36.4A and B: (A) Ceiling mounted, (B) Wall mounted endomicroscope

c. For patient education by videos.
d. For documentation for legal purposes
e. For teaching programs by video libraries
f. For marketing dental practice
g. For providing reports to insurance companies

## How does Surgical Operating Microscope Work?

*It is discussed under four headings:*

a. Magnification
b. Illumination
c. Documentation
d. Accessories

a. **Magnification:** Magnification is determined by:
   i. Power of eyepiece
   ii. Focal length of binoculars
   iii. Focal length of objective lens
   iv. Magnification change factor

   i. **Power of eyepiece:** Eyepiece has diopter settings ranging from –5 to +5. These are used to adjust for accommodation, which is ability to focus the lens of eyes.

   ii. **Focal length of binoculars:** Binoculars hold the eyepieces. The interpupillary distance is set by adjusting the distance between binocular tubes. While adjusting focal length, one should remember that longer the focal length, greater is the magnification, and narrower the field of view (Fig. 36.6).

   iii. **Focal length of objective lens:** Focal length of objective lens determines the operating distance between the lens and surgical field. If objective lens is removed, the microscope focuses at infinity and performs as pair of field binoculars.

   For SOM, variety of objective lenses are available with focal length ranging from 100 to 400 mm.

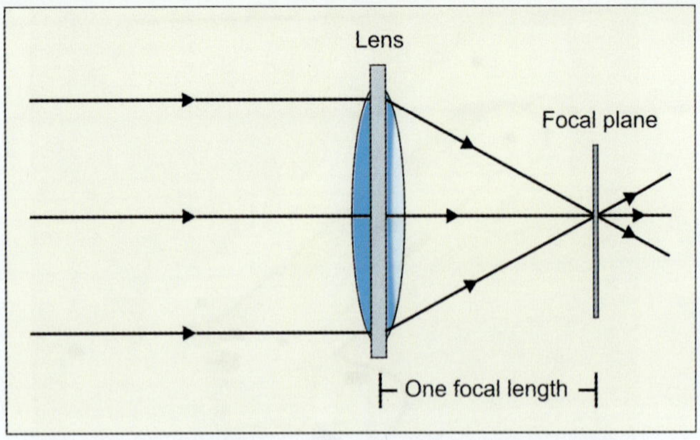


**Fig. 36.6:** Focal lenght is the between principal focus and the optical center of lens

iv. **Magnification changers:** These are available as 3- or 5-step manual changers or power zoom changers. These are located within the head of microscope, the manual step changers consist of lenses which are mounted on a turret which is jointed to a dial. The dial positions one lens in front of other within the changer to produce a fixed magnification values.

b. **Illumination:** Commonly used light source is 100 watt Xenon halogen bulb. The intensity of light can be controlled by rheostat. This light is reflected through condensing lens to a series of prisms and then through objective lens to surgical field area. On reaching surgical field, it is again reflected back through objective lens through magnification changer lenses, through binoculars and then exits to eyes as two separate beams of light. This results in stereoscope effect which allows the clinician to see depth of the field.

   Illumination with operating microscope is coaxial with line of sight. This means that light is focused between the eyepieces such that a dentist can look at surgical site without seeing the shadow.

c. **Documentation:** The ability to produce quality video slides is directly related to magnification and illumination system. The adapter attaches video camera to beam splitter. It also provides the necessary focal length to that camera.

   Records an image with same magnification and field of view as seen by operator.

d. **Accessories**

   *Different accessories used in SOM are:*

   a. Bicycle style handles attached at bottom of head to facilitate movement during surgery.
   b. Eyepiece with reticle field for alignment during videotaping and photography
   c. Observation ports for helping in teaching situations.
   d. LCD screen so as to provide view to patient as well as to assistant.

**Fundamental requisites to be met before using microscope:**

*Following fundamental requirements need to be met before having optimal use of microscope.*

a. *Vision*: with microscope, it is almost impossible to do endodontic treatment using direct vision. So, front surface good quality mirror which is silvered on the surface of glass should be used for having best quality undistorted reflected image.
b. *Lightening*: Adequate lightening is also mandatory for using a microscope. Built-in lightening system is usually present in microscope, but if necessary an auxillary light can also be used. This can be placed perpendicular to long axis of the tooth at the level of pulp chamber.

**Patient compliance:** Patient compliance is must for use of microscope. Even a slight movement of patient's head can affect field of vision adversely. For optimal view through microscope, patient needs to have extended neck. This can be achieved by providing a U-shaped inflatable pillow.

**Cooperation from dental assistance:** Dental assistant can also help in increasing the efficiency of clinician. Use of secondary eyepiece from microscope provide better view of root canals. A dental assistant should be given adequate training for use of microscope.

**Prerequisites for use of microscope:**

1. *Rubber dam placement:* Rubber dam placement is necessary with microscope because direct viewing with microscope is difficult. So if mirror is used without using rubber dam, due to exhalation of patient, mirror would fog immediately. This would affect visualization. For absorbing bright reflected light and to accentuate tooth structure, use of blue or green rubber dam sheet is recommended.
2. *Mouth mirror placement:* Mouth mirror should be placed slightly away from the tooth. If it is placed close to tooth, it will make use of endodontic instruments difficult.
3. *Indirect view and patient head position:* Mirror should be placed at 45° to the microscope. For indirect viewing, patient's head should be positioned such that it form 90° angle between binocular and the maxillary arch.
4. *Instruments:* Clinician should use specially designed micro-instruments for locating canals. Use of files called micropeners (by maileffer), micromirrors and other microinstruments is recommended.

## Uses of SOM

SOM is useful in all aspects of endodontic therapy from diagnosis to evaluation of final obturation.

1. *Diagnosis*
   a. SOM allows calcified, irregularly positioned or accessory canals to be found with ease and thereby increasing the success rate and decreasing stress.
   b. SOM helps to detect microfractures which are not visible with naked eye.
   c. Missing canals (most common MB2 of maxillary molar) can be successfully located by use of endomicroscope.
2. Removal of foreign materials like cast post and cement filling material, can be easily accomplished by its use.

3. The endodontic retreatment involving the removal of screw posts, separated instruments, silver points can be guided by use of endomicroscope.
4. Perforation repair can be precisely done by use of SOM by accurate placement of the repair material and by précised manipulation of the tissue.
5. Evaluation of the canal preparation can be accurately done by use of endomicroscope.
6. SOM is also useful in evaluation of the final obturation of root canals. With the help of SOM one can assess the irregularly shaped and poorly obturated canals, and quality of apical seal.
7. Intracanal isthmus communication can be well assessed by use of endomicroscope.

## ENDOSCOPE

It was introduced in endodontics in 1979. Endoscope consists of glass rods, camera, light source and a monitor. Endoscope offers a better magnification than loupes or a microscope. It is mainly used during surgical endodontic treatment.

### Advantage

Provides better view to surgical site in non-fixed field of vision.

### Disadvantage of Endoscope

Requires hemostasis of operating field.

## ORASCOPE

Orascope is a fiberoptic endoscope. Since fiberoptics are made up of plastics, so they are small, flexible and light weight. It is mainly used for intracanal visualization. An orascope consists of 10,000 parallel visual fibers. Quality of image produced by orascope is directly related to number of fibers.

### Advantage

Better imaging of apical third of canal.

### Disadvantages

1. Canal must be enlarged to number 90 file in coronal 15 mm of canal
2. Presence of sodium hypochlorite blurs the image.

## QUESTION

**Q. Write short notes on:**

a. Endomicroscope
b. Loupes

## BIBLIOGRAPHY


1. Carr GB. Microscopes in endodontics. J Calif Dent Assoc 1992;20:55-61.
2. Coeth de CArvalho MC, Zuolo ML. Orifice locating with a microscope. J Endod 2000;26:532-34.
3. Kanca J, Jordan PG. Magnification systems in clinical dentistry. J can Dent Assoc 1995;61:851-56.
4. Kim S, Kratchman S. Modern endodontic surgery concepts and practice. A review. J Endod 2006;32(7):601-23.
5. Kim S. Microscope in endododntics. Dent Clin North Am 1997;41:481-97.
6. Kim S, Rethnam S. Haemostasis in endodontic microsurgery. Dent Clin North Am 1997;41:499-511.
7. Kim S. The microscope and endodontis. Dent Clin North Am 2004;48:11-18.
8. Louis J Buhrley, Micheal J, Barrows MS, Ellen A BeGole, Christopher S Wenckus. Effect of magnification on locating the MB2 canal in maxillary molars. J Endod 2002;28: 324-27.
9. Pecora G, Andreana S. Use of dental operating microscope in endodontic surgery. Oral Surg. Oral Med Oral Pathol 1993;75:751-58.
10. Pecora G, Baek SH, Rethnam S, Kim S. Barrier membrane technique in endodontic microsurgery. Dent Clin North Am 1997;41(3):585-602.
11. Rubinstein R. The anatomy of the surgical operating microscope and operating positions. Dent Clin North Am 1997;41:391-94.

# Tissue Engineering

CHAPTER 37



Every year millions of Indians suffer from some type of tissue loss or end-stage organ failure which can be due to inherited disorders, trauma, and neoplastic or infectious diseases. Tissue engineering is expected to solve many such problems by the use of stem cells.

Stem cell is a special kind of cell that has a unique capacity to renew itself and to give rise to specialized cell types. Although most cells of the body, such as heart cells or skin cells, are committed to perform a specific function, a stem cell is uncommitted and remains uncommitted, until it receives a signal to develop into a specialized cell.

One novel approach to restore tooth structure is based on biology: "Regenerative Endodontics" procedures by application of tissue engineering. Regenerative endodontics is a biological procedure designed to replace the diseased, missing, and traumatized tissue including dentin and root structures as well as cells of pulp-dentin complex.

## CURRENT STRATEGIES FOR TREATMENT OF LOST TISSUE

Currently, the replacement of lost or deficient tissues involves prosthetic materials, drug therapies, and tissue and organ transplantation. However, all of these have limitations, including the inability of synthetic prostheses to replace the structural functions of a tissue.

It includes:

1. Autografts
2. Allografts
3. Synthetic materials (Xenografts)

But all these materials have their own limitations. Therefore, the gold standard to replace a lost or damaged tissue is the same natural healthy tissue, which has led to the concept of regenerating new tissue from pre-existing tissue.

### Tissue Engineering

Tissue engineering is a multidisciplinary field. Tissue engineering is the use of a combination of cells, engineering materials, and suitable biochemical factors to improve or replace biological functions.

Probably the first definition of tissue engineering was by Langer and Vacanti who stated it to be *"an interdisciplinary field that applies the principles of engineering and life sciences towards the development of biological substitutes that restore, maintain, or improve tissue function or a whole organ"*.

MacArthur and Oreffo defined tissue engineering as *"understanding the principles of tissue growth, and applying this to produce functional replacement tissue for clinical use"*.

## STRATEGIES OF STEM CELL TECHNOLOGY

There are three strategies to stem cell technology (Figs 37.1A to C)

- Conductive
- Inductive
- Cell base transplantation

These approaches all typically utilize a material component, although with different goals.

### Conductive

Conductive approaches utilize biomaterials in a passive manner to facilitate the growth or regenerative capacity of existing tissue.

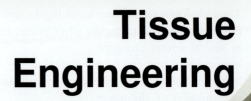

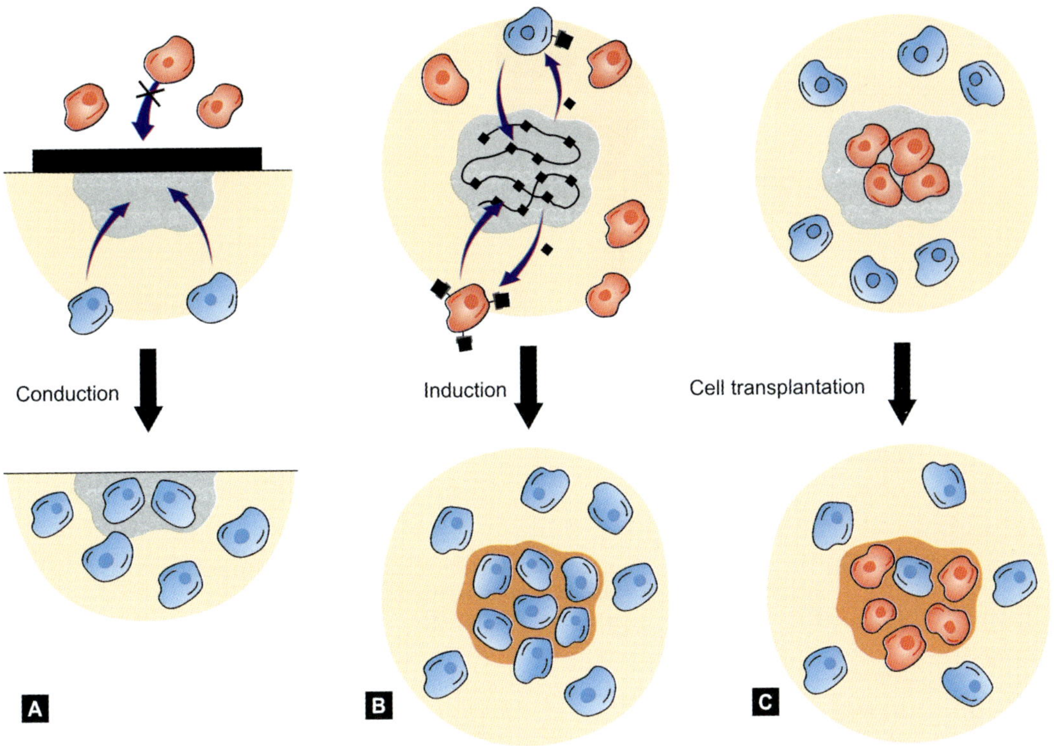


**Figs 37.1A to C:** Strategies of tissue engineering: (A) Conduction; (B) Induction; (C) Cell transplantation

An example of this is guided tissue regeneration in which the appropriate use of barrier membranes promotes predictable bone repair and new attachment with new formation of cementum and periodontal ligament fibers. Conductive approach utilizes biomaterial in a passive manner to facilitate the growth or regenerative capacity of existing tissue.

*Example*: Application of $Ca(OH)_2$ uses conductive approach. Limitation of conductive approach is that it is not predictable.

### Inductive

The second major tissue engineering strategy (induction) involves activating cells in close proximity to the defect site with specific biological signals like BMPs.

Urist first showed that new bone could be formed at nonmineralizing, or ectopic, sites after implantation of powdered bone (bone demineralized and ground into fine particles). Contained within the powdered bone were proteins (BMPs), which turned out to be the key elements for inducing bone formation.

Limitation of this technique is that the inductive factor for a particular tissue may not be known.

### Cell Transplantation (Fig. 37.2)

This approach involves direct transplantation of cells grown in the laboratory.

## TRIAD OF TISSUE ENGINEERING (FIG. 37.3)

Tissue engineering employs use of three materials:

1. Stem cells/progenitor cells: These are capable of differentiating into specialized cells and are able to respond to morphogens by dividing or specializing
2. Morphogens/signaling molecules: These are the biological factors that regulate stem cells to form desirable cell type, e.g. BMPs, which are major morphogens family for tooth regeneration
3. Scaffold/matrix: It provides a biocompatible 3-dimensional structure for cell adhesion and migration. It can be
   - Biological scaffolds (e.g. collagen, glycosaminoglycan)
   - Artificial scaffolds (e.g. PLA, PGA, PLGA).

### Stem Cells/Progenitor Cells

Adult stem/progenitor cells reside in a variety of tissues. Tissues are composed of cells, insoluble extracellular matrix (ECM) and soluble molecules that serve as regulators of cell function.

Stem cells are undifferentiated cells which divide and respond into specialized cell on response to morphogens (Fig. 37.4).

Stem cells are commonly defined as either *embryonic/fetal* or *adult/postnatal*. The term *embryonic* is preferred to *fetal*, because the majority of these cells are embryonic and the term *postnatal* is preferred to *adult* because these same cells are present in babies, infants and children.

The differentiation between embryonic and postnatal is because these cells have different potential for developing into various specialized cells (i.e. plasticity). Studies indicate that postnatal stem cells are more plastic than the embryonic stem cells.

### *Unique Characteristics of Stem Cells*

a. They exist as undifferentiated cells and maintain this phenotype by the environment and/or the adjacent cell populations until they are exposed to and respond to the appropriate signals.

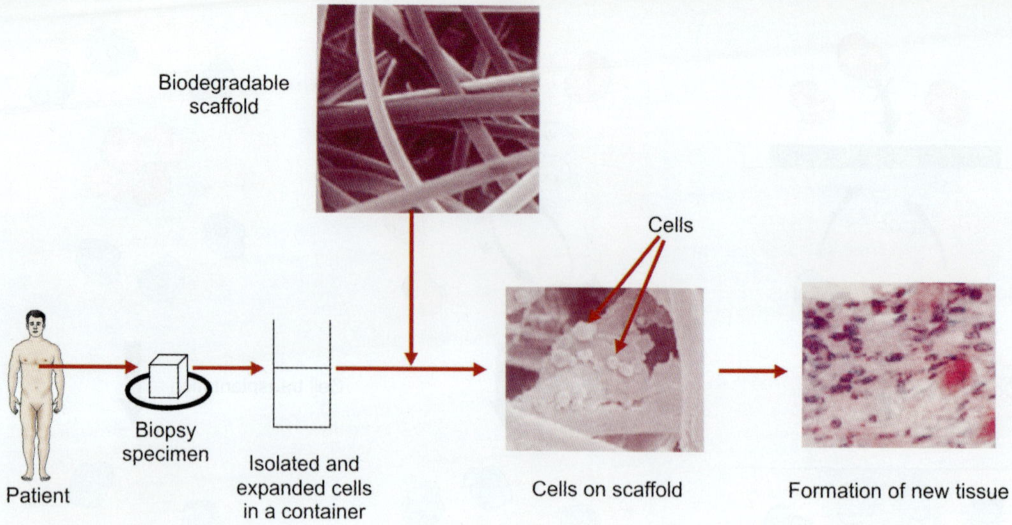


**Fig. 37.2:** Cell transplantation – an approach of tissue engineering in which cultured cells and biodegradable scaffolds can be used to form new tissue

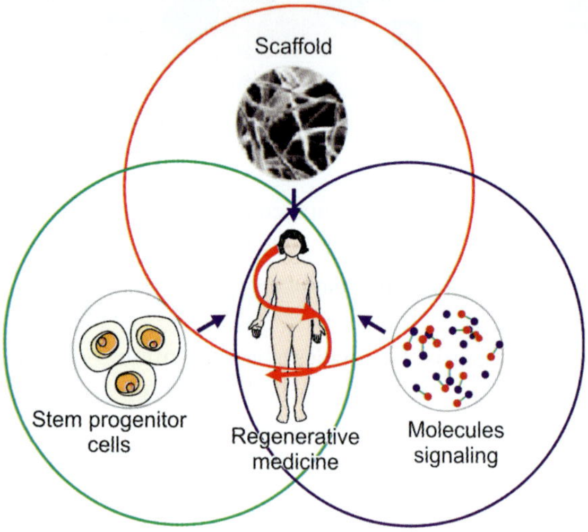


**Fig. 37.3:** Triad of tissue engineering

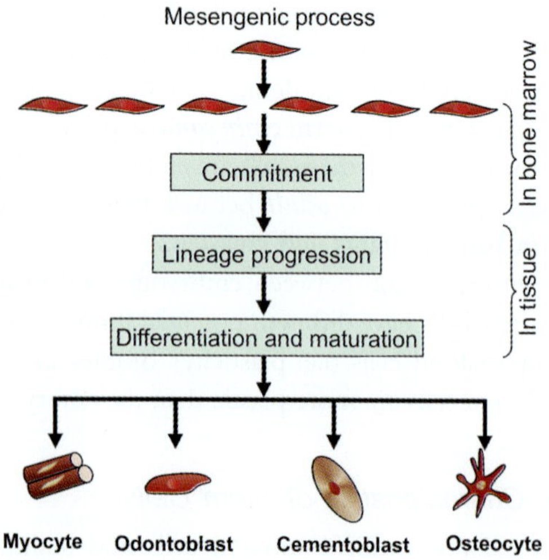


**Fig. 37.4:** Lifecycle of stem cells differentiating into various other type of cells, i.e. myocyte, stromal cell, cementoblasts, etc.

b. Ability to self replicate for prolonged periods
c. Maintain their multiple differentiation potential throughout the life of the organism.

## Stem Cells are Often Categorized by Their Source

1. *Autologous cells* are obtained from the same individual to whom they will be reimplanted. Advantage of autologous stem cells is that they have minimum problems with rejection and pathogen transmission, however, the disadvantage is limited availability.
2. *Allogenic cells* are obtained from the body of a donor of the same species.
3. *Xenogenic cells* are those isolated from individuals of another species. In particular animal cells have been used quite extensively in experiments aimed at the construction of cardiovascular implants.
4. *Syngeneic* or *isogenic cells* are isolated from genetically identical organisms, such as twins, clones, or highly inbred research animal models.
   – Primary cells are from an organism.
   – Secondary cells are from a cell bank.

## Progenitor Cells (Fig. 37.5)

These cells retain the differentiation potential and high proliferation capability but have lost the self-replication property unlike stem cells.

## Types of Stem Cells

1. Embryonic stem cells (pluripotent)
2. Fetal stem cells (multipotent)
3. Adult stem cells (multipotent)

Embryonic stem cells can be isolated from normal blastocyst, the structures formed at about 32 cell stage during embryonic development.

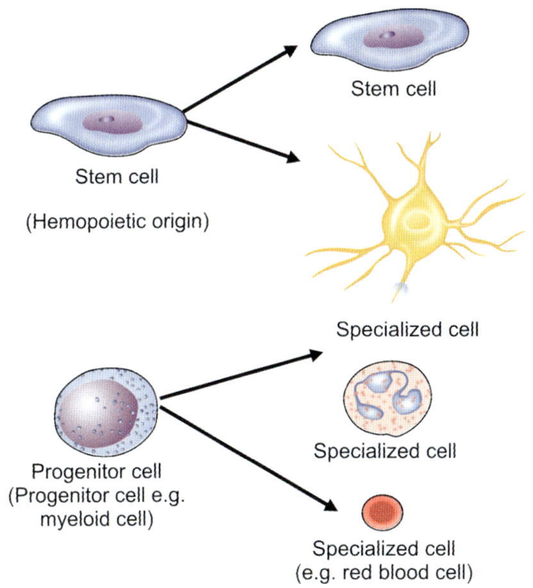


**Fig. 37.5:** Different features of progenitor/precursor cells

Adult stem cells can be collected directly from the bone narrow, from umbilical cord blood and from circulating blood of individuals receiving cytokines which mobilizes stem cells.

Stem cells defined by their capacity for asymmetric division, where in a single cell division results in one cell identical to mother cell and another more differentiated cell, thus maintaining the stem cell population even after differentiation.

## DENTAL PULP STEM CELLS (DPSCs)

Although the regenerative capacity of the human dentin-pulp complex is not well understood, it is known that, upon injury, reparative dentin is formed as a protective barrier for the pulp. Accordingly, one might anticipate that dental pulp contains the dentinogenic progenitors, i.e dental pulp stem cells (DPSCs) that are responsible for dentin repair.

The most striking feature of DPSCs is their ability to regenerate a dentin-pulp like complex that is composed of mineralized matrix with tubules lined with odontoblasts, and fibrous tissue containing blood vessels in an arrangement similar to the dentin-pulp complex found in normal human teeth.

Stem cell properties of human dental pulp stem cells:

1. Self-renewal capability.
2. Multilineage differentiation capacity.
3. Clonogenic efficiency of human dental pulp stem cells (DPSCs).
4. DPSCs were capable of forming ectopic dentin and associated pulp tissue *in vivo*.

## STEM CELLS FROM HUMAN EXFOLIATED DECIDUOUS TEETH (SHED)

The exfoliated deciduous tooth contains living pulp remnants consisting of connective tissue, blood vessels, and odontoblasts. This tissue contains special kind of cells known as SHED (stem cells from human exfoliated deciduous teeth). SHED can differentiated into odontoblast-like cells that form small dentin-like structures. SHEDs are distinctive from DPSCs with respect to odontogenic differentiation and osteogenic induction.

## PERIODONTAL LIGAMENT STEM CELLS (PDLSCs)

The periodontal ligament (PDL) connects the cementum to alveolar bone, and functions primarily to support the tooth in the alveolar socket. A recent report identified stem cells in human PDL (PDLSCs) and found that PDLSCs implanted into nude mice generated cementum/PDL-like structures that resemble the native PDL as a thin layer of cementum that interfaced with dense collagen fibers, similar to Sharpey's fibers. Thus, the PDLSCs have the ability of forming periodontal structures, including the cementum and PDL.

## STEM CELL MARKERS, ISOLATION

Every cell in the body are coated with specialized proteins on their surface, called receptors that have the capability of selectively binding or adhere to other "signaling" molecules. Normally, cells use these receptors and the molecules that bind to them as a way of communicating with other cells and to carry out their proper functions in the body.

The stem cell markers are similar to these cell surface receptors. Each cell type, for example, a liver cell, has a certain combination of receptors on their surface that makes them distinguishable from other kinds of cells. Researchers use the signaling molecules that selectively adhere to the receptors on the surface of the cell as a tool that allows them to identify stem cells. The signaling molecules have the ability to fluoresce or emit light energy when activated by an energy source such as an ultraviolet light or laser beam (Fig. 37.6).

Thus, stem cell markers help in identification and isolation of stem cells.

### Isolation of Stem Cells

Stem cells can be identified and isolated from mixed cell population by four commonly used techniques:

- By staining the cells with specific antibody markers and using a flow cytometer. This process is called fluorescent antibody cell sorting (FACS).
- Physiological and histological criteria. This includes phenotype, chemotaxis, proliferation, differentiation, and mineralizing activity.
- Immunomagnetic bead selection.
- Immunohistochemical staining.

Tooth bud tissues containing stem cells are dissociated enzymatically and mechanically and filtered to remove even small clumps of cells, generating single cell suspensions. The tissue is then plated *in vitro* and cultured to eliminate differentiated cell types. The resultant culture contains enriched dental stem cell population (Fig. 37.7).

## MORPHOGENS/SIGNALING MOLECULES

Morphogens are extracellularly secreted signals governing morphogenesis during epithelial-mesenchymal interactions.

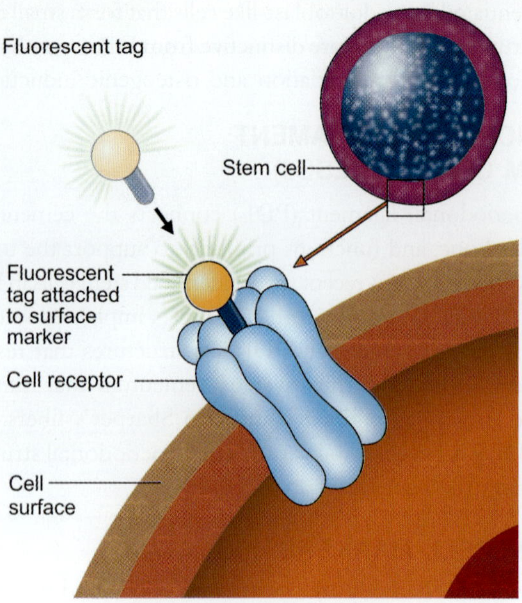


**Fig. 37.6:** Identification of cell surface markers using fluorescent tags

These are biological factors that regulate stem cells to form the desirable cell type. They are injected alone or bound to a biomaterial used as delivery system.

### Functions

1. To stimulate division of neighboring cells and those infiltrating the defect (Example: Growth factors - *PDGF*)
2. To stimulate the differentiation of certain cells along a specified pathway (Example: Differentiation factors - *BMP*)
3. To stimulate angiogenesis
4. To serve as chemoattractants for specific cell types.

*Different types of morphogens are*:

1. Bone morphogenic proteins (*BMPs*) } Embryonic tooth development
2. Fibroblast growth factors (FGFs) } Embryonic tooth development
3. Wingless and intrelated proteins (*Wnts*)
4. Hedgehog proteins (*Hhs*)
5. Tumor necrotic factor (*TNF*)
6. Transforming growth factor (TGF)
7. Insulin-like growth factor (IGF)
8. Colony stimulating factor (CSF)
9. Epidermal growth factor (EGF)
10. Interleukins (IL)
11. Platelet-derived growth factor (PDGF).
12. Nerve growth factor (NGF)

These families exhibit signaling, each with distinct expression during initiation, pattern formation and morphogenesis, and cytodifferentiation. These can be used to control stem cell activity, such as by increasing the rate of proliferation, inducing differentiation of cells into another tissue type, or stimulating stem cells to synthesize and secrete mineralized matrix.

Dentin contains many proteins capable of stimulating tissue responses. Demineralization of dental tissues leads to the release of growth factors following the application of cavity etching agents, restorative materials and even caries. Indeed, it is likely that much of the therapeutic effect of calcium hydroxide may be because of its attraction of growth factors from the dentin matrix.

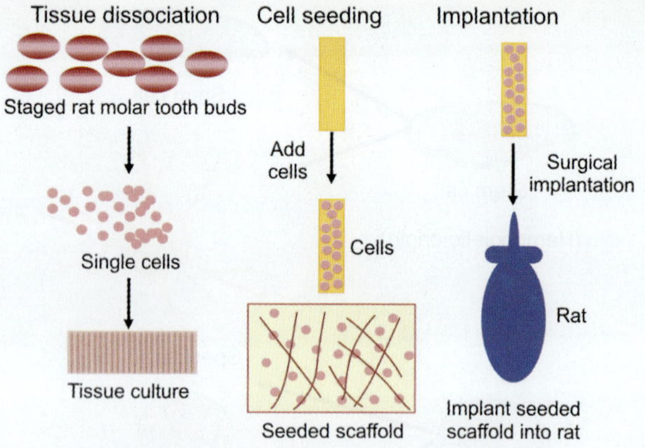


**Fig. 37.7:** Tooth tissue engineering

## SCAFFOLD/MATRIX

The scaffold provides a physicochemical and biological three-dimensional microenvironment for cell growth and differentiation, promoting cell adhesion and migration. The scaffold serves as a carrier for morphogen and for cells.

Natural scaffold are proteic materials such as collagen or fibrin, and polysaccharide materials, like chitosan or glycosaminoglycans which offer good biocompatibility and bioactivity, and synthetic scaffold can elaborate physicochemical features such as degradation rate, microstructure, and mechanical strength.

Commonly used synthetic materials are polylactic acid (PLA), polyglycolic acid (PGA), and their copolymers, polylactic-co-glycolic acid (PLGA) and polycaprolactone (PCL). Synthetic hydrogels include poly ethylene glycol (PEG) based polymers. Scaffolds containing inorganic compounds such as hydroxyapatite and calcium phosphate are used to enhance bone conductivity (Fig. 37.8).

### Requirements of a Scaffold

1. It should be effective for transport of nutrients, oxygen, and waste.
2. It should be gradually degraded and replaced by regenerative tissue, retaining the feature of the final tissue structure.
3. It should be biocompatible, nontoxic, and should have proper physical and mechanical strength.
4. Easy cell penetration, distribution and proliferation.
5. Permeability of culture medium.
6. *In vivo* vascularization (once implanted).
7. Maintenance of osteoblastic cell phenotype.
8. Adequate mechanical stiffness.
9. Ease of fabrication.

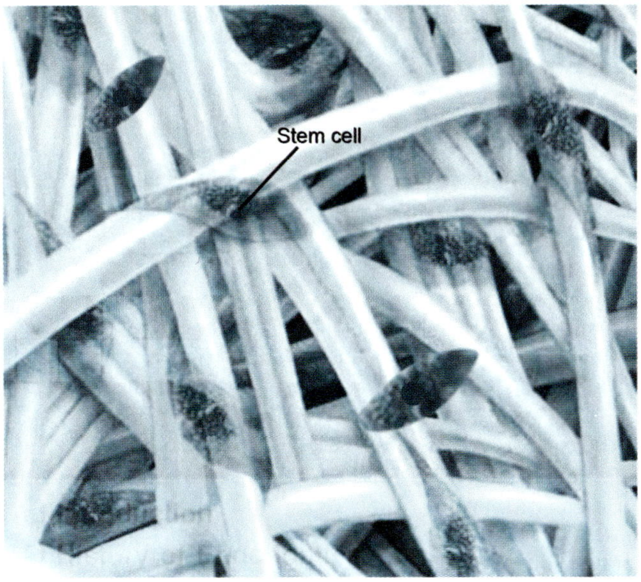


Fig. 37.8: Scaffold with stem cells

## APPROACHES TO STEM CELL TECHNOLOGY

### Cell Therapy

Adult stem cells are prime candidates for cell therapy. *Two approaches of cell therapy.*

- *In vitro*
- *In vivo*

1. *In vitro*
   Tissue or organ regenerated in culture room by combining three elements (Scaffold/matrix, signaling molecules and cells) before transplanting tissue engineered organ into patients.
2. *In vivo*
   Intrinsic healing activity is induced at site of tissue defect using these three elements (i.e. stem cells, scaffold and morphogens).

### *Gene Therapy and Protein Delivery (Fig. 37.9)*

In the presence of vital responsive cells in the target tissue - the signaling molecule (Protein) can be delivered through two approaches.

### Gene Delivery

Gene therapy is recently used as a means of delivering genes for growth factors, morphogens, transcription factors, extracellular matrix molecules locally to somatic cells of individuals with a resulting therapeutic effect. The gene can stimulate or induce a natural biological process by expressing a molecules involved in regenerative response for the tissue of interest. Both an *in vivo* and an *in vitro* approach can be used for gene therapy (Fig. 37.10).

1. *In vivo*
   In the *in vivo* approach, the gene is delivered systemically into the bloodstream or locally to target tissues by injection or inhalation. Scaffold then implanted into tissue defect,

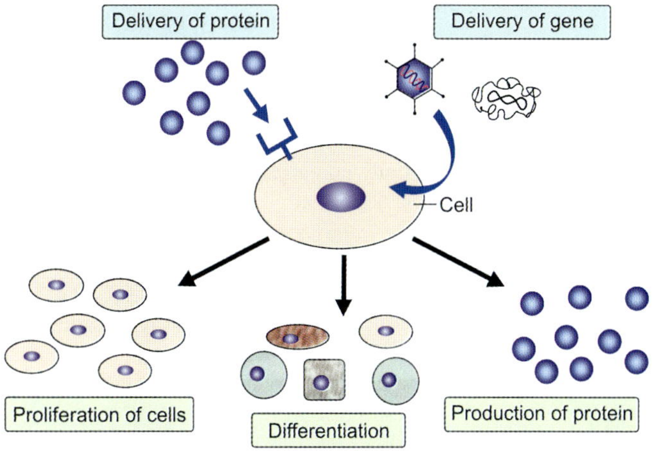


Fig. 37.9: Gene therapy and protein delivery

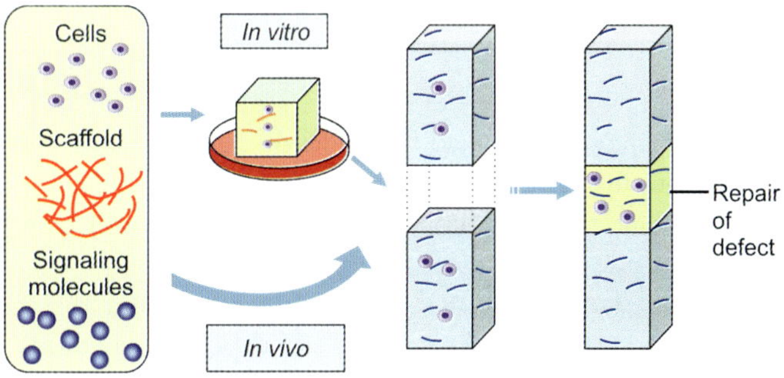


Fig. 37.10: Gene delivery by both approach i.e. *in vitro* and *in vivo*

   the host cells migrate into the implant, take up the gene construct and start to produce the encoded protein.
2. *In vitro*
   The ex vivo approach involves genetic manipulation of cells *in vitro*, which are subsequently transplanted to the regeneration site. The cells play a role not only in the repair process but also in secretion of growth factors locally to stimulate host cell.

### Protein Delivery

Therapeutic proteins are applied locally that bind to appropriate receptors displayed at cell surface. Subsequently, cells are activated and undergo proliferation or differentiation.

### *Stem Cell Engineering of Biomimetic Material*

It is always problematic to regenerate the lost tooth structure. Now a days, the latest concept of transplantation of natural tooth substance has gained wide popularity.

### Harvesting Teeth Created by Tissue Engineering

Many researches have been conducted in tissue engineering therapies so as to develop a synthetic tooth. All these approaches employ the use of existing developmental tooth structures as a template and attained partial success.

| Summary of tooth injury and possible applications of tissue-engineering approaches to aid healing | | | | | |
|---|---|---|---|---|---|
| *Degree of tooth injury* | *Minimal* | *Severe* | *Some loss of vital tissue* | *Large loss of vital tissue* | *Complete loss of vital tissue* |
| Example of dental problem | Early non-arrested caries lesion | Arrested deep-penetrating caries lesion | Arrested or slowly progressing caries lesion extending to pulp tissue | Partially decayed or fractured tooth | Decayed tooth, or accidentally evulsed tooth. |
| Common current restorative therapy | Seal fissure or excavate caries and apply restorative materials. | Excavate caries and apply restorative materials. | Stepwise excavation of caries lesion, or pulp capping | Pulp capping, endodontic treatment, or tooth extraction | Remove injured tissue and place implant or prosthetic teeth. |
| Likely objective of tissue engineering in restorative therapy | Alter oral bacterial DNA to arrest and prevent subsequent enamel and dentin caries demineralization. | Stimulate pulp-dentin healing with growth factors. | Regenerate lost tissues and dentin repair with growth factors. | Implant progenitor cells to regenerate lost tissue and tooth mineralized structure. | Use progenitor cells and growth factors in three-dimensional tissue culture to harvest artificial teeth for implantation. |

Chair side technique for developing a synthetic tooth:

1. Create a computer aided biomodel of the oral cavity and evaluate the existing teeth.
2. Make blue print for designing a replacement tooth from sizes, shapes and esthetics using database.
3. Biomanufacture the tooth using a scaffold and three-dimensional cell pattern printing and deposition methods.
4. Cut the slabs of biosynthetic enamel and dentin according to shape of tooth.
5. Implant the tooth surgically into the socket and connect it with blood vessels, nerves and periodontal ligament.

## Bioengineered Teeth From Tooth Bud Cells (Fig. 37.11)

Using tissue engineering approach, a highly mineralized anatomically correct replacement of tooth tissue can be done from tooth bud cells.

Here the immature tooth bud tissue supplemented with dental progenitor cells were used to seed biodegradable scaffolds. These were then implanted in a host animal to provide enough vascularization of bioengineered tissues. When the implants were harvested and evaluated after 6-7 months of growth, the tooth bud cells had attained the anatomically correct tooth crowns with rudimentary tooth root structures.

### *Bioactive Molecules in Restorative Dentistry*

- For years, dental surgeons have used a limited number of capping agents to keep teeth alive. The most efficient was calcium hydroxide.
- Extracellular matrix molecules/Bioactive molecules pave the road for controlled tissue repair and regeneration.
- Promotes healing or regeneration of dental pulp by forming a barrier of limited sizes and induces extensive mineralization area, with the prospect of filling the crown and root pulp partially or totally.

## Calcium Hydroxide

1. As direct capping agent induces formation of reparative dentinal bridge
2. As indirect capping agent, it brings about formation of reactionary dentin.

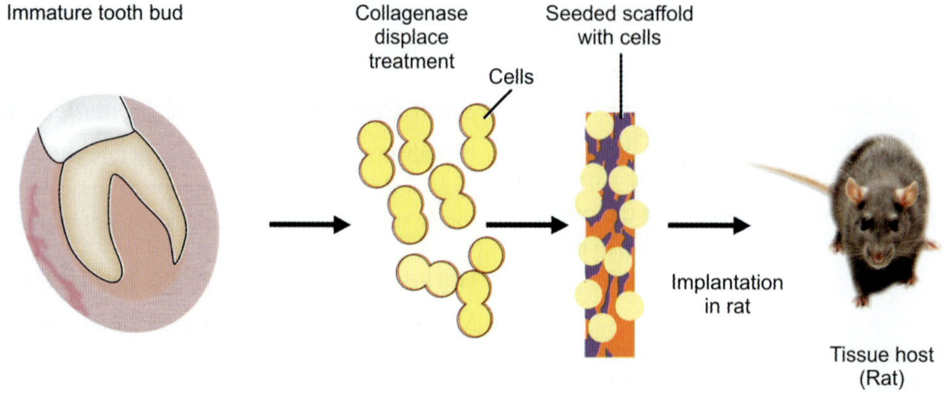


**Fig. 37.11:** Bioengineered teeth from immature tooth bud

Biologic properties of $Ca(OH)_2$

↓

High alkaline pH induces burn of limited amplitude at surface of exposed pulp

↓

Below the scar, once inflammatory process has resolved - reparative cells are recruited in central part of pulp

↓

Migration to the site

↓

Proliferation and differentiation

### New Bioactive Molecules

1. Bone sialoprotein
2. BMP-7
3. Amelogenin gene splice products A M + 4, A – 4.
4. Dentin phosphoprotein (DPP)
5. Dentin matrix protein (DMP – 1)

These stimulate the formation of thick homogenous dentinal bridge in contrast to dentinal bridge after $Ca(OH)_2$ pulp capping (Fig. 37.12).

## Different Strategies Used for Regenerative Endodontics

### Definition

Regenerative endodontic procedures are biologically based procedures designed to replace damaged structures, including dentin and root structures, as well as cells of the pulp-dentin complex. Regenerative dental procedures have a long history, originating around 1952, when Dr BW Hermann reported on the application of $Ca(OH)_2$ in a case report of vital pulp amputation. Subsequent regenerative dental procedures include the development of guided tissue or bone regeneration (GTR, GBR) procedures and distraction osteogenesis; the application of platelet rich plasma (PRP) for bone augmentation, Emdogain for periodontal tissue regeneration, and recombinant human bone morphogenic protein (rhBMP) for bone augmentation; and preclinical trials on the use of fibroblast growth factor 2 ($FGF_2$) for periodontal tissue regeneration.

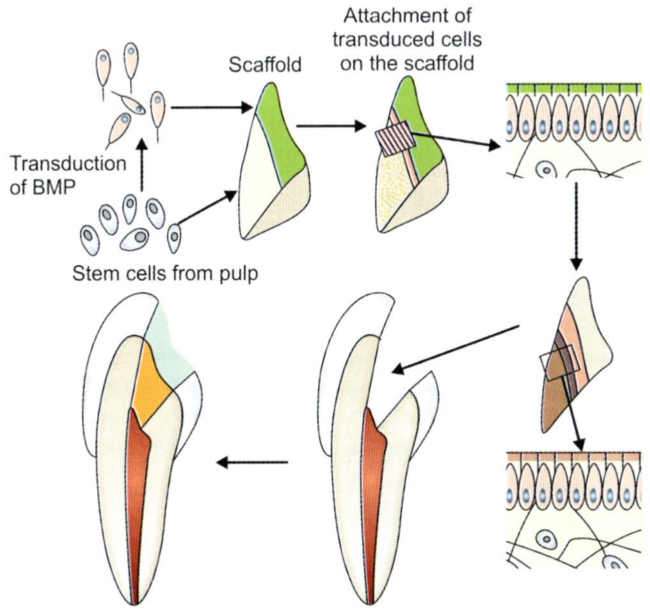


**Fig. 37.12:** Regeneration of dentin from stem cells from pulp

Several major areas of research that might have application in the development of regenerative endodontic techniques. These techniques are:

a. Root canal revascularization via blood clotting,
b. Postnatal stem cell therapy,
c. Pulp implantation,
d. Scaffold implantation,
e. Injectable scaffold delivery,
f. Three-dimensional cell printing, and
g. Gene delivery.

## REVASCULARIZATION TO INDUCE APEXIFICATION/APEXOGENESIS IN INFECTED, NONVITAL, IMMATURE TOOTH

Trauma to teeth during development may lead to open apex and blunderbuss canals. If vital pulp is present, apexogenesis is the best option. But if teeth are nonvital, several treatment challenges are there:

I. Adequate mechanical cleaning/shaping of tooth
II. Thin, fragile lateral dentinal walls may fracture during mechanical filing
III. Large amount of necrotic debris in a wide root canal is difficult to disinfect.
IV. Obturation is problematic
V. Surgical procedures with retrograde filling may leave the tooth with an unfavorable crown root ratio.

## Apexification

It is the method used to induce a calcified barrier in nonvital immature teeth that serves as a matrix against which the root filling material is compacted.

Conventional materials used for apexification are $Ca(OH)_2$, $Ca(OH)_2$ in combination with CMCP, cresanol, saline or local anesthetic solution, ZnO, Tricalcium phosphate, collagen, calcium phosphate gel, osteogenic protein I and II, MTA, etc.

## Calcium Hydroxide

It has been the most often advocated material for this purpose.

### Disadvantages

i. Variability of treatment time
ii. Patient compliance for attending the recalls
iii. Although the open apex might be "closed" by a calcific barrier, apexification does not promote the continued development of the root.

iv. Because the pulp canal space is physically occupied by the material, there is no room for vital tissue to proliferate
v. Calcium hydroxide treatment will have short roots with thin dentinal walls and a high risk of fracture
vi. Its high pH may cause necrosis of tissues that can potentially differentiate into new pulp
vii. May make teeth brittle because of its proteolytic and hygroscopic properties
viii. Barrier formation is often porous and noncontinuous.

## Mineral Trioxide Aggregate

A new technique has been proposed to decrease the time to create a bridge at the apex. After disinfection of the canal, MTA is placed in the apical third of the immature root to create a stop for the filling material. This technique will also not allow new tissue to grow into the root canal, and the root remains thin and weak.

Hence, apexification would not lead to continued root formation or thickening of the root canal wall, leading to the risk of an undesirable side effect of a short and weakened root that is susceptible to fracture. An alternative treatment regime is preferred to overcome these problems, i.e. pulp revascularization.

## Pulp Revascularization

### Definition

Revascularization is the procedure to re-establish vitality in a nonvital tooth to allow repair and regeneration of tissue.

### Advantages

Revascularization will allow further development of root and dentin structure with a better long-term prognosis.

It is favored when apical foramen is not completely formed and the apical diameter exceeds 1 mm.

## Pulp Revascularization in Replanted Teeth

This is affected by certain factors

i. *Extraoral time:* The extraoral timing and storage medium appear to affect potential pulp revascularization. Prognosis is favorable if the time of replantation is no longer than 45 minutes post-avulsion.

   Revascularization following dry storage usually occurs in about half of the cases when the storage period is less than 5 minutes. Further, the frequency of revascularization drops to about one-third in the period from 6 to 20 minutes, and then continues to decrease consistently with the increase in drying periods. Thereafter, radiographic controls should be carried out after 2, 3 and 4 weeks in order to demonstrate signs of pulp necrosis, such as periapical radiolucency and/or inflammatory root resorption.

ii. *Presence or absence of bacteria:* Cvek et al showed that pulp revascularization is highly dependent upon the presence or absence of bacteria in the pulpal lumen. It is possible that the movement of bacteria from the oral cavity or from contaminated root surfaces can occur during extraoral time. Bacterial penetration into the pulp canal space seems to be the cause of revascularization failure in the majority of the cases. This leads to pulp necrosis and inflammatory root resorption, if endodontic treatment is delayed or pulp and dentin infection is severe.

The time needed for the initial healing of the periodontal ligament under normal conditions is approximately 10 days after replantation. The process of revascularization is observed within 7 days and is completed after 4-5 weeks after the replantation of immature teeth.

## Pulp Revascularization in Immature Teeth

Once the canal infection is controlled, it resembles avulsed tooth that has a necrotic but sterile pulp canal space. Blood clot is then introduced so as to mimic the scaffold that is in place with ischemic necrotic pulp as in avulsed tooth and access cavity is restored with a bacteria tight seal. In teeth with open apices and necrotic pulp, it is possible that some vital pulp tissue and Hertwig's epithelial root sheath remain. When canal is disinfected, inflammatory process reverses and these tissues may proliferate. It depends mainly on:

i. Disinfection of root canal.
ii. Placement of matrix in canal for tissue ingrowth.
iii. Bacteria tight seal of access opening.

### Indications

- The teeth that present with symptoms of acute or chronic apical periodontitis (i.e. pain, diffuse facial and/or mucosal swelling, tenderness to percussion, or intraoral sinuses).
- Radiographically, the tooth had an immature apex, either blunderbuss or in the form of a wide canal with parallel walls and an open apex. On electric pulp test the affected tooth is nonvital.

### Techniques

- The tooth is anesthetized with a local injection with epinephrine and is isolated with rubber dam.
- The access cavity is prepared with a round diamond and Endo-Z bur
- The canal is gently flushed with 20 mL of 5.25% sodium hypochlorite (NaOCl) solution.

A. For teeth with chronic apical periodontitis (vital pulp)

   i. The canal is dried with sterile paper points and etching and dentin bonding agent light curing is done followed by application of a flowable composite. A mixture of ciprofloxacin 250 mg, metronidazole 250 mg, and minocycline 250 mg, is placed in the sterile root canal 2 mm from the working length and left for 7 days.
   ii. In the next visit, the antibiotic dressing material is removed by rinsing with 5.25 percent NaOCl, if the tooth is symptom free. The canal is dried with sterile paper points and is confirmed to have no exudate.
   iii. A size #40 K-file is introduced into the root canal until vital tissue is felt, and this instrument is used to irritate this tissue to create some bleeding into the root canal.

iv. The bleeding is allowed to reach a level 3 mm below the cementoenamel junction, and tooth is left for 15 minutes so that a blood clot is formed. Then a grey mineral trioxide aggregate is placed over the clot carefully upto the level of CEJ followed by a wet cotton pellet and restored with a temporary dressing material.

B. For teeth with an acute apical abscess (nonvital pulp)
  i. The tooth is left open to drain for 3 days by packing the pulp chamber with cotton pellets, after which the canal is similarly dressed with the antibiotic mixture for 1 week.
  ii. Steps ii, iii, iv is same as above.
    - One week later, the tooth is restored with a dentin-bonded resin composite restoration, and the patient is scheduled for recall to check vitality/radiological finding
    - For teeth with persistent infection, or where the canal could not be dried, the triple antibiotics mixture dressing is repeated at one week interval until no symptom or exudation is present.
    - Patients are recalled after a minimum of 1 year. The criteria of success are
      - Lack of symptoms
      - Radiographic evidence of increased root length
      - Radiographic evidence of increased root canal thickness.

## Mechanism of Revascularization

i. Few cells remain at the apical end of the root canal. These cells might proliferate into the newly formed matrix and differentiate into odontoblasts under the organizing influence of cells of Hertwig's epithelial root sheath, which are quite resistant to destruction, even in the presence of inflammation. The newly formed odontoblasts can lay down a tubular dentin at the apical end, causing apexogenesis as well as on lateral aspects of dentinal walls of the root canal, reinforcing and strengthening the root.

ii. Continued root development due to multipotent dental pulp stem cells, which are present in permanent teeth and might be present in abundance in immature teeth. These cells from the apical end might be seeded onto the existing dentinal walls and might differentiate into odontoblasts and deposit tertiary or atubular dentin.

iii. Stem cells in the periodontal ligament can proliferate, grow into the apical end and within the root canal, and deposit hard tissue both at the apical end and on the lateral root walls.

iv. Root development could be attributed to stem cells from the apical papilla or the bone marrow. Instrumentation beyond the confines of the root canal to induce bleeding can also transplant mesenchymal cells from the bone into the canal lumen. These cells have excellent proliferative capacity. Transplantation studies have shown that human stem cells from bone marrow can form bone or dentin *in vivo*.

v. Blood clot itself being a rich source of growth factors could play important role regeneration. These include platelet-derived growth factor, vascular factor, tissue growth factor and could stimulate differentiation, growth and maturation of fibroblasts, odontoblasts, cementoblasts, etc. from the immature undifferentiated mesenchymal cells in the newly formed tissue matrix.

## Advantages of Revascularization Procedure

1. Short treatment time.
2. The approach is technically simple and can be completed using currently available instruments and medicaments without expensive biotechnology.
3. The regeneration of tissue in root canal systems by a patient's own blood cells avoids the possibility of immune rejection and pathogen transmission from replacing the pulp with a tissue engineered construct.
4. Cost-effective.
5. Obturation of canal not required.
6. Continued root development and strengthening.

## Limitations of Revascularization Procedure

1. The case reports of a blood clot having the capacity to regenerate pulp tissue are exciting, but caution is required, because the source of the regenerated tissue has not been identified. Generally, tissue engineering does not rely on blood clot formation, because the concentration and composition of cells trapped in the fibrin clot is unpredictable. This is a critical limitation to a blood clot revascularization approach; because tissue engineering is founded on the delivery of effective concentrations and compositions of cells to restore function. It is very possible that variations in cell concentration and composition, particularly in older patients (where circulating stem cell concentrations may be lower) may lead to variations in treatment outcome.
2. Enlargement of the apical foramen is necessary to promote vascularizaton and to maintain initial cell viability via nutrient diffusion. Related to this point, cells must have an available supply of oxygen; therefore, it is likely that cells in the coronal portion of the root canal system either would not survive or would survive under hypoxic conditions before angiogenesis. Interestingly, endothelial cells release soluble factors under hypoxic conditions that promote cell survival and angiogenesis, whereas other cell types demonstrate similar responses to low oxygen availability.
3. Crown discoloration, development of resistant bacterial strains and allergic reactions to intracanal medications. Access opening may be sealed with dentin bonding agents and flowable composite to avoid contact of triantibiotic paste with dentin.
4. Canal may get calcified compromising esthetics and not allowing post placement.

It is accepted that in luxated or avulsed teeth with open apices and apical periodontitis, revascularization is a possibility. The explanation for this positive outcome is that although the pulp is devitalized after avulsion, it will stay free of bacteria for sometime. If, in this time, the new vital tissue fills the canal space, the ingress of bacteria will be stopped. Thus, the disinfection relies solely on irrigants and intracanal medications and formation of a blood clot in the canal after disinfection. This blood clot acts as a matrix for the growth of new tissue into the pulp space. An interesting question is the origin of the new pulp tissue. Based on the fact that the root continued to grow, and that the walls of the root appeared to thicken in a conventional manner, it is likely that the tissue is in fact pulp with functioning odontoblasts. Therefore, even though a large apical lesion is present, it is probable that some vital pulp tissue and Hertwig's epithelial root sheath remained. When the canal is disinfected and the inflammatory conditions reversed, these tissues can proliferate. However, the predictability of this procedure and the type of tissue that develops in these cases are still to be studied. The benefit is so great compared with leaving a root with a thin and fracture-susceptible wall that, in our opinion, it is worth attempting. If no root development can be seen within 3 months, the more traditional apexification procedures can then be started.

We have entered an exciting era where the diverse fields of stem cell biology tissue engineering, nanotechnology, and material science have converged synergistically to characterize and manipulate signaling cascades regulating tissue and organ regeneration. The field of tissue engineering is certainly the one in which there are more questions than answers. From the conceptual standpoint, there is little doubt that the best material to replace tooth structure is tooth structure.

## QUESTIONS

**Q. Define tissue engineering? What are different approaches to stem cell therapy?**

**Q. Explain revascularization in detail with its advantages and limitations.**

## BIBLIOGRAPHY


1. Baum BJ, Mooney DJ. The impact of tissue engineering on dentistry. JADA 2000;131:309-18.
2. Freitas RA Jr. Nanodentistry. JADA 2000;131:1559-65.
3. Hochman R. Neurotransmitter modulator (TENS) for control of dental operative pain. JADA 1988;116:208-12.
4. West JL, Halas NJ. Applications of nanotechnology to biotechnology. Curr Opin Biotechnol 2000;11(2):215-17.

# CHAPTER 38

# Ethics in Endodontics



## INTRODUCTION

Ethics is a moral concept which has been considered worthy of major contemplation since the begining of human life on the earth.

The word "ethics" is derived from a Greek word "Ethos" meaning custom or character.

### Nature of Ethics

1. It is related with evaluation of human conduct and standards for judging whether actions performed are right or wrong.
2. It is philosophy of human conduct, away from stating and evaluating principles by which problems of behavior can be solved.
3. It is an attempt to determine the goals of living.

## PRINCIPLES OF ETHICS

The principles of ethics for dental profession should be considered as guidelines for the dentist in treating patients. The dentist has obligation to work on some principles for providing service to the patient, community and his profession.

### Related to Patient

Primary duty of dentist is to provide proper care to patients irrespective of nationality, socioeconomic status or race, etc.

- Dentist should not hesitate in referring specialist for treatment of patient.
- Dentist should tell all the possible treatment options available to patient.
- Proposed treatment plan and option should be explained to the patient before starting the procedure.
- Any complication which may occur during or after the dental procedure should be explained to the patient.

### Related to Community

- Dentist should provide knowledge about prevention, prophylaxis and treatment of dental diseases.
- Dentists may advance their reputation through professional services to patients and to society and assume a responsible role in the community.

### Related to Profession

- Dentist should update his knowledge and skill by continuing education.
- Dentist should maintain honor, morality and integrity of profession and should avoid any misconduct.
- Dentist should have obligation to support advancement of their profession through membership at scientific and professional organization.

## ROOT CANAL ETHICS

In present situation, patients really want to know what the problems are, and their solutions. Before commencing a treatment, the dentist should take treatment records as well as informed consent of the patient. These two, treatment records and informed consent are most important tools in prevention and/or defense of dental malpractice claim.

### Treatment Records

Each dentist should have standardized protocol for diagnosis and management of pulpal and periapical diseases. In addition to established standardized protocol, the endodontist should have the habit of recording written documentation of treatment provided. It include the following procedure:

1. A detailed written medical history should be taken if medical consultation is required, then consultant's remarks should be recorded in the file.

2. The chief complaint of patient should be recorded in his or her own words and treatment should be planned according to that.
3. The dental history of the patient should also be recorded. If any treatment previously given, affects the present outcome of the treatment, it should be explained to the patient. It should also be recorded in the performa.
4. The extraoral and intraoral examination should be conducted and recorded in the performa.
5. An important part of performa, i.e. examination of affected tooth/teeth should be done thoroughly. Both subjective and objective tests related to diagnosis and treatment should be done and recorded in the performa. If required, a dental specialist can be referred. Radiographs of good diagnostic quality should be taken and interpreted. The dentist should record the findings of radiographs in the performa.
6. A detailed pulpal and periodontal examination should be done and recorded in the performa.
7. A proposed treatment plan and provisional diagnosis should be presented to the patient. It should be recorded in the performa also.
8. The medication if prescribed should also be recorded in the dental performa.
9. The informed consent regarding the treatment outcomes should be recorded and included in the performa.
10. The dentist should always sign the performa.

### Common Elements of Negligence and Malpractice

1. Failure to meet the standard of care.
2. Failure to diagnose properly.
3. Failure to refer.
4. Use of poor standard dental materials.
5. Practice beyond scope of license.
6. Performing procedure not up to the mark.

### Common Malpractice Errors Against Endodontics

1. Failure to meet the standard of care.
2. Instrument separation.
3. Treating a wrong tooth.
4. Performing procedure not upto mark.
5. Failure to get informed consent.
6. Paresthesia.

## INFORMED CONSENT

As a general rule, the information presented to a patient must be presented in a terminology that is easily understood by the patient. The dentist should tell advantages, risks, and cost related to patient's problems. Informed consent should also be duly signed by the patient and date should also be recorded. Failure to provide the adequate information to the patient is also breach in the code. In the written informed consent should include the following:

1. The diagnosis for each affected tooth should be recorded.
2. The treatment plan should be recorded in brief.
3. The date in which consent is taken, should be recorded in consent form.
4. The potential complication which may occur during or after the treatment should be written in consent form.
5. The success rate of treatment should also be mentioned in the consent form.
6. Alternative treatment options such as tooth extraction or no treatment should be told to patient and it should also be mentioned in the consent form.
7. The patient or his/her guardians should sign the consent form along with date.

No specific form should be used in every case. In endodontics, the incidence of complications is relatively low if done by specialist. The endodontist should tell the patient about the following facts:

1. Despite best efforts by endodontist few cases of root canal failure are reported.
2. Sometimes overextensions occur in root canal therapy. If it is minor, then no treatment is required because these cases heal well and remain asymptomatic.
3. Slight to moderate pain may occur after root canal therapy.
4. A file may break in canal during root canal therapy, then, patient should be informed about this occurrence.
5. Perforation may also occur during root canal therapy. Tell the patient about the perforation and explain him/her that it can be repaired with newer materials.

## DENTAL NEGLIGENCE

Dental negligence is defined as a violation of the standards of care. In a layman term, malpractice means negligence. Dental negligence occur mainly due to two reasons either a clinician does not possess a required qualification or despite of qualification he or she acts carelessly.

### Related to Local Anesthesia

There are certain problems which can occur while injecting local anesthesia in the patient. Some cases which can give rise to allegations of negligence are:

1. Syncope (fainting)
2. Fracture of the needle in site.
3. Hematoma
4. Trismus
5. Drug allergy
6. Injection of incorrect solution
7. Infection
8. Injection of expired solution.

### Syncope (fainting)

**Syncope** can be seen usually occurs in the dental clinic. But this can be reduced if proper counseling of the patient is done before initiating treatment.

Doctor should explain patient about each and every step of dental procedure which he is doing on the patient.

If at all it happens even after taking proper care, the clinician and his assistant should be ready to manage the situation effectively.

### Fracture of the Needle *In Situ*

Incidence of fracture of the needle has been reduced in modern era because of wider availability of disposable needles and syringes. In past, reuse of the needles and syringes was the main reason for this problem.

Several other conditions such as hematoma, trismus and drug allergy, may also make the conditions worse for dentist in the dental clinic. So, good communication and rapport between the practitioner and the patient is key in these circumstances to prevent the allegation of negligence.

The injection of an incorrect or expired solution causing harm is considered as an indefensible action. Such occurrences should be avoided in the dental office or extra care should be taken during injection of local anesthetic.

### Thermal or Chemical Burns

Both thermal or chemical burns are also part of dental negligence.

#### *Thermal Burns*

Thermal burns can occur due to overheated instruments such as handpieces or when instruments are insufficiently cooled after sterilization. These can cause burns on the lips, oral mucosa and the lips. To prevent or minimize such occurrences.

1. All instruments such as handpiece should be properly maintained and oiling of the handpiece should be done regularly.
2. Burs used in these handpieces should be new and sharp.
3. Excessive pressure should not be applied during cutting.
4. Irrigation with normal saline should be done all the way during cutting of bone.

Any instrument which appears warm to the operator's hands is likely to retain some heat which can cause problem when applied to oral structure immediately. It is usually found that claims based on these findings are difficult to defend. So, these circumstances should be avoided.

#### *Chemical Burns*

Chemical burns are also common in the dentists clinic. These can be avoided by following steps:

1. Provide proper training of dental assistants.
2. Avoid use of strong chemicals in the oral cavity.
3. Avoid overuse of chemicals.
4. Avoid carrying the chemicals over patient's face.
5. Accidental ingestion or inhalation.

Sometimes incidents such as accidental ingestion or inhalation of certain objects may occur for example:

- A portion of tooth.
- Burs
- Endodontic instruments such as file or reamer.
- Bridge

It is on dentist's part to make all provisions so that no instrument or object is ingested or inhaled. To prevent this dentist should take following precautions:

1. Use of rubber dam
2. Use of floss to tie endodontic instruments and rubber dam clamps.

If claims are made for these negligence, heavy compensation has to paid because these cases are truly a case of negligence on the part of dentist.

### Poor Quality of Radiographs

An improper radiographic film or poorly developed film can also lead to allegation of negligence which is difficult to refute. So, treatment provided on the basis of poor quality of radiographs should be repeated.

Since radiographs are only two-dimensional view of three-dimensional objects, in some cases it becomes necessary to take different radiographs in different angulations. Unable to take the radiographs is also liable to cause allegation of negligence.

### Failure to Provide Adequate Care

Failure to provide adequate care and treatment to a patient is also the part of dental negligence. Commonly seen cases of dental negligence performed by most of dentist in practice are:

1. Failure to use rubber-dam while doing endodontics.
2. Failure to take good quality radiographs.
3. Failure to periodically check the water unit connected to dental unit.
4. Failure to record and probe the periodontal pockets.
5. Failure to follow barrier technique such as use of sterilized gloves, face masks, instruments, use of protective eye shields and disposal of waste.

### Negligence Related to Patient

Patient also has to follow some rules of behavior while undergoing treatment. In accepting treatment, the patient should:

1. Cooperate during and after treatment.
2. Follow home care instructions given by dentist.
3. Immediately inform any change in health status.
4. Pay his/her bills timely.

Depending upon treatment, additional warranties may exists. If patient does not follow any of these instructions or instruction given by dentist, these should be recorded in patient's record.

## MALPRACTICE AND THE STANDARD OF CARE

Good endodontic practice is defined as standard of reasonable care legally to be performed by a reasonably careful clinician.

A careful clinician always keeps records. Records are considered as a single most evidence which a dentist can present in the court.

The law recognized that there are differences in the abilities of doctors with same qualification as there are also differences in the abilities of people engaged in different activities. To practice the profession, the clinician does not require extraordinary skills. In providing dental services to the community, the doctor is entitled to use his/her brain for judgement of cases and providing optimal care. For preventing malpractice, certain guidelines should be followed:

1. Do not provide treatment beyond your ability even if patient insist.
2. In patients where speciality care is required, refer the patient to specialist.
3. In patients where certain diagnostic tests are required for his/her care, if he/she refuses for that, clinician should not undertake treatment otherwise the clinician will be at risk.

### Standard of Care Set by Endodontics

Endodontists set a high standard of care as compared to general dentist. Endodontists should not forget their general dentist norms as these are required during care of endodontic treatment also.

After referrel from the patient thoroughly take new radiographs if required for starting procedure.

Endodontists should not provide rubber stamp treatment for what the clinician has asked. He/she should record complete medical and dental history before doing a thorough clinical examination. Endodontist should examine specific tooth/teeth along with general oral condition of the patient.

An endodontist should expose a new radiograph to know the status of tooth/teeth before starting a treatment.

### Standard of Care as Set by Endodontist

1. Take complete dental and medical history.
2. Thoroughly examine the oral cavity along with affected tooth/teeth.
3. Expose new radiograph before commencing the treatment.
4. Analyze the previous treatment plan.
5. Inform patient about the status of affected and adjacent tooth/teeth.

## ABANDONMENT

By initiating endodontic treatment the dentist has taken the legal responsibility to complete the case or the case can further be referred to a specialist. He should also be responsible for postoperative emergency care. If the dentist fails to comply with his or her obligation to complete treatment, he/she can be exposed to liability on the basis of abandonment. A dentist/endodontist if wants to ends his or her treatment obligation may have several reasons like patient:

1. Failed to keep appointments
2. Failed to cooperate.
3. Failed to follow home care instructions.
4. Failed to give payment at time.

To avoid abandonment claim, several precautionary measures need to be taken. These are:

1. No law can force the dentist to do all patients despite severe pain, infection or any other emergency condition. A dentist can do the emergency treatment, if patient and dentist both are interested but dentist should write clearly in the patient's record that he has given emergency treatment only.
2. Reasonable notice should be given to patient if patient is willing to seek endodontic treatment from somewhere else. The dentist should provide copies of treatment record and radiographs.
3. Once treatment is complete and any complication or emergency situation develops not related to the treatment given by the dentist, then there is no law which can force dentist to continue treatment.

Regardless of the justification given for treatment cessation, a dentist/endodontist who fails to follow the proper procedures may incur liability on the ground of abandonment. For prevention of abandonment claim, reasonable notice should be given to the patient. Reasonable notice would be considered valid only when no immediate threat to patient's medical and dental health is found evident. The following points should be taken care of while preparing a notice:

1. Notify the patient that he/she plans to terminate the treatment.
2. Give in detail the reason for not continuing the treatment for example, if patient is not following instruction properly, the notice should include instruction in writing.
3. Give reasonable time to patient to locate a new dentist/endodontist. Time given is usually one month. In rural areas, time limit may be prolonged due to lesser number of dentists available.
4. Provide all details about the treatment, i.e. treatment records and diagnostic radiographs.
5. Dentist should provide emergency care during the intermediate time.
6. A patient can contact any time regarding previous treatment given by dentist.
7. The notice should be certified by the dentist himself mentioning the date and signature.

## MALPRACTICE CASES

### Injury from Slips of the Drill

A slip of the drill is usually the result of operator's error. It can cause injury to tongue oral mucosa and lips. To avoid malpractice claim the dentist should follow these steps:

1. Inform the patient about incident and explain that he/she feels sorry for this incident.
2. Refer the patient to an oral and maxillofacial surgeon or plastic surgeon.
3. Dentist should bear the expenditure.
4. Call the patient for periodic check-up.

### Inhalation or Ingestion of Endodontic Instruments

Rubber dam should be used in every conditions and its use is mandatory for endodontic work. It not only reduces the chances of aspirating or swallowing endodontic instruments but also reduces the microbial contamination. If patient swallows or aspirates dental instrument, it is operator's fault. He should follow the following steps:

1. Inform the patient about the incident and should regret what has happened.
2. Refer the patient immediately for medical care.
3. Pay all the bills of patient.
4. Record the findings in treatment records of the patient.
5. Assure that it can be quickly repaired with newer materials.
6. Follow-up the case regularly.

## Broken File

These incidents usually occur in routine endodontic practice. But to avoid malpractice claims, you have to follow some guidelines. Before going into discussion about these guidelines consider some facts about broken or separated instruments:

1. Multiple use can result in fatigue of the instruments which further lead to failure of the these instruments.
2. Failure to follow the manufactures's instructions regard-ing use of the instruments can lead to failure.
3. Manufacturing defect may also lead to failure.
4. Teeth with separated files may remain asymptomatic and functional for years.

When an instrument gets separated in a tooth, dentist should follow some guidelines which are as follows:

1. Explain the patient about the incident.
2. Show the remaining part of endodontic instruments to the patient and assure that tooth will remain asymptomatic.
3. Dental assistant should place the part of endodontic instrument and radiographs in the treatment record for future reference.
4. Dentist should reassure the patient that he/she would follow this case closely.

## Perforations

Any dentist who is performing endodontic treatment can cause perforation. It usually occurs in or around furcal floor. Despite getting panic at the time of incident dentist should follow some basic steps:

1. Explain the patient about the incident that despite of best effort, perforation has occurred.
2. Record the findings in treatment records of the patient.
3. Assure that it can be quickly repaired with newer materials.
4. Follow-up the case regularly.

## Overextensions

Overextensions of obturation usually happen to every dentist. The irony about overextensions is that no one agree on exactly where the overextensions begin. Does it begin at the apex? 1 mm beyond the apex or 2 mm?

Rather than going into controversial discussion, we should follow some basic steps which are as follows:

1. Explain the incident to the patient mention the patient that some of the biocompatible material is gone beyond the end of the root.
2. There can be little more soreness for few days.
3. Mostly these cases heal asymptomatically.
4. Follow-up the case closely.

## QUESTIONS

**Q. What are principles of endodontic ethics?**
**Q. Mention different malpractice cases.**

## BIBLIOGRAPHY


1. Bailey B. Informed consent in dentistry. J Am Dent Assoc 1985;110:709.
2. Cohen S, et al. Endodontics and the law. Calif Dent Assoc J 1985;13:97.
3. Cohen S, et al. Endodontic complications and the law. J Endod 1987;13:191.
4. Row AHR. Damage to the inferior alveolar nerve during or following endodontic treatment. Br Dent J 1983;153:306.
5. Weichman JA. Malpractice prevention and defense. Calif Dent Assoc 1975;3:58.

# INDEX

## D

## M



## N



## O

## Q



## R



## S